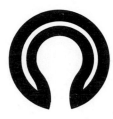

OSTEOARTHRITIS

Diagnosis

and

Management

ROLAND W. MOSKOWITZ, M.D.
Professor of Medicine
Case Western Reserve University
School of Medicine
Director, Division of Rheumatic Diseases
University Hospitals
Cleveland, Ohio

DAVID S. HOWELL, M.D.
Professor of Medicine
Director, Arthritis Division
University of Miami School of Medicine
Staff Physician
Veterans Administration Hospital
Miami, Florida

VICTOR M. GOLDBERG, M.D.
Professor of Orthopaedics
Case Western Reserve University
School of Medicine
Attending Orthopaedist
University Hospitals and Veterans Administration Hospital
Cleveland, Ohio

HENRY J. MANKIN, M.D.
Edith M. Ashley Professor of Orthopaedic Surgery
Harvard Medical School
Chief of Orthopaedic Service
Massachusetts General Hospital
Boston, Massachusetts

1984
W. B. Saunders Company

PHILADELPHIA   LONDON   TORONTO
MEXICO CITY   RIO DE JANEIRO   SYDNEY   TOKYO

W. B. Saunders Company: West Washington Square
                           Philadelphia, PA   19105

                           1 St. Anne's Road
                           Eastbourne, East Sussex BN21 3UN, England

                           1 Goldthorne Avenue
                           Toronto, Ontario M8Z 5T9, Canada

                           Apartado 26370—Cedro 512
                           Mexico 4, D.F., Mexico

                           Rua Coronel Cabrita, 8
                           Sao Cristovao Caixa Postal 21176
                           Rio de Janeiro, Brazil

                           9 Waltham Street
                           Artarmon, N.S.W. 2064, Australia

                           Ichibancho, Central Bldg., 22-1 Ichibancho
                           Chiyoda-Ku, Tokyo 102, Japan

Library of Congress Cataloging in Publication Data

Main entry under title:

Osteoarthritis, diagnosis and management.

1. Osteoarthritis.   I. Moskowitz, Roland W.
   [DNLM: 1. Osteoarthritis. WE 348 0848]

RC931.067088   1984   616.7'22   83–20054

ISBN 0–7216–6571–3

Osteoarthritis: Diagnosis and Management   ISBN 0–7216–6571–3

Last digit is the print number: 9   8   7   6   5   4   3   2   1

DEDICATION

This textbook is respectfully dedicated to Drs. Leon Sokoloff, Jonas H. Kellgren, and John S. Lawrence in recognition of the fundamental contributions they have made and continue to make to our understanding of osteoarthritis, and to our wives, Peta, Margaret, Harriet, and Carole, for their patience and support.

CONTRIBUTORS

ROY D. ALTMAN, M.D.
Professor of Medicine, University of Miami School of Medicine; Chief, Arthritis Division, Veterans Administration Medical Center, Miami, Florida

HARLAN C. AMSTUTZ, M.D.
Professor and Chief, Division of Orthopaedic Surgery, UCLA School of Medicine and UCLA Hospital and Clinics, Los Angeles, California

GEORGE J. ANNAS, J.D., M.P.H.
Edward Utley Professor of Health Law, Boston University Schools of Medicine and Public Health, Boston, Massachusetts

RODNEY BLUESTONE, M.B., F.R.C.P.
Clinical Professor of Medicine, UCLA School of Medicine; Attending Physician, Cedars-Sinai Medical Center, Los Angeles, California

HENRY H. BOHLMAN, M.D.
Associate Professor, Department of Orthopedic Surgery, Case Western Reserve University School of Medicine and University Hospitals of Cleveland; Chief, Acute Spinal Cord Injury Service, Veterans Administration Medical Center, Cleveland, Ohio

ROBERT E. BOOTH, Jr., M.D.
Associate Professor of Orthopaedic Surgery, University of Pennsylvania School of Medicine; Attending Orthopaedic Surgeon and Chief, Section of Physical Medicine and Rehabilitation, Pennsylvania Hospital; Attending Orthopaedic Surgeon, Hospital of the University of Pennsylvania, Philadelphia, Pennsylvania

KENNETH D. BRANDT, M.D.
Professor of Medicine and Chief, Rheumatology Division, Indiana University School of Medicine; Attending Physician, University Hospital, Indiana University Medical Center; Consulting Physician, Richard L. Roudebush Veterans Administration Medical Center, Indianapolis, Indiana

GILLIAN BROOKE, B.Sc.
Research Associate, Department of Pathology, University of Liverpool, Liverpool, England

JOHN J. CALABRO, M.D., F.A.C.P.
Professor of Medicine and Pediatrics, University of Massachusetts Medical School; Director of Rheumatology, Saint Vincent Hospital, Worcester, Massachusetts

ROBERT A. COLYER, M.D.
Associate Professor of Orthopaedic Surgery, Indiana University School of Medicine; Attending Orthopaedic Surgeon, Indiana University Hospitals, Indianapolis, Indiana

GEORGE E. EHRLICH, M.D.
Visiting Professor of Clinical Medicine, New York University Medical Center; Vice President, Development, Anti-Inflammatory/Endocrine, Pharmaceuticals Division, Ciba-Geigy Corporation, New York, New York

ROSE SPITZ FIFE, M.D.
Assistant Professor of Medicine, Division of Rheumatology, Indiana University School of Medicine; Attending Physician, University Hospital, Indiana University Medical Center; Consulting Physician, Wishard Memorial Hospital, Indiana University Medical Center, and Richard L. Roudebush Veterans Administration Hospital, Indianapolis, Indiana

LYNN H. GERBER, M.D.
Chief, Department of Rehabilitation Medicine and Clinical Center, National Institutes of Health, Bethesda, Maryland; Associate Clinical Professor of Medicine, George Washington University School of Medicine, Washington, D.C.

VICTOR M. GOLDBERG, M.D.
Professor of Orthopaedic Surgery, Case Western Reserve University School of Medicine; Associate Orthopaedist, University Hospitals of Cleveland; Consultant, Veterans Administration Hospital and Cleveland Metropolitan General Hospital, Cleveland, Ohio

v

ROBERT G. GRAY, M.D.
Assistant Clinical Professor of Medicine, Tufts University School of Medicine, Boston, and Baystate Medical Center, Springfield, Massachusetts

WALTER GURALNICK, D.M.D.
Professor of Oral and Maxillofacial Surgery, Harvard School of Dental Medicine; Visiting Oral and Maxillofacial Surgeon, Massachusetts General Hospital, Boston, Massachusetts

JEANNE E. HICKS, M.D.
Deputy Chief, Department of Rehabilitation Medicine and Clinical Center, National Institutes of Health, Bethesda, Maryland; Adjunct Assistant Professor of Medicine, George Washington University School of Medicine, Washington, D.C.

DAVID S. HOWELL, M.D.
Professor of Medicine, and Director, Arthritis Division, University of Miami School of Medicine; Medical Investigator, Veterans Administration Medical Center; Full-Time Staff, Jackson Memorial Hospital, University of Miami Clinics, and Veterans Administration Medical Center, Miami, Florida

DAVID S. HUNGERFORD, M.D.
Associate Professor, Department of Orthopaedic Surgery, The Johns Hopkins University School of Medicine; Chief, Division of Arthritis Surgery, The Good Samaritan Hospital, Baltimore, Maryland

DAVID A. KEITH, B.D.S., F.D.S.R.C.S.
Assistant Professor of Oral and Maxillofacial Surgery, Harvard School of Dental Medicine; Assistant Oral and Maxillofacial Surgeon, Massachusetts General Hospital, Boston, Massachusetts

CARY S. KELLER, M.D.
Director, Denali Sports Medicine Center, Fairbanks Clinic; Team Physician, University of Alaska; Director of Sports Medicine, Fairbanks North Star Borough Public Schools; Attending Orthopedic Surgeon, Fairbanks Memorial Hospital, Fairbanks, Alaska; Staff Orthopedic Surgeon, Deaconess Hospital, Cincinnati, Ohio

DONALD B. KETTELKAMP, M.D.
Professor and Chairman, Department of Orthopaedic Surgery, Indiana University School of Medicine; Head, Orthopaedic Surgery, Indiana University Hospitals, Indianapolis, Indiana

WILLIAM C. KIM, M.D.
Assistant Professor, Division of Orthopaedic Surgery, UCLA School of Medicine, Harbor-UCLA Medical Center, and UCLA Hospitals and Clinics, Los Angeles, California

DENNIS W. LENNOX, M.D.
Assistant Professor, Department of Orthopaedic Surgery, The Johns Hopkins University School of Medicine; Attending Orthopaedic Surgeon, The Johns Hopkins Hospital and Good Samaritan Hospital, Baltimore, Maryland

HENRY J. MANKIN, M.D.
Edith M. Ashley Professor of Orthopaedics, Harvard Medical School; Orthopaedist-in-Chief, Massachusetts General Hospital, Boston, Massachusetts

ROGER A. MANN, M.D.
Associate Clinical Professor of Orthopaedic Surgery, University of California, San Francisco, School of Medicine, San Francisco; Chief, Division of Foot Surgery, Samuel Merrit Hospital and Children's Hospital of the East Bay, Oakland, California

GEORGE MEACHIM, M.A., M.D., F.R.C.Path.
Reader in Pathology, University of Liverpool; Consultant Pathologist, Royal Liverpool Hospital, Liverpool, England

ROLAND W. MOSKOWITZ, M.D.
Professor of Medicine, Case Western Reserve University School of Medicine; Director, Division of Rheumatic Diseases, University Hospitals of Cleveland, Cleveland, Ohio

DAVID H. NEUSTADT, M.D.
Clinical Professor of Medicine, University of Louisville School of Medicine; Attending Rheumatologist, Jewish Hospital; Consulting Rheumatologist, Veterans Administration Hospital, Louisville, Kentucky

ALEX NORMAN, M.D.
Professor of Radiology, Mount Sinai School of Medicine of the City University of New York; Director of Radiology, Hospital for Joint Diseases Orthopaedic Institute, New York, New York

JACQUES G. PEYRON, M.D.
Attending Physician, Centre de Rhumatologie, Hôpital Tenon, Paris, France

ERIC L. RADIN, M.D.
Professor and Chairman, Department of Orthopedic Surgery, West Virginia University Medical Center, Morgantown, West Virginia

RICHARD H. ROTHMAN, M.D., Ph.D.
Professor of Orthopedic Surgery, University of Pennsylvania School of Medicine; Chief of Orthopedic Surgery, Pennsylvania Hospital, Philadelphia, Pennsylvania

H. RALPH SCHUMACHER, Jr., M.D.
Professor of Medicine, University of Pennsylvania School of Medicine; Director, Arthritis-Immunology Center, Veterans Administration Medical Center; Staff Rheumatologist, Hospital of The University of Pennsylvania, Philadelphia, Pennsylvania

RICHARD J. SMITH, M.D.
Clinical Professor of Orthopaedic Surgery, Havard Medical School; Chief, Hand Surgery, Department of Orthopaedics, Massachusetts General Hospital, Boston, Massachusetts

S. DAVID STULBERG, M.D.
Associate Professor of Orthopaedic Surgery, Northwestern University Medical School; Associate Attending Physician, Northwestern Memorial Hospital, Chicago, Illinois

THOMAS R. F. TAYLOR, M.D.
Professor of Orthopaedics and Traumatic Surgery, University of Sydney and Royal North Shore Hospital, St. Leonards, New South Wales, Australia

PETER D. UTSINGER, M.D.
Professor of Clinical Medicine, Temple University School of Medicine; Director of Immunology and Chief of Research and Development, Germantown Hospital and Medical Center, Philadelphia, Pennsylvania

ALAN H. WILDE, M.D.
Chairman, Department of Orthopaedic Surgery, Cleveland Clinic Foundation, Cleveland, Ohio

FOREWORD

There is a lot to be said for a Foreword of four words, that is, "I recommend this book," but today, such laconic *ex cathedra* statements need to be amplified and, indeed, reasoned and justified. Despite the 39 expert authors and the 33 up-to-date chapters, as well as a wide-ranging introduction and a very modest preface, there is still a need, as I see it, for a brief historical background and, having lived through 50 years of cartilage research (and this is what it is all about), I am glad to supply that.

Osteoarthrosis or *osteoarthritis* arguments betray terminologic decrepitude. Too many flatulent words have been written on the subject (and still are), resulting only in rude and unnecessary noise. Wisely, this has been here avoided.

If there is any new disease, it is osteoarthritis. It is not *really* new; indeed, it is one of the oldest in man's history and in other vertebrates before him, but it is new in the sense that it is much more prevalent, obvious, and significant today with our hitherto unprecedented years of survival. Today, osteoarthritis is one of man's major problems because of the relative lack of healing; this is in contrast to most diseases characteristic of the first 50 years of life in which inflammatory or traumatic lesions heal. Degenerative joint disease was not catered for by evolution and the mechanisms of selection, except perhaps in a negative sense, and does not heal without artificial aid. (In the same way but on a more domestic scale, increased height due to better nutrition was not envisaged by the builders of Elizabethan doorways, with resultant sore heads.)

The recognition of osteoarthritis as a separate type of chronic arthritis at the end of the nineteenth century was an enormous step forward, and the history of its development as a concept has been recounted many times. However, there is still a great deal of argument about this so-called "entity." Most people seem to agree that this present age, with increased longevity due to better social measures and to antibiotics, has given it much more importance not only for conjecture, speculation, and research but also for practical measures of support, if not cure. Prevention is always the flaming beacon on the horizon, much like the quest for eternal youth and immortality. It does not seem likely to me that either cure or prevention will be achieved, because aging and death are part of life and are essential for the survival of every known species. However, we are now able to mitigate not only environmental diseases but also those that are inborn or are entailed in our way of life. Therefore, this book manages to end as it has begun, with some hope. The only viewpoint not represented here is that of the individual articulate but "misarticulated" or "disarticulated" patient, either before or after artificial articulation, but that view is implicit in the text.

We now realize that osteoarthritis is the end result of use and abuse and trauma, acting on a basic background of genetic, metabolic, developmental, and other faults, contributing to what, in a simplistic view, would be attributed to aging and the wear and tear of a lifetime.

This timely (because it is needed now), up-to-the-moment review covers all the known options as well as many of the unknown ones and, in actually three words instead of four, is "to be recommended."

When I first began to work on cartilage as a young research fellow in 1935, it was a totally neglected tissue, an apparently passive and inert covering for the evolutionary emergence of bones, serving a role in heavy leverage and movement. We have begun to realize that bone is essentially a late insertion into primeval cartilage, a necessity for those ancestral Reptilia who crawled out from the water onto dry land and into the field of terrestrial gravity. The spine, for instance, which distinguishes the Vertebrata, is essentially a cartilaginous tube built around the notochord and protecting our infolded nervous system; bone was later built into it to ensure stability and strength.

The evolution of our views on cartilage as a tissue and, indeed, of the actual concept of "osteoarthrosis or osteoarthritis" (essentially a cartilage-concerned change) occupies a much shorter time, perhaps 200 years, However, it is most relevant to today's problems of an increasingly aged population and the where-withal to care for it with dignity, both for our aging selves and for mankind, and we must remember that aging starts when growth stops.

For every extra noncontributory year of life that we survive, society has to pay in one way or another. But what is noncontributory? Today, the population of nursing homes, old peoples' homes, and senior citizen refuges (and a whole range of other terms to avoid that prejudicial and pejorative word "senile") is greater than ever before but has to be weighed against what a number of people beyond three score years and ten can and do now continue to contribute to the cultural aspects of human life.

I know of no statistical comparison with age-related cultural contributions to life, for example, in the 1920's or even in the Victorian age. There were giants then who continued to contribute well into their old age, but as I see it, there are now more of them, although not necessarily giants, just a lot of old people who are still useful. The retiring age of 70 would be ridiculous in a fully employed and producing society but is probably necessary at this time of unfortunately increased unemployment.

For the purposes of this book, which addresses much longer-term problems, osteoarthritis is a major factor influencing survival in an affluent society, thanks to the skill and continuing technologic research of orthopedic surgeons. The damaged hip is the main functional limitation of osteoarthritis, followed perhaps by knee problems, and both joints today can be replaced, provided the resources are available.

I am glad for two reasons to write a Foreword to this multiauthored text concerned with our own aging society and, indeed, with ourselves: first, to say how much I think such a gathering together of widely diversified studies is needed at this point in historical development, when the diseases associated with the aging population have reached, at least in the developed countries, an all-time high, and because of the problems this has brought to economists, politicians, health workers, bureaucrats, and indeed the whole of society; and second, because I would like to pay tribute not only to the 39 distinguished authors and their spirited editors but also to my three outstanding colleagues in the United Kingdom and the United States who first put this area of enquiry forward onto a sound scientific basis, Jonas Kellgren, John Lawrence, and Leon Sokoloff, who from varying angles imparted such an impetus to a previously neglected subject that it has now become a major concern of governments, economists, and ordinary people.

The diseases, disabilities, and handicaps associated with prolonged survival are creating year by year more and more problems for the individual, for the health services, and for society as a whole. The processes involved are usually obscure and the residual disability cumulative, exposing the patients progressively in their turn to further health hazards, such as osteoporosis and fractures or inanition.

This landmark book deals with one of the most interesting of such processes, that affecting predominantly joint cartilage and underlying bone and thus mobility. Although the centuries have depicted old age with a stoop and a stick, it was not until the early years of the century that osteoarthritis was "put on the map," first of all by the pathologists, and of these Nichols and Richardson in 1909 were the most cogent in distinguishing "chronic inflammatory arthritis," which we now call "rheumatoid arthritis," from this degenerative noninflammatory condition. Roentgenography had by then come into regular use, and the differences between these two entities became roentgenologically visible. Although Dr. J. Kent Spender was the first to use the term "osteoarthritis" as a title for a book in 1889, the use of the term "arthritis deformans," confounding both inflammatory and noninflammatory chronic joint disease, continued well into the 1930's. In the 1931 edition of Osler's "The Principles and Practice of Medicine," edited by Thomas McCrae, it was stated that "there is a difference of opinion as to whether there are two distinct diseases or varying forms of the same disease included under this heading. Those who hold the former view consider that in one disease the synovial membranes and the periarticular tissues are particularly affected (rheumatoid arthritis) and in the other disease the cartilage and bone (osteoarthritis). The disease is common and to it belong many of the cases termed 'chronic rheumatism.'" The section then continues to deal with them as one disease.

By 1949, however, Douglas Collins, from Leeds, England, one of the most perspicacious and percipient of the few pathologists ever interested in joint disease, dealt fully and in a very modern way with osteoarthritis in his book "The Pathology of Articular Spinal Diseases." He was followed by Leon Sokoloff ("The Biology of Degenerative Joint Disease" published in 1969), who had developed the experimental and comparative anatomic approach. It is perhaps ironic that a process such as aging (associated with degenerative joint change) is common to all vertebrates and can be experimentally studied prospectively and experimentally (in contrast to rheumatoid arthritis, for which we still have no experimental models) and yet we are still uncertain how much genetically determined biochemical constitution contributes to the generalized tendency in a particular species for the development of osteoarthritis. On the other hand, we know very well that overuse, abuse, or bad use produces this and that in underused joints, such as those on the paralyzed side in hemiplegic man, degenerative joint disease does not occur.

When does a *process* like aging become a *disease*? Presumably, it does so when it produces symptoms, but a process has to have other triggering factors to make it become a disease. In the same way, is senile skin a process, a change, or a disease depending partly upon how much sunlight we have been exposed to? Is there really a primary osteoarthritis in man apart from the cumulative troubles of his morphologic genes and his accident-prone life? Certainly cartilage ages, even in the ribs or disks, but these are protected areas. Even in the hereditary anomaly of progeria with so many other accompaniments of old age, the joints remain free of osteoarthritis, as I have determined by personal study at postmortem examination.

The pioneering studies of rheumatic diseases in rural and urban populations in 1948 by Kellgren and Lawrence from Manchester began this distinction between process, complaint, and disease; Philip Wood, who succeeded John Lawrence in the Arthritis and Rheumatism Field Unit (now the ARC Epidemiological Research Unit), similarly has pioneered the distinction between impairment, disability, and handicap. However, cost and resource considerations for society may serve to limit fulfillment for a large number of potentially contributory citizens. Total joint replacement can be a "rejuvenating miracle," but regrettably cost will play a major role in the availability of such new procedures for those who could benefit from them, as in so many other fields. Societies will have to decide how to spend limited resources; cost-effectiveness must include personal satisfaction and social productivity. Advances in medical research and treatment in many fields, including osteoarthritis (as detailed in this text), have made it even more urgent for those responsible to determine priorities—among basic research, delivery of care, and other needs of society at all levels, including those of defense and possible survival.

ERIC G. L. BYWATERS, C.B.E., M.D., F.R.C.P.

Emeritus Professor of Rheumatology
in the University of London, at the
Royal Postgraduate Medical School

PREFACE

Osteoarthritis is the most common form of rheumatologic disease. Although it is fortunately a benign disease in many patients, its frequency and potential for severe progressive joint destruction result in its ranking high as a cause of disability with profound socioeconomic impact. Discussion of this disorder is appropriately routinely included in major rheumatology textbooks and has been the subject of numerous published basic and clinical reviews. Nevertheless, it is surprising that for a disease of such import no one textbook has been forthcoming to serve as a comprehensive resource volume to bring together investigational and clinical aspects of this common and important disorder. The editors of this book, all of whom have had a longstanding interest in studies of basic cartilage metabolism and osteoarthritis, have taken upon ourselves the challenge to fill this void for a book "whose time had come."

The contents of this text are designed to be of value to both the researcher and the clinician. For the researcher, the chapters on basic investigation will serve to update and coordinate current concepts in the field; clinically oriented chapters will allow the basic scientists to relate their investigations to important clinical aspects of the disease with which they may be unfamiliar. Conversely, the detailed clinical information provided in the text will allow clinicians to expand their knowledge of diagnostic and management aspects of this disease; the basic science chapters will provide a sounder understanding of pathophysiologic mechanisms on which clinical and therapeutic aspects of the disorder are based. The text has been written to be comprehensive and yet not exhaustive. It is designed to be practical in both content and size, serving to answer questions as they arise on a day-to-day basis with respect to all aspects of the disease.

The text is divided into five major sections: basic considerations; general aspects of diagnosis; general aspects of management; regional considerations, including diagnosis, differential diagnosis, medical and surgical management, outcomes, and prognosis; and a general section that addresses such aspects as industrial and medicolegal considerations, investigations related to attempts at specific therapy, and the interrelationships of exercise and sports in osteoarthritis. The section on basic considerations addresses epidemiology, pathology, biochemistry and metabolism of cartilage, immunology of cartilage, biomechanical considerations, experimental models of osteoarthritis, and concepts of etiopathogenesis. The section on general aspects of diagnosis reviews in detail symptoms and signs, roentgenologic diagnosis, laboratory findings, concepts of disease subsets such as erosive inflammatory osteoarthritis, generalized osteoarthritis, chondromalacia patellae, and DISH syndrome, and general aspects of differential diagnosis. The section on general aspects of management includes discussions of physical and adjunctive therapy, drug therapy, intra-articular steroid use, and general surgical considerations.

Clinical aspects of specific disease involvement are addressed in the section on regional considerations and detailed discussion of orthopedic surgical management is provided. These chapters are divided primarily into discussions of osteoarthritis as it involves specific joints of the upper extremity, lower extremity, and spine. Newer concepts of involvement of the temporomandibular joint are discussed. In the final section of the text, the interrelationships of occupation, exercise, and sports, which are so important in the pathogenesis of the disease and its clinical manifestations, are reviewed in detail. Medicolegal considerations, which have an important bearing on disease research and management, are outlined. A chapter on investigational therapy directed toward evaluation of specific agents to reverse, retard, or prevent the disease provides insights into the potential for delineation of more effective therapeutic agents based on vastly expanding knowledge about disease pathophysiology.

The contributors to this volume represent individuals who are regarded as leaders in their field. Chapter content based on extensive reviews of the literature is additionally flavored by factual information, hypotheses, and speculations based on each author's own involvement and contributions to the field of expertise about which he or she is writing. It was the consensus of all contributors involved in the text that this was an essential, needed addition to the literature, worthy of their involvement despite already heavy schedules related to research and contributions to other textbooks and reviews in this area of study. Any initial reticence to take on a new added commitment was quickly superseded by a desire to be included in this effort to fill the void previously noted.

Although no text is totally complete, it was the goal of the editors that this volume be worthy of this disease. As individuals who have spent major segments of our lifetimes in studies attempting to decipher the basic and clinical facets related to a better understanding of osteoarthritis, we are hopeful that this text will serve as a basic functional resource volume to all interested investigators and clinicians.

ROLAND W. MOSKOWITZ, M.D.
DAVID S. HOWELL, M.D.
VICTOR M. GOLDBERG, M.D.
HENRY J. MANKIN, M.D.

ACKNOWLEDGMENTS

Our deep thanks go to Mr. John Hanley, President of the W. B. Saunders Company, for his guidance and support throughout the preparation and culmination of this text. The knowledgeable guidance of Mr. John Dyson, Associate Medical Editor of W. B. Saunders Company, in the completion of this text is further gratefully acknowledged. We further acknowledge our deep and sincere thanks to those personnel who worked with us on a day-to-day basis in the preparation and editing of the volume. In particular, Ms. Connie McSweeney, our Editorial Assistant, brought expertise and calm that served to provide equanimity and reassurance when references, figures, manuscripts, and submission deadlines made us wonder whether all this was necessary! Ms. Bonnie Langevin played an essential role in editor/author communications early in the inception of the book and provided invaluable typing assistance.

ROLAND W. MOSKOWITZ, M.D.
DAVID S. HOWELL, M.D.
VICTOR M. GOLDBERG, M.D.
HENRY J. MANKIN, M.D.

CONTENTS

INTRODUCTION 1
Roland W. Moskowitz, M.D.

SECTION 1
BASIC CONSIDERATIONS 7

1
THE EPIDEMIOLOGY OF OSTEOARTHRITIS 9
Jacques G. Peyron, M.D.

2
THE PATHOLOGY OF OSTEOARTHRITIS........................... 29
George Meachim, M.A., M.D., and Gillian Brooke, B.Sc.

3
BIOCHEMISTRY AND METABOLISM OF CARTILAGE IN
OSTEOARTHRITIS 43
Henry J. Mankin, M.D., and Kenneth D. Brandt, M.D.

4
THE IMMUNOLOGY OF ARTICULAR CARTILAGE................ 81
Victor M. Goldberg, M.D.

5
BIOMECHANICAL CONSIDERATIONS............................... 93
Eric L. Radin, M.D.

6
EXPERIMENTAL MODELS OF OSTEOARTHRITIS 109
Roland W. Moskowitz, M.D.

7
ETIOPATHOGENESIS OF OSTEOARTHRITIS........................ 129
David S. Howell, M.D.

SECTION 2
GENERAL ASPECTS OF DIAGNOSIS 147

8
OSTEOARTHRITIS—SYMPTOMS AND SIGNS 149
Roland W. Moskowitz, M.D.

9
ROENTGENOLOGIC DIAGNOSIS 155
Alex Norman, M.D.

10
LABORATORY FINDINGS IN OSTEOARTHRITIS 185
Roy D. Altman, M.D., and Robert G. Gray, M.D.

11
EROSIVE INFLAMMATORY AND PRIMARY GENERALIZED
OSTEOARTHRITIS 199
George E. Ehrlich, M.D.

12
CHONDROMALACIA PATELLAE 211
David S. Hungerford, M.D., and Dennis W. Lennox, M.D.

13
DIFFUSE IDIOPATHIC SKELETAL HYPEROSTOSIS (DISH,
ANKYLOSING HYPEROSTOSIS) 225
Peter D. Utsinger, M.D.

14
SECONDARY OSTEOARTHRITIS 235
H. Ralph Schumacher, Jr., M.D.

15
THE ETIOLOGY AND NATURAL COURSE OF OSTEOARTHRITIS
OF THE HIP (COXARTHROSIS) 265
S. David Stulberg, M.D.

16
GENERAL ASPECTS OF DIFFERENTIAL DIAGNOSIS 275
Rodney Bluestone, M.B., F.R.C.P.

SECTION 3
GENERAL ASPECTS OF MANAGEMENT 285

17
REHABILITATON IN THE MANAGEMENT OF PATIENTS
WITH OSTEOARTHRITIS 287
Lynn H. Gerber, M.D., and Jeanne E. Hicks, M.D.

18
PRINCIPLES OF DRUG THERAPY 317
John J. Calabro, M.D.

19
INTRA-ARTICULAR STEROID THERAPY 333
David H. Neustadt, M.D.

20
SURGERY IN OSTEOARTHRITIS: GENERAL
CONSIDERATIONS 351
Victor M. Goldberg, M.D.

SECTION 4
REGIONAL CONSIDERATIONS (INCLUDING DIAGNOSIS,
DIFFERENTIAL DIAGNOSIS, MEDICAL AND SURGICAL
MANAGEMENT, OUTCOMES, AND PROGNOSIS) 361

21
OSTEOARTHRITIS OF THE HAND AND WRIST 363
Richard J. Smith, M.D.

22
OSTEOARTHRITIS OF THE SHOULDER AND ELBOW 377
Alan H. Wilde, M.D.

23
OSTEOARTHRITIS OF THE FOOT AND ANKLE 389
Roger A. Mann, M.D.

24
OSTEOARTHRITIS OF THE KNEE 403
Donald B. Kettelkamp, M.D., and Robert A. Colyer, M.D.

25
OSTEOARTHRITIS OF THE HIP 423
Harlan C. Amstutz, M.D., and William C. Kim, M.D.

26
OSTEOARTHRITIS OF THE CERVICAL SPINE 443
Henry H. Bohlman, M.D.

27
OSTEOARTHRITIS OF THE THORACIC SPINE 461
Thomas K. F. Taylor, M.D.

28
OSTEOARTHRITIS OF THE LUMBAR SPINE, DISK DISEASE 473
Robert E. Booth, Jr., M.D., and Richard H. Rothman, M.D., Ph.D.

29
OSTEOARTHRITIS OF THE TEMPOROMANDIBULAR JOINT.... 523
Walter Guralnick, D.M.D., and David A. Keith, B.D.S., F.D.S.R.C.S.

SECTION 5
OTHER CONSIDERATIONS... 531

30
INDUSTRIAL CONSIDERATIONS 533
George E. Ehrlich, M.D.

31
MEDICOLEGAL CONSIDERATIONS.................................. 541
George J. Annas, J.D., M.P.H.

32
EXPERIMENTAL MODES OF THERAPY IN
OSTEOARTHRITIS 549
Rose Spitz Fife, M.D., and Kenneth D. Brandt, M.D.

33
EXERCISE AND OSTEOARTHRITIS 561
S. David Stulberg, M.D., and Cary S. Keller, M.D.

INDEX 569

Introduction

Roland W. Moskowitz, M. D.

Osteoarthritis (OA) is the most common of the various articular disorders affecting man. It has been described in other vertebrates and in all mammalian species and spares no race or geographic area. Only as recently as the early 1900's was a distinction made between hypertrophic (degenerative joint disease) and atrophic (rheumatoid) arthritis, and osteoarthritis defined as a clinical entity.[1, 2] The evolution of osteoarthritis has been characterized by a number of myths that persist even now, namely that OA is an inevitable disease of aging, that it is a benign disorder leading to minimal disability, and that it represents a disorder for which little can be done therapeutically even when the diagnosis has been made. Expanded research has demonstrated significant differences between the aging process and osteoarthritis. Although osteoarthritis occurs more frequently in older people, it is incorrect to infer that it is a simple "wear and tear" process of cartilage breakdown. The belief that OA is an inevitable disease of aging, analogous to graying of the hair or senescent changes in the skin, is simplistic and incorrect. The observed increased frequency and severity of the disease in older populations are likely the result of prolonged exposure to pathophysiologic processes that occur much earlier in life.

Although it is true that the majority of patients with osteoarthritis, particularly those in younger age groups, will have mild and relatively asymptomatic disease, data have demonstrated significant disabilities associated with this disorder in patients in older age groups, in which the disease is eventually almost universal.[3] As the single most frequent cause of rheumatic symptoms, it results in major losses of time from work and carries with it an overall significant socioeconomic impact.[4, 5] Finally, as will be evidenced by the information contained in the chapters related to therapy, much can already be done to help relieve symptoms related to osteoarthritis, although at present therapy remains symptomatic rather than specific. Current knowledge of basic science and clinical aspects of OA are detailed in this text. This introductory chapter summarizes some of the highlights contained in these presentations so as to provide a broad background to familiarize the reader with concepts and terminology.

Epidemiology. Numerous epidemiologic surveys have been performed to characterize the prevalence and clinical characteristics of osteoarthritis.[3, 6–11] Observed differences in findings are most likely related to variations in analytic techniques and populations studied. For example, studies that utilize autopsy analysis[9] will define disease earlier than will clinical studies in which pathologic changes are insufficient to cause significant symptoms. Furthermore, clinical surveys will elicit varying results depending on differences in disease definition and the use of prospective or retrospective techniques. Results based on roentgenographic studies[10] will vary depending on the number and location of joints analyzed. Despite these caveats, epidemiologic studies have defined a number of important characteristics of this disorder. There is general concurrence that osteoarthritis increases in prevalence in parallel with age. Although degenerative changes in joints can be shown to occur as early as the second decade of life in autopsy studies[9] and some pathologic abnormalities in weight-bearing joints can be demonstrated in almost all persons by age 40, the rate of frequency of osteoarthritis increases progressively, so that in individuals over age 75 it is almost universal.[3] The disease affects both men and women, with the prevalence being greater in men under age 45 and in women over age 55.[7, 10] When all ages are considered, men and women are equally affected. Racial differences in the presence of osteoarthritis have been noted, particularly when patterns of joint involvement are reviewed.[6, 11] Variations in occupation and life style existing in different populations may have an impact on these findings attributed to racial and hereditary influences.

Osteoarthritis has been noted to occur in all climates, and no specific differences in disease frequency on a climatic basis have been unquestionably defined.[6, 12, 13] Although intuitively it would appear that obesity would represent a major factor in relation to osteoarthritis, the role of obesity as an etiologic factor has been the subject of conflicting findings.[14–18] Nevertheless, given the important proposed role for biomechanical influences in the initiation or augmentation of osteoarthritic changes, weight reduction is usually advised. The role of chronic stress related to either occupation or sports injury has been similarly evaluated with varying results. For example, an increased frequency in the severity of osteoarthritis of the right hand as compared with the left hand in right-handed people has been noted,[19] and an increased frequency of OA is seen in association with long-standing internal derangements of the knee. Prolonged overuse of any joint or group of joints has been related to an increased frequency of osteoarthritis in coal miners,[20] bus drivers,[8] and foundry workers.[21] Other studies performed in individuals such as pneumatic hammer drillers[22] and long-distance running champions[23] have revealed no increase in osteoarthritis as compared with matched controls.

Definition and Classification. Clinical and research observations in osteoarthritis have been confounded by differences in disease definition. There is increasing acceptance that osteoarthritis may represent not one specific disorder but rather a series of disease subsets that lead to similar clinical and pathologic alterations. Difficulties in disease classification have led to the recent appointment of a subcommittee of the American Rheumatism Association to evaluate and define an all-encompassing valid concept of classification of osteoarthritis. Osteoarthritis is usually classified as primary (idiopathic) and secondary.

The disease is characterized as primary when it occurs in the absence of any known underlying predisposing factor. Secondary osteoarthritis, on the other hand, can be defined as that form of the disease that has an important, clearly defined, underlying condition contributing to its etiology. Even this simple classification, however, may be artificial at times. Studies on osteoarthritis of the hip, for example, have shown that many cases of "primary" osteoarthritis are actually secondary to anatomic abnormalities that result in articular incongruity and premature cartilage degeneration, such as variable degrees of childhood disorders such as congenital hip dysplasia and a slipped capital femoral epiphysis[24, 25] (see Chapter 15). The concept of osteoarthritis subsets is supported by the existence of variant forms of the disease that are sufficiently different in clinical, roentgenologic, and pathologic findings to warrant consideration as being distinct symptom complexes. In particular, these subsets relate to the existence of primary generalized osteoarthritis,[26] erosive inflammatory osteoarthritis,[27–29] diffuse idiopathic skeletal hyperostosis,[30] and chondromalacia patellae (see Chapters 11, 12, 13). Whether these symptom complexes represent disease subsets or merely reflect one end of the clinical spectrum of disease severity has yet to be determined. A suggested classification of osteoarthritis based on anatomic and etiologic mechanisms and that includes most of the known forms of the disease is provided in Table 1.

Pathology. Joint articular cartilage and subchondral bone are the sites of major abnormalities in the osteoarthritic process. It should be noted that two primary pathologic responses are seen. One response is characterized by a structural breakdown of cartilage that leads to development of erosions that involve focal and, later, diffuse areas of the cartilage surface. On histopathologic study, it is noted that the cartilage surface becomes uneven as fissuring and pitting develop. Progression of disease is characterized by the appearance of gross ulcerations. A second pathologic response, which contrasts with the structural loss just noted, is characterized by proliferation of new bone and cartilage at the joint periphery, leading to osteochondrophyte spur formation. Osteochondrophytes are characterized by a central core of new bone capped by hyaline and fibrocartilage. Although osteophyte spur formation is usually considered a characteristic component of the osteoarthritic process, recent studies challenge this con-

Table 1. CLASSIFICATION OF OSTEOARTHRITIS

Primary (idiopathic)
  Peripheral joints (single versus multiple joints)
    Interphalangeal joints (nodal) (e.g., DIP, PIP)
    Other small joints (e.g., first CMC, first MTP)
    Large joints (e.g., hip, knee)
  Spine
    Apophyseal joints
    Intervertebral joints
  Variant subsets
    Erosive inflammatory osteoarthritis (EOA)
    Generalized osteoarthritis (GOA)
    Chondromalacia patellae
    Diffuse idiopathic skeletal hyperostosis (DISH, ankylosing hyperostosis)
Secondary
  Trauma
    Acute
    Chronic (occupational, sports, obesity)
  Other joint disorders
    Local (fracture, avascular necrosis, infection)
    Diffuse (rheumatoid arthritis, hypermobility syndrome, hemorrhagic diatheses)
  Systemic metabolic disease
    Ochronosis (alkaptonuria)
    Hemochromatosis
    Wilson's disease
    Kashin-Beck disease
  Endocrine disorders
    Acromegaly
    Hyperparathyroidism
    Diabetes mellitus
  Calcium crystal deposition diseases
    Calcium pyrophosphate dihydrate
    Calcium apatite
  Neuropathic disorders (Charcot joints) (e.g., tabes dorsalis, diabetes mellitus, intra-articular steroid overuse)
  Bone dysplasias (multiple epiphyseal dysplasia, spondyloepiphyseal dysplasia)
  Miscellaneous
    Frostbite
    Long-leg arthropathy

Abbreviations: DIP = distal interphalangeal joint; PIP = proximal interphalangeal joint; CMC = carpometacarpal joint; MTP = metatarsophalangeal joint

cept.[31–33] These studies noted that structural cartilage loss did not inevitably follow the appearance of osteophytes, even over a period of many years; their presence as a manifestation of aging was suggested. At present, most workers still consider osteophytes to be manifestations of the degenerative disease process, although developing via a different pathophysiologic process from erosions. The presence of both structural cartilage loss and proliferative new bone and cartilage formation is of clinical significance in that medications that might become available to specifically stimulate cartilage to heal erosions may inadvertently aggravate the disease process by stimulating osteochondrophyte spurs as well. Conversely, agents that inhibit spur formation may aggravate and enhance cartilage breakdown.

Significantly expanded research efforts and the introduction of new methodologies have led to major advances in understanding the pathophysiology of osteoarthritis.[34] The availability of new study technologies such as cell culture techniques and the development of experimental animal models that simulate the human disorder have allowed extensive advances in knowledge of basic cartilage metabolism and the underlying OA disease process. It has been hypothesized that some primary insult(s) results in chondrocyte release of proteolytic and collagenolytic enzymes that degrade matrix proteoglycan and collagen. Biomechanical abnormalities, either chronic and subtle or more overt, may result in early cell breakdown; other primary insults such as chemical, inflammatory, or immunologic abnormalities cannot be excluded. Cartilage breakdown is followed by attempts at repair characterized by chondrocyte proliferation and increased synthesis of matrix proteoglycan and collagen. When reparative processes fail to keep pace with degenerative change, osteoarthritis ensues. The prevalence of osteoarthritis late in life and its slowly progressive course may reflect the slow rate at which chondrocytes release matrix-digesting enzymes, with cartilage failure resulting only when reparative efforts fail. More recent studies suggest that immunologic factors may play a role in the perpetuation and acceleration of osteoarthritic damage.[35] Exposed cartilage, normally "isolated" from body tissue, may lead to stimulation of humoral and cell-mediated immune mechanisms with release of antibodies (complexes) and lymphokine mediators that accelerate cartilage destruction on the basis of immune interplays. Although the term osteoarthritis implies a significant role for inflammation in this disorder, it is generally conceded that the inflammation commonly present represents a secondary factor in disease etiopathogenesis. Studies that suggest a role for calcium mineral deposition in cartilage[36] and genetic predispositions to disease development[7, 8, 26] add to the complexities of etiopathogenesis of this disorder. Concepts of etiopathogenesis based on recent research findings are well defined in Chapter 7.

Diagnosis. In many patients, the clinical and roentgenologic findings are sufficiently characteristic to allow a secure diagnosis of osteoarthritis on a positive basis. In some patients, however, the disease shows variations that are sufficient in degree to provide difficulties in differential diagnosis. Symptoms of pain, stiffness, and limitation of motion and signs that include tenderness, crepitus, joint enlargement, and joint limitation are not specific and may be seen in a number of other rheumatologic disorders. Difficulties in diagnosis are further compounded by the fact that osteoarthritis is an ubiquitous disease; accordingly, roentgenologic evidence of osteoarthritis does not exclude another disorder as the cause of the patient's primary presenting problem. Differential diagnosis can be especially confusing when osteoarthritis presents in atypical fashion such as involvement of joints not usually affected by primary osteoarthritic disease (for example, the shoulder or elbow) or when secondary structures such as nerve roots are involved and suggest another primary disorder.

There are no specific diagnostic laboratory abnormalities that will define the presence of osteoarthritis; laboratory studies are performed primarily to exclude other disease states. Examination of synovial fluid is helpful because findings are normal or only slightly deranged; significant abnormalities of an inflammatory nature serve to assist in excluding OA as the primary problem. Roentgenographic examination is the major diagnostic study used to confirm the diagnosis.

Treatment. Although treatment of osteoarthritis is symptomatic and nonspecific at present, much can be done to provide relief in many patients (see Chapters 17 to 20). Current therapy involves a baseline approach that includes patient understanding of the disease, appropriate rest for localized joint involvement, correction of factors causing excess strain, and physical therapy and rehabilitation measures. Restorative goals should be based on realistic use of available modalities; patient motivation and acceptance should be defined for each individual case. Drug therapy is an important mainstay in the treatment of osteoarthritis, but many patients can be effectively managed for long periods of time without the use of these agents. In other patients, analgesic and anti-inflammatory medications are extremely helpful. The short-term goal of most patients is relief of pain and localized stiffness. Primary long-term goals similarly include relief of pain and stiffness but are also strongly directed toward prevention of deformity and associated limitation of motion. In addition, maintenance of activities of daily living, job performance capabilities, and a functional independent role in family and community units needs to be addressed. The most

elusive long-term goal is the development of medical or surgical techniques that can prevent or consistently retard or reverse the disease.

As noted, at present there are no specific agents for use in the treatment of osteoarthritis that will prevent, retard, or reverse the disease. Nevertheless, a number of agents that have been studied in experimental models lead to the suggestion that the disease might be amenable to specific therapeutic management. Agents that inhibit proteolytic and collagenolytic enzymes may lessen or prevent matrix degradation; conversely, agents that stimulate chondrocyte proliferation or proteoglycan and collagen synthesis might be beneficial by stimulating repair (see Chapter 32).

Orthopedic procedures are important in the management of osteoarthritis and should not be reserved only for late severe disease. Disease progression may be retarded by correction of malalignment, which produces abnormal joint stresses such as genu varum (bowleg) or genu valgum (knock-knee) deformities of the knee. Tibial or femoral osteotomy, which redistributes stresses across the joint, may provide gratifying relief of pain by bringing healthy articular cartilages into apposition. Joint fusion, although less frequently used, particularly in weight-bearing joints, may still be indicated in certain patients for relief of pain in the presence of severe disease. Partial and total joint prosthetic replacements represent advances that provide a quantum improvement in the overall quality of life desired by any given patient, with marked relief of pain and improvement in limitation of motion. Significant complications related to these procedures such as early and late infection, venous thrombosis and pulmonary embolism, loosening of the prosthesis, and prosthesis fracture represent areas requiring further research. Rapidly developing advances in surgical techniques and management and the introduction of new prosthesis designs are targeted toward reducing the complication and failure rate of these procedures. Newer procedures utilizing biomaterials such as ceramics, and fixation of the prosthesis without the need for cement are promising alternatives to currently available methodologies.

Further Investigations. Research studies will be important in defining and clarifying questions that are basic to a further understanding of osteoarthritis. Of particular importance with respect to further investigations are studies defining (1) disease frequency; (2) disease susceptibility; (3) disease subsets; (4) the role of age, sex, race, heredity, obesity, and occupation; and (5) reasons for specific joint localization. A number of significant questions related to osteoarthritis remain to be considered. For example, why do so-called "nonprogressive" lesions of cartilage similar to lesions seen early in osteoarthritis fail to go on to produce clinically significant disease? How can differences in disease frequency and joint localization seen in males and females best be explained? Why do certain individuals respond differently to the same basic insult, with some individuals developing osteoarthritis and others not? How do we explain variations in rates of disease progression with obvious differences in the ability of cartilage in certain individuals to resist breakdown? Do genetic predispositions operate via specific factors such as excessive enzyme production or relative lack of enzyme inhibitors, decreased capability of cells to replicate or synthesize collagen and proteoglycan, or primary alterations in proteoglycan or collagen composition that make them more susceptible to damage?

As noted, further resolution of the concept that osteoarthritis represents a number of disease subsets that lead to similar clinical and pathologic end results, the final common pathway of the disease, needs to be delineated. Clinical and epidemiologic investigations, coupled with other avenues of basic research in cartilage pathophysiology, should allow a clearer delineation of clinical and pathogenic characteristics related to this ubiquitous disease.

References

1. Goldthwait JE: The differential diagnosis and treatment of the so-called rheumatoid diseases. Boston Med Surg J 151:529–534, 1904.
2. Garrod AE: Rheumatoid arthritis, osteoarthritis, arthritis deformans. In Allbutt TC, Radleston HD (eds.): A System of Medicine. New ed. London, Macmillan & Company, 1910, Vol. 3, 3–43.
3. Lawrence JS, Bremner JM, Bier F: Osteo-arthrosis. Prevalence in the population and relationship between symptoms and x-ray changes. Ann Rheum Dis 25:1–24, 1966.
4. Lawrence JS: Surveys of rheumatic complaints in the population. In Dixon ASJ (ed.):Progress in Clinical Rheumatology. London, J. and A. Churchill, 1966, p. 1.
5. Wood PHN: Rheumatic complaints. Br Med Bull 27:82–88, 1971.
6. Bremner JM, Lawrence JS, Miall WE: Degenerative joint disease in a Jamaican rural population. Ann Rheum Dis 27:326–332, 1968.
7. Kellgren JH, Lawrence JS, Bier F: Genetic factors in generalized osteoarthrosis. Ann Rheum Dis 22:237–255, 1963.
8. Lawrence JS: Generalized osteoarthrosis in a population sample. Am J Epidemiol 90:381–389, 1969.
9. Lowman EW: Osteoarthritis. JAMA 157:487–488, 1955.
10. Roberts J, Burch TA: Prevalence of osteoarthritis in adults by age, sex, race, and geographic area, United States—1960–1962. (National Center for Health Statistics: Vital and Health Statistics: Data from the National Health Survey.) Washington, D.C.: U.S. Government Printing Office. U.S. Public Health Service Publication 1000, Series 11, No. 15, 1966.
11. Solomon L, Beighton P, Lawrence JS: Rheumatic disorders in the South African Negro. Part II. Osteoarthrosis. S Afr Med J 49:1737–1740, 1975.
12. Blumberg BS, Bloch KJ, Black RL, Dotter C: A study of the prevalence of arthritis in Alaskan Eskimos. Arthritis Rheum 4:325–341, 1964.
13. Lawrence JS, DeGraff R, Laine VAI: Degenerative joint disease in random samples and occupational groups. In Kellgren JH, Jeffrey MR, Ball J (eds): The Epidemiology of Chronic Rheumatism, Vol 1. Oxford, Blackwell, 1963, pp. 98–119.
14. Goldin RH, McAdam L, Louie JS, et al.: Clinical and radiological survey of the incidence of osteoarthrosis among obese patients. Ann Rheum Dis 35:349–353, 1976.
15. Leach RE, Baumgard S, Broom J: Obesity: Its relationship to osteoarthritis of the knee. Clin Orthop 93:271–273, 1973.
16. Saville PD, Dickson J: Age and weight in osteoarthritis of the hip. Arthritis Rheum 11:635–644, 1968.
17. Silberberg M, Silberberg R: Osteoarthritis in mice fed diets enriched with animal or vegetable fat. Arch Pathol 70:385–390, 1960.
18. Sokoloff L, Mickelsen O, Silverstein E, Jay GE Jr, Yamamoto RS: Experimental obesity and osteoarthritis. Am J Physiol 198:765–770, 1960.
19. Acheson RM, Chan YK, Clemett AR: New Haven survey of joint diseases. XII. Distribution and symptoms of osteoarthrosis in the hands with reference to handedness. Ann Rheum Dis 35:274–278, 1976.
20. Kellgren JH, Lawrence JS: Osteo arthrosis and disk degeneration in an urban population. Ann Rheum Dis 17:388–397, 1958.
21. Mintz G, Fraga A: Severe osteoarthritis of the elbow in foundry workers. Arch Environ Health 27:78–80, 1973.
22. Burke MJ, Fear EC, Wright V: Bone and joint changes in pneumatic drillers. Ann Rheum Dis 36:276–279, 1977.
23. Puranen J, Ala-Ketola L, Peltokallio P, et al.: Running and primary osteoarthritis of the hip. Br Med J 2:424–425, 1975.
24. Murray RO: The aetiology of primary osteoarthritis of the hip. Br J Radiol 38:810–824, 1965.
25. Solomon L: Patterns of osteoarthritis of the hip. J Bone Joint Surg 58B:176-183, 1976.
26. Kellgren JH, Moore R: Generalized osteoarthritis and Heberden's nodes. Br Med J 1:181–187, 1952.
27. Crain DC: Interphalangeal osteoarthritis. JAMA 175:1049–1053, 1961.
28. Peter JB, Pearson CM, Marmor L: Erosive osteoarthritis of the hands. Arthritis Rheum 9:365–388, 1966.
29. Ehrlich GE: Osteoarthritis beginning with inflammation: Definitions and correlations. JAMA 232:157–159, 1975.

30. Resnick D, Shapiro RF, Wiesner KB, et al.: Diffuse idiopathic skeletal hyperostosis (DISH) (ankylosing hyperostosis of Forestier and Rotes-Querol). Semin Arthritis Rheum 7:153–187, 1978.

31. Danielsson LG, Hernborg J: Morbidity and mortality of osteoarthritis of the knee (gonarthrosis) in Malmo, Sweden. Clin Orthop 69:224–226, 1970.

32. Danielsson LG, Hernborg J: Clinical and roentgenologic study of knee joints with osteophytes. Clin Orthop 69:302–312, 1970.

33. Hernborg J, Nilsson BE: The relationship between osteophytes in the knee joint, osteoarthritis and aging. Acta Orthop Scand 44:69–74, 1973.

34. Howell DS, Moskowitz RW: Symposium on osteoarthritis: A brief review of research and definitions of future investigations. Arthritis Rheum 20(Suppl):S96–S103, 1977.

35. Herman JH, Carpenter BA: Immunobiology of cartilage. Semin Arthritis Rheum 5:1–40, 1975.

36. Malemud CJ, Moskowitz RW: Physiology of articular cartilage. Clin Rheum Dis 7:29–55, 1981.

BASIC
CONSIDERATIONS

Henry J. Mankin, M.D.
Section Editor

SECTION
1

1

The Epidemiology of Osteoarthritis

Jacques G. Peyron, M.D.

Epidemiology, usually defined as the study of diseases in groups or populations, is a powerful tool for uncovering significant clusters of cases and disclosing their correlations with etiologic factors or pathophysiologic mechanisms. For these reasons, epidemiology is potentially a very promising way of approaching study of a condition such as osteoarthritis that is widespread, has numerous variations with respect to clinical features, and is clearly multifactorial in origin.

HISTORY AND METHODS

The first epidemiologic studies of osteoarthritis (OA) appeared in the 1920's and endeavored to evaluate incapacity and invalidism in patients with this disorder who appeared for medical care. These early studies had obvious limitations in design, but in the 1950's more thorough population sample surveys were conducted to include people not limited to those seeking medical advice, thus permitting the evaluation of the overall prevalence of this and other rheumatic conditions. Lawrence, Kellgren, and colleagues, in Manchester, England, conducted many of these enquiries, the conclusions of which have been collected in two recent publications.[1, 2]

When questionnaires and clinical examination were the only methods used, considerable difficulty arose regarding diagnostic reliability and/or classification of the disease state. Systematic use of roentgenograms for detection of OA was introduced in 1956.[3] Given the discrepancy between clinical findings and roentgenologic changes and the relatively low predictive value of clinical signs for the presence of roentgenologic changes of OA (27% to 48%[4]), systematic roentgenologic surveys represented a substantial improvement on clinical screening. Conversely, it must be kept in mind that 15% or more of individuals with roentgenologic signs of joint degeneration are, on careful study, asymptomatic.[4]

The existence of these latent cases and of many "formes frustes" made it necessary to establish a roentgenologic grading system. In 1963, the Atlas of Standard Radiographs of Arthritis was published,[5] in which pictorial references allowed cases of osteoarthritis to be classified into four more or less distinct grades (Grade 1: small osteophytes of doubtful significance; Grade 2: definite osteophytes but joint space not impaired; Grade 3: moderate diminution of the joint space; and Grade 4: extensive loss of joint space with sclerosis of subchondral bone). It should be pointed out, however, that the presence of osteophytes cannot always be equated with the existence of OA or predictive of its appearance in the future.[6] Such a seemingly pathognomonic sign as isolated narrowing of the hip joint on roentgenogram has been shown to be of limited predictive value.[7] However, those roentgenograms that clearly demonstrate the criteria for Grades 3 and 4 are almost surely an indication of definite OA.

Another issue in any population survey is the joints studied. Some variation may be noted when hands or feet, the cervical spine (lateral view in flexion to visualize the interapophyseal joints), the knees (anteroposterior) and, in certain studies and after menopause in women, the pelvis and lumbar spine are utilized. Most authorities agree, however, that the roentgenograms should be read "blind" and by different independent observers. When studying a defined population sample, it is estimated that the sample size should be at least 85% of the individuals at risk so that the survey may be considered significant.[1]

Another method sometimes used is the clinical assessment of the presence of Heberden's nodes of the distal interphalangeal joints, because early physical findings may precede roentgenologic change, especially on anteroposterior views (the first osteophyte is often located dorsally and is seen only on lateral views).

It should be pointed out that one area of continued confusion is the definition of "generalized osteoarthritis," a clinical type described by Kellgren and Moore in 1952.[8] By arbitrary convention, this term is usually applied to individuals who display involvement of three or more joints or joint groups (the interphalangeals being considered a joint group).

Another type of survey is based on examination of the pathology of joints in systematic autopsy studies. Classic examples of these are the large series of Heine in 1926[9] on 1000 cases and the well-known, careful analysis of material by Bennett, Wayne, and Bauer in 1942,[10] in which the authors presented the gross and microscopic findings in 63 knee joints from individuals between 20 and 80 years of age.

The finding of late changes, such as full-thickness cartilage erosion, is rather straightforward and is clearly indicative of the disease; limited changes such as discoloration, fibrillation, or focal malacia of cartilage, however, can be much more difficult to evaluate. To further confuse the issue, it is apparent that in some large joints, "nonprogressive lesions" may be present that may not necessarily represent an early stage of typical OA.[11] An example of such confusion can be found in two recent gross studies of the knee joint in autopsy series. In the first one, in 300 subjects above age 50, lesions of the patella were found in 38% of the subjects, with similar findings in the femoral condyles in 23%.[12] The second report analyzed 66 subjects with a mean age above 70 and described osteoarthritic patellofemoral joints in 60% of the males and 72% of the females, with figures for the incidence in the tibiofemoral joints of 55% and 69%, respectively.[13]

Surveys of hospitalized patients are much more narrow in scope. Although unsuitable for estimating the overall prevalence of OA, they may be useful in individualizing certain subgroups and studying their significance or in comparing etiologic profiles of conditions occurring in the same age range (e.g., osteoporosis or calcium pyrophosphate deposition disease).

GENERAL PREVALENCE OF OSTEOARTHRITIS

It is clearly evident from the data shown in Table 1–1 that OA is present, in at least one joint, in a large proportion of individuals of different ethnic groups living in varied geographic locations. The values were collected by dissimilar techniques, so that they cannot really be compared with one another. They do, however, bear testimony to the indisputable fact that in any population over 35 years of age, OA will be present in one to two individuals out of three.

The weight of OA as a social and economic burden is also difficult to evaluate, chiefly because governmental agencies that collect such data usually do not single out OA in the

Table 1–1. PREVALENCE OF OA IN DIFFERENT POPULATIONS

	Age (years)	Female (%)	Male (%)
English population*[14]	35 and over	70	69
U.S. whites[15]	40 and over	44	43
Alaskan Eskimos[15]	40 and over	24	22
Jamaican rural population[16]	35–64	62	54
Pima Indians[17]	30 and over	74	56
Blackfeet Indians[17]	30 and over	74	61
South African blacks[18]	35 and over	53	60
Mean of 17 populations†[2]	35 and over	60	60

*Data from Lawrence JS, Bremner JM, Bier F: Ann Rheum Dis 25:1–24, 1966.
†Nine white, four black, four Indian.

"rheumatic disease" or "arthritis" groups. However, fragmentary evidence derived mostly from social agency statistics discloses alarmingly high figures. Evidence from British studies shows that in 1974 2.3% of the men and 1.3% of the women in the working population had to retire from employment because of OA or allied conditions; the total loss of work days for that year amounted to 4.7 million.[19] In individuals 55 to 64 years of age, 5% are required to leave their employment for 3 or more months because of peripheral OA.[14]

Figures from the United States reveal that in 1973 OA was the second ranking cause (after cardiovascular disease) of permanent incapacity in people over 50 years of age. Based on surveys, OA incapacitates two[20] to six[1] subjects out of 1000 in a general population.

OA of the hip strikes about 5% of the population above 55 years of age, and it is likely that about half of these patients will require hip surgery.[21] It was estimated that in 1975, 1.7 million individuals in the United States would benefit by hip arthroplasties and 4.6 million from knee arthroplasties.[22] In France, a 1975 survey of 2527 general practitioners revealed that 2.3% of their activity was addressed to peripheral OA.[23] Based on these surveys, there is no doubt that OA is a very major cause of incapacity, economic loss, and social disadvantage in all the world's populations over age 50.

Table 1–2. PREVALENCE OF OA (GRADES 3 AND 4) WITH ADVANCING AGE*

	15–44 years	45–64 years	65 years and over
Males	3%	25%	58%
Females	2%	30%	68%

*Data from Lawrence JS, Bremner JM, Bier F: Ann Rheum Dis 25:1–24, 1966.

INFLUENCE OF AGE

In all epidemiologic studies, the relationship of OA to aging is perhaps its most striking feature. In studies of an English population comprising more than 2000 individuals of mixed urban and rural origin, Lawrence and associates[14] found a marked increase in the frequency of severe OA (Grades 3 and 4) with advancing age (Table 1–2). The arrangement of the detailed figures along a curve clearly shows that the correlation is nonlinear and that the age-related increase appears exponential after 50 years of age (Fig. 1–1). The same trend is apparent from a review of several other studies, even taking into account variations between methods and examiners (Table 1–3). Heberden's nodes, for instance, have a prevalence of 29% in individuals between the ages of 59 and 69, but the prevalence increases to 69% in the 75-year-old and over age group.[28] Several studies have shown that the age-related

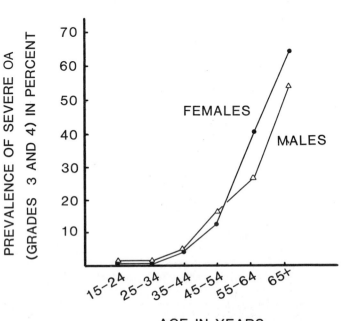

Figure 1–1. Correlation with age of the prevalence of OA in at least one joint in males and females from two English population samples. (Data from Lawrence JS: Rheumatism in Populations. London, William Heinemann Medical Books, 1977.)

Table 1–3. PREVALENCE OF OA IN WHITE POPULATIONS (PERCENTAGE)
RELATED TO AGE (OA IN AT LEAST ONE JOINT)

Author(s)	Age (years)	Females (%)	Males (%)	Both sexes (%)
Tzonchev et al.[24] (d)	15–24			0.8
Mikkelsen et al.[25] (b)	16–24			0.0
Gordon[26] (b)	18–24			4
Lawrence et al.[14] (a)	15 and over	22	19	
Gordon[26] (a)	18–79			37
Blumberg et al.[15] (c)	40 and over	44	43	
Kellgren and Lawrence[27] (d)	55–64	87	83	
(in 3+ joints)		47	25	
Gordon[26] (b)	65 and over	87	78	
Tzonchev et al.[24] (d)	65 and over			37
Mikkelsen et al.[25] (b)	65 and over	90	78	

a = roentgenograms of hands, feet, and cervical spine
b = roentgenograms of hands and feet
c = roentgenograms of hands
d = mixed clinical and roentgenologic assessment

increment in the prevalence of OA applies particularly to multiarticular involvement in women over age 55.[1, 25, 26]

Lawrence has shown that the age-related increase appears linear for OA cases of Grades 2 to 4 but that if one studies only individuals with OA of Grades 3 and 4, which are the cases most likely to be expressed clinically, the increase is exponential (Fig. 1–1). This feature is found in both British and United States studies, applies equally to both sexes, and is the same for groups of differing socioeconomic status.[1]

It has been suggested that the exponential increase in the frequency of OA seen in advanced age groups may be explained by a mutation in recognition of autologous cartilage proteins by cells of the immune system, which, because of the isolation of the cartilage from the blood system, are viewed by the immune cells as "foreign."[29] Alternatively, the finding may simply represent an effect of increasing secondary mechanical instability superimposed on degenerated cartilage over a period of years.[1]

The specific joints affected by OA appear to vary somewhat depending on the age group studied. The site where OA is seen earliest is the first metatarsophalangeal joint, with significant numbers of cases present in individuals over 25 years of age. From age 35 on, OA begins to appear in the wrist and the spine. In subjects 45 years of age, the distal interphalangeal joints are likely to be involved, usually the index finger first, followed by other small joints of the hand (first carpometacarpal, metacarpophalangeal, and proximal interphalangeal joints). Localization of the process in the knees, especially in women, seems to appear somewhat later in life, and the hip is statistically the joint to be involved latest.

AGING AND THE PATHOPHYSIOLOGY OF OSTEOARTHRITIS

The mechanisms by which the process of aging relates to the onset of OA is at present poorly understood. Factors possibly operative include minute anatomic changes of the joints, or biochemical or biomechanical alterations in the articular cartilage, which in turn compromise its mechanical properties.

Anatomic Joint Changes

Most joints are obviously incongruent, even the ankle joint,[30] a feature only partially compensated for in some of them by fibrocartilaginous menisci or labra. Several studies have shown that in the unloaded hip, the contact zone is in the shape of a horseshoe, sagittally crossing the femoral upper pole and leaving a shallow space between the femoral apex and the acetabulum.[31, 32] Because of cartilage deformability, this contact area increases under load, thus maintaining the pressure per unit area within physiologic limits. This incongruity seems to be maintained throughout life by an active process that is pressure-dependent and occurs as a result of slow remodeling of the osteochrondal junction.[33] In elderly people, however, the joints seem to become more congruent, a fact that has been demonstrated at the hip[34] and at the radiohumeral joints.[35]

The cause of this increased incongruity is not known, but it has been speculated that it results from an imperfect remodeling process.[36, 37] The end result, however, appears to render the protective mechanism described above less efficient.

Structural changes that have been related to age occur mostly in the superficial layer of cartilage. Scanning electron microscopy has disclosed an uncovering of superficial collagen bundles that seem less coated with matrix and are torn off in places, with fibrils floating in the joint cavity.[38] Age-related changes in cell density have also been described.[39] Some age-related *changes in the mechanical properties* of articular cartilage have been documented.[40] The compression stress-strain curve and the tensile stiffness under weak force (5 MN/m²) do not vary with age,[40, 41] but under strong stresses (10 MN/m²) the tensile stiffness decreases in an age-related way.[40] It is of interest that compression strain and low stress tensile properties are related essentially to protease-sensitive components of the matrix, i.e., proteoglycan concentration, whereas the high stress tensile properties (as well as the fracture stress) are dependent on the collagen content, as shown by dramatic alterations after collagenase treatment.[42] Increased compliance due to age would allow increased contact area of articular surfaces under load.[43]

The fibrous network of articular cartilage appears to become increasingly prone to fatigue failure with advancing age, i.e., the number of repeated stresses necessary to rupture a piece of cartilage stretched parallel to its superficial fibers decreases very significantly with the advancing age of the individual from whom the specimen was obtained.[44, 45] The mechanism of this change is not known. It has been postulated that the alteration results from a slow change in the perifibrillar coating material (a part of the matrix about which very little is known), a progressive disruption of intermolecular crosslinks between collagen monomers, and/or changes in fibrillar hydration. In this respect, the recent description of a hydroxy-pyridinium-derived bond and a peculiar packing of molecules in Type II collagen is of interest and importance.[46] Changes in the staining properties of the superficial layer of articular cartilage with advancing age have suggested that in specimens from older individuals, keratan sulfate (as well as perhaps an amyloid-like substance), usually found mostly in the deep layers, is found near the surface.[47]

With regard to *biochemical changes,* the alterations that might be relevant to the inception of OA are those that will occur between early adulthood and approximately 50 to 60 years of age, thus excluding the changes related to growth and maturation of the skeleton. Moreover, one must be certain to study only histologically normal (nonfibrillated) cartilage. Although these changes have been extensively reviewed recently,[48] it is apparent that full agreement about them has not been reached.

The water content of articular cartilage shows a small but significant decrease with age, from approximately 75% to 70%, especially in the deeper layers.[49] This is in sharp contrast to the findings in OA in which an increase in water content has been consistently reported.

The total glycosaminoglycan content, evaluated by fixed-charge density, shows a small increment with age, mostly in the deep layer, essentially thought to arise as a result of the increased concentration of keratan sulfate.[49–52] Old cartilage is richer in chondroitin 6-sulfate at the expense of chondroitin 4-sulfate,[50] perhaps through a shift in synthesis by older chondrocytes.[53] Hyaluronic acid concentration has been reported to rise from 1% to 6% between skeletal maturity and age 60.[43]

Collagen shows a slight decrease on a dry weight basis with age, roughly parallel to the fall in water content, so that its wet weight ratio stays unchanged at approximately 20%. Cartilage collagen, which is relatively insoluble in salt and acid solutions in the young adult, becomes even less soluble in older subjects, possibly owing to a change in the nature of its crosslinks.[46, 54]

The proportion of relatively small-density proteoglycan monomers appears to increase significantly in aging dog[55] and human[56] cartilages. The linear length of the macromolecules is shortened, primarily at the expense of the chondroitin sulfate–rich region, thus demonstrating a relative increase in the ratio of keratan sulfate to chondroitin sulfate, and protein.[55, 57] Among the different populations of proteoglycan monomers, a subset made up of small units with a distinct electrophoretic migration has been shown to disappear in the cartilage of subjects more than 40 years old.[58]

The aggregating capacity between hyaluronic acid and proteoglycans extracted from the femoral head cartilage of elderly people has been reported to be impaired,[59] a defect that might compromise the mechanical properties of older cartilage.

Finally, there is some evidence from cell

culture experiments that "older" chondrocytes (i.e., those studied after several cell passages) display an increased catabolic activity.[60]

In general, it is difficult to assess how these age-related changes in the biochemistry of articular cartilage could predispose to OA, because the biochemical alterations seen in aging and OA are markedly different, except perhaps for diminished size of the monomer and decreased proteoglycan aggregation. Collagen properties and collagen-proteoglycan-water interactions are currently the central foci of considerable research interest.

ROLE OF SEX AND HORMONES

The relation of sex to the prevalence of OA is mostly noticeable in the second half of adult life. Up to 45 years of age, OA is globally rare and slightly more prevalent in males. Between the ages of 45 and 55 years, it is found with equal frequency in both sexes, but over the age of 55, the disease occurs significantly more frequently in women (Fig. 1–1).[25, 61, 62] Osteoarthritis in females occurs not only more frequently but is also more severe, as shown by the steeper increase in the severity index of OA of the fingers in women between 45 and 55 years of age when compared with that for men in the same age group.[63] Multiple involvement is also a feature more prevalent in OA in women, with 1.8% of women over 15 years of age displaying five or more joints involved, compared with 0.5% of men.[14] In the 55- to 64-year-old age group, four or more involved joints are noted in 47% of women but in only 29% of men.[14]

Sex also appears to influence the pattern of distribution of OA. While involvement of the interphalangeal joints (especially the distal ones), the first carpometacarpal joint, and the knee joints constitutes the most frequent pattern for women, localization of the disease to the metacarpophalangeal joints and to the hips is more common in men. In general, OA tends to be more widespread and more severe in women from age 50 on.

Some experimental data have been reported that suggest that estrogens may have a protective effect against OA. In strains of mice that spontaneously develop OA, the prevalence is more marked in males that can be partially protected by orchiectomy or by estrogens. On the other hand, testosterone and progesterone somewhat increase the expression of OA in male and spayed female animals.[64–67] In other

OA-prone strains, however, Sokoloff and associates failed to observe a similar sex hormone–directed sparing or enhancing effect.[68, 69] In a study of postmenopausal women, no significant difference was found in urinary excretion of gonadotropic hormones between those with OA and normal controls.[70] In an experimental partial-meniscectomy model in the rabbit, estrogens appeared to exert no preventive or ameliorative effect on joint degeneration.[71] On the contrary, in this study, estrogens appeared to accentuate the frequency and severity of degenerative changes; tamoxifen, an estrogen antagonist, ameliorated osteoarthritic findings.

In a clinical study, protracted estrogen therapy started 1 year after menopause in a group of women with OA of the proximal and distal interphalangeal joints did not prevent progression of the disease or alter the severity of the lesion grade.[63] In consideration of these data, it has been suggested that sex hormones have less effect on joint structures than on bony tissue and that if such hormones are operative in the disease, they may act through the modulation of genetic factors.[67, 68, 72]

Enlargement of joints and development of osteophytes are constant features of acromegalic arthropathy. Growth hormone levels studied in women with OA at the time of menopause were found to be approximately twice those of matched control subjects with normal joints.[73] The comparison of the histologic pattern is not entirely valid, however, because thickening of the cartilage and diffuse chondrocytic proliferation typical of acromegaly are not regularly noted in histologic study of cartilage from osteoarthritic joints.

MECHANICAL FACTORS IN OSTEOARTHRITIS

Studies of comparative series in selected groups of subjects can help to disclose some putative relationships between abnormal or excessive physical stress on joints and the prevalence of OA.

Joint Hyperlaxity

In one study, ligamentous laxity was found to be associated with postmenopausal joint degeneration in 11% of 250 cases;[74] in another report, evidence of generalized OA was present in 11 of 16 patients with joint hyperlaxity (three of whom had had recurrent joint luxation), whereas among 21 age- and sex-matched controls only two cases of generalized OA were revealed.[75] Patients with OA were shown to have a higher prevalence of generalized hyperlaxity than controls matched for age and sex.[76] The most striking feature of the syndrome of hypermobile joints, however, is the remarkable frequency of synovial effusions and chondrocalcinosis.[75, 77] Some of these joints with calcified cartilages may go on to develop florid degenerative changes.

The explanation of the association of hypermobility and OA has to date been less than clear. Joint hypermobility is well known to be associated with disorders such as recurrent dislocation of the shoulder or the patella[78] or with recurrent effusion of the knee or the hip joint.[79] It has been speculated that such chronic recurrent injuries to joints may, over time, favor the inception of OA. Of interest in this regard, however, is a recent discussion of hypermobility associated with inherited connective tissue disorders or neuromuscular disease of infancy in which it was concluded that precocious OA is not a commonly observed feature of these conditions.[80] Finally, it remains to be established if hypermobile joints favor the onset of classic OA or, instead, lead to the "arthritis of hypermobility," a particular pattern of joint damage characterized by traumatic synovitis and chondrocalcinosis.[75]

Effect of Mechanical Overuse

Over the years, numerous surveys have been made of groups exposed to prolonged and/or excessive stresses to certain joints (see Chapters 30 and 33). In a study of skeletal remains of contemporary white and black Americans, twelfth-century Pueblo Indians, and protohistorical Alaskan Eskimos,[61] the last group, believed to have sustained the heaviest physical strain, consistently displayed the earliest and most severe joint lesions. The prevalence of shoulder OA in the males of this group was particularly striking, possibly implicating occupational factors such as boating and fishing. The joints of black individuals, whose occupations tend to be more heavily weighted toward physical labor than those of whites, showed a more severe involvement. In all groups, lesions were more marked in right elbows than in the left ones, indicating the possible effect of handedness.

Numerous studies have been conducted on selected occupational groups and on athletes. A review of cases seen in a French rheumatologic clinic, when compared with regional population surveys, showed that farmers had a higher prevalence of OA of the hip, that the syndrome appeared somewhat earlier (mean 54 years versus 58 years of age) and was more often of the primary type (i.e., without joint anatomic defect), and that it was noted in a higher proportion of males than in the controls.[81] These data suggested that joint "overuse" might have a significant influence on the development of OA. Confirmatory evidence for these findings has been reported from Austria[82] and in another French study,[83] which disclosed primary OA in 33% of farmers but in only 19% of controls. In a Swedish geographic survey,[84] the highest prevalence of OA in general was noted in regions where farming and forestry were the leading occupations.

Along similar lines, a European study of retired athletes showed a particularly high percentage of subjects with OA of the hip (52%) of early onset (42 years of age) and predominating on the left side (usually the driving or kicking limb).[85] Of some significance in considering this association is the fact that intensive sports training often begins at about 14 years of age in many individuals, prior to skeletal maturity. It could be speculated that such early activity could lead to a slight posterior slip of the capital femoral epiphysis, eventually resulting in a dysplastic joint and osteoarthritis in later life.[86] In a recent study in which matched groups of patients seeking advice for musculoskeletal problems were compared with individuals with nonmusculoskeletal disorders,[87] a higher prevalence of a past history of sports participation, especially rugby and soccer, was reported in the "rheumatologic" patients.

Among industrial workers, miners have been most extensively studied. Several series have shown that the incidence of OA in miners, when compared with that in porters or clerks, is considerably greater in the hips (43% for miners, 28% for porters), in the knees (46% versus 32%), and in the shoulders (52% versus 12%).[88] The figures for involvement of the shoulder, an ordinarily infrequent site for the development of OA, are particularly suggestive of the possibility that injuries to the rotator cuff caused by the peculiarities of working in the mine may play an initiating role in the pathogenesis of OA.

Lawrence[89] found a high proportion of severe OA of the knees in mine roadway workers

(10%), which he felt was most likely related to the frequency of work-related injuries to the menisci. Similarly, dock workers showed a higher prevalence of OA in fingers, elbows, and knees (mean of 21.3%) when compared with age-matched civil servants (mean of 9.4%).[90] In general, however, the prevalence of OA is higher in miners than in dockyard workers.[91]

Increased involvement of the right hand of subjects when compared with the left has been amply documented in the literature.[1, 92] In cotton factory workers, the joints of the hand, particularly the distal interphalangeal joints, are frequently affected.[93] In women working in a weaving factory for over 20 years, a detailed study of groups of workers involved in three distinct stereotypic, repetitive types of handwork confirmed that the right hand was more severely involved; this study also disclosed a pattern of hand and finger lesions that could be directly related to the type of work done by each group (with the joints most repetitively taxed being the most involved).[94]

Other investigators, however, have failed to demonstrate a clear relationship between mechanical overuse and the development of osteoarthritis. In a survey of a group of 364 female physical education teachers, aged 45 to 60 years and active in their profession for 15 to 30 years, OA of the knee was found in only 8% and OA of the hip in 7.7%, figures that were comparable to those of the same age group in the general population.[76] Of some note in this series, however, was the high correlation of knee OA with previous meniscectomy. Pneumatic drilling has been stated to favor the development of degenerative lesions in the elbow,[95] but in a recent survey of 34 pneumatic drill operators, only two cases of moderate osteoarthritis of this joint were found.[96] Of some interest was the finding of spurs in the triceps insertions in 9 subjects and mild OA of the hands in 17.

As noted above and in other studies,[97, 98] OA affecting the lower limb has been found with excessive frequency in athletes, but the issue has recently been questioned.[99] Wright[76] examined 66 professional soccer players and found OA of the knee in only 10.6%, a prevalence that the author feels would be expected in the general population.

The ankle joint, for reasons not completely defined, appears to be "immune" to OA, even in the elderly population[100] or in face of overuse,[101] as long as the bony and ligamentous structures of the joint are intact. It is likely that earlier studies claiming ankle vulnerability in soccer players accepted as a roentgenologic criterion of OA the presence of nonprogressive periarticular spurs, which probably arise in response to repeated local stresses.

In their study, Puranen and associates[102] found fewer cases of OA of the hip in 74 professional runners than in a group of matched controls. A recent evaluation of the knee joints of 15 veteran marathon runners confirmed the relative absence of OA in this group.[103] In a study of 100 patients with osteoarthritis of the hip who were sufficiently disabled to require surgery, no association was found with prior athletic activity.[104]

The interpretation of epidemiologic studies that have attempted to relate OA to mechanical stress is not a simple problem. If joint overuse began prior to complete skeletal maturity, epiphyseal injuries and slight joint deformations that could cause a subsequent secondary OA might have occurred. Alternatively, the excessive rate of OA in certain groups at risk might be primarily due to an increased rate of joint injuries (e.g., meniscal or ligamentous damage). Finally, the criteria chosen to define the presence of OA in such groups must be quite strict and should certainly include evidence of progressive changes in the joint and indisputable cartilage damage.

In general, a review of the data available suggests that normal joints have a remarkable tolerance to mechanical wear and that as long as the usage (or even abuse) does not exceed their normal anatomic and physiologic ranges, joints probably do not "wear out," even under very severe and chronic stress. It should be emphasized, however, that the periarticular structures (ligaments, capsule, and muscular attachments) are of the utmost importance in this respect and that damage (traumatic or surgical) to these parts of the joint may lead to an accelerated degeneration of the joint (see Chapter 33). Under these circumstances, it is probably true that repetitive mechanical stresses can materially influence the distribution and pattern of OA.[91, 93, 94]

Bone Density

Ample evidence now exists to support the concept that bone density bears a relationship to the development and extent of OA. In a roentgenographic evaluation of the bone trabecular pattern (and, hence, bone density) in the femoral head, a diminished bony mass was associated with fractures of the femoral neck, whereas increased bone mass, not only in the femur but also in the second metacarpal, showed a distinct positive correlation with OA of the hip.[105] These data were confirmed by a study using photon absorbtiometry.[106] Solomon,[107] in comparing 60 individuals with "primary OA" of the hip with 63 patients with fractures of the femoral neck, showed an above-average bone density in the group with OA and a statistically significant decrease in the group with the fractures.

The same concept was supported when a similar study was performed using a reverse analytic system. When the OA index for finger involvement was assessed in postmenopausal women, the value was found to fall considerably below the average in subjects who had sustained a fracture of the femoral neck or vertebral body but was increased to values above the average in those patients with OA of the hip.[63] Analysis of the digital bone mass of the group of subjects with OA was at least one standard deviation above the mean, confirming the findings now generally accepted—that individuals with OA and those with fractures due to osteopenia make up two statistically exclusive populations.

The nature of this inverse correlation has not been established, but it has been postulated that a reduced bone mass increases the vibration-absorbing capacity of the juxta-articular bone and thus protects articular cartilage against peak stresses. Conversely, increase in bone density in the subchondral region may increase the forces acting on the cartilage and thus predispose the individual to osteoarthritic change.

Obesity

Based on logic, it would be anticipated that obesity would inflict increased stress on weight-bearing joints and lead to increased prevalence of osteoarthritis. Indeed, in a survey of British patients, Lawrence[1] found a significant association of obesity with OA of the knees in females in the 55- to 64-year-old age group and a lesser correlation with OA of the hips in males. In another investigation, 100 patients with OA of the hips referred for surgery were found to have a marked tendency toward obesity, with more than 60% being above ideal body weight.[104] In a French study, 27% of postmenopausal women with OA were found to be overweight.[74]

The correlation was not entirely clearly defined by these studies, however, because patients with OA of weight-bearing joints tend to exercise less than their counterparts with healthy joints. As possible evidence for this point is the fact that when the converse study was performed, a group of severely obese patients between 25 and 34 years of age did not display an increased prevalence of OA in the lower limbs (or in the wrists and fingers).[108] Finally, in a survey of 121 orthopedic patients with OA of the hip, no difference in height/weight ratio was shown when compared with that of normal controls.[109]

As indicated above, the relationship between obesity and OA might not be a simple mechanical one but may involve associated systemic or physiologic factors. It is certainly possible that genetics may play a significant role as well.

Several studies have attempted to define an association of OA with somatotypes. In 1975, Acheson and Collart[62] noted that the prevalence of OA was greater in stout individuals than in thin ones, and they described an inverse correlation with the height/weight ratio, even when the main location of the disease was in the digits. In 1981, Solomon and associates[110] compared the somatotypes of 105 patients with OA of the hip with those of 100 patients with fracture of the femoral neck and found that 96% of those in the group with OA were endomorphic mesomorphs, whereas 75% of the group with the fracture displayed features of ectomorphy.

ASSOCIATION WITH SOME SYSTEMIC FACTORS

A variety of systemic disorders have been found to be statistically associated with the presence of OA. In terms of laboratory abnormalities, elevated levels of serum uric acid, antistreptolysin O, C-reactive protein, and acute-phase reactants have been described in a comprehensive survey of 685 individuals in New Haven, Connecticut.[62] These factors correlate with single-digit OA as well as with polyarticular disease and with weight-bearing as well as with non–weight-bearing joint involvement. The correlation for women was significantly greater than that for men. The association of OA with an increased serum uric acid level was confirmatory of a prior study performed by Lawrence in 1969.[111] These systemic factors, suggestive of some past or present low-grade inflammatory process, seem to correlate particularly well with generalized OA occurring in the absence of Heberden's nodes (non-nodal generalized OA).

Hypertension, defined as a diastolic blood pressure greater than 100 mm Hg, has been found to be significantly associated with generalized OA in elderly male patients.[112] The OA in the hypertensive group was found primarily in the hips, knees, carpometacarpal joints, and metatarsophalangeal joints and appeared to be independent of obesity.

INFLUENCE OF CLIMATE

Climatic conditions do not appear to have any influence on the prevalence of OA. Comparison of figures for populations living in very different parts of the world show no correlation with latitude or with any type of climate (see Table 1–1).

Roentgenograms of the hands and feet were compared for two groups of American Indians of the same ethnic descent but living in a cold mountain region and a hot desert, respectively, and no differences were noted.[17] In an extensive survey by Lawrence and Sebo,[2] a comparison was made among roentgenograms of hands and feet for 17 different European, African, and American populations, all living from 54 degrees North to 26 degrees South latitude. Nine of these groups were white, four black, and four American Indian; six lived in urban areas, and 11 lived in rural settings. No significant differences were noted in the prevalence of OA among the different groups.

In a Swedish questionnaire survey conducted in 1975 and 1976, the highest prevalence of OA was found in the southeastern and midnorthern regions of the country and seemed to be considerably more closely correlated with occupation (farming and forestry) than with climatic variations.[84]

PATTERN OF MULTIPLE JOINT INVOLVEMENT: GENERALIZED OSTEOARTHRITIS

Multiple Joint Involvement: Generalized Osteoarthritis

Since the first report by Haygarth in 1805[113] of OA involvement in several joints simulta-

neously in the same subject, the pattern has been observed frequently. Cecil and Archer[114] noted polyarticular nodal (i.e., in association with Heberden's nodes) disease in 145 subjects out of a total of 182. In 1952, Kellgren and Moore[8] studied 391 subjects with OA and, on the basis of their findings, coined the term "generalized osteoarthritis" for those individuals who manifested involvement of three or more joints or groups of joints outside the spine.

The first issue in relation to this category of disease is the question of the validity of the pattern: Is generalized OA part of a progressive, age-related, random extension of the OA process, or does it, in fact, stand apart as a recognizable constellation of joint involvement with special features in terms of its pattern and its associated processes? The implication of an affirmative answer to the latter part of this question is that generalized OA is somehow a systemic disease.

In a study of OA of the hand and fingers performed in the United States, it was concluded that cases with multiple joint involvement were not a discrete group but merely the extreme end of a continuum.[115] However, in a European multicenter study of 178 case records, it was concluded that multiple joint involvement of a particular pattern of distribution is sufficiently discrete to make generalized OA a clinical entity.[116] Support for this concept was noted when the cases of the British surveys were plotted according to the number of joints involved. In the 55- to 64-year-old age group, a bimodal distribution was noted, with peaks at one and three joints in females.[1] If only cases involving five or more joints are included, generalized OA stands out even more strikingly as a specific, discrete syndrome.[117]

The most commonly observed constellation of generalized OA consists of involvement of interphalangeal, first metatarsophalangeal, and first carpometacarpal joints. Then, in order of decreasing frequency, the process involves the knees, cervical and lumbar spine, metacarpophalangeal joints, hips, and wrists. The involvement of the joints of the fingers is a pivotal and characteristic feature of generalized OA. Differences in clinical features have been noted if the disease principally affects the distal rather than the proximal interphalangeal joints, although the groups show considerable overlap.[118] The distal type (associated with Heberden's nodes and, hence, "nodal") characteristically displays a strong familial history and occurs predominantly in women. In the "non-nodal" type (proximal interphalangeal joint involvement), the familial tendency is less striking and the syndrome seems to predominate (if it does so at all) in males (9% versus 8%). In patients with non-nodal disease, a history of episodes of transient, seronegative, inflammatory polyarthritis and the occurrence of roentgenologic juxta-articular bony erosions are encountered in a highly significant proportion of the cases (especially in women).[8, 117] Despite these findings, no relationship has been noted with rheumatoid arthritis.[1] Indeed, recent reappraisals of the clinical presentation of OA have revealed that 73% of cases of OA of the knees and 18% of cases involving the distal interphalangeal joints display local inflammatory signs.[119] However, these features are thought to be secondary to degeneration of joint tissues.

Relation to Ethnic Groups

Differences in the pattern of presentation and joint involvement have been noted in different ethnic groups. A South African rural population displayed approximately one-third the frequency of multiple joint involvement (three or more joints) than seen in most European surveys, a feature considered to be related to the rarity of inflammatory polyarthritis in Africans.[18] Localization of the disease to the first metatarsophalangeal joint, the first carpometacarpal joint, and the hips is common in white populations but rare in blacks and American Indians.[2]

Heberden's nodes are rare in all the black populations of South Africa, Nigeria, Liberia, Jamaica, and the United States.[1, 18, 120] The average values for prevalence for subjects over 35 years of age in white populations is 21.3% in females and 17.3% in males, whereas in blacks the values are 2.2% to 8% in females and 2.7% to 5% in males. There is a greater prevalence in American Indians than in blacks, but investigators have indicated that the prevalence in some populations may be influenced by occupational factors, especially in males.

Differences appear to exist among the various ethnic populations as well. In English surveys, the prevalence of Heberden's nodes and nodal generalized OA is lower in the populations of Welsh stock than in groups of Anglo-Saxon or Viking descent.[2] Non-nodal generalized OA, which is common in white and rare in all black and Indian populations, occurs as frequently in Jamaicans as in European whites. In contrast, the same disorder is rare in white patients in Czechoslovakia.[2]

The prevalence of OA of the hips is noticeably greater in white populations and is considerably diminished in frequency in black and American Indian populations. In subjects above 55 years of age, OA of the hip was noted in 3% to 9% of males and 2% to 11% of females in six European population samples and in 0% to 2% of males and 0% to 4% of females in three black African samples.[2] The prevalence of OA of the hip in the Chinese population in Hong Kong 54 years of age and older has been found to be 1.2% in males and 0.8% in females.[121] Similar values were noted in the Japanese population.[122] The rarity of OA of the hip in Asian populations stands in sharp contrast to a prevalence of distal interphalangeal joint involvement, which is similar to that for Europeans. A major factor in hip involvement probably lies in the decreased frequency of congenital hip dysplasia in many of the nonwhite populations,[18, 121, 122] thus drastically reducing the cases secondary to anatomic defects.

Study of OA of the knees shows considerably less difference among the ethnic groups. The frequency of OA of the knees in South Africans and Jamaicans does not differ significantly from that for white populations. In a recent study from Greenland,[123] it was shown that the prevalence of knee OA was significantly higher in women of the western coast (36%) (from a mixed Eskimo-European stock) than in women of the eastern coast (13%) (from a pure Eskimo population). However, occupational factors might have played a role in this difference.

HEREDITY

The approaches to the possible hereditary factors operative in OA have been mainly along two lines.[80] The first follows the classic epidemiologic methods of evaluating the prevalence of the different types of the disease in the families of the patients (especially in twins) or searching for significant associations with known hereditary characteristics such as blood or tissue types. The second technique uses the study of models in which the number of variables can be expected to be lower than in the naturally occurring condition. These models may be found in some animal strains, or in certain hereditary diseases of connective tissues in which degenerative arthritis is a particularly prominent feature.

Heberden's Nodes

Heberden's nodes, a disease state with an extraordinarily strong familial tendency and known to be extremely rare in the black races,[18, 120] is a type of OA in which the influence of heredity is the most obvious. Stecher[120] noted that Heberden's nodes occurred three times more frequently in the sisters of affected women than in the general population and hypothesized that the disorder is transmitted as a simple, autosomal dominant genetic error in females and as a recessive one in males. This view is supported by studies by McKusick,[124] who postulated that expression was long delayed, with clinical manifestations peaking at approximately 70 years of age, at which age 27% of women and 3% of men would manifest the trait. Data from British studies[1] showed that Grades 3 and 4 nodal disease could be found in 38% of females aged 75 or more but also in 31% of males of the same age. Although these data are compatible with the hypothesis advanced by Stecher[120] and McKusick,[124] the "fit" would be somewhat better for a disorder of polygenic heredity with a higher threshold of expressivity in males.[1]

In British twin studies, Heberden's nodes were observed in 60% of monozygous and 39% of dizygous co-twins of probands, and in 13% and 18%, respectively, of co-twins of subjects without nodes.[1] However, hereditary predisposition to Heberden's nodes would seem to be obvious in only about half the observed cases, and it is likely that a sizable proportion of the cases are of traumatic origin.[1]

Generalized Osteoarthritis

The genetics of the disorder described as generalized OA are far less clear. The condition shows a familial aggregation, being distinctly more common in the first-degree relatives of patients with generalized OA. Thirty-six per cent of the relatives of men with nodal generalized OA and 49% of the kin of women with the disorder showed the disease, with the expected values for the same age group of the general population being 17% and 26%, respectively.[117] If only female relatives are studied, the value is increased, with 45% of first-degree relatives of nodal probands showing nodal generalized OA. Spouses of the probands showed no increased incidence of osteoarthritis over the level of the general population.

The aforementioned figures appear to apply only to patients with multiple joint involvement, because among patients with only one or two locations of the disease, there is not a significant increase in the frequency of the process in their relatives. Thus, it seems that it is the polyarticular feature that is transmitted, and study of these patients discloses that most of the involved joints occur in the upper limb and non–weight-bearing segments.

If cases of generalized OA are broken down into nodal and non-nodal types, close relatives of patients with nodal disease develop the nodal variant of generalized OA (more frequently in women and about three times the expected frequency). Conversely, families of patients with non-nodal disease tend to have mostly non-nodal generalized OA; strikingly, the prevalence of Heberden's nodes is no more than that of the general population, except, remarkably, in the female relatives of male probands (2.5 times the expected rate). An increase in metacarpophalangeal joint and wrist involvement is also noticeable, suggesting the possibility that the disorder may be associated with a polyarticular inflammatory factor.

Twin studies have also confirmed the influence of a hereditary factor in the familial trend for generalized OA, especially in cases involving five or more joints in women. Concordance was noted in 57% of monozygous and 33% of dizygous co-twins, whereas the values for control subjects without OA were 0% and 14%, respectively.

If the hereditary data for the two clinical forms of generalized OA are considered, it appears that nodal disease has a high rate of hereditary transmission, whereas the non-nodal form may well be associated with a polyarticular inflammatory factor.

No correlation has been found between the prevalence of OA and that of the main blood groups[1] or with HLA tissue types.[125]

Animal Studies

Epidemiologic studies of animal populations with spontaneous OA have, for the most part, used certain inbred strains of mice[126–129] (see Chapter 6). In general, the breeding experiments point to a polygenic type of heredity, often displaying a recessive behavior. In some strains, the distribution of OA seems to be sex-linked, with most cases occurring in males. Differentiation from a hereditarily transmitted joint dysplasia that, over time, leads to a secondary type of OA is not always clear.[130] Moreover, comparison of the process to human OA must sometimes be critically viewed, particularly for such species as the STR/1N strain of mice, in which detachment of articular cartilage occurs without fibrillation.[131]

Hereditary Connective Tissue Diseases

There are numerous hereditary disorders that affect the connective tissues and have osteoarthritis as a prominent feature. Such diseases include the mucopolysaccharidoses, alkaptonuric ochronosis, hereditary chondrocalcinosis, dysplasia epiphysealis multiplex, the spondyloepiphyseal dysplasias, pseudoachondroplasia, and the various Ehlers-Danlos syndromes, to mention a few (see Chapter 14). Most of these syndromes are transmitted by a single gene, usually autosomal (except certain types of spondyloepiphyseal dysplasias and Hunter's disease), sometimes dominant, and occasionally recessive.[80] The pathogenesis of the joint lesions is not always clearly defined for most of these conditions, and the question of whether the OA is due to joint deformation or malfunction or results from some primary alteration in articular cartilage biochemistry has not really been answered. The possibility of this latter mechanism is supported by certain cases of apparently primary and precocious OA with no systemic involvement but with histologic lesions suggestive of primary chondrocyte storage dysfunction.[132]

OSTEOARTHRITIS AND INFLAMMATION

Generalized Relationships

The relationship of OA to inflammation is a subject about which studies based on large series of patients have disclosed some interesting correlations. Classically, OA is considered to be a noninflammatory type of arthritis (as opposed to rheumatoid arthritis [RA]), although it is apparent, as mentioned earlier,

that prior inflammatory episodes in certain subsets may play a role in the pathogenesis of the disease. In fact, however, several recent evaluations of rather large series of patients have shown that signs of local joint inflammation are frequently seen in patients with OA. In a review of 100 consecutive patients with classic OA without roentgenographic evidence of juxta-articular erosions such as are seen in rheumatoid arthritis, 55% had polyarticular disease (three or more joints involved), 71% experienced morning stiffness of more than 5 minutes' duration, 73% of involved knees displayed effusions, and 26% of the knees were warm.[119] Compared with the clinical picture of 100 patients with rheumatoid arthritis, the patients with OA were found to have fewer involved joints (OA—two to four joints; RA—six to ten joints). Disease progression in OA was much slower, with a mean delay between involvement of the first and second joint of 48 months in OA, as compared with 11 months in RA. Both disorders showed an identical tendency toward symmetry.

Synovial fluid and synovial membranes in OA often display mild inflammatory features,[133–136] and histobiochemical study of synovial tissue has shown a significant increase in lysosomal enzyme activity.[137, 138] Rheumatologists have recognized for some time that the majority of (but not all) osteoarthritic patients respond to nonsteroidal anti-inflammatory drugs. In a study of 366 patients with OA, 306 had relief of symptoms by such therapy, and the mean erythrocyte sedimentation rate for this group fell from 27 to 17 mm/hr (p < 0.001). In the 60 nonresponders, the mean sedimentation rate did not change (25 to 22 mm/hr N.S.).[139] In a histochemical study of synovial membranes resected at the time of hip surgery for OA, 80% were found to show mild inflammatory change, while 20% displayed features of marked inflammation comparable to those seen in RA.[140] In another similar study performed recently, 8.6% of patients were found to have a high-grade inflammatory change in resected synovium.[141]

A variant form of osteoarthritis, variously described as "interphalangeal osteoarthritis,"[142] "osteoarthrosis of the fingers with ankylosis,"[143] "erosive OA of the hands,"[144] "inflammatory OA,"[145] and "erosive inflammatory osteoarthritis,"[146] has been separated out as a subset of OA due to marked inflammatory features (see Chapter 11). Symptoms usually involve the distal and proximal interphalangeal joints of the hands. Attacks of mild to moderate painful synovitis are followed by eventual joint deformity and sometimes by ankylosis. The disease is seen most frequently in postmenopausal women. Acute flares of inflammation may occur periodically over a number of years, after which the joints become essentially pain-free. Gelatinous cysts are prominent. Roentgenographic examination reveals prominent bony erosions in addition to loss of joint space and osteophyte formation. Bony ankylosis is a notable finding.

Chondrocalcinosis

Chondrocalcinosis is known to occur frequently in elderly people[147–150] (see Chapter 14). Its prevalence is age-related, as has been confirmed by a recent long-term longitudinal study of patients with chondrocalcinosis, in whom new calcifications were seen to appear with advancing years.[151] OA is also common in elderly persons and is clearly age-related, and the presence of calcific deposits in joints with classic OA is not rare. The question arises as to whether the two conditions are coincidental or causally related.

The pattern of joint involvement in the two disorders is somewhat different. The sporadic form of chondrocalcinosis is frequently located in the wrist, the metacarpophalangeal joints, and the patellofemoral compartment of the knee.[152] In the chronic polyarticular type ("pseudo-osteoarthritis"), wrists, metacarpophalangeal joints, shoulders, and elbows are often affected, thus differing from the general pattern of OA.[153]

In a study of 272 hospital patients over 50 years of age, it was found that the prevalence of both chondrocalcinosis and OA increased with advancing age, but no statistically significant correlation could be found between the two conditions. Osteoarthritis of the joints commonly affected by chondrocalcinosis (trapezioscaphoid, the first carpometacarpal, and knee joints) was not discovered to occur more frequently in patients with chondrocalcinosis than in those without it, even when the calcific diathesis was of the destructive type.[150] It should be noted, however, that in another study that centered on the knee joint, it was disclosed that of 116 patients with chondrocalcinosis, 33.6% also had OA, whereas only 11% of controls showed the same changes.[154] In a survey of 72 patients with generalized OA (six or more joints), 20.8% were found to have chondrocalcinosis on roentgenogram. The mean age (75.6 and 77.4 years, respectively), sex ratio, prevalence of destructive arthritis, or presence of erosive OA was not significantly different between those with and those without chondrocalcinosis.[155]

Dieppe[156] compared the findings in 100 patients presenting with OA with those in 100 patients with pyrophosphate arthritis and found no striking clinical differences between the two groups. Calcium pyrophosphate deposition may, on the other hand, be associated at times with a severely destructive "pseudo-neuropathic" type of OA, which is seen more commonly in elderly women. He concluded that chondrocalcinosis could be a secondary event in OA, possibly related to such factors as hypermobility, steroid therapy, or thyroid dysfunction.

Hydroxyapatite crystals have been described in synovial fluid and synovium from patients with acute synovitis with and without osteoarthritis and may account for some of the acute inflammatory flares previously attributed to primary OA.[157] According to recent surveys, the presence of roentgenographically evident calcium hydroxyapatite deposits in and around the joint does not seem to correlate with the presence of inflammatory signs or with a more rapid progression of the disease.[156, 158]

PROTECTIVE FACTORS

That a paralyzed limb is spared by OA is a well-documented phenomenon, whether the motor impairment results from hemiplegia[159] or anterior poliomyelitis.[160] Studies of several series have shown that lower limb amputees display significantly less OA of the remaining joints of the amputated limb as compared with the opposite side.[161, 162] A recent survey of 44 such cases confirmed the absence of OA of the hip on the amputated side and also demonstrated an osteoporosis of the hip region and associated narrowing of the joint space in 25 of the patients.[163] These changes were interpreted as a regional adaptation to the regressive state of the limb.

In all these conditions, the protective factors seem to be mainly the absence of mechanical stress related to muscle contraction, and osteoporosis of the subchondral bone.

Finally, one cannot help but comment on significant differences in the role of various etiologic factors known or suspected in OA according to specific joints involved (Table 1–4).[164] These differences favor the concept that

Table 1–4. MAIN FACTORS IN PATHOGENESIS ACCORDING TO OSTEOARTHRITIS LOCATION*

	Intrinsic Factors					Extrinsic Factors		
	Age	Female Sex	Heredity	Obesity	Inflammation	Trauma	Minor Mechanical Disturbances	Dysplasia or Angulation
Fingers: Distal interphalangeal joints and nodal generalized OA	+	+ +	+ +					
Fingers: Proximal interphalangeal joints and non-nodal generalized OA	+			+	+ +			
First carpometacarpal joint	+	+						
First metatarsophalangeal joint	(+)						+	
Hip	(+)							+ +
Knee	(+)	+		+			+	+ +
Shoulder	(+)					+	+	
Ankle						+		
Wrist						+		

*From Peyron JG: Semin Arthritis Rheum 8:288–306, 1979.

we are dealing with a heterogeneous group of related conditions of multifactorial origin. Awareness of differing etiopathogenic pathways and disease subsets is essential to efforts to further clarify the causality of this disorder.[165] For instance, the separation of OA of the hip into subsets with localized narrowing of the joint space as opposed to cases with concentric narrowing disclosed that only the latter type was significantly related to OA of the fingers, thereby suggesting some systemic factor in this particular subset.[166] Another example is provided by a longitudinal study of OA of the fingers[167] that revealed a more protracted progression of Heberden's nodes in contrast to a more limited evolution of OA of the proximal interphalangeal joints, confirming the likelihood that they represent two different processes. Thus, the recognition of significant subsets of OA is likely to allow epidemiologic studies to bring about their most fruitful results, hitherto somewhat obscured by "background noise."

References

1. Lawrence JS: Rheumatism in populations. London, William Heinemann Medical Books, 1977.
2. Lawrence JS, Sebo M: The geography of osteoarthritis. *In* Nuki G (ed.): The Aetiopathogenesis of Osteoarthrosis. Tunbridge Wells, Pitman Medical Publishing Co., 1981, pp. 155–183.
3. Kellgren JH, Lawrence JS: Radiological assessment of OA. Ann Rheum Dis 16:494–502, 1957.
4. Valkenburg HA: Clinical versus radiological osteoarthrosis in the general population. *In* Peyron JG (ed.): Epidemiology of osteoarthritis. Paris, Geigy, 1981, pp. 53–58.
5. Atlas of Standard Radiographs, Vol 2, The epidemiology of chronic rheumatism. Oxford, Blackwell Scientific Publications, 1963.
6. Danielsson L, Hernborg J: Clinical and roentgenological study of knee joints with osteophytes. Clin Orthop 69:302–312, 1970.
7. Kashimoto T, Friedenberg ZB: A study of radiographic variations of the hip joint. Acta Orthop Scand 48:487–493, 1977.
8. Kellgren JG, Moore R: Generalized osteoarthritis and Heberden's nodes. Br Med J 1:181–187, 1952.
9. Heine J: Über die Arthritis Deformans. Ark Pathol Anat 260:521–663, 1926.
10. Bennett GA, Wayne H, Bauer W: Changes in the Knee Joint at Various Ages. Boston, Commonwealth Fund, 1942.
11. Byers P, Contepomi CA, Farkas TA: Post-mortem study of the hip joint. Ann Rheum Dis 29:15–31, 1970.
12. Cascclls SW: Gross pathologic changes in the knee joint of the aged individual. A study of 300 cases. Clin Orthop 132:227–232, 1978.
13. Stankovic A, Mitrovic D, Ryckewaert A: Prevalence of the degenerative lesions in articular cartilage of the human knee joint. Relationship with age. *In* Peyron JG (ed.): Epidemiology of Osteoarthritis. Paris, Geigy, 1981, pp. 94–98.
14. Lawrence JS, Bremner JM, Bier F: Osteoarthrosis. Prevalence in the population and relationship between symptoms and x-ray changes. Ann Rheum Dis 25:1–24, 1966.
15. Blumberg BS, Bloch KJ, Black RL, Dotter C: A study of the prevalence of arthritis in Alaskan Eskimos. Arthritis Rheum 4:325–341, 1961.
16. Bremner JM, Lawrence JS, Miall WE: Degenerative joint disease in a Jamaican rural population. Ann Rheum Dis 27:326–332, 1968.
17. Bennet PH, Burch TA: Osteoarthrosis in the Blackfeet and Pima Indians. *In* Bennet PH, Wood PHN (eds.): Population Studies of the Rheumatic Diseases. Amsterdam, Excerpta Medical Foundation, 1968, pp. 407–412.
18. Solomon L, Beighton P, Lawrence JW: Osteoarthrosis in a rural South African Negro population. Ann Rheum Dis 35:274–278, 1976.

19. Wood PHN, McLeish CL: Statistical appendix. Digest of data on the rheumatic diseases. 5: Morbidity in industry and rheumatism in general practice. Ann Rheum Dis 33:93–105, 1974.

20. Edstrom G: Cited in Lawrence JS: Rheumatism in Populations. London, William Heinemann Medical Books, 1977.

21. Wilcock JK: The prevalence of osteoarthritis of the hip requiring total hip replacement in the elderly. Int J Epidemiol 8:247–250, 1979.

22. Kelsley JL, Patides H, Bisbee GE, White AA: Musculo-skeletal disorders. Their frequency of occurrence and their impact on the population of the United States. New York, Prodist, 1978.

23. Guidevaux M, Colvez A, Michel E, Hatton F: Les malades en médecine libérale, qui sont-ils? De quoi souffrent-ils? Monographie. Paris, INSERM, 1975.

24. Tzonchev VT, Pilosoff T, Kane VK: Prevalence of osteoarthrosis in Bulgaria. *In* Bennett PH, Wood PHN (eds.): Population Studies of the Rheumatic Diseases. Amsterdam, Excerpta Medica Foundation, 1968, pp. 413–416.

25. Mikkelsen WN, Duff IF, Dodge HJ: Age and sex specific prevalence of radiographic abnormalities of the joints of the hands, wrist and cervical spine of adult residents of the Tecumseh, Michigan, community health study area, 1962–1965. J Chronic Dis 23:151–159, 1970.

26. Gordon T: Osteoarthrosis in U.S. adults. *In* Bennet PH, Wood PHN (eds.): Population Studies of the Rheumatic Diseases. Amsterdam, Excerpta Medica Foundation, 1968, pp. 391–397.

27. Kellgren JH, Lawrence JS: Osteoarthrosis and disk degeneration in an urban population. Ann Rheum Dis 17:388–397, 1958.

28. Yazici H, Saville PD, Salvati EA, et al.: Primary osteoarthrosis of the knee or hip: Prevalence of Heberden's nodes in relation to age and sex. JAMA 231:1256–1260, 1975.

29. Burch TA: Cited in Lawrence JS: Rheumatism in Populations. London, William Heinemann Medical Books, 1977, p. 112.

30. Greenwald AS, Matejczyk MB: Articular cartilage contact areas of the ankle. (Abstract.) Ann Rheum Dis 37:482, 1978.

31. Bullough P, Goodfellow J, Greenwald AS, O'Connor J: Incongruent surfaces in the human hip joint. Nature 217:1290, 1968.

32. Byers PD, Afoke NYP, Hutton WC: A test of the Freeman hypothesis. *In* Peyron JG (ed.): Epidemiology of Osteoarthritis. Paris, Geigy, 1981, pp. 87–89.

33. Goodfellow J, Mitsou A: Joint surface incongruity and its maintenance. An experimental study. J Bone Joint Surg 59A:446–451, 1977.

34. Bullough P, Goodfellow J, O'Connor J: The relationship between degenerative changes and load bearing in the human hip. J Bone Joint Surg 55B:746–758, 1973.

35. Goodfellow J, Bullough P: The pattern of ageing of the articular cartilage of the elbow joint. J Bone Joint Surg 49B:175–181, 1967.

36. Johnson LC: Kinetics of osteoarthritis. Lab Invest 8:1223–1241, 1959.

37. Lane LB, Villacin A. Bullough PG: The vascularity and remodelling of subchondral bone and calcified cartilage in adult human femoral and humeral heads. J Bone Joint Surg 59B:272–278, 1977.

38. Longmore RB, Gardner DL: Development with age

39. Vignon E, Arlot M, Patricot LM, Vignon G: The cell density of human femoral head cartilage. Clin Orthop 121:303–308, 1976.

40. Kempson GE: Mechanical properties of articular cartilage and their relation to matrix degradation and age. Ann Rheum Dis 34 (Suppl 2):111–113, 1975.

41. Sokoloff L: Elasticity of ageing cartilage. Fed Proc 25:1089–1095, 1966.

42. Kempson GE: The mechanical properties of articular cartilage. *In* Sokoloff L (ed.): The Joints and Synovial Fluid. New York, Academic Press, 1980, pp. 177–238.

43. Gardner DL, Elliott RJ, Armstrong CG, Longmore RB: The relationship between age, thickness, surface structure, compliance and composition of human femoral head articular cartilage. *In* Nuki G (ed.): The Aetiopathogenesis of Osteoarthrosis. Tunbridge Wells, Pitman Medical Publishing Co., 1980, pp. 65–83.

44. Weightman BO, Freeman MAR, Swanson SAV: Fatigue of articular cartilage. Nature 244:303–304, 1973.

45. Freeman MAR: The fatigue of cartilage in the pathogenesis of osteoarthrosis. Acta Orthop Scand 47:323–328, 1975.

46. Eyre DR, Oguchi H: The hydroxypyridinium cross-links of skeletal collagens: Their measurement, properties and a proposed pathway of formation. Biochem Biophys Res Commun 92:403–410, 1980.

47. Stockwell RA: Change in the acid glycosaminoglycan of the matrix of ageing human articular cartilage. Ann Rheum Dis 29:509–515, 1970.

48. Bayliss MT, Venn M: Chemistry of human articular cartilage. *In* Maroudas A, Holborow EJ (eds.): Studies of Joint Disease. I. Tunbridge Wells, Pitman Medical Publishing Co., 1980, pp. 2–58.

49. Venn MF: Variation of chemical composition with age in human femoral head cartilage. Ann Rheum Dis 37:168–174, 1978.

50. Hjertquist SO, Lemperg R: Identification and concentration of the glycosaminoglycans of human articular cartilage in relation to age and osteoarthritis. Calcif Tissue Res 10:223–237, 1972.

51. Kuhn R, Leppelmann HJ: Der Hexosamingehalt des Knorpels in Abhangigkeit vom Lebensalter. Liebigs Annalen Der Chemie 607:202–206, 1957.

52. Vignon E, Chapuy MC, Arlot M, et al.: Étude de la concentration en glycosaminoglycans du cartilage de la tête femorale humaine normale et arthrosique. Pathol Biol 23:283–289, 1975.

53. Mankin HJ, Zarins TA: Variation in rates of glycosaminoglycan synthesis in rabbit cartilage with aging. (Abstract.) J Bone Joint Surg 57A:575, 1975.

54. Fujii K: Aging of the collagen in human joint components: Changes in the reducible cross-links and solubilities. J Jpn Orthop Assoc 49:145–155, 1975.

55. Inerot S, Heinegaard D, Audell L, Olsson EE: Articular cartilage proteoglycans in aging and osteoarthritis. Biochem J 169:143–156, 1978.

56. Bayliss MT, Ali S: Age-related changes in the composition and structure of human articular cartilage proteoglycans. Biochem J 176:683–693, 1978.

57. Heinegaard D, Axelsson I: The distribution of keratan sulfate in cartilage proteoglycans. J Biol Chem 252:1971–1979, 1977.

58. Peyron JG, Stanescu R, Stanescu V, Maroteaux P:

Distribution électrophoretique particulière des populations de proteoglycanes dans les zones de régénération du cartilage arthrosique et étude de leur collagene. Rev Rhum Mal Osteoartic 45:569–575, 1978.

59. Perricone E, Palmoski MJ, Brandt KD: Failure of proteoglycans to form aggregates in morphologically normal aged human hip cartilage. Arthritis Rheum 20:1372–1380, 1977.

60. Evans CH, Georgescu HI, Mazzocchi RA: Does cellular aging of chondrocytes engender primary osteoarthritis? Trans Orthop Res Soc 6:153, 1981.

61. Jurmain RD: Stress and the etiology of osteoarthritis. Am J Phys Anthropol 46:353–366, 1977.

62. Acheson RM, Collart AB: New Haven survey of joint diseases. XVII. Relationship between some systemic characteristics and osteoarthrosis in a general population. Ann Rheum Dis 34:379–387, 1975.

63. Dequeker J, Burssens A, Creytens G, Bouillon R: Le vieillissement de l'os. Relation avec l'ostéoporose et l'ostéoarthrose chez les femmes á la post-ménopause. Les oestrogenes à la post-ménopause. Front Recherche Hormonale. Basel, Karger 3:120–135, 1975.

64. Silberberg R, Thomasson R, Silberberg M: Degenerative joint disease in castrate mice. II. Effect of orchiectomy at various ages. Arch Pathol 65:442–444, 1958.

65. Silberberg M, Silberberg R: Modifying action of estrogen on the evolution of osteoarthrosis in mice of different ages. Endocrinology 72:449–451, 1963.

66. Silberberg M, Silberberg R: Role of sex hormones in the pathogenesis of osteoarthrosis of mice. Lab Invest 12:285–289, 1963.

67. Silberberg R, Silberberg M: Aging changes and osteoarthrosis in castrate mice receiving progesterone. J Gerontol 20:228–232, 1965.

68. Sokoloff L: Failure of orchiectomy to affect degenerative joint disease in STR/1N mice. Proc Soc Exp Biol Med 108:792–793, 1961.

69. Sokoloff L, Varney DA, Scott JF: Sex hormones, bone changes and osteoarthritis in DBA/2JN mice. Arthritis Rheum 8:1027–1038, 1965.

70. Rogers FB, Lansbury J: Urinary gonadotropin excretion in osteoarthritis. Am J Med Sci 232:419–420, 1956.

71. Rosner IA, Malemud CJ, Goldberg VM, et al.: Pathologic and metabolic responses of experimental osteoarthritis to estradiol and an estradiol antagonist. Clin Orthop 171:280–286, 1982.

72. Dequeker J, Burssens A, Greytens G: Are osteoarthrosis and osteoporosis the end result of normal ageing or two different disease entities? Acta Rheumatol Belgica 1:46–57, 1977.

73. Franchimont P, Denis F: Détermination du taux de somatotrophine et des gonadotrophines dans des cas d'arthrose apparaissant lors de la ménopause. J Belge Rhumatol Med Phys 23:59–64, 1968.

74. Rubens-Duval A, Villiaumey J, Kaplan G, Brondani JC: Aspects cliniques de la maladie arthrosique. Rev Rhum Mal Osteoartic 37:129–137, 1970.

75. Bird HA, Tribe CR, Bacon PA: Joint hypermobility leading to osteoarthrosis and chondrocalcinosis. Ann Rheum Dis 37:203–211, 1978.

76. Wright V: Biomechanical factors in the development of osteoarthrosis: epidemiological studies. In Peyron JG (ed.): Epidemiology of Osteoarthritis. Paris, Geigy, 1981, pp. 140–146.

77. Kirk JA, Ansell BM, Bywaters EGL: The hyper-mobility syndrome. Ann Rheum Dis 28:419–425, 1967.

78. Carter C, Sweetnam R: Recurrent dislocation of the patella and the shoulder. Their association with familial joint laxity. J Bone Joint Surg 40B:664–667, 1958.

79. Sutro CJ: Hypermobility of knees due to overlength capsular and ligamentous tissues. Surgery 21:67–78, 1947.

80. Harper P, Nuki G: Genetic factors in osteoarthrosis. In Nuki G (ed.): The Aetiopathogenesis of Osteoarthrosis. Tunbridge Wells, Pitman Medical Publishing Co., 1980, pp. 184–202.

81. Louyot P, Savin R: La coxarthrose chez l'agriculteur. Rev Rhum Mal Osteoartic 33:625–632, 1966.

82. Frank O, Klemmayer K: Die Coxarthrose bie der Landbevolkerung. Z Rheumatol 27:371–379, 1968.

83. Pommier L: Contribution à l'étude de la coxarthrose chez l'agriculteur. Profil clinique et étiologique. À propos de 245 dossiers de coxarthrose chirurigicale. Thèse Med. Tours, 1977.

84. Bjelle A: Osteoarthrosis and back disorders in Sweden. In Peyron JG (ed.): Epidemiology of Osteoarthritis. Paris, Geigy, 1981, pp. 17–29.

85. Desmarais Y: La hanche du sportif. Thèse. Paris, 1971.

86. Murray RO, Duncan C: Athletic activity in adolescence as an etiological factor in degenerative hip disease. J Bone Joint Surg 53B:406–415, 1971.

87. Boyer T, Delaire M, Beranek L, et al.: Un antécédent de practique sportive: est-il plus fréquent chez les sujets atteints d'arthrose? Une étude controlée. In Peyron JG (ed.): Épidémiologie de l'Arthrose. Paris, Geigy, 1981, pp. 156–163.

88. Schlomka G, Schroter G, Ocherwal A: Über der bedeutung der beruflischer Belastung fur die entsehung der degenerativen Gelenkleiden. Z Gesamte Inn Med 10:993, 1955.

89. Lawrence JS: Rheumatism in coal miners. III. Occupational factor. Br J Ind Med 12:249–251, 1955.

90. Partridge REH, Duthie JJR: Rheumatism in dockers and civil servants: A comparison of heavy manual and sedentary workers. Ann Rheum Dis 27:559–568, 1968.

91. Duthie JJR: Rheumatism in the working population. In Second Nuffield Conference on Rheumatism. London, The Nuffield Foundation, 1964.

92. Acheson RM, Chan YK, Clemett AR: New Haven survey of joint diseases. XII. Distribution and symptoms of osteoarthrosis in the hands with reference to handedness. Ann Rheum Dis 29:275–286, 1970.

93. Lawrence JS: Rheumatism in cotton operatives. Br J Ind Med 18:270–276, 1961.

94. Hadler NM, Gillings DB, Imbus HR, et al.: Hand structure and function in an industrial setting. Influence of three patterns of stereotyped repetitive usage. Arthritis Rheum 21:210–220, 1978.

95. Radin EL, Paul IL, Rose RM: Role of mechanical factors in pathogenesis of primary osteoarthrosis. Lancet 1:519–521, 1972.

96. Burke MJ, Fear EC, Wright V: Bone and joint changes in pneumatic drillers. Ann Rheum Dis 36:276–279, 1977.

97. Brodelius A: Osteoarthrosis of the talar joints in footballers and ballet dancers. Acta Orthop Scand 30:309–314, 1961.

98. Solonen KA: The joints of the lower extremities of football players. Ann Khir Gyn Fenn 55:176–180, 1966.

99. Roass A: Degenerative phenomena in the knee joint of football players. Geneesk Sport 8:32–34, 1975.
100. Cassou B, Camus JP, Peyron JG, et al.: Recherche d'une arthrose primitive de la cheville chez les sujets de plus de 70 ans. *In* Peyron JG (ed.): Epidemiologie de l'Arthrose. Paris, Geigy, 1981, pp. 180–184.
101. Funk FJ Jr: Osteoarthritis of the foot and ankle. *In* American Academy of Orthopedic Surgeons (ed.): Symposium on Osteoarthritis. St. Louis, C. V. Mosby, 1976, pp. 287–301.
102. Puranen J, Alaketola L, Reltokalio P, Saarela J: Running and primary osteoarthritis of the hip. Br Med J 276:424–425, 1975.
103. Nettles JL, Whelan E, Filson E: Does long term long distance running cause osteoarthritis. (Abstract.) XV Congress Internat Rhum. Rev Rhum Mal Osteoartic 1981, special No. abstract 794.
104. Kraus JF, D'Ambrosia RD, Smith EG, et al.: Epidemiological study of severe osteoarthritis. Orthopedics 1:37–42, 1978.
105. Foss MVL, Byers PD: Bone density, osteoarthrosis of the hip and fracture of the upper end of the femur. Ann Rheum Dis 31:259–264, 1972.
106. Roh YS, Dequeker J, Mulier JC: Bone mass in osteoarthrosis, measured in vivo by photon absorption. J Bone Joint Surg 56:587–591, 1974.
107. Solomon L: Osteoarthritis of the hip and femoral neck fracture. A mutually exclusive diad. *In* Arthritis and Rheumatism Council (ed.): Studies in Joint Diseases. London, 1978.
108. Goldin RH, McAdam L, Louie JS, et al.: Clinical and radiological survey of the incidence of osteoarthritis among obese patients. Ann Rheum Dis 35:349–353, 1976.
109. Saville PD, Dickson J: Age and weight in osteoarthritis of the hip. Arthritis Rheum 11:635–644, 1968.
110. Solomon L, Schnitzler C, Browett J: Osteoarthritis of the hip. The patient behind the disease. *In* Peyron JG (ed.): Epidemiology of Osteoarthritis. Paris, Geigy, 1981, pp. 40–52.
111. Lawrence JS: Generalized osteoarthritis in a population sample. J Epidemiol 90:381–389, 1969.
112. Lawrence JS: Hypertension in relation to musculoskeletal disorders. Ann Rheum Dis 74:451–456, 1976.
113. Haygarth J: A Clinical History of Diseases. London, Cadwell and Davies, 1805.
114. Cecil RL, Archer BH: Classification and treatment of chronic arthritis. JAMA 87:741–746, 1926.
115. O'Brien WM, Clemett AR, Acheson RM: Symptoms and patterns of OA of the hand in the New Haven Survey of joint diseases. *In* Bennett PH, Wood PHN (eds.): Population Studies of the Rheumatic Diseases. Amsterdam, Excerpta Medica Foundation, 1968, pp. 398–406.
116. Benn T, Wood PHN: Generalized osteoarthrosis. A problem of definition. (Abstract.) Ann Rheum Dis 34:466, 1975.
117. Kellgren JH, Lawrence JS, Bier F: Genetic factors in generalized osteoarthrosis. Ann Rheum Dis 22:237–255, 1963.
118. Lawrence JS, DeGraaf R, Laine VAI: Degenerative joint disease in random samples and occupational groups. *In* Kellgren JH, Jeffrey MR, Ball J (eds.): The epidemiology of chronic rheumatism. Oxford, Blackwell Scientific Publications, 1963, pp. 98–119.
119. Huskisson EC, Dieppe PA, Tucker AK, Cannell LB:

Another look at osteoarthritis. Ann Rheum Dis 38:423–428, 1979.
120. Stecher RM: Heberden's nodes. A clinical description of osteoarthritis of the finger joints. Ann Rheum Dis 14:1–10, 1955.
121. Hoaglund FT, Yau ACMC, Wong WL: Osteoarthritis of the hip and other joints in southern Chinese in Hong Kong: Incidence and related factors. J Bone Joint Surg 55A:545–557, 1973.
122. Ota H, Schichkawa K, Tsusimoto M, et al.: Prevalence of osteoarthrosis of the hips in Japanese people. (Abstract.) XIV International Congress of Rheumatology, San Francisco, 1977, Abstract 1122.
123. Anderson S: The epidemiology of primary osteoarthrosis of the knee in Greenland. Scand J Rheumatol 7:109–112, 1978.
124. McKusick V: Genetic factors in disease of connective tissue: A survey of the present state of knowledge. Am J Med 2:283–302, 1959.
125. Colombo B, Panajotopoulos N: Sistema HLA et artrosi primaria. Reumatismo 29:125–128, 1977.
126. Sokoloff L: Osteoarthritis in laboratory animals. Lab Invest 8:1209–1217, 1959.
127. Sokoloff L, Crittenden LB, Hamamoto RS, Jay GE: The genetics of degenerative joint disease in mice. Arthritis Rheum 5:531–546, 1962.
128. Walton M: Naturally occurring osteoarthrosis in the mouse and other animals. *In* Ali SY, Elves MW, Leaback DH (eds.): Normal and Osteoarthrotic Articular Cartilage. London, Institute of Orthopaedics, 1974, pp. 285–298.
129. Wigley RD, Couchman KJ, Maul R, Reay BR: Degenerative arthritis in mice. Study of age and sex frequency in various strains with a genetic study of NZB/B1, NZY/B1, and hybrid mice. Ann Rheum Dis 36:249–253, 1977.
130. Walton M: Patella displacement and osteoarthrosis of the knee joint in mice. J Pathol 127:165–172, 1979.
131. Sokoloff L: Comparative pathology of degenerative joint disease. *In* Peyron JG (ed.): Epidemiology of Osteoarthritis. Paris, Geigy, 1981, pp. 81–86.
132. Stanescu R, Stanescu V, Maroteaux P, Peyron JG: Constitutional articular cartilage dysplasia with accumulation of complex lipids in chondrocytes and precocious arthrosis. Arthritis Rheum 24:965–968, 1981.
133. Lloyd-Roberts GC: The role of capsular changes in osteoarthritis of the hip joint. J Bone Joint Surg 35B:627–642, 1953.
134. Guiraudon C, Delbarre F, Coste F: Aspects anatomopathologiques des synoviales arthrosiques. Rev Rhum Mal Osteoartic 37:125–127, 1970.
135. Soren A, Klein W, Hulth F: Microscopic comparison of the synovial changes in post-traumatic synovitis and osteoarthritis. Clin Orthop 121:191–195, 1976.
136. Meachim G, Whitehouse GH, Pedley RB, et al.: An investigation of radiological, clinical and pathological correlations in osteoarthrosis of the hip. Clin Radiol 31:565–574, 1980.
137. Waxman BA, Sledge GB: Correlation of histochemical, histologic and biochemical evaluations of human synovium with clinical activity. Arthritis Rheum 16:376–382, 1973.
138. Kar NC, Cracchiolo A, Mirra J, Pearson CM: Acid, neutral, and alkaline hydrolases in arthritis synovium. Am J Clin Pathol 65:220–228, 1976.
139. Peltier AP, Rivet JP: Effet du traitement anti-inflammatoire par le Diclofenac sur la vitesse de sédi-

mentation, en particulier au cours des arthroses. Rev Rhumat 45:367–372, 1978.

140. Salvati EA, Granda JL, Mirra J, Wilson PD: Clinical, enzymatic and histological study of synovium in coxarthrosis. Int Orthop 1:39–42, 1977.

141. Bullough P: Synovial and osseous inflammation in osteoarthritis. Semin Arthritis Rheum 11 (Suppl 1):146, 1981.

142. Crain DC: Interphalangeal osteoarthritis. JAMA 175:1949–1953, 1961.

143. McEwen C: Osteoarthritis of the fingers with ankyloses. Arthritis Rheum 11:734–744, 1968.

144. Marmor L, Peter JB: Osteoarthritis of the hand. Clin Orthop 64:164–174, 1969.

145. Ehrlich G: Inflammatory osteoarthritis. I. The clinical syndrome. J Chronic Dis 25:317–328, 1972.

146. Utsinger PD, Resnick D, Shapiro RF, Wiesner KB: Roentgenologic, immunologic and therapeutic study of erosive (inflammatory) osteoarthritis. Arch Intern Med 138:693–697, 1978.

147. McCarty DJ, Hogan JM, Quatter RA, Grossman MM: Studies on pathological calcifications in human cartilage. I. Prevalence and types of crystal deposits in the menisci of two hundred fifteen cadavers. J Bone Joint Surg 48A:309–325, 1966.

148. Ellman MH, Levin B: Chondrocalcinosis in elderly persons. Arthritis Rheum 18:43–47, 1975.

149. DeLauche MC, Stehle B, Cassou B, et al.: Fréquence de la chondrocalcinose radiologique après 80 ans. Rev Rhum Mal Osteoartic 44:559–564, 1977.

150. Leonard A, Solnica J, Cauvin M, Houdent G, et al.: La chondrocalcinose. Étude de sa fréquence radiologique et de ses rapports avec l'arthrose. Étude du taux de la parathormone. Rev Rhum Mal Osteoartic 44:559–564, 1977.

151. Hamilton EDB: Chondrocalcinosis and osteoarthritis. In Peyron JG (ed.): Epidemiology of Osteoarthritis. Paris, Geigy, 1981, pp. 109–112.

152. Resnick D, Ninayama G, Goergen TG, et al.: Clinical, radiographic and pathological abnormalities in calcium pyrophosphate dihydrate deposition disease: Pseudogout. Radiology 122:1–16, 1977.

153. McCarty DJ: Pyrophosphate dihydrate crystal deposition disease (pseudogout syndrome). Clinical aspects. Clin Rheum Dis 3:61–89, 1977.

154. Morlock G, Sany J, Serre H: Relation entre chondrocalcinose articulaire. érosions fémorales sus-trochléennes, et arthropathies destructrices de genou. Nouv Presse Med 5:1145, 1976.

155. Gerster JC, Vischer TL, Fallet GH: Destructive arthropathy in generalized osteoarthritis with articular chondrocalcinosis. J Rheumatol 2:265–269, 1975.

156. Dieppe P: Calcium phosphate crystal deposition and clinical subsets of osteoarthritis. In Peyron JG (ed.): Epidemiology of Osteoarthritis. Paris, Geigy, 1981, pp. 71–80.

157. Schumacher HR: Arthritis associated with apatite crystals. Ann Intern Med 87:411, 1977.

158. Huskisson EC: The clinical features of osteoarthritis. Evidence of inflammation and crystal deposition. In Peyron JG (ed.): Epidemiology of Osteoarthritis. Paris, Geigy, 1981, pp. 62–70.

159. Coste F, Forestier J: Hémiplégie et nodosités d'Heberden controlatérales. Bull Soc Med Hop Paris 51:772–777, 1935.

160. Glynn JH, Sutherland I, Walker JF, Young AC: Low incidence of osteoarthritis of hip and knee after anterior poliomyelitis: A late show. Br Med J 2:739–742, 1966.

161. Hungerford OS, Cockin J: The fate of the retained lower limb in World War II amputees. (Abstract.) Br Orthop Assoc, Autumn Meeting, 1974.

162. Burke MJ, Roman V, Wright V: Bone and joint changes in lower limb amputees. Ann Rheum Dis 37:252–254, 1978.

163. Benichou C, Wirotius JM: Articular cartilage atrophy in lower limb amputees. Arthritis Rheum 25:80–82, 1982.

164. Peyron JG: Epidemiologic and etiologic approach of osteoarthritis. Semin Arthritis Rheum 8:288–306, 1979.

165. Ilardi CF, Sokoloff L: The pathology of osteoarthritis: Ten strategic questions for pharmacologic management. Semin Arthritis Rheum 11(Suppl 1):3–7, 1981.

166. Marks JS, Stewart IM, Hardinge K: Primary osteoarthrosis of the hip and Heberden's nodes. Ann Rheum Dis 38:107–111, 1979.

167. Plato CC, Norris RR: Osteoarthritis of the hand. Longitudinal studies. Am J Epidemiol 110:740–746, 1979.

2

The Pathology of Osteoarthritis

George Meachim, M.A., M.D.,
Gillian Brooke, B.Sc.

The term osteoarthritis (OA), or its synonym osteoarthrosis, is used by clinicians and radiologists as a diagnostic label for a degenerative disease of synovial joints. In secondary osteoarthritis, the degenerative process develops in a joint with a pre-existing abnormality, such as rheumatoid arthritis or congenital dislocation. In idiopathic (primary) osteoarthritis, no predisposing local cause is found.

In our study of the pathology of this disease in man, an empirical approach was used. The study was made on a random series of 450 surgical excision specimens that had been submitted to our laboratories in Liverpool accompanied by a clinical diagnosis of osteoarthritis. Thus, the material was from patients requiring treatment for joint changes that orthopaedic surgeons had labeled "osteoarthritic" because of the clinical and roentgenologic features they had found. We were able to detect a basic morphologic theme in this series of specimens from joints with symptomatic disease and to look for variations on the basic theme. The study also drew our attention to the difficulty of defining the initial morphologic change in human osteoarthritis.

PRECLINICAL STAGE OF OSTEOARTHRITIS

Cartilage degeneration is extremely common in asymptomatic adult synovial joints in the general population. It increases in amount with increasing age but varies in its potential to progress to clinically significant disease.[1, 2] Therefore, study of mild forms of cartilage degeneration in joints obtained from random necropsies gives no guarantee that such lesions truly represent the early stage of osteoarthritis. Specimens from patients with clinical joint disease are a more valid source of material. However, joints are symptom-free during the initial morphologic changes of osteoarthritis, and therefore, surgical excision specimens for laboratory examination are not available. Thus, the initial changes in an osteoarthritic joint are still the subject of speculation (see Chapter 7). Current hypotheses include the following:

Change in Cartilage Collagen Framework. Freeman and Meachim[3] have suggested that the initial lesion is in the collagen fiber framework of the articular cartilage, causing an abnormally wide separation of the fibers, a deterioration in the mechanical strength of the matrix, and thus an increased susceptibility to further structural damage during subsequent use of the joint. In man, such a lesion is known to occur at an early stage of cartilage degeneration, as seen in joints obtained from random necropsies.[4]

Collagen framework damage might be caused by fatigue failure. In fatigue failure, a material fails after repetitive loading, the failure occurring under loading of an amount previously withstood without damage. Should this phenomenon occur in cartilage, it could loosen the chemical or physical bonding of the fiber framework or cause ultrastructural breaks in the collagen fibers. Another possibility[4] is that a cartilage collagen lesion might be caused by abrasive wear (i.e., from rubbing between apposing articular surfaces) or by adhesive wear (i.e., from "sticking" between apposing surfaces). A further possibility is shearing damage.[5] In shearing, splitting develops between the uncalcified cartilage and its calcified base. This comes about because the uncalcified cartilage is more able to flow laterally under load. Stress is thereby caused at the interface between the two materials and can result in microtrauma to the fibers bridging the calcified to the uncalcified matrix.[6]

Change in Cartilage Proteoglycan Synthesis. Biochemical[7] and physicochemical research[8] has underlined the importance of proteoglycan in giving cartilage its special properties as a material and in protecting the collagen fiber framework from damage during use of a joint. Because of this, a reduction in the quantity or quality of the matrix proteoglycan could cause harm to the collagen framework. A change in proteoglycan synthesis by chondrocytes is known to occur at an early stage of experimentally induced osteoarthritis in dogs[9] and is accompanied by an ultrastructural deterioration in the collagen framework of the articular cartilage, giving an abnormally wide separation of the fibers.[10]

Enzymatic Degradation of Cartilage. Another biochemical hypothesis suggests that the initial event may be an enzymatic degradation of the cartilage collagen by collagenase activity, or an enzymatic degradation of the proteoglycan resulting in loss of its protective effect against collagen framework damage. Such degradation could be caused if there was excessive release of lysosomal or nonlysosomal enzymes, either from the articular chondrocytes (perhaps stimulated by microstresses) or from the synovial tissue, or it could be caused if there was a failure of the inhibitors that normally keep degradative activities in check. Cartilage matrix degradation from intra-articular injection of papain leads to experimentally induced osteoarthritis in animals.[11]

Crystal Deposition in Cartilage. It has been suggested that osteoarthritis in man is sometimes due to an excessive deposition of hydroxyapatite crystals within normally uncalcified layers of articular cartilage.[12] Because of the crystal deposits, the matrix would then be more susceptible to mechanically induced damage. (A similar explanation accounts for osteoarthritis secondary to pyrophosphate crystal arthropathy and for osteoarthritis secondary to pigment deposition in ochronosis.)

Disturbance at the Cartilage-Bone Interface. Johnson[13] has suggested that the initial event in osteoarthritis is a pathologic disturbance in tissue remodeling activity at the cartilage-bone interface, with this disturbance in some way predisposing to cartilage destruction. Goodfellow[14] favors a similar hypothesis and suggests that remodeling could lead to a loss of the normal "physiologic incongruity" of apposing articular surfaces, and thus predispose to degeneration of the joint.

Change in Subchondral Bone Resilience. Radin[15, 16] has pointed out that resilience in subchondral bone will permit it to deform under load, thus reducing the stress on the overlying cartilage. A decrease in bone resilience might therefore predispose to cartilage degeneration. Radin suggests that forces acting on a joint can cause microfractures of its bony trabeculae, which heal by microcallus. Because each microcallus would thicken the trabecula on which it forms, a gradual accumulation of microfractures could increase bone density, reduce bone resilience, and promote cartilage wear.

Defect in Synovial Fluid. Synovial fluid may contain substances that bond physically or chemically with the surface of articular cartilage and thus protect the cartilage against wear. A defect in the quantity or quality of such substances might predispose to cartilage degeneration. It should be noted that the wear-protective property postulated here may be unrelated to the "slipperiness" of synovial fluid as measured in coefficient of friction studies.

Because osteoarthritis is clinically due to a number of different causes, the above hypotheses for its initial pathologic event are not mutually exclusive. Moreover, there are close functional interdependences among synovial fluid, articular cartilage, and subchondral bone, between cartilage matrix and chondrocytes, and between matrix proteoglycan and matrix collagen. Thus, the initial event, whatever it may be, is likely soon to be accompanied by other changes, so that several of the phenomena mentioned above become present together in the same joint (Fig. 2–1). For example, in intermediate-stage osteoarthritis, the cartilage shows changes in its collagen framework, matrix proteoglycan, and cells; in late-stage osteoarthritis, abrasive wear of exposed bone becomes apparent. One can speculate about the exact time sequence of events during the initiation of cartilage degeneration and about the relative merits of mechanical and biochemical hypotheses, but one also needs to investigate what combination of me-

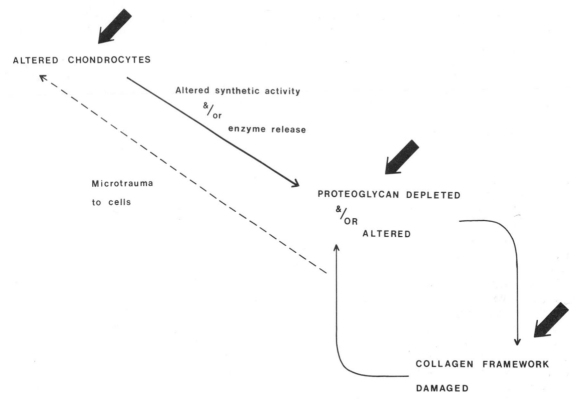

Figure 2–1. The potential for a vicious cycle in articular cartilage degeneration. The broad arrows indicate possible modes of entry, not mutually exclusive, into the cycle.

chanical and biochemical factors determines whether the cartilage changes will or will not progress to clinically significant disease.

The site of a cartilage lesion is one of the factors that influences its progression. For example, cartilage degeneration on the zenith of the femoral head is more likely to become truly osteoarthritic than is a lesion inferomedial to the fovea.[1] In the case of the patella, the potential to progress to osteoarthritic bone exposure is greater in lateral and central lesions compared with medial lesions.[17, 18] This influence of site may be attributable to local topographic variation in the amount of loading on the cartilage and perhaps also to topographic variation in the degree of resilience of the subchondral bone.[18]

Radin[15] has pointed out that the amount of loading on cartilage is influenced not only by body weight but also by the magnitude of muscle forces acting on the articulation. This may explain why roentgenologic changes of osteoarthritis (Heberden's and Bouchard's nodes) are common[19] at the interphalangeal joints of the hand, although these are classified as "non–weight-bearing." In contrast, osteoar-

thritis of the ankle, a "weight-bearing" joint, is uncommon in the absence of a predisposing local disease or abnormality, such as rheumatoid arthritis, neurologic defect, or previous fracture.[20]

INTERMEDIATE AND LATE STAGES OF OSTEOARTHRITIS

Although the nature of the morphologic changes in preclinical osteoarthritis is still debatable, it has been possible to observe in man the pathology of the intermediate and late stages of the disease. A series of 450 surgical excision specimens from osteoarthritic joints has been studied in Liverpool, using histologic examination and slab radiology for study. Most of the specimens were femoral heads; others were from osteoarthritic knees or hands. Both idiopathic (primary) and secondary osteoarthritis were represented. The cartilage and bone changes were similar in "weight-bearing" compared with "non–weight-bearing" (i.e., hand) joints and in idiopathic compared with secondary osteoarthritis. Thus, although the initial events in human osteoarthritis probably differ according to the clinical cause, they all lead to similar pathologic changes in the intermediate and late stages of the disease.

Intermediate-Stage Osteoarthritis

In a minority of the surgical excision specimens, it has been possible to study osteoarthritic cartilage destruction at its intermediate stage, prior to that of calcified tissue exposure. Affected cartilage segments show one or more of the following lesions:

1. *Fibrillation*, characterized by splitting extending tangentially, obliquely, and then vertically into the uncalcified layers of the articular cartilage, along the alignments of its collagen fiber framework (Fig. 2–2). Fibrillated cartilage has a reduced content of proteoglycan and an increased water content. Superficial fibrillation is accompanied by necrosis of chondrocytes in the superficial layer of the cartilage; in deep fibrillation, there can be both cell necrosis and proliferation of other, viable cells to form rounded clusters. Metabolic activity is altered in fibrillated cartilage. The nature and cause of the metabolic changes have recently been reviewed by Mitrovic and associates.[21] In intermediate-stage osteoarthritis, the vertical extension of fibrillation downward into the cartilage, with progressive tissue destruction, is probably dependent on the combined action of several of the phenomena already mentioned when discussing various hypotheses about the initial lesion in this disease. The reduced content of proteoglycan in the matrix can be attributed to factors such as altered synthetic activity by the chondrocytes, enzymatic degradation, and physical leakage from a damaged collagen fiber framework no longer able to entrap the proteoglycan molecules. The defect in proteoglycan content will potentiate further damage to the collagen fiber framework from microstresses during use of the joint, and this, in turn, will potentiate further proteoglycan loss. In fibrillation, whether it be due initially to a hypothetical fatigue failure of the material or to some other cause, there is thus the possibility of a vicious cycle (see Figure 1–1) of proteoglycan depletion and collagen framework disintegration causing tissue destruction.

2. *Horizontal splitting at the interface between the uncalcified cartilage and its calcified zone* (Figs. 2–2 and 2–3). This type of splitting is due to shearing damage.

3. *Cartilage thinning* from grinding damage

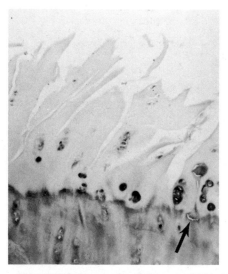

Figure 2–2. Photomicrograph of deep vertical splitting (fibrillation) of articular cartilage on an osteoarthritic femoral head. Note also the tiny horizontal split (arrow) at the interface between the uncalcified and calcified cartilage. (× 100.)

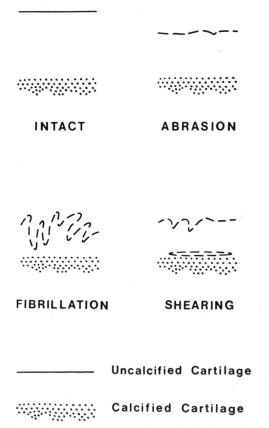

INTACT ABRASION

FIBRILLATION SHEARING

———— Uncalcified Cartilage

Calcified Cartilage

Figure 2–3. Various forms of cartilage destruction in osteoarthritis. More than one form can occur in the same cartilage segment.

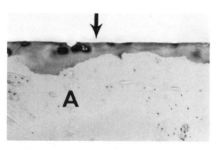

Figure 2–4. In this area on an articular surface, osteoarthritic cartilage destruction has exposed the calcified zone of the cartilage (arrow) but has not yet exposed the underlying bone (A). Further development of the tissue destruction from the appearance shown here is thought to be by abrasive wear of the calcified cartilage and then of its underlying bone. (Photomicrograph, hematoxylin and eosin stain, × 60.)

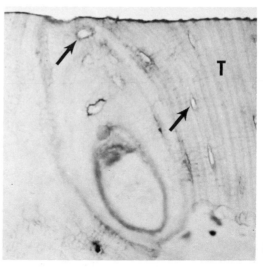

Figure 2–6. Characteristic histologic appearance of an exposed bone surface in osteoarthritis. Note the empty osteocyte lacunae beneath the surface (arrows). Note also the transected lamellar system (T). (Photomicrograph, × 375.) (See also Figure 2–7.)

due to abrasive wear. This lesion is characterized by destructive loss of uncalcified cartilage to a variable depth from the original articular surface, with the matrix that remains presenting a comparatively smooth appearance at its synovial interface (Fig. 2–3).

These intermediate-stage lesions of fibrillation, shearing damage, and abrasive wear cause disintegration and destruction of the uncalcified articular cartilage by a splitting and grinding process. In osteoarthritic cartilage degeneration, they progress to focal exposure of the underlying calcified cartilage and bone (Figs. 2–4 and 2–5).

Late-Stage Osteoarthritis

In most of the surgical excision specimens, the osteoarthritis had already reached the stage

where there is a region of calcified tissue exposure on part of the joint surface. In pathologic terms, such specimens represent the late stage of the disease. Osteoarthritic bone exposure has a characteristic histologic appearance in vertical section (Figs. 2–6 and 2–7). Its surface shows a "clean-cut" transection across lamellar systems, and beneath the synovial interface there are a few rows of empty osteocyte lacunae. The subarticular bone shows excessive osteoblastic and osteoclastic activity (Fig. 2–8), giving a roentgenologic picture of osteosclerosis, often interspersed with osteolytic foci or "cysts" (Figs. 2–9 to 2–12). Occasionally a cyst is so large that it may repre-

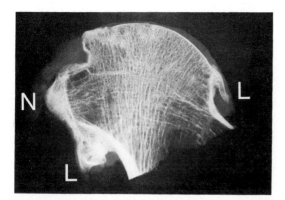

Figure 2–5. Midcoronal slab radiograph of an osteoarthritic femoral head on which cartilage thinning on the superior aspect has not yet led to destructive loss of bony height. The inferomedial segment is expanded by new bone (N), in continuity with inferomedial osteophytic lipping (L). Osteophytic lipping (L) is also seen at the lateral periphery.

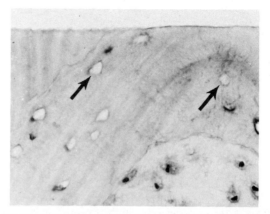

Figure 2–7. Characteristic histologic appearance of an exposed bone surface in osteoarthritis. Note the empty osteocyte lacunae beneath the surface (arrows). (Photomicrograph, × 375.) (See also Figure 2–6.)

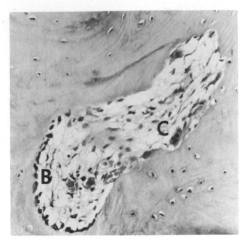

Figure 2–8. Photomicrograph from subarticular bone plate beneath osteoarthritic bone exposure (not shown) and from a site unrelated to a bone cyst. There is osteoblastic (B) and osteoclastic (C) remodeling activity. (× 150.)

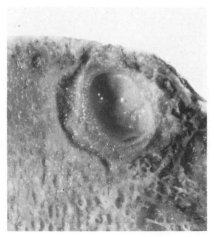

Figure 2–10. Subarticular bone cyst in an osteoarthritic femoral head. (Photograph of a coronal slab, × 2.)

sent a pre-existing lesion (Fig. 2–13) and may not simply be a consequence of the osteoarthritis.

The mechanism responsible for the shallow band of osteocyte necrosis is unknown. Possible explanations would include (1) loss of the protective effect of articular cartilage, thus causing microtrauma acting directly on the bone cells or indirectly by impeding their blood supply; and (2) a cytotoxic chemical action by synovial fluid seeping into the uncovered bone.

In a minority of specimens, there are surface segments where bone necrosis extends more deeply. The mechanism responsible is again unknown. On femoral heads, some of these small segments of deeper osteonecrosis (3 to 20 mm in surface length and 1 to 10 mm in depth) are topographically related to the roof of a subarticular bone cyst (Fig. 2–14), whereas others are not.

The osteosclerotic and osteolytic remodeling activity of bone that has lost the protective effects of its overlying articular cartilage may be an attempt to adjust to local changes in the magnitude and alignment of stresses on the bone trabeculae, with a response to trabecular microfractures as a possible contributory factor. An appearance seen in microfocal slab roentgenograms suggests that there may also be an actual crushing of bony tissue at the exposed surface.

Having lost its protective cover of articular cartilage, the region of exposed bone surface undergoes osteoarthritic wear from abrasive

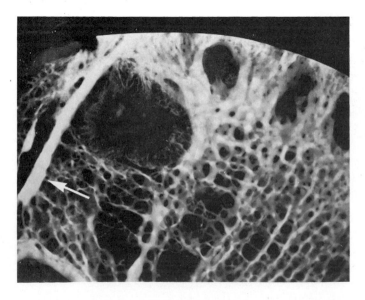

Figure 2–9. Microfocal slab radiograph of part of an osteoarthritic femoral head. Beneath the exposed bone surface, there is osteosclerosis interspersed with osteolytic foci and "cyst" formation (see also Figure 2–15). The line of the original inferomedial articular surface (arrow) is apparent. (Courtesy of Dr. William Park.)

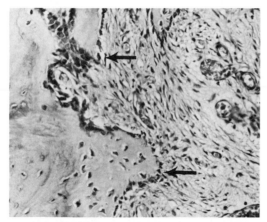

Figure 2–11. Photomicrograph of osteoblastic activity (arrows) at the periphery of an osteoarthritic bone "cyst" (× 150).

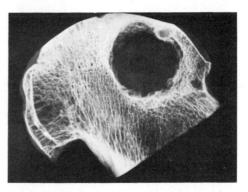

Figure 2–13. Midcoronal slab radiograph of an unusually large subarticular bone cyst in association with osteoarthritis of the femoral head. Note also the subarticular osteosclerosis.

damage by grinding during joint movement which in turn causes destruction of bony tissue. Loss of bony height can occur, e.g., on the zenith of the femoral head (Fig. 2–15), because of abrasive bone destruction and perhaps also to trabecular collapse from microfractures. At the same time the area occupied by the region of bone exposure gradually enlarges, as a result of continued destruction of more and more of the cartilage that still remains in the affected joint. The exposed bone surface is often interspersed with plugs of new fibrous or chondroid tissue that extend to the synovial interface through gaps in the subarticular bone plate (Fig. 2–16).

In joints where movement is or has become uniaxial, track markings can develop on exposed bone and adjacent cartilage.

On a surgical specimen showing a region of osteoarthritic bone and cartilage destruction, sites of remodeling activity are often evident elsewhere on the same specimen (see Figures 2–5 and 2–15). New bone can form in a plane vertical to that of the original chondro-osseous junction (Fig. 2–17), giving a region of expansive remodeling, e.g., on the inferomedial segment of an osteoarthritic femoral head.[22] Outgrowths of new bone can form beyond the original perimeter of the articular surface, giving osteophytic lipping (see Figures 2–5 and 2–15). The new bone is covered by a layer of new fibrous or chondroid tissue.

The significance of osteophytosis as a diagnostic feature in osteoarthritis merits discussion. Our observations on surgical excision specimens indicate that osteoarthritic tissue destruction can occur in the absence of any major element of bony expansive remodeling or osteophytic lipping. Conversely, our observations on joints at necropsy indicate that, at

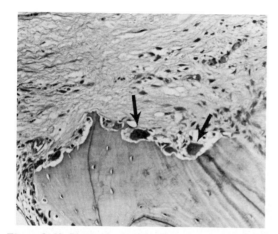

Figure 2–12. Photomicrograph of osteoclastic remodeling activity (arrows) at the periphery of an osteoarthritic bone "cyst" (× 150).

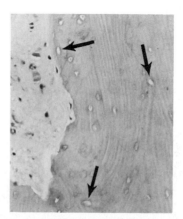

Figure 2–14. Photomicrograph of necrotic bone in the roof of an osteoarthritic bone "cyst." Note the empty osteocyte lacunae (arrows) (× 150).

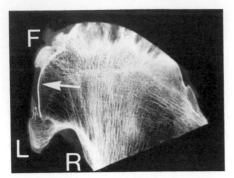

Figure 2–15. Midcoronal slab radiograph of an osteoarthritic femoral head, showing flattening from destructive loss of bony height on the superior and lateral aspects (compare with Figure 2–5). Note the subarticular osteosclerosis, interspersed with small osteolytic foci, beneath the exposed bone on this part of the femoral head. In contrast, there is bony expansion around the fovea (F) and inferomedially, with osteophytic lipping (L); the line of the inferomedial original chondro-osseous junction is readily apparent (arrow). Note also the new bone on the external aspect of the inferior cortex of the femoral neck (R).

least in males, osteophytes can occur in the absence of osteoarthritis.[17]

The mechanism responsible for expansive bony remodeling is unknown. Possible explanations include (1) osteophytosis as a fundamental event in the initiation of osteoarthritis in some patients; (2) stimulation of synovial osteochondrogenesis by debris released from the articular surface; (3) adjustment to altered contours in the articulation; and (4) an attempt to counteract the destructive process by spontaneously reproducing the effects of an osteotomy.

In some osteoarthritic hips, flattening of the femoral head zenith from destructive loss of

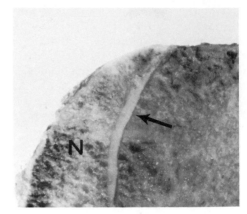

Figure 2–17. New bone (N) external to the original inferomedial articular cartilage (arrow) of an osteoarthritic femoral head. (Coronal slab, × 2).

bony height can, when accompanied by expansive bony remodeling of the inferomedial segment, give rise to an appearance spuriously suggestive of a pre-existing "tilt deformity." This is because the osteoarthritic changes have caused a medial shift in the apparent (but not the true) position of the center of the femoral head.[23]

Synovial and Capsular Changes

In osteoarthritic joints, the synovial and capsular changes can include one or more of the following features: fibrosis; adherence and entrapment of bony and other debris (Fig. 2–18), sometimes with a multinucleate giant cell reaction to this; multilayering of the synovial

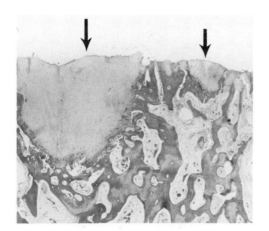

Figure 2–16. Photomicrograph showing plugs of nonosseous tissue (arrows) at an osteoarthritic exposed bone surface (× 10).

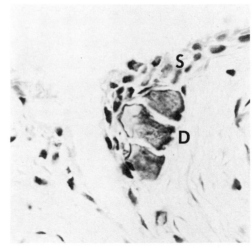

Figure 2–18. Photomicrograph of calcified debris (D) entrapped just beneath the surface cell layer (S) of synovial membrane from an osteoarthritic joint (× 600).

lining (intima) cells; and/or mild or moderate infiltration by lymphocytes and plasma cells beneath the synovial surface (subintima) and in the deeper fibrofat.

The synovial or capsular surface may show changes attributable to the effects of chronic microtrauma, with surface fraying and foci of superficial frond necrosis. An alteration of cell morphology to a chondroid appearance is sometimes seen.

We have assessed the amount of lymphocytic and plasma cell infiltration in hip synovial membrane from 52 patients treated surgically for idiopathic osteoarthritis of the hip. Subintimal (i.e., just beneath the surface) infiltration by lymphocytes and plasma cells was minimal or absent in 18 patients, minor in 24 patients, and of moderate intensity in 10 patients (19%); none showed an infiltrate of severe degree. In the 10 patients in whom the synovitis was of moderate intensity, there was no clinical or roentgenologic evidence of rheumatoid disease. Thus, our findings indicate that there is an element of active synovitis in some patients with idiopathic osteoarthritis. This inflammatory component has been attributed to a response to debris released into the joint cavity from the degenerating articular surface.[24] Such debris could contain chemical degradation products from cartilage, fragments of cartilage and bone, and hydroxyapatite crystals. It is possible that it might set up an immunologic reaction in synovial membrane and that there is an immunologic component in the pathogenesis of osteoarthritis (see Chapter 4).

ARTICULAR SURFACE REPAIR IN OSTEOARTHRITIS

In osteoarthritis, new bone and new fibrous or chondroid tissue can form as part of the remodeling process already described. These new tissues are topographically separate from the region of tissue destruction and do not contribute to its repair. In untreated osteoarthritis of the hip, any attempt at repair of the femoral tissue destruction on or near the zenith is usually overwhelmed or severely counteracted by the osteoarthritic wear process. The same probably holds true for the acetabulum (although surgical specimens of osteoarthritic acetabula suitable for adequate laboratory examination are not readily available).

There is clinical and roentgenologic evidence that osteotomy can relieve the effects of osteoarthritis of the hip. How may it do so? The relationship between clinical features in osteoarthritic patients and morphologic features in their tissues is difficult to analyze. However, at least three suggestions, not mutually exclusive, can be made:

1. Excessive vascular engorgement in osteoarthritic femoral heads may be one cause of pain in the diseased hip. Osteotomy, by interrupting the blood supply, could reduce vascular engorgement and might thus relieve pain.

2. If osteotomy were in some way to reduce the amount of osteoarthritic wear at the articular surface, it would lessen the amount of debris released into the joint cavity and might thereby relieve the synovitis.

3. Laboratory examination of femoral heads excised during hip replacement after previous osteotomy sometimes shows that the region of tissue destruction has been partly or completely re-covered by new bone-based chondroid or fibrous tissue (Fig. 2–19). This new articular surface tissue represents a repair process.[25] It protects the underlying bone against further wear. In addition, the subarticular osteosclerosis and focal osteolysis seen before osteotomy tend to diminish.

What is the source of the surface repair tissue, chondroid or fibrous, found after osteotomy for osteoarthritis of the hip in man? The chondrocytes of adult human articular cartilage have only a limited potential to form new tissue.[26] In response to cartilage damage, the cells can multiply and can manufacture matrix proteoglycans, but they seem to have difficulty in forming a new matrix collagen framework (at least in the absence of hormone or drug treatment). Thus, any of the original articular cartilage that still remains on an osteoarthritic femoral head is unlikely to be a source of repair tissue. Instead, there is evidence that the new tissue is formed by cells originating from the subarticular bone plate, and perhaps also by cells originating from the synovial membrane.

We suggest that surface repair by cells of subarticular origin comes about in the following way. The exposed bone surface of late-stage osteoarthritis is often interspersed with plugs of chondroid or fibrous tissue. The plugs extend to the synovial interface through gaps in the subarticular bone plate (see Figure 2–16). In untreated patients, any further proliferation of tissue from the plugs is usually inhibited by the action of the osteoarthritic wear process at the articular surface. Osteot-

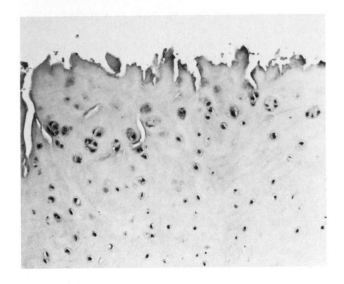

Figure 2–19. Photomicrograph showing new chondroid tissue at the articular surface following osteotomy for osteoarthritis of the hip (× 150).

omy may create a more favorable mechanical environment for the new tissue, thus allowing it to spread out over adjacent exposed bone and to re-cover the bone with a new surface of chondroid or fibrous repair (Fig. 2–20). A similar morphologic process may account for occasional reports of repair in osteoarthritic joints where there has been no osteotomy.

In summary, there is histologic evidence that surface repair can occur following osteotomy for osteoarthritis in man. Experimental evidence supports the suggestion that the repair

tissue is of subarticular origin.[27] However, having shown that repair can occur, it is also important to consider its quantity and quality. Our findings indicate that the following questions are useful when assessing a specimen for the effectiveness of articular surface repair:

1. What percentage of the total surface area of tissue destruction has been re-covered by a new surface layer of chondroid or fibrous tissue?

2. What are the relative amounts of bone-based chondroid tissue and of fibrous tissue in

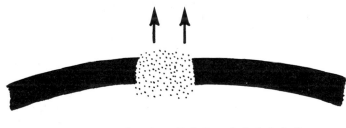

POTENTIAL FOR REPAIR

Figure 2–20. Diagram indicating a potential mechanism for surface re-covering of exposed bone by a plug (see Figure 2–16) of new fibrous or chondroid tissue of "extrinsic" subarticular origin that has gained access to the articular surface.

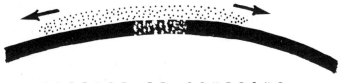

SURFACE RE-COVERING

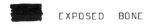   EXPOSED BONE

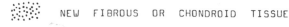   NEW FIBROUS OR CHONDROID TISSUE

the surface repair? Where chondroid, is the new tissue fibrocartilaginous or hyaline in texture and collagen type?

3. What is the thickness of the new surface cover, and what is its ability, in the long term, to resist wear?

SECONDARY OSTEOARTHRITIS

Osteoarthritis has multiple causes.[28] In some patients, it is secondary to a pre-existing abnormality of the same joint or of the contralateral articulation (see Chapter 14). Examples of such "local" causes are presented in Table 2–1. More general, "constitutional" factors, such as age, sex, body weight, and height, have been omitted intentionally, but this does not imply that we discount their possible importance in the epidemiology of osteoarthritis.

When discussing the pathogenesis of osteoarthritis, the term "trauma," if used without further qualification, causes semantic confusion. Acute trauma causing a macroscopic fracture can result in an abnormality of a joint and can lead to a secondary osteoarthritis. This is a separate question from that of whether or not chronic repetitive trauma may, perhaps by causing microfractures in bone or stresses in cartilage, predispose to osteoarthritis of the sort at present classified as idiopathic. A distinction between acute major and repetitive minor trauma is also pertinent when investigating occupational and sporting activities as possible factors in the etiopathogenesis of degenerative joint disease.

Secondary Osteoarthritis of the Hip

A combined clinical, roentgenologic, and pathologic assessment has recently been made in Liverpool of 100 patients requiring surgical treatment (joint replacement) for osteoarthritis of the hip. Most of the patients were from North Wales, U.K. In 70 of the 100 patients (70%), no predisposing cause for the hip osteoarthritis was found. The other 30 patients (30%) were excluded from the idiopathic group. The grounds for exclusion were as follows, but this does not imply the conditions listed were necessarily the basic "cause" of the hip osteoarthritis in all these patients:

Rheumatoid disease	6
Chronic juvenile polyarthritis	1
Previous abnormality of the same hip	10

Table 2–1. CAUSES OF SECONDARY OSTEOARTHRITIS

Rheumatoid disease; chronic juvenile polyarthritis
Ankylosing spondylitis
Dislocation (congenital of hip; recurrent of patella)
Slipped upper femoral epiphysis; Perthes' disease of hip; acetabular dysplasia; protrusio acetabuli
Previous avascular bone necrosis (post-traumatic; renal disease; alcohol)
Neurologic defect
Paget's disease of bone
Abnormality of contralateral joint (e.g., fusion)
Pyrophosphate arthropathy (chondrocalcinosis); ochronosis
Bleeding disorder (e.g., Christmas disease)
Previous fracture

Previous abnormality of the opposite hip	3
Previous avascular bone necrosis	3
Neurologic defect	2
Chondrocalcinosis	4
Christmas disease	1

The age range of the 70 patients requiring surgery for idiopathic osteoarthritis of the hip was from 57 to 82 years (with a median age of 69 years for women and 67 years for men) and that of the 30 "excluded" patients was from 23 to 78 years. Thus, the "excluded" patients tended to be younger than those in the idiopathic category, although there was considerable overlap between the ages of the two groups.

For the reasons discussed elsewhere[19] the percentage of patients excluded from the idiopathic group in the Liverpool multidisciplinary study was considerably less than in the Johannesburg study reported by Solomon.[29] Even so, the Liverpool study confirms that osteoarthritis of the hip is not a single disease but, instead, can result from a number of initially different pathologic processes (see Chapter 15). The most appropriate method of prophylaxis and treatment might therefore differ from patient to patient, according to the predisposing cause.

In secondary osteoarthritis, is the local abnormality sufficient in itself to cause secondary degenerative disease, or will it sometimes do so only if there is also a constitutional predisposition to osteoarthritis? For example, in patients who develop osteoarthritis of the hip following a hip abnormality in childhood, is there also a generalized abnormality of their articular cartilage (i.e., an "osteoarthritic diathesis")?

Rheumatoid Disease

In surgical excision specimens from late-stage osteoarthritis, there is overlap between the histologic appearances of idiopathic osteoarthritis and those of osteoarthritis secondary to rheumatoid disease. Both can show "pannus" on part of the articular surface,[30] focal infiltrates of lymphocytes and plasma cells in marrow spaces, and an active synovitis of moderate intensity. Moreover, there is some overlap between the mid-coronal slab radiograph patterns found in idiopathic osteoarthritis and in osteoarthritis associated with rheumatoid disease.[19]

We therefore believe that a conclusive choice between these two diagnostic possibilities is often not possible if based solely on laboratory examination of a surgical excision specimen from a joint in late-stage disease. Byers has also investigated this diagnostic problem and reached a similar opinion.[31]

Avascular (Nonseptic) Bone Necrosis

As mentioned previously, small segments of subarticular osteonecrosis are found in a minority of specimens from osteoarthritic joints and appear to be a consequence of late-stage disease. However, in some patients, an infarct affecting most of the femoral head, or a sizable segment of it, antedates the osteoarthritic change and predisposes to its development. Trabecular collapse develops in the osteonecrotic zone, with flattening of the bony contour at the site of the lesion (Fig. 2–21). At this stage, the overlying articular cartilage may still be intact, but it is unable fully to adjust its rounded shape to the abnormal contour of its bony base. A gap opens just below the chondro-osseous junction at the site of the infarct (Fig. 2–21), and eventually a flap of articular cartilage, with a microscopic layer of subchondral bone attached to it, separates off from the infarct by a dissecting process similar to that of osteochondritis dissecans. Osteoarthritic wear can then develop as a consequence of these events. In some surgical excision specimens from patients with hip osteoarthritis secondary to this cause, the infarct is still present as a diagnostic feature on laboratory examination. However, occasional specimens show flattening that could be due either to osteoarthritis secondary to an infarct no longer demonstrable on histologic examination (because the necrotic bone has "worn away") or to an idiopathic osteoarthritis with unusually severe bone destruction.

CORRELATION OF MORPHOLOGIC WITH CLINICAL FEATURES

From laboratory studies, it is possible to describe the morphologic features of osteoarthritis and to correlate them with the findings in roentgenograms. However, an important limitation of descriptive osteoarticular pathology becomes apparent when one attempts to relate clinical symptoms to morphologic changes. At present, there is insufficient knowledge of the mechanisms whereby structural changes in tissues affect the physiology and neurophysiology of joints and thus cause clinical effects. In this context, more data are also needed on the comparative frequency of symptomatic and of clinically silent osteoarthritis.

SUMMARY AND CONCLUSIONS

Osteoarthritis has many clinical causes. The nature of its initial morphologic event is still debatable and probably varies according to the cause (see Chapter 7). However, the intermediate and late stages of the disease show a basic morphologic theme. There is a progressive destruction of articular cartilage leading to exposure of bone at a site where the bone will then be subjected to abrasion and other damage. A cartilage segment undergoing os-

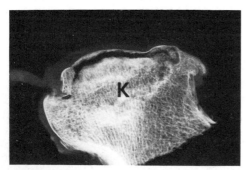

Figure 2–21. Midcoronal slab radiograph of a femoral head with flattening due to a bone infarct (K). The overlying articular cartilage and its calcified base have separated from the main mass of the infarct by a horizontal split. This splitting can lead to the cartilage dissecting away from the femoral head, thus exposing the underlying bone and eventually resulting in superimposed osteoarthritic wear.

teoarthritic destruction shows one or more of the following features: fibrillation, abrasion, and/or shearing. A segment of exposed bone showing osteoarthritic wear has a characteristic appearance in histologic sections: a "clean-cut" surface at the synovial interface; empty osteocyte lacunae for a few rows beneath the surface; and osteoblastic and osteoclastic activity, producing subarticular osteosclerosis interspersed with osteolytic foci. This characteristic histologic lesion is found in both "weight-bearing" and "non–weight-bearing" joints and in both idiopathic and secondary osteoarthritis.

Contrasting with the destructive lesion of osteoarthritis and topographically distinct from it, there is formation of new bone and of new fibrous or chondroid tissue elsewhere at the joint surface. Remodeling by new bone formation often leads to a variable amount of localized expansion of the original bony contour and to osteophytic lipping, but these features are not essential in diagnosis of the disease.

Some patients with idiopathic (primary) osteoarthritis have an active synovitis, with infiltration of the synovial membrane by lymphocytes and plasma cells.

In patients with osteoarthritis secondary to a pre-existing abnormality of the joint, such as rheumatoid disease or a hip disorder of childhood, diagnostic differentiation from idopathic osteoarthritis is not always possible solely from laboratory examination of a surgical excision specimen.

In late osteoarthritis, there is a potential for reparative re-covering of the exposed bone surface by new fibrous or chondroid tissue originating from gaps in the continuity of the subarticular bone plate at the sites of the destructive lesions. The potential for repair (as distinct from surface remodeling elsewhere in the joint) is, however, usually overwhelmed by the osteoarthritic destructive process. When in vogue as a method of treatment, osteotomy was observed to release some of this potential to re-cover previously exposed bone.

References

1. Byers PD, Contepomi CA, Farkas TA: A post-mortem study of the hip joint. Ann Rheum Dis 29:15–31, 1970.
2. Meachim G: Articular cartilage lesions in the Liverpool population. Ann Rheum Dis 34(Suppl 2):122–124, 1975.
3. Freeman MAR, Meachim G: Ageing and degeneration. In Freeman MAR (ed.): Adult Articular Cartilage. 2nd ed. Tunbridge Wells, Pitman Medical Publishing Co., 1979, pp. 487–543.
4. Meachim G, Denham D, Emery IH, Wilkinson PH: Collagen alignments and artificial splits at the surface of human articular cartilage. J Anat 118:101–118, 1974.
5. Meachim G, Bentley G: Horizontal splitting in patellar articular cartilage. Arthritis Rheum 21:669–674, 1978.
6. Sokoloff L: A note on the histology of cement lines. In Kenedi RM (ed.): Perspectives in Biomedical Engineering. New York, Macmillan, 1973, pp. 135–138.
7. Muir IHM: Biochemistry. In Freeman MAR (ed.): Adult Articular Cartilage. 2nd ed. Tunbridge Wells, Pitman Medical Publishing Co., 1979, pp. 145–214.
8. Maroudas A: Physicochemical properties of articular cartilage. In Freeman MAR (ed.): Adult Articular Cartilage. 2nd ed. Tunbridge Wells, Pitman Medical Publishing Co., 1979, pp. 215–290.
9. McDevitt CA, Muir H: Biochemical changes in the cartilage of the knees in experimental and natural osteoarthritis in the dog. J Bone Joint Surg 58B:94–101, 1976.
10. Stockwell RA: Private communication, 1980.
11. Bentley G: Papain-induced degenerative arthritis of the hip in rabbits. J Bone Joint Surg 53B:324–337, 1971.
12. Ali SY: Mineral-containing matrix vesicles in human osteoarthritic cartilage. In Nuki G (ed.): The Aetiopathogenesis of Osteoarthritis. Tunbridge Wells, Pitman Medical Publishing Co., 1980, pp. 105–116.
13. Johnson LC: Kinetics of osteoarthritis. Lab Invest 8:1223–1241, 1959.
14. Goodfellow JW: Private communication, 1977.
15. Radin EL, Paul IL, Rose RM: Role of mechanical factors in the pathogenesis of primary osteoarthritis. Lancet 1:519–522, 1972.
16. Townsend PR, Rose RM, Radin EL, Raux P: The biomechanics of the human patella and its implications for chondromalacia. J Biomech 10:403–407, 1977.
17. Emery IH, Meachim G: Surface morphology and topography of patello-femoral cartilage fibrillation in Liverpool necropsies. J Anat 116:103–120, 1973.
18. Pedley RB, Meachim G: Topographical variation in patellar subarticular calcified tissue density. J Anat 128:737–745, 1979.
19. Meachim G, Whitehouse GH, Pedley RB, et al.: An investigation of radiological, clinical and pathological correlations in osteoarthritis of the hip. Clin Radiol 31:565–574, 1980.
20. Meachim G: Cartilage fibrillation at the ankle joint in Liverpool necropsies. J Anat 119:601–610, 1975.
21. Mitrovic D, Gruson M, Demignon J, et al.: Metabolism of human femoral head cartilage in osteoarthritis and subcapital fracture. Ann Rheum Dis 40:18–26, 1981.
22. Harrison MHM, Schajowicz F, Trueta J: Osteoarthritis of the hip: A study of the nature and evolution of the disease. J Bone Joint Surg 35B:598–626, 1953.
23. Meachim G, Hardinge K, Williams DR: Methods for correlating pathological and radiological findings in

osteoarthrosis of the hip. Br J Radiol 45:670–676, 1972.

24. Huskisson EC, Dieppe PA, Tucker AK, Cannell LB: Another look at osteoarthritis. Ann Rheum Dis 38:423–428, 1979.

25. Meachim G, Osborne GV: Repair at the femoral articular surface in osteoarthritis of the hip. J Pathol 102:1–8, 1970.

26. Stockwell RA, Meachim G: The chondrocytes. *In* Freeman MAR (ed.): Adult Articular Cartilage. 2nd ed. Tunbridge Wells, Pitman Medical Publishing Co., 1979, pp. 69–144.

27. Meachim G, Roberts C: Repair of the joint surface from subarticular tissue in the rabbit knee. J Anat 109:317–327, 1971.

28. Sokoloff L: The pathology of osteoarthritis and the role of ageing. *In* Nuki G (ed.): The Aetiopathogenesis of Osteoarthrosis. Tunbridge Wells, Pitman Medical Publishing Co., 1980, pp. 1–15.

29. Solomon L: Patterns of osteoarthritis of the hip. J Bone Joint Surg 58B:176–183, 1976.

30. Meachim G: Articular cartilage lesions in osteo-arthritis of the femoral head. J Pathol 107:199–210, 1972.

31. Byers PD, Roper BA, Glennie B: Attempt to classify patients with arthritis of the hip suitable for prosthetic replacement, and their femoral heads. Ann Rheum Dis 34:298–302, 1975.

3

Biochemistry and Metabolism of Cartilage in Osteoarthritis*

Henry J. Mankin, M.D.
Kenneth D. Brandt, M.D.

It is clear from the gross and histologic descriptions of osteoarthritic joints (see Chapter 2) that although alterations in the capsule, synovium, and subchondral bone may be present (and indeed are considered to be characteristics of the disease), the major and central changes occur in the hyaline articular cartilage. In fact, most investigators believe osteoarthritis to be a true cartilage disease. Over the past four decades, a small but steadily increasing number of investigators have studied the cartilage from patients and from animal models of osteoarthritis and have defined, first, the histologic changes and, subsequently, the biochemical and metabolic changes seen in this tissue. These alterations have been recognized to be of paramount importance in the pathogenesis of the disease. As will be discussed later, the chemical and metabolic alterations may well be the key to defining the etiology of this common and often devastating disease and to advancing a system for its prevention and/or cure.

It should be apparent that if we are to discuss the changes in biochemistry and metabolism in osteoarthritic articular cartilage, we must first briefly describe these features in normal cartilage, not only to provide a basis for comparison, but also to indicate how even minor derangements in the cartilage might interfere with its resiliency and the almost frictionless movement essential for normal function of the diarthrodial joint.

THE NUTRITION OF ARTICULAR CARTILAGE

Cartilage from mature animals is totally avascular, aneural, and alymphatic.[1] The surface is not covered by a perichondrium, nor has a synovial layer or reflection been observed.[2-8] Electron microscopic studies have failed to show any form of limiting membrane other than the "lamina splendens" described by Collins,[9] which conforms well to the 10 nm fine-fibered filamentous layer, as described by Weiss and associates,[8] and Meachim and Roy[5] (Fig. 3–1).

The source of nutritive materials for the cartilaginous surfaces is an ancient puzzle. Because the tissue is avascular in adult life, the earliest investigators thought that the nutritive materials diffused through the matrix either from the synovial fluid that bathes the surface of the cartilage or from the underlying bone.[9-12] In 1920, Strangeways[11] reported an experiment suggesting that the synovial route is the only source of nutrients for adult cartilage. Subsequent dye diffusion studies by Brower and colleagues[13] and studies using other substrates or hydrogen gas have confirmed this point of view.[14-18] In the past 30 years, experimental evidence has been presented that suggests that in immature animals at least a portion of the substrates enter the articular cartilage by diffusion from the underlying bony endplate[19-24] but that in the adult, with the appearance of the tidemark and heavy deposition of apatite in the calcified zone, this type of diffusion disappears or becomes severely limited.

*Supported in part by grants AM#16265-09 and AM#37075 from N.I.A.M.D.D.

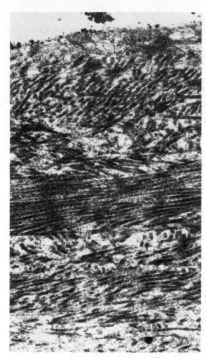

Figure 3-1. The surface of normal human articular cartilage is covered by a fine-fibered filamentous layer corresponding to the "lamina splendens" seen on light microscopy. Collagen fibers of the superficial zone (the "skin") are arranged in closely packed bundles that run parallel to the surface. (× 28,000.) (Courtesy of Charles Weiss, M.D.)

Synovial fluid, then, appears to serve as the primary source of nutrition for the articular chondrocyte. The fluid itself arises by diffusion from the synovial vascular network and represents a diffusate of plasma (without fibrinogen and with somewhat diminished levels of urea, glucose, and plasma protein) to which the synoviocytes have added hyaluronate and some additional proteins.[25, 26] The synovial fluid is sparse in quantity in normal joints,[25, 26] but sufficient quantities of nutrients and oxygen reach the chondrocytes, presumably by diffusion through the cartilage matrix. Extensive studies performed by Maroudas[27–29] have shown that the diffusion of nutrients through the matrix of the cartilage is not unrestricted and is limited by the size and charge of the molecule, and perhaps also by steric configuration. Until recently, the "pore size" was thought to be 6.8 nm (large enough to admit a hemoglobin molecule), but a recent study of Maroudas[17] suggests that larger molecules (such as albumin) may enter the cartilage under special circumstances.

Presumably because it facilitates the passage of nutrient molecules from the synovial fluid into the cartilage and of catabolites from the cartilage into the fluid, joint movement is essential for maintenance of normal articular cartilage. Thus, when knee joints of normal dogs were immobilized in casts for only a few weeks, the articular cartilage rapidly underwent atrophy.[30] Notably, the cartilage atrophy under these conditions was rapidly reversible if the cast was removed after 6 to 12 weeks and the dog was then permitted to ambulate "on all fours" within the confines of its pen.[31] However, the cartilage did *not* recover from the degenerative changes within this period if, after cast removal, the dog was placed on a treadmill exercise program.[32] Because changes of cartilage atrophy indistinguishable from those induced by casting occurred in the cartilage of the ipsilateral knee of nonimmobilized dogs after transection of the distal paw when the knee retained a reasonable arc of motion, it appears that the cartilage degeneration that occurs with casting is not due merely to a lack of oscillatory motion of the joint but to a reduction in loading of the cartilage that normally occurs with contraction of the quadriceps and hamstrings and stabilizes the knee in the stance phase of gait.[30]

It is intriguing to consider that normal articular cartilage "lives in isolation." Humoral messages, such as are given to other organs by rapid transit of information peptides and proteins, may not be transmitted through cartilage because of a diffusion barrier, or, if transport of such messenger does occur, it may be considerably slower than in more vascular tissue. Furthermore, neural impulses, which regulate many of the body processes, cannot provide information to cartilage because it has no nerve supply, and cellular and humoral immune responses are likely not to occur in cartilage because the size of lymphocytes and immunoglobulins tends to exclude them from the tissue. In theory at least, the chondrocytes can receive only limited information regarding the rest of the body state by the standard neural, lymphatic, or humoral pathways. On the other hand, if the cell is pressure-sensitive, it may in fact derive considerable information by alteration in the physical state of the tissue resulting from loading, unloading, or movement.

THE CHEMISTRY OF ARTICULAR CARTILAGE

Considering the sparse cellularity of articular cartilage, it is apparent that, for the most part, the chemistry of articular cartilage reflects the composition of the matrix.[33-35] Cartilage is a hyperhydrated tissue with values for water ranging from 60% to almost 80% of the total wet weight.[36-40] The remaining 20% to 30% of the wet weight of the tissue is principally accounted for by two macromolecular materials: collagen, which composes up to approximately 60% of the dry weight, and proteoglycan, which accounts for a large part of the remainder[36, 38, 41] (Table 3–1). The ash content has been estimated to be approximately 6%, and the residue is composed of trace amounts of lipid, phospholipid, lysozyme, and an as yet uncharacterized component that is believed to be glycoprotein[37, 38, 41] or possibly a "matrix protein" with a molecular weight of 200,000 to 300,000 daltons.[42]

Water

The water content of articular cartilage is extraordinarily important in maintaining the resiliency of tissue, as well as contributing to the almost frictionless movement associated with a boundary lubrication system.[17, 43-45] The water content is highest at birth, with only a modest decrease in adult tissues[34, 36, 39, 46-49] and a further slight diminution with advanced age.[34, 40, 50] An increase in total water content has been noted with immobilization,[31] with denervation,[51] and with joint motion without weight bearing.[30]

The mechanism of water binding within cartilage is not entirely understood. Because most of the extracellular matrix consists of collagen and proteoglycan and because gel formation occurs when water is in contact with either of these macromolecules,[52-56] this process is considered to be the major mechanism by which the tissue holds water.[57-60] The water of the gel, although unable to "flow," is believed to be freely exchangeable with that of fluids on the other side of the gel membrane and is subject to all of the physicochemical laws that govern osmotic solutions or membrane theory.[17, 27, 28, 58, 59, 61] Only a small portion of the water (<5%) remains tightly bound, and it cannot be removed by heating or desiccation. The nature of this binding is not well understood.[61]

Proteoglycans

Proteoglycans are complex macromolecules that consist of a linear protein core to which are linked long-chain polysaccharide moieties (glycosaminoglycans). The glycosaminoglycans are polyanionic in charge, owing to the regular occurrence of carboxyl and sulfate groups along the macromolecules. (Proteoglycans were formerly called protein-polysaccharides or chondromucoproteins, and glycosaminoglycans were formerly termed mucopolysaccharides.) The standard model for the steric and chemical structure of the proteoglycans is that of a "test tube brush" (Fig. 3–2), with the central core of the molecule consisting of a linear protein, to which are linked numerous glycosaminoglycan chains, radiating from the core at right angles and stiffly extending in space (presumably through the entire 360 degrees).[62] This model has been partially confirmed by the elegant studies of Rosenberg and

Table 3–1. APPROXIMATE BIOCHEMICAL COMPOSITION OF ADULT ARTICULAR CARTILAGE

Water	66%–79%	
Solids	21%–34%	
Inorganic		
Ash		5%–6%
Organic		
Collagen		48%–62%
Protein		8%–15%
Glycosaminoglycan		14%–23%
Hyaluronate		<1%
Sialic Acid		< 1%
Lipid		< 1%
Lysozyme		< 1%
Glycoprotein		?

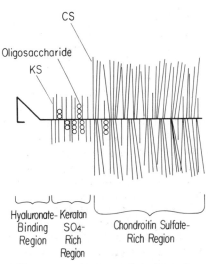

Figure 3–2. Diagram of the proposed structure of the proteoglycan subunit (PGS). As can be noted, the subunit is not structurally homogeneous, and there are three distinct portions: the protein-rich hyaluronate attachment region (left); a keratan-rich region adjacent to it; and a chondroitin sulfate–rich region containing some keratan sulfate (right) (see text).

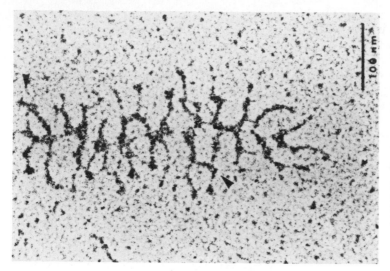

Figure 3–3. Electron micrograph of a clearly defined molecule (long form) of the kind from which measurements of the lengths of the polypeptide chain (long axis), lengths of the chondroitin sulfate side chains, and the number of apparent side chains per macromolecule were made. Some side chains appear to be intertwined with a neighboring chain; other side chains are bridged by short strands that run perpendicular from the middle of one chondroitin sulfate chain to another (arrow). (× 270,000.) (From Rosenberg L, et al.: J Biol Chem 245:4123, 1980.)

coworkers,[63] who performed ultrahigh-power electron microscopy of mixed proteoglycan–cytochrome c monolayers (Fig. 3–3).

The glycosaminoglycan molecules consist of long-chain, unbranched repeating polydimeric saccharides, and only three of these have been found in the proteoglycan subunit: chondroitin 4-sulfate; its stereoisomer, chondroitin 6-sulfate; and keratan sulfate[60, 64, 65] (Fig. 3–4). The chondroitin sulfates are the most prevalent glycosaminoglycans in cartilage and account for 55% to over 90% of the total glycosaminoglycans, depending principally on the age of the subject.[41] The repeating disaccharide units of chondroitin sulfate are *N*-acetylgalactosamine and glucuronic acid, linked by a 1:4 linkage. The position of the sulfate on the *N*-acetylgalactosamine defines the isomer. When the sulfate is present on the fourth carbon, the molecule is called chondroitin 4-sulfate, and when it is linked to the sixth carbon, it is called chondroitin 6-sulfate (Fig. 3–4). The average chain weight for chondroitin sulfate in articular cartilage is about 15,000 to 20,000 daltons, so that 25 to 30 repeating disaccharide units compose each chain.[64–66]

The keratan sulfate constituent of articular cartilage is not as well defined as the chondroitin sulfates. A number of species of keratan sulfate occur in various body sites. The composition and degree of sulfation of keratan sulfate from human articular cartilage are variable and may be considerably altered with the age of the individual.[67] The repeating structure for the keratan sulfate molecule consists of galactose linked by a 1:4 O-glycoside bond to 2-acetamidoglucosamine, with a sulfate moiety linked to the sixth carbon[64] (Fig. 3–4). Keratan sulfate chains of proteoglycans from human

articular cartilage are believed to be shorter than those of chondroitin sulfates. They consist of only five to six repeating dimeric units, so

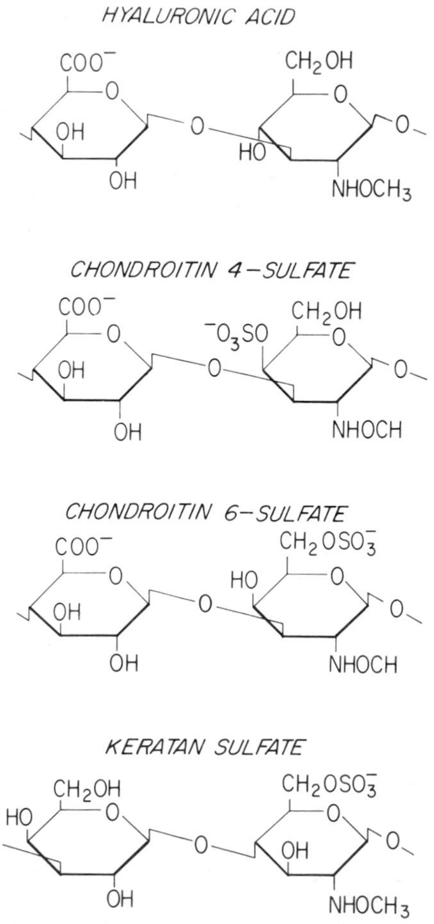

HYALURONIC ACID

CHONDROITIN 4–SULFATE

CHONDROITIN 6–SULFATE

KERATAN SULFATE

Figure 3–4. Biochemical structural formulas for the dimeric units of the four major glycosaminoglycans of articular cartilage (see text).

that the molecular weight of the entire chain is between 2300 and 2600 daltons.[68, 69]

The combination of the glycosaminoglycans and a protein constitutes the proteoglycan subunit. The core protein of the molecule is rich in serine, glutamic acid, proline, and glycine. The proteoglycan subunit measures approximately 180 to 210 nm in length and has a molecular weight of 1.5 to 4.0 × 10⁶ daltons.[49, 63–65, 69, 70] The glycosaminoglycan chains are covalently attached to the protein at specific amino acid sites.[71] The linkage region for the chondroitin sulfates consists of a galactosyl-galactosyl-xylosyl bridge bonded to serine.[72–75] Most investigators believe the keratan sulfate is bonded to threonine[76] or, as has been suggested recently, to glutamic acid.[68, 69] The linkage region includes also a neuraminylgalactosyl disaccharide or galactosamine; the presence of sialate and small quantities of mannose or fucose distinguishes the keratan sulfate linkage region from that of chondroitin sulfate, which has only xylose and galactose as unique sugar components. Recently, several investigators have described oligosaccharide components, quite distinct from the glycosaminoglycans that attach to the core protein, mostly in the keratan sulfate–rich region (see below). These consist of short-chain sugars that are free of keratan and chondroitin sulfates and contain small quantities of sialic acid and even smaller concentrations of the neutral sugars mannose and fucose.[77–79] Their significance is as yet unknown.

Extensive chemical studies of the proteoglycan subunit have demonstrated that the glycosaminoglycan chains are not uniformly distributed along the entire length of the core protein (see Fig 3–2).[68, 69, 80] At one end (the hyaluronate binding region [see below]), the macromolecule has few or no polysaccharide chains. Adjacent to this section is a linear segment (the keratan sulfate–rich segment) to which are attached principally keratan sulfate moieties and a few oligosaccharide chains. Attached to the remainder of the macromolecule are long chondroitin sulfate chains and a smaller number of shorter keratan sulfate chains. The asymmetric nature of the proteoglycan subunit probably accounts for the puzzling finding reported by earlier investigators of fairly marked variation in the concentrations of the glycosaminoglycans (chondroitin 4-sulfate, chondroitin 6-sulfate, and keratan sulfate) at different ages, in different sites, and, indeed, in different zones of the articular cartilage. Based on recent studies by a number of

investigators, it is most likely that the differences in the macromolecule result from variations in the length of the chondroitin sulfate–rich region (as a result of either altered synthesis or partial degradation)[81–86] or possibly from altered chain lengths of its polysaccharides.[85, 87, 88] However, evidence presented by Stanescu and associates[89] and Swann and coworkers[90] suggests that more than one species of proteoglycan subunit exist and that these vary with respect to peptide composition, binding regions, and associated glycoprotein fractions.

From data reported by several research groups, it is evident that only a small fraction of the proteoglycan exists as the free subunit in articular cartilage.[69–71, 82, 91–93] The majority of the macromolecular material forms high-order aggregates, which contain many subunits and have molecular weights of 60 to 150 × 10⁶ daltons.[64, 69] These complex materials, together with their gel-trapped water, occupy enormous domains that, because of the polyanionic nature of the glycosaminoglycans, are strongly electronegative and evoke a resistance to compressive force, which contributes materially to the resiliency of the tissue.[91] Studies have now established that the major aggregating factor is hyaluronic acid, which forms a filamentous backbone for the aggregate.[94–97] Hyaluronate exists in the aggregate as a long, filamentous strand, 40,000 to 420,000 nanometers in length, to which monomeric (or conceivably dimeric) subunits are linked at regular intervals at approximately right angles[69] (Fig. 3–5). Proteoglycan subunits bind to the filament at their protein-rich terminal adjacent to the keratan sulfate–rich portion of the macromolecule. The average interval between proteoglycan subunits on the filamentous hyaluronate backbone has been calculated to be 2400 to 2600 nanometers.[63]

Although hyaluronate is clearly the major factor in the aggregation of proteoglycan subunits, protein constituents, known as link proteins, have been found as components of the proteoglycan aggregates from every cartilage examined thus far.[64, 69, 91, 98–104] Two link proteins with molecular weights of approximately 44,000 and 48,000 daltons, respectively, have been isolated in a sufficiently purified state to raise specific antibody.[105, 106] Chemical studies of the link proteins have indicated that the larger link protein contains a considerable percentage of carbohydrate and, hence, is thought to be a glycoprotein in nature.[69, 100] The smaller link protein has a similar amino acid compo-

PROTEOGLYCAN AGGREGATE

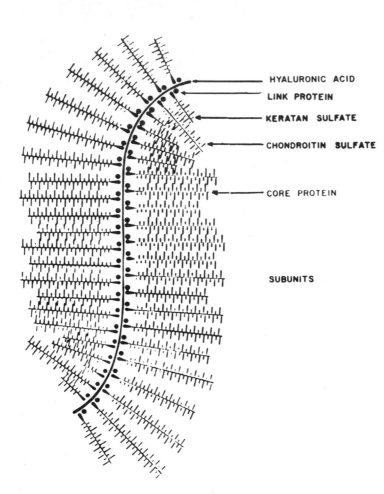

HYALURONIC ACID

LINK PROTEIN

KERATAN SULFATE

CHONDROITIN SULFATE

CORE PROTEIN

SUBUNITS

Figure 3–5. Model of the proteoglycan aggregate. The lengths of hyaluronic acid filaments and the PGS core proteins and the spacing between the subunits have been drawn to scale based on the measurements of electron micrographs of proteoglycan aggregates from bovine articular cartilage. The lengths of the chondroitin sulfate chains have been reduced about 1.5 times to avoid entanglement with the neighboring subunits. As can be noted, proteoglycan subunits attach at their protein-rich terminal end to a long core filament of hyaluronic acid. Adjacent to the binding sites are molecules of link protein. The proteoglycan subunits may vary considerably in length. The entire molecule may be as large as 160×10^6 daltons. (From Rosenberg L: Dynamics of Connective Tissue Macromolecules. New York, American Elsevier Publishing Co., 1975, p. 105.)

sition but is devoid of carbohydrate and may be a breakdown product of the larger link molecule.

The proteoglycans have a number of physical and chemical properties considered to be important to the resiliency of articular cartilage, and they probably aid materially in providing water for surface lubrication.[17, 45, 107] These properties are related to viscosity, water binding capacity, and the polyelectrolytic character of this complex macromolecule.[28] The proteoglycans are closely associated with collagen and may serve to direct or maintain the spatial position of the fibrous protein, influence fibril formation, and possibly prevent calcification.[64, 108–114]

Another property imparted to the cartilage by the proteoglycan is that of metachromatic staining. Dyes such as toluidine blue, azure A, crystal violet, and others serve as counterions (cations) to the polyanionic glycosaminogly-

cans.[115] Minute crystals of dye polymerize in a spatial relationship dictated by the loci of available sulfate and carboxyl groups. When a critical concentration is reached, the arrangement changes the spectrum of transmitted light from the "orthochromatic" to the "metachromatic" color.[115, 116] This phenomenon, known as metachromasia, is reasonably specific for glycosaminoglycans (and hence, proteoglycans) and is of great value as a qualitative and semiquantitative indicator of the concentration and distribution of these molecules within the cartilage. Rosenberg[117] reintroduced the use of safranin-O, an aniline dye, which interacts with chondroitin sulfate or keratan sulfate in solution. The orthochromatic and metachromatic absorption spectra for this material suggest that in permanently mounted sections, safranin-O binds only to tissue polyanions and not to the collagen. In solutions, its relationship in the orthochromatic spectrum is essentially 1:1 with the negatively charged groups of the proteoglycans, although this may not be so in tissue sections.

The proteoglycans of articular cartilage are not homogeneously distributed throughout the depth of the tissue.[118–121] The surface zone is rich in collagen and relatively poor in proteoglycan.[8, 119, 121–125] In the transitional zone, the concentration of proteoglycans increases, and they are homogeneously distributed, as demonstrated by histochemical staining,[126, 127] measurements of fixed charged density,[125, 128] biochemical analysis,[118–121] and immunofluorescent antibody techniques.[105, 129, 130] In the radial zone, the distribution is more variable,[119–121] with some increase in the chondrocyte territorial areas as compared with the interterritorial areas.[127, 131]

Collagen

Well over 50% of the dry weight of adult articular cartilage consists of collagen.[34, 36, 37, 41, 132] For many years, the collagen of cartilage was considered to be similar, and perhaps identical, to that isolated from skin, bone, and other body tissues, but as described below, compelling evidence now exists to indicate that cartilage collagen is a different genetic species. Collagen fibers of articular cartilage are thinner than those seen in tendon or bone and are less soluble. They have an organization and structure that were thought initially to be in the form of tension-resisting arcades but have recently been shown to be more a random distribution, at least in the middle zones of the cartilage[133] (Fig. 3–6).

Collagen is the most prevalent protein in the human body and, by definition, is the major organic component of the structural and support systems of the body.[134, 135] The simplest unit of extracellular collagen is the tropocollagen molecule,[99] which measures approximately 1.5 nm in diameter and 300 nm in length.[134, 136–139] Each of these molecules consists of three polypeptide chains coiled in a rigid, left-handed, helical structure.[133, 137, 140] Collagens from skin and bone (Type I) consist of two identical $\alpha 1$ chains and a single $\alpha 2$ chain, which are quite similar in structure but have differences in amino acid composition, so that they can be separated and independently assayed.[133, 134, 137, 141, 142] Each chain contains about 1000 to 1050 amino acids, with a total molecular weight of less than 100,000 daltons.[107, 130, 135, 140, 143] The molecular weight of the tropocollagen molecule is estimated to

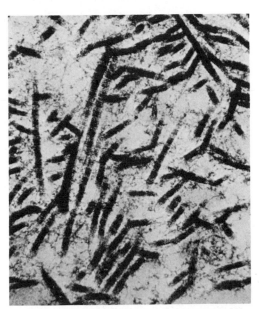

Figure 3–6. Electron photomicrograph of the interterritorial zone and the middle zone of articular cartilage. Note that the collagen fibers appear to be randomly distributed. The fibers show a characteristic 64-nanometer banding and are approximately 16 nanometers in diameter. Fine fibers fill the interfibrillar space. ($\times$ 30,000.) (Courtesy of Charles Weiss, M.D.)

range between 270,000 and 300,000 daltons.[136, 137, 143] In terms of the molecular conformation of the tropocollagen molecule, each of the three α chains consists of a major central region (approximately 95% of the molecule) in which the amino acid sequence is a repetition of glycine-x-y triplets, where x is frequently proline and y is less frequently hydroxyproline.[135, 142] The stability of the triple helix results, in large measure, from the distribution of its imino acids, proline and hydroxyproline, which allows an orderly arrangement of interchain hydrogen bonds.[144] Purified collagens contain both glucose and galactose, covalently linked to hydroxylysine either as single galactose residues or as glucopyranosylgalactose disaccharide units.[145, 146]

Tropocollagen molecules are ordered to form fibrils, and the fibrils are then ordered to form fibers,[141, 142, 147–151] which are stabilized by interfibrillar crosslinks. The fibers in articular cartilage, as seen with the electron microscope, may vary in width from 10 to 100 nanometers (see Figure 3–6), and as has been reported by Weiss,[152] this value may be exceeded in aging or osteoarthritis.

By electron microscopy, the collagen of cartilage is similar to that of other body tissues. In 1973, Igarashi and coworkers[146] pointed out that the optical rotary dispersion, intrinsic viscosity, and thermal stability of cartilage collagen are essentially identical to those of collagen from skin or bone. Cartilage collagen, however, is considerably less soluble than most other collagens and is not extractable in cold salt or acid solutions.[134, 135, 153, 154] The major differences, however, were pointed out by Miller and Matukas,[155] who, in 1969, demonstrated that the amount of α2 chain present in the tropocollagen molecule was insignificant, suggesting that the cartilage collagen is a different genetic species, consisting of three identical α1 chains.[155–158] Of perhaps more interest was the additional finding that the α1 chains of cartilage collagen have a different biochemical composition than those of skin or bone collagen.[141, 155, 156].

Collagen from cartilage has now been designated as Type II collagen, and the tropocollagen molecular structure is abbreviated as $\alpha1(II)_3$ (as opposed to that from skin and bone, which is designated by the formula $[\alpha1(I)]_2\alpha2$.[141] On amino acid analysis, the two types of α1 chains are shown to exhibit relatively large differences in their contents of glutamic acid, alanine, and leucine.[141, 155, 156] Of perhaps greater importance in terms of crosslinking is a fivefold increase in the extent of hydroxylation of the lysyl residues in the Type II chain[141] and a ninefold increase in the content of hydroxylysine-linked carbohydrate.[157–159]

The importance of these observations has been made clear by subsequent studies by several investigators, indicating that there is a rather large variation in the type of crosslinks found in Type II collagen as compared with Type I.[160–165] The crosslinks possibly result in greater structural stability,[166] less susceptibility to calcification, and more availability of the collagen for proteoglycan linkage and for gel formation to maintain the high water content of articular cartilage. The variation in crosslinking may also account for the smaller size of the collagen fibers of cartilage than those of bone and the frequent difficulty in observing the periodic banding.[167] An observation by Bruns and coworkers[168] has indicted a staggered substructure of reconstituted fibrils, with perhaps a different ordering in the native state.

In the past few years, considerable evidence has been introduced to suggest that other forms of collagen may be present in hyaline articular cartilage. Burgeson and Hollister[169] have described collagenous proteins in normal articular cartilage that are distinct from the α1(II) chain of Type II collagen. Some appear to contain disulfide bonds.[170] In 1976, Stanescu and coworkers[171] demonstrated the presence of Type I collagen in the superficial layers of articular cartilage, and more recently, Gay and associates[172] have reported the finding of collagen Types A and B in the pericellular regions of cartilage.[173] Under certain circumstances, chondrocytes in tissue culture may synthesize Type I or Type III collagen.[87, 174, 175] Nimni and Deshmukh[176] suggested that Type I collagen is synthesized by chondrocytes from osteoarthritic joints (see below). Similarly, when aspirin was fed to normal dogs in which atrophy of knee cartilage had been induced by casting, Type I collagen synthesis by the chondrocytes could be shown, although the bulk of the cartilage collagen remained Type II. In contrast, no Type I collagen could be demonstrated in the atrophic cartilage of dogs not given aspirin, or after aspirin administration to normal dogs.[177]

Other Materials

An "adhesive" protein, chondronectin, has been recently found in articular cartilage and is presumed to be responsible for establishing a relationship between the collagen fibrils and the chondrocytes.[178, 179] Lipids, which form 1% or less of the wet weight of human adult articular cartilage,[180] are found both in the cells[181] and in the matrix.[35, 39, 182] They may be revealed by lipid stains and vary considerably, depending on the site and the individual studies.[183–185] Extracellular lipid is found in the pericellular region of the cartilage from younger individuals and more frequently in the superficial zone. With aging, the lipid may be diffusely distributed throughout the matrix. Only limited information regarding the nature of the lipid is available. Studies by Bonner and associates[186] and by Rabinowitz and coworkers[180] show similar values, suggesting that neutral lipids (triglycerides, cholesterol, and glycolipids) account for 60% to 70% of the material and that phospholipids account for the remainder. Among the neutral fats, triglycerides and cholesterol account for the greatest percentages and almost no free fatty acids are detectable. A broad range of phospholipids, including gangliosides, are present.[180]

Ali[183, 187] has described pericellular osmiophilic matrix vesicles measuring 50 to 250 nm in size and containing apatitic calcific modules. The bodies have a double membrane and are more prevalent in the radial zone. They are noted with increased frequency in osteoarthritic cartilage.

Lysozyme, an enzyme that hydrolyzes the 1:4 linkage between N-acetylmuramic acid and N-acetylglucosamine, has been found in high concentration in epiphyseal cartilage,[188–190] and studies suggest that it is present in other cartilages as well.[191–192] There are no known substrates present within the articular cartilage that could yield to the action of the enzyme, and its extracellular location has been somewhat of a puzzle.[191]

Muir and coworkers[41, 193] and Maroudas and associates[38] have indicated that a glycoprotein, as yet poorly defined, may be present in considerable concentration in cartilage. This material is distinct from the link glycoprotein present in proteoglycan aggregates. Its chemical composition and sugar content are unknown, but it is believed to have a relatively low concentration of sugar and separates readily from the highly glycosylated proteoglycans. The material might be identical to the "matrix protein" with a molecular weight of 200,000 to 300,000 daltons recently described by Paulsson and Heinegard.[42]

METABOLISM OF ARTICULAR CARTILAGE

Over the past 30 years, there has been ample demonstration of a surprisingly active level of metabolism in articular cartilage, and it is now clear that the chondrocytes, despite their effete appearance in adult cartilage, synthesize and assemble the matrix components and direct their distribution within the tissue. The synthetic apparatus is complex, because not only are proteins (core protein of the proteoglycan, collagen, glycoproteins, enzymes, and so on) synthesized by the standard genetic pathway, but also sugars are assembled into glycosaminoglycans, linked to the protein, and sulfated. All of these actions take place under avascular and, at times, anaerobic conditions, with considerable variation in local pressure and physicochemical state. What is even more striking, however, is that the chondrocyte also directs an active internal remodeling system for at least portions of the proteoglycan and probably the collagen by means of an elaborate series of degradative enzymes.

Glycolysis and Energy Production

One of the factors that led to the general impression that articular cartilage was inert was the early demonstration that although articular cartilage had a well-defined glycolytic system, oxygen utilization was considerably lower than that in other tissues.[194] In 1937, Bywaters[195] presented data suggesting that glycolysis in articular cartilage is unvaried in the presence or absence of oxygen and that the QO_2 for articular cartilage is less than 0.1 mm^3/ mg of dry weight/hour. This value is about one fiftieth of that of other adult tissues and is comparable only to the QO_2 of non-nucleated red blood cells. In several later appraisals of these data, it was pointed out that the rate of oxygen consumption per unit mass was indeed low, but because of the sparse cell population, the rate per cell approached that seen for other relatively avascular body tissues.[196–198]

Despite the latter observation, there remains little doubt that articular cartilage utilizes principally the anaerobic pathway for energy production. Articular cartilage is relatively tolerant to high concentrations of potassium cyanide but is very sensitive to moniodoacetate,[19] and lactate concentration is high and remains unchanged, despite deprivation of oxygen.[197, 200] The lactic hydrogenase isoenzyme pattern for articular cartilage from rabbit, cow, and man has been shown to contain mostly LDH_4 and LDH_5,[200] which are thought to be facilitators of anaerobic glycolysis.[201, 202] Further confirmation for anaerobic activity was provided by the studies of Marcus,[203] who demonstrated that metabolic activities were unaffected by oxygen concentrations as low as 6.8%.

Proteoglycan Synthesis

Since the earliest studies by Böström[204] and by Dziewiatkowski and Campo,[205, 206] many investigators have clearly demonstrated that the chondrocyte is responsible for the synthesis, assembly, and sulfation of the proteoglycan molecule.[207–211] At the molecular level, this activity begins with the synthesis of a protein at the ribosome as dictated by a "message" carried from the nuclear DNA by messenger RNA. Autoradiographic studies with tritiated amino acids have demonstrated intracytoplasmic localization of the grains within the chondrocyte within minutes of intra-articular administration of the isotope and subsequent discharge of the grains from the cell into the surrounding territorial matrix (Fig. 3–7).[212, 213] The process varies depending on the isotope utilized, and there is autoradiographic,[213] histochemical,[214] and, most recently, metabolic[215]

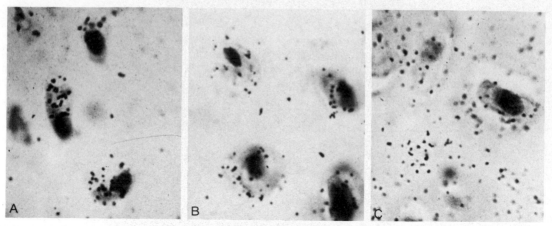

Figure 3–7. High resolution of autoradiographs of rabbit articular cartilage, 30 minutes (*A*), 1 hour (*B*), and 4 hours (*C*) after intra-articular administration of ³H-glycine. Grains are initially seen overlying the cytoplasm but rapidly move out of the cell, at first close to its margins (1 hour [*B*]) and subsequently widely scattered throughout the matrix (4 hours [*C*]). (× 1000.)

evidence to suggest that the chondrocytes are metabolically heterogeneous in the sense that some cells incorporate and export their proteoglycan substrate precursors more rapidly than others (and may, in fact, synthesize different materials).

Synthesis of the proteoglycan by the chondrocyte appears to occur at a rapid rate and is affected by numerous endogenous and exogenous environmental alterations.[216] Radioisotope tracer studies both in vivo and in vitro have demonstrated that such diverse physical and pathologic states as lacerative injury,[217] osteoarthritis,[212, 216] altered hydrostatic pressure,[218] varied oxygen tension,[197, 219–221] pH alteration,[222] calcium concentration,[223] substrate or serum concentration,[220, 224, 225] growth hormone,[226–229] ascorbate,[229, 230] vitamin E,[231] cortisol,[232–234] prostaglandins,[235–237] diphosphonates,[238] salicylates[239] and several other non-steroidal anti-inflammatory drugs,[240, 241] hyaluronate,[242, 243] uridine diphosphate,[244] xyloside,[245] synovial tissue,[246] and a variety of other factors have significant effects on the rate of synthesis of the proteoglycan.[212, 216] These data suggest that the control mechanisms for proteoglycan synthesis are extraordinarily sensitive to stimuli of a biochemical, mechanical, and physical nature.

The formation of O-glycoside bonds between unmodified sugars requires a large amount of free energy.[65] The standard mechanism by which sugar polymerization occurs in living tissue involves the utilization of sugar-nucleotides as glycosyl donors, a process in which energy exchange is considerably lessened.[247, 248] The process by which polymeriza-

tion occurs for chondroitin 4-sulfate or chondroitin 6-sulfate in articular cartilage utilizes a series of uridine diphosphate (UDP) intermediaries. All of the substrates arise from glucose in one of two pathways: conversion of glucose-1-phosphate to uridine diphosphate-*N*-acetyl-glucosamine by a series of reactions involving fructose; or conversion of glucose-1-phosphate to UDP-glucose, which is then further converted to UDP-glucuronic acid, UDP-galactose, or UDP-xylose by a series of enzymatically catalyzed reactions (Fig. 3–8).[65, 242, 249–251] The "primer" for chain assembly, at least for chondroitin sulfate, appears to be the presence of an appropriate serine-glycine group on the protein core.[249, 252]

This synthetic process is unusual in that the assembly of the polymer occurs within the Golgi apparatus of the cell and appears to be independent of the ribosome.[139, 253, 254] Once the chain has reached appropriate length, sulfation occurs, utilizing an adenosine nucleotide carrier for donation of the sulfate[255–259] (Fig. 3–9). Our current understanding suggests that sulfation occurs only when the chondroitin chain has reached a moderately large size and perhaps serves to limit the length of the chain.[251, 260] The enzymes for this process are microsomal in origin and are probably specific for the C4 and C6 position.[259]

Perhaps one of the areas of most interest and controversy in articular cartilage is the problem of "turnover" of proteoglycan. In 1952, Böström[204] demonstrated a half-life of 17 days for ³⁵SO₄ incorporated into costal cartilage of adult rats. Subsequent demonstrations of short half-lives for isotope-labeled proteo-

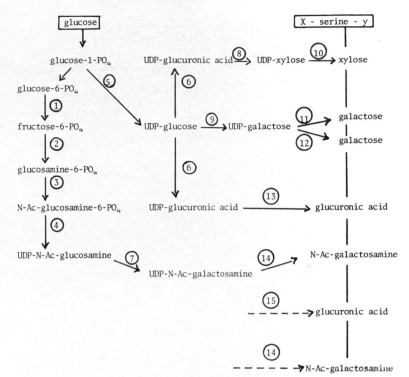

Metabolic Pathways in the Synthesis
of Chondroitin

Figure 3–8. Metabolic pathways in the synthesis of chondroitin. As can be noted, all of the substrates arise from glucose by two pathways: conversion of glucose-1-phosphate to uridine diphosphate-*N*-acetylglucosamine by a series of reactions involving fructose; and conversion of glucose-1-phosphate to UDP-glucose, which is then further converted to UDP-glucuronic ,acid, UDP-galactose, or UDP-xylose by a series of enzymatically catalyzed reactions. The "primer" for chain assembly appears to be the presence of an appropriate serine-glycine group on the protein core.

Enzyme catalysts
1. phosphoglucoisomirase 2. L-glutamine:D-fructose-6-phosphate-aminotransferase
3. acetyl CoA:2 amino-L-deoxy-D glucose-6-phosphate-N-acetyltransferase
4. N-acetyl-glucosamine-phosphate-nucleotidyltransferase 5. glucose-1-phosphate-nucleotidyltransferase 6. UDP-glucose: NAD oxireductase 7. UDP-N-acetyl-glucosamine-4-epimerase 8. UDP-glucuronic acid-carbonic-lyase 9. UDP-glucose-4-epimerase 10. xylosyltransferase 11. galactosyltransferase I 12. galactosyltransferase II 13. glucuronyltransferase I 14. N-acetyl-galactosaminyltransferase 15. glucuronyltransferase II

glycans by Schiller and associates[261] and Gross and coworkers[262] clearly indicated that the proteoglycan macromolecule is not inert. These data have since been confirmed by a number of investigators, and half-life values range from 3.5 to 20 days for various tissues and species[263–265] (Fig. 3–10). None of these studies, however, clearly defined whether the entire proteoglycan pool was turning over or whether the data reflected only a metabolically active portion. In 1963, Davidson and Small[263] performed a study on labeled intervertebral disk tissue and demonstrated that the proteoglycan pool was not homogenous and that considerable difference existed between the turnover rates for the soluble and insoluble fractions. Since then, several studies by other investigators have demonstrated evidence for multiple pools and

support the concept of metabolic heterogeneity.[122, 152, 265–268] The rapidity of turnover of a small proportion of the total proteoglycan population ("fast fraction") and, indeed, the turnover of additional fractions, seems to indicate a rate of proteoglycan metabolism far in excess of that necessary merely to compensate for any attrition that may occur in cartilage in a joint that operates in an almost frictionless state. Because the rapid disappearance of the isotopic tracer appears to be uniform throughout the articular cartilage mass on autoradiographs[264, 269] there is no evidence that focal loss occurs or that the cartilage surface is being "shed" in a manner analogous to that seen in skin. These data strongly suggest the presence of an enzymatic internal remodeling system that has the proteoglycans as its sub-

Metabolic Pathway for Sulfation
of Chondroitin

sulfate + ATP ——①——→ adenosine 5'-phosphosulfate (APS) + PPi

APS + ATP ——②——→ 3'-phosphoadenosine-5'-phosphosulfate (PAPS) + ADP

chondroitin + PAPS ——③——→ chondroitin sulfate + phospho AMP

Enzyme catalysts:

① ATP: sulfate adenyltransferase

② ATP: adenylsulfate-3'-phosphotransferase

③ sulfotransferase ?

Figure 3–9. Mechanism for sulfation of glycosaminoglycan chains. Once the chain has reached appropriate length, sulfation occurs. Sulfate and ATP combine to form adenosine 5'-phosphosulfate (APS). In the presence of additional ATP, an "active" sulfate (3'-phosphoadenosine-5'-phosphosulfate) is formed that serves as the donor of sulfate through either the fourth or sixth carbon of chondroitin in the presence of a specific sulfotransferase.

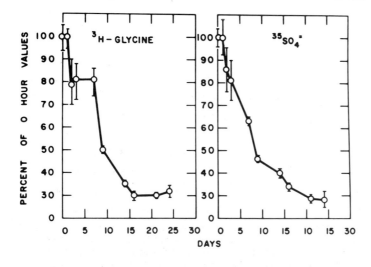

DEGRADATION RATE OF INCORPORATED ^{3}H-GLYCINE
AND ^{35}SO$_4^=$ INTO ADULT ARTICULAR CARTILAGE

Figure 3–10. The rate of disappearance of intra-articularly administered ^{3}H-glycine and ^{35}SO$_4$ from adult rabbit articular cartilage. Animals were killed serially up to 24 days, and the retained isotopic substrate was assayed by liquid scintillation spectrometry. Both isotopes appear to have an 8-day half-life. (From Mankin HJ: Bull Rheum Dis 17:447, 1967.)

strate and presumably is dictated by circumstances other than attrition.

Collagen Synthesis

The collagen of articular cartilage is considered to be much more stable than the proteoglycan, and until recently, there was little evidence for metabolic activity of the collagen. The appearance of this material on light and electron microscopy, its relative insolubility, and the failure to find a collagenase in normal cartilage supported the contention that the collagen of cartilage turns over very slowly, if at all. In 1972, however, Repo and Mitchell[270] reported an experiment that demonstrated a slow but measurable turnover of the collagen of articular cartilage in adult rabbits and a modest increase in the turnover rate in animals in which the cartilage surfaces had undergone lacerative injury.

The synthesis of collagen in cartilage is believed to be similar to that in other connective tissues, but it has been suggested that, in contradistinction to the collagen of skin and bone, in which two different chains are synthesized, presumably under the control of two separate genes, only one gene is responsible for the synthesis of the Type II collagen of cartilage.[114] (This hypothesis has been challenged recently by the findings of several dissimilar $\alpha 1(II)$ chains in cartilage.[271]) Synthesis occurs on polyribosomes in which up to 60 ribosomes are linked by messenger RNA.[135, 249, 272] The specific code sequences for collagen synthesis are as yet unknown.

The primary collagen product at the ribosome levels is called procollagen,[273-278] which, in cartilage, consists of three $\alpha 1(II)$ chains. These are larger than the $\alpha 1$ chains of the final exported product[279] and demonstrate some variation in the proline-hydroxyproline ratio.[280, 281] Enzymatic activity is necessary to convert procollagen to collagen during or after export,[274, 275, 279] and some of the procollagen (or fragments of it) remains intracellular[281, 282] and is subsequently degraded (Fig. 3–11).

Two processes occur during the intracellular synthesis of procollagen, during or just after its assembly on the ribosomes. The first of these is hydroxylation of proline and lysine to produce the amino acids hydroxyproline and hydroxylysine, which are almost unique to collagen.[274] This process requires specific enzymes (proline hydroxylase, lysine hydroxylase)[283, 284] and, as cofactors, molecular oxygen, ferrous iron, α-ketoglutarate (which is metabolized to succinate during the process), and a reducing agent, such as ascorbic acid.[284-286] The

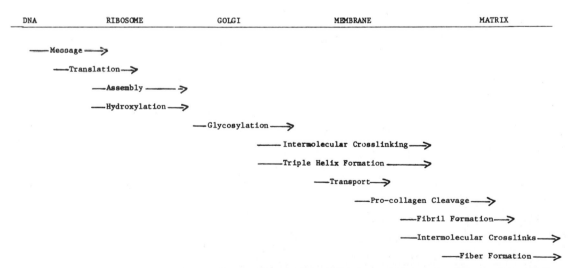

Figure 3–11. A scheme for the synthesis of collagen. Message from DNA is translated at the ribosome by messenger RNA to assemble the proteins of collagen. At almost the same time, hydroxylation occurs in the presence of ferrous iron, α-ketoglutarate, oxygen, and ascorbic acid. Glycosylation takes place at the Golgi apparatus, and the entire molecule is transferred to the cell membrane, where intermolecular crosslinking and triple helix formation occur. Transport of the procollagen molecule to the matrix occurs, and the ends are "clipped." Fibers are formed, and intermolecular crosslinking and fiber formation occur.

second process, the synthesis of hydroxylysyl glycosides,[145, 154, 156, 157] is dependent on the presence of galactose and glucose in the form of UDP-derivatives and two specific transfer enzymes.

Once assembled, the procollagen molecule undergoes enzymatic conversion to native collagen during or following export,[176] but to date the exact site and nature of both this conversion and the method by which the molecule is extruded from the cell are not clearly understood. The remaining processes affecting collagen occur in the matrix and consist of crosslink formation, which provides intramolecular links between the chains of the tropocollagen molecule, intrafilament crosslinks between the tropocollagen molecules composing the primary unit, and interfilament crosslinks between the primary filaments making up the fibril.[135, 287]

The Degradation Enzymes of Articular Cartilage

It has been known for years that certain degradative enzymes act on articular cartilage to destroy the matrix. Papain, a material extracted from the papaya plant, was noted to cause a loss of basophilia and metachromasia on histologic study and a profound depletion of the glycosaminoglycans on biochemical analysis, presumably by cleavage of the core protein of the proteoglycan.[288, 289] In 1960, Fell and Thomas[288] noted that administration of vitamin A in large doses caused a similar chondrolytic action. Subsequent studies suggested that vitamin A caused an activation or

release of potent autolytic enzymes contained within the chondrocyte but ordinarily stored in an "inactive" form.[290, 291] The bodies in which these enzymes are stored are known as lysosomes, and the enzymes are known as lysosomal enzymes.[292, 293] Lysosomal bodies have been observed on electron microscopic studies of articular cartilage[8, 294] (Fig. 3–12), and analyses of cartilage for "lysosomal marker enzymes," such as acid phosphatase or β-glucuronidase, have shown them to be present in very low concentration in normal tissue. They may be increased in amount by chemical maneuvers such as acidification or treatment with detergents, both of which destroy the envelope of lysosomal bodies.[295, 296]

If one considers the classes of lysosomal enzymes, only two could act to degrade the intact proteoglycan. The first is a hyaluronidase, which could lyse the hyaluronate "backbone" of the proteoglycan aggregate and also the chondroitin sulfate chains (keratan sulfate is resistant to most hyaluronidases).[64, 297] Studies by Bollet and coworkers[298] have failed to demonstrate evidence for a hyaluronidase in normal articular cartilage or in cartilage from severely arthritic joints. Recently, however, with a viscometric technique that has greater sensitivity than the colorimetric methods previously employed, heat-stable hyaluronidase activity has been found in normal articular cartilage. The activity appears to be related to the concentration of cyclic adenosine monophosphate in the cartilage.[299]

The second type of enzyme is a cathepsin, which would attack the core protein.[297, 300–302] Fessel and Chrisman[303] and Tourtelotte and associates[304] independently demonstrated that

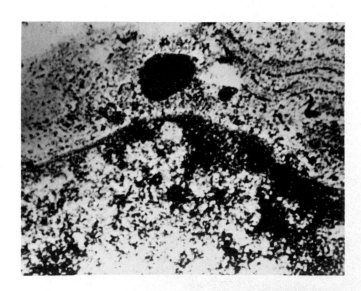

Figure 3–12. Electron micrograph of a chondrocyte showing a densely stained body believed to be a lysosome. The membrane-bound sac contains numerous proteolytic and other types of enzymes responsible for matrix degradation. (× 46,000.) (Courtesy of O.D. Chrisman, M.D.)

proteoglycan could be enzymatically degraded by an extract of cartilage, and in 1964 Ali[305] first demonstrated the presence of a lysosomal acid protease that could cleave the protein of the proteoglycan. Subsequent studies of Ali and coworkers,[306, 307] Woessner,[308, 309] and others[297, 310–312] have identified these materials as cathepsins D and B, and both are known to occur in articular cartilage, although the evidence for the action of cathepsin B in normal and osteoarthritic cartilage is limited and its presence in significant amounts is doubtful.[307, 313]

Of considerable concern to investigators has been the low pH optima at which acid cathepsins act. It seems unlikely that pH's of 5.5 or less occur extracellularly in normal cartilage, except perhaps in the immediate pericellular zone. This suggests the possibility that another enzyme, a neutral proteoglycanase, is operative in the tissues.[297] Sapolsky and colleagues[314] and Ehrlich and coworkers[315, 316, 317] have independently described a metal-dependent enzyme, as yet only partially purified, that degrades proteoglycan subunit at a neutral pH.[318, 319]

Collagenase that is active at neutral pH has been demonstrated in numerous body tissues, and the pattern of degradation of the collagen molecule is well established.[320–324] Most mammalian collagenases act on the substrate to cleave it into two fragments, which represent approximately three fourths and one fourth, respectively, of the length of the intact molecule.[320–324] The degraded material is soluble and can be further degraded by the action of other proteases.[324] Although Ehrlich and associates[325] were able to demonstrate an endogenous collagenase in osteoarthritic human articular cartilage, to date no direct evidence exists for the presence of a collagenase in normal joint cartilage. The turnover rate for collagen, as has been recently described,[294] is sufficient, however, to require some form of enzymatic degradative system for this otherwise insoluble material, and the recent observations by Pelletier and associates suggest that a small amount of collagenolytic action may be observed in normal cartilage.[326]

IMMATURE ARTICULAR CARTILAGE AND THE EFFECTS OF AGING

Unlike many other body tissues, immature articular cartilage differs considerably from adult articular cartilage. On gross inspection, the cartilage from an immature animal appears blue-white in color (presumably because of the reflection of the vascular structures in the underlying immature bone) and is considerably thicker on cut section.[327] As will be discussed, however, the thickness is primarily a function of the dual nature of the cartilage mass; it serves not only as a cartilaginous articular surface for the joint but also as a microepiphyseal plate for endochondral ossification of the underlying bony nucleus of the epiphysis.

On histologic examination, it is apparent that immature articular cartilage is considerably more cellular than the adult tissue, and numerous studies have corroborated the increased number of cells per unit volume or mass[35, 67, 195, 212, 328] (Fig. 3–13). The hypercellularity appears fairly uniform throughout the cartilage, and little variation is noted in cell density. The structural organization of the tis-

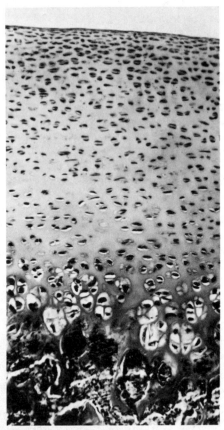

Figure 3–13. Low-power photomicrograph of the articular cartilage of an immature (2-month-old) rabbit. Note the increased cellularity and the structural heterogeneity. In the lower zones, the orientation differs markedly from that of an adult. About halfway from the surface, the chondrocytes are arranged in irregular columns, and at further depth, the columniation becomes more evident. The cells in these columns show characteristics consistent with those of chondrocytes of an epiphyseal plate. (Iron hematoxylin-safranin-O-fast green stain, × 200.)

sue also differs from that of adult cartilage in that the zonal characteristics show major variation, particularly in the lower zones.[329, 330] The gliding or tangential layer remains evident in immature cartilage, although the surface cells are somewhat larger and less discoid than those seen in adult cartilage. The midzone is wider and contains a larger number of randomly arranged cells. In the lower zones, however, the orientation differs markedly; at about the halfway mark in the distance from the surface to the underlying bone, the chondrocytes are arranged in irregular columns, and at further depth the columniation becomes more evident. The cells in these columns show characteristics consistent with those of chondrocytes of the epiphyseal plate.[331] In the uppermost portion of the column, the chondrocytes are round or flat or occasionally triangular in shape, indicating their participation in the process of diagonal division.[331] With further distance from the surface, the cells are increased in size and show shrunken pyknotic nuclei and large intracytoplasmic vacuoles that have been demonstrated to contain glycogen. Vascular buds from the underlying bone invade the cartilage columns in a pattern resembling the zone of provisional calcification of the epiphyseal plate[329] (Fig. 3–13).

When immature articular cartilage is examined by light microscopy, mitotic figures are readily noted and all stages of mitosis can be seen.[328, 329, 332, 333] Cell replication is not uniformly present throughout the tissue, however. In the very young animal, the mitotic activity occurs in two distinct zones. One lies subjacent to the surface and presumably accounts for the growth of the cellular complement of the articular portion of the cartilage mass; the second lies below this region and consists of a narrow band of cells that morphologically resemble the proliferative zone of the microepiphyseal plate for the subjacent bony nucleus[329, 333, 334] (Fig. 3–14). As the animal ages and approaches maturity, the pattern of cell replication changes. The mitotic index is diminished, and mitotic activity is confined to the area just above the zone of vascular invasion in the lowermost portion of the cartilage, which now demonstrates a diffuse calcification. No evidence for cell replication can be found in the more superficial regions.

In the adult animal, mitotic activity ceases with the development of a well-defined calcified zone, a tidemark, and, in some species, with closure of the epiphyseal plate.[328, 329, 335–338] Careful search of normal articular cartilage from adult animals of numerous species has

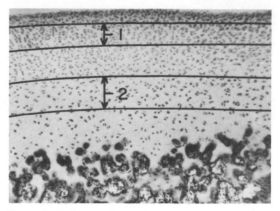

Figure 3–14. Zones of cell division indicated on a low-power photomicrograph from an immature rabbit (2 months of age). The superficial zone (1) lies subjacent to the gliding surfaces and is considered to contribute to the growth of the cartilage mass. The deeper layer (2) lies in proximity to the underlying bony epiphysis and is thought to be the proliferative zone of a microepiphyseal plate for endochondral ossification of the epiphyseal nucleus. (Hematoxylin and eosin stain, × 150.) (From Mankin HJ: AAOS Instructional Course Lecture 14:204, 1970.)

failed to demonstrate mitotic figures, and ^{3}H-thymidine studies have not demonstrated grains over the nucleus indicating DNA replication.[335, 336, 338] Although it has been suggested that the chondrocyte may divide by amitotic division, there is only limited evidence for such an activity, and cytophotometry and cytofluorometry have failed to demonstrate evidence of nuclear polyploidy in the adult tissue.[332, 339, 340]

In recent years, investigations have provided data regarding variation of the chemistry of articular cartilage with advancing age. Water content appears to be increased in immature animals and slowly diminishes to a standard figure that remains constant throughout most of adulthood.[34, 46–49, 341] The collagen content of fetal articular cartilage is considerably lower than that of mature animals.[47, 342] Once the value climbs to the adult values (shortly after birth), the concentration is maintained throughout the life of the animal.

The principal chemical changes in articular cartilage matrix with advancing age appear to be in the proteoglycan molecule. Proteoglycan content in articular cartilage is highest at birth and diminishes slowly through the period of immaturity.[85] The length of the protein is diminished in immature animals, but polymerization of the glycosaminoglycan is greater.[66, 85, 132, 342, 343] As the animal approaches adolescence and maturity, the proteoglycan core becomes longer and the glycosaminoglycan chain lengths, particularly those of chondroitin sulfate, diminish. Although the concentration of chondroitin 4-sulfate has been noted to be extraordinarily high in immature animals, a fairly rapid diminution in this value is noted with aging.[85, 88, 238, 343–346] Furthermore, with advancing age, the total chondroitin sulfate concentration falls and that of keratan sulfate increases until at approximately age 30 in humans, keratan sulfate represents 25% to 50% of the total glycosaminoglycan. This value then remains constant through old age.[119, 347–351] Inerot and coworkers[82] have shown a decrease in the size of the core protein of proteoglycan subunit with advancing age and have suggested that the loss of the chondroitin sulfate–rich terminal end of the macromolecule explains the altered glycosaminoglycan distribution seen with advancing years.

BIOCHEMICAL ALTERATIONS IN THE CARTILAGE IN OSTEOARTHRITIS

Before considering the biochemical or metabolic alterations of articular cartilage from osteoarthritic human joints or animal models, several important qualifying remarks must be introduced in order to at least partially explain divergent views that have appeared in the literature in recent years. There is the problem of "controls." If one seeks to determine an abnormality in a chemical constituent of the articular cartilage, it is logical to have as a comparison normal tissue that comes from a corresponding site of the corresponding joint from an individual of the same age, sex, body habitus, and so on. Although this is a logical application of the scientific method, it is frequently difficult or impossible to achieve in studies of osteoarthritis. As noted previously, the biochemical composition of articular cartilage may vary considerably from species to species, individual to individual, joint to joint, and site to site within a joint and with the depth of the cartilage from surface to calcified zone. Diffusion of materials through the cartilage may vary, depending on the thickness of the tissue studied and the integrity of the collagenous "skin"; cell density may vary widely in small segments of cartilage adjacent to one another. Furthermore, there is ample reason to believe that there may be significant differences between the biochemical abnormalities seen in osteoarthritic cartilage recovered at autopsy from asymptomatic individuals and cartilage involved with "end-stage disease" obtained at the time of surgical extirpation of the joint.[352, 353] Drawing conclusions

regarding the nature of a process on the basis of the latter specimens (which are readily obtainable in current orthopaedic practice) may lead to erroneous conclusions (and frequently has).

Current animal models of osteoarthritis (see Chapter 6), although accepted as demonstrating facets of the disease, may differ considerably from the human or naturally occurring mammalian condition, depending on the nature of the insult utilized to cause the disease, the species and age of the animal, and so on. Immobilization osteoarthritis[354, 355] differs in its gross and microscopic characteristics from that seen in the partial meniscectomy model[45, 356] or from the dog model in which the anterior cruciate has been severed.[357] Furthermore, in models of osteoarthritis that depend on mechanical instability, the degree of usage of the unstable joint will affect development of the disease. Thus, in dogs that had undergone transection of the anterior cruciate ligament, no evidence of osteoarthritis was present 12 weeks later (when typical changes of disease are usually obvious), if the unstable knee was maintained in a cast postoperatively.[358]

Lesions resulting from chemical insults may vary widely from those occurring as a result of mechanical conditions. The naturally occurring hip dysplasia model reported by Lust and coworkers[359, 360] in the dog seems to be an appropriate model for the human disease, but all of the animals studied in their experiments were 5 to 8 months of age (still immature, with open epiphyseal plates). Similarly, the fidelity of models of naturally occurring osteoarthritis in rodents may be questioned because of differences in biochemical features of the cartilage and the persistence of open epiphyseal plates throughout the lifetime of the animal.[151]

All of the factors cited above make interpretation of biochemical data complicated. Perhaps even more important, they make it very difficult to find alterations that are reproducible from one species to another or from site to site. Nevertheless, some features of osteoarthritis are widely agreed upon and have been utilized by a number of investigators to attempt to establish a pathogenic mechanism for the disorder.

DNA Content

Cell counts and measurements of the quantity of DNA per unit tissue show considerable variation in osteoarthritis, depending on the site tested and the degree of the disease[361–364]

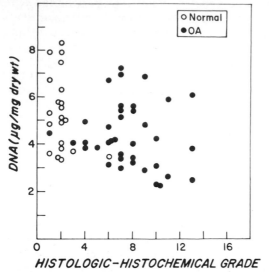

Figure 3–15. Graphic representation of variation of DNA content of normal and osteoarthritic cartilage with histologic-histochemical grade. As can be noted, there is little variation between the DNA content of normal cartilage and osteoarthritic cartilage. This does not alter with degree of the disease, although there is a tendency to have a diminished concentration of DNA with advancing disease.

(Fig. 3–15). Examination of histologic sections and the ultrastructural studies of Weiss and Mirow[365] confirm the fact that cellularity is highly variable. Usually, however, DNA concentrations have been reported to be near normal and occasionally increased in osteoarthritis. This supports the concept that despite a reduction in the volume of tissue, the cell count is maintained reasonably well.[362, 366] Some of the chondrocyte clones show intense activity when studied autoradiographically using ^{3}H-cytidine.[367] It is probably these active cells that Mitchell and Shepard[368] have shown electron microscopically to have an increased collar of proteoglycan with special stains. Other cells, and indeed entire clones, may show little or no evidence of RNA metabolism and are probably dead or dying.[367] As the disease worsens, the tissue becomes hypocellular, and eventually all cellular substance is lost.

Water

The water content of osteoarthritic articular cartilage has been the subject of a number of studies in the past few decades. In 1966, Bollet and Nance[46] found a significant increase in the water content of articular cartilage from chondromalacic patellae when compared with normal tissues, a finding that seemed inconsistent with the fact that the concentration of "hydrophilic" proteoglycans, which constitute almost 50% of the dry weight of normal cartilage, is significantly reduced in osteoarthritic articular cartilage (see below). This apparent paradox suggested that the water content of articular cartilage may be independent of the concentration of proteoglycan. In 1975, Mankin and Thrasher[49] reported a study in which fresh articular cartilage was obtained from osteoarthritic and "normal" femoral heads (the former obtained at the time of total hip replacement and the latter at the time of insertion of an Austin Moore prosthesis for fracture of the neck of the femur). Cartilage slices were incubated for 5 minutes in medium with tritiated water, and an attempt was made to assess the water content, the number of counts of newly administered water (tritiated) that were incorporated, and the binding of newly administered water (in the form of tritiated water) by heating the cartilage samples at 60° C to assess the quantity of the labeled material driven off. The study demonstrated a statistically significant increase in the quantity of water contained in osteoarthritic human cartilage as compared with normal human cartilage (Fig. 3–16). The 9% increase found in the study was comparable to that previously reported by Bollet and

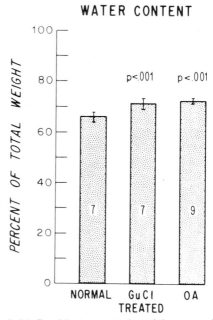

Figure 3–16. Graphic representation of the comparison of the water content in normal cartilage (left bar), osteoarthritic cartilage (right bar), and cartilage treated with guanidine hydrochloride (center bar). As can be noted, there is a small but statistically significant increase in the water content of both the osteoarthritic and guanidine hydrochloride–treated cartilage as compared with normal.

Nance[46] and analogous to that subsequently reported by Maroudas and Venn,[40, 369] McDevitt and associates,[357] and Sweet and colleagues.[370] No increase was noted in the quantity of tritiated water that was incorporated in the osteoarthritic samples as compared with the normal ones, but the osteoarthritic samples apparently held the newly administered tritiated water with greater avidity (12.1% increase in retention). Of perhaps greater significance was the finding that when the proteoglycan was removed from normal articular cartilage by treatment with 4 M guanidine hydrochloride, the changes seen in osteoarthritis could be reproduced (Fig. 3–16). Thus, removing the proteoglycan increased the concentration of water within the cartilage and also the apparent "avidity" with which newly administered water was held to the tissue.

These data suggested that removal of the proteoglycan either by natural means (osteoarthritis) or artificially (4 M guanidine hydrochloride) did not reduce the concentration of water but actually allowed it to increase and perhaps caused the water to be more tightly bound to the tissue. Several possible explanations were offered for this observed change. The first of these suggested that perhaps removal of the proteoglycan opened up binding sites on the collagen that were otherwise obscured and that held water with greater avidity than the proteoglycan-collagen gel. A second and more logical possibility, in view of the work of Maroudas and Venn,[369] is that removal of the proteoglycan allows the remainder of the material to uncoil and increase its negatively charged domain and its hydrophilic character. The studies of Maroudas and Venn[369] failed to demonstrate a greater avidity for water (presumably because the experiment was done in a different way), which lent further support to the concept that in both osteoarthritic and normal cartilage, the water is held in the form of a freely exchangeable gel.

Perhaps the more important finding in the studies of Maroudas and Venn[40, 369] was the increased swelling of cartilage seen in osteoarthritis as compared with normal tissues. The swelling pressure observed in their samples was significantly different from that in normal controls and implied some alteration in the collagen network. Electron microscopic studies by them and by Weiss and Mirow[365] supported the concept that the collagen network was probably defective in osteoarthritis and that the spaces between the collagen fibers were materially enlarged, allowing the tissue to "swell" in the presence of increased water

(probably independent of the proteoglycan concentration). Treatment of normal cartilage with collagenase produced a similar change, supporting the concept that intrinsic abnormality in the collagen network may be a very significant part of the osteoarthritic lesion. This may account for the alteration in swelling and may provide an explanation for the increase in water content that is noted in the face of a decreased concentration of proteoglycan in osteoarthritis.

Proteoglycan

The proteoglycans of osteoarthritic articular cartilage have received the greatest amount of investigative attention. In 1944, on the basis of an alteration in the color seen when cartilage was exposed to a variety of basic dyes, Hirsch[371] suggested that osteoarthritis articular cartilage undergoes a progressive depletion of the ground substance. These studies were subsequently confirmed by the biochemical analyses of Bollet and associates[372] and other investigators.[40, 357, 361, 362, 364, 366, 370, 373–376] It has now been well established that the protcoglycan content of osteoarthritic cartilage is diminished. The decrease appears to be directly proportional to the severity of the disease[289] (Fig. 3–17), as determined by a histologic-

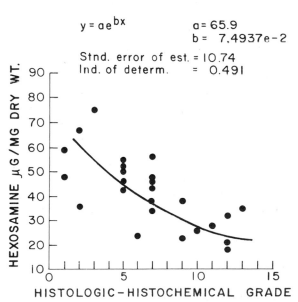

Figure 3–17. Variation in the concentration of hexosamine (an indicator of proteoglycan concentration) with severity of osteoarthritis, as measured by a histologic-histochemical grading system (see Table 3–2). Note that as the process worsens, the concentration of hexosamine diminishes. (From Mankin HJ, et al.: J Bone Joint Surg 53A:523, 1971.)

Table 3–2. HISTOLOGIC-HISTOCHEMICAL GRADING SYSTEM FOR OSTEOARTHRITIS*

	Grade
I. Structure	
a. Normal	0
b. Surface irregularities	1
c. Pannus and surface irregularities	2
d. Clefts to transitional zone	3
e. Clefts to radial zone	4
f. Clefts to calcified zone	5
g. Complete disorganization	6
II. Cells	
a. Normal	0
b. Diffuse hypercellularity	1
c. Cloning	2
d. Hypocellularity	3
III. Safranin-O staining	
a. Normal	0
b. Slight reduction	1
c. Moderate reduction	2
d. Severe reduction	3
e. No dye noted	4
IV. "Tidemark" integrity	
a. Intact	0
b. Crossed by blood vessels	1

*Adapted from Mankin HJ, et al.: Bone Joint Surg 53A:523, 1971.

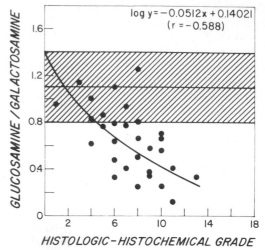

Figure 3–18. Variation of glucosamine/galactosamine ratio (an indicator of relative concentration of keratan sulfate and chondroitin sulfates) with histologic-histochemical grade (see Table 3–2). Note the rapid decline in the ratio with advancing severity of the process. The shaded areas represent the normal range. (From Mankin HJ, et al.: J Bone Joint Surg 63A:131, 1981.)

histochemical grading system (Table 3–2). These biochemical data have been further confirmed by Maroudas and coworkers,[40, 377] who have shown a decrease in fixed charge density that closely parallels the glycosaminoglycan depletion in both early and late lesions.

Since these initial studies, additional investigations have been performed to attempt to define the nature of the proteoglycan macromolecule that is present in osteoarthritic articular cartilage, particularly in relation to aggregation, glycosaminoglycan chain length, and distribution of the glycosaminoglycans. A report by Mankin and Lippiello in 1971[349] detailed experimental evidence that suggested an altered glycosaminoglycan pattern in osteoarthritis, in which the percentage of chondroitin 4-sulfate was markedly increased and that of keratan sulfate diminished. These findings were in part confirmatory of those of Bollet and Nance[46] and Bjelle and coworkers,[119] McDevitt,[37] Mankin and associates,[362] and Brocklehurst and Maroudas,[376] who have found a similar alteration. For the most part, the data suggest that in osteoarthritic cartilage, keratan sulfate is diminished, whereas chondroitin sulfate either remains the same or increases. There is thus a resultant decrease in the concentration of glucosamine (with no change in galactosamine) and, therefore, a fall in the glucosamine/galactosamine ratio[378] (Fig.

3–18). One explanation for this alteration is that the articular chondrocyte in osteoarthritic cartilage is synthesizing an "immature" proteoglycan that is characterized by an increased concentration of chondroitin 4-sulfate and a diminished concentration of keratan sulfate.[375] The other explanation is the possibility that there is an asymmetric degradation of the proteoglycan moiety that could, as suggested by Inerot and associates,[82] selectively attack the hyaluronate binding region of the macromolecule or possibly the keratan sulfate chains. This latter finding is in part supported by the recent observation of Ehrlich and colleagues[317] that suggests the presence of a keratanase in osteoarthritic articular cartilage.

As indicated earlier, the proteoglycans of articular cartilage, which consist of core protein and glycosaminoglycan side chains (proteoglycan subunit), are usually found as aggregates in which the subunits are linked at specific binding sites to a long-chain filament of hyaluronic acid in the presence of link proteins. As noted previously, the core protein consists of three portions: a hyaluronate binding region, a keratan sulfate–rich region, and a chondroitin sulfate–rich terminal region that is probably variable in length (the first two are reasonably stable in length and chemical configuration) (see Figure 3–2). In recent years, the attention of proteoglycan chemists has shifted to the physical conformation of the macromolecule and its various species. Studies by Brandt in 1974[379] demonstrated that proteoglycan appeared to be considerably more extractable from osteoarthritic articular cartilage than from normal articular cartilage. Subsequent studies by Brandt and coworkers[380] and others[82, 357, 381] have shown that in osteoarthritis, a higher percentage of the cartilage proteoglycan exists in the form of proteoglycan subunit and that only a small proportion is aggregated. In review of these data, Muir[375] has proposed three possible explanations: (1) an abnormality of the hyaluronate binding region of the core protein; (2) an alteration in the quantity of hyaluronate; and (3) a reduction in the quantity of link protein present in the osteoarthritic tissue.

In 1976, Brandt and coworkers[380] were able to demonstrate that proteoglycan subunit isolated from bovine osteoarthritic articular cartilage interacted with hyaluronic acid in vitro in a fashion similar to that of the normal subunit isolated from nonosteoarthritic tissue. The same investigators,[382] however, studied the cartilage from a human with osteoarthritis and demonstrated that in a less diseased area, the aggregating ability was normal but in an extensively diseased area, subunits could not aggregate in vitro in the presence of hyaluronic acid. In 1978, Inerot and coworkers[82] demonstrated that proteoglycans extracted from osteoarthritic dog cartilage were smaller than those extracted from normal cartilage of animals of the same age and seemed to have a smaller chondroitin sulfate–rich region. Some of the molecules also appeared to lack the hyaluronate binding region. On the basis of these studies, it was postulated that increasing proteolytic activity first attacked the free terminal end of the subunit and then the protein-rich portion. Several other investigators have demonstrated that the chain length of chondroitin sulfate was diminished in proteoglycans from osteoarthritic cartilage,[66, 373, 383] and Sweet and coworkers[370] showed a decrease in hyaluronic acid. These data suggest that the concentration of hyaluronate or the nature of the hyaluronate produced in osteoarthritis may limit the amount of aggregation that occurs, causing a serious weakening of the structure of the proteoglycan aggregate in the articular cartilage. In late cases, however, sufficient injury occurs to the proteoglycan subunit to damage the hyaluronate binding region of the core protein, so that even if additional hyaluronate is added, no aggregation occurs.

To date, few studies have been performed to identify whether glycoprotein link is present in sufficient quantity. Treadwell and associates[103] have demonstrated the synthesis of normal link proteins (identifiable by specific antibody) in a messenger-directed cell–free system in which the messenger RNA was obtained from osteoarthritic chondrocytes. Their presence, however, does not necessarily imply that they function normally in stabilizing the proteoglycan-hyaluronate interaction.

Collagen

The collagen of articular cartilage from osteoarthritic joints may show some marked variations in the size and arrangement of the fibers.[40, 365, 384] In a number of studies in which the concentration of collagen in normal and osteoarthritic tissue has been assessed by measurements of hydroxyproline and hydroxylysine content,[357, 361, 366, 374, 375, 385, 386] the data have failed to demonstrate a significant alteration in the amount of collagen per unit weight of tissue or per unit of DNA, suggesting that the concentration of collagen within the cartilage remains stable. In severe disease, when the cartilage is almost totally destroyed, the collagen content must fall (along with that of the other constituents), but the relative concentration in relation to total mass (wet weight, dry weight, and per microgram of DNA) is not altered materially until the end stages of the process.

One of the questions that has arisen in recent years has been whether the collagen of osteoarthritic cartilage remains as Type II. In 1973, Nimni and Deshmukh[176] reported that osteoarthritic chondrocytes in an in vitro system appeared to synthesize not only Type II collagen but also substantial amounts of Type I. This suggested that despite gross maintenance of the collagen content in osteoarthritic cartilage, the chondrocytes renew the collagen by synthesizing collagen more closely resembling that found in fibrocartilage. Although a report by Gay and coworkers[387] suggest that minute quantities of Type I collagen may exist in osteoarthritic cartilage, a study by Lippiello and associates[385] failed to show a significant change in the hydroxyproline/hydroxylysine ratio, and studies by Eyre and colleagues[388] and by Floman and coworkers[374] demonstrated no evidence of a shift from Type II to Type I collagen synthesis in osteoarthritic cartilage from an animal model. As has been noted by a number of investigators, collagen production by cells in tissue culture may be significantly affected by the environment or the concentration of various substances in the medium.[87, 172, 174, 175] It is possible that under certain circumstances, Type I collagen might be synthesized by chondrocytes in vivo in osteoarthritic tissue.

Other Materials

In considering some of the chemical agents that cause osteoarthritis, it is apparent that the presence of certain metabolic products that may occur in articular cartilage under special circumstances may lead to rapid cartilage degradation. The most clearly defined of these disorders is a genetic one, alkaptonuric ochronosis, in which patients who lack homogentisic acid oxidase deposit large quantities of brown pigment in the cartilage. The pigment exists in relation to the collagen fiber, effectively "tanning" it by increasing the crosslinking.[389–392] The cartilage alterations in ochronotic arthropathy are quite pronounced, and osteoarthritis occurs much more rapidly than is seen in other forms of the disease. A similar alteration may be observed in hemochromatosis.[392–394] A more subtle form of chemical disorder has been suggested recently by Howell[395] and by Dieppe and coworkers,[396, 397] based on the observation of McCarty and colleagues,[398] pointing out the increased frequency of joint cartilage calcification (chondrocalcinosis articularis) in osteoarthritis. A considerable body of data has evolved that has demonstrated increased pyrophosphate in the joint,[395, 399–402] increased prevalence of membrane-bound calcium-containing vesicles,[183, 187] and increased alkaline phosphatase concentration in cartilage from some patients with osteoarthritis.[403] Recent studies by Ryan and associates[404] have failed to show a significant increase in the serum concentrations of phosphate or alkaline phosphatase, but localized changes in the cartilage may be quite significant, particularly if they occur in the middle zone, decreasing the resistance of the region to mechanical shearing forces.[402]

THE METABOLISM OF OSTEOARTHRITIC CARTILAGE

Perhaps the most controversial issue in the biochemical analysis of the cartilage in osteoarthritis has been the assessment of the metabolic rate of the tissue as compared with that of normal tissue. The early concept of the disease suggested that the process consisted of a passive mechanical erosion by "wear and tear" of a relatively inert tissue. It would, therefore, seem logical that the cells would show signs of degeneration and of decreased synthetic activity as the disease progressed. It was with some surprise, then, that scientists greeted the observation by Collins and McElligott[181] in 1960 that articular cartilage from osteoarthritic human joints was considerably more active metabolically than normal articular cartilage. The investigators used a radioisotopic tracer technique employing $^{35}SO_4$, which is an excellent indicator of proteoglycan synthesis in cartilage. Subsequent studies on human and experimental animal models of osteoarthritis by Meachim and Collins,[363] Meachim,[405] Bollet,[406] Bollet and Nance,[46] Ehrlich and associates,[356] McDevitt and coworkers,[407] Mayor and Moskowitz,[408] Jacoby and Jayson,[409] Thompson and Oegema,[364] Mitrovic and coworkers,[410] and Eronen and colleagues[373] have supported this finding, and until recently, the concept that cartilage showed increased metabolic activity appeared to be fairly universally accepted. Ultrastructural study of the chondrocytes has revealed findings consistent with a very high level of cell activity, including a well-developed endoplasmic reticulum, secretory vesicles, and a prominent Golgi apparatus.[365] Recent autoradiographic studies with proteoglycan precursors by Mitrovic and associates[410] showed a marked increase in grains over the osteoarthritic cell as compared with the normal, a finding that coincides nicely with electron microscopic data of Mitchell and Shepard[368] showing an increased amount of proteoglycan (newly formed?) immediately around the cell in osteoarthritic cartilage.

Two groups, however, one in Australia and another in London, have cast some doubt on the view that the metabolic rate of osteoarthritic chondrocytes is increased. Studies by Ghosh and coworkers[411] and McKenzie and associates[412] supported those by Maroudas,[268] Byers and colleagues,[413] and Brocklehurst and Maroudas[376] that suggested that there was essentially no change in the rate of synthesis of osteoarthritic articular cartilage as compared with that of normal cartilage. Recent studies by Moskowitz, Goldberg, and Malemud[413a] demonstrated that chondrocyte activity did not increase in parallel with degenerative change in an experimental model of osteoarthritis in rabbits. Rather, cell replication and proteoglycan synthesis were reduced at times of maximal

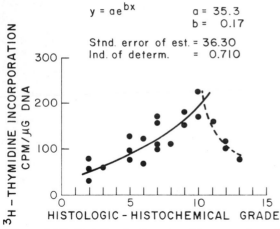

Figure 3–19. Variation in the rate of incorporation of $^{35}SO_4$ (an indicator of matrix synthesis) with severity of the osteoarthritic process, as measured by the histologic-histochemical grade (see Table 3–2). Note that the sulfate incorporation increases with advancing severity up to a point of 10 on the scale and then appears to fall off, possibly indicating the beginning of "end-stage" disease. (From Mankin HJ, et al.: J Bone Joint Surg 53A:523, 1971.)

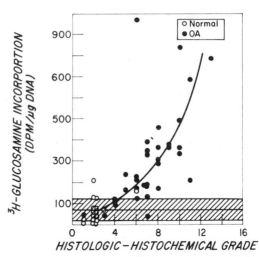

Figure 3–20. Graphic demonstration of the increasing rate of incorporation of ^{3}H-glucosamine into articular cartilage with increasing severity of the disease process, as measured by the histologic-histochemical grade. These data firmly support the concept of the hypermetabolic state of the chondrocyte in osteoarthritis. (From Mankin HJ, et al.: J Bone Joint Surg 63A:131, 1981.)

pathology. Because the experimental techniques differed in these various studies, there is probably little reason to suggest that one or the other group is in error, but the reader should be aware of the controversy.

As indicated previously, there is clear evidence based on numerous studies (with only a few groups dissenting) that proteoglycan is being synthesized more rapidly than normal in articular cartilage from osteoarthritic joints. Regardless of whether $^{35}SO_4$ (Fig. 3–19) or ^{3}H-glucosamine (Fig. 3–20) is used as substrate, the rate of incorporation not only is higher but appears to parallel the severity of the disease process.[362] The increase in proteoglycan synthesis in osteoarthritic cartilage from knees rendered unstable by cruciate ligament transection can be prevented by immobilization of the limb, which in itself decreases the rate of proteoglycan synthesis to subnormal level.[358]

Notably, aspirin, when fed to dogs with osteoarthritis of the knee secondary to cruciate ligament transection in doses sufficient to maintain a serum salicylate level of 20 to 25 mg/dl, suppressed the augmented level of proteoglycan synthesis in the diseased cartilage so that it was no greater than that in control cartilage. In vitro, the inhibition of proteoglycan synthesis in organ cultures of osteoarthritic cartilage was much greater than that in organ cultures of normal cartilage,[414] presumably because of greater diffusion of the drug through

the matrix of the diseased cartilage, in which the proteoglycan content was diminished. Similarly, the inhibitory effect of salicylate on proteoglycan synthesis in atrophic knee cartilage from dogs that had borne leg casts for 6 weeks was much greater than the effect of the drug on normal cartilage from the same animals.[415]

The drug's effects in vitro were also more marked on cartilage from habitually unloaded regions of normal canine femoral condyles (in which the proteoglycan content was lower) than they were on cartilage from habitually loaded regions of the same condyle in which the proteoglycan content was higher.[416] Furthermore, indomethacin, which had no effect on cartilage from the habitually loaded areas, suppressed proteoglycan synthesis in cartilage from the unloaded sites by 30%. Whether these agents have a similar effect in vivo on the relatively unloaded regions of normal joints (which are frequently the site of nonprogressive, age-related degeneration[352, 417]) is not known.

A study by Mankin and associates[362] has demonstrated a significant increment in the rate of incorporation of ^{3}H-glucosamine into both the glucosamine and galactosamine fractions of proteoglycan in osteoarthritic cartilage. Of considerable interest, however, was that the ratio of tritiated glucosamine to tritiated galactosamine after administration of radioisotope-labeled glucosamine was unaltered as compared with normal articular cartilage. These data suggest that although the rate of synthesis of proteoglycan is increased in osteoarthritis, the product synthesized is probably normal in terms of its proportions of keratan sulfate (^{3}H-glucosamine incorporation) and chondroitin sulfates (^{3}H-galactosamine incorporation). In a more recent study, hyaluronate synthesis was found to be excessively increased as compared with the synthetic rate for proteoglycan subunit,[418] a finding that at first appears to be puzzling in view of the discovery by Brandt and coworkers[380, 382] that aggregation is diminished or absent in osteoarthritic cartilage. Considering the data, it seems reasonable either that the hyaluronate that is synthesized is abnormal and hence does not allow aggregation or that the excess synthesis is in response to a rapid degradation of the synthesized product.

Collagen Synthesis

The collagen of articular cartilage is considered to be much more stable than the proteoglycan, but a metabolic study by Lippiello, Hall, and Mankin[385] showed that collagen synthesis in osteoarthritic human cartilage, as measured by incorporation of ^{3}H-proline into hydroxyproline, was greater than normal and that the rate of collagen synthesis seemed to vary with the severity of the disease, as determined by histologic-histochemical grading (Fig. 3–21). At the peak value for synthesis (at a grade of 7 on the arbitrary histologic-histochemical grading scale), the rate appeared to be at least five times that in normal cartilage. Recently, Floman and coworkers[374] performed a similar study on an animal model of osteoarthritis and demonstrated a similar increment in the rate of collagen synthesis as compared with the normal control. Their data also demonstrated that the majority of the collagen synthesized was Type II rather than Type I, supporting the concept that the "repair tissue" in osteoarthritis is hyaline cartilage rather than fibrocartilage.

DNA Synthesis

Hulth, Telhag, and coworkers[289, 367, 419, 420] and Rothwell and Bentley[421] have studied DNA synthesis in osteoarthritic articular cartilage and have demonstrated evidence for mitotic activity and ^{3}H-thymidine incorpora-

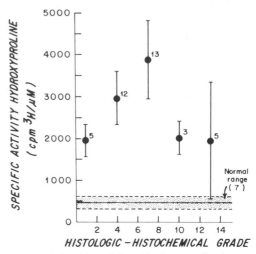

Figure 3–21. Specific activity of hydroxyproline in normal and osteoarthritic human cartilage after administration of ^{3}H-proline in an ex vivo system. The shaded area represents the range for the normal cartilage. Note the marked increase in the rates of incorporation of the isotopic tracer, particularly in the mid-range of the osteoarthritis. The severity was assessed by the histologic-histochemical grading system shown in Table 3–2. (From Lippiello L, et al.: J Clin Invest 59:5903, 1977.)

tion in a rabbit model of osteoarthritis as well as in human osteoarthritic lesions and cartilage from patellar chondromalacia. The studies showed labeled cells in chondrocyte clones, suggesting mitotic activity and supporting an earlier finding by Mankin and Lippiello[366] of increased incorporation of ^{3}H-thymidine into articular cartilage from osteoarthritic human hip joints (Fig. 3–22). Weiss and Mirow[365] found evidence for replicative activity in their electron microscopic studies of osteoarthritic chondrocytes. All of these data point to the likelihood that the articular chondrocyte in osteoarthritis "turns on the switch" for DNA synthesis and makes new cells that presumably become metabolically active. The rate of DNA synthesis appears to vary directly with the morphologic severity of the process up to a point of "failure," after which the rate falls.[361]

DEGRADATIVE ENZYMES IN OSTEOARTHRITIC ARTICULAR CARTILAGE

If, in fact, osteoarthritis is a disorder in which the cartilage is slowly degraded and if, as indicated earlier, it is universally agreed that a progressive decrease in the content of proteoglycan occurs, the findings that the rates for synthesis of proteoglycan, collagen, and DNA are all increased would seem to indicate that catabolic activity of the tissue is extraor-

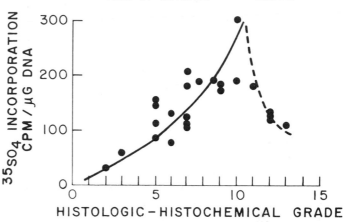

$$y = x/a + bx \qquad a = 6.6323e\text{-}2$$
$$b = -2.7088e\text{-}3$$

Stnd. error of est. = 41.24
Ind. of determ.   = 0.879

Figure 3–22. Graphic representation of the variation of ³H-thymidine incorporation into osteoarthritic human articular cartilage with severity of the disease process. Note that as the disease becomes more severe, the rate of DNA synthesis increases until a grade of 10 is reached and the response falls off. This may indicate failure of the reparative mechanism. (From Mankin HJ, et al.: J Bone Joint Surg 53A:523, 1971.)

dinarily high. Although "wear" may be a factor in the loss of articular cartilage, there is now strong evidence to support the concept that lysosomal and extralysosomal enzymes account for the majority of the loss of substance.

Over the past few years, there have been numerous demonstrations of proteolytic enzymes within the cells and matrix of articular cartilage in health and in certain pathologic states (see above). Although either a hyaluronidase or a protease theoretically could act on proteoglycan to initiate degradation, there is little evidence for the presence of the former. On the other hand, a number of studies have shown that acid cathepsins present in the lysosome of the chondrocytes have a powerful hydrolytic action on the protein core of the macromolecule. In 1964, Ali[305] first described the presence of a lysosomal acid protease in cartilage that could cleave the protein of the proteoglycan. Subsequent studies by Ali and coworkers,[306] and Woessner,[308, 309, 422] and others have identified these materials as cathepsins D and B. Cathepsin D levels are elevated in osteoarthritic articular cartilage,[308, 313] and acid phosphatase activity is markedly increased and varies with the severity of the disease[295] (Fig. 3–23). The findings of a neutral proteoglycanase by Sapolsky and coworkers[312, 423] and Ehrlich and associates[317] have explained at least in part the enigma posed by the pH optimum for the acid cathepsins, which is far lower than that likely to be present even in osteoarthritic tissues, except within the cell in the immediate pericellular area. Neutral pro-

teoglycanase, a metal-dependent enzyme, is present in increased concentrations in articular cartilage from osteoarthritic joints and may be the principal agent in the degradation of proteoglycan. In 1977, Ehrlich and colleagues,[325] using a 7-day culture technique and brief exposure to trypsin to remove inhibitors, demonstrated the presence of a collagenase in osteoarthritic cartilage. The data obtained in this study suggested that the concentration of collagenase appeared to increase with the advancing severity of the disease[325, 424] and probably accounted for the destruction of collagen in the disorder. A recent report by Pelletier and associates on an animal model supported these findings.[326] It is obvious that cathepsins, neutral proteoglycanase, and collagenase are present in normal as well as osteoarthritic articular cartilage, but they are probably controlled by potent inhibitors in normal tissue. Stephens and coworkers[425] have proposed a theory that osteoarthritis may result from an interference with the inhibitor enzyme.

THE BIOCHEMICAL PATHOGENESIS OF OSTEOARTHRITIS

Although Radin[426, 427] has suggested that the primary lesion in osteoarthritis may be in the subchondral bone, the majority of investigators feel that the disorder begins in the cartilage. Even if Radin has correctly implied that stiffening of the underlying bone is a major factor in producing the cartilage change, one must still consider cartilage loss central to the

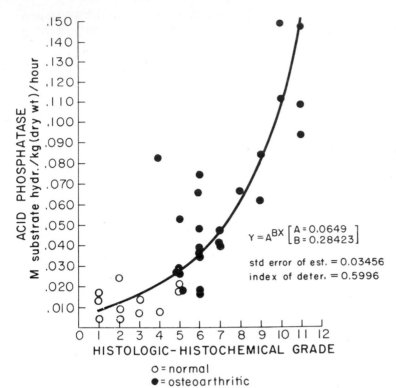

Figure 3–23. Variation in acid phosphatase concentration in human articular cartilage with severity of osteoarthritis. The open circles represent normal specimens; the dots represent osteoarthritic specimens. As the process becomes more severe, more and more of the lysosomal marker enzyme is present. (From Ehrlich MG, et al.: J Bone Joint Surg 55A:1068, 1973.)

process. Understanding of the pathogenesis of the changes in the cartilage may lead to important discoveries in regard to techniques of chemical management or ways of preventing the disease.

In summary, the cartilage changes in osteoarthritis consist of a slowly progressive loss of articular cartilage, which is associated biochemically with an early loss of proteoglycan, increased water, and no alteration in collagen content but a probably highly significant change in the arrangement and size of the collagen fibers, particularly in the middle zone. Of considerable importance is the reduction of proteoglycan aggregation. It is probable that an alteration occurs in the hyaluronate concentration or perhaps in the hyaluronate binding region of the proteoglycan subunit that decreases the number of aggregates formed.

The mechanisms by which these changes occur are likely to be partially mechanical, but there is strong support for enzymatic alteration. Lysosomal and extralysosomal enzymes, particularly cathepsins D and B, neutral proteoglycanase, and collagenase, are present in increased amounts in osteoarthritic cartilage and probably account for the alterations in both collagen and proteoglycan. If the enzyme activity were unopposed, cartilage degradation would be very rapid, but there is ample evidence for a reparative response. The chondrocytes undergo cell replication to produce new cells, some of which appear to be very active metabolically, producing increased quantities of proteoglycan, collagen, and hyaluronic acid. These new materials are probably abnormal in the sense that they do not aggregate well, and there is a significant alteration in the glycosaminoglycan distribution within the newly synthesized proteoglycans. Despite this, however (and probably the reason why the disease may take so long to evolve), the repair process appears to keep pace with the disease, and the response may be sufficiently brisk to maintain the joint in a marginal state of cartilage "health," possibly for many years. Eventually, at least in some cases, the degradative process far exceeds the reparative one, and the individual progresses to "end-stage" disease, with total loss of cartilage, eburnation of bone, and severe clinical symptoms. The relationship of biochemical alterations and other factors in pathogenesis of OA are reviewed in further detail in Chapter 7.

References

1. Barnett CH, Davies DV, MacConnaill MS: Synovial Joints: Their Structure and Mechanics. Springfield, Illinois, Charles C Thomas, 1961.

2. Davies DV, Barnett CH, Cochrane W, Palfrey AJ: Electron microscopy of articular cartilage in the young adult rabbit. Ann Rheum Dis 21:11–22, 1962.

3. Ghadially FN: Fine structure of joints. In Sokoloff L (ed.): The Joints and Synovial Fluid, Vol. I. New York, Academic Press, 1978, pp. 105–176.

4. Meachim G, Ghadially FN, Collins DH: Regressive changes in the superficial layer of human articular cartilage. Ann Rheum Dis 24:23–30, 1965.

5. Meachim G, Roy S: Surface ultrastructure of mature adult human articular cartilage. J Bone Joint Surg 51B:529–539, 1969.

6. Redler I: A scanning electron microscope study of human normal and osteoarthritic articular cartilage. Clin Orthop 103:262–268, 1974.

7. Silberberg R: Ultrastructure of articular cartilage in health and disease. Clin Orthop 57:233–257, 1968.

8. Weiss C, Rosenberg L, Helfet AJ: An ultrastructural study of normal young adult human articular cartilage. J Bone Joint Surg 50A:663–674, 1968.

9. Collins DH: The Pathology of Articular and Spinal Disease. London, Arnold and Company, 1949.

10. Hunter W: Of the structure and diseases of articulating cartilage. Philos Trans R Soc Lond 42:514–521, 1943.

11. Strangeways TSP: Observations in the nutrition of articular cartilage. Br Med J 1:661–663, 1920.

12. Virchow R: Die Krankhaften Geschwulste, I. Berlin, 1863. Cited by Ekholm R: Acta Anat 11(Suppl): 15–2, 1–76, 1951.

13. Brower TD, Akahoshi Y, Orlic P: Diffusion of dyes through articular cartilage in vivo. J Bone Joint Surg 44A:456–463, 1962.

14. McKibben B, Maroudas A: Nutrition and metabolism. In Freeman MAR (ed.): Adult Articular Cartilage. 2nd ed. New York, Grune and Stratton, 1979, pp. 461 ff.

15. Mankin HJ: Localization of tritiated cytidine in articular cartilage of immature and adult rabbits after intra-articular injection. Lab Invest 12:543–548, 1963.

16. Maroudas A, Bullough P, Swanson SAV, Freeman MAR: The permeability of articular cartilage. J Bone Joint Surg 50B:166–177, 1968.

17. Maroudas A: Physical chemistry of articular cartilage and the intervertebral disc. In Sokoloff L (ed.): The Joints and Synovial Fluid, Vol. II. New York, Academic Press, 1980, pp. 239–291.

18. Ogston A: On articular cartilage. J Anat Physiol (Lond) 10:49–74, 1875.

19. Agata K, Whiteside LA, Lesker PA: Subchondral route for nutrition of articular cartilage in the rabbit. Measurement of diffusion with hydrogen gas in vitro. J Bone Joint Surg 60A:905–910, 1978.

20. Ekholm R: Articular cartilage nutrition. Acta Anat 11(Suppl):15–2, 1–76, 1951.

21. Greenwald AS, Haynes DW: A pathway for nutrients from the medullary cavity to the articular cartilage of the human femoral head. J Bone Joint Surg 51B:747–753, 1969.

22. Holmdahl DE, Ingelmark BE: The contact between the articular cartilage and the medullary cavities of the bone. Acta Orthop Scand 20:156–165, 1950.

23. Ingelmark BE, Saaf J: Über die Ernahrung des gelenknorpels und die Bildung der Gelenkflussigheit unter verscheidenen funktionellen Verhaltnissen. Acta Orthop Scand 17:303–357, 1948.

24. McKibben B, Holdsworth FS: The nutrition of immature joint cartilage in the lamb. J Bone Joint Surg 48B:793–803, 1966.

25. Ropes MW, Bauer W: Synovial Fluid Changes in Joint Disease. Cambridge, Harvard University Press, 1953.

26. Swann DA: Macromolecules of synovial fluid. In Sokoloff L (ed.): The Joints and Synovial Fluid, Vol. I. New York, Academic Press, 1978, pp. 407–432.

27. Maroudas A: Distribution and diffusion of solutes in articular cartilage. Biophys J 10:365–379, 1970.

28. Maroudas A: Physiochemical properties of articular cartilage. In Freeman MAR (ed.): Adult Articular Cartilage. New York, Grune and Stratton, 1973, pp. 131–170.

29. Maroudas A: Transport of solutes through cartilage: permeability to large molecules. J Anat 122:335–347, 1976.

30. Palmoski MJ, Coyler RA, Brandt KD: Joint motion in the absence of normal loading does not maintain normal articular cartilage. Arthritis Rheum 23:325–334, 1980.

31. Palmoski M, Perricone R, Brandt KD: Development and reversal of a proteoglycan aggregation defect in normal canine knee cartilage after immobilization. Arthritis Rheum 22:508–517, 1979.

32. Palmoski MJ, Brandt KD: Running inhibits the reversal of atrophic changes in canine knee cartilage after removal of a leg cast. Arthritis Rheum 24:1329–1337, 1981.

33. Kempson EG, Muir H, Pollard C, Tuke M: The tensile properties of the cartilage of human femoral condyles related to the content of collagen and glycosaminoglycans. Biochim Biophys Acta 297:465–472, 1973.

34. Miles JS, Eichelberger J: Biochemical studies of human cartilage during the aging process. J Am Geriatr Soc 12:1–20, 1964.

35. Stockwell RA, Meachim G: The chondrocytes. In Freeman MAR (ed.): Adult Articular Cartilage. New York, Grune and Stratton, 1973, pp. 51–99.

36. Campo RD, Tourtelotte DC: The composition of bovine cartilage and bone. Biochim Biophys Acta 141:614–624, 1967.

37. McDevitt CA: Biochemistry of articular cartilage: Nature of proteoglycans and collagen of articular cartilage and their role in aging and in osteoarthrosis. Ann Rheum Dis 32:364–378, 1973.

38. Maroudas A, Bayliss MT, Venn MF: Further studies on the composition of human femoral head cartilages. Ann Rheum Dis 39:514–523, 1980.

39. Meachim G, Stockwell RA: The matrix. In Freeman MAR, (ed.): Adult Articular Cartilage. New York, Grune and Stratton, 1973, pp. 1–50.

40. Venn MF, Maroudas A: Chemical composition and swelling of normal and osteoarthritic femoral head cartilage. I. Chemical composition. Ann Rheum Dis 36:121, 1977.

41. Muir H: Biochemistry. In Freeman MAR (ed.): Adult Articular Cartilage. New York, Grune and Stratton, 1973, pp. 100–131.

42. Paulsson M, Heinegard D: Matrix proteins bound to associatively prepared proteoglycans from bovine cartilage. Biochem J 183:539–545, 1979.

43. Linn FC: Lubrication of animal joints. I. The arthrotripsometer. J Bone Joint Surg 48A:1079–1098, 1967.

44. McCutchen CW: Lubrication of joints. In Sokoloff L (ed.): The Joints and Synovial Fluid, Vol. I. New York, Academic Press, 1978, pp. 438–483.

45. Mow VC, Lai VM: Recent developments in synovial joint biomechanics. SIAM Rev 22:275–317, 1980.

46. Bollet AJ, Nance JL: Biochemical findings in normal

and osteoarthritic articular cartilage. II. Chondroitin sulfate concentration and chain length, water and ash content. J Clin Invest 45:1170–1177, 1966.

47. Eichelberger L, Akeson WH, Roma M: Biochemical studies of articular cartilage. I. Normal values. J Bone Joint Surg 40A:142–162, 1958.

48. Lindahl O: Über den wassergehalt des knorpels. Acta Orthop Scand 17:134–136, 1948.

49. Mankin HJ, Thrasher ZA: Water content and binding in normal and osteoarthritic human cartilage. J Bone Joint Surg 57A:76–80, 1975.

50. Amado R, Werner G, Neukom H: Water content of human articular cartilage and its determination by gas chromatography. Biochem Med 16:169–172, 1976.

51. Palmoski M, O'Connor B, Brandt KD: Interruption of articular nerves impairs macromolecular organization of articular cartilage. Arthritis Rheum 22:644, 1979.

52. Balazs EA, Bloom GD, Swann DA: Fine structure and glycosaminoglycan content of the surface layer of articular cartilage. Fed Proc 25:1813–1816, 1966.

53. Berendson HJC, Michelsen D: Hydration structure of fibrous macromolecules. Ann NY Acad Sci 125:365–379, 1965.

54. Clarke IC: Surface characteristics of human articular cartilage—a scanning electron microscope study. J Anat 108:23–30, 1971.

55. Laurent TC: Physicochemical characteristics of the acid glycosaminoglycans. Fed Proc 25:1037–1038, 1966.

56. McCall JG: Ultrastructure of human articular cartilage. J Anat 104:586–587, 1969.

57. Ling GN: The physical state of water in biological systems. Food Technol 22:1254–1258, 1968.

58. Maroudas A, Muir H: The distribution of collagen and glycosaminoglycans in human articular cartilage and the influence on hydraulic permeability. In Balazs EA (ed.): Chemistry and Molecular Biology of the Intercellular Matrix, Vol. 3. London, Academic Press, 1970, pp. 1381–1387.

59. Ogston AG: When is pressure osmotic? Fed Proc 25:1112–1114, 1966.

60. Schubert M, Hamerman D: A Primer on Connective Tissue Biochemistry. Philadelphia, Lea and Febiger, 1968.

61. Jaffe FF, Mankin HJ, Weiss C, Zarins A: Water binding in the articular cartilage of rabbits. J Bone Joint Surg 56A:1031–1039, 1974.

62. Mathews MB, Lozaityte I: Sodium chondroitin sulfate protein complexes of cartilage. II. Molecular weight and shape. Arch Biochem Biophys 74:158–174, 1958.

63. Rosenberg L, Hellman W, Kleinschmidt AK: Electron microscopic studies of proteoglycan aggregates from bovine articular cartilage. J Biol Chem 250:1877–1883, 1975.

64. Muir H, Hardingham TE: Structure of proteoglycans. In Whelan WJ (ed.): MTP International Review of Science, Biochemistry Series One, Vol. 5: Biochemistry of Carbohydrates. Baltimore, University Park Press, 1975, pp. 153–222.

65. Serafini-Fracassini A, Smith JW: The Structure and Biochemistry of Cartilage. London, Churchill Livingstone, 1974.

66. Hjertquist S-O, Wasteson A: The molecular weight of chondroitin sulphate from human articular cartilage: Effect of age and osteoarthritis. Calcif Tissue Res 10:31–37, 1972.

67. Stockwell RA: The inter-relationship of cell density and cartilage thickness in mammalian articular cartilage. J Anat 109:411–421, 1971.

68. Heinegard D: Hyaluronidase digestion and alkaline treatment of bovine tracheal cartilage proteoglycans. Isolation and characterizaiton of different keratan sulfate proteins. Biochim Biophys Acta 285:193–207, 1972.

69. Rosenberg L: Structure of cartilage proteoglycan. In Burleigh PMC, Poole AR (eds.); dynamics of Connective Tissue Macromolecules. New York, American Elsevier Publishing Co., 1975, pp. 105–128.

70. Hascall VC, Sajdera SW: Physical properties and polydispersity of proteoglycans from bovine nasal cartilage. J Biol Chem 245:4920–4930, 1970.

71. Rosenberg L, Pal S, Beale RJ: Proteoglycans from bovine proximal humeral articular cartilage. J Biol Chem 248:3681–3690, 1973.

72. Helting T, Rodén L: The carbohydrate-protein linkage region of chondroitin 6-sulfate. Biochim Biophys Acta 170:301–308, 1968.

73. Lindahl U, Rodén L: The chondroitin 4-sulfate–protein linkage. J Biol Chem 241:2113–3119, 1966.

74. Rodén L, Armand G: Structure of chondroitin 4-sulfate-protein linkage region. Isolation and characterization of the disaccharide 3-O-beta-D-glucuronosyl-D-galactose. J Biol Chem 241:65–70, 1966.

75. Rodén L, Smith R: Structure of the neutral trisaccharide of the chondroitin 4-sulfate protein linkage region. J Biol Chem 241:5949–5954, 1966.

76. Bray BA, Lieberman R, Meyer K: Structure of human skeletal keratan sulfate. The linkage region. J Biol Chem 242:3373–3380, 1967.

77. DeLuca S, Lohmander LD, Nilsson B, Hascall VC, Caplan AI: Proteoglycans from chick limb bud chondrocyte cultures. Keratan sulfate and oligosaccharides which contain mannose and sialic acid. J Biol Chem 255:6077–6083, 1980.

78. Lohmander S, DeLuca S, Nilsson B, Hascall VC, Caputo CB, Kimura HJ, Heinegard D: Oligosaccharides of proteoglycans from the Swarm rat chondrosarcoma. J Biol Chem 255:6084–6091, 1980.

79. Thonar EJ, Sweet MB: An oligosaccharide component in proteoglycans of articular cartilage. Biochim Biophys Acta 584:353–357, 1979.

80. Heinegard D, Hascall VC: Aggregation of proteoglycan. II. Characteristics of the proteins isolated from trypsin digests of aggregates. J Biol Chem 249:4250–4256, 1974.

81. Bayliss MT, Ali SY: Age related changes in the composition and structure of human articular cartilage proteoglycans. Biochem J 176:683–693, 1978.

82. Inerot S, Heinegard D, Andell L, Olsson S-E: Articular cartilage proteoglycans in aging and osteoarthritis. Biochem J 169:143–156, 1978.

83. Rosenberg L, Wolfenstein-Todel C, Maroudas R, Pal S, Strider W: Proteoglycans from bovine proximal humeral articular cartilage. Structural basis for the polydispersity of proteoglycan subunit. J Biol Chem 251:6439–6444, 1976.

84. Roughley PJ: A comparative study of the glycosaminoglycan peptides obtained after degradation of cartilage proteoglycan by different proteinases and their use in the characterization of the different proteoglycans. Connect Tissue Res 6:145–153, 1978.

85. Roughley PJ, White RJ: Age related changes in the structure of the proteoglycan subunits from human articular cartilage. J Biol Chem 255:217–224, 1980.

86. Sweet MBE, Thonar EJ, Marsh J: Age related changes in proteoglycan structure. Arch Biochem Biophys 198:439–448, 1979.

87. Benya PD, Padilla SR, Nimni ME: The progeny of rabbit articular chondrocytes synthesize collagen types I and III and type I primer but not type II: Verifications by cyanogen bromide peptide analysis. Biochemistry 16:805–872, 1977.

88. Murata K, Bjelle AO: Age dependent constitution of chondroitin sulfate isomers in cartilage proteoglycans under associative conditions. J Biochem (Tokyo) 86:371–376, 1979.

89. Stanescu V, Maroteaux P, Sobczak E.: Proteoglycan population of baboon *(Papio papio)* articular cartilage. Biochem J 163:103–105, 1977.

90. Swann DA, Powell S, Sotman S: The heterogeneity of cartilage proteoglycans. Isolation of different types of proteoglycans from bovine articular cartilage. J. Biol Chem 254:945–954, 1979.

91. Muir IHM: The chemistry of ground substance of joint cartilage. *In* Sokoloff L (ed.): The Joints of Synovial Fluid, Vol. II. New York, Academic Press, 1980, pp. 27–94.

92. Rosenberg L, Pal S, Beale RJ, Schubert M: A comparison of protein-polysaccharides of bovine nasal cartilage isolated and fractionated by different methods. J Biol Chem 245:4112–4122, 1970.

93. Sajdera SW, Hascall VC: Protein-polysaccharide complex from bovine nasal cartilage: A comparison of low and high shear extraction procedures. J Biol Chem 244:74–87, 1969.

94. Hardingham TE, Muir H: The specific interaction of hyaluronic acid with cartilage proteoglycans. Biochim Biophys Acta 279:401–405, 1972.

95. Hardingham TE, Muir H: Hyaluronic acid in cartilage. Biochem Soc Trans 1:282–284, 1973.

96. Hascall VC, Heinegard D: Aggregation of cartilage proteoglycans. I. The role of hyaluronic acid. J Biol Chem 249:4232–4241, 1974.

97. Hascall VC, Heinegard D: Aggregation of cartilage proteoglycans. II. Oligosaccharide competitors of the proteoglycan-hyaluronic acid interaction. J Biol Chem 249:4242–4249, 1974.

98. Baker JR, Caterson B: The isolation of link protein from bovine nasal cartilage. Biochim Biophys Acta 532:249–258, 1978.

99. Hardingham TE: The role of link protein in· the structure of cartilage proteoglycan aggregate. Biochem J 177:237–247, 1979.

100. Hascall VC, Sajdera SW: Protein-polysaccharide complex from bovine nasal cartilage. The function of glycoprotein in the formation of aggregates. J Biol Chem 244:2384–2396, 1969.

101. Oegema TR, Brown M, Dziewatkowski DD: The link protein proteoglycans from Swarm rat chondrosarcoma. J Biol Chem 252:6470–6477, 1977.

102. Tang LH, Rosenberg L, Reiner A, Poole RA: Proteoglycans from bovine nasal cartilage: Properties of a soluble form of link protein. J Biol Chem 254:10523–10531, 1979.

103. Treadwell BV, Mankin DP, Ho PK, Mankin HJ: Cell-free synthesis of cartilage proteins: Partial identification of proteoglycan core and link proteins. Biochemistry 19:2269–2275, 1980.

104. Treadwell BV, Shader L, Towle CA, Mankin DP, Mankin HJ: Purification of the link proteins from bovine articular cartilage and comparison with link proteins from nasal septum. Biochem Biophys Res Commun 94:159–166, 1980.

105. Poole AR, Pidoux I, Reinier A, Tang LH, Choi H, Rosenberg L: Localization of proteoglycan monomers and link protein in the matrix of bovine articular cartilage: An immunohistochemical study. J Histochem Cytochem 28:621–635, 1980.

106. Wieslander J, Heinegard D: Immunochemical analysis of cartilage proteoglycans. Radioimmunoassay of the molecules and the substructures. Biochem J 187:867–694, 1980.

107. Piez KA, Lewis MS, Martin GR, Gross J: Subunits of the collagen molecule. Biochim Biophys Acta 53:596–598, 1961.

108. Brandt KD, Muir HJ: Heterogeneity of protein-polysaccharides of porcine articular cartilage. The chondroitin sulphate proteins associated with collagen. Biochem J 123:747–755, 1971.

109. Gelman RA, Blackwell J: Interaction between collagen and chondroitin 6-sulfate. Connect Tissue Res 2:31–35, 1973.

110. Laros GS, Cooper RR: Electron microscopic visualization of protein polysaccharides. Clin Orthop 84:179–192, 1972.

111. Mathews MB: The interaction of collagen and acid mucopolysaccharides. A model for connective tissue. Biochem J 96:710–716, 1965.

112. Serafini-Fracassini A, Smith JW: Observations on the morphology of the protein polysaccharide complex of bovine nasal cartilage and its relationship to collagen. Proc R Soc Lond 165:440–449, 1966.

113. Shepard N, Mitchell N: The localization of proteoglycan by light and microscopy using safranin O. J Ultrastruct Res 54:451–460, 1976.

114. Shepard N, Mitchell N: The isolation of articular cartilage proteoglycan by electron microscopy. Anat Rec 187:463–476, 1977.

115. Quintarelli G: Methods for the histochemical identification of acid mucopolysaccharides: A critical evaluation. *In* Quintarelli G (ed.): The Chemical Physiology of Mucopolysaccharides. Boston, Little, Brown and Co., 1968, pp. 199–215.

116. Scott JE: Affinity, competition and specific interactions in the biochemistry and histochemistry of polyelectrolytes. Biochem Soc Trans 1:787–806, 1973.

117. Rosenberg L: Chemical bases for the histological use of safranin-O in the study of articular cartilage. J Bone Joint Surg 53A:69–82, 1971.

118. Bjelle AO: Variations in content and composition of glycosaminoglycans within the articular cartilage of the lower femoral epiphysis of an adult. Scand J Rheumatol 3:81–88, 1973.

119. Bjelle AO, Antonopoulos CA, Engfeldt B, Hjertquist S-O: Fractionation of the glycosaminoglycans of human articular cartilage on ecteolacellulose in aging and in osteoarthrosis. Calcif Tissue Res 8:237–246, 1972.

120. Bjelle AO, Gardell S, Heinegard D: Proteoglycans of articular cartilage from bovine lower femoral epiphysis. Extraction and characterization of proteoglycans from two sites within the same joint. Connect Tissue Res 2:111–116, 1974.

121. Lemperg RK, Larsson SE, Hjertquist S-O: The glycosaminoglycans of bovine articular cartilage. I. Concentration and distribution in different layers in relation to age. Calcif Tissue Res 15:237–251, 1974.

122. Bentley JP, Rokosova B: The metabolic heterogeneity of rabbit ear cartilage chondroitin-sulfate. Biochim J 116:329–336, 1970.

123. Lipshitz H, Etheredge R III, Glimcher MJ: *In vitro* wear of articular cartilage. J Bone Joint Surg 57A:527–534, 1975.

124. Lipshitz H, Etheredge R, Glimcher MJ: Changes in hexosamine content and swelling ratio of articular cartilage as a function of depth from the surface. J Bone Joint Surg 58A:1149–1153, 1976.

125. Maroudas A, Evans H, Almeida L: Cartilage of the hip joint: Topographical variation of glycosaminoglycan content in normal and fibrillated tissue. Ann Rheum Dis 32:1–9, 1973.

126. Stockwell RA: Biology of Cartilage Cells. Cambridge, Cambridge University Press, 1979.

127. Stockwell RA, Scott JE: Distribution of acid glycosaminoglycans in human articular cartilage. Nature 215:1376–1378, 1967.

128. Maroudas A, Muir H, Wingham J: The correlation of fixed negative charge with glycosaminoglycan content of human articular cartilage. Biochim Biophys Acta 177:492–500, 1969.

129. Barland P, Janis R, Sandson J: Immunofluorescent studies of human articular cartilage. Ann Rheum Dis 25:156–163, 1966.

130. Hamerman D, Sandson J: Antigenicity of connective tissue components. Mt Sinai J Med 37:453–465, 1970.

131. Stockwell RA: Structural and histochemical aspects of the pericellular environment in cartilage. Philos Trans R Soc Lond B271:243–245, 1975.

132. Anderson CD, Ludoweig J, Haper HA, Engleman EP: The composition of organic component of human articular cartilage. J Bone Joint Surg 46A:1176–1183, 1964.

133. Lane JM, Weiss C: Current comment: Review of articular cartilage collagen research. Arthritis Rheum 18:553–562, 1975.

134. Fietzik PT, Kahn K: The primary structure of collagen. Int Rev Connect Tissue Res 7:1–60, 1976.

135. Miller EJ: The collagen of joints. *In* Sokoloff L (ed.): The Joint and Synovial Fluid, Vol. I. New York, Academic Press, 1978, pp. 205–224.

136. Elden HR: Physical properties of collagen fibers. *In* Int Rev Connect Tissue Res 4:283–288, 1968.

137. Harrington WF, von Hippel PH: The structure of collagen and gelatin. Adv Protein Chem 16:1–138, 1961.

138. Hodge AJ: Structure at the electon microscopic level. *In* Ramachandran BM (ed.): Treatise on Collagen, Vol. I: Chemistry of collagen. New York, Academic Press, 1967, pp. 185–205.

139. Horwitz AL, Dorfman A: Subcellular sites for synthesis of chondromucoprotein of cartilage. J Cell Biol 38:358–368, 1968.

140. Piez K, Eigner EA, Lewis MS: The chromatographic separation and amino acid composition of the subunits of several collagens. Biochemistry 2:58–66, 1963.

141. Miller EJ: A review of biochemical studies in the genetically distinct collagens of the skeletal system. Clin Orthop 92:260–280, 1973.

142. Miller EJ, Martin GR: The collagen of bone. Clin Orthop 59:195–232, 1953.

143. Piez K: Cross-linking of collagen and elastin. Ann Rev Biochem 37:547–570, 1968.

144. Ramachandran GN: Structure of collagen at the molecular level. *In* Ramachandran GN (ed.): Treatise on Collagen, Vol. I. New York, Academic Press, 1967, pp. 103–183.

145. Butler WT, Cunningham LW: Evidence for the linkage of a disaccharide to hydroxylysine in tropocollagen. J Biol Chem 24:3882–3888, 1966.

146. Igarashi J, Trelstad RL, Kang AH: Physical chemical properties of chick cartilage collagen. Biochim Biophys Acta 295:514–519, 1973.

147. Bailey AJ, Fowler LJ, Peach CM: Identification of two interchain crosslinks of bone and dentine collagen. Biochem Biophys Res Commun 34:663–671, 1969.

148. Bailey AJ, Peack CM: Isolation and structural identification of a labile intermolecular crosslink in collagen. Biochem Biophys Res Commun 33:812–819, 1968.

149. Fowler LJ, Bailey AJ: Current concepts of the cross-linking in bone collagen. Clin Orthop 86:193–206, 1972.

150. Siegel RC, Pinnell SR, Martin GR: Cross-linking of collagen and elastin. Properties of lysyl oxidase. Biochemistry 9:4480–4492, 1970.

151. Sokoloff L: Natural history of degenerative joint disease in small laboratory animals. I. Pathologic anatomy of degenerative joint disease in mice. Arch Pathol 62:118–128, 1956.

152. Weiss C: Ultrastructural characteristics of osteoarthritis. Fed Proc 32:1459–1466, 1973.

153. Seyer JM, Brickley DM, Glimcher MJ: The identification of two types of collagen in the articular cartilage of postnatal chickens. Calcif Tissue Res 17:43–55, 1974.

154. Spiro RG: Characterization and quantitative determination of hydroxylysine-linked carbohydrate units in several collagens. J Biol Chem 244:602–612, 1969.

155. Miller EJ, Matukas VJ: Chick cartilage collagen: A new type of 1 chain not present in bone or skin or the species. Proc Natl Acad Sci USA 64:1264–1268, 1969.

156. Miller EJ: Isolation and characterization of a collagen from chick cartilage containing three identical chains. Biochemistry 10:1652–1658, 1971.

157. Strawick E, Nimni ME: Properties of a collagen molecule containing three identical components extracted from bovine articular cartilage. Biochemistry 10:3905–3911, 1971.

158. Trelstad RL, Kang AH, Igaraski S, et al.: Isolation of two distinct collagens from chick cartilage. Biochemistry 9:4993–4998, 1970.

159. Blumenkrantz N, Prockop DJ: Variations in the glycosylation of the collagen synthesized by chick embryo cartilage. Effects of development and several hormones. Biochim Biophys Acta 208:461–466, 1970.

160. Deshmukh K, Nimni ME: Isolation and characterization of cyanogen bromide peptides from the collagen of bovine articular cartilage. Biochem J 133:615–622, 1973.

161. Eyre DR, Muir H: Characterization of the major CNBr-derived peptides of porcine type II collagen. Connect Tissue Res 3:105–170, 1975.

162. Fugimoto D, Motiguchi T: Pyridinoline, a non-reducible cross-link of collagen. J Biochem 83:863–867, 1978.

163. Miller EJ: Collagen cross-linking: Identification of two cyanogen bromide peptides containing sites of

intermolecular cross-link formation in cartilage collagen. Biochem Biophys Res Commun 45:444–451, 1971.

164. Miller EJ: Isolation and characterization of the cyanogen bromide peptides from the α1(II) chain of chick cartilage collagen. Biochemistry 10:3030–3035, 1971.

165. Miller EJ, Lunde LG: Isolation and characterization of the cyanogen bromide peptides from the alpha 1(II) chain of bovine and human articular cartilage collagen. Biochemistry 12:3153–3159, 1973.

166. Robertson PB, Miller EJ: Cartilage collagen: Inability to serve as a substrate for collagenase active against skin and bone collagen. Biochim Biophys Acta 289:247–250, 1972.

167. Trelstad RL, Kang AH, Toole BP: High resolution and separation of native [alpha₁(I)]₂ alpha₂ and [alpha₁(II)]₃ and their component alpha chains. J Biol Chem 247:6469–6473, 1972.

168. Bruns R, Trelstad RL, Gross J: Cartilage collagen: A staggered substructure in reconstituted fibrils. Science 181:269–172, 1973.

169. Burgeson RE, Hollister DW: Collagen heterogeneity in human cartilage: Identification of several new collagen chains. Biochem Biophys Res Commun 87:1124–1131, 1979.

170. Shimokomaka M, Duance VS, Bailey AJ: Identification of a new disulphide bonded collagen from cartilage. FEBS Lett 121:51–54, 1980.

171. Stanescu V, Stanescu R, Maroteaux P: Répartition différente du collagene de type I et du collagene de type II dans la zone superficielle et dans la zone intermédiare du cartilage articulaire. CR Hebd Seances Acad Sci Ser D 283:279–282, 1976.

172. Gay S, Gay R, Miller EJ: The collagen of the joint. Arthritis Rheum 23:937–941, 1980.

173. Rhodes RK, Miller EJ: Physicochemical characterization and molecular organization of the collagen A and B chains. Biochemistry 17:3447–3448, 1978.

174. Mayne R, Vail MS, Mayne PM, Miller EJ: Changes in type of collagen synthesized as clones of chick chondrocyte grow and eventually lose division capacity. Proc Natl Acad Sci USA 73:1674–1678, 1976.

175. Norby DP, Malemud CJ, Sokoloff L: Differences in the collagen types synthesized by lapine articular chondrocytes in spinner and monolayer culture. Arthritis Rheum 20:709–716, 1977.

176. Nimni M, Deshmukh K: Differences in collagen metabolism between normal and osteoarthritic human articular cartilage. Science 181:751–752, 1973.

177. Gay S, Gay R, Brandt K, Palmoski M: Aspirin causes chondrocytes in atrophic articular cartilage to synthesize type I collagen in vivo. Arthritis Rheum 25:540, 1982.

178. Hewitt AT, Kleinman HK, Pennypacker JP, Martin GR: Identification of an adhesion factor for chondrocytes. Proc Natl Acad Sci USA 77:385–388, 1980.

179. Kleinman HK, Hewitt AT, Murray JS, Liotta LA, Rennard SE, Pennypacker JP, McGoodwin EM, Martin GR, Fishman PH: Cellular and metabolic specificity in the interaction of adhesion proteins with collagen and with cells. J Supramol Struct 11:69–78, 1979.

180. Rabinowitz SL, Gregg JR, Nixon JE, Schumacher HR: Lipid composition of tissue of human knee joints. Clin Orthop 143:260–265, 1973.

181. Collins DH, McElligott TF: Sulfate (³⁵SO₄) uptake by chondrocytes in relation to histological changes in osteoarthritic human articular cartilage. Ann Rheum Dis 19:330, 1960.

182. Ghadially FN, Meachim G, Collins DH: Extracellular lipids in the matrix of human articular cartilage. Ann Rheum Dis 27:136–146, 1965.

183. Ali SY: Mineral containing matrix vesicles in human osteoarthritic cartilage. In Nuki G (ed.): Aetiopathogenesis of Osteoarthritis. Tunbridge Wells, Pitman Medical Publishing Co., 1980, pp. 105–116.

184. Stockwell RA: Lipid content of human costal and articular cartilage. Ann Rheum Dis 26:481–486, 1967.

185. Stockwell RA: The lipid and glycogen content of rabbit articular and non-articular hyaline cartilage. J Anat 102:87–94, 1967.

186. Bonner WM, Jonsson H, Malanos C, Bryant M: Changes in the lipids of human articular cartilage with age. Arthritis Rheum 18:461–473, 1975.

187. Ali SY: Matrix vesicles and apatitic modules in arthritic cartilage. In Willoughby DA, Girard JP, Velo GP (eds.): Perspectives on Inflammation. Lancaster, MTP Press, 1977, pp. 211–223.

188. Guenther HL, Sorgente N, Guenther HE, Eisenstein R, Kuettner K: Lysozyme in preosseous cartilage. VI. Purification, characterization and localization of mammalian cartilage lysozyme. Biochim Biophys Acta 372:321–334, 1974.

189. Kuettner KE, Soble LW, Guenther HL, Croxen RL, Eisenstein R: Lysozyme in epiphyseal cartilage. I. The nature of the morphologic response of cartilage in culture to exogenous lysozyme. Calcif Tissue Res 5:56–63, 1970.

190. Kuettner KE, Sorgente N, Croxen RL, Howell DS, Pita JC: Lysozyme in preosseous cartilage. VII. Evidence for physiological role of lysozyme in normal and endochondral calcification. Biochim Biophys Acta 372:335–344, 1974.

191. Kuettner KE, Eisenstein R, Sorgente N: Lysozyme in calcifying tissues. Clin Orthop 112:316–339, 1975.

192. Sorgente N, Hascall VC, Kuettner KE: Extractability of lysozyme from bovine nasal cartilage. Biochim Biophys Acta 284:441–450, 1972.

193. Muir H, Bullough P, Maroudas A: The distribution of collagen in human articular cartilage with some of its physiological implications. J. Bone Joint Surg 52B:554–563, 1970.

194. Lutwak-Mann C: Enzymes in articular cartilage. Biochem J 34:517–527, 1940.

195. Bywaters ECL: The metabolism of joint tissues. J Pathol Bacteriol 44:247–268, 1937.

196. Dickens F, Weil-Malherbe H: Metabolism of cartilage. Nature 138:126, 1936.

197. Lane JM, Brighton CT, Minkowitz BT: Anaerobic and aerobic metabolism in articular cartilage. J Rheumatol 4:334–342, 1977.

198. Rosenthal O, Bowie MA, Wagoner G: Studies on the metabolism of articular cartilage. I. Respiration and glycolysis in relation to age. J Cell Comp Physiol 17:221–233, 1941.

199. Mankin HJ, Orlic PA: A method estimating the "health" of rabbit articular cartilage by assays of ribonucleic acid and protein synthesis. Lab Invest 13:465–475, 1964.

200. Tushan FS, Rodnan GP, Altman M, Robin ED:

Anaerobic glycolysis and lactate dehydrogenase LDH isoenzymes in articular cartilage. J Lab Clin Med 73:549–656, 1969.

201. Vessel ES: Lactate dehydrogenase isozyme patterns of human platelets and bovine lens fibers. Science 150:1735–1736, 1965.

202. Vessel ES, Poole PE: Lactate and pyruvate concentrations in exercised ischemic canine muscle: Relationship of tissue substrate level to lactate dehydrogenase isozyme pattern. Proc Natl Acad Sci USA 55:756–762, 1966.

203. Marcus RE: The effect of low oxygen concentration on growth glycolysis and sulphate incorporation by articular chondrocytes in monoculture. Arthritis Rheum 16:646–656, 1973.

204. Böström H: On the metabolism of the sulfate group of chondroitin sulphuric acid. J Biol Chem 196:477–481, 1952.

205. Dziewiatkowski DD: Effect of age on some aspects of sulfate metabolism in the rat. J Exp Med 99:283–298, 1954.

206. Dziewiatkowski DD: Some aspects of the metabolism of chondroitin sulfate-S^{35} in the rat. J Biol Chem 223:239–249, 1956.

207. Campo RD, Dziewiatkowski DD: Intracellular synthesis of protein polysaccharides by slices of bovine costal cartilage. J Clin Invest 55:1373–1381, 1975.

208. Coelho RR, Chrisman OD: Sulphate metabolism in cartilage. II. S35-sulphate uptake and total sulphate in cartilage slices. J Bone Joint Surg 42A:165–172, 1960.

209. Collins DH, Meachim G: Sulphate (^{35}SO$_4$) fixation by human articular cartilage compared in the knee and shoulder joint. Ann Rheum Dis 20:117–122, 1961.

210. Schwartz ER, Kirkpatrick PR, Thompson RC: Sulfate metabolism in human chondrocyte cultures. J Clin Invest 54:1056–1063, 1974.

211. Shulman JH, Meyer K: Protein polysaccharide of chicken cartilage and chondrocyte cell cultures. Biochem J 120:689–697, 1970.

212. Mankin HJ: The metabolism of articular cartilage in health and disease. *In* Burleigh PMC, Poole AR (eds.): Dynamics of Connective Tissue Macromolecules. New York, American Elsevier Publishing Co., 1975, pp. 327–353.

213. Weiss C, Mankin HJ, Zarins A: Autoradiographic studies of matrix synthesis in articular cartilage. Surg Forum 24:485–487, 1973.

214. Kincaid SA, VanSickle C, Wilsman NJ: Histochemical evidence of a functional heterogeneity of the chondrocytes of adult canine articular cartilage. Histochem J 4:237–243, 1972.

215. Trippel SB, Ehrlich MG, Lippiello L, Mankin HJ: Characterization of chondrocytes from bovine articular cartilage. I. Metabolic and morphological studies. J Bone Joint Surg 62A:816–819, 1980.

216. Mankin HJ: The reaction of articular cartilage to injury and osteoarthritis. N Engl J Med 291:1285–1291, 1335–1340, 1974.

217. Mankin HJ, Boyle CJ: The acute effects of lacerative injury on DNA and protein synthesis in articular cartilage. *In* Bassett CAL (ed.): Cartilage Degradation and Repair. Washington, D.C., NAS-NRC, 1967, pp. 185–199.

218. Numata T, Deutsch S: Effect of hydrostatic pressure on the metabolism of chondrocytes. Unpublished material.

219. Bergenholtz A, Lemperg RK: Calf articular cartilage in organ culture in a chemically defined medium. I. Autoradiographic study after [^{35}S]-sulfate labeling. In Vitro 11:286–230, 1975.

220. Brighton CT, Lane JM, Koh JK: *In vitro* rabbit articular cartilage organ model. II. ^{35}S incorporation at various oxygen tensions. Arthritis Rheum 17:245–252, 1974.

221. Lemperg RK, Bergenholtz A, Smith TWD: Calf articular cartilage in organ culture in a chemically defined medium. II. Concentrations of glycosaminoglycans and [^{35}S]-sulfate incorporation at different oxygen tensions. In Vitro 11:291–301, 1975.

222. Schwartz ER, Kirkpatrick RR, Thompson TC: The effect of environmental pH on glycosaminoglycan metabolism by normal human chondrocytes. J Lab Clin Med 87:198–205, 1976.

223. Palmoski J, Brandt KD: Effect of calcipenia on proteoglycan metabolism and aggregation in normal articular cartilage *in vitro*. Biochem J 182:399–406, 1979.

224. Choi YC, Morris GM, Lev FS, Sokoloff L: The effect of serum on monolayer culture of mammalian articular chondrocyte. Connect Tissue Res 7:105–112, 1980.

225. Sandy JD, Brown HL, Lowther DA: Control of proteoglycan synthesis. Studies on the activation of synthesis observed during culture of articular cartilage. Biochem J 188:119–130, 1980.

226. Mankin HJ, Thrasher AZ, Weinberg EH, Harris WH: Dissociation between the effect of bovine growth hormone in articular cartilage and in bone of the adult dog. J Bone Joint Surg 60A:1071–1075, 1978.

227. Phillips LS, Herington AC, Daughaday WH: Somatomedin stimulation of sulfate incorporation in porcine costal cartilage discs. Endocrinology 94:856–863, 1974.

228. Smith TWD, Duckworth T, Bergenholtz A, Lemperg RK: Role of growth hormone in glycosaminoglycan synthesis by articular cartilage. Nature 253:269–271, 1975.

229. Malemud CJ, Norby DP, Sokoloff L: Explant culture of human and rabbit articular chondrocytes. Connect Tissue Res 6:171–179, 1978.

230. Schwartz ER, Adamy L: Effect of ascorbic acid on arylsulfate activities and sulfated proteoglycan metabolism in chondrocyte cultures. J Clin Invest 60:96–106, 1977.

231. Brighton CT, Shadle CA, Jiminez SA, Irwin JT, Lane JM, Lipton M: Articular cartilage preservation and storage. I. Application of tissue culture techniques in the storage of viable articular cartilage. Arthritis Rheum 22:1093–1101, 1979.

232. Mankin HJ, Conger KA: The acute effects of intra-articular hydrocortisone on articular cartilage in rabbits. J Bone Joint Surg 48A:1383–1388, 1966.

233. Mankin HJ, Conger KA: The effect of cortisol on articular cartilage of rabbits. I. Effect of a single dose of cortisol on glycine-C14 incorporation. Lab Invest 15:794–800, 1966.

234. Mankin HJ, Zarins A, Jaffe WL: The effect of systemic corticosteroids on rabbit articular cartilage. Arthritis Rheum 15:593–599, 1972.

235. Kent L, Malemud CJ, Moskwitz RW: Differential response of articular chondrocyte population to thromboxane B$_2$ and analogs of prostaglandin cyclic endoperoxidases. Prostaglandins 19:391–406, 1980.

236. Lippiello L, Yamamoto K, Robinson D, Mankin HJ:

Involvement of prostaglandins from rheumatoid synovium in inhibtion of articular cartilage metabolism. Arthritis Rheum 21:908–917, 1978.

237. Malemud DJ, Sokoloff L: The effect of prostaglandins on cultured lapine articular chondrocytes. Prostaglandins 13:845–860, 1977.

238. Palmoski MJ, Brandt KD: Effects of disphosphonates on glycosaminoglycan synthesis and proteoglycan aggregation in normal adult articular cartilage. Arthritis Rheum 21:942–949, 1978.

239. Murata K, Bjelle AO: Constitutional variations of acidic glycosaminoglycans in normal and arthritic bovine articular cartilage proteoglycans at different ages. Connect Tissue Res 7:143–156, 1980.

240. Palmoski MJ, Brandt KD: Effects of some nonsteroidal anti-inflammatory drugs on proteoglycan metabolism and organization in canine articular cartilage. Arthritis Rheum 23:1010–1020, 1980.

241. Palmoski MJ, Brandt KD: Benoxaprofen stimulates proteoglycan synthesis in normal articular cartilage. Arthritis Rheum 25:S29, 1982.

242. Silbert JE: Incorporation of ^{14}D and ^{3}H from nucleotide sugars into a polysaccharide in the presence of a cell-free preparation from cartilage. J Biol Chem 239:1310–1315, 1964.

243. Wiebkin OW, Muir H: Synthesis of proteoglycans by suspensions and monolayer cultures of adult chondrocytes and *de novo* cartilage nodules: The effect of hyaluronic acid. J Cell Sci 27:199–211, 1977.

244. Ehrlich MG, Mankin HJ, Treadwell BV, Jones H: Uridine diphosphate (UDP) stimulation of protein-polysaccharide production: A preliminary report. J Bone Joint Surg 56A:1239–1245, 1974.

245. Schwartz NB, Galligani L, Ho PL, Dorfman A: Stimulation of synthesis of free chondroitin sulfate chains α-D-xylosides in cultured cells. Proc Natl Acad Sci USA 71:4047–4051, 1974.

246. Jubb RW, Fell HB: The effect of synovial tissue on the synthesis of proteoglycan by the articular cartilage of young pigs. Arthritis Rheum 23:545–555, 1980.

247. Caputto R, Barra HS, Cumar FA: Carbohydrate metabolism. Ann Rev Biochem 36:211–246, 1967.

248. Leloir LF, Cabib E: The enzymic synthesis of trehalose phosphate. J Am Chem Soc 75:5445–5446, 1953.

249. Baker JR, Roden L, Stoolmiller AC: Biosynthesis of chondroitin sulfate proteoglycan. Xylosyl transfer to Smith-degraded cartilage proteoglycan and other exogenous acceptors. J Biol Chem 247:3838–3847, 1972.

250. Pawloski PJ, Gillette MT, Martinelli J, Lukens LN, Furthmayer H: Identification and purification of collagen-synthesizing polysomes with anti-collagen antibodies. J Biol Chem 250:2135–2142, 1975.

251. Rosen L, Schwartz NB: Biosynthesis of connective tissue proteoglycans. *In* Whelan WJ (ed.): MTP International Review of Science, Biochemistry, Series One, Vol. 5: Biochemistry of Carbohydrates. Baltimore, University Park Press, 1975, pp. 95–152.

252. Leloir LF, Cardini CE: Biosynthesis of glycogen from uridine diphosphate glucose. J Am Chem Soc 79:6340–6341, 1957.

253. Godman GC, Lane N: On the site of sulfation in the chondrocyte. J Cell Biol 21:353–366, 1964.

254. Young RW: The role of the Golgi complex in sulfate metabolism. J Cell Biol 57:175–189, 1973.

255. D'Ambramo R, Lipmann F: The formation of adenosine-3-phosphate-5-phosphosulfate in extracts of chick embryo cartilage and its conversion into chondroitin sufate. Biochim Biophys Acta 25:211–213, 1957.

256. Pasternak CA: The synthesis of 3'-phosphoadenosine 5'-phosphosulfate by mouse tissues: Sulfate activation *in vitro* and *in vivo*. J Biol Chem 235:438–442, 1960.

257. Robinson HC: The sulphation of chondroitin sulphate in embryonic chicken cartilage. Biochem J 113:543–549, 1969.

258. Suzuki S, Strominger JL: Enzymatic sulfation of mucopolysaccharides in hen oviduct. I. Transfer of sulfate from 3'-phosphoadenosine-5'-phosphosulphate to mucopolysaccharide. J Biol Chem 235:257–266, 1960.

259. Suzuki S, Trenn RH, Strominger JL: Separation of specific mucopolysaccharide sulfo-transferases. Biochim Biophys Acta 50:169–170, 1961.

260. Eichelberger L, Roma M, Moulder PV: Biochemical studies of articular cartilage. III. Values following the immobilization of an extremity. J Bone Joint Surg 41A:1127–1142, 1959.

261. Schiller S, Mathews MB, Cifonelli JA, Dorfman A: The metabolism of mucopolysaccharides in animals. III. Further studies on skin utilizing C^{14} glucose, C^{14} acetate and S^{35} sodium sulfate. J Biol Chem 218:139–145, 1956.

262. Gross J, Mathews MB, Dorfman A: Sodium chondroitin sulphate–protein complexes of cartilage. II. Metabolism. J Biol Chem 235:2889–2892, 1960.

263. Davidson FA, Small W: Metabolism *in vivo* of connective tissue mucopolysaccharides. III. Chondroitin sulfate and keratosulfate of cartilage. Biochim Biophys Acta 69:459–463, 1963.

264. Mankin HJ, Lippiello L: The turnover of adult rabbit articular cartilage. J Bone Joint Surg 63A:131–134, 1981.

265. Rokosova B, Bentley JP: The uptake of (^{14}C)glucose into rabbit ear cartilage proteoglycans isolated by differential extraction and by collagenase digestion. Biochim Biophys Acta 297:493–495, 1973.

266. Hardingham TE, Muir H: Biosynthesis of proteoglycans in cartilage slices. Biochem J 126:791–803, 1972.

267. Lohmander S, Antonopoulos CA, Friberg U: Chemical and metabolic heterogeneity of chondroitin sulfate and keratan sulfate in guinea pig cartilage and nucleus pulposus. Biochim Biophys Acta 304:430–448, 1973.

268. Maroudas A: Glycosaminoglycan turnover in articular cartilage. Philos Trans R Soc Lond B271:292–323, 1975.

269. Mankin HJ, Hall D, Lippiello L: The turnover of rabbit articular cartilage. II. ^{3}H-glucosamine studies. In press.

270. Repo RU, Mitchell N: Collagen synthesis in mature articular cartilage of the rabbit. J Bone Joint Surg 53B:541–548, 1971.

271. Butler WT, Finch JE Jr, Miller EJ: The covalent structure of cartilage collagen: Evidence for sequence heterogeneity of bovine α1(II) chains. J Biol Chem 252:639–643, 1977.

272. Manner G, Kretsinger RH, Gould BS, Rich A: The polyribosomal synthesis of collagen. Biochim Biophys Acta 134:411–429, 1967.

273. Bellamy G, Bornstein P: Evidence for procollagen, a biosynthetic precursor of collagen. Proc Natl Acad Sci USA 68:1138–1141, 1971.

274. Dehm P, Prockop DJ: Biosynthesis of cartilage procollagen. Eur J Biochem 35:159–166, 1973.

275. Fessler LI, Morris NP, Fessler HJ: Procollagen.

Biological scission of amino carboxyl extension peptides. Proc Natl Acad Sci USA 72:4905–4909, 1975.

276. Grant ME, Prockop DJ: The biosynthesis of collagen. N Engl J Med 268:194–199, 242–249, 291–300, 1972.

277. Grant ME, Schofield JD, Kefalides S, Prockop DJ: The biosynthesis of basement membrane collagen in embryonic chick lens. II. Intracellular formation of the triple helix and the formation of aggregates through disulfide bonds. J Biol Chem 28:7432–7437, 1973.

278. Prockop DJ: The intracellular biosynthesis of collagen: Some possible implications for diseases of bone and other connective tissues. Arch Intern Med 124:563–570, 1969.

279. Church RL, Pfeifer SE, Tanzer ML: Collagen biosynthesis and secretion of a high molecular weight collagen precursor (procollagen). Proc Natl Acad Sci USA 68:2638–2642, 1971.

280. Bekhor I, Bavetta LA: Evidence for a low-molecular-weight collagen precursor. Proc Natl Acad Sci USA 58:2351–2358, 1967.

281. Bhatnagar RS, Prockop DJ, Rosenblum J: Intracellular pool of unhydroxylated polypeptide precursors of collagen. Science 158:491–494, 1967.

282. Pontz BF, Muller PK, Miegel WN: A study of the conversion of procollagen: Release and recovery of procollagen peptides in the culture medium. J Biol Chem 248:7558–7564, 1973.

283. Kivirikko KI, Bright HJ, Prockop DJ: Kinetic patterns of protocollagen hydroxylase and further studies on the polypeptide substrate. Biochim Biophys Acta 151:538–567, 1968.

284. Kivirikko KI, Prockop DJ: Purification and partial characterization of the enzyme for the hydroxylation of proline in protocollagen. Arch Biochem Biophys 118:611–618, 1967.

285. Hutton JJ, Tappel AL, Undenfriend S: Cofactor and substrate requirements of collagen proline hydroxylase. Arch Biochem Biophys 118:231–240, 1967.

286. Prockop DJ: Role of iron in the synthesis of collagen in connective tissue. Fed Proc 30:984–990, 1971.

287. Kivirikko KI, Risteli: Biosynthesis of collagen and its alteration in pathological states. Med Biol 54:159–186, 1976.

288. Fell HB, Thomas L: Comparison of the effects of papain and vitamin A on cartilage. II. The effects on organ cultures of embryonic skeletal tissue. J Exp Med 111:719–744, 1960.

289. Lund F, Telhag H: Content and synthesis of nucleic acids in the cartilage in chondromalacia patellae. Acta Orthop Scand 49:535–541, 1978.

290. Fell HB, Dingle JT: Studies on the mode of action of excess of vitamin A. 6. Lysosomal protease and the degradation of cartilage matrix. Biochem J 87:403–408, 1963.

291. Lucy JA, Dingle JT, Fell HB: Studies on the mode of action on excess of vitamin A. 2. A possible role of intracellular proteases in the degradation of cartilage matrix. Biochem J 79:500–508, 1961.

292. DeDuve C: A new group of cytoplasmic particles. In Hyashi T (ed.): Subcellular Particles. New York, Ronald Press Co. 1959, pp. 128–169.

293. DeDuve C, Wattiaux R: Functions of lysosomes. Ann Rev Physiol 28:435–492, 1966.

294. Roy S, Meachim G: Chondrocyte ultrastructure in adult human articular cartilage. Ann Rheum Dis 27:544–558, 1968.

295. Ehrlich MG, Mankin JH, Treadwell BV: Acid hydrolase activity in osteoarthritic and normal human cartilage. J Bone Joint Surg 55A:1068–1076, 1973.

296. Thompson RC, Clarke I: Acid hydrolases in slices of articular cartilage and synovium from normal and abnormal joints. Proc Soc Exp Biol Med 133:1102–1108, 1970.

297. Barrett AJ: The enzymatic degradation of cartilage matrix. In Burleigh RMC, Poole AR (eds.): Dynamics of Connective Tissue Macromolecules. New York, American Elsevier Publishing Co., 1975, pp. 189–215.

298. Bollet AJ, Bonner WM, Nance JL: The presence of hyaluronidase in various mammalian tissues. J Biol Chem 238:3522–3527, 1963.

299. Stack MT, Brandt KD: Identification and characterization of articular cartilage hyaluronidase. Arthritis Rheum 25:S100, 1982.

300. Roughley PJ: Degradation of cartilage by proteinases. Proteoglycan heterogeneity and the pathway of proteolytic degradation. Biochem J 167:639–646, 1977.

301. Roughley PJ, Barrett AJ: The degradation of cartilage proteoglycans by tissue proteinases. Proteoglycan structure and its susceptibility to proteolysis. Biochem J 167:629–637, 1977.

302. Sandy JD, Brown HL, Lowther DA: Degradation of proteoglycan in articular cartilage. Biochim Biophys Acta 543:535–544, 1978.

303. Fessel JM, Chrisman OD: Enzymatic degradation of chondromucoprotein by cell-free extracts of human cartilage. Arthritis Rheum 7:398–405, 1964.

304. Tourtelotte DC, Campo RD, Dziewiatkowski DD: Degradation of chondromucoprotein by an enzyme extracted from cartilage. Fed Proc 223:413, 1963.

305. Ali SY: The degradation of cartilage matrix by an intercellular protease. Biochem J 93:611–618, 1964.

306. Ali SY, Evans L, Stainthorpe E, Lack DH: Characterization of cathepsins in cartilage. Biochem J 105:549–557, 1967.

307. Bayliss MT, Ali SY: Studies on cathepsin B in human articular cartilage. Biochem J 171:149–154, 1978.

308. Woessner JF Jr: Acid cathepsins of cartilage. In Basset CAL (ed.): Cartilage Degradation and Repair. Washington, D. C., NAS-NRC, 1967, pp. 96–106.

309. Woessner JF Jr: Cartilage cathepsin D and its action on matrix components. Fed Proc 32:1485–1488, 1973.

310. Mitchell N, Shepard N: The resurfacing of adult rabbit articular cartilage by multiple perforations through the subchondral bone. J Bone Joint Surg 58A:230–233, 1976.

311. Poole AR: Immunocytochemical studies on the secretion of a proteolytic enzyme, cathepsin D_1 in relation to cartilage breakdown. In Burleigh PMC, Poole AR (eds.): Dynamics of Connective Tissue Macromolecules. New York, American Elsevier Publishing Co., 1975, pp. 357–359.

312. Sapolsky AI, Altman RD, Woessner JF Jr, Howell DS: The action of cathepsin D in human articular cartilage on proteoglycans. J Clin Invest 52:624–633, 1973.

313. Ali SY, Evans L: Enzymatic degradation of cartilage in osteoarthritis. Fed Proc 32:1494–1498, 1973.

314. Sapolsky AI, Howell DS, Woessner JF Jr: Neutral proteinases and cathepsin D in human articular cartilage. J Clin Invest 53:1044–1053, 1974.

315. Ehrlich MG, Armstrong AL, Newman RG, et al.: Patterns of proteoglycan degradation by a neutral

protease from human growth plate epiphyseal cartilage. J Bone Joint Surg 64A:1350–1354, 1982.

316. Ehrlich MG, Armstrong A, Mankin HJ: Isolation and partial purification and characterization of growth plate neutral proteoglycanase. Trans Orthop Res Soc 6:109, 1981.

317. Ehrlich MG, Mankin HJ, Davis NM: Human epiphyseal plate proteoglycanases and degradation patterns. Trans Orthop Res Soc 4:139, 1979.

318. Malemud CJ, Janoff A: Identification of neutral protease in human neutrophil granules that degrade articular cartilage proteoglycan. Arthritis Rheum 18:361–368, 1975.

319. Malemud CJ, Weitzman GA, Norby DP, Sapolsky AI, Howell DS: Metal-dependent neutral proteoglycanase activity from monolayer-cultured lapine articular chondrocytes. J Lab Clin Med 93:1018–1030, 1979.

320. Eisen AZ, Jeffery JJ, Gross J: Human skin collagenase: Isolation and mechanism of attack on the collagen molecule. Biochim Biophys Acta 151:637–645, 1968.

321. Harris ED Jr: Role of collagenase in joint destruction. *In* Sokoloff L (ed.): The Joints and Synovial Fluid, Vol. I. New York, Academic Press, 1978, pp. 243–272.

322. Harris ED Jr, Krane SM: Collagenases. N Engl J Med 291:557–563, 605–609, 652–661, 1974.

323. Lazarus GS, Daniels JR, Brown RS, Bladen HA, Fullmer HM: Degradation of collagen by a human granulocyte collagenolytic system. J Clin Invest 47:2622–2629, 1968.

324. Woessner JF Jr: Mammalian collagenases. Clin Orthop 96:310–326, 1973.

325. Ehrlich MG, Mankin HJ, Jones H, Wright R, Crispen C, Vigliani G: Collagenase and collagenase inhibitors in osteoarthritic and normal human cartilage. J Clin Invest 59:226–233, 1977.

326. Pelletier JP, Martel-Pelletier J, Altman RD, et al.: Collagenolytic activity and collagen matrix breakdown of the articular cartilage in the Pond-Nuki model of osteoarthritis. Arthritis Rheum 26:866–874, 1983.

327. Meachim G: Effect of age on the thickness of adult articular cartilage at the shoulder joint. Ann Rheum Dis 30:43–46, 1971.

328. Mankin HJ: The effect of aging on articular cartilage. Bull Acad Med 44:545–552, 1968.

329. Mankin HJ: The calcified bone (basal layers) of articular cartilage of rabbits. Anat Rec 145:73–78, 1963.

330. Ogston A: On the growth and maintenance of the articular ends of adult bones. J Anat Physiol 12:503–517, 1878.

331. Ham AW: Histology. 5th ed. Tunbridge Wells, Pitman Medical Publishing Co., 1965, p. 377.

332. Elliott HC: Studies on articular cartilage. I. Growth mechanisms. Am J Anat 58:27–145, 1936.

333. Mankin HJ: Localization of tritiated thymidine in articular cartilage of rabbits. I. Growth in immature cartilage. J Bone Joint Surg 44A:682–688, 1962.

334. Mankin HJ: Localization of tritiated thymidine in articular cartilage of rabbits. II. Repair in immature cartilage. J Bone Joint Surg 44A:668–692, 1962.

335. Dustmann HO, Puhl W, Krempien B: Das phanomen der cluster in arthrosseknorpel. Arch Orthop Unfall Chir 79:321–333, 1974.

336. Mankin HJ: Localization of tritiated thymidine in articular cartilage in rabbits. III. Mature articular cartilage. J Bone Joint Surg 45A:529–540, 1963.

337. Telhag H: DNA synthesis in degenerated and normal joint cartilage in full-grown rabbits. Acta Orthop Scand 44:604–610, 1973.

338. Telhag H, Hardrup T: Nucleic acids in articular cartilage from rabbits of different ages. Acta Orthop Scand 46:185, 1975.

339. Clarke IC: Human articular surface contours and related surface depression frequency studies. Ann Rheum Dis 30:15–23, 1971.

340. Imerlishivili IA: Experimental study of joint cartilage regeneration. Akh Anast Moskva 34:58–71, 1957.

341. Ruttner JR, Spycher AM, Werner G, Amado R: Biochemische und morphologische befunde am knorpel des femurkopfes. Verh Dtsch Ges Pathol 58:392–394, 1974.

342. Simunek Z, Muir H: Changes in the protein-polysaccharides of pig articular cartilage during prenatal life, development and old age. Biochem J 126:515–523, 1972.

343. Hjertquist S-O, Lemperg R: Identification and concentration of the glycosaminoglycans of human articular cartilage in relation to age and osteoarthritis. Calcif Tissue Res 10:223–237, 1972.

344. Bayliss MT, Ali SY: Isolation of proteoglycans from human articular cartilage. Biochem J 169:112–132, 1978.

345. Elliott RJ, Gardner DL: Changes with age in the glycosaminoglycans of human articular cartilage. Ann Rheum Dis 38:371–377, 1979.

346. Kuhn K, Leppelmann HJ: Galaktosamin und glucosamin im knorpel in abhangigkeit von lebensalter. Justus Liebigs Ann Chem 611:254–258, 1958.

347. Benmaman JD, Ludoweig JJ, Anderson CE: Glucosamine and galactosamine distribution in human articular cartilage: Relationship to age and degenerative joint disease. Clin Biochem 2:461–464, 1969.

348. Loewi G: Changes in the ground substance of aging cartilage. J Pathol Bacteriol 65:381–388, 1953.

349. Mankin HJ, Lippiello L: The glycosaminoglycans of normal and arthritic cartilage. J Clin Invest 50:1712–1719, 1971.

350. Mathews MB, Glagov S: Acid mucopolysaccharide patterns in aging human cartilage. J Clin Invest 45:1103–1111, 1966.

351. Stidworthy G, Masters YF, Shetlar MR: The effect of aging on mucopolysaccharide composition of human costal cartilage as measured by hexosamine and uronic acid content. J Gerontol 13:10–13, 1958.

352. Byers PD, Contepomi CA, Farkas TA: A post mortem study of the hip joint including the prevalence of the features on the right side. Ann Rheum Dis 29:15–31, 1970.

353. Sokoloff L: The Biology of Degenerative Joint Disease. Chicago, University of Chicago Press, 1969.

354. Langenskiold A, Michellsson JC, Videman TS: Osteoarthritis of the knee in the rabbit produced by immobilization. Arch Orthop Scand 50:1–14, 1979.

355. Thaxter TH, Mann RA, Anderson CE: Degeneration of immobilized knee joints in rats. J Bone Joint Surg 47A:567–585, 1965.

356. Ehrlich MG, Mankin HJ, Jones H, Grossman A, Crispin C, Ancona D: Biochemical confirmation of an experimental model for osteoarthritis. J Bone Joint Surg 57A:392–396, 1975.

357. McDevitt CA, Gilbertson F, Muir H: An experimental model of osteoarthritis: Early morphological

and biochemical changes. J Bone Joint Surg 59B:24–35, 1977.

358. Palmoski MJ, Brandt KD: Immobilization of the knee prevents osteoarthritis after anterior cruciate ligament transection. Arthritis Rheum 25:1201–1208, 1982.

359. Lust G, Pronsky W, Sherman DM: Biochemical and ultrastructural observations in normal and degenerative canine articular cartilage. Am J Vet Res 33:2429–2440, 1972.

360. Wiltberger H, Lust G: Ultrastructure of canine articular cartilage: Comparison of normal and degenerative (osteoarthritic) hip joints. Am J Vet Res 36:727–739, 1975.

361. Mankin HJ, Dorfman H, Lippiello L, Zarins A: Biochemical and metabolic abnormalities in articular cartilage from osteoarthritic human hips. II. Correlation of morphology with biochemical and metabolic data. J Bone Joint Surg 53A:523–537, 1971.

362. Mankin HJ, Johnson ME, Lippiello L: Biochemical and metabolic abnormalities in articular cartilage from osteoarthritic human hips. II. Distribution and metabolism of amino sugar containing macromolecules. J Bone Joint Surg 51A:1591–1600, 1969.

363. Meachim G, Collins DH: Cell counts of normal and osteoarthritic cartilage in relation to the uptake of sulfate ($^{35}SO_4$) in vitro. Ann Rheum Dis 221:45–50, 1962.

364. Thompson RC Jr, Oegema TR Jr: Metabolic activity of articular cartilage in osteoarthritis. An in vitro study. J Bone Joint Surg 61A:407–416, 1979.

365. Weiss C, Mirow S: An ultrastructural study of osteoarthritic changes in articular cartilage of human knees. J Bone Joint Surg 54A:954–972, 1971.

366. Mankin HJ, Lippiello L: Biochemical and metabolic abnormalities in articular cartilage from osteoarthritic human hips. J Bone Joint Surg 52A:424–434, 1970.

367. Telhag H: Nucleic acids in human normal and osteoarthritic articular cartilage. Acta Orthop Scand 47:585–587, 1976.

368. Mitchell N, Shepard N: Pericellular proteoglycan concentrations in early degenerative arthritis. In press.

369. Maroudas A, Venn M: Chemical composition and swelling of normal and osteoarthritic femoral head cartilage. II. Swelling. Ann Rheum Dis 36:399–406, 1977.

370. Sweet MBE, Thonar EJ, Immelman AR, Solomon L: Biochemical change in progressive osteoarthrosis. Ann Rheum Dis 36:387–398, 1977.

371. Hirsch C: A contribution to the pathogenesis of chondromalacia of the patella: A physical, histologic and chemical study. Acta Chir Scand 83(suppl):5–106, 1944.

372. Bollet AJ, Handy JR, Sturgill BC: Chondroitin sulfate concentration and protein-polysaccharide composition of articular cartilage in osteoarthritis. J Clin Invest 42:853–859, 1963.

373. Eronen I, Videman T, Freeman MAR, Michelsson JE: Glycosaminoglycan metabolism in experimental osteoarthritis caused by immobilization. Acta Orthop Scand 49:329–334, 1978.

374. Floman Y, Eyre DR, Glimcher MJ: Induction of osteoarthrosis in the rabbit knee joint: Biochemical studies on the articular cartilage. Clin Orthop 147:278–288, 1980.

375. Muir H: Molecular approach to the understanding of osteoarthritis. Ann Rheum Dis 36:199–208, 1977.

376. Lust G, Pronsky W: Glycosaminoglycan content of normal and degenerative articular cartilage from dogs. Clin Chim Acta 39:281–286, 1972.

377. Brocklehurst R, Maroudas A: Comparative studies of the composition and sulphate uptake of normal and osteoarthritic cartilage from the knee, the hip and the ankle. In Peyron JG (ed.): Epidemiology of Osteoarthritis. Paris, Geigy, 1981, pp. 124–135.

378. Lippiello L, Mankin HJ: Thin-layer chromatographic separation of the isometric chondroitin sulfates, dermatan sulfate and keratan sulfate. Anal Biochem 39:54–58, 1971.

379. Brandt KD: Enhanced extractability of articular cartilage proteoglycans in osteoarthritis. Biochem J 143:475–478, 1974.

380. Brandt KD, Palmoski MJ, Perricone E: Aggregation of cartilage proteoglycans. I. Evidence for the presence of a hyaluronate binding region in proteoglycans from osteoarthritic cartilage. Arthritis Rheum 19:1308–1314, 1976.

381. Moskowitz, RW, Howell DS, Goldberg VM, Muniz O, Pita JC: Cartilage proteoglycan abnormalities in an experimentally induced model of rabbit osteoarthritis. Arthritis Rheum 22:155–163, 1979.

382. Palmoski MJ, Brandt KD: Hyaluronate binding by proteoglycans: Comparison of mildly and severely osteoarthritic regions of the human femoral cartilage. Clin Chim Acta 79:87–95, 1976.

383. Bjelle AO: Glycosaminoglycans in human articular cartilage of the lower femoral epiphysis in osteoarthritis. Scand J Rheum 6:37–44, 1977.

384. Minns RJ, Stevens FS, Harding K: Osteoarthrotic articular cartilage lesions of the femoral head. J Pathol 122:63–70, 1977.

385. Lippiello L, Hall D, Mankin HJ: Collagen synthesis in normal and osteoarthritic human cartilage. J Clin Invest 59:593–600, 1977.

386. Miller DR, Lust G: Accumulation of procollagen in the degenerative articular cartilage of dogs with osteoarthritis. Biochim Biophys Acta 583:218–231, 1979.

387. Gay S, Muller PK, Lemmen C, Remberger K, Matzen K, Kuhn K: Immunohistological study on collagen in cartilage-bone metamorphoses and degenerative arthritis. Klin Wochenschr 54:969–976, 1976.

388. Eyre DR, McDevitt CA, Muir H: Experimentally induced osteoarthritis in the dog collagen. Biosynthesis in control and fibrillated cartilage. Ann Rheum Dis 34(suppl):138–140, 1975.

389. Gardner DL: Pathology of the Connective Tissue Disease. Baltimore, Williams and Wilkins Company, 1965, pp. 243–244.

390. Jaffe HL: Metabolic Degenerative and Inflammatory Diseases of Bones and Joints. Philadelphia, Lea and Febiger, 1972.

391. Milch RA: Studies of alcaptonuria: Mechanisms of swelling of homogentisic acid-collagen preparations. Arthritis Rheum 4:153–267, 1961.

392. Schumacher HR: Ochronosis, hemochromatosis and Wilson's disease. In McCarty D (ed.): Arthritis. 9th ed. Philadelphia, Lea and Febiger, 1979, pp. 1262–1275.

393. Dymock IW, Hamilton EBD, Laws JW, Williams R: Arthropathy of haemochromatosis: Clinical and radiological analysis of 63 patients with iron overload. Ann Rheum Dis 29:469–476, 1970

394. Hamilton E, Williams R, Barlow KA, et al.: The

arthropathy of idiopathic haemochromatosis. Q J Med 37:171–182, 1968.

395. Howell DS: Osteoarthritis: Speculation on some biochemical factors of possible aetiological nature including cartilage mineralization. *In* Nuki G (ed.): Aetiopathogenesis of Osteoarthritis. Tunbridge Wells, Pitman Medical Publishing Co., 1980, pp. 83–104.

396. Dieppe PA: Calcium phosphate crystal deposition and clinical subsets of osteoarthritis. *In* Peyron JG (ed.): Epidemiology of Osteoarthritis. Paris, Geigy, 1981, pp. 71–80.

397. Dieppe PA, Huskisson EC, Crocker P, Willoughby DA: Apatitic deposition diseases: A new arthropathy. Lancet 1:266–268, 1976.

398. McCarty DJ, Hogan JM, Gatter RA, Grossman MM: Studies in pathological calcifications in human cartilage. I. Prevalence and types of crystal deposits in the menisci of two hundred and fifteen cadavers. J Bone Joint Surg 48A:309–325, 1966.

399. Camerlain M, McCarty DJ, Silcox DC et al.: Inorganic pyrophosphate pool size and turnover rate in arthritic joints. J Clin Invest 55:1373–1381, 1975.

400. Howell DS, Muniz OE, Morales S: 5'-Nucleotidase and pyrophosphate (PPi) generating activities in articular cartilage extracts of calcium pyrophosphate deposition disease (CPDD). *In* Peyron JG (ed.): Epidemiology of Osteoarthritis. Paris, Geigy, 1981, pp. 99–112.

401. Howell DS, Muniz OE, Pita JC, Enis JE: Extrusion of pyrophosphate into extracellular media by osteoarthritic cartilage incubates. J Clin Invest 56:1473–1480, 1975.

402. Howell DS, Woessner JF Jr, Jiminez S, Seda H, Schumacher HR Jr: A view on the pathogenesis of osteoarthritis. Bull Rheum Dis 29:996–1001, 1978-9.

403. Howell DS, Muniz OE, Pita JC, Arsenes C: Preliminary observations on phosphatases in articular cartilage. Arthritis Rheum 19:495–498, 1976.

404. Ryan LM, Kozen F, McCarty DJ: Quantification of human plasma inorganic pyrophosphate. I. Normal values in osteoarthritis and calcium pyrophosphate dihydrate crystal deposition disease. Arthritis Rheum 22:886–891, 1979.

405. Meachim G: Sulfate metabolism of articular cartilage after surgical interference with the joint. Ann Rheum Dis 23:372–380, 1964.

406. Bollet AJ: Connective tissue polysaccharide metabolism and pathogenesis of osteoarthritis. Adv Intern Med 13:33–60, 1967.

407. McDevitt CA, Eyre DR, Muir H: Altered metabolism of proteoglycans and collagen in early experimental osteoarthrosis. Scand J Rheumatol 4(Suppl):8, 1975.

408. Mayor MB, Moskowitz RW: Metabolic studies on experimentally induced degenerative disease in the rabbit. J Rheumatol 1:17–23, 1974.

409. Jacoby RK, Jayson MIV: The organ culture of adult articular cartilage from patients with osteoarthrosis. Rheumatol Rehabil 16:116–122, 1976.

410. Mitrovic D, Gruson M, Demignon J, Mercier P, Aprile F, DeSeze S: Metabolism of human femoral head cartilage in osteoarthrosis and subcapital fracture. Ann Rheum Dis 40:18–26, 1981.

411. Ghosh P, Taylor TKF, McKenzie LS, Horsburgh BA: Comparison of the synthesis levels of glycosaminoglycans in aged and osteoarthritic hips. Trans Orthop Res Soc 2:9, 1977.

412. McKenzie LS, Horsburgh BA, Ghosh P, Taylor TKF: Sulphated glycosaminoglycan synthesis in normal and osteoarthritic hip cartilage. Ann Rheum Dis 36:369–373, 1977.

413. Byers PD, Maroudas A, Ozlop F, Stockwell RA, Venn MF: Histological and biochemical studies on cartilage from osteoarthritic femoral heads with special reference to surface characteristics. Connect Tissue Res 5:41–49, 1977.

413a. Moskowitz RW, Goldberg, VM, Malemud CJ: Metabolic responses of cartilage in experimentally induced osteoarthritis. Ann Rheum Dis 40:584–592, 1981.

414. Palmoski MJ, Colyer RA, Brandt KD: Marked suppression by salicylate of the augmented proteoglycan synthesis in osteoarthritic cartilage. Arthritis Rheum 23:83–91, 1980.

415. Palmoski MJ, Brandt KD: Aspirin aggravates the degeneration of canine joint cartilage caused by immobilization. Arthritis Rheum 25:1333–1342, 1982.

416. Palmoski MJ, Brandt KD: Knee cartilage from unloaded sites is more vulnerable than cartilage from loaded areas to the effects of salicylate on glycosaminoglycan synthesis. Arthritis Rheum 25:S129, 1982.

417. Bullough PG, Goodfellow JW, O'Connor J: The relationship between degenerative changes and load-bearing in the human hip. J Bone Joint Surg 55B:746–758, 1973.

418. Ryu J, Treadwell BV, Mankin HJ: Biochemical and metabolic abnormalities in normal and osteoarthritic human cartilage. Arthritis Rheum 27:49–57, 1984.

419. Hulth A, Lindberg L, Telhag H: Mitosis in human osteoarthritic cartilage. Clin Orthop 84:197–199, 1972.

420. Telhag H, Gudmundson C: Nucleic acids in degenerative joint disease. Clin Orthop 88:247–251, 1972.

421. Rothwell AG, Bentley G: Chondrocyte multiplication in osteoarthritic articular cartilage. J Bone Joint Surg 55B:588–594, 1973.

422. Woessner JF Jr: Purification of cathepsin D from cartilage and uterus and its action on the protein-polysaccharide complex of cartilage. J Biol Chem 248:1634–1642, 1973.

423. Sapolsky A, Howell DS: Proteolytic enzymes in human cartilage: The pathogenesis of osteoarthritis. Comp Ther 2:33–40, 1976.

424. Ehrlich MG, Howle PA, Vigliani G, Mankin HJ: Correlation between articular cartilage collagenase activity and osteoarthritis. Arthritis Rheum 21:761–766, 1978.

425. Stephens RW, Ghosh P, Taylor TK: Pathogenesis of osteoarthrosis. Med Hypotheses 5:809–816, 1979.

426. Radin EL: Aetiology of osteoarthrosis. Clin Rheum Dis 2:509–522, 1976.

427. Radin EL, Paul IL, Rose RM: Role of mechanical fractures in the pathogenesis of primary osteoarthrosis. Lancet 1:519–522, 1976.

4

The Immunology of Articular Cartilage

Victor M. Goldberg, M.D.

The structural elements of cartilage have been extensively discussed in the basic science sections of this text. At first glance, it may appear that the primary etiology of osteoarthritis is unrelated to an immune mechanism. Recent reports, however, have implicated an inflammatory response as part of the ongoing process of the disease.[1-9] The components of articular cartilage provide fertile sites for antigenic determinants and the possible immune responses to these antigens. For many years, cartilage was believed to be a "privileged site" in transplantation immunology.[10-19] Its apparent weak antigenicity was attributed to its relative isolation from lymphatic and vascular structures as well as the protective properties of its matrix. However, reports have shown that cartilage is immunogenic, and this property has been used recently to further delineate structural characteristics of the matrix components.[3, 17, 20]

Although it is beyond this chapter to discuss immunology in depth, a brief review of the principles of immunology will be discussed and the present place of immunobiology as it applies to cartilage and osteoarthritis will be reviewed.

PRINCIPLES OF IMMUNOBIOLOGY

A basic review of some immune principles is necessary to appreciate the possible role of this system in the physiology of articular cartilage and the pathology of osteoarthritis. The reader is referred to more complete texts referenced at the end of this chapter for more in-depth discussions of the immune system.[21-23]

The two basic reactions of the immune response against foreign antigens are cellular and humoral. The characteristics of each are shown in Table 4–1. The immune response is initiated by stimulation of specific lymphocytes referred to as "T" and "B" cells. Both cells are derived from a basic bone marrow stem cell. The T cells, which are primarily responsible for cellular immunity, develop under the influence of the thymus. The B lymphocytes mature under the direction of the bursa of Fabricius in chickens or bursal equivalents in higher mammals (Fig. 4–1). These latter cells orchestrate humoral immune responses and become plasma cells, which also secrete antibodies. However, it is somewhat artificial to discuss these two cell lines separately, as evidence indicates a close interaction between the two systems in a response to any antigen.

Recent studies have elucidated two subpopulations of T cells. One is a suppressor cell that appears to inhibit antibody production by B cells, and the other is a helper cell that enhances humoral responses.[22-24] In addition to the interaction of lymphocytes in an immune reaction, foreign material must be processed for a reaction to occur. This event requires the phagocytosis of antigen by macrophages, which can then pass the information derived from the immunogenic breakdown fragments of the foreign protein to T and B cells. There are also a small number of monocytes present in the circulation that are neither T nor B lymphocytes but are called "null" cells. Their exact role is as yet ill defined.

Antibodies are immunoglobulins that are produced by mature B cells and plasma cells and are the hallmark of the humoral response.

Table 4–1. CHARACTERISTICS OF THE IMMUNE SYSTEM

		Humoral Immunity	Cell-Mediated Immunity
Response		Rapid	Delayed
Primary cell		"B" lymphocyte; plasma cell	"T" lymphocyte
Transfer of immunity		Immunoglobulins (antibody)	Lymphocyte (lymphokines)
Examples		*Anaphylaxis*	*Tuberculin type*
		Virus and toxin neutralization	*Delayed hypersensitivity*
			Allograft rejection

They have been subdivided into five classes because of different physiochemical properties: IgG, IgM, IgA, IgE, and IgD. However, they all share common structural subunits consisting of two light and two heavy peptide chains, linked by a disulfide bond (Fig. 4–2). The light chains (L) have a molecular weight of approximately 25,000 daltons each. The heavy chains (H) each have a molecular weight of between 50,000 and 75,000 daltons. There are two groups of light chains—kappa and lambda. Sixty-five per cent of the immunoglobulins of normal serum contain kappa chains, and the remaining contain lambda chains. Studies using antisera prepared against heavy chains have identified five separate classes, as noted above, which give rise to the five major divisions of immunoglobulins. Therefore, although each immunoglobulin subclass contains a special heavy chain, they all have either kappa or lambda light chains.

The amino acid sequence within each immunoglobulin class has terminal regions of both the heavy and light chains that are variable (V_h, V_l), whereas the remaining part of the polypeptide chains is constant. It is the variable portion that gives the immunoglobulin the specificity to bind antigen. The constant portion has varying properties, depending on the immunoglobulin class, and requires antigen binding for activation. Papain cleaves immunoglobulins at the hinge regions to produce two identical antigen-binding fragments, F_{ab}, and a third component F_c. Pepsin digestion results in a single bivalent antigen-binding fragment $(F_{ab})_2$. The F_{ab} is the antigen-binding portion of the molecule and the F_c fragment retains the ability to fix complement, cross the placenta, and bind to macrophages (see Figure 4–2).

Each immune globulin has specific biologic functions. The reader is referred to the excellent references at the end of this chapter for greater detail. IgG is the most abundant immunoglobulin in the extravascular space. It has a sedimentation coefficient of 7S and a

ORIGINS OF IMMUNOCOMPETENT CELLS

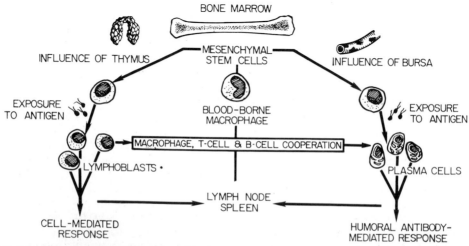

Figure 4–1. Schematic diagram of the origins of both "arms" of immunity. Both types of immunocompetent cells are derived from basic bone marrow mesenchymal cells.

THE IMMUNOGLOBULIN MOLECULE

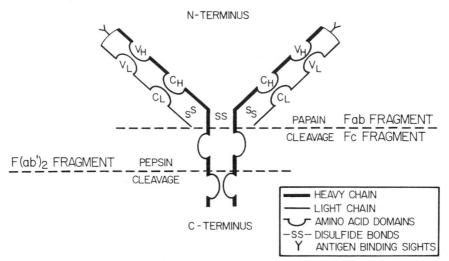

Figure 4–2. The structure of the immunoglobulin molecule.

molecular weight of about 150,000 daltons. IgG fixes complement, binds to macrophages, crosses the placenta, and combats most infectious organisms and toxins. IgM has a pentameric structure, with a sedimentation coefficient of 19S and a molecular weight of 900,000 daltons. It appears first after an antigenic stimulus. Because of its structure, it is well suited to its role as a bacterial agglutinator and complement mediator. IgA, found in both monomeric and polymeric forms, is seen mostly in seromucous secretions, where it is the major defense against bacteria. IgD is most likely an antigen receptor on the surface of lymphocytes. IgE is concerned with parasitic infection and mediates many allergic reactions, e.g., atopic allergy.

The Immune Response

The two basic immune reactions to any antigen are humoral and cellular.[22, 23] The former is concerned with the synthesis and secretion of antibody to directly neutralize bacterial toxins and the bacteria in order to expedite their clearance (Fig. 4–3). Cellular immune mechanisms depend on the production of specific sensitized lymphocytes that have immunoglobulins on their surface. These cells secrete small effector molecules called lymphokines and are responsible for transplantation immunity and "delayed hypersensitivity" (Fig. 4–4).

The small lymphocyte is important in order for both cellular and humoral reactions to occur. If the small lymphocyte is removed from the circulation, one cannot mount a primary antibody response to antigens, such as tetanus toxoid. In addition, these lymphocytes carry the memory for the first contact with antigen. When these cells are transferred to an animal that has not had contact with a specific antigen, the animal, after exposure to this antigen, responds with the production of a high titer of antibody (secondary response). There is a time lapse in a primary response before the host produces antibodies at a detectable level, whereas in the secondary response there is a rapid high-level reaction.

The first step in any immune response is antigen recognition and processing (afferent limb). Macrophages phagocytize the antigen, which is usually cleaved to immunogenic fragments. These molecules may interact with RNA and form substances capable of carrying immunologic information to lymphocytes or are actually transmitted as modified antigens to either B or T cells, depending on the specific antigen. Cooperation of all these cells is important in the afferent arc of the immune response.

The humoral immune reaction depends on B-cell antigenic stimulation. Nonsensitized cells respond to antigens by undergoing a morphologic and metabolic change called blastogenesis. This process does require the participation of a subpopulation of T cells, helper

HUMORAL ANTIBODY–MEDIATED RESPONSE

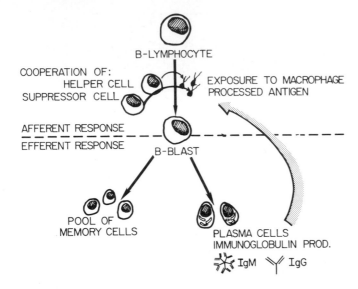

Figure 4–3. Outline of the humoral immune reaction that depends on "B" lymphocytes.

cells, for enhancement. The B lymphoblast may then become a plasma cell, whose primary purpose is the production of a specific immunoglobulin. In addition, the B blast cell may also become a memory cell. This phase of the response is known as the efferent arc. Specific antibody is the effector molecule that neutralizes the specific antigen, usually with the involvement of the complement system (see Figure 4–3).

Cell-mediated reactions are a delayed type of response to, for example, organ allografts. The T cell is the primary cell that both re-

sponds to the antigen and acts as the effector arm. Specific antigens stimulate T cells to undergo blastogenesis, which may evolve into either effector cells or memory cells (see Figure 4–4). Macrophages also appear to be involved in both the afferent and efferent part of this system. The role of the B cells in this response is not yet well defined. The responding effector T cells can become K cells or cytotoxic. These latter cells secrete low–molecular-weight peptides known as lymphokines, which may inhibit macrophages (macrophage inhibition factor [MIF]) and influence

CELL–MEDIATED RESPONSE

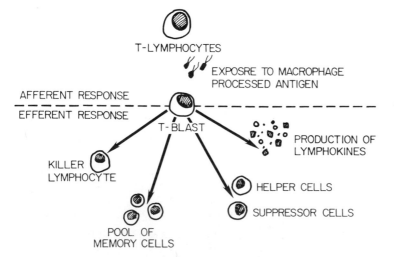

Figure 4–4. Summary of the cell-mediated response to specific antigens.

lymphocytes (transfer factor) or other targets such as viruses (interferon). T cells also help regulate B-cell functions, as described previously. It is evident from this brief description that the immune system is a finely balanced tool of biologic surveillance. This entire system is under the direction of genetic factors that determine cell surface antigens, the ability to respond to specific antigens, and the alloantigenic differences between serum immunoglobulins.

In Vitro Tests of Humoral and Cell-Mediated Immunity

In order to understand some of the aspects of immune reactions as they pertain to the physiology of cartilage and the pathophysiology of osteoarthritis, a brief description of some of the techniques used to identify the in vitro interaction of antigen and antibody is important.[21-23] The formation of a *precipitate* when multivalent antigens are mixed with bivalent antibodies can be studied in solutions or visualized in gels. In the double *immunodiffusion* method of *Ouchterlony,* antigen and antibody are placed in adjacent agar gel wells and migrate toward each other to form opaque lines that precipitate at the region where each is present in equivalent or optimal proportions (Fig. 4–5). *Single radial immunodiffusion* is a technique in which antigen diffuses into an agar that contains diluted antiserum. At the level of optimal proportions, a ring forms, so that different concentrations of antigen can be quantified by the size of the precipitant ring. The reaction of antibody with cell surface antigen leads to an agglutination reaction, which is a lattice effect and can be visually identified and quantified.

OUCHTERLONY METHOD OF IMMUNODIFFUSION

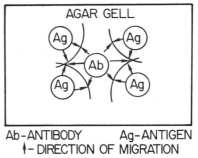

Figure 4–5. The Ouchterlony immunodiffusion method is used to detect antibody and antigen interaction in vitro.

Immunoelectrophoresis identifies antigens by their electrophoretic mobility. Semiquantitative information about immunoglobulins may be obtained by this technique (Fig. 4–6). *Counterelectrophoresis* is the migration of antigens to the positive pole in agar. *Rocket electrophoresis* is a quantitative technique whereby antigen migrates into a gel with antibody using electrophoretic principles. The precipitant arcs look like "rockets," and again, the antigen moves to the positive pole. There are *radioisotopic assays* for analyzing the antibody concentration in serum using radioisotope-labeled antigen and estimating its binding to antibody by ammonium sulfate precipitation or by measuring the concentration of antibody binding to insoluble antigen by the addition of a labeled anti-immunoglobulin.

Immunofluorescence utilizes the concept that antibodies can be tagged with fluorescent dyes and still combine with antigen. This allows localization of antigens in tissues within or on cells. Labeled antibody reacts directly with the tissue, and ultraviolet light microscopy is used

IMMUNOELECTROPHORESIS

Figure 4–6. Immunoelectrophoresis identifies antigens by their ability to migrate in an electrically charged field.

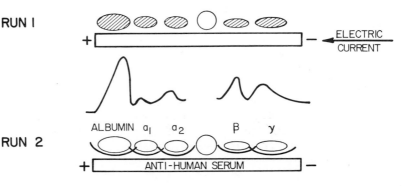

to identify complexes bound to antigen. In the indirect test, the label is bound to an anti-immunoglobulin used as a second amplifying antibody.

There are additional in vitro assays that can specifically identify T cells by their ability, for example, to form spontaneous rosettes with sheep red blood cells. Techniques have been developed that quantify the humoral and cell-mediated immune response by using cytotoxicity assays directed toward isotope-labeled target cells. In addition, *lymphoblast transformation* may be identified by monitoring the protein and DNA synthesis of responding lymphocytes using tritiated thymidine. *Lymphokine* production from activated lymphocytes may be identified by assaying, for example, the function of the macrophage inhibition factor. This may be used as a measure of in vitro cell-mediated immunity.

Tolerance and Autoimmunity

The gradual recognition of immune pathways as a major force in the pathophysiology of many connective tissue diseases has implicated the concept of autoantigenicity. In order to understand this process, some understanding of the breakdown of tolerance and the emergence of autoimmunity is important.[17, 22–24] As will be discussed, there is a gradual accumulation of information that seems to implicate similar mechanisms in osteoarthritis.

Tolerance is immunologic unresponsiveness to autoantigens. This appears to be a natural phenomenon that develops during fetal life and depends on the ability of immunocompetent lymphocytes to recognize "self." Tolerance may be induced by the exposure of the lymphocytes to antigens during embryonic development or by the administration of high doses of antigen during adulthood. Maintenance of tolerance depends on the contribution of both the lymphocyte population T and B cells and the interactions of suppressor and helper T cells. The breakdown of tolerance results in autoimmunity. The exact defect that results in loss of self-recognition has not been identified, but several concepts have been proposed.[23, 24] One mechanism suggests the exposure of sequestered antigens that were not encountered by lymphocytes during fetal life, thereby causing these lymphocytes to respond as they would to a foreign protein. Nucleoprotein, antigenic determinants hidden within protein structures, and chondrocytes are so-called immunologically privileged structures that may

become exposed as a result of adjunctive disease processes.

Autoimmunity may also result if previously tolerated antigens are altered by, for example, interaction with viral material or other exogenous factors so that lymphocytes no longer recognize the protein as "self." A similar mechanism is cross-reactivity, in which a foreign antigen is structurally close to a native antigen, so that antibodies directed against the exogenous antigen cross-react and destroy native, previously tolerated antigen. If a mutation occurs during the lifetime of a normal lymphocyte, the mutant cells may not be capable of normal surveillance, so that it interacts with normal proteins and produces autoantibodies. Lastly, with the delineation of subpopulations of T cells charged with the responsibility of suppressing and checking immune responses, it is possible that these suppressor cells may develop defective functions. As a result, helper T cells are unrestrained and result in the unchecked stimulation of antibody production, which may include autoantibodies. Whatever the mechanism that causes the loss of tolerance, the result is the production of immune destructive mechanisms directed against "self-antigens."

IMMUNOGENICITY OF CARTILAGE

Although cartilage seems to enjoy the status of immunologic privilege by virtue of its anatomic structure, studies have identified antigenic determinants present within each component of articular cartilage.[3, 17, 25] If there is a role for the immune system in the pathogenesis of osteoarthritis, further delineation of the immunogenicity of cartilage components must be determined.

Proteoglycan

The results of early studies of the antigenic capacity of proteoglycan were somewhat equivocal.[26–36] However, recent studies have utilized antigenic determinants of proteoglycans to learn more structural detail of these molecules.[13, 17, 20, 37–43] Glynn and Holborow,[44] Loewi and Muir,[31] and others[17, 45, 46] were not able to elicit antibody responses to chondroitin sulfate alone. Later studies using chemically isolated proteoglycan as the immunizing agent did demontrate its antigenicity by using a precipitant technique.[27, 45–53] When the glycosaminoglycans were removed by the action of hyaluronidase, the reaction was not abolished.[33, 49, 51, 54] The major antigenic determinants therefore appear to reside in the central core protein of the molecule or at the link-protein region. This antigenicity is destroyed by papain digestion.[3, 46, 55]

Mechanical disruption of the cartilage proteoglycans produces two fractions: PP-L, the light portion, and PP-H, the heavy portion. Antibodies have been detected to each of these crude extracts using immunoprecipitin and hemagglutination techniques.[27, 33, 35, 46–48, 56] DiFerrante immunized rabbits with extracts of bovine nasal cartilage and found antibodies to the PP-L fraction, but not with papain-treated material. The antibodies were specific for the bovine material but did not cross-react with other species.[27] DiFerrante and Pauling later reported the identification of cross-reactive antibodies against bovine PP-L with human or porcine PP-L.[47, 48] According to these techniques, two forms of antigen therefore seem to be present—one is species-specific and is associated with the glycoprotein link region; the other, a species-common determinant, is present on the proteoglycan subunits.[49–51] The strongest species–cross-reacting determinants were shown by Keiser and associates to be located in the keratan sulfate region, whereas the weakest were seen about the chondroitin sulfate chains.[57–60] In addition, species-specific sites have been associated with link protein, which shows no cross-reactivity with the core protein molecule.[37, 39] It appears, then, that proteoglycans are weakly antigenic and that these determinants reside on the core protein and link protein of the molecule. Trypsin or papain destroys this antigenicity, whereas treatment of proteoglycan with hyaluronidase enhances it. If one removes all the chondroitin sulfate or keratan sulfate chains, leaving an intact protein core, the antigenicity is unaffected. There remain some topics that must be addressed—namely, the cross-reactivity with different species of many antisera used in these studies and the fact that proteoglycans do share common antigens with other tissues as well as with bacteria.[17, 61, 62] New knowledge about these issues may have important overtones in the pathophysiology of many diseases.

Collagen

As discussed in Chapter 3, the structure of collagen is complex and consists of three polypeptide chains coiled to form a triple helix. Although antigenic sites have been identified on the triple helix, collagen is only weakly immunogenic. The immunogenicity of collagen has usually been studied using collagen from noncartilaginous sources.[63–70] Three major antigenic sites have been identified using either the hemaglutination or complement fixation tests. These include the terminal regions, the helical region, and the central sites of the alpha chains.[3, 17]

Using cyanogen bromide cleavage techniques, Timpl and colleagues[71, 72] and Lindsley and associates[67] demonstrated antigenic determinants present on the N- and C-terminal ends of the molecule. These antigenic determinants were shown by Pontz and coworkers[69] and Timpl and colleagues[73, 74] to be mostly species-specific, with only weak cross-reactivity.

Early studies did not show antigenic determinants on the helical region. Using immunoadsorbent techniques, however, investigators were able to demonstrate major immunogenicity associated with the helical sites in rat, mouse, and chicken systems.[64, 75–79] Hahn and Timpl[77] developed artificial helices and confirmed a distinct anticollagen antibody comparable to those directed against separated alpha chains. These helical antigens also appear to be species-specific.

The central antigen determinants are not species-specific and have been identified after removal of the terminal ends of the alpha chains. They appear to be present only on alpha chains from denatured collagen and not on the native molecule.[73, 80–82] Timpl and associates also used cyanogen bromide–isolated peptides and showed that alpha chains may vary in the degree of immunogenicity, depending on the species used.[72]

The immunogenicity of collagen and its role in articular disease is still fertile ground for investigation; both cell-mediated and humoral responses to the molecule have been demonstrated.

Chondrocytes

There is no question that the surface of chondrocytes has antigens that are controlled by the genes of the major histocompatibility locus. However, the difficulty in identifying these antigens may lie in the protection afforded by the surrounding matrix. Langer and colleagues used the lymphocyte migration inhibition test to demonstrate cell-mediated responses to cartilage allografts exchanged between rats that were disparate at the major histocompatibility locus.[83, 84] Only when isolated chondrocytes were devoid of their surrounding matrix and then transplanted did a cell-mediated response result. A similar response was also seen in a syngeneic system, which suggested an unmasking of sequestered surface antigens. In other studies using cartilage allografts, varying results have been reported, depending on the circumstances of the experimental design.[10–16, 18] Heyner demonstrated in a rat system that after trypsin and collagenase digestion, allogenic chondrocytes produced an immune response not seen with intact cartilage grafts.[85] Presensitization of the host did ultimately result in the resorption of even the intact grafts. Heyner was not able to demonstrate a response with syngeneic cells that Langer attributed to the use of trypsin digestion, which he felt might have altered the chondrocyte surface.

Elves demonstrated cell surface antigens on sheep articular chondrocytes that were shared by peripheral lymphocytes. However, there also remained antigens that appeared to be specific for chondrocytes.[14] Gertzbein and associates used a mixed lymphocyte-chondrocyte culture technique and reported a lymphoblast transformation when the cells were from disparate animals. They also reported similar findings when a syngeneic system was used, suggesting organ-specific antigenic determinants.[86, 87]

In summary, there appear to be cell surface antigens on chondrocytes that are both species-specific and tissue-specific. The apparent immune privilege enjoyed by these cells seems to be the result of the protection afforded by the surrounding matrix.

THE ROLE OF IMMUNITY IN OSTEOARTHRITIS

At first glance, a disease that progresses by mechanical and biochemical pathways would not appear to be immunologically mediated. However, recent evidence indicates some role for both inflammation and the immune response in the pathophysiology of osteoarthritis (OA).[1–7, 9, 88] Peyron has pointed to the inflammatory symptoms that are present in most cases of osteoarthritis.[6, 7] One may see an abrupt, painful swelling, with redness as well as morning stiffness and rest pain. The synovial fluid of these patients often demonstrates an increased mononuclear count and an increase in protein, immunoglobulins, and complement. The synovial membrane may also show an infiltrate of mononuclear cells as well as

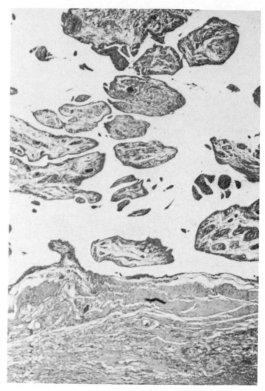

Figure 4–7. A photomicrograph of a synovial membrane removed at the time of total hip arthroplasty for severe primary osteoarthritis demonstrating a moderate inflammatory response (hematoxylin and eosin stain, × 100).

vascular engorgement (Fig. 4–7). The subchondral marrow spaces often acquire an increased vascularity with the presence of plasma cells and lymphocytes.[89] Furthermore, the level of lysosomal enzymes such as cathepsin D is elevated and has been correlated with the inflammation present.[8] This inflammatory response appears to be related to a heightened progression of joint destruction. Many times the erythrocyte sedimentation rate is also elevated in these patients, and its reduction coincides with the remission of articular symptoms. The initiating factors that lead to the inflammatory response may well be the degradative products of the cartilage and their sequestered antigenic sites. Of particular interest in this regard is the subset of osteoarthritis that has been described as involving primarily the hip and proximal interphalangeal joints. These patients usually present with a rapidly destructive process of the hips with many of the inflammatory hallmarks discussed as well as an elevated erythrocyte sedimentation rate.[9, 90] The role of a true immune response in the pathophysiology of OA will be discussed further below.

Although a large body of knowledge has accumulated that indicates the essential role of autoimmunity in rheumatoid arthritis and other diseases,[3, 5, 17, 91–94] there are still few reports that point to the role of the immune response in OA. It is apparent that whatever the initiating factor of cartilage destruction in osteoarthritis, ultimately the process may unmask the immunogenic determinants of chondrocytes, proteoglycan, and collagen. These sequestered antigens of cartilage that have been "tolerated" may well act as autoantigens after being unmasked and evoke an immune response. These antigens have been detected at times in synovial fluid in patients with OA as well as within immunocompetent cells in the fluid.[95–100] Barland and coworkers have demonstrated an increased immunofluorescence to antigenic determinants of proteoglycan in cartilage from patients with degenerative joint disease.[54] Steffen and associates have shown the presence of anticollagen antibodies in some patients with OA.[100] Cracchiolo and colleagues demonstrated antibodies to collagen in synovial effusions from patients with traumatic effusions, which suggested a possible role for humoral immunity in nonrheumatoid articular destructive processes.[96] Andriopoulis and coworkers also identified synovial fluid antibodies to Type I collagen in 30% of patients with OA.[95] Endler and colleagues[101] and Stuart and associates[102] demonstrated cell-mediated immunologic responses to collagen in patients with osteoarthritis.

Herman and coworkers were unable to detect antibodies against proteoglycans in synovial fluid or serum from patients with OA using the crudely separated proteoglycan or PP-L fraction.[3, 41] When they used the antigen obtained from a 4 M guanidine hydrochloride separation technique, a positive hemagglutination test was found in the serum of some patients with severe OA.[3, 103] They further reported positive responses to crudely prepared human cartilage proteoglycan (PP-L) and products of chondrocyte synthesis in 9 of 22 patients with OA using a lymphotoxin release assay. The response to this in vitro measure of cell-mediated immunity was not as great as that seen from patients with rheumatoid arthritis.[4, 103] Stastny and colleagues used a lymphocyte migration inhibitory test, an in vitro assay for cell-mediated immunity, and detected positive responses when synovial fluid from patients with OA was used in the assay.[104]

Cooke and associates used immunofluorescent techniques to study articular tissue obtained from 114 patients with OA and noted that in over one third of the patients, immunoglobulin and complement deposition was seen in the collagenous tissue.[1] The distribution and intensity of the staining were similar to rheumatoid arthritis in those patients with generalized osteoarthritis affecting hips and proximal interphalangeal joints (Fig. 4–8). They were unable to find any correlation between the intensity of immunoglobulin deposition and the inflammatory changes or histologic grade of the cartilage. They did not identify immune complex aggregates by electron microscopy. These studies suggest that primary or idiopathic OA may have several subsets, some of which are similar to rheumatoid arthritis (RA) and may be immunologically mediated. Herman and colleagues recently indicated a role for lymphokines in OA.[4] They showed that lymphokines secreted by mitogen-stimulated lymphocytes could modify

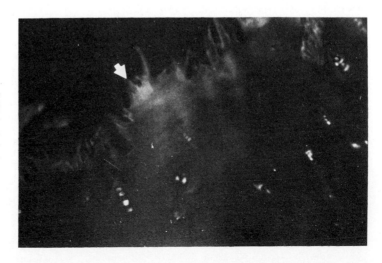

Figure 4–8. A photomicrograph section of hyaline cartilage removed at the time of total hip arthroplasty for severe primary osteoarthritis demonstrating positive immunofluorescence against IgA (arrow) (hematoxylin and eosin stain, × 100). (Courtesy of Dr. T. D. Cooke.)

chondrocyte functions in vitro and induce proteoglycan degradation. It appeared that the response may have been mediated through a monocyte proteoglycanase. Further studies demonstrated a significant suppression of glycosaminoglycan, protein, RNA, and DNA synthesis by chondrocytes in explant cultures after the addition of a lymphokine-containing supernatant derived from a mitogen-stimulated T cell. Herman feels that this evidence mandates additional studies to clarify the role of lymphokines in the pathophysiology of OA.

There have been almost no experimental studies investigating the role of the immune system in animal models. However, in a rabbit model of osteoarthritis induced by partial meniscectomy, Champion and Poole showed cellular immunity using blastogenic responses to proteoglycan and rabbit type I, II, and III collagen.[88] The immune response to collagen was seen after both partial meniscectomy and sham operations and appeared as a nonspecific response to surgically induced tissue damage. Type III collagen peptides gave the greatest responses and may have cross-reacted with Types I and II to cause that response. Immunity to proteoglycan occurred primarily in the animals that had undergone partial meniscectomy and correlated significantly with the severity of the OA lesions produced.

The concept of autoimmunity as part of the destructive mechanism causing the progression of the degeneration of articular structures in osteoarthritis is also appealing considering the increased incidence of the disease with advancing age. The immune surveillance that is critical for the maintenance of health does deteriorate with age, so that if the normal suppressor mechanisms that protect the antigenic determinants of cartilage are lost, another pathway of cartilage destruction in OA could become operative. Most important, because OA appears to be a complex disease, further studies of the relationship between the immune system and OA might identify important subsets of the disease with different destructive pathways. This might then help in the development of new therapeutic modalities and preventive measures.

References

1. Cooke TD, Bennet EL, Ohno O: Identification of immunoglobulins and complement components in articular collagenous tissues of patients with idiopathic osteoarthrosis. *In* Nuki G: The Aetiopathogenesis of Osteoarthrosis. Tunbridge Wells, Pitman Medical Publishing Co., 1980, pp. 144–155.
2. Dieppe P: Calcium phosphate crystal deposition and clinical subsets of osteoarthritis. *In* Peyron JG: Proceedings of a Symposium of Epidemiology of Osteoarthritis. Paris, CIBA Geigy, 1980.
3. Herman JH, Carpenter BA: Immunobiology of cartilage. Semin Arthritis Rheum 5:1–40, 1975.
4. Herman JH Mowery HS, Koo KH, Dennis NV: Lymphokines: Potential role in the immunopathogenesis of osteoarthritis. Semin Arthritis Rheum 11(Suppl 1):104–107, 1980.
5. Huskisson EC, Dieppe PA, Scott J: Inflammatory polyarthritis in osteoarthritis. Ann Rheum Dis 37:571–572, 1978.
6. Peyron J: Inflammation in osteoarthritis (OA): Review of its role in clinical picture, disease progress, subsets, and pathophysiology. Semin Arthritis Rheum 11(Suppl 1):115–116, 1980.
7. Peyron J: Epidemiologic and etiologic approach of osteoarthritis. Semin Arthritis Rheum 8:288–306, 1979.
8. Salvati E, Granda JL, Mirra J, Wilson PD: Clinical enzymatic and histological study of synovium in coxarthrosis. Int Orthop 1:39–42, 1977.
9. Solomon L: Patterns of osteoarthritis of the hip. J Bone Joint Surg 58:176–183, 1976.
10. Bentley G, Greer RB: Homotransplantation of isolated epiphyseal and articular cartilage chondrocytes into joint surfaces of rabbits. Nature 230:385–388, 1971.
11. Chalmers J: Transplantation immunity in bone homografting. J Bone Joint Surg 41B:160–179, 1959.
12. Craigmyle MGL: An autoradiographic and histochemical study of long term cartilage grafts in the rabbit. J Anat 92:467–471, 1958.
13. Elves MW: Immunological studies of the osteoarticular allograft. *In* Ingwersen DS (ed.): The Knee Joint. Amsterdam, Excerpta Medica, 1973, pp. 183–192.
14. Elves MW: A study of the transplantation antigens on chondrocytes from articular cartilage. J Bone Joint Surg 56B:178–185, 1974.
15. Elves MW, Zervas J: An investigation into the immunogenicity of various components of osteoarticular grafts. Br J Exp Pathol 55:344–351, 1974.
16. Elves MW: New knowledge of the immunology of bone and cartilage. Clin Orthop Rel Res 120:2327, 1976.
17. Elves MW: The joints and synovial fluid. *In* Sokoloff L (ed.): The Immunobiology of Joints and Synovial Fluid. New York, Academic Press, 1978, p. 331.
18. Gibson R: Bone and cartilage transplantation. *In* Rappaport FT, Dausset J: Human Transplantation. New York, Grune and Stratton, 1968, p. 313.
19. Stjernsward J: Studies in the transplantation of allogeneic cartilage across known histocompatibility barriers. Proceedings of the 10th Congress of the International Society of Blood Transfusions, 1964, pp. 197–202.
20. Wieslander J, Heinegard D: Immunochemical analysis of cartilage proteoglycans. Antigeneic determinants of substructures. Biochem J 179:35–45, 1979.
21. Bloom BR, David J: In Vitro Methods in Cell Mediated and Tumor Immunity. New York, Academic Press, 1976.
22. Friedlaender G: Immunology. *In* Albright J, Brand R: The Scientific Basis of Orthopaedics. New York, Appleton-Century-Crofts, 1979, pp. 437–479.
23. Roitt I: Essentially Immunology. 3rd ed. London, Blackwell Scientific Publications, 1977.
24. Allison AC, Denman AM, Barnes RD: Cooperating and controlling function of thymus derived lym-

phocytes in relationship to autoimmunity. Lancet 1:135, 1971.

25. McDevitt CA: Biochemistry of articular cartilage. Nature of proteoglycans and collagen of articular cartilage and their role in ageing and in osteoarthritis. Ann Rheum Dis 32:364–378, 1973.

26. Boake WC, Muir H: The non-antigenicity of chondroitin sulphate. Lancet 2:1222–1223, 1955.

27. DiFerrante N: Production of precipitins in the rabbit by protein-polysaccharide complex from bovine nasal septum. Fed Proc, Fed Am Soc Exp Biol 22:498, 1963.

28. Hamerman D, Rojkind M, Sandson J: Protein bound to hyaluronate: Chemical and immunological studies. Fed Proc 25:1040–1045, 1966.

29. Hamerman D, Sandson J: Antigenicity of connective tissue components. Mt Sinai J Med 37:453–465, 1970.

30. Loewi G: Localisation of chondromucoprotein in cartilage. Ann Rheum Dis 24:528–535, 1965.

31. Loewi G, Muir H: The antigenicity of chondromucoprotein. Immunology 9:119–127, 1965.

32. Pankovich AM, Korngold L: Comparison of the antigenic properties of nucleus pulposus and cartilage protein polysaccharide complexes. J Immunol 99:431–437, 1967.

33. Sandson J, Rosenberg L, White D: The antigenic determinants of the protein-polysaccharides of cartilage. J Exp Med 123:817–828, 1966.

34. Saunders AM, Mathews MB, Dorfman A: Antigenicity of chondroitin sulfate. Fed Proc 21:26, 1962.

35. White D, Sandson J, Rosenberg L, et al: The antigenicity of the protein polysaccharides of human cartilage. J Clin Invest 42:992–993, 1963.

36. Quinn RW, Cerroni R: Antigenicity of chondroitin sulfate. Proc Soc Exp Biol 96:268–269, 1957.

37. Baker J, Caterson B: The isolation of link protein from bovine nasal cartilage. Biochim Biophys Acta 532:249–259, 1966.

38. Brandt KD, Tsiganos CP, Muir H: Immunological relationships between proteoglycans of different hydrodynamic size from articular cartilage of foetal and mature pigs. Biochim Biophys Acta 320:453–468, 1973.

39. Caterson B, Baker MD, Levitt D, Paslay JE: Radioimmunoassay of the proteins associated with bovine nasal cartilage proteoglycan. J Biol Chem 254:2394–2399, 1979.

40. Heingard D, Axelsson I: The distribution of keratan sulfate in cartilage proteoglycans. J Biol Chem 252:1971–1978, 1977.

41. Herman JH, Dennis MW: Polydispersity of human articular cartilage amorphous matrix antigens. Clin Res 22:642A, 1974.

42. Oegema TR, Brown M, Dziewiatkowski DD: The link protein in proteoglycan aggregates from the rat chondrosarcoma. J Biol Chem 252:6470–6477, 1977.

43. Tang LH, Rosenberg L, Reiner A, Poole RA: Proteoglycans from bovine nasal cartilage. Properties of a soluble form of link protein. J Biol Chem 254:10523–10531, 1979.

44. Glynn LE, Holborow EJ: Conversion of tissue polysaccharides to auto-antigens by group-A beta-haemolytic streptococci. Lancet 2:449–451, 1952.

45. Baxter E, Muir H: The antigenicity of cartilage proteoglycans. Biochim Biophys Acta 279:276–281, 1972.

46. White D, Sandson J, Rosenberg L, et al.: The role of the protein moiety in the antigenicity of chondromucoprotein. Arthritis Rheum 6:305, 1963.

47. DiFerrante N: Precipitins in the rabbit produced by protein-polysaccharide from bovine nasal cartilage. Science 143:250–251, 1964.

48. DiFerrante N, Pauling M: Properties of antibodies to a protein-polysaccharide from bovine nasal cartilage. J Lab Clin Med 63:945–952, 1964.

49. DiFerrante N, Donnelly PV, Gregory JD, et al.: Antigenic determinants of two components of proteoglycan complex from bovine cartilage. FEBS Lett 9:149–151, 1970.

50. DiFerrante N, Donnelly PV, Sajdera SW: A segregated antigen in cartilage matrix. J Lab Clin Med 80:364–372, 1972.

51. Donnelly PV, DiFerrante N, Hrgovcic R: Antigenicity of protein-polysaccharide complexes from cartilage. Immunochemistry 6:353–360, 1969.

52. Tsiganos CP, Muir H: Studies on protein-polysaccharides from pig laryngeal cartilage. Heterogeneity, fractionation and characterisation. Biochem J 113:885–894, 1969.

53. Tsiganos CP: Immunologic differences of proteoglycans of cartilage. Z Klin Chem Klin Biochem 9:83, 1971.

54. Barland P, Janis R, Sandson J: Immunofluorescent studies of human articular cartilage. Ann Rheum Dis 25:156–164, 1966.

55. Sanderson J, Damon H, Mathews MB: Molecular localization of a cross-reactive antigenic determinant of cartilage proteoglycan. Chem Mol Biol Intercell Matrix Adv Study Inst 3:1563–1567, 1970.

56. Sandson J, Hamerman D, Janis R, Rojkind J: Immunologic and chemical similarities between the streptococcus and human connective tissue. Trans Assoc Am Physicians 81:249–257, 1968.

57. Keiser H, Shulman HJ, Sandson J: Immunochemistry of cartilage proteoglycan: Immunodiffusion and gel electrophoretic studies. Biochem J 126:163–169, 1972.

58. Keiser H, Sandson J: Immunology of cartilage proteoglycan. Fed Proc 32:1474–1477, 1973.

59. Keiser H, Sandson J: Immunodiffusion and gel electrophoretic studies of human articular cartilage proteoglycan. Arthritis Rheum 17:218–228, 1974.

60. Keiser H: Immunological studies of bovine nasal cartilage proteoglycan "link" proteins. Biochemistry 14:5304–5307, 1975.

61. Hamerman D, Sandson J: Immunologic cross-reactions between streptococcal hyaluronic acid and proteoglycans of human connective tissue. Chem Mol Biol Intercell Matrix Adv Study Inst 3:1537–1549, 1969.

62. Janis R, Sandson J, Smith C: Synovial cell synthesis of a substance immunologically like cartilage protein polysaccharide. Science 158:1464–1467, 1976.

63. Adelmann BC, Kirrane J: The structural basis of cell mediated immunological reaction of collagen. The species specificity of the cutaneous delayed hypersensitivity reaction. Immunology 25:123–130, 1973.

64. Beil W, Furthmayr H, Timpl R: Chicken antibodies to soluble rat collagen. I. Characterisation of the immune response by precipitation and agglutination methods. Immunochemistry 9:779–799, 1972.

65. Brown PC, Glynn LE: The antigenicity of sequential polypeptides. II. The antigenicity of some sequential polymers including several related to collagen. Immunology 25:251–260, 1973.

66. Jasin HE, Glynn LE: The antigenic properties of some synthetic poly-iminoacids. II. The antigenicity of polypeptides related to collagen peptides containing hydroxyproline and acetylhydroxyproline. Immunology 8:260–269, 1965.

67. Lindsley H, Mannik M, Bornstein P: The distribution

of antigenic determinants in rat skin collagen. J Exp Med 133:1309–1324, 1971.

68. Michaeli D, Martin GR, Kettman J, et al.: Localization of antigenic determinants in the polypeptide chains of collagen. Science 166:1522–1524, 1969.

69. Pontz B, Meigel W, Rauterberg J, Kuhn K: Localisation of two species-specific antigenic determinants on the peptide chains of calf-skin collagen. Eur J Biochem 16:50–54, 1970.

70. Wolff I, Wick G, Furthmayr H, et al.: Immunogenicity and specificity of collagen. VIII. Studies on the antigenic structure of soluble fish collagen. Immunology 18:843–847, 1970.

71. Timpl R, Furthmayr H, Beil W: Maturation of the immune response to soluble rat collagen: Late appearance of antibodies directed to N-terminal sites of the 2-chain. J Immunol 108:119–125, 1972.

72. Timpl R, Wick G, Gay S: Antibodies to distinct types of collagens and procollagens and their application in immunohistology. J Immunol Methods 18:165–182, 1977.

73. Timpl R, Wolff I, Furthmayr H, Steffen C: Immunogenicity and specificity of collagen. VI. Separation of antibody fractions with restricted specificity from anti-collagen sera using an immunoadsorbent technique. Immunology 15:145–151, 1968.

74. Timpl R, Wolff I, Wick G, et al: Immunogenicity and specificity of collagen. VII. Differences between various collagens demonstrated by cross reaction studies. J Immunol 101:725–729, 1968.

75. Furthmayr H, Beil W, Timpl R: Different antigenic determinants in the polypeptide chains of human collagen. FEBS Lett 12:341–344, 1971.

76. Furthmayr H, Stoltz M, Becker U, et al.: Chicken antibodies to soluble rat collagen. II. Specificity of the reaction with individual polypeptide chains and cyanogen bromide peptides of collagen. Immunochemistry 9:789–798, 1972.

77. Hahn E, Timpl R: Involvement of more than a single polypeptide chain in the helical antigenic determinants of collagen. Eur J Immunol 3:442–446, 1973.

78. Hahn E, Timpl R, Miller EJ: The production of specific antibodies to native collagens with the chain compositions (alpha 1(I)3, (alpha 1(II)3, and (alpha 1(I))2 alpha 2. J Immunol 113:421–423, 1974.

79. Nowack H, Hahn E, Timple R: Specificity of the antibody response in inbred mice to bovine type I and type II collagen. Immunology 29:621–628, 1975.

80. Steffen C, Timpl R, Wolff I: Immunogenitat und spezifitat von kollagen. 3. Erzeugugng und nachwies von antikollagen-antikorpern und serologischer vergleich non nativern und denaturiertem loslicher kollagen. Z Immunitatsforsch Allerg Klin Immunol 134:91–107, 1967.

81. Steffen C, Timpl R, Wolff I: Immunogenicity and specificity of collagen. V. Demonstration of three different antigenic determinants on calf collagen. Immunology 15:135–144, 1968.

82. Steffen C, Dichtl M, Knapp W, Brunner H: Immunogenicity and specificity of collagen. XII. Demonstration by immunofluorescence and haemagglutination of antibodies with different specificity to human collagen. Immunology 21:649–657, 1971.

83. Langer F, Gross AE, Greaves MD: The autoimmunogenicity of articular cartilage. Clin Exp Immunol 12:31–37, 1972.

84. Langer R, Gross AE: Immunogenicity of allograft articular cartilage. J Bone Joint Surg 55A:297–304, 1974.

85. Heyner S: The significance of the inter-cellular matrix in the survival of the cartilage allografts. Transplantation 8:666–677, 1969.

86. Gertzbein SD, Lance EM: The stimulation of lymphocytes of chondrocytes in mixed cultures. Clin Exp Immunol 24:102–109, 1976.

87. Gerzbein SD, Tait JH, Devlin SR, Argue S: The antigenicity of chondrocytes. Immunology 33:141–151, 1977.

88. Champion BR, Poole AR: Immunity to homologous type III collagen after partial meniscectomy and sham surgery in rabbits. Arthritis Rheum 25:274–285, 1972.

89. Jaffe HL: Degenerative Joint Disease in Metabolic, Degenerative and Inflammatory Diseases of Bones and Joints. Philadelphia, Lea and Febiger, 1972.

90. Kellgren JH, Moore R: Generalized osteoarthritis and Heberden's nodes. Br Med J 1:181–187, 1952.

91. Cooke TD, Hurd ER, Ziff M, Jasin HE: The pathogenesis of chronic inflammation in experimental antigen-induced arthritis. J Exp Med 135:323–338, 1972.

92. Herman JH, Hess EV: Immunopathologic studies in relapsing polychondritis. Arthritis Rheum 14:166, 1971.

93. Rajapakse DA, Bywaters EGL: Cell mediated immunity to cartilage proteoglycan in relapsing polychondritis. Clin Exp Immunol 16:497–502, 1974.

94. Steffen C: Relationship between collagen immunology and pathogenesis of rheumatoid arthritis. *In* Muller W, Harwerth HG, Fehr K (eds.): Rheumatoid Arthritis. New York, Academic Press, 1972, pp. 411–423.

95. Andriopoulos NA, Mestecky J, Miller EJ, Bennett JC: Antibodies to human native and denatured collagens in synovial fluids of patients with rheumatoid arthritis. Clin Immunol Immunopathol 6:209–212, 1976.

96. Cracchiolo A, Michaeli D, Goldberg LS, Fudenberg HH: The occurrence of antibodies to collagen in synovial fluids. Clin Immunol Immunopathol 3:567–574, 1975.

97. Menzel J, Steffen C, Kolarz R, et al.: Demonstration of antibodies to collagen and of collagen-anticollagen immune complexes in rheumatoid arthritis synovial fluids. Ann Rheum 35:446–450, 1976.

98. Michaeli D, Fudenberg HH: Incidence of antibodies to denatured collagen in rheumatoid arthritis. Arthritis Rheum 14:404, 1971.

99. Steffen C, Knapp W, Thumb N, et al.: Demonstration of collagen in synovial fluid cells of rheumatoid arthritis by immunofluorescence. Zlummunforsch 143:252, 1972.

100. Steffen C, Ludwig H, Knapp W: Collagen-anticollagen immune complexes in rheumatoid arthritis synovial fluid cells. Z Immunitatsforsch 147:229–235, 1974.

101. Endler AT, Zielinski C, Menzel EJ, et al: Leukocyte migration inhibition with collagen type I and collagen type III in rheumatoid arthritis and degenerative joint disease. Z Rheumatol 37:87–92, 1978.

102. Stuart JM, Postlethwaite AE, Townes AS, Kang AH: Cell mediated immunity to collagen and collagen chains in rheumatoid arthritis and other rheumatic diseases. Am J Med 69:13–18, 1980.

103. Herman JH, Houk JL, Dennis MV: Cartilage antigen dependent lymphotoxin release. Immunopathological significance in articular destructive disorders. Ann Rheum Dis 33:446–452, 1974.

104. Stastny P, Rosenthal M, Andreis M, et al.: Lymphokines in the rheumatoid joint. Arthritis Rheum 16:572, 1973.

5

Biomechanical Considerations*

Eric L. Radin, M.D.

It should not be surprising that the compressive stress under which joints function is considerably higher than might be first imagined, because muscle contracture is responsible for creating an equilibrium of moments and stability about a loaded joint. The major joints of the lower extremity—the knee, hip, and ankle—usually function under loads approximating 2.5 to 10 times the body weight.[1-3] Similar compressive stresses approximating 14 to 35 $\times$ 0.05 N/m² (200 to 500 lbs/inch²) are seen in the joints of the upper extremity. The load on joints is intermittent in nature, and activities of daily living create very high peak dynamic loads. Joint motion is characterized by frequent shut-downs and start-ups. It is remarkable that under such potentially punishing mechanical conditions, most joints function throughout the life of the individual without evidence of destruction of their major load-bearing areas. In this chapter, I will relate the structural characteristics of joints to their mechanical function and will attempt to explain the design characteristics that provide for an unusually long bearing service life under such adverse conditions.

GENERAL DESIGN

Each joint is unique in its configuration. The wide variation in configuration, considered on an individual joint basis, achieves maximum contact area for the most usual positions of loading, a desired range of motion, and stability.[4] Each joint has somewhat different load and positional requirements, and its individual

design reflects that. If a joint becomes unstable, it loses its fulcrum, and the muscles that move it can no longer act with maximum leverage. Thus, momentary displacement of a joint under load, subluxation, seriously decreases the acceleration that the limb segments can achieve about that joint. Stability in the joint is provided by ligaments, thickenings of the capsule, surrounding muscles, and the bony configuration of the joint itself.

The most proximal appendicular joints, the shoulder and the hip, have wide ranges of motion and are basically of a ball-and-socket design. Much of the stability about these joints is created by muscles that surround them, providing control and stability in all degrees of freedom. The specialized upper extremity requires an especially great range of motion at its base for optimal function, and the shoulder joint is a ball on a disk (Fig. 5–1A), creating little if any bony impingement and thus allowing a very wide range of motion. This range is further enhanced by mounting this joint on a movable platform, the scapula, which in turn articulates with the chest wall. It was initially taught that the first 90 degrees of shoulder motion was glenohumeral and that all subsequent forward flexion and abduction occurred between the scapula and the thorax. A group of investigators at the University of California[5] demonstrated that this concept was incorrect and that once 30 degrees of forward flexion had been achieved, the relationship of the scapulothoracic motion to the glenohumeral motion remained remarkably constant at a ratio of 2 to 1. In a subsequent analysis of 61 subjects, Freedman and Munro[6] found the ratio to be 2 degrees of scapulothoracic motion for each 3 degrees of glenohumeral motion,

*Supported by Grant AM-27127, NIH, USPHS

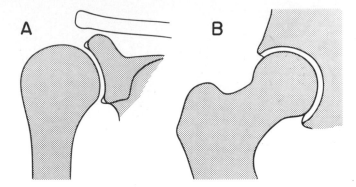

Figure 5–1. The lack of bony constraints about the shoulder joint *(A)* allows it a much greater range of motion than the hip joint *(B)*. It should be noted that in the absence of bony stability, as in the shoulder, the joint is dependent on muscles and ligaments for its stability.

but they noted a wide range of individual variation among subjects.

The ligaments and surrounding muscles play an important role in providing stability around the shoulder. The glenoid, with which the humeral head articulates, rarely exceeds a diameter of 3 to 4 cm, and the joint gains most of its stability from the surrounding heavy musculature.[7] Muscles require considerable space for origins, and for the shoulder, they utilize all available bony sites, including the chest wall, scapula, and clavicle.[8]

The other proximal appendicular ball-and-socket joint is the hip, which, unlike the shoulder, is primarily concerned with stance and in serving as the fulcrum for the body weight during those moments of single-leg stance that occur in ambulation. The hip has a well-developed bony socket (Fig. 5–1*B*). Inman[1] pointed out that in the frontal plane, the abductors have a moment arm that is approximately one-third as long as that of the body weight; thus, the abductors must generate a force approximating twice the body weight in order to obtain a torque equilibrium about the hip (Fig. 5–2). This means that the overall load in the joint approximates 3 times the body weight. Inman's work has been repeated by McLeish and Charnley[9] in live subjects rather than cadavers, and these investigators estimate that with limbs symmetrically disposed in the normal walking attitude, the muscle force ranged from 1 to 1.8 times the body weight and the joint forces from 2 to 7 times the body weight. The effects of sparing the hip joint with canes and similar supports are nicely discussed by Denham.[10] Friedrich Pauwels, a biomechanician, pointed out that it is possible for bony operations to alter the leverage through which the abductor muscles act and thus significantly change the

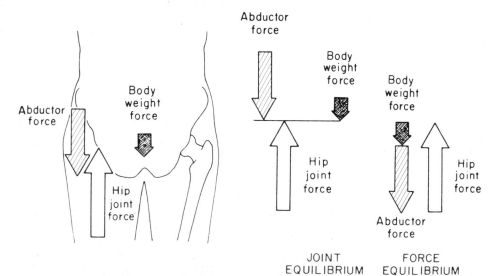

JOINT EQUILIBRIUM   FORCE EQUILIBRIUM

Figure 5–2. In order to maintain stability about the hip in single-leg stance, the abductors must generate a force approximating twice the body weight. (From Radin EL, Simon SR, Rose RM, Paul IL: Practical Biomechanics for the Orthopedic Surgeon. New York, John Wiley & Sons, Inc., 1979.)

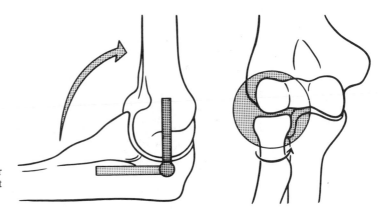

Figure 5–3. In the elbow, the humeroulnar joint acts as a hinge. Rotation occurs about the humeroradial joint.

load on the hip joint.[11] Such changes can theoretically exert profound effects on the metabolism of cells in both the cartilage and the subchondral bone.

The middle appendicular linkages in the limbs, the knee and the elbow, are both hinges that allow axial rotation. The elbow allows a freer range of axial rotation (160 degrees to 180 degrees) than does the knee. In general, joints of the lower extremity are more stable than are joints in the upper extremity. Compared with the knee, the elbow is a relatively unstable joint and basically has its hinge and rotatory functions separated, with the radius rotating on the humerus and the ulna, acting through its joint with the humerus, serving as the hinge (Fig. 5–3). Many of the studies of the biomechanics of the elbow involve injuries sustained from repeated high-acceleration activities such as throwing,[12–14] but kinematic studies of this joint have been published.[15, 16]

The knee is a very stable joint, and consequently, complete or even partial dislocations are rare. The knee resembles a rounded, condylar, cam-shaped bearing that allows rota-

tion—a hinge with rounded-off edges[17] (Fig. 5–4). The rounded-off edges allow the hinges to rotate axially. The space created by the curved periphery is filled by fibrocartilaginous menisci, which act as washers, provide stability, and prevent limited central point contact of the articular surfaces (Fig. 5–4). The initial suggestion made in 1942[18] that the menisci bear load has since been confirmed experimentally.[19–21] The forces across the knee joint have been extensively studied by several authors[22–24] and have been simulated in vitro.[25] This latter study determined that the force required by the quadriceps musculature to stabilize the knee in the sagittal plane rose from 75% of the load on the hip at 15 degrees of knee flexion to 410% at 60 degrees of knee flexion, with the stresses in the tibiofemoral and patellofemoral (kneecap) joint surfaces increasing in the same fashion. The maximum joint force is said to vary between 2 and 4 times the body weight. Reilly and Martens,[26] on the basis of free body diagrams, calculated that the patellofemoral joint reaction force obtained a level of approximately 3.5 times

Figure 5–4. The knee resembles a rounded, condylar, cam-shaped bearing that has rounded-off edges to allow rotation. The menisci of the knee act as washers to maintain stability. (From Radin EL: Biomechanics of the knee joint. Orthop Clin North Am 4:541, 1973.)

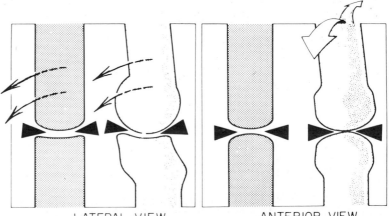

LATERAL VIEW   ANTERIOR VIEW

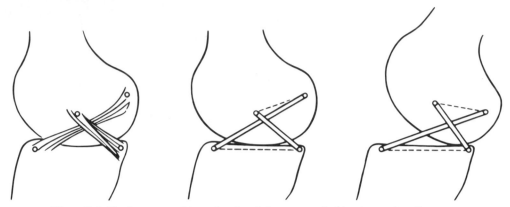

Figure 5–5. The knee resembles a four-bar linkage controlled by the cruciate ligaments.

the body weight. The torque created by the quadriceps in the sagittal plane can be significantly increased by altering the length of the lever arm through which it acts.[27]

The patella acts to increase the leverage of the quadriceps muscle. Patellectomy creates an almost 50% reduction in quadriceps strength.[28] In the frontal plane, the body weight, acting through its lever arm medial to the knee, is balanced by the lateral muscles and ligaments, which are balanced by a shorter lever arm.[24]

The combination of rolling and sliding motion that occurs in the sagittal plane makes the knee resemble a four-bar linkage*[29] (Fig. 5–5) controlled by the cruciate and collateral ligaments.[30] This creates a series of instant centers of rotation in the sagittal plane, which were first described by Fick[31] in 1910. Although it has been suggested that alterations in the path of the instant centers might have diagnostic significance in cases of internal derangement of the knee,[32] Walker has subsequently shown that the medial and lateral parts of the joint, because of the significant difference in their diameters, create their own individual paths of instant centers. Furthermore, he reports that the variation from subject to subject is too great to allow reproducible measurement.[33]

The relative contributions of the various ligamentous and capsular structures to knee stiffness and laxity have been studied extensively.[34–48] The conclusions are contradictory, and much controversy still exists. One of the problems is that when studies are performed in vitro, active muscle contraction is eliminated

and abnormal motions can occur. With the few in vivo studies that have been performed, it is impossible to control all the possible variables. Needless to say, the knee is probably the most complicated joint in the body;[49] however, newer approaches using finite-element analysis to study ligamentous function[50] and to calculate the joint contact stresses[51] hold considerable promise.

The concept of conservation of energy dictates that the diameter of both the upper and lower limbs diminishes as one moves distal to the center of gravity, so that only the joints closest to the trunk can have a ball-and-socket design that requires stabilization from all sides with bulky muscles. The wrist and foot, which cannot be as totally surrounded by muscles as the more centrally placed joints, are stabilized mainly by ligaments and bony configuration. Thus, the more peripheral joints—the wrist, ankle, and hindfoot—depend more on bony impingement for stability. The ankle is a very complexly shaped mortised hinge. Together with the hindfoot joints, it manages to summate several separate hinge motions at angles to one another to create the effect of universal bearing just at the base of the touch-down area of the lower limb[52] (Fig. 5–6). Kinematic studies of the ankle, performed initially by Braune and Fischer[53] in 1895 and more recently by the Case Western Reserve University group, confirm this theoretical observation.[54]

The earliest recorded measurements of pressure distribution in the foot were made in 1882 by Beely,[55] when he had a patient step on a thin bag filled with plaster of Paris. Morton[56] was the first to use corrugated rubber mats overlaid with inked fabric; various modifications of the mat technique were later developed and are still in current use, including the utilization of pressure transducers placed into

---

*Although only two bars of the "four-bar" system are rigid (the other two being ligamentous), the shape of the articulating surfaces is such that the ligaments are always under considerable tension, thus causing them to act as rigid members.

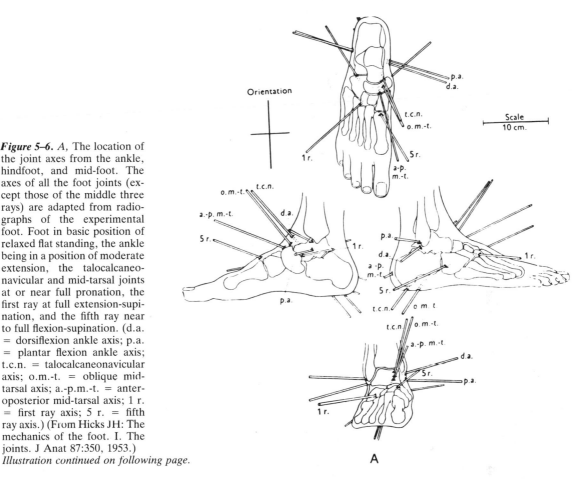

Figure 5–6. *A,* The location of the joint axes from the ankle, hindfoot, and mid-foot. The axes of all the foot joints (except those of the middle three rays) are adapted from radiographs of the experimental foot. Foot in basic position of relaxed flat standing, the ankle being in a position of moderate extension, the talocalcaneonavicular and mid-tarsal joints at or near full pronation, the first ray at full extension-supination, and the fifth ray near to full flexion-supination. (d.a. = dorsiflexion ankle axis; p.a. = plantar flexion ankle axis; t.c.n. = talocalcaneonavicular axis; o.m.-t. = oblique mid-tarsal axis; a.-p.m.-t. = anteroposterior mid-tarsal axis; 1 r. = first ray axis; 5 r. = fifth ray axis.) (From Hicks JH: The mechanics of the foot. I. The joints. J Anat 87:350, 1953.)

Illustration continued on following page.

A

shoes.[57] The study techniques have included deformation of Perspex rods photographed as the subject walked over them[58]; analysis of data from pressure transducers attached to the sole of the bare foot[59]; calculation of forces transmitted to stress-sensitive force plates during gait[60, 61]; and analysis of patterns seen with pressure-sensitive dye-filled microcapsules.[62] All authors conclude that initial pressure is on the heel at foot-strike and moves across the lateral aspect of the sole and then medially again across the ball of the foot, with the final push-off occurring by action of the flexor pollicis longus at the great toe. The arch of the foot, in normal patients, is non–weight-bearing.

The biomechanics of the hand have been studied extensively. Because the hand represents a highly specialized appendage combining both fine motion (for dexterity) and considerable strength in grasp, care of patients with hand problems and study of the functional anatomy and engineering principles have evolved into a subspecialized discipline. The interested reader is referred to many fine reviews of this subject.[63–69]

JOINT COMPOSITION

The materials that compose human joints are universal throughout vertebrates. The articulating joints are all surfaced with articular cartilage, the base of which is calcified. This calcified cartilage rests on a subchondral bony plate, which is in turn supported by spongy bone (Fig. 5–7). The cartilage is bathed in a lubricant, synovial fluid, which also serves as the source of nutrition. The joint space is enclosed by a fibrous capsule; the innermost lining, the synovium, serves as a filter for diffusion of materials into the synovial fluid and also adds several major constituents. The joint is held together by ligaments and is traversed by tendons and, in some instances, by muscles as well.

Articular Cartilage

The chemical composition and structure of articular cartilage are described in considerable detail in Chapter 3. Cartilage is composed of a systematically oriented fibrous network of

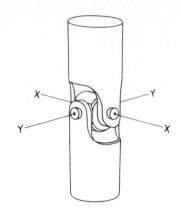

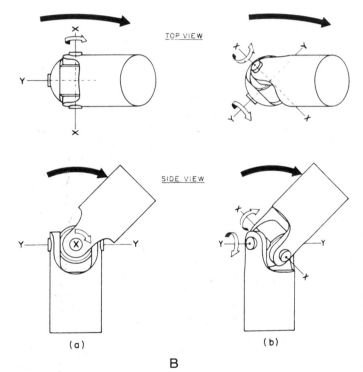

PLANE OF MOTION
PERPENDICULAR TO X-AXIS

PLANE OF MOTION
PERPENDICULAR TO NEITHER AXIS

TOP VIEW

SIDE VIEW

(a)

(b)

B

Figure 5–6 (Continued). B, A universal joint showing that these joints collaborate to always keep the foot flat on the ground in spite of uneven terrain. (From Wright DC, Desai SM, Henderson WH: Action of the subtalar and ankle-joint complex during the stance phase of walking. J Bone Joint Surg 46A:363, 1964.)

collagen that entraps large, highly negatively charged proteoglycan macromolecular aggregates.[70] The collagen fibers at the surface are tangential, forming a skin-like enclosure; those at the base are arranged perpendicular to the bone, acting to anchor the interface; the fibers in the middle zone of the cartilage appear to be randomly oriented. The collagen-proteoglycan structure traps or binds large amounts of water (up to 80% by weight) and small solutes. As in any living tissue, cells are present to maintain and replace the structural molecules as necessary. Because articular cartilage is avascular, these cells, the chondrocytes, re-

ceive their nutrition by diffusion from the synovial fluid. The avascularity of articular cartilage is a functional necessity, because the tissue can be expected to deform with strains exceeding 40% under normal service conditions. One can imagine what would happen to the flow of blood through small vessels subjected to such compression! It has been calculated, on the basis of measurements of the diffusion rates through cartilage and the metabolic requirements of the cells, that the maximal tolerable cartilage thickness for continued chondrocyte life is 6 mm.[71] Anatomically, that turns out to be the case. Such a thin layer

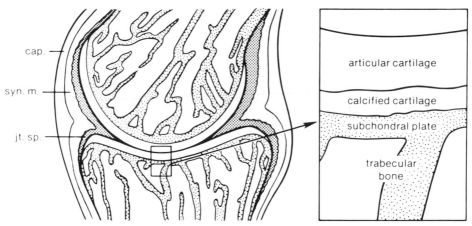

Figure 5–7. The articular cartilage rests on calcified cartilage that sits on the subchondral plate, which is supported by spongy bone. The joint is surrounded by a fibrous capsule (cap.) and lined by a synovial membrane (syn. m.), which creates the lubricant in the joint space (jt. sp.).

probably has a limited role as a peak dynamic force attenuator or shock absorber, suggesting that the principal role for articular cartilage is as a bearing surface; its quite remarkable lubricating characteristics keep the coefficient of friction in joints very low.

Denuded of their articular cartilage, the subchondral bony plates of a joint do not precisely fit. It is the relatively compliant articular cartilage that acts to provide the maximum surface contact area. Cartilage thickness is not related to stress but rather to the degree of underlying bony congruity; it is maximal in joints with the poorest bony "fit" and least in joints with relatively good bony congruity. Articular cartilage in compression has a modulus of elasticity approximating 7×10^6 N/m^2 (10,000 psi). Articular cartilage is highly confined, owing to its generally ordered fibrous component, its skin-like surface, and its very firm attachment to its underlying bed. These rather strong restrictions to unlimited deformation make the tissue very anisotropic in behavior. For these reasons, the data obtained in tests performed on specimens of cartilage cut from joints and attempts to measure the Poisson's ratio of articular cartilage must be considered subject to error. Cartilage deformation is strain-rate related, and its viscoelastic behavior has been well studied[72]; within the physiologic range, under high strain rates, cartilage probably acts elastically.

Coefficients of friction of animal joints have been measured as low as 0.002,[73] half that of rubber on steel and one-tenth that of an ice skate on ice. Two hydrated cartilage surfaces will contain a fluid film between them under all conceivable conditions of service.[74] Because

of its highly charged proteoglycan phase, cartilage is not very permeable to water.[75] The ability of articular cartilage to maintain a squeeze film under a wide variety of conditions lies principally in the extrusion of water that occurs as cartilage compresses under load. Thus, with compression, fibrous and proteoglycan phases remain unchanged, but the observed deformation largely results from the movement of water.[76] Because in the adult the underlying bony bed on which the articular cartilage rests is impervious to fluid flow and the cartilage matrix is moderately dense, fluid flow within the substance of the cartilage is limited. The water, displaced by cartilage compression, will preferentially flow in the path of least resistance, which is out onto the surface of the cartilage. The precise flow depends on the local pressure gradient at the surface but mainly occurs peripheral to the zone of impending contact. In a moving joint, under most physiologic conditions and under usual loads, the water tends to be pushed just in front of the zone of impending contact.[77] When the compression is released, cartilage regains its original height. The trapped proteoglycan within the compressed cartilage contains enough of a fixed charge, now depleted of its balanced counterions, which flow out with the water, to osmotically suck the water and small solutes back into the matrix.[78]

As mentioned, the collagen in the mid-zone of the articular cartilage appears at the ultrastructural level to be randomly oriented. However, under compression perpendicular to the surface, mid-zone collagen tends to orient preferentially in opposition to the stress.[79] The junction between cartilage and its underlying calcified cartilage and the subchondral plate under it undulates. Such a configuration tends to transform shear stress into compressive stress and aids in keeping the articular cartilage from being sheared off its bony backing.[80] The modulus of elasticity of the underlying calcified cartilage lies somewhere between that of cartilage (7×10^6 N/m^2 [10,000 psi]) and cancellous bone (70×10^6 N/m^2 [100,000 psi]).[81] The calcified cartilage thus acts to minimize stress concentrations at the bone-cartilage interface.

The spring effect of the mid-zone collagen is augmented by the inherent property of the proteoglycans to maintain a maximal domain because of repulsion of like charges both intramolecularly and intermolecularly. Unconstrained proteoglycan molecules will bind or trap thousands of times their own weight in water, as will collagen.[82]

Subchondral Bone

The calcified cartilage sits on a thin subchondral plate of bone that rests on an area of spongy or cellular bone. (The word "cellular" as used here is defined in an engineering sense as "containing chambers or cells.") Spongy or "cancellous" bone has a volume fraction of usually less than 50% and a modulus of elasticity of about one-tenth to one-twentieth that of the bone in the shaft.[81] The overlying cartilage acts to transmit load. It appears to have little effect in distributing that load.[83] There is evidence to suggest that deformation of the subchondral bone is mainly responsible for maximal joint fit under high loads.[84] It has been found that for joints to conform fully under maximal loads, they must be slightly incongruous in the unloaded state.[85] Because of the compliance of spongy bone, if one starts with a congruous situation and then loads the joint, high spots occur, with resultant areas of stress concentration (Fig. 5–8). Deformation of subchondral bone is therefore of great importance to the effective distribution of stress within a joint. A low frequency of microfracture of the cancellous subchondral bone occurs physiologically.[86] It has been suggested that overstraining of the sheets and interconnecting sheets and struts that make up this bone results in microfracture, with the plates healing in a preferential trajectory direction. Such a mechanism may, to a large extent, be responsible for the resultant organization of the trabecular bone in a trajectoral pattern relative to its most usual stress distribution as well as the

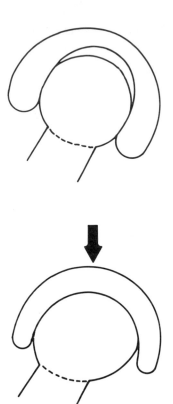

Figure 5–8. Placing a joint under load creates a primary deformation of subchondral cancellous bone that determines the contact area of the joint. Although articular cartilage is deformable, it is much too thin a layer to significantly deform. Decreasing deformability or compliance of subchondral bone decreases the contact area of the joint and will dramatically increase the stress on the articular cartilage. (From Radin EL, Paul IL, Rose RM, Simon SR: The mechanism of joints as it relates to their degeneration. *In* American Academy of Orthopedic Surgeons: Symposium on Osteoarthritis. St. Louis, C. V. Mosby Co., 1976.)

mechanism of the strengthening of bone consistently subjected to moderate loading.[87] The microfractures heal with a callous scaffolding, causing a reduction in the contiguity of the intertrabecular spaces, an increase in the volume fracture of the material, and a stiffening of the subchondral bone, which, depending on the stress history, may be transient or permanent.

Ligaments

Ligaments are fibrous structures that act to maintain joint stability and to guide joint motion. Most joint motion is a combination of sliding and rolling. The advantage of this combined movement is to maintain, in any particular orientation, maximum lever arms through which the force couple stabilizing the joint can act.[88] The greater the lever arm, the less the force required to create a moment, resulting in the lowest possible compressive stress on the joint. The ligaments are mostly collagenous and have very complicated fibrous arrangements, so that certain parts of the ligament are in tension throughout the range of motion of a particular joint.[34] Not all the ligaments are extra-articular; some are intra-articular. In the knee, for example, the intra-articular cruciate ligaments function as two parts of the four-bar linkage that dictate the precise combination of rolling and sliding motion between the articular surfaces of the knee and knee flexion, as discussed above. Because ligaments function as tension bands, their point of attachment to bone is a "stress riser," and attempts to repair ligament-bone junctions with screws or staples are frequently unsuccessful for this reason. Anatomically, the ligament-bone junction is a fairly complex, widespread area.

Menisci

Intra-articular fibrocartilages or menisci exist in several human joints. It would appear as if the menisci primarily function as washers to enable joints that are basically hinge joints to rotate by rounding off their edges.[51] Without washers, these joints would have fairly small articular cartilage contact areas. Thus, the menisci are clearly load-bearing and also act to spread the load. The stresses in the menisci-containing joints are not greater than those in other joints, and menisci would not seem to be essential for shock-absorbing purposes, but if present, they can help in this regard. Tears within the substance of the menisci or rips in their moorings can result in displacement of these washers and can cause derangements of motion as well as areas of stress concentration on the articular cartilage surfaces.[89] The suggestion that menisci are important in lubrication is difficult to substantiate.

Synovial Fluid and Joint Lubrication

The main difference between synovial fluid and serum (aside from the absence of certain proteins such as fibrinogen) is that synovial fluid contains a large sugar-protein complex, hyaluronate. It is this molecule that is responsible for the characteristic non-Newtonian behavior of synovial fluid. It was these flow characteristics that led early investigators to assume that joints were lubricated hydrodynamically. However, joints are obviously intermittently oscillating and not constantly rotating bearings and are therefore unsuited to hydrodynamic lubrication. The major evidence destroying the concept that hydrodynamic mechanisms were important in joint lubrication was the finding that the coefficient of friction of joints lubricated with synovial fluid was unaltered by enzymatic destruction of its viscosity.[90] Hydrodynamic lubrication plays no significant conceptual role in joint lubrication, although at some instant of time, in mid-cycle, there may indeed be a thin layer of motion induced between the articulating surfaces.

This does not mean to imply that the presence of hyaluronate, which is responsible for the viscosity of joint fluid, is unimportant. Most of the resistance to joint motion, well over 99% of it, comes from periarticular soft tissues and resistance of muscle.[91] Less than 1% of the frictional resistance comes from cartilage-on-cartilage friction. Soft tissues actually make up the largest proportion of the rubbing area within a joint. The inner lining, the synovial membrane, in order to allow large amounts of motion, is expansive and folded on itself. Upon motion of the joint, this membrane must move both upon itself and upon articular cartilage. Most of the so-called noncontact area of the articular surface is actually involved in synovium-on-cartilage lubrication. There is no area in any joint where synovium articulates directly on the bone. It is hyaluronate that lubricates this soft tissue system.[92] Such lubrication by hyaluronate makes joint fluid viscous and thixotropic, tends to keep some fluid pooled in the outer recesses of the joint, and gives the synovial fluid a great adhesive quality. Hyaluronate solutions are difficult to rub off one's fingers or to wash off synovium. One cannot pat or sponge it off. Synovium-on-synovium and synovium-on-cartilage surfaces are usually lightly loaded in contrast to the cartilage-on-cartilage surfaces. Certain places where tendons cross joints would subject this local area of soft tissue to a high load. Nature has provided, in just these places of high stress, either special sheaths for the tendons to slide through or small bones within the substance of the tendon, sesamoid bones. These small bones have articular cartilage surfaces and convert potential soft-tissue lubricating surfaces into cartilage-on-cartilage ones. The patella is the most obvious example of a sesamoid bone. Sesamoid bones also act

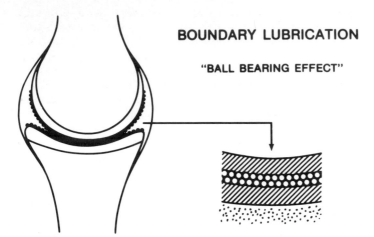

BOUNDARY LUBRICATION

"BALL BEARING EFFECT"

Figure 5–9. Articular cartilage is lubricated by a boundary phenomenon under all but heavy loads.

to increase the lever arm and thus the torque of the muscles that contain them.

Cartilage-on-cartilage lubrication under light loads is handled by a boundary lubricating mechanism (Fig. 5–9).[93] The molecule responsible for this is not hyaluronate, but another glycoprotein molecule,[94] which may have some components contributed by the cartilage itself. It is this glycoprotein that provides the lubricating advantage of synovial fluid over buffer in the cartilage-on-cartilage system. This boundary mechanism is, of course, most effective under light loads.[74] At high loads, the boundary molecules tend to be abraded off the surface. Saline solution lubricates cartilage-on-cartilage systems almost as well as synovial fluid, with a remarkably low coefficient of friction.[95] This coefficient decreases with increasing load, suggesting a fluid film mechanism. The film is contributed by two sources. One is the lubricant already in the joint space, which is entrapped as the relatively deformable articular surfaces come together. The other source of the fluid in the film is the cartilaginous interstitial fluid, which is forced onto the surface peripheral to the zone of impending contact by deformation of the cartilage. In a sliding or rolling joint, this fluid will be naturally included in future fluid films. Elastohydrodynamic effects tend to narrow the intracartilaginous space at the periphery of the zone of contact and help trap this fluid film. The viscosity of the fluid does not seem to play a key role, because fluid films are still maintained under maximal loads with nonviscous saline solution as the lubricant. The pressurization of the interstitial fluid within the cartilage helps trap the fluid, as does the shutdown of permeability secondary to cartilage deformation.[27] Fluid cannot flow into the cartilage

and has difficulty running out into the zone of impending contact. This hydrostatic mechanism will improve as the pressure increases up to the point at which the underlying bone grossly fractures. The hydrostatic mechanism will not function well at low pressure, and under mild loads the boundary or surface lubricating mechanism will predominate. The combination of the boundary and hydrostatic lubricating mechanisms provides the joint with ideal lubrication throughout a wide range of loading conditions, even with frequent shutdown and start-up. Joint motion under high load from a stopped position does not increase the coefficient of friction by more than about 20% and does so only for a brief interval of the first cycle.[96]

WEAR AND TEAR

It is obvious that the continued function of the lubricating system within joints depends to a great extent on the integrity of the articular cartilage.[97] When this bearing surface is worn away, "degenerative joint disease,"* or osteoarthrosis, is said to be taking place.

The conditions under which joints are normally asked to function would be punishing for any bearing. There are several natural protective mechanisms that normally function to insure a long service life for the joint. First, articular cartilage is almost shear-free. It rubs with an extremely low coefficient of friction at the surface under all conditions, and any shear stress within the cartilage is normally trans-

---

*This is generally considered to be a poor term, as such arthritis is characterized at the cellular level by a proliferative rather than a degenerative response.[33]

formed to compressive stress at the calcified cartilage junction.[80] The compressive stress is borne mainly by the pressurized water and is passed through onto the underlying bony bed. Making cuts with a scalpel or knife perpendicular to the surface of the articular cartilage does not cause the cartilage to wear and does not cause arthritis.[98] The lubricating systems are sufficient to function even in the presence of significant local loss of pressurization.[99] Perhaps the widespread contact areas play a role in this regard. Removing all the cartilage in the weight-bearing areas will lead to significant stress concentration and joint wear.[100] One cannot wear out intact articular cartilage or even scarified articular cartilage by simple oscillation of the joint, even under high loads. It is necessary to create an internal shear stress by imparting a peak impulsive load during the cycle.[8] This wear process can be speeded up by locally stiffening the underlying subchondral bone. If the bone is stiffer and less able to conform, a stiffness gradient is created under the cartilage, probably creating significant shear stresses within the cartilage. Experimentally, animals subjected to impulsive loads while their legs are moving develop osteoarthrosis of their knees.[101] The subchondral bone is noted to be significantly stiffer before any mechanical deterioration can be detected in the cartilage. Examination of this bone reveals a higher-than-normal incidence of healing trabecular microfractures.[86]

Such observations suggest that the attenuation of peak dynamic force is important if cartilage is to survive intermittent loading during joint motion, a very frequent physiologic activity. The mechanisms that protect the articular cartilage are several. First, there is the conformation of the underlying bony bed, in which the relatively compliant subchondral bone plays a measurable role.[84] Deformation of bone protects its overlying cartilage. The subchondral bone exists in sufficiently deep layers so that its ability to deform, in terms of joint conformation, can be significant. Furthermore, we know that patients with fairly deformable bone are spared osteoarthrosis and are instead plagued by numerous clinical fractures.[102] Fracture in and of itself is an elegant attenuator of peak dynamic force. Physiologically, small numbers of microfractures of the underlying cancellous structure occur. If the impulsive load is high enough, grossly evident macrofracture results. Such injuries, if they fail to disturb the integrity of the joint itself, actually spare the cartilage. As long as the

bones heal without malalignment of the joint, there is no problem. If a malalignment occurs, however, the stress distribution is altered and the joint may well be subjected to secondary trauma.

In the intact animal, the major shock-absorbing mechanisms are probably musculoskeletal and involve reflexual activity. Joint motion associated with the stretching of muscles that are under tension can absorb vast amounts of energy.[103] That is how we "prepare" to land from a fall or jump. We can sustain considerable impacts without damage if we are ready at the time we land. We prepare by positioning our joints and tensing appropriate muscles so that as we come down, we move the joint and pull on the tensed muscles.[104] The major jolts or damage we sustain occurs after falls that exceed the capability of our musculoskeletal system to attenuate them (such as a road accident or falls from a substantial height) or when we do not have time to prepare (as in unexpectedly stepping off a curb) or do not know when to prepare (as in a free-falling elevator).

Periarticular soft tissue and bone attenuate physiologically reasonable peak dynamic forces most effectively in the higher frequency ranges. These components tend to complement the stretching of muscle and joint motion, which appears to be more effective at low frequencies. Structures such as the heel pad have been shown to contribute to peak force attenuation over the whole possible frequency spectrum.[105]

REPAIR OF JOINTS

All living tissue has the potential to repair, but clearly not all organs and structures perform this step necessary to restore continuity. Damage confined to the articular cartilage in adult animals usually is not repaired. Although the cells under such circumstances are metabolically very active, actually undergo a proliferative response, and appear to be producing molecules that would be expected to participate in the repair process,[106] the repair usually does not succeed. In order to achieve repair, the stress on the cartilage must be reduced. It has been shown that reducing the stress either by decreasing the overall force on the joint by lengthening the muscles, or by surgically increasing the weight-bearing area of a joint to allow for greater conformation under load (as by an appropriate osteotomy)[11] is associated with clinical remissions of severely osteoarthritic joints.[107, 108] Therefore, the process of joint wear should not be thought of as one of unremitting progressive deterioration, although it can be and, untreated, frequently is. If it is kept in mind that the connective tissue cells are controlled by hormones, metabolic stimuli, and mechanical stimuli, one can understand how the changes of osteoarthritis can be reversed by mechanical means acting through altering cellular metabolism. Fractures can be made to heal faster under the influence of mechanical[109] or electromagnetic and electric energy.[110] It has been shown experimentally that fibrocartilage will form in the presence of hydrostatic pressures.[111] A better understanding of the relationship between cellular metabolism and mechanical stress will enable us to suggest more appropriate methods to stimulate joint healing.

Present concepts of the pathogenesis of osteoarthritis (see Chapter 7) suggest a major role for abnormal stresses on cartilage as key factors in disease initiation. Epidemiologic studies (see Chapters 1, 30, and 33) have demonstrated the importance of chronic injury to the induction of osteoarthritis in association with occupational or athletic overuse of joints. An increased incidence of osteoarthritis in individuals with an endomorphic mesomorphic somatotype may be related to increased biomechanical stresses in such individuals. Solomon[113] compared individuals with primary osteoarthritis of the hip with patients with fractures of the femoral neck; he demonstrated an above-average bone density in the group with osteoarthritis, with a statistically significant decrease in the group with fractures. These findings may be related to differences in resorption of forces across subchondral bone and cartilage in these two different populations.

Studies in our laboratories have suggested that the primary lesion in osteoarthritis may be in subchondral bone.[114, 115] When the knee joints of rabbits were exposed to repetitive impulsive loading, increased subchondral bone stiffness was associated with slight surface loss of proteoglycan and no change in collagen content. More striking were the findings of cell proliferation and increased synthesis of proteins and proteoglycan. Stiffening of subchondral bone associated with metabolic changes seen in osteoarthritis suggested that trabecular microfractures may occur early as part of the initial change of the osteoarthritic lesion. In further studies pursuing the same concept,

comparisons were made between joints of sheep subjected to daily walking on concrete and those of control sheep that were walked on compliant woodchip surfaces. Significant metabolic changes in articular cartilage and alterations in subchondral trabecular bone of the knee joints of the hard-surface walkers were noted. Contrary findings relative to the response of rabbit subchondral bone to repetitive impact loading were reported by Serink and colleagues.[116] Subchondral bone cores from impacted tibiae revealed progressive increased deformability under a constant force. These changes were considered consistent with bone softening. It was suggested that decreased mechanical support by softened subchondral bone contributed to cartilage degeneration. Other experimental studies have demonstrated a relationship between degenerative changes in joints and biomechanical alterations[117, 118] (see Chapter 6). In particular, valgus angular osteotomy of the tibia was associated with degenerative changes analogous to human osteoarthritis. Rats experimentally induced to be bipedal developed significant osteophyte formation at or around spinal curvatures where pressures were greatest, similar to osteophyte formation at concavities of the spine seen in humans with scoliosis.

Although a role for abnormal biomechanical stresses in the etiology of secondary osteoarthritis can be easily conceptualized, the role of biomechanical alterations in the etiology of primary osteoarthritis is more difficult to define. Extensive investigations have been and are being performed to determine how the effect of abnormal biomechanical stresses is translated into biochemical and metabolic changes in cartilage that ultimately lead to classic osteoarthritic lesions. Further details regarding the role of biomechanical stresses in osteoarthritis are described in the chapters on epidemiology (see Chapters 1, 30, and 33), experimental models (see Chapter 6), and etiopathogenesis (see Chapter 7) in this text.

References

1. Inman VT: Functional aspects of the abductor muscles of the hip. J Bone Joint Surg 29:607–619, 1947.
2. Maquet P: Biomechanics and osteoarthritis of the knee. Proc SICOT 11:317–357, 1969.
3. Stauffer RN, Chao EYS, Brewster RC: Force and motion analysis of the normal, diseased and prosthetic ankle joint. Clin Orthop 127:189–196, 1977.

4. Barnett CH, Davies DV, MacConaill MA: Synovial Joints: Their Structure and Mechanics. Springfield, Illinois, Charles C Thomas, 1961.

5. Inman VT, Dec JB, Saunders M, Abbott LC: Observations on the function of the shoulder joint. J Bone Joint Surg 26:1–30, 1944.

6. Freedman L, Munro RR: Abduction of the arm in the scapular plane: Scapular and glenohumeral movements. J Bone Joint Surg 48A:1503–1510, 1966.

7. Jones L: Shoulder joint: Anatomy and physiology with analysis of reconstructive operation following extensive injury. Surg Gynecol Obstet 75:433, 1942.

8. Radin EL: Biomechanics and functional anatomy. In Post M (ed.): Shoulder, Surgical and Nonsurgical Management. Philadelphia, Lea and Febiger, 1978, pp. 44–49.

9. McLeish RD, Charnley J: Abduction forces in the one-legged stance. J Biomech 3:191–209, 1970.

10. Denham RA: Hip mechanics. J Bone Joint Surg 41B:550–557, 1959.

11. Pauwels F: Biomechanics of the Normal and Diseased Hip. New York, Springer-Verlag, 1976.

12. Woods GW, Tullos HS, Wiking J: The throwing arm: Elbow joint injuries. J Sports Med 1(Suppl):43–47, 1973.

13. Nirschl RP: Tennis elbow. Orthop Clin North Am 4:787–800, 1973.

14. Priest JD, Jones HH, Chinn CJ, Nagel DA: The elbow and tennis: A study of expert players. Orthop Dig 3:9–17, 1975.

15. Morrey BF, Askew LJ, An KN, Chao EY: A biomechanical study of normal functional elbow motion. J Bone Joint Surg 63A:872–877, 1981.

16. London JT: Kinematics of the elbow. J Bone Joint Surg 63A:529–535, 1981.

17. Radin EL: Biomechanics of the knee joint. Its implications in the design of replacements. Orthop Clin North Am 4:539–546, 1973.

18. Bennett GA, Waine H, Bauer W: Changes in the Knee Joint at Various Ages with Particular Reference to the Nature and Development of Degenerative Joint Disease. New York, The Commonwealth Fund, New York Academy of Medicine, 1942.

19. Kettelkamp DB, Jacobs AW: Tibiofemoral contact area—determination and implications. J Bone Joint Surg 54A:349–356, 1972.

20. Maquet PG, Van de Berg AJ, Simonet JC: Femorotibial weight-bearing areas. Experimental determination. J Bone Joint Surg 57A:766–771, 1975.

21. Walker PS, Erkman MJ: The role of the menisci in force transmission across the knee. Clin Orthop 109:184–192, 1975.

22. Morrison JB: The mechanics of the knee joint in relation to normal walking. J Biomech 3:51–61, 1970.

23. Perry J, Antonelli D, Ford W: Analysis of knee-joint forces during flexed-knee stance. J Bone Joint Surg 57A:961–967, 1975.

24. Maquet P: Biomechanics of the Knee. Berlin, Springer-Verlag, 1976.

25. Engin AE, Korde MS: Biomechanics of normal and abnormal knee joint. J Biomech 7:325–334, 1974.

26. Reilly DT, Martens M: Experimental analysis of the quadriceps muscle force and patello-femoral joint reaction force for various activities. Acta Orthop Scand 43:126–137, 1972.

27. Maquet P: Un traitment biomécanique de l'arthrose fémoro-patellaire. L'avancement du tendon rotulien. Rev Rhum 30:779–783, 1963.

28. Sutton FS, Thompson CH, Lipke J, Kettelkamp DB: The effect of patellectomy on knee function. J Bone Joint Surg 58A:537–540, 1976.

29. Huson A: The functional anatomy of the knee joint: The closed kinematic chain as a model of the knee joint. In Ingwersen OS, Van Linge B, Van Rens TJG, et al. (eds.): The Knee Joint. Amsterdam, Excerpta Medica, 1974, pp. 163–168.

30. Menschik A: Mechanik des Kniegelenkes. II. Teil: Schlussrotation. Z Orthop 113:338–400, 1975.

31. Fick R: Handbuch der Anatomie und Mechanik der Gelenke. Jena, G. Fischer, 1910.

32. Frankel VH, Burstein AH, Brooks DB: Biomechanics of internal derangement of the knee. J Bone Joint Surg 53A:945–962, 1971.

33. Walker PS, Shoji H, Erkman MJ: The rotational axis of the knee and its significance to prosthesis design. Clin Orthop 89:160–170, 1972.

34. Brantigan OC, Voshell AF: The mechanics of the ligaments and menisci of the knee joint. J Bone Joint Surg 23:44–66, 1941.

35. Slocum DB, Larson RL: Rotatory instability of the knee. Its pathogenesis and a clinical test to demonstrate its presence. J Bone Joint Surg 50A:211–225, 1968.

36. Kennedy JC, Fowler PJ: Medial and anterior instability of the knee. An anatomical and clinical study using stress machines. J Bone Joint Surg 53A:1257–1270, 1971.

37. Roberts TDM: Standing with a bent knee. Nature 230:499–501, 1971.

38. White AA, Raphael IG: The effect of quadriceps loads and knee position on strain measurements of the tibial collateral ligament. Acta Orthop Scand 43:176–187, 1972.

39. Wang CJ, Walker PS: The effects of flexion and rotation on the length patterns of the ligaments of the knee. J Biomech 6:587–596, 1973.

40. Kennedy JC, Weinberg HW, Wilson AS: The anatomy and function of the anterior cruciate ligament. J Bone Joint Surg 56A:223–235, 1974.

41. Noyes FR, DeLucas JL, Torvik PJ: Biomechanics of anterior cruciate ligament failure: An analysis of strain-rate sensitivity and mechanisms of failure in primates. J Bone Joint Surg 56A:236–253, 1974.

42. Shaw J, Murray DG: The longitudinal axis of the knee and the role of the cruciate ligaments in controlling transverse rotation. J Bone Joint Surg 56A:1603–1609, 1974.

43. Warren LF, Marshall JL, Girgis F: The prime static stabilizer of the medial side of the knee. J Bone Joint Surg 56A:665–674, 1974.

44. Girgis FG, Marshall JL, Al Monajem ARS: The cruciate ligaments of the knee joint. Clin Orthop 106:216–231, 1975.

45. Furman W, Marshall JL, Girgis FG: The anterior cruciate ligament. J Bone Joint Surg 58A:179–185, 1976.

46. Hughston JC, Andrews JR, Cross MJ, Moschi A: Classification of knee ligament instabilities. Part I. The medical compartment and cruciate ligaments. J Bone Joint Surg 58A:159–172, 1976.

47. Kennedy JC, Hawkins RJ, Willis RB, Danylchuk KD: Tension studies of human knee ligaments. J Bone Joint Surg 58A:350–355, 1976.

48. Markolf KL, Mensch JS, Amstutz H: Stiffness and

laxity of the knee—the contributions of the supporting structures. J Bone Joint Surg 58A:583–594, 1976.

49. Radin EL: Our current understanding of normal knee mechanics and its implications for successful knee surgery. *In* McCollister Evarts C (eds.): AAOS Symposium on Reconstructive Surgery of the Knee. St. Louis, C. V. Mosby, 1978, pp. 37–46.

50. Crowninshield R, Pope MH, Johnson RJ: An analytical model of the knee. J Biomech 9:397–405, 1976.

51. Chand R, Haug E, Rim K: Stresses in the human knee joint. J Biomech 9:417–422, 1976.

52. Wright DG, Desai SM, Henderson WH: Action of the subtalar and ankle-joint complex during the stance phase of walking. J Bone Joint Surg 46A:361–382, 1964.

53. Braune W, Fischer O: Der Gang des Menschen. I. Teil. Versuche am Unbelasteten und Belasteten Menschen. Abhandld Math-Phys Cldk Sachs, Gesellsch Wissensch 21:153–332, 1895.

54. Sammarco GJ, Burstein AH, Frankel VH: Biomechanics of the ankle: A kinematic study. Orthop Clin North Am 4:75–96, 1973.

55. Beely F: Zur Mechanik des Stehens. Über die Bedeutung des Fussgewölbes beim Stehen. Langenbecks Arch Klin Chir 27:457–471, 1882.

56. Morton DJ: The Human Foot. New York, Columbia University Press, 1935.

57. Holden TS, Muncey RW: Pressures on the human foot during walking. Aust J Appl Sci 4:405, 1953.

58. Barnett CH: A plastic pedograph. Lancet 2:267–273, 1954.

59. Schwartz RP, Heath AL: The oscillographic recording and quantitative definition of functional disabilities of human locomotion. Arch Phys Med 30:568–578, 1949.

60. Hutton WC, Drabble GE: An apparatus to give the distribution of vertical load under the foot. Rheumatol Phys Med 11:313–317, 1972.

61. Grundy M, Tosh PA, McLeish RD, Smidt L: An investigation of the centres of pressure under the foot while walking. J Bone Joint Surg 57B:98–103, 1975.

62. Brand PW, Ebner JD: Pressure sensitive devices for denervated hands and feet. J Bone Joint Surg 51A:109–116, 1969.

63. Boyer, JH: Bunnel's Surgery of the Hand. 5th ed. Philadelphia, J. B. Lippincott, 1965.

64. Brand PW: Biomechanics of tendon transfer. Orthop Clin North Am 5:205–230, 1974.

65. Flatt AE: Kinesiology of the hand. AAOS Instructional Course Lectures 18:266–281, 1961.

66. Kaplan EB: Functional and Surgical Anatomy of the Hand. 2nd ed. Philadelphia, J. B. Lippincott, 1965.

67. Napier J: Functional aspects of the anatomy of the hand. *In* Rob C, Smith R (eds.): Clinical Surgery. London, Butterworth, 1966, pp. 1–3.

68. Steindler A: Kinesiology of the Human Body Under Normal and Pathological Conditions. Springfield, Illinois, Charles C Thomas, 1955, pp. 516–540.

69. Smith RJ: Balance and kinetics of the fingers under normal and pathological conditions. Clin Orthop 104:92–111, 1974.

70. Mankin HJ, Radin EL: Structure and function of joints. *In* McCarty DJ (eds.): Arthritis and Allied Conditions. 9th ed. Philadelphia, Lea and Febiger, 1979.

71. Maroudas A: Distribution and diffusion of solutes in articular cartilage. Biophys J 10:365–379, 1970.

72. Hayes WC, Mockros LF: Viscoelastic properties of human articular cartilage. J Appl Physiol 31:562–568, 1971.

73. Radin EL, Paul IL: Response of joints to impact loading. I. In vitro wear. Arthritis Rheum 14:356–362, 1971.

74. Radin EL, Paul IL, Pollock D: Animal joint behavior under excessive loading. Nature 226:554–555, 1970.

75. Edwards J: Physical characteristics of articular cartilage. *In* Lubrication and Wear in Living and Artificial Human Joints. London, Institute of Mechanical Engineering, 1967, p. 16.

76. Ekholm R, Norback B: On the relationship between articular changes and function. Acta Orthop Scand 21:81–98, 1951.

77. Mow VC, Mansour JM: The nonlinear interaction between cartilage deformation and interstitial fluid flow. J Biomech 10:31–39, 1977.

78. Linn FC, Sokoloff L: Movement and composition of interstitial fluid of cartilage. Arthritis Rheum 8:481–494, 1965.

79. McCall J: Load deformation response of microstructure of articular cartilage. *In* Wright V (ed.): Lubrication and Wear in Joints. Philadelphia, J. B. Lippincott, 1969, pp. 39–48.

80. Redler I, Mow VC, Zimny ML, Mansell J: The ultrastructure and biomechanical significance of the tidemark of articular cartilage. Clin Orthop 112:357–362, 1975.

81. Radin EL, Paul IL, Lowy M: A comparison of the dynamic force transmitting properties of subchondral bone and articular cartilage. J Bone Joint Surg 52A:444–456, 1970.

82. Tanford C: Physical Chemistry of Macromolecules. New York, John Wiley and Sons, 1961.

83. Radin EL, Paul IL: Does cartilage compliance reduce skeletal impact loads? The relative force-attenuating properties of articular cartilage, synovial fluid, periarticular soft tissues and bone. Arthritis Rheum 13:139–144, 1970.

84. Mital MA: Human Hip Joint. M. S. Thesis. Glasgow, University of Strathclyde, 1970.

85. Bullough P, Goodfellow J, O'Connor J: The relationship between degenerative changes and load-bearing in the human hip. J Bone Joint Surg 55B:746–758, 1973.

86. Radin EL, Parker GH, Pugh JW, et al.: Response of joints to impact loading. III. Relationship between trabecular microfractures and cartilage degeneration. J Biomech 6:51–57, 1973.

87. Pugh JW, Rose RM, Radin EL: A possible mechanism of Wolff's law: Trabecular microfractures. Arch Int Physiol Biochim 81:27–40, 1973.

88. O'Connor JJ: Personal communication, 1981.

89. Fairbank TJ: Knee joint changes after meniscectomy. J Bone Joint Surg 30B:664–670, 1948.

90. Linn FC, Radin EL: Lubrication of animal joints. III. The effect of certain chemical alterations of the cartilage and lubricant. Arthritis Rheum 11:674–682, 1968.

91. Johns RJ, Wright V: Relative importance of various tissues in joint stiffness. J Appl Physiol. 17:824–828, 1962.

92. Radin EL, Paul IL, Swann DA, Schottstaedt ES: Lubrication of synovial membrane. Ann Rheum Dis 30:322–325, 1971.

93. Swann DA, Radin EL, Nazimiec M, et al.: Role of hyaluronic acid in joint lubrication. Ann Rheum Dis 33:318–326, 1974.

94. Swann DA, Radin EL: The molecular basis of articular lubrication. I. Purification and properties of a lubricating fraction from bovine synovial fluid. J Biol Chem 247:8069–8073, 1972.

95. Linn FC: Lubrication of animal joints. J Bone Joint Surg 49A:1079–1098, 1967.

96. Simon SR, Paul IL, Rose RM, Radin EL: "Stiction-friction" of total hip prostheses and its relationship to loosening. J Bone Joint Surg 57A:226–230, 1975.

97. Mow VC, Lai WM: Recent developments in synovial joint biomechanics. SIAM Review 22(3):275–317, 1980.

98. Meachim G: The effect of scarification on articular cartilage in the rabbit. J Bone Joint Surg 45B:150–161, 1963.

99. Radin EL, Swann DA, Paul IL, McGrath PJ: Factors influencing articular cartilage wear in vitro. Arthritis Rheum 25:974–980, 1982.

100. Kettunen KO: Skin arthroplasty: In the light of animal experiments with special reference to functional metaplasia of connective tissue. Acta Orthop Scand Suppl 29:9–75, 1958.

101. Simon SR, Radin EL, Paul IL, Rose RM: The response of joints to impact loading. II. In vivo behavior of subchondral bone. J Biomech 5:267–272, 1972.

102. Foss MVL, Byers PD: Bone density osteoarthrosis of the hip, and fracture of the upper end of the femur. Ann Rheum Dis 31:259–264, 1972.

103. Hill AV: Production and absorption of work by muscle. Science 131:897–903, 1960.

104. Radin EL, Paul IL, Rose RM, Simon SR: The Mechanics of Joints as It Relates to Their Degeneration. AAOS Symposium on Osteoarthritis. St. Louis, C. V. Mosby, 1976, pp. 34–43.

105. Paul IL, Munro M, Abernethy PJ, et al.: Musculoskeletal shock absorption: Relative contribution of bone and soft tissues at various frequencies. J Biomech 11:237–239, 1978.

106. Radin EL, Maquet P, Parker H: Rationale and indications for the "Hanging Hip" procedure. A clinical and experimental study. Clin Orthop 112:221–230, 1975.

107. Storey GO, Landells JW: Restoration of the femoral head after collapse in osteoarthrosis. Ann Rheum Dis 30:406–412, 1971.

108. Perry GH, Smith MJG, Whiteside CG: Spontaneous recovery of the joint space in degenerative hip disease. Ann Rheum Dis 31:440–448, 1972.

109. Dehne E: Treatment of fractures of the tibial shaft. Clin Orthop 66:159–173, 1969.

110. Friedenberg ZB, Harlow MC, Brighton CT: Healing of nonunion of the medial malleolus by means of direct current: A case report. J Trauma 11:883–885, 1971.

111. Bassett CAL: Current concepts of bone formation. J Bone Joint Surg 44A:1217–1244, 1962.

112. Solomon L, Schnitzler C, Browett J: Osteoarthritis of the hip. The patient behind the disease. In Peyron JG (eds.): Epidemiology of Osteoarthritis. Paris, Geigy, 1981, pp. 40–52.

113. Solomon L: Osteoarthritis of the hip and femoral neck fracture. A mutually exclusive diad. In Arthritis and Rheumatism Council (ed.): Studies in Joint Diseases. London, 1978.

114. Radin EL, Ehrlich MG, Chernak R, et al.: Effect of repetitive impulsive loading on the knee joints of rabbits. Clin Orthop 131:288–293, 1978.

115. Radin EL: Mechanical factors in the etiology of osteoarthrosis. In Peyron JG (ed.): Epidemiology of Osteoarthritis (Proceedings of Symposium). Paris, 1980, pp. 136–139.

116. Serink MT, Nachemson A, Hansson G: The effect of impact loading on rabbit knee joints. Acta Orthop Scand 48:250–262, 1977.

117. Reimann I: Experimental osteoarthritis of the knee in rabbits induced by alteration of the load-bearing. Acta Orthop Scand 44:496–504, 1973.

118. Gloobe H, Nathan H: Osteophyte formation in experimental bipedal rats. J Comp Pathol 83:133–141, 1973.

6

Experimental Models of Osteoarthritis*

Roland W. Moskowitz, M.D.

Significant advances have been made over the past several decades in our understanding of the basic pathologic, biomechanical, biochemical, and pathophysiologic processes associated with degenerative joint disease.[1, 2] Data suggest that osteoarthritis (OA) is not an inevitable concomitant of aging but develops rather as a result of definable alterations in biomechanical and biochemical mechanisms. Based on newly derived information, reasonable hypotheses and schemata of pathogenesis have evolved. Unfortunately, despite these significant research advances and the availability of an augmented number of interested investigators, the specific pathogenesis of osteoarthritis remains unknown.

Further understanding of osteoarthritis would be significantly aided by the availability of experimental models that faithfully simulate the human disease.[3-5] Translation of results must take into account the complicating fact that various forms of human osteoarthritis likely represent subsets of the disorder, with major differences in the roles played by age, sex, biomechanical alteration, hormones, inflammatory mediators, and the immune process.

Experimental models of osteoarthritis offer distinct advantages over the use of human materials. Use of the latter is associated with difficulties in standardizing and grading pathologic change, inaccuracies in quantitation of disease duration, and the inability to define results at serial timed intervals during disease development. Experimental models, on the other hand, allow accurate definition of the time of disease induction and critical assessment of disease severity and progress on a detailed temporal basis. In addition, control tissues are readily available for study, both from contralateral joints of the same animal and from joints of nonoperated normal animals; metabolic changes based on in vivo radioactive labeling are feasible; environmental, dietary, and physical activity parameters can be controlled; and studies of therapeutic agents and related toxicity can be performed free of concerns that would apply to the evaluation of similar agents in humans.

In addition to the requirement that experimental models represent a reasonable reproduction of the disease as it occurs in humans, a number of practical factors must be taken into account when such models are considered for study. Important in such considerations are disease reproducibility, ease of animal handling, and cost. In some models, for example, pathologic changes occur too infrequently to be of value for statistical purposes. Experimental models utilizing dogs or pigs involve limitations related to the high cost of animal purchase and daily boarding for extensive studies. The utility of experimental models developed in small animals such as mice or guinea pigs is limited by the relatively small amount of joint cartilage available for study for parallel evaluations of cartilage pathologic and biochemical responses.

Experimental models that induce changes simulating limited components of the osteoarthritic process are available. These models are

*Supported by grants AM 30134 and AM 20618, NIH, USPHS.

based on hypotheses suggested by clinical and experimental observations. Those techniques that only incompletely reproduce selected components of the pathologic and pathophysiologic process such as degeneration of matrix and cells, regenerative repair characterized by chondrocyte proliferation and replacement of cartilage matrix components, or secondary synovial proliferative and inflammatory responses are nevertheless of value in studying basic cartilage responses to various pathogenic stimuli. Other models that simulate the human disease more completely are obviously of greater advantage in studying the total disease process. Both the incomplete and complete models provide opportunity for assessment of therapeutic interventions to possibly prevent, retard, or reverse the disease process.

This chapter provides a review of the many models of experimentally induced degenerative joint disease currently available. Special emphasis will be given to those commonly used models that more completely reproduce the disease counterpart as seen in the human. The understanding of the validity and value of these models will be enhanced if the reader has familiarized himself with the fundamental concepts of the osteoarthritic process detailed in the basic science chapters of this text.

Although studies derived from experiments utilizing animal models must always be viewed with caution, given differences between species, significant gains in understanding parallel pathophysiologic changes in the human can nevertheless be achieved. Recognition of the limitations inherent in the use of such models coupled with caution as to the relevance of such findings as they relate to human disease will obviate many of the concerns related to their use.

MODELS BASED ON METABOLIC AND ENDOCRINE MANIPULATION

Degenerative changes in cartilage have been described in association with fasting,[6] diabetes mellitus,[7] somatotrophin deficiency,[8] and adrenal corticosteroid administration.[9, 10] Injections of insulin together with dextrose, or dextrose alone produced swelling and hypertrophy and stimulation of organellar development in articular chondrocytes of young dwarf mice.[11] Somatotrophin (STH, growth hormone) has been shown to stimulate chondrocytes and to accelerate organellar development and hypertrophy of cytoplasm.[8] A lack of STH, on the other hand, is associated with retardation of organellar development.

Cortisone acetate administered to weanling mice produced signs of chondrocyte regression and eventual cell death.[9] Intra-articular injection of adrenal corticosteroids into rabbit knees was associated with degeneration of chondrocyte nuclei, cyst formation, and fibrillation and thinning of cartilage (Fig. 6–1).[10] The localization of degenerative changes to the medial tibial plateau was striking and appeared likely to be related in some way to the normal increased cellularity of medial plateau cartilage as compared with cartilage of the lateral tibial plateau and femoral condyles.

Daily injection of pharmacologic doses of triamcinolone diacetate, 1.5 mg/kg of body weight for 8 consecutive weeks, induced degenerative changes in the temporomandibular joints of mice.[12] Histopathologic changes in-

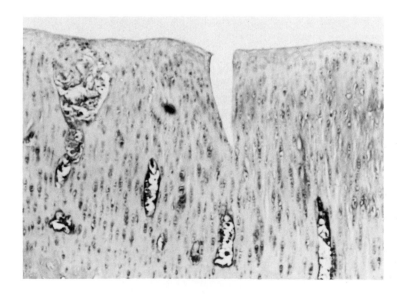

Figure 6–1. Rabbit knee cartilage, medial tibial plateau, after six intra-articular injections of triamcinolone acetonide, 3 mg. Chondrocyte nuclei have undergone degenerative change. Numerous cysts of varying size contain dying or dead chondrocytes and fibrillar detritus. (H and E stain, × 300.)

cluded cartilage fibrillation, shredding of degenerated cartilage into the articular space, and obliteration of the joint cavity by fibrous adhesions. Clustering of chondrocytes was frequently observed. Hypertrophied empty lacunae appeared to coalesce and form large empty cavities within the damaged cartilage.

Although the preceding manipulations are associated with limited pathophysiologic responses, knowledge gained may be used to selectively study components of the degenerative process.

MODELS OF OSTEOARTHRITIS RESULTING FROM INTRA-ARTICULAR INJECTION OF VARIOUS MATERIALS INTO JOINTS

Pathologic changes induced by intra-articular injection of a number of agents have been described. Studies of these responses, which are qualitatively and quantitatively similar at times to various components of the osteoarthritic process, may shed light on degenerative mechanisms.

Homogenous Cartilage and Bone Fragments. Injection of homogenous cartilage and bone fragments into rabbit knees resulted in synovial hyperplasia and fibroblastic change after only one injection.[13] Later studies revealed development of synovitis following repeated injections of various chondroitin sulfates into rabbit knees.[14] Repeated injections of sterile autogenous cartilage homogenates into the knee joints of dogs produced not only synovitis but also marginal exostoses and marginal cyst formation.[15] It was suggested that these exostoses resulted from an increased concentration of cartilage nutrients.

Papain. Injection of a solution of crude papain, a proteolytic enzyme, into rabbit knee joints resulted in degradation of articular cartilage.[16] Elevation and loosening of cartilage in weight-bearing areas were followed by thinning and fibrillation of the remaining articular cartilage surface. Superficial cartilage layers were lost, and cartilage adjacent to subchondral bone was disrupted. Surviving cells were frequently grouped in clusters. The late appearance of thin fibrillated fibrocartilage represented attempts at repair. Similar changes that mimic naturally occurring osteoarthritis have been described by other investigators in joints other than the knee. Serial studies of hip changes in rabbits following multiple injections of papain demonstrated fibrillation, loss of matrix proteoglycan and chondrocyte nu-

clear stain, and, within 24 hours, disorganization and death of chondrocytes.[17] Deep chondrocytes were affected more extensively than superficial ones. Sparing of chondrocytes at the surface may reflect dilution of papain by synovial fluid or an increased vulnerability of deep, more metabolically active chondrocytes to degeneration. Later responses included erosion of articular cartilage, subchondral sclerosis, and osteophyte formation. New blood vessels were seen to invade the base of articular cartilage at the periphery of the femoral head and the acetabulum. Synovial membrane hyperplasia was marked. Eventually, articular cartilage of the femoral head was denuded down to the calcified zone of cartilage. The sequence of findings suggested that osteoarthritis developed from primary changes induced in the articular cartilage matrix, with a secondary response in subchondral bone.

It was initially suggested that chondrocyte clusters that formed soon after papain injection represented a simple aggregation of chondrocytes following loss of matrix.[17] Studies by Havdrup and Telhag, however, demonstrated the ability of these chondrocytes in clusters to incorporate radioactive thymidine, suggesting that they evolved from active division and not by a simple "floating together."[18]

The effects of intra-articular injections of concentrated versus dilute (20%) solutions of papain were compared.[18] Although notable degenerative changes were observed after a single dose of either concentration, the effects of concentrated papain were, as expected, more marked. The lesions seen with papain in lower concentration more closely simulated those observed in human osteoarthritis, however, and provided a better model for study of early changes of degradation and repair.

Vitamin A. Intra-articular injections of large doses of vitamin A into rabbit knees resulted in progressive changes in articular cartilage that closely resembled human osteoarthritis.[19] Abnormalities included fibrillation, fraying, and erosions accompanied by marginal proliferation with osteophyte formation. Subchondral sclerosis was observed. Examination of synovial membrane revealed mild hypervascularity and pannus, which showed little tendency to invade articular cartilage, however. Studies suggested that the initial lesion was due to lysosomal activation from chondrocytes with depletion of matrix. The lesions then became progressive and self-perpetuating. The similarity of response to changes induced by papain suggests similar mechanisms of disease induction.

Filipin. Intra-articular injections of filipin, a polyene antibiotic capable of lysosome disruption, induce joint changes that simulate some components of the pathologic picture of osteoarthritis.[20] Specific findings include loss of matrix proteoglycan, cartilage fibrillation and fissuring, and proliferation of chondrocytes in clusters. The marked synovial hyperplasia and fibroblastic pannus seen with injection of this agent, however, may play a primary role in the cartilage response, and therefore, caution is suggested in the use of this model in studies of osteoarthritis.

Sodium Iodoacetate. Intra-articular injections of sodium iodoacetate into hen knees have been shown to produce rapidly progressive changes in cartilage that resemble osteoarthritis.[21] The degenerative process begins with small erosions and thinning of the cartilage and progresses to deeper ulceration and destruction, with involvement of subchondral bone as the lesions advance. Histologic evaluation of lesions reveals reduced metachromatic staining of cartilage and a progressive unmasking of collagen fibers. Within 8 to 12 weeks, there is severe destruction of the cartilage surface and lamina splendens, and deep ulcerations are observed. Chondrocyte proliferation in clusters, newly formed granulation tissue, and subchondral cystic bone changes are seen. Biochemical studies reveal a marked lowering of the proteoglycan content of cartilage. Similar lesions have been demonstrated to occur following the injection of sodium iodoacetate intra-articularly into guinea pigs.[22, 23] Joints from animals sacrificed after 3 weekly injections showed cartilage fibrillation, chondrocyte death, loss of matrix proteoglycans, and osteophyte formation. It was of interest that immobilization of the leg following injection of sodium iodoacetate prevented the formation of osteophytes and fibrillation but did not prevent cell death or loss of safranin-O orthochromatic staining. Experimental data suggest that disturbances of anabolic activity of cartilage cells induced by the sodium iodoacetate were responsible for alterations in structural composition and functional performance of cartilage, with resultant progressive degeneration.

EXPERIMENTAL MODELS BASED ON INDUCTION OF FOCAL CARTILAGE DEFECTS

Degenerative changes associated with local resection of cartilage or of cartilage and bone from joints in various animal species have been described. In studies of knee joints of adult dogs sacrificed up to 28 weeks following surgery, defects in cartilage alone underwent only incomplete attempts at repair characterized by proliferation of cartilage cells.[24] Defects extending down to the subchondral bone exhibited more complete evidence of repair, consisting of fibrous tissue, fibrocartilage, and, later, formation of an imperfect hyaline cartilage. The fibrous tissue appeared to originate from several sources, including bone marrow, connective tissue, marginal synovial membrane, and, in some instances, articular cartilage cells. Joint pathologic changes were limited to the area of the defect itself. Similar studies in which a circular reamer was used to create cartilage defects of varying depth down to the subchondral bone in young dogs were described by other investigators.[25] Varying degrees of repair of the defect resulted from proliferation of cells from the superficial cartilage layer, ingrowth of granulation tissue from subchondral bone, and formation of new hyaline cartilage; a sequence of metaplasia from fibrous tissue to fibrocartilage and finally to hyaline cartilage was observed.

Degenerative and regenerative responses were also noted in studies of rabbit patellar cartilage, in which a central defect was produced by paring off a thin chip of cartilage deep into the radial zone without penetrating the subchondral bone.[26] Degenerative changes, seen predominantly at the central aspect of the patella, were characterized by nuclear pyknosis and reduced stainability of cells; on autoradiographic study, little or no $^{35}SO_4$ was shown to be incorporated. Regenerative changes, characterized by clusters of chondrocytes that incorporated increased amounts of $^{35}SO_4$, were seen more frequently in the better-nourished peripheral cartilage away from the defect.

Salter and colleagues studied the effects of immobilization, active motion, and passive motion on the healing of 1-mm diameter full-thickness articular cartilage defects that penetrated the subchondral bone of rabbit knee joints.[27] In both adolescent and adult animals, healing of defects was more rapid and complete when the knees were exposed to continuous passive motion as opposed to either immobilization or intermittent active motion. Neochondrogenesis seen in the healing of these defects appeared to occur through differentiation of pluripotential cells of subchondral tissues to chondrocytes as a result of stimulation provided by continuous passive motion. Degenerative changes and the structural integrity of the repair tissue stimulated by continuous passive motion were re-evaluated at the end of 1 year. Although not completely normal, the tissue produced under conditions of continuous passive motion was superior with respect to histologic abnormalities as compared with repair tissue exposed initially to immobilization or active motion.[28]

Histologic and biochemical changes associated with healing of surgically induced defects in rabbit hyaline cartilage have been evaluated by other investigators.[29, 30] Furukawa and coworkers noted that the main collagen in repair tissue after 3 weeks was Type I.[29] By 6 to 8 weeks, Type II collagen had become predominant and continued to be enriched up to 1 year. Type I collagen persisted in significant amount, however, so that repair cartilage never fully resembled normal articular cartilage. In contrast, Cheung and associates[30] noted only Type II collagen in repair tissue at 10 weeks. Differences in findings may be related to differences in experimental methods and sampling.

Studies of the response of articular cartilage to multiple scarification have been described.[31, 32] Following arthrotomy, appropriate areas of the cartilage are lightly scarified by multiple cuts with a sharp scalpel. Care must be taken not to penetrate through cartilage to the underlying bone if the reaction of cartilage alone to injury is to be evaluated. The pathologic response to scarification is characterized by fibrillation, variable reduction or enhancement of matrix metachromatic staining in neighboring cells, and, later, proliferating clusters of chondrocytes. Joint lesions remain localized to the traumatized areas of cartilage, and no progressive erosive lesions characteristic of generalized osteoarthritis are noted. Bone changes and joint remodeling with ostephytes are not observed. This localization of lesions to traumatized areas and lack of remodeling changes represent significant differences in the lesions of this model from osteoarthritis. The absence of progressive disease suggests that articular cartilage has an injury threshold whereby chondrocytes are capable of repairing surface injury if the damage is not massive or repetitive. The finding that cartilage aryl sulfatase activity returns to normal after a transient elevation following scarification is consistent with this recovery process.[32]

Freezing of a localized area of articular hyaline cartilage was associated with minimal degenerative response when followed up to 6 months after the freezing injury.[33] The frozen cartilage surface appeared grossly smooth and intact. Histologic study revealed variable degrees of chondrocyte death manifested by loss of nuclear staining, and segmental loss of metachromasia. When animals were studied 12 months following freezing, however, progressive degenerative changes were observed, still limited to the area of the initial freezing injury.[34] Horizontal tears involved the surface layers, and vertical clefts extended down into subchondral bone. Subchondral bone itself was built up in an irregular fashion, and from it clusters of chondrocytes, visible in otherwise acellular regions, were surrounded by increased metachromatic staining for proteoglycans. The normal alignment of collagen fibers was disrupted, with collagen now arranged in whorls. Chemical assays revealed diminished hexosamine content of experimental cartilage but normal hydroxyproline concentration.

MODELS RELATED TO PRIMARY ALTERATION OF JOINT FORCES

Current concepts of the pathogenesis of osteoarthritis suggest that abnormal stresses on cartilage due to abnormal forces, or to normal forces abnormally directed, may be key factors in disease initiation. Osteoarthritis develops when joints are unable to cope with mechanical stresses produced by activities of daily living or when mechanical stresses on the joint become excessive.[35] Epidemiologic studies have demonstrated the importance of trauma to the induction of osteoarthritis related to occupational or athletic overuse of joints. These observed relationships between biomechanical abnormalities and joint degeneration have led to the development of experimental models based on variations in joint load.

Pathologic and metabolic changes similar to those seen in early osteoarthritis were described by Radin and colleagues in the knee joints of rabbits exposed to repetitive impulsive loading.[36] In these studies, the right foot of adult rabbits was subjected to repetitive impact loading for up to 40 minutes a day either daily for variable numbers of days or with intermittent rest periods. Increased subchondral bone stiffness was associated with slight surface loss of proteoglycan, confirmed by a slight fall in hexosamine, and no change in collagen content. More striking was that cell proliferation and protein and glycosaminoglycan formation were increased, as studied by ^{3}H-thymidine, ^{3}H-glycine, and $^{35}SO_4$ incorporation, respectively. The severity of responses paralleled the number of days of repetitive loading. When loading was followed by 4 weeks of rest, bone stiffness returned to normal, but metabolic effects persisted, although to a lesser degree. The stiffening of subchondral bone associated with metabolic changes seen in early osteoarthritis suggested that trabecular microfractures may occur early as part of the sequence of pathophysiologic change.

In a subsequent study performed on adult sheep, Radin and coworkers investigated the effects of prolonged activity on hard surfaces.[37] Sheep in the experimental group were subjected to daily walking on concrete, with routine housing on tarmac. Control sheep were walked on compliant woodchip surfaces and pastured. When studied after 2.5 years, significant changes were seen in both articular cartilage and subchondral trabecular bone of the knee joints of the hard-surface walkers. The hexosamine content of the articular cartilage in the hard-surface walkers was lower, with the decrease being more marked in the weight-bearing areas. Increased cortical thickness and alterations in the trabecular pattern of the subchondral bone acted to stiffen the tibiofemoral joint. Gross pathologic changes of osteoarthritis were not evident in any of the animals, however.

In further studies investigating the relationship between stiffening of underlying subchondral bone and deterioration of overlying articular cartilage, the effect of chrome-cobalt metal plugs placed in drill holes directly under the subchondral plate of the medial tibial plateau of adult sheep was evaluated.[37] The contralateral medial tibial plateau was utilized as a control, with insertion of a porous polyethylene plug of equal dimensions inserted into the subchondral area. Preliminary results in 3 months showed fibrillation and loss of hexosamine in the articular cartilage overlying the metal plugs but no change over the porous polyethylene plugs.

Contrary findings relative to the response of rabbit subchondral bone to repetitive impact loading were reported by Serink, Nachemson, and Hansson.[38] Subchondral bone cores from impacted tibiae revealed progressive increased deformability under a constant force, consistent with bone softening. Concurrent degenerative changes in the articular cartilage included fibrillation, cleft formation, and variable depletion of matrix substance. Increased vascularity of subchondral bone with invasion of blood vessels into cartilage was noted. It was suggested that decreased me-

chanical support by softened subchondral bone may contribute to cartilage degeneration.

Although repetitive loading models provide interesting data for the study of the trauma component of the suggested hypothesis of osteoarthritis, the nonphysiologic nature of lesion induction requires that findings be viewed with great caution prior to translating them to the human process.

Joint responses to alterations in load bearing have also been studied following valgus angular osteotomy of the tibia.[39] Valgus angulation of 30 degrees was induced by wedge osteotomy, and the operated animals were observed for up to 3 months after surgery. Although no roentgenologic signs of osteoarthritis were observed, and gross changes of degeneration were only rarely noted, histologic evidence of degenerative abnormalities was present in all of a small number of animals studied. Cartilage changes were characterized by loss of metachromasia, fibrillation, clefts and flaking in the superficial layers, and loss of nuclear staining. Moderate subchondral sclerosis was seen, but osteophyte formation was absent. Degenerative changes were limited to the lateral tibial and femoral condyles. This model, based on experimentally induced alteration of load bearing, appeared to induce degenerative changes analogous to human osteoarthritis.

Rats experimentally induced to be bipedal represent another model in which degencrative changes resulting from altered mechanical loads can be studied.[40] Normal rats are converted to bipedal rats by removing their forelegs. To encourage bipedalism, food and water are placed near the top of high cages made especially for this purpose, thus obliging the animals to adopt an upright position for nourishment. Significant osteophyte formation occurs at or around spinal curvatures, where pressures are greatest, similar to osteophyte formation at concavities of the spine in humans with scoliosis. Osteophyte formation was higher in males, likely related to the heavier male bodies, with accordingly greater pressure exerted on the vertebral column. This model is somewhat unique in the formation of osteophytes with little or no demonstrable structural cartilage breakdown.

Recently, a new model of experimental OA in guinea pigs has been developed that utilizes an extra-articular surgical technique to modify joint forces.[41] Guinea pigs with diets supplemented with vitamin C were subjected to unilateral resection of the origin of the gluteal muscles of the sacrum and/or sectioning of the infrapatellar ligament. Roentgenologic studies showed joint space narrowing and early osteophytes in hips and in some knee joints. Gross examination revealed thinning, roughening, and pitting of cartilage, especially that of femoral heads and tibial plateaus. Histopathologic studies demonstrated cartilage thinning, chondrocyte proliferation, and loss of metachromatic staining in most specimens at 12 to 16 weeks. Changes were observed both in ipsilateral and contralateral joints. No evidence of inflammation was seen. Cartilage water content was increased in the osteoarthritic hips as compared with controls. This model affords opportunity to study OA events without violation of the joint space.

LIMB DENERVATION MODEL

Loss of sensation in an extremity is frequently associated with degenerative joint changes. Unilateral sensory denervation of the hind limb was produced in rabbits by posterior nerve root section.[42] Chondrocyte degenerative changes occurred earliest in the middle cartilage layers, suggesting impaired nutrition. Protection of the limb in a plaster cast did not materially alter the response to denervation, suggesting that trauma is not the primary factor in the deterioration of anesthetic joints, although it likely remains an important contributory factor.

Palmoski, O'Connor, and Brandt investigated the effect of sectioning the posterior and medial articular nerves of the knees of normal dogs.[43] This study was designed to evaluate cartilage response following interference with mechanoreceptor function. Mechanoreceptors, highly specialized nerve endings within the joint that are sensitive to joint position, initiate reflexes that control muscle tone around the joint to check excessive movement, thereby protecting the joint from the microtrauma of daily activity. It was postulated that diminished mechanoreceptor function could result in excess muscle tone, which, by increasing the load on the joint, could lead to cartilage breakdown. Sectioning of the nerves led to increased cartilage water content and proteoglycan synthesis. Cartilage showed loss of metachromatic staining and loss of thickness. Proteoglycan extractability was increased, although proteoglycan aggregation was not affected. Data suggested that nerve sectioning profoundly disrupted the macromolecular organization of joint cartilage. Whether this would eventually lead to osteoarthritis was not determined.

SPONTANEOUSLY OCCURRING ANIMAL MODELS

Degenerative joint disease has been described in various strains of small laboratory animals such a mice, hamsters, and guinea pigs. Several strains of mice with spontaneously occurring disease have been reported in detail. C57BL[44–49] and STR/1N[50, 51] strains have been especially analyzed and utilized in studies of the pathogenesis of OA. Degenerative changes are characterized by fraying and ulceration of cartilage, subchondral bony sclerosis, and proliferative osteophyte-like changes. Lesions occur with variable frequency, depending on the mouse strain used, reaching a 50 to 93% incidence in some strains. Degenerative lesions are manifested only after many months, with maximal frequency and severity occurring after 15 to 17 months of age. The lesions of degenerative arthritis must be differentiated from aging changes characterized by nonspecific regressive changes in cells and matrix. Differences in sex-linked incidence and modes of genetic transmission among the various strains have been identified. Estradiol administration was shown to lessen the incidence of OA lesions in C57BL animals studied.[46–48] The rate of lesion development, frequency, and severity were significantly increased when the animals were fed a diet enriched with lard, or animal fat.[52] Conversely, the course of OA was not adversely affected by administration of cottonseed oil, a vegetable fat.[45]

High frequencies of osteoarthritis have been described in NZY/B1 and PN mouse strains, which are predisposed to the development of autoimmune disease.[53] Degenerative lesions were unrelated to associated immune phenomena such as antinuclear antibodies, glomerulitis, and arteritis.

In another study of blotchy mice (BLO strain), which carry a gene causing inadequate crosslinking of collagen, 88% of the animals studied were shown to develop osteoarthritic lesions.[54] It was suggested that the lesions might result from mechanical trauma due to decreased ligament and capsule strength as a result of defective collagen crosslinking. Alternatively, osteoarthritic changes might result from abnormalities in collagen/proteoglycan complexing in the cartilage. This model might be particularly useful in studies of the role of collagen in the pathogenesis of osteoarthritis.

In contrast to mice, rats display an unexplained marked resistance to development of osteoarthritis.[55] Increased general activity of mice with greater opportunity to drop from heights within the confined space of the cage may play a role.

Osteoarthritis has also been shown to occur spontaneously in domestic animals, including horses, swine, cattle, and dogs.[56] Joint laxity and degenerative changes of the hip joint in dogs have been particularly studied as a model of degenerative joint disease.[57–60] Although these are associated with hip dysplasia in many breeds, German shepherds and Labrador retrievers are commonly affected. Gross cartilage abnormalities, seen as early as 3 months of age, are characterized by softening and dulling of cartilage, flaking, erosions, and fibrillation. The connecting round ligament of the femoral head becomes frayed and, at times, totally severed. Similar findings of fibrillation and ulceration are noted on histologic study. Loss of proteoglycan results in decreased uptake of metachromatic stain. In general, increased chondrocyte cellularity is not observed. Biochemical studies reveal normal or slightly lowered DNA content.[59] Glycosaminoglycans, as measured by hexosamine and uronic acid, are decreased. Isotope incorporation studies reveal normal or slightly decreased DNA synthesis, decreased protein synthesis, and slightly increased glycosaminoglycan synthesis. Procollagen accumulation in involved cartilage has been described, in the presence of normal total collagen content and rate of collagen synthesis.[60] A partial defect in conversion of procollagen to collagen has been suggested.

It is unresolved whether joint laxity appears first in dogs with hip dysplasia or whether cartilage or ligament abnormalities are primary.[61] Joint instability is accompanied by an increased volume of synovial fluid and of the ligamentum teres (increased total intra-articular volume). Injection of buffered solutions of hyaluronic acid into nonsubluxated hip joints increases subluxation, whereas withdrawal of synovial fluid from a severely subluxated joint reduces the degree of subluxation. These studies suggest that joint instability in these animals may be related to increased intra-articular volume.

The pathologic and biochemical findings seen in the hip dysplasia model in dogs have many of the characteristics of OA in humans.

In contrast to human degenerative arthritis, however, cloning-type hypercellularity is uncommon, and the overall rate of DNA synthesis is reduced.

The use of animals undergoing spontaneous osteoarthritis for experimental purposes is limited by considerations of disease reproducibility, ease of handling, and, particularly, cost. In some animals, such as the dog, the disease occurs too infrequently to be of value for statistical purposes. In other species, such as the mouse, large numbers of animals may be required for study to demonstrate statistically significant differences between affected and control groups under analysis; a significant mortality rate compounds the problem. The long time lapse, measured in months and, at times, years between birth and the development of osteoarthritis, represents an additional disadvantage to the use of any of these spontaneous animal models.

DEGENERATIVE CHANGES AFTER EXPERIMENTAL RELEASE OF JOINT CONTACT

Clinical studies have shown that cartilage degeneration may be related to non–pressure-bearing areas rather than to areas of abnormally increased pressure. These findings suggest that cartilage apposition and weight bearing of adjoining articular surfaces are important in the maintenance of proper cartilage nutrition. Accordingly, experimental models of OA have been developed based on experimental relief of joint contact.[62–64]

In studies in rats and rabbits, degenerative changes in the knee were described following resection of the lateral femoral condyle, which prevented contact of the lateral aspect of the femur with the lateral tibial plateau. Sham surgery without condylar resection was performed for control purposes. Degenerative changes were noted primarily on the lateral tibial plateau. The absence of significant abnormalities in the medial compartment of the knee was striking, despite the fact that the medial femoral condyle was likely transmitting more weight than normal. Cartilage degenerative changes were characterized by progressive loss of metachromasia and nuclear staining, gradual cellular disorganization with formation of clones of chondrocytes, fibrillation, fissuring, and ulcer formation. Osteophyte formation was uncommon. Subchondral bone thickening deep to advanced lesions was noted in rats; this contrasted with the subchondral bone thinning and vascular hyperplasia found in rabbits. Pannus formation was occasionally observed at the joint periphery. Degenerative changes occurred in both mature and immature animals.

The changes observed following experimental relief of joint contact bear a strong resemblance to human osteoarthritis and suggest that absence of weight bearing plays a role in the induction of degenerative changes. Certain aspects of interpretation of this model must be viewed with caution, however. Although postoperative stress maneuvers and roentgenograms were performed to demonstrate that condylar resection was associated with loss of contact of apposing surfaces,[63] repeat maneuvers to demonstrate continued lack of joint contact at various stages of disease development were not performed. Eventual contact of presumably unapposed joint surfaces might have occurred after a period of time. Furthermore, pannus formation in response to surgery and joint manipulation cannot be excluded as a cause of some of the phenomena observed.

IMMOBILIZATION AND COMPRESSION-IMMOBILIZATION MODELS

Degenerative changes secondary to immobilization with or without compression have been evaluated in rats, rabbits, and dogs by a number of investigators.[65–78] Lesions are generally similar, regardless of the species studied. Certain of these models are designated as immobilization models, because no definitive efforts to provide compression were performed.[65, 68, 70–73, 75–78] In many of these experiments, however, some degree of at least intermittent compression of contact areas was likely, depending on the position of the joint in the immobilized state. In other experiments, definitive compressive forces were built into the experimental methodology.[66, 67, 69] For purposes of this presentation, immobilization and compression-immobilization models will be discussed separately, based on the primary intent of the experimental design.

Immobilization Models. Prolonged immobilization leads to restricted motion, as a result of capsular and pericapsular contractures.[65, 68, 70] Eventually, intra-articular ankylosis ensues. Progressive contracture of the capsule and the pericapsular structures is associated with intra-articular encroachment on the joint by fibrofatty connective tissue, with eventual obliteration of the joint cavity. The initially fairly distinct interface between the fibrofatty tissue and hyaline cartilage is eventually replaced with mature fibrous connective tissue. Synovial hyperplasia may be prominent. Cartilage degenerative changes are characterized by loss of metachromasia, fibrillation, and erosion. Invasion of the subchondral bony plate by proliferating mesenchymal tissue from the marrow space replaces the deeper layers of articular cartilage. Proliferative changes at the synovium-cartilage junction lead to lipping and osteophyte formation. Degenerative changes in contact areas of cartilage appear to be largely due to mechanical compression, which produces damage directly by pressure and indirectly by prevention of diffusion of synovial fluid into compressed cartilage.[71, 72] Degeneration of contact-free areas may result from lack of cartilage nutrition as a result of reduced synovial fluid diffusion related to joint limitation, and from diminished synovial fluid production by atrophic synovial membrane. Remobilization failed to reverse any of the major pathologic cartilage alterations induced by immobilization.[65]

Weight bearing, absence of weight bearing, and rigidity of fixation have been evaluated as variables related to degenerative changes induced by immobilization. The effects of immobilization with weight bearing, immobilization without weight bearing, and immobilization without weight bearing and with neurectomy were compared.[70] Changes in the immobilized weight-bearing and immobilized non–weight-bearing groups were similar and characteristic of degenerative responses described in previous immobilization studies. The similarity of changes between the two groups demonstrated that degenerative changes can occur in immobilized joints in the absence of weight bearing. Less extensive degenerative changes were noted in the immobilized denervated non–weight-bearing group. This finding suggested that static compression as a result of muscle contraction contributes to articular degeneration in immobilized joints.

Ultrastructural studies of the response of articular cartilage to experimental immobilization have been performed using electron microscopy.[71] Degeneration and necrosis of chondrocytes occurred not only in areas of cartilage compression but also in contact-free areas. The changes in the contact areas, however, appeared earlier and were more severe, resulting in early onset of necrosis. Lesions seen included swelling of mitochondria, dilatation of cisternae of the rough endoplasmic reticulum, and accumulation of fine filamentous fibers, lipids, and lysosomal bodies. Similar changes have been described in human osteoarthritis.

Metabolic and biochemical responses to immobilization have also been investigated.[73, 75, 77] Oxytetracycline labeling was utilized to evaluate changes in bone formation during immobilization of rabbit knees.[75] There was an increased turnover of bone tissue in the immobilized knee as compared with the contralateral knee. In another study in rabbits, the periarticular connective tissues of immobilized knees revealed marked reduction in water concentration, hyaluronic acid, and chondroitin 4- and 6-sulfates.[73] Dermatan sulfate and total collagen content were not appreciably altered. The total hexosamine content of articular cartilage and menisci in the immobilized joint was significantly reduced; total collagen content was unchanged.

The biochemical responses to immobilization were also evaluated in the hind limbs of mature dogs.[77] The right hind limbs of the dogs were immobilized with a light cast against the trunk, with 90 degrees of flexion of the hip and knee. The dogs were able to ambulate on three legs but bore no weight on the immobilized extremity for 6 days, 3 weeks, 6 weeks, or 8 weeks until time of sacrifice. No gross lesions were discernible in any of the animals at time of study. Histologic evaluation, however, revealed progressive loss of cartilage metachromatic staining and a significant decrease in cartilage thickness in the immobilized knees. In addition, examination of immobilized knee cartilage revealed fewer cells per unit area than cartilage in control knees. Removal of cast restraint was followed in 2 to 4 weeks by resolution of histologic degenerative changes and a regaining of cartilage thickness almost to control levels. Biochemical studies of cartilage of the immobilized knees revealed increased water content and decreased uronic acid content. Proteoglycan synthesis by cartilage of the restrained knee was markedly reduced as early as 6 days after immobilization. After 3 weeks of immobilization, proteoglycan aggregation was no longer demonstrable. The aggregation defect was rapidly reversible, with normal aggregates seen as early as 2 weeks following cast removal.

Further studies using this same dog knee immobilization model evaluated the effect of treadmill running on immobilization-induced atrophic changes in cartilage.[79] Daily treadmill running after cast removal inhibited the reversal of the atrophic changes described above. Cartilage continued to exhibit decreased thickness, decreased metachromatic staining, and decreased uronic acid content compared with control cartilage from the contralateral nonimmobilized knee. Defects in proteoglycan aggregation persisted. These studies suggest that cartilage whose integrity has been diminished by immobilization may be vulnerable to loading during subsequent exercise, with decreased capacity for repair.

Compression-Immobilization Models. Joint degeneration observed in humans following orthopedic immobilization of joints in a forced position has led to the development of models that combine immobilization with variable degrees of compression.[66, 67, 69, 70] Different methods have been used to induce compression and immobilization in several species of animals, including rabbits, monkeys, and rats. In some studies, compression was performed using stainless-steel pins drilled transversely through the distal femur and the proximal tibia in a coronal plane, followed by application of a Charnley compression clamp. A cylindrical plaster cast was applied to maintain the various forced positions of the knee. In other studies, plaster casts or splints were utilized to immobilize the joint under study in forced positions. Progressive cartilage degenerative changes ensued. Loss of normal cartilage luster and translucency occurred early. The cartilage became yellow-white and soft to the touch. Focal lesions occurred at sites of cartilage apposition. Histologic studies revealed loss of staining power of chondrocyte nuclei in the superficial and transitional zones of cartilage, with varying degrees of cartilage degeneration in deeper areas. Fibrillation (Fig. 6–2A) and loss of matrix metachromasia were noted. Partial- and then full-thickness erosions of cartilage followed, with exposure of subchondral bone in the center of the lesion (Fig. 6–2B). Chondrocyte proliferation with clone formation was observed at the margins of ulcerative lesions. Attempts at fibrous repair of extensive lesions were also observed. Hypertrophic eburnation of subchondral bone was associated with vascular penetration of cartilage. Cartilage regeneration was prominent at times. Osteophytes were noted occasionally. Lesions were consistent with pressure necrosis of cartilage as a consequence of interference with diffusion of nutrients.

Studies of glycosaminoglycan metabolism were performed on cartilage from rabbit knees

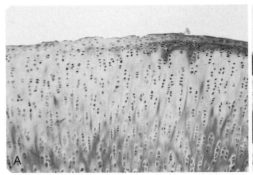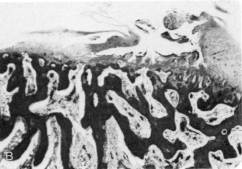

Figure 6–2. Compression-immobilization model using overlapping plaster splints in the rabbit, right knee femoral cartilage. *A,* Three-day compression. Fibrillation and irregularity of the joint surface are noted. (H and E stain, × 100.) *B,* Twenty-one–day compression. Partial- to full-thickness erosion is noted, with exposure to subchondral bone. Chondrocyte proliferation with clone formation was evident at the periphery of the lesion. (H and E stain, × 60.) (From Moskowitz RW: Semin Arthritis Rheum 2:95, 1972.)

that had been immobilized by application of a plastic splint followed by bandaging of the knee region.[76] Although described as an immobilization model, this technique likely allows considerable compression, at least on an intermittent basis, on the knee joint as the animal ambulates with the leg in an extended position. Accordingly, the results are described under compression-immobilization effects. Studies revealed an increased rate of synthesis of sulfated glycosaminoglycans (GAGs) from all cartilage sites examined. However, loss of GAG content as measured by hexosamine and uronic acid was noted in tibial weight-bearing and femoral condylar cartilage, in contrast to tibial marginal areas, where it was increased at the sites of osteophyte formation. These results, which demonstrated that GAG degradation exceeded synthesis in weight-bearing areas, simulated findings reported in human osteoarthritis.

Compression-immobilization studies utilizing somewhat lesser forces of compression have been reported.[69] Rat knees were immobilized using wire fixation, and the knees were extended without applying undue force. Study of knees at sacrifice after various intervals revealed extensive degenerative changes in both contact and noncontact areas. Pressure-bearing areas revealed death of cartilage cells, loss of matrix staining, fissure formation, and thickening of the subchondral plate. Non–pressure-bearing areas revealed increased size and number of cells, increased nuclear chondrocyte staining, and hyperplastic overgrowth of synovium in peripheral areas. It was concluded that severe force was not necessary to induce pathologic changes.

The aforementioned models in which carti-lage degenerative changes result from immobilization or compression-immobilization have been utilized by a number of investigators to study degenerative joint disease. Although many of the lesions observed resemble various components of the osteoarthritic process, prominent proliferative changes and marked differences in response between apposing and nonapposing joint surfaces suggest caution in using these models as representative of human osteoarthritis. Induction of lesions related to pressure necrosis and nutritional deficiency represent etiologic pathways that appear to be significantly different from those hypothesized for spontaneous osteoarthritis.

PATELLECTOMY AND PATELLAR DISLOCATION MODELS

Patellectomy, performed occasionally as a clinical therapeutic procedure, may be followed by persistent knee pain and weakness and degenerative joint breakdown. Experimental studies of patellectomy have investigated the biomechanical and degenerative changes associated with this procedure. Total patellectomy in rabbits resulted in degenerative ulceration of articular cartilage of the patellar surface of the femur with exposure of subjacent bone.[80] Further studies compared the effects of partial and total patellectomy in young and adult rabbits, with sacrifice 10 to 12 months after surgery.[81] Degenerative changes seen in adult rabbits that had undergone total patellectomy were characterized by chondrocyte cloning, irregularity of cartilage margins, vascularization, and fibrillation. Erosions and complete denudation of cartilage were seen.

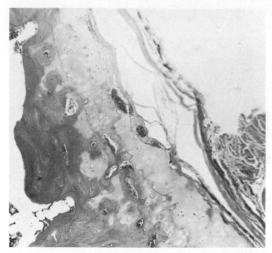

Figure 6–3. Rabbit right knee cartilage 14 weeks after patellectomy. A pannus of granulation and fibrous tissue invades the cartilage surface. Underlying cartilage is ulcerated. (H and E stain, × 120.) (From Garr EL, et al.: Clin Orthop 92:296, 1973.)

Fibrous layers over hyaline cartilage were a constant finding. Changes were seen mainly in the patellofemoral region; tibias were usually normal. Partial patellectomy produced similar but less severe changes. In young rabbits, pathologic changes were less severe in both the total and partial patellectomy models. Degenerative changes following patellectomy may well be due to subluxation of the normally lax and unstable extensor apparatus of the rabbit knee.

Serial studies of the response to total patellectomy in rabbits were also reported.[82] Sacrifices were performed at intervals from 1 to 27 weeks. Controls included sham patellectomized and normal knees. The earliest changes noted were those of synovial inflammation and proliferation with development of a pannus of inflammatory, granulation, and fibrous tissue (Fig. 6–3). These changes were associated with generalized loss of metachromasia in superficial layers of cartilage. Later, there were chondrocyte degeneration, fibrillation, fissure formation, cyst formation, and eventual ulceration of cartilage. Cartilage changes were seen primarily in areas associated with pannus invasion. Spur formation was seen, but the spurs were limited in size and number.

To obviate some of the criticisms that might pertain to studies of patellectomy in knees of rabbits whose extensor apparatus is relatively unstable, De Palma and Flynn investigated the effects of partial and total patellectomy in the dog, whose extensor apparatus is very stable.[83]

In these animals, the patella is firmly supported on the anterior surface of the femur and is dislocated only with great force. Groups studied included animals that underwent total patellectomy, animals that underwent partial patellectomy in the sagittal plane, and animals in which either the superior or inferior half of the patella was excised. Although abnormalities were noted in all groups, degenerative changes were most marked following total patellectomy and partial patellectomy in the sagittal plane. An intense hyperplastic fibrous and fibrocartilaginous response associated with large clusters of synovial villi was observed in all animals. The articular surface of cartilage became frayed, pitted, and fibrillated; erosions and loss of cartilage layers were common. Marginal osteophytes were observed.

Degenerative lesions of cartilage observed after patellectomy appear to represent a secondary response to the prominent synovial inflammation and pannus formation observed early in the course of joint reaction following surgery. Additional factors possibly involved in the induction of pathologic changes include the direct mechanical effect of the roughened surgical surface, deranged biomechanics induced by alteration of the normal quadriceps mechanism, and lack of normal nutrition due to loss of normal apposition of articular cartilage surfaces.

Osteoarthritis occurs spontaneously in man following chronic recurrent subluxation of the patella. Similar degenerative changes have been noted in animal models in which patellar subluxation develops spontaneously or is a complication of an experimental procedure. Bennet and Bauer,[24] in studies of patellar dislocation in dogs, demonstrated marked changes, including pannus formation, hypertrophic villous synovitis, and formation of "joint mice" consisting of cartilage-bone fragments. Subchondral bone reaction was noted. These findings bear strong resemblance to lesions induced by patellectomy, and the possible role of subluxation of the quadriceps mechanism in the latter model in rabbits has been noted previously.

MODELS BASED ON SECTION OF CRUCIATE LIGAMENTS

Knee degeneration has been demonstrated clinically when joint instability follows cruciate ligament rupture. Based on these observations, models in which osteoarthritis has been induced by surgical section of the cruciate ligaments have been studied in various species of animals.[84–89] Most of these investigations involve sectioning of the anterior cruciate ligament, either by exposure at arthrotomy or by blind closed section. Joint instability appears to be the initiating factor in the induction of observed degenerative lesions. Detailed studies of the pathologic and biochemical alterations associated with this model have been reported, particularly in the dog.[84–88] Gross examination of cartilage at serial intervals following surgery reveals softening, fibrillation, and erosions. Lesions were most severe and prominent at the medial aspect of the medial tibial plateau; lesions noted in the lateral tibial plateau and femoral condyles were somewhat less severe. Histologic study revealed fibrillation and deep cartilage clefts, leading to eventual formation of erosions. Loss of cartilage metachromatic staining was observed only in severely fibrillated areas. Cell density increased progressively with time; the cartilage matrix became highly cellular, and clones of two or more cells were abundant, particularly around severely fibrillated sites. Synovial vascular proliferation with villous folds and adhesions was observed. Meniscal fibrillation and tears, particularly of the medial meniscus, occurred in the majority of animals.

Osteophyte formation was prominent and was noted at the proximal limit of the femoral trochlea as early as 2 weeks after cruciate section.[86] The number and size of osteophytes increased progressively with time, with involvement of tibial, patellar, and femoral cartilages. Detailed studies of the development of these osteophytes were performed using sequential bone labeling with fluorochromes, microangiography, and microradiography.[86] Osteophytes developed most commonly at the marginal zone where synovial membrane merges with fibrocartilage. They appeared to begin as a deposition of mineral outside the existing femoral bone cortex. Formation of a mature osteophyte developed as deposition of new bone and resorption led to remodeling. Bone changes were not confined to development of the osteophyte. The whole distal end of the femur revealed a marked increase in bone turnover. Dye injection techniques demonstrated an increase in vascularity in association with this development of new bone.

Biochemical studies of cartilage in this dog model revealed increased water content; proteoglycans were more easily extracted and had higher galactosamine:glucosamine molar ratios. The latter finding suggested that the chondrocytes synthesized proteoglycans containing more chondroitin sulfate relative to keratan sulfate, similar to immature articular cartilage. It was notable that biochemical alterations were present throughout all regions of the cartilage of joints operated on and that they occurred prior to any grossly observable degenerative lesions.

Degenerative lesions of articular cartilage were also shown to follow transection of the anterior cruciate ligament in the rat.[89] Lesions included surface disruptions; a reduction in matrix proteoglycans, as evidenced by loss of metachromatic staining; loss of cells; and occasional cell cloning. No osteophytes were seen. Lesions were observed more frequently in animals exercised on a treadmill following ligament section. These studies suggested that the rat knee joint may be useful in studies of the effects of mechanical derangement on articular tissues.

Degenerative joint lesions have also been demonstrated following posterior cruciate ligament section in the rabbit.[90] Findings resulting from complete and incomplete sectioning of the ligament and the effects of sham operation were compared. Degenerative changes following complete and incomplete section were qualitatively similar. Cartilage pitting and ulceration were observed. Loss of safranin-O stain was seen primarily in areas of ulceration. Chondrocyte degeneration and proliferation occurred together. Osteophyte formation was prominent and occurred primarily on the tibial plateaus (Fig. 6–4).

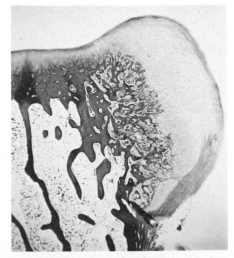

Figure 6–4. Right tibia, inner rim of medial plateau, 12 weeks following posterior cruciate ligament section. Osteophyte formation is marked by bony proliferation with hyaline and fibrocartilage capping. (H and E stain, × 45.)

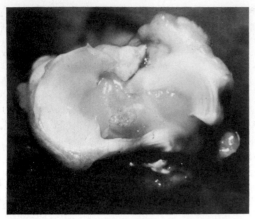

Figure 6–5. Right tibia of rabbit, partial meniscectomy model. The anterior 30% of the medial meniscus has been excised. (From Moskowitz RW, et al.: Arthritis Rheum 16:397, 1973.)

MENISCECTOMY MODELS

Extensive studies of experimental osteoarthritis have been performed by Moskowitz and coworkers utilizing a rabbit model of osteoarthritis in which degenerative changes follow partial resection of the medial meniscus.[91–93] This model was based on the clinical observation that degenerative joint disease is not an uncommon sequela in humans following meniscus injury. In this model, approximately one fourth to one third of the anterior aspect of the medial meniscus is excised (Fig. 6–5).[91] Pathologic lesions begin within several weeks following surgery. Changes include cartilage pitting and ulceration, fissuring, cyst formation, and diminished concentration of matrix proteoglycans[91] (Fig. 6–6). Proliferation of chondrocytes in clones represents efforts at repair. Pitting and erosions (Fig. 6–7) occur primarily on the medial femoral condyle and, at 12 weeks, are seen in 70% and 30% of animals, respectively. Osteochondrocytes, seen on both the medial femoral condyle and at the inner aspect of the medial tibial plateau (Fig. 6–8), occur in approximately 75% of femurs and 95% of tibias studied.

Biochemical studies of cartilage responses in this model have been performed. In one such study, autoradiographic techniques were utilized to assess metabolic activity following in vivo intra-articular injections of ^{3}H-glycine, ^{35}SO$_4$, and ^{3}H-thymidine.[94] Proteoglycan and protein synthesis was shown to be increased throughout the 12-week period of study (Fig. 6–9). Cell replication was increased early in cartilage and subchondral bone but was later diminished to control levels despite progression of degeneration. The finding of cell replication early in subchondral bone was of interest, lending some support to the hypothesis that early changes in osteoarthritis involve subchondral bone. Surprisingly contrasting results were obtained when cartilage metabolism was studied using in vitro organ culture techniques.[95] Cell replication and protein synthesis were shown to be stimulated early but were decreased at later periods of sacrifice when pathologic changes were maximal. Proteoglycan synthesis, as measured by sulfate incorporation, was reduced throughout the entire 12-week span of study. Accordingly, and in contrast to the autoradiographic studies performed on this same model, metabolic parameters of cartilage activity were not increased in

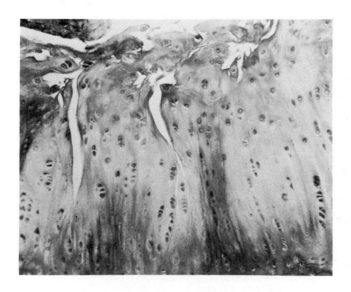

Figure 6–6. Degenerative changes in a rabbit medial femoral condyle 12 weeks following partial medial meniscectomy. Fibrillation and fissuring are associated with chondrocyte proliferation in the area of gross erosive change. (H and E stain, × 350.)

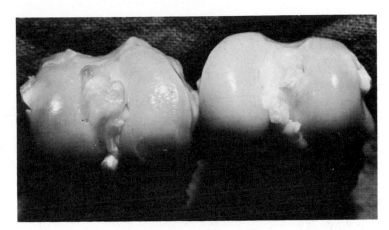

Figure 6–7. Right femur of rabbit 12 weeks following partial meniscectomy is compared with an unoperated contralateral left knee. Pitting and ulceration are most marked in the medial femoral condyle. (From Moskowitz RW: Arthritis Rheum 20:S104, 1977.)

parallel with the development of degenerative joint disease.

Additional studies revealed complete loss of proteoglycan aggregates in the partial meniscectomy osteoarthritic knee, whether cartilage was removed from ulcer, cartilage rim around ulcer, or distant normal-appearing cartilage. Proteoglycan was more readily extractable from operated knee cartilage.[93] Weight average sedimentation constants of proteoglycan subunits, 15S, were similar to those of normal controls.

Analysis of the partial meniscectomy rabbit model demonstrated that degenerative changes were seen more frequently and to a greater extent in younger, lighter animals (weight range: 1500 to 2250 grams) as compared with older, heavier rabbits (weight range: 2300 to 3600 grams). It was suggested that the greater number of lesions seen in the younger, lighter animals was related to an increased sensitivity of young, mitotically active chondroblasts to damage following biomechanical alterations.

This model was also used to study synovitis as a manifestation of degenerative joint disease. Although mild focal synovial reaction was seen in experimentally induced osteoarthritis alone, moderate to severe synovitis was induced in animals only after combined partial meniscectomy and treadmill running.[96] A statistically significant increase in synovial cathepsin-D activity seen in the partial meniscectomy animals with running confirmed the inflammatory reaction seen histologically. Studies of various therapeutic agents in this model revealed that salicylates did not affect the histopathologic findings.[97] Temporary inhibition of ulcer induction was, however, noted with chloroquine and with Rumalon, an extract derived from calf cartilage and bone marrow.[92] Tamoxifen, an estrogen inhibitor with weak estrogenic activities, was shown to decrease the severity of pathologic lesions.[98]

A rabbit model in which osteoarthritis is induced by resection of small portions of the fibular collateral and sesamoid ligaments of

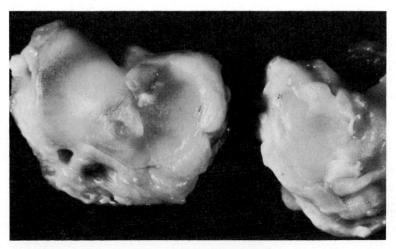

Figure 6–8. Right and left rabbit tibias. Osteophyte formation is seen along the entire rim of the medial tibial plateau of the right tibia 12 weeks after partial medial meniscectomy. The left knee shows normal soft synovial reflection.

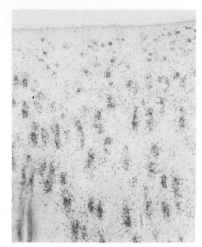

Figure 6–9. $^{35}SO_4$-labeled tibial cartilage, 5 weeks following partial medial meniscectomy. Dense uptake of the isotope is seen maximally over the chondrocytes, with spread to the surrounding matrix. ($\times$ 250.) (From Mayor MB, et al.: J Rheumatol 1:17, 1974.)

the rabbit knee in association with removal of a portion of the lateral meniscus has been described.[99] This model is included here under meniscectomy rather than "combined" models because only minimal degenerative lesions were noted when ligaments alone were cut but the meniscus was left intact. Gross degenerative lesions included cartilage deterioration on the lateral and medial condyles of the tibia, and ulcerations, exposure of subchondral bone, and osteophyte formation on the articular surfaces of the femurs. Histologic studies revealed loss of cartilage layers, cartilage fissuring and ulceration, clusters of chondrocytes in clones, and invasion of the calcified cartilage layer by proliferating bone and capillaries. A marked decrease in cartilage metachromasia identified loss of matrix proteoglycan. In pilot studies using this model, lesions were diminished in animals receiving low-dose systemic administration of glucocorticoids; pirprofen, a nonsteroidal anti-inflammatory agent; and tribenoside, a glucofuranoside derivative.[100]

Elmer, Moskowitz, and Frankel studied the effects of complete excision of the medial meniscus in rabbits and dogs.[101] Degenerative changes were seen most frequently in those animals in which there was absence of meniscal regeneration. Degenerative lesions included pitting and fibrillation of the articular surface and medial tibial osteophyte formation. Safranin-O stain was almost completely lost within the hyaline cartilage.

Pathologic and biochemical changes following total meniscectomy and meniscal lesions in rabbits were further evaluated by other investigators.[102, 103] In one group of animals, medial meniscectomy was performed. In a second group, the meniscus was retained but a large C-type bucket-handle lesion was created. Degenerative changes noted after meniscectomy and after induction of meniscal injury were similar in both severity and progression. These changes, limited almost exclusively to the medial tibia, were characterized by loss of surface luster, fissure and cleft formation, chondrocyte proliferation in clones, and diminished matrix metachromasia. Peripheral osteophytes were noted. It is of interest that the surgical lesions in the tear created in the meniscus never healed; the inner and outer portions of the meniscus remained completely separate. Biochemical studies performed on the articular cartilage in these animals revealed similar findings in the two groups.[102] In vivo measurements of ^3H-proline incorporation into ^3H-hydroxyproline demonstrated a several-fold increase in collagen synthesis. The newly made collagen was predominantly Type II.

The degenerative effects of partial and total resection of the medial meniscus were studied in dog knees by Cox and coworkers.[104] One group of animals underwent total excision of the medial meniscus at its periphery; another group had excision of the medial portion of the medial meniscus composing one third to two thirds of the width of the meniscus, leaving an intact peripheral rim. Degenerative changes were most marked in the knees in which total meniscectomy had been performed. Synovial fluid was increased, and synovial inflammation and thickening were noted. Varying degrees of pitting, erosion, and fibrillation of the articular cartilage of the medial femoral condyle and medial tibial plateau were observed. The knees in which the medial meniscus was partially removed revealed changes that varied from a normal gross appearance to variable amounts of degenerative change. The amount of change appeared to be directly proportional to the amount of meniscus removed. It is of interest that the lateral compartments of all knees, regardless of whether they had undergone total or partial meniscectomy, were essentially normal in appearance, even when knees revealed severe changes in the medial compartment.

EXPERIMENTAL OSTEOARTHRITIS FOLLOWING EXTENSIVE SURGICAL MANIPULATION OF THE JOINT

Degenerative lesions induced by surgical manipulations that result in marked joint laxity have been described.[105–111] These procedures involve various combinations of excision of collateral ligaments, cruciate ligaments, and menisci. In a well-defined model, severe degenerative joint lesions were rapidly induced in rabbit knees following excision of the medial collateral ligament, the medial meniscus, and both cruciate ligaments.[105–110] Gross joint instability was associated with frequent tibiofemoral and patellofemoral subluxation and occasionally with dislocation. Degenerative lesions produced were characterized by cellular degeneration, flaking of the superficial cartilage layer, fissure, fibrillation, loss of metachromasia, a disturbed arrangement of cells with formation of cell clusters, "blistering" of cartilage, and penetration of the calcified layer by subchondral capillaries. Cartilage thinning led to focal erosions. Osteophytes were seen on both the patella and the patellar surface of the femoral condyles. Increased deoxyribonucleic acid synthesis by cartilage was observed using autoradiographic localization of ^{3}H-thymidine uptake.[107]

Expanded biochemical studies of the cartilage response utilizing this model were performed by Ehrlich and colleagues.[108] Operated joints revealed a decrease in proteoglycan, an increase in acid phosphatase, and increases in the rates of synthesis of protein and glycosaminoglycan. No significant changes in hydroxyproline content or ^{3}H-thymidine uptake were observed. These biochemical data simulated those seen in human osteoarthritis.

Similar degenerative changes have been described in rabbits in studies utilizing slight variations in technique from that described above.[109, 110] In one such variation, the medial collateral and the two cruciate ligaments were sectioned. The peripheral margin of the anterior two thirds of the medial meniscus was then cut in a crescent-like shape and the meniscus allowed to float free within the medial compartment.[110] This additional local factor further enhanced the internal derangement. Degenerative changes were characterized by loss of joint space, loss of metachromasia, severe fibrillation and necrosis of articular cartilage, osteophyte formation, exposure of subchondral bone to the joint space, and marked sclerosis of eburnated bone.

Conversely, Bohr studied the effects of increasing the stability of this model following section of the collateral and cruciate ligaments and meniscectomy.[109] The medial collateral ligament was resutured, and more sutures were placed in the fascia. Pathologic findings were essentially unchanged, however. Microangio-

graphic and scintigraphic investigations demonstrated increased vascular flow to the operated joint.

Combined surgical manipulations were utilized to induce osteoarthritis in guinea pigs.[111] Osteoarthritis was induced by several methods. In the first series of animals, degenerative changes followed transection of the anterior cruciate ligament and the major portion of the medial collateral ligaments. A second series of animals had similar transection of the anterior cruciate and medial collateral ligaments, but partial meniscectomy was added. Degenerative changes occurred in both series but were more rapid in onset and progression in the group of animals receiving the partial meniscectomy. Qualitative pathologic changes induced by either surgical procedure were characteristic of those seen in other animal models of osteoarthritis as well as those seen in human disease. Joint cartilage lesions were characterized by fibrillation, pitting, ulceration, and subchondral eburnation. Histopathologic studies demonstrated loss of safranin-O stain and irregular cell arrangement with clusters of chondrocytes in clones. Osteophyte formation was noted. Operated joints contained significantly more total cartilage than contralateral normal joints in the same animals. New cartilage formation reflected attempts at repair; found particularly around the periphery of the structural surfaces, it was similar in appearance to the original hyaline cartilage. Although the DNA content of cartilage of the operated knees was unaltered, DNA synthesis, as measured by ^{3}H-thymidine uptake, was increased. Elevations of lysosomal enzymes, including acid phosphatase, arylsulfatase A, and beta-glucuronidase, were noted. Administration of vitamin C had a protective effect on cartilage degenerative changes.

It is apparent that a number of experimental models that variably simulate human osteoarthritis with respect to pathology, biochemistry, and pathogenesis are already available. Although many of these models reproduce the disease only incompletely, they are still of value in investigations of various facets of disease pathogenesis and pathology. Certain models, such as the cruciate ligament section models, the various partial and total meniscectomy models, and the combined ligament/meniscus resection models, more completely simulate the human disease; for this reason, they are more currently in vogue as models for study. These latter models are reasonably consistent in reproducibility, and the exact time of induction of joint derangement leading to degenerative change can be accurately identified. They simulate naturally occurring clinical sequences in the human that lead to degenerative change. Although it might be criticized that these models represent a traumatic secondary osteoarthritis, interpretations based on these models can be transferred with some degree of assurance to the naturally occurring human disease. Models utilizing small animals such as mice, guinea pigs, and rabbits are more attractive with regard to cost than models that utilize larger animals such as dogs. The availability of the models described in this chapter has already led to an augmented understanding of the pathology, biochemical alterations, and pathogenesis of osteoarthritis.

References

1. Howell DS, Moskowitz RW: Introduction: Symposium on osteoarthritis. A brief review of research and directions of future investigation. Arthritis Rheum 20:S96–S103, 1977.
2. Howell DS, Sapolsky AJ, Pita JC, et al.: The pathogenesis of osteoarthritis. Semin Arthritis Rheum 5:365–383, 1976.
3. McDevitt CA: Towards an Understanding of Osteoarthritis: The Contribution of Experimental Models. *In* Veys EM, Verbruggen G (eds.): Amsterdam, Excerpta Medica, 1982.
4. Moskowitz RW: Experimental models of degenerative joint disease. Semin Arthritis Rheum 2:95–116, 1972.
5. Troyer H: Experimental models of osteoarthritis: A review. Semin Arthritis Rheum 11:362–374, 1982.
6. Silberberg R: *In* Current concepts of degenerative joint disease (osteoarthritis). Bull Rheum Dis 17:459, 1967.
7. Waine H: *In* Current concepts of degenerative joint disease (osteoarthritis). Bull Rheum Dis 17:459, 1967.
8. Silberberg M, Hasler M, Silberberg R: Articular cartilage of dwarf mice: Submicroscopic effects of somatotrophin. Pathol Microbiol 29:137–155, 1966.
9. Silberberg M, Silberberg R, Hasler M: Fine structure of articular cartilage in mice receiving cortisone acetate. Arch Pathol 82:569–582, 1966.
10. Moskowitz RW, Davis W, Sammarco J, et al.: Experimentally induced corticosteroid arthropathy. Arthritis Rheum 13:236–243, 1970.
11. Silberberg R, Hasler M, Silberberg M: Response of articular cartilage of dwarf mice to insulin: Electromicroscopic studies. Anat Rec 155:577–589, 1966.
12. Silbermann M: Experimentally induced osteoarthrosis in the temporomandibular joint of the mouse. Acta Anat 96:9–24, 1976.
13. Lloyd-Roberts G: The role of capsular changes in osteoarthritis of the hip joint. J Bone Joint Surg 35B:627–642, 1953.
14. George RC, Chrisman OD: The role of cartilage polysaccharides in osteoarthritis. Clin Orthop 57:259–265, 1968.
15. Chrisman OD, Fessel JM, Southwick WD: Experimental production of synovitis and marginal articular exostoses in the knee joints of dogs. Yale J Biol Med 37:409–412, 1965.
16. Murray DG: Experimentally induced arthritis using intra-articular papain. Arthritis Rheum 7:211–219, 1964.
17. Bentley G: Papain-induced degenerative arthritis of the hip in rabbits. J Bone Joint Surg 53B:324–337, 1971.
18. Havdrup T, Telhag H: Papain-induced changes in the knee joints of adult rabbits. Acta Orthop Scand 48:143–149, 1977.
19. Lenzi L, Berlanda P, Flora A, et al.: Vitamin A induced osteoarthritis in rabbits: An experimental model for the study of human disease. *In* Articular Cartilage. Proceedings of the Symposium Held at the Institute of Orthopaedics, November, 1973. London, Institute of Orthopaedics, 1974, pp. 243–257.
20. Weissman G, Pras M, Rosenberg L: Arthritis induced by filipin in rabbits. Arthritis Rheum 10:325–336, 1967.
21. Kalbhen DA: *In* Nuki G (ed.): Aetiopathogenesis of Osteoarthritis. Tunbridge Wells, Pitman Medical Publishing Co., 1980, pp. 123–138.
22. Williams JM, Brandt KD: Iodo-acetate (IA) causes osteoarthritis in guinea pigs. (Abstract.) Anat Rec 202:201A, 1982.
23. Williams JM, Brandt KD: Effect of immobility on formation of osteophytes after intra-articular injection of iodo-acetate. Clin Res 30:810A, 1982.
24. Bennett GA, Bauer W: A study of the repair of the articular cartilage and the reaction of normal joints of adult dogs to surgically created defects of articular cartilage, "joint mice," and patellar displacement. Am J Pathol 8:499–524, 1932.
25. Calandruccio RA, Gilmer WS Jr: Proliferation, generation and repair of articular cartilage of immature animals. J Bone Joint Surg 44A:431–455, 1962.
26. Carlson H: Reactions of rabbit patellar cartilage following operative defects: A morphological and autoradiographic study. Acta Orthop Scand 28(Suppl):1–104, 1957.
27. Salter RB, Simmonds DF, Malcolm BW, et al.: The biological effect of continuous passive motion on the healing of full-thickness defects in articular cartilage. J Bone Joint Surg 62A:1232–1251, 1980.
28. Salter RB, Minster RR, Bell RS, et al.: Continuous passive motion and the repair of full-thickness articular cartilage defects—a one year follow-up. Trans Orthop Res Soc 7:167, 1982.
29. Furukawa T, Eyre D, Koide S, et al.: Biochemical studies on repair cartilage resurfacing experimental defects in the rabbit knee. J Bone Joint Surg 62A:79–89, 1980.
30. Cheung HS, Fynch KL, Johnson RP, et al.: In vitro synthesis of tissue-specific type II collagen by healing cartilage. Arthritis Rheum 23:211–219, 1980.
31. Meachim G: The effect of scarification on articular cartilage in the rabbit. J Bone Joint Surg 45B:150–161, 1963.
32. Thompson RC Jr: An experimental study of surface injury to articular cartilage and enzyme responses within the joint. Clin Orthop 107:239–248, 1975.
33. Simon WH, Green WT Jr: Experimental production of cartilage necrosis by cold injury: Failure to cause degenerative joint disease. Am J Pathol 64:145–153, 1971.

34. Simon WH, Richardson S, Herman W, et al.: Long-term effects of chondrocyte death on rabbit articular cartilage "in vivo." J Bone Joint Surg 58A:517–526, 1976.

35. Pauwels F: Biomechanics of the Normal and Diseased Hip: Theoretical Foundation, Technique and Result of Treatment: An Atlas. Berlin and New York, Springer-Verlag, 1976.

36. Radin EL, Ehrlich MG, Chernack R, et al.: Effect of repetitive impulsive loading on the knee joints of rabbits. Clin Orthop 131:288–293, 1978.

37. Radin EL: Mechanical factors in the etiology of osteoarthrosis. In Peyron JG (ed.): Epidemiology of Osteoarthritis. Proceedings of a Symposium. Paris, France, 1980, pp. 136–139.

38. Serink MT, Nachemson A, Hansson G: The effect of impact loading on rabbit knee joints. Acta Orthop Scand 48:250–262, 1977.

39. Reimann I: Experimental osteoarthritis of the knee in rabbits induced by alteration of the load-bearing. Acta Orthop Scand 44:496–504, 1973.

40. Gloobe H, Nathan H: Osteophyte formation in experimental bipedal rats. J Comp Pathol 83:133–141, 1973.

41. Arsever CL, Bole G, Van Natter S, et al.: Induction of experimental osteoarthritis (OA) by selective myectomy and tendotomy. Arthritis Rheum 26(Suppl):S22, 1983.

42. Finsterbush A, Friedman B: The effect of sensory denervation on rabbits' knee joints: A light and electron microscopic study. J Bone Joint Surg 57A:949–956, 1975.

43. Palmoski M, O'Connor B, Brandt K: Interruption of articular nerves impairs macromolecular organization of articular cartilage. (Abstract.) Arthritis Rheum 22:644, 1979.

44. Silberberg M, Silberberg R: Age changes of bones and joints in various strains of mice. Am J Anat 68:69–95, 1941.

45. Silberberg M, Silberberg R: Osteoarthritis in mice fed diets enriched with animal or vegetable fat. Arch Pathol 70:385–390, 1960.

46. Silberberg M, Silberberg R: Modifying action of estrogen on the evolution of osteoarthritis in mice of different ages. Endocrinology 72:449–457, 1963.

47. Silberberg M, Silberberg R: Effect of castration and intermittent administration of estrogen on knee joints and femoral shafts of mice. Pathol Microbiol (Basel) 33:274–286, 1969.

48. Silberberg M, Silberberg R: Age-linked modification of the effect of estrogen on joints and cortical bone of female mice. Gerontologia 16:201–211, 1970.

49. Wilhelmi G, Faust R: Suitability of the C57 black mouse as an experimental animal for the study of skeletal changes due to ageing, with special reference to osteo-arthrosis and its response to tribenoside. Pharmacology 14:289–296, 1976.

50. Sokoloff L: Natural history of degenerative joint disease in small laboratory animals. I. Pathological anatomy of degenerative joint disease in mice. Arch Pathol 62:118–128, 1956.

51. Sokoloff L, Gay GE Jr: Natural history of degenerative joint disease in small laboratory animals. II. Epiphyseal maturation and osteoarthritis of the knee of mice of inbred strains. Arch Pathol 62:129–135, 1956.

52. Silberberg M, Silberberg R: Effects of a high fat diet on the joints of aging mice. Arch Pathol 50:828–846, 1950.

53. Wigley RD, Couchman KG, Maule R, et al.: Degenerative arthritis in mice: Study of age and sex frequency in various strains with a genetic study of NZB/B1, NZY/B1, and hybrid mice. Ann Rheum Dis 36:249–253, 1977.

54. Silberberg R: Epiphyseal growth and osteoarthrosis in blotchy mice. Exp Cell Biol 45:1–8, 1977.

55. Sokoloff L, Jay GE Jr: Natural history of degenerative joint disease in small laboratory animals. IV. Degenerative joint disease in the laboratory rat. Arch Pathol 62:140–142, 1956.

56. Sokoloff L: The Biology of Degenerative Joint Disease. Chicago, Illinois, University of Chicago Press, 1969, pp. 18–21.

57. Schnell GB: Canine hip dysplasia. Lab Invest 8:1178–1189, 1959.

58. Lust G, Miller DR: Biochemical changes in canine osteoarthrosis. In Nuki G (ed.): The Aetiopathogenesis of Osteoarthrosis. Tunbridge Wells, Pitman Medical Publishing Co., 1980, pp. 47–51.

59. Lust G, Pronsky W, Sherman DM: Biochemical and ultrastructural observations in normal and degenerative canine articular cartilage. Am J Vet Res 33:2429–2440, 1972.

60. Miller DR, Lust G: Accumulation of procollagen in the degenerative articular cartilage of dogs with osteoarthritis. Biochim Biophys Acta 583:218–231, 1979.

61. Lust G, Beilman WT, Dueland DJ, et al.: Intra-articular volume and hip joint instability in dogs with hip dysplasia. J Bone Joint Surg 62A:576–582, 1980.

62. Hall MC: Cartilage changes after experimental relief of contact in knee joint of the mature rat. Clin Orthop 64:64–76, 1969.

63. Thompson RC Jr, Bassett CAL: Histological observations on experimentally induced degeneration of articular cartilage. J Bone Joint Surg 52A:435–443, 1970.

64. Engh GA, Chrisman OD: Experimental arthritis in rabbit knees: A study of relief of pressure on one tibial plateau in immature and mature rabbits. Clin Orthop 125:221–226, 1977.

65. Evans EB, Eggers GW, Butler JK, et al.: Experimental immobilization and remobilization of rat knee joints. J Bone Joint Surg 42A:737–758, 1960.

66. Salter RB, Field P: The effects of continuous compression on living articular cartilage: An experimental investigation. J Bone Joint Surg 42A:31–49, 1960.

67. Trias A: Effect of persistent pressure on the articular cartilage: An experimental study. J Bone Joint Surg 43B:376–386, 1961.

68. Hall MC: Cartilage changes after experimental immobilization of the knee joint of the young rat. J Bone Joint Surg 45A:36–44, 1963.

69. Hall MC: Articular changes in the knee of the adult rat after prolonged immobilization in extension. Clin Orthop 34:184–195, 1964.

70. Thaxter TH, Mann RA, Anderson CE: Degeneration of immobilized knee joints in rats: Histological and autoradiographic study. J Bone Joint Surg 47A:567–585, 1965.

71. Roy S: Ultrastructure of articular cartilage in experimental immobilization. Ann Rheum Dis 29:634–642, 1970.

72. Enneking WF, Horowitz M: The intra-articular effects of immobilization on the human knee. J Bone Joint Surg 54A:973–985, 1972.

73. Akeson WH, Woo SLY, Amiel D, et al.: The

connective tissue response to immobility: biochemical changes in periarticular connective tissue of the immobilized rabbit knee. Clin Orthop 93:356–362, 1973.

74. Troyer H: The effect of short-term immobilization on the rabbit knee joint cartilage: A histochemical study. Clin Orthop 107:249–257, 1975.

75. Michelsson J-E, Videman T, Langenskiöld A: Changes in bone formation during immobilization and development of experimental osteoarthritis. Acta Orthop Scand 48:443–449, 1977.

76. Eronen I, Videman T, Friman C, et al.: Glycosaminoglycan metabolism in experimental osteoarthrosis caused by immobilization. Acta Orthop Scand 49:329–334, 1978.

77. Palmoski M, Perricone E, Brandt KD: Development and reversal of a proteoglycan aggregation defect in normal canine knee cartilage after immobilization. Arthritis Rheum 22:508–517, 1979.

78. Langenskiöld A, Michelsson J-E, Videman T: Osteoarthritis of the knee in the rabbit produced by immobilization: Attempts to achieve a reproducible model for studies on pathogenesis and therapy. Acta Orthop Scand 50:1–14, 1979.

79. Palmoski MJ, Brandt KD: Running inhibits the reversal of atrophic changes in canine knee cartilage after removal of a leg cast. Arthritis Rheum 24:1329–1337, 1981.

80. Bruce J, Walmsley R: Excision of the patella; some experimental and anatomical observations. J Bone Joint Surg 24:311–325, 1942.

81. Cohn BNE: Total and partial patellectomy; experimental study. Surg Gynecol Obstet 79:526–536, 1944.

82. Garr EL, Moskowitz RW, Davis W: Degenerative changes following experimental patellectomy in the rabbit. Clin Orthop 92:296–304, 1973.

83. De Palma AF, Flynn JJ: Joint changes following experimental partial and total patellectomy. J Bone Joint Surg 40A:395–413, 1958.

84. Marshall JL: Periarticular osteophytes: Initiation and formation in the knee of the dog. Clin Orthop 62:37–47, 1969.

85. Pond MJ, Nuki G: Experimentally-induced osteoarthritis in the dog. Ann Rheum Dis 32:387–388, 1973.

86. Gilbertson EMM: Development of periarticular osteophytes in experimentally induced osteoarthritis in the dog: A study using microradiographic, microangiographic, and fluorescent bone-labelling techniques. Ann Rheum Dis 34:12–25, 1975.

87. McDevitt CA, Muir H: Biochemical changes in the cartilage of the knee in experimental and natural osteoarthritis in the dog. J Bone Joint Surg 58B:94–101, 1976.

88. McDevitt C, Gilbertson E, Muir H: An experimental model of osteoarthritis; early morphological and biochemical changes. J Bone Joint Surg 59B:24–35, 1977.

89. Williams JM, Felton DL, Peterson RG, et al.: Effects of surgically induced instability on rat knee articular cartilage. J Anat 134:103–109, 1982.

90. Davis W, Moskowitz RW: Degenerative joint changes following posterior cruciate ligament section in the rabbit. Clin Orthop 93:307–312, 1973.

91. Moskowitz RW, Davis W, Sammarco J, et al.: Experimentally induced degenerative joint lesions following partial meniscectomy in the rabbit. Arthritis Rheum 16:397–405, 1973.

92. Moskowitz RW: Osteoarthritis—studies with experimental models. Arthritis Rheum 20:S104–S108, 1977.

93. Moskowitz RW, Howell DS, Goldberg VM, et al.: Cartilage proteoglycan alterations in an experimentally induced model of rabbit osteoarthritis. Arthritis Rheum 22:155–163, 1979.

94. Mayor MB, Moskowitz RW: Metabolic studies in experimentally-induced degenerative joint disease in the rabbit. J Rheumatol 1:17–23, 1974.

95. Moskowitz RW, Goldberg VM, Malemud CJ: Metabolic responses of cartilage in experimentally induced osteoarthritis. Ann Rheum Dis 40:584–592, 1981.

96. Moskowitz RW, Goldberg VM, Berman L: Synovitis as a manifestation of degenerative joint disease: An experimental study. (Abstract.) Arthritis Rheum 19:813, 1976.

97. Moskowitz RW, Davis W, Jones W, et al.: Effects of salicylates on an experimentally induced model of osteoarthritis. (Abstract.) Arthritis Rheum 15:447–448, 1972.

98. Rosner IA, Malemud CJ, Goldberg VM, et al.: Pathologic and metabolic responses of experimental osteoarthritis to estradiol and an estradiol antagonist. Clin Orthop 171:280–286, 1982.

99. Colombo C, Butler M, O'Byrne E, et al.: I. Development of knee joint pathology following lateral meniscectomy and section of the fibular collateral and sesamoid ligaments. Arthritis Rheum 26:875–886, 1983.

100. Steinetz BG, Colombo C, Butler MC, et al.: Animal models of osteoarthritis: Possible applications in a drug development program. Curr Ther Res 20(Suppl):S60–S75, 1981.

101. Elmer RM, Moskowitz RW, Frankel VH: Meniscal regeneration and postmeniscectomy degenerative joint disease. Clin Orthop 124:304–310, 1977.

102. Floman Y, Eyre DR, Glimcher MJ: Induction of osteoarthrosis in the rabbit knee joint: Biochemical studies on the articular cartilage. Clin Orthop 147:278–286, 1980.

103. Shapiro F, Glimcher MJ: Induction of osteoarthrosis in the rabbit knee joint: Histologic changes following meniscectomy and meniscal lesions. Clin Orthop 147:287–295, 1980.

104. Cox JS, Nye CE, Schaefer WW, et al.: The degenerative effects of partial and total resection of the medial meniscus in dogs' knees. Clin Orthop 109:178–183, 1975.

105. Hulth A, Lindberg L, Telhag H: Experimental osteoarthritis in rabbits: Preliminary report. Acta Orthop Scand 41:522–530, 1970.

106. Telhag H, Lindberg L: A method for inducing osteoarthritic changes in rabbits' knees. Clin Orthop 86:214–229, 1972.

107. Telhag H: Mitosis of chondrocytes in experimental "osteoarthritis" in rabbits. Clin Orthop 86:224–229, 1972.

108. Ehrlich MG, Mankin HJ, Jones H, et al.: Biochemical confirmation of an experimental osteoarthritis model. J Bone Joint Surg 57A:392–396, 1975.

109. Bohr H: Experimental osteoarthritis in the rabbit knee joint. Acta Orthop Scand 47:558–565, 1976.

110. Mendes DG, Gotfried Y, Hamburger S, et al.: Induction of the three grades of osteoarthritis in rabbit's knee. Orthop Rev 10:113–116, 1981.

111. Schwartz ER, Oh WH, Leveille CR: Experimentally induced osteoarthritis in guinea pigs: Metabolic responses in articular cartilage to developing pathology. Arthritis Rheum 24:1345–1355, 1981.

7

Etiopathogenesis of Osteoarthritis

David S. Howell, M.D.

Most etiopathogenic pathways suggested to explain cartilage degradation and associated phenomena during the last two decades are based on tissue responses of an extremely complex nature. Those biochemical and biomechanical processes on which most emphasis has been placed during recent years have already been discussed in prior chapters from the viewpoint of epidemiology, pathology, biochemistry, and animal models. The goal of this chapter is to survey and interrelate some of these hypotheses from a personal approach.

DEFINITION OF TERMS

Briefly reviewed, a *pathogenic mechanism* describes a related series of events manifested as a number of biomechanical and inflammatory phenomena as the host body responds to a noxious agent.

Etiologic agent refers, of course, to the primary inciting cause. Etiologic and pathogenic pathways may closely interrelate and overlap where etiologic factors of aging, environmental trauma, or hereditary defects in a tissue are involved. On the other hand, etiologic and pathogenic pathways may be widely separated in their characteristics, as, for example, in the case of staphylococcal septic arthritis leading to tissue destruction and secondary osteoarthritis.

Primary versus secondary osteoarthritis has been the subject of changing definitions through the years. I prefer to define secondary osteoarthritis as that form of the disease that has an important, clearly defined, underlying disease contributing to its causation. When it is of totally unknown cause, the disease is considered to be primary osteoarthritis. If osteoarthritis is affected by a variety of important *conditioning factors* the disease is considered secondary but of multifactorial origin. *Osteoarthritis* is defined here as a characteristic picture of cartilage degradation with variable amounts of hypertrophic cartilage and bony remodeling—that is, the broadest use of the term, a pathologic rather than clinical entity. Subclassifications of osteoarthritis into symptomatic, asymptomatic, and progressive versus nonprogressive erosive disease are all definable characteristics within the overall definition.

BUILDING AN ETIOLOGIC HYPOTHESIS

The value of a hypothesis on the etiopathogenesis of osteoarthritis must be based on its powers of predictability for natural events. The hypothesis must be sufficiently precise to be testable, and as long as it holds up in the face of critical experiments, it remains a useful description of nature. As propounded by the British philosopher, Karl Popper, a hypothesis that tries to explain too wide a series of events has no value because it can be either supported or rejected by proper experimentation.[1] With each advance in the understanding of the biomechanical properties of joints, their biochemical structure, and changes in disease, more sensible, detailed hypotheses with greater predictability can be derived to replace the older hypotheses. Certain treatises cover various as-

FLOW DIAGRAM INDICATING ETIOPATHOGENIC FACTORS INVOLVED IN
OSTEOARTHRITIS

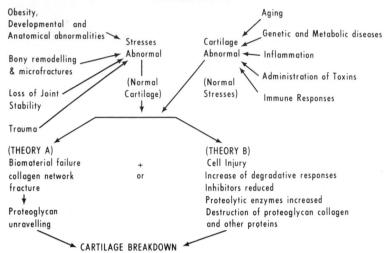

Figure 7–1. Flow diagram indicating etiopathogenic factors involved in osteoarthritis.

pects of recent advances in the field of osteoarthritis, cartilage degradation, and repair.[2-7]

A simplified flow diagram combining certain pathogenic theories is shown in Figure 7–1. The building blocks of these theories include joint geometry, congruity or lack of it, the quality of the cartilage, the load on the cartilage (normal, reduced, or excessive), and adjacent bone degradative as well as reparative mechanisms. Most of the events in this diagram would have to be modified into a series of more precise statements to be suitable for scientific testing. Information from previously rejected hypotheses may still be useful in evolving important answers.[8]

THREE MAJOR TYPES OF ETIOPATHOGENESIS

In the search for the etiology of osteoarthritis, there are currently three major categories of theories. One of these is based on the major role of physical forces and biomaterial failure of articular cartilage. The second attributes a major part of the disease to failing articular chondrocytic responses involving both degradation and repair (Figs. 7–1 and 7–2). A third group of views of the disease considers bony remodeling, synovial responses, microfractures, vascular changes, and other extracartilaginous factors as primary problems, with

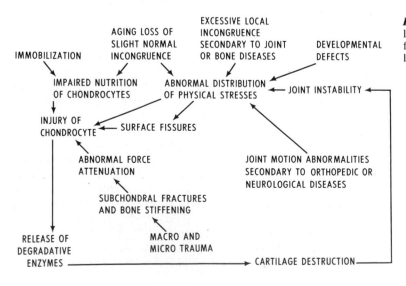

Figure 7–2. Schema of pathophysiologic interrelationships of physical forces and chondrocyte responses leading to cartilage destruction.

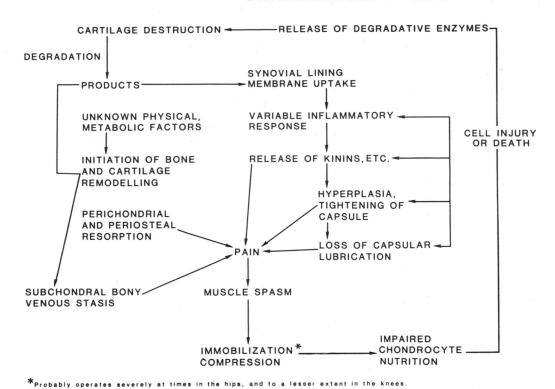

Figure 7–3. Interrelationships of bony remodeling, synovial responses, vascular changes, and extracartilaginous factors in etiopathogenesis.

cartilage changes being secondary (Figs. 7–2 and 7–3). There is a likelihood of multiple etiologic subsets, and important effects of aging on all of them seem certain.[9, 10]

Biomaterial Failure

The overall viewpoint embodied in this group of theories, as I interpret the proponents' views, is either a defective biomaterial that gradually disintegrates in the face of normal wear as a function of aging, or a normal biomaterial that fails in response to single or multiple excessive traumatic events. This biomaterial viewpoint includes subsets of theories that point to (1) abnormal or unequal growth plate function during growth and development, leading to an abnormal weight distribution carried through that joint; (2) failure of collagen fibril or fiber formation in respect to crosslinking, or errors of proteoglycan or glycoprotein metabolism to the extent that these bond the collagen network; or (3) failure in the final complex basket weave of the tissue caused by unknown cellular functions during the formation of the matrix. Factors that will influence the time of joint failure, that is, the time when progressive deep carti-

lage erosions lead to final joint instability and other phenotypic expressions of disease, would depend on the component deviations in respect to wear properties, abnormalities in joint configuration and alignment due to bone and cartilage growth during development, and the type of trauma in terms of quantity and quality that historically afflicts a given joint. Examples of such disturbances would be multiple changes in growth plates and adult remodeling, which might contribute to formation of the so-called pistol-grip deformity,[11] the acetabular bone thickening described by Day and associates,[12] and tibial bowing. Shallowness of the acetabulum[11] and tilted position of the femoral head on the femoral neck[13] (femoral neck diaphyseal angle $> 135°$) may be important factors with osteoarthritis-producing action.

The controversial effects of various forms of sport and industrial activities have been reviewed by Radin.[14] Most researchers feel that these factors are so important that once a given link in the chain, such as mild acetabular dysplasia,[13] is identified, it would indicate that the ensuing osteoarthritis is secondary. Still, it will be necessary to show with adequate controls what happens in different population groups to evaluate the importance of such circumstantial evidence observed post hoc at hip surgery, as discussed by Byers and associates.[15, 16]

One step in this direction preliminary to a matched control study is the development of detailed criteria for assessment of the disease, as illustrated in the studies of Altman and colleagues.[17] An epidemiologic prospective study to establish this theory requires decades for completion and is almost always beyond the realm of current attainment in most centers. Yet, such controlled studies are precisely what are needed. How many patients with bowlegs, pistol-grip or femoral neck valgus deformities, or acetabular dysplasia in the population survive to old age without osteoarthritis? Obviously, there must also exist a wide variation in biomaterial durability in a general population. Furthermore, a role for an aging loss of normal joint incongruity has been postulated.[18]

The stiffening of subchondral bone through microfractures as an initiator of osteoarthritis exemplifies use of the Popper[1] approach by Radin. His initial hypothesis is that subchondral bone fractures from inadvertent weight-bearing trauma stiffen the bone and throw an additional stress on the cartilage; conversely, the critical level of damage to the collagen network in a highly stressed histologic area of cartilage may be the key factor in starting the progressive lesions.

The concept of the tight and loose collagen network has derived support largely from the studies from Maroudas' laboratory.[19–21] The molecules, which are partly in the form of subunits and aggregates, occupy large domains up to 50 ml/gm of dry weight when fully extended in solution.[21, 22] In hyaline cartilage, it is proposed that these molecules are probably constrained to much smaller volumes by a collagen network.[20, 23] In those sites, they are so concentrated as to constitute viscoelastic gels. Because of their high glycosaminoglycan content, these molecules exert a very low hydraulic permeability and the amount of interstitial fluid loss from the surface of cartilage in vivo is limited under compressive loads. Whatever lymph is extruded reassociates within the proteoglycans when this load is removed. Constraints on water uptake are imposed by the collagen network, which causes at least three atmospheres of positive pressure when the cartilage is unloaded. The osmotic pressure increases proportionally to proteoglycan concentration as it, in turn, increases during loading.[21, 24, 25]

As indicated by Maroudas, a tight collagen network is probably needed to create this elastic mechanism in cartilage. The mechanism is demonstrable by the lack of swelling and lack of imbibition of water in experiments in which cubes of fresh normal articular cartilage are placed in physiologic saline solution.[21] In contrast, normal invertebral disk contents imbibe water under the same experimental conditions, indicating a lack of a tight collagen network in the latter tissue.[21] It has been theorized that differences in articular cartilage from that of the nucleus pulposus are due to the finding that proteoglycans are confined by the annulus fibrosis laterally, and above and below by the vertebral end plates under considerable normal pressure of body weight and muscle tone. Such a rigid boundary framework would hypothetically seem to cause the same sort of restraint on the proteoglycans on a macro scale, as seen in articular cartilage. Consistent with such a framework is data of Harris and associates,[26] who showed that selective loss of proteoglycans from cartilage eradicates its elastic properties, but a collagen framework preserves articular shape.

Although much of the increased water content in osteoarthritic tissue relates to the proteoglycans unraveling, there is still considerable uptake of water into cartilage collagen,[27] and a role for this tissue in the elastic properties has been explained in the kinetic biomaterial studies of Mow and colleagues.[28, 29] Certainly, other phenomena are probably operative in explaining water imbibition by osteoarthritic cartilage. Disruption of collagen bundles may open up sites where proteoglycans and other proteins tightly bound to the fibers either change their conformation or become partially degraded, with a consequent shift of water into the collagen bundles, as postulated by Mankin and Thrasher.[27] How the collagen network and proteoglycan form a theoretical junction at an ultramicroscopic level to provide shear moduli at orders of magnitude larger than those of equally concentrated gels of proteoglycans alone is a burning unanswered question.

Some insights into what etiologic agent might be involved might be based on the location of the earliest injury. So far, no single site can be found.[30] Possibly the first change is a deepening of cleavages in the cartilage surface cracks; alternatively, a deep separation of collagen bundles within their insertion into calcified cartilage has been described by Meachim and Bentley.[30, 31] There are likely varying initiation sites. Studies on histologic layers tangentially sectioned from human osteoarthritic cartilage were performed by Maroudas' group. These studies suggest that the collagen network becomes damaged early, and water content rises to the highest levels in the upper radial zone or transitional zone of osteoarthritic cartilage.[32] Cystic lesions have occasionally been observed in such a central location in early osteoarthritic disease. It seems that inasmuch as the tangential zone is braced to resist tensile forces, vulnerability to biomaterial failure might become apparent at the interface of these zones following various stresses. Our electron-microscopic findings in the Pond-Nuki dog model of osteoarthritis of swelling of fibers around the chondrocyte, cell injury, and edema fit this viewpoint.[33]

Another site of initial vulnerability might be the territorial matrix or surface zone if there were a peculiar error in formation of these matrices. Several studies indicate that proteoglycan (PG) aggregates (hyaluronic acid, PG subunit, link protein complexes) are anchored within the interterritorial region between the latticework of the vertically oriented collagen bundles. Link proteins have been associated with proteoglycans in this histologic region as detected on transmission electron microscopy by labeled antibody techniques from Poole's laboratory.[34] In contrast, link proteins were arrayed differently in the tangential zone and territorial matrix around chondrocytes; link proteins were not demonstrated to be associated with proteoglycans here but were irregularly spaced on the collagen fibers.[34] The association of link proteins with collagen fibers in irregular array suggests a different relationship to proteoglycans. Some of the proteoglycans there are also resistant to extraction except by extreme methods and are bound in some manner within the collagen bundles, especially in the territorial matrix.

How the collagen network is held together is totally unknown. It might be joined simply by basket weave. On the other hand, it might be held together by crosslinks of the hydroxypyridinium type or by extraneous compounds.[35–37] At least 24 protein bands have been found by Rosenberg in the A5 and A6 fractions of bovine growth embryonic cartilage.[38] Is it possible that one or more such proteins, particularly chondronectin,[39] a high–molecular-weight (over 180,000 daltons) glycoprotein, or perhaps the 148,000-dalton protein of Paulsson and Heinegård,[40] compose a glue to attach the corners of the module constituting the collagen network? No data to support such a view have yet been accrued; so far, all data indicate only cell adherence at sites of new tissue growth or remodeling. An-

other glycoprotein of particular interest from this standpoint is one found in sponge biopsy connective tissue by Mejer and Noble.[41] This one contained a hydroxyproline peptide and weighed about 20,000 daltons; it has not been sought in cartilage. Thus, there might be either biomaterial failure of collagen fibers per se etiologically, or there might be a failure of chemicals that could hypothetically glue the collagen network together. Following failure of such a collagen network, or the "glues," proteoglycans would no longer be confined but would take up water and, like the ticking within a mattress, uncoil and unravel through erosions and fissures to the joint surface.

During the last 10 years, interesting data have been obtained concerning the resistance to wear of cartilage as a function of aging. In two separate studies, resistance to wear was shown to decline significantly between the ages of 40 and 90 years.[42, 43] One system of biomaterial measurement involved time-to-break; the other involved indentation. Admittedly, insufficient data of this type have been obtained to firmly establish these effects of aging. Yet, such data are provocative and suggest a biochemical failure beyond the increasing wear properties of such aging cartilage. Another type of threat to biomaterial integrity is a postulated overcrosslinking of collagen, as seen as a result of homogentisic acid oxidation to benzoquinone in ochronosis.[44] Experimental demonstration of increased vulnerability of tissue to fatigue failure in experimental animal models would be consistent with such overcrosslinking. It also is possible that the increased fatigue failure of aging is a result of less rigid or less hydrophilic proteoglycan constituents. Keratan sulfate, enriched in cartilage during aging, is a more "flaccid" molecule than the chondroitin sulfates, based on hydrogen bonding between acetamino and adjacent carboxyl groups in the latter but not the former molecular class.[45]

Cartilage Degradation and Repair

Role of Repair Mechanisms in the Etiology of Osteoarthritis

It is difficult to assign a primary *etiologic* role for repair failure in the production of osteoarthritis. Such a role might exist if normal control repair mechanisms failed to maintain pace with minor degradative effects that otherwise would not lead to an irreversible osteoarthritic lesion. Failure to maintain the integrity of the collagen fibers at the cartilage surface might, for example, lead to more extensive degenerative change. Failure of repair may play a more definitive role in disease *pathogenesis,* as contrasted to primary etiology. Deep cartilage lesions that fail to penetrate bone marrow show poor repair. With erosion through to the bone marrow, layers of fairly presentable–looking repair cartilage are seen by light microscopy in both animals and humans; however, mechanical properties of this cartilage formed through subchondral vascular invasion have been considered to be inadequate. Abnormal and accelerated repair within and surrounding erosive sites is an osteoarthritic phenomenon studied extensively by Mankin and colleagues.[46–49] Other possible cellular phenomena leading to eventual matrix injury might be (1) stimulated phagocytosis by cartilage cells and (2) the effects of cellular proliferation and brood capsule formation on the integrity of existing cartilage matrix structures. No hard data support these latter contentions.

The Concept of the Role of Cellular Intervention in Progressive Lesions

According to this group of theories (see Fig. 7–1), cartilage degradation, whether in an etiologic or pathogenic pathway, is intimately involved, not simply during formation of the cartilage in development and growth but throughout a lifetime.

Cellular intervention based on prompt healing of minor surface erosions of cartilage might therefore be important in the prevention of progressive lesions. Postulations based on years of study suggest that changes in the cartilage surface occur with normal aging; osteoarthritis develops when failure of repair occurs at some critical point followed by progression of erosion. As mentioned previously, evidence against this viewpoint has been the undisputed frequent finding at autopsy of erosions in non–weight-bearing sites of knees and hips that apparently have not progressed over many years and are presumably asymptomatic.[10] This has led many researchers to the view that simple breaks or erosions in the surface are probably insufficient to initiate osteoarthritis in a normal joint. Further support for this view is found from studies in which the surface of cartilage abraded with Carborundum particles in vivo failed to produce osteoarthritis.[50] Loss of surface cellularity[51] and increased size of tertiary hollows,

controversially attributed to cells beneath the surface layer of cartilage as a function of aging,[9] would fit possibly as initiating events in some cases. How the cellular loss could lead to clefts and deep progressive erosions in some cases and not others remains unexplained.

Degradative Enzyme Theories

In these views, the thesis is held that cellular products have an important influence on cartilage breakdown in osteoarthritis. Implicit in this view is the chance that medical therapy that regulates cartilage degeneration by chondrocytes may effect improvement in the disease. The rapid overnight loss of collagen and proteoglycans seen when incubates of cartilage matrix are treated in vitro with catabolin, mononuclear cell factor, or retinol[52–57] indicates the potentially deleterious effects of degradative enzymes released by chondrocytes, which, in adulthood, occupy 5% to 10% of the volume of cartilage.[56] Obviously, mechanisms must normally exist to safeguard against the enzymes contained within the cells (cathepsins B, D, and F, neutral metalloproteoglycanase, neutral serine protease, and collagenase) to protect the matrix against devastating destruction in vivo.

Over several years of osteoarthritic cartilage alterations, destruction of cartilage may be influenced by cellular degradation of an extremely focal and locked-in nature, with respect to both histologic location and time. This would make the process extremely difficult to study except in animal models. This viewpoint could partly explain the wide differences in data among laboratories on turnover rates in osteoarthritic hip and knee cartilage samples incubated in vitro.[58, 59] In clinically manifested human osteoarthritis that comes to surgery, the disease is, of course, so advanced that one may be dealing with varying amounts of new fibrocartilage at sites of sampling as opposed to the original cartilage.

Neutral proteoglycanase and collagenase in chondrocytes might be liberated from their inhibitors into the adjacent matrix, where they act at neutral pH to break down cartilage components to a limited extent, with these breakdown products being carried to the cell margins.[60, 61] One might then visualize uptake of these partially degraded products into the chondrocyte lysosomes, with further breakdown by acid proteases within the chondrocytes. Failure, most of the time, to find breakdown products of proteoglycans in the cartilage has been interpreted by some groups[5, 58] as evidence against the theory altogether, but it has been interpreted by others as indicating only that the products are removed almost as rapidly as they are formed.[60]

Cartilage is normally protected against the acid protease action of chondrocytes by their enclosure within lysosomal membranes. If, however, the cells die and release these cathepsins from the lysosomes or other compartments of the chondrocytes, widespread coronal matrix damage is seen, as observed in heated samples of cartilage.[57] Acid proteases probably do not act outside the cells,[57] as demonstrated by the fact that the potent inhibitor pepstatin, which works on cathepsin D, and inhibitors that work on cathepsins B[62] and F are unable to block retinol-provoked chondrocyte matrix degradation. These inhibitors do not penetrate cells readily and are therefore unable to reach the intracellular site of major degradation.

In osteoarthritis, a diffuse loss of proteoglycans over a wide area of matrix between cells is commonly observed. How this matrix is broken down is an enigma. At any one level in the osteoarthritic cartilage, both at the margin and in the depths of the erosions, the profile of proteoglycans does not seem abnormal.[63] This supports the concept of rapid removal of degradation products. In in vitro models, rapid removal of degradation products from cartilage in organ culture has been found; there was almost no evidence of breakdown products inside the cartilage per se. Rapid liberation of partially degraded proteoglycan subunits into the surrounding medium has been noted in previous studies.[64] Possibly, free radical formation, as so extensively demonstrated in leukocytes, could be involved in the degradation.[65]

Another possible route for enzymatic breakdown relates to the elaboration of a neutral metalloprotease. Such neutral metalloproteases of human cartilage have been studied by us and by Ehrlich and coworkers over the last 10 years.[60, 61] In our hands, one such enzyme has a monomeric weight of 13,000 daltons, with a probable dimer form weighing 26,000 daltons.[60, 66] These enzymes have been demonstrated to diffuse rapidly through cartilage and are capable of causing proteoglycan breakdown.[60] Further evidence indicates that they are for the most part bound to an inhibitor of low molecular weight.[67] It is possible that under conditions of inadequate weight-bearing forces, immobilization, or other noxious stimuli, an imbalance of this enzyme in relation to its inhibitor might lead to proteoglycan degradation. Tiny concentrations of this neutral protease have been found to clip proteoglycan subunits preferentially in the hyaluronic acid (HA) binding region,[66] as also noted by Roughley and associates for some other proteases.[68] Evidence for chondrocytic origin of these neutral proteases has been shown in tissue culture studies performed by investigators from Case Western Reserve University in collaboration with our laboratory group.[67] Elevated levels of cathepsin B,[62] acid phosphatase,[69, 70] and, recently, active and latent collagenase assayed in osteoarthritic human cartilage cell cultures[71, 72] and samples of cartilage taken in vivo[73] strongly suggest that focal areas of tissue are undergoing degradation.

The presence of TCA and TCB peptide fragments in the cartilage containing collagenolytic activity strongly suggests that collagen cleavage has taken place in these osteoarthritic samples.[73] Inasmuch as cells are multiplying in these tissues to form brood capsules, it cannot be excluded, of course, that such evidence of protease increase is related to remodeling rather than to pathologic gross tissue destruction. Nevertheless, the evidence that these enzymes are deeply involved in either remodeling or degradation is currently a hypothesis that has survived critical attack over the last 10 years and has allowed more intelligently based modifications in experimentation in line with concepts espoused by Popper.[1] Despite these experimental approaches with respect to both etiologic and pathogenic pathways, the role of these enzymes still remains controversial. A role in etiology seems more remote than one in pathogenesis.

Tissue Mediators and Chondrocyte-Derived Proteolysis

It was stated by Bennett, Waine, and Bauer that the synovial membrane should not be neglected as having potential etiologic and pathogenic roles in osteoarthritis.[74] Certainly, with regard to pathogenesis, there is still little question that marginal bony remodeling occurs at an extremely early stage in the Pond-Nuki model of osteoarthritis in dogs.[75] It is uncertain whether this stimulation in such models is due to microscopic bruising of ligament at attachment sites, stirring up a local cellular response, or whether cartilage wear particles trapped in the sulcus of the synovial membrane adjacent to these remodeling sites might cause the reaction, as demonstrated in normal joints by Chrisman.[76] Lust and colleagues found intense synovial effusions in canine dysplastic hip joints as an early sign of disability and postulated a role for synovium in the development of joint dislocation.[77] Arnoldi and Reimann attributed some cases of osteoarthritis of the hip to noxious effects of synovial effusion on joint nutrition.[78] Clinically, a great deal of ligamentous injury is seen throughout adolescence and into adulthood related to sports trauma without invocation of an osteoarthritic response. Simply, the injection of cartilage products into a joint has not resulted in a completely reproducible osteoarthritis model, despite the hypertrophic marginal changes mentioned above.[76] Traumatic synovial injury in dogs fails to lead to osteoarthritis and synovial injury, i.e., a sham operation is used as a control in many studies. Thus, it would seem that in these models the noxious influences of an inflamed synovial membrane were insufficient to produce osteoarthritis.

Do synovial enzymes produced by inflammation ever account for cartilage damage in osteoarthritis? Even where the membranes become inflamed, as in the presence of rheumatoid arthritis lesions or septic arthritis, the enzymes elaborated by inflammatory cells are immediately taken up by α_2 macroglobulin, with only slight residual unneutralized activity (either by this or by the α_1 and α_2 proteinase inhibitors).[57] However, of great interest is the presence of high synovial fluid levels of active collagenase in the "Milwaukee shoulder" syndrome, which could theoretically lead to the observed disintegration of cartilage and a pseudotabes–like picture in the shoulder.[79] Studies to date indicate a low level of synovial α_2 macroglobulin in Milwaukee shoulder, so that decreased inhibition of activated collagenase might occur in these cases. Under such situations, activated collagenase derived from synovium could diffuse into cartilage and would theoretically bind to cartilage collagenase inhibitors.[79] Traces of residual, incompletely neutralized collagenase activity could slowly destroy the cartilage, thus providing a role for exogenously derived synovial enzymes rather than implicating cartilage proteases.[79] Could there be an imbalance between synovial cell and inflammatory cell enzymes and inhibitors in the etiology of some forms of osteoarthritis in the same way that has been postulated above for cartilage-derived enzymes?

A third route of cartilage degradation that must be considered in both pathogenesis and etiology might be the initiation of cartilage breakdown by factors derived from phagocytes in synovial lining membranes. Thus, the lymphocyte activating factor (LAF),[80] catabolin,[52] interleukin I, and mononuclear cell factor (MCF)[80] have all been studied in synovial cultures.[52–54, 80] These factors are believed to share a similar structure, with molecular weights in the order of 20,000 to 30,000 daltons, which allows for rapid permeation of cartilage. The characteristic of such mediators as studied on cartilage incubates is the initiation of protease degradation of the matrix by chondrocytes. Regulators and inhibitors of the factor are unknown, so far, at least to me. Again, whether such a factor (are they the same factor?) might be involved in the pseudotabes type of destructive arthropathies occasionally seen with osteoarthritis remains to be determined. Furthermore, a relationship to the osteoarthritis secondary to mineral crystal production, as found in "Milwaukee shoulder" syndrome, requires further study, as discussed below.

In any event, the early loss of surface cartilage wear particles during microtraumatic or macrotraumatic abrasion is followed by engulfment of such particles in floating and fixed lining macrophages. The possible role of the activation of inflammatory pathways in augmenting the clinical expression of osteoarthritis has been discussed elsewhere. The direct effect of possible MCF release has also been speculated as a possible etiologic factor, but the possibility of a variable secondary pathogenic role is more likely. The same tempered view applies, so far, to the role of immunologic responses.

Role of Immunologic Responses

Both cartilage cell surface antigens and matrix components are believed to be shielded for the most part from the immune system during embryonic and postnatal development. Considerable study by Herman and associates,[81–84] Glant and coworkers,[85] Gertzbein and colleagues,[86] and Cooke and associates[87] has been directed toward possible humoral and cell-mediated immune responses engendered in patients with osteoarthritis or degenerative disk disease when sporadically exposed to multiple cartilage antigens. Thus far, evidence for a humoral immune response as a pathogenic factor has been limited. In a substantial percentage of patients with osteoarthritis of the hip studied by Cooke and coworkers, IgG, IgA, IgM, and C^1 were detectable in cartilage.[87] The fact that such patients had a higher frequency of polyarthritis than those without such immunohistologic deposits was suggestive of an etiopathologic immune response in at least one or more subsets of osteoarthritis,[87] but one that probably is not operative in the majority of patients with osteoarthritis.

Herman and colleagues have found variable evidence for activation of cell-mediated immune responses to proteoglycans by mononuclear cells from osteoarthritic patients, as evidenced by release of lymphokines as well as mitogenic responses.[82] The subject is difficult to study; if only local synovial cells are activated, there are usually too few cells to harvest from osteoarthritic synovial membranes. Most studies involve peripheral circulating mononuclear cells tested directly or grown in tissue culture. One lymphokine from such a study in humans appears to depress cartilage cell synthesis of proteoglycans and could have an etiopathogenic role.[83]

Role of Mineral Production

Recently, there has been much interest in a possibly important role in the production of osteoarthritis by calcium mineral salts in articular cartilage, particularly by calcium pyrophosphate dihydrate crystals in the middle zone of cartilage in chondrocalcinosis and by hydroxyapatite in the deep radial zone as a secondary response to remodeling of subchondral bone. These minerals are postulated to have a noxious action on chondrocytes following sufficient accumulation in cartilage.[88] In addition, hydroxyapatite crystal aggregates and calcium pyrophosphate crystals have been found to be phlogistic in both in vivo animal studies and in vitro cell culture studies.[89]

The Possible Relationship of Hydroxyapatite and Other Minerals to Osteoarthritis

Calcium pyrophosphate dihydrate ($Ca_2P_2O_7 \cdot 2H_2O$) is not the exclusive mineral detected in synovial fluid and synovial membranes associated with secondary osteoarthritis. Hydroxyapatite ($Ca_{10}[PO_4]_6[OH]_2$) or a prototype of this mineral has been incriminated as a cause of crystal-induced synovitis. In cases of subacute or acute synovitis and osteoarthritis, as reported by Dieppe and associates, detectable hydroxyapatite appeared in the pellet derived from knee effusions following centrifugation of samples removed by aspiration.[90] This mineral was also detected in the inflammatory cells. Findings of a similar nature were also recorded by Schumacher and colleagues[91] in patients who appeared to be osteoarthritic on clinical grounds. Thereafter, Schumacher and coworkers injected canine joints in vivo with a solution containing a suspension of synthetic hydroxyapatite.[92] The injections produced heat and swelling in the animal joints that were reminiscent of crystal-induced synovitis[92] caused by calcium pyrophosphate. Polymorphonuclear leukocytes from synovial effusions were studied by electron probe analysis and were found to contain a high concentration of calcium and phosphate, consistent with the presence of amorphous calcium phosphate or apatite. Analogous studies were conducted by Dieppe.[93] As Wilkens and associates recently reported, several such patients suffered from severe osteoarthritis, and the association with destructive lesions was also recorded.[94]

Overall, these findings render likely the role of hydroxyapatite aggregates per se in the invocation of serious joint disease similar to that of calcium pyrophosphate deposition disease (Fig. 7–4). Additional experience from McCarty's laboratory supports this viewpoint.[79] A group of patients with glenohumeral osteoarthritis and bilateral rotator cuff defects, joint stiffness, and instability were studied. These patients presented with interesting synovial fluid findings: hydroxyapatite crystals in clumps, active synovial collagenase, neutral proteases, and the presence of collagen Types I, II, and III in an almost acellular synovial fluid.[79] Synovial tissue from these joints showed typical chondromatosis. Transmission electron-microscopic views revealed clumps of crystals leaking into the joint space through histologic regions denuded of synoviocytes. Some crystal aggregates were found within the synovia per se. The cartilage and bony destruction, synovial proliferation, and tendon erosion are not unlike the arthropathy with chondrocalcinosis described by Menkes and coworkers.[95] Instead of bands of calcium-mineral deposits confined to articular cartilage, however, there were exuberant deposits of mineral in the capsule. The cases reported by McCarty and colleagues, designated "Milwaukee shoulder," manifested roentgenographic evidence of upward dislocation of the humeral head against the acromion or downward dislocation on hyperextension. Both types of arthropathy, i.e., "Milwaukee shoulder" and the arthropathy described by Menkes and associates,[95] are characterized by mineral deposition in joint tissues, chronic proliferative synovitis, cartilage degeneration, and tendon erosion.

HYPOTHETICAL SCHEME RELATING MINERAL DEPOSITION TO DESTRUCTIVE ARTHROPATHY*

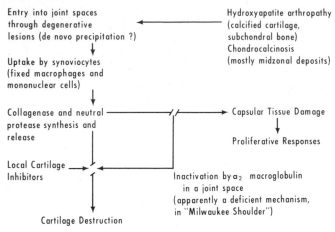

Figure 7–4. Hypothetical scheme relating mineral deposition to destructive arthropathy.

* So far mononuclear cell factor (or catabolin) has not yet been reported present in chondrocalcinosis or hydroxyapatite arthropathy. If present, such factors could lead to intrinsic cartilage destruction.

A feature shared by "Milwaukee shoulder,"[79] hydroxyapatite arthropathy,[90] and non-familial calcium pyrophosphate deposition disease[96] is the presence of concurrent osteoarthritis in the same and other joints. Inasmuch as histologic evidence of tissue breakdown may antedate roentgenologic or clinical signs, most cases of chondrocalcinosis might have this association. Could it be that in all three of these disorders (and possibly in multiple subsets not yet studied in detail) osteoarthritis may precede apatite deposition or chondrocalcinosis, with mineral formation a consequence of disarrayed cartilage metabolism, thus representing a secondary effect of osteoarthritis? Consistent with this viewpoint have been the data accrued by Schumacher and coworkers, in which over half the individuals studied in an autopsy series revealed osteoarthritic lesions by light microscopy, with signs of mineral deposition in the deep radial zone of articular cartilage.[97] They found a positive correlation between the severity of osteoarthritic lesions and the presence of mineral. Howell and colleagues, employing block Kashiwa methods, showed that 16 of 40 patients with osteoarthritis had evidence of phosphate attributed to mineral collections surrounding the chondrocytes in the deep radial zone of ulcerated osteoarthritic cartilage.[98] Bjelle[99] and Bullough[100] have observed the frequent presence of birefringent crystals indicative of scattered calcium pyrophosphate crystals in autopsy samples of human osteoarthritic cartilage. These deposits probably would be undetectable in clinical roentgenologic studies. Such

deposits are usually localized close to or at Nélaton's line or the tidemark. This site has been demonstrated by Lane and associates to undergo intense remodeling after the age of 50 years, with alternation of joint contours as a result.[101] This sort of subchondral remodeling of an osteoarthritic site has been postulated to be the source of mineral particles detected in the synovial fluid in hydroxyapatite arthropathy.[90] Once an osteoarthritic erosion has enlarged to expose calcified cartilage, the abrasion of joint surfaces at this stage could generate further release of mineral particles into the synovial fluid. This type of remodeling of cartilage is heralded by capillary invasion up to the tidemark, production of new bone salts by the chondrocytes in the deep radial zone, and expansion of subchondral bone toward the joint surface.[90] To what extent this process perpetuates or is etiologically concerned in osteoarthritis is unknown.[102] Similar remodeling was demonstrated beneath the shallow artificial excavation of the articular cartilage produced by Lemperg and coworkers in normal sheep.[103]

Another origin of mineral commonly observed in calcium pyrophosphate deposition disease involves the "switch on" of middle-layer chondrocytes to form a mineral phase. In almost all instances, this mineral phase is calcium pyrophosphate dihydrate, although calcium hydrogen phosphate and some hydroxyapatite deposits have been shown by x-ray diffraction in recent studies. Why these middle-layer chondrocytes are the principal site of calcium mineral salt deposition is unknown, but the same site is afflicted in experimental chondrocalcinosis produced by high-dose vitamin D administration in rabbits.[104] The localization does not seem to be dependent on pyrophosphate metabolism because the mineral phase in aged rabbits with chondrocalcinosis is hydroxyapatite.[105] In the rabbit model of chondrocalcinosis caused by corticosteroid administration, there is loss of metachromasia surrounding the cartilage cells, formation of cysts, and deposition of minerals, all occurring sequentially.[106] Altogether, it seems likely that centrally located chondrocytes are particularly prone to modulate and to calcify. Large aggregates or granular deposits of mineral are found in human chondrocalcinosis, with signs of cellular necrosis along the margins of these large deposits. There is probably also proliferation of crystals into sites of surviving chondrocytes. Rims of mineral surround some of the cells in early deposits.[96] Such rims are believed to indicate a primary role of chondrocytes in initiation of the mineral phase.

The results reported for the rabbit models did not address the question of whether enzymes degradative to the matrix are elaborated prior to or following mineral generation. In contrast to calcified subhyaline cartilage, chondrocytes fail to survive within calcified matrix of chondrocalcinosis. Such deposits expand and are destructive to living cells in their path, as indicated previously. Furthermore, in contrast to growth plate cartilage calcification, capillaries are not invasive about the tidemark and do not ossify in relationship to chrondrocalcinotic deposition. Thus, in this respect, the lesions resemble an ectopic calcification much more. The central location of chondrocalcinotic mineral deposition may have implications of a more general nature; namely, there is a pericellular loss of proteoglycan staining in the mid-zonal regions in certain histologic studies of animal models of osteoarthritis. This is a major site of response in the Moskowitz rabbit model, as mentioned earlier.[106] Hypothetically, preferential degradation of proteoglycans at this site might explain loss of control against mineral crystal proliferation. This view is based on studies demonstrating the importance of intact proteoglycan aggregates to block mineral growth in cartilage.[107, 108] In addition, latent and active collagenases are increased in human and dog osteoarthritic cartilage according to recent studies.[73] Possibly, the aforementioned postulated breakdown of collagen bundles and increased water uptake by cartilage could result from release of this latent enzyme in active form. Regardless of whether it is due

purely to physical trauma or is enzymatic in origin, the site of initial collagen network breakdown frequently seems to be the central zone, i.e., those sites in which bone salts are deposited in chondrocalcinosis. Possibly, in addition to loss of proteoglycans, the breakdown of the collagen network might permit improved special conditions for crystal growth and proliferation. Thus, these central regions in human osteoarthritic cartilage have been thought by several workers to be prone to earlier deterioration and would, at least in some patients with osteoarthritis, fit the findings of animal models.

It is possible but unlikely that mineral is formed either at the surface or in the tidemark region and then transported to the central sites in chondrocalcinosis. Considerable evidence for elaboration of pyrophosphate ion by osteoarthritic and even normal cartilage has accrued.[109, 110] These studies provide a reasonable explanation, but not proof, for the development of the unique mineral calcium pyrophosphate dihydrate. Clearly, concretions of calcium phosphate and pyrophosphate can grow relentlessly in a precisely adjusted physical environment[111-113] and alter unfavorably the biophysical properties of overlying cartilage as well as probably cause vertical fissure formation. Possibly, these fissures could precede deposition and be part of an etiologic or pathologic process involved in the production of at least some subsets of osteoarthritis. On the other hand, a passenger effect of the mineral deposition is a viable alternative. No research findings can securely discriminate between them at present.

PRIMARY GENERALIZED AND EROSIVE INFLAMMATORY OSTEOARTHRITIS

Some forms of more generalized osteoarthritis suggest that some patients with osteoarthritis may suffer from a generalized metabolic defect. In primary generalized osteoarthritis, as described by Kellgren and Moore,[114] involvement of the distal and proximal interphalangeal joints of the hands, the first carpometacarpal joints, the knees, the hips, the first metatarsophalangeal joints, and the spine is common. Inflammatory reactions are not uncommon. So far, no specifically determined errors in cartilage metabolism of a genetic nature have been demonstrated.

Considerable circumstantial evidence indicates that there is a separate subtype (or separate subtypes) of osteoarthritis of the hip if one separates those patients in whom cartilage was shown roentgenographically to be degraded in a concentric rather than a focal manner (see Chapters 1 and 15). This concentricity of wear favors a metabolic error or at least a generalized matrix disturbance.[115] The etiology of the inflammatory proximal interphalangeal arthropathy (erosive inflammatory osteoarthritis) described early by Crain[116] and later by Ehrlich is unknown.[117, 118] No animal model of this disease has been made, and it has been very difficult to frame a hypothesis that could be tested to explain the destructive arthropathy with synovial hyperplasia and giant cells. Ehrlich described what he considered to be a special subgroup of osteoarthritis; namely, a group of 170 patients, mostly women at the menopause, with symmetric polyarthritis afflicting both the distal and proximal finger joints, the base of the thumb, the neck, the hip, and the knee.[118] In most of these patients, Ehrlich described an abrupt, relatively explosive onset with considerable pain, redness, swelling, heat, and functional deficiency. Some of the patient's conditions progressed to ankylosis of the fingers, including both the proximal and distal joints. About 15% of these patients eventually developed rheumatoid arthritis. By Ehrlich's concept (as well as those of many other investigators), each joint location may entail a separate etiology and even variations in pathogenesis. Each given location reflects identifiable motions and stresses, so that the arthritis is a consequence of the special problems there. Several pathogenic aspects of the disease, Ehrlich also notes, would be serving a reparative function. The osteophytes may be conceived of as internalized orthoses directed toward reduction of motion and amelioration of inflammation. Similarly, thickening of subchondral bone might be considered in the same light. The inflammatory stage might be a secondary event. This concept constitutes reasonable teleology but is very difficult to test experimentally.

ETIOLOGY OF SECONDARY FORMS OF OSTEOARTHRITIS

Because this subject is discussed by Schumacher (see Chapter 14), remarks here will be confined more or less to the personal views of the author. One can classify the secondary forms of OA in terms of relative importance of etiologic factors and certainty of their involvement, as indicated in Table 7–1. Clearly defined etiologies of secondary osteoarthritis are exemplified by destructive processes such as gouty tophi or cysts of hyperparathyroidism involving subchondral bone or, alternatively, traumatic injury to articular surfaces with resultant disturbances in weight-bearing force distribution. Certainly, the various inflammatory responses characteristic of fungal and bacterial infection that lead to destruction of cartilage will lead in the same way to remodeling of the joint indicative of secondary osteoarthritis. Furthermore, clearly isolated phenomena such as Legg-Calvé-Perthes disease, slipped capital femoral epiphysis, severe hip dysplasia, severe valgus deformities of the femoral head,[14] and other conditions mentioned in the introduction may cause the development of osteoarthritis on a one-to-one basis. The effects of ochronosis were mentioned previously in the discussion of the collagen network. Similarly, it is likely that in hydroxyapatite arthropathy and severe chondrocalcinosis, a direct secondary effect of the presence of a mineral layer might be to destroy the biomaterial properties of cartilage as well as injure local cells. As already noted, however, minor developmental defects in growth might have a less certain role in etiology and might require other abnormalities or conditions to be fulfilled in order to produce osteoarthritis. Thus, there is a no man's land between the definite etiologic agent and the conditioning factors that are only partially involved in the production of osteoarthritis. Other less clearly defined influences such as joint laxity, endocrine effects, diet, obesity, and toxic chemical poisons probably fit into this category. Well-conducted epidemiologic studies have directed attention to joint laxity as a possible conditioning factor for osteoarthritis.[119] Despite the anecdotal nature of the evidence, increased frequency of osteoarthritis in Ehlers-Danlos syndrome and other heritable disorders has been postulated. Opposing views as to the role of joint laxity[120] have been reviewed by Peyron (see Chapter 1). To what extent joint laxity represents joint instability, as seen in various animal models of osteoarthritis, is unknown. Excessive noxious stimuli in the form of physical forces could lead to cartilage loss, but there is also evidence that chondrocalcinosis and calcium pyrophosphate deposition in man ensues as a secondary effect of joint laxity.[121, 122]

Hormones

The role of growth hormone or related polypeptides in the production of osteoarthritis[123] remains enigmatic. Elevated levels of growth hormone in postmenopausal patients with os-

Table 7–1. ETIOLOGIC FACTORS RELATED TO SECONDARY OSTEOARTHRITIS

1. *Post-traumatic Injury*
   A. Chronic excessive joint usage (e.g., industrial hand syndrome)
   B. Acute injury
   Meniscal loss
   Ligamentous tears
   Bone or cartilage defects, fractures
2. *Injury Due to Primary Diseases or Vascular Impairment*
   A. Postseptic arthritis
   B. Post–rheumatoid arthritis or variants
   C. Loss of subchondral bone support— hyperparathyroidism, cysts, Paget's disease, bone tumors
   D. Vascular impairment—avascular necrosis of the hip or knee, sickle cell disease, caisson disease
   E. Maldistribution of weight
   Scoliosis, other spinal weight shifts
   Shortened (or lengthened) limbs secondary to spinal arthritis or bone disease
3. *Iatrogenic Causes*
   A. Limb atrophy—casts, followed by overexercise
   B. Overadministration of joint corticosteroids
   C. ? Systemic medications affecting cartilage
4. *Obesity*
   A. Weight distribution
   a. Production of genu valgum by adipose thighs
   b. Quantitative effects of overweight combined with excessive exercise
5. *Developmental or Abiotrophic Effects*
   A. Hip osteoarthritis
   a. Legg-Calvé-Perthes disease—congenital hip dysplasia
   b. Slipped capital femoral epiphysis
   c. Biomaterial normal, joint weight-bearing alignment or architecture abnormal
   1) Mild dysplasia—acetabulum
   2) Cock-up deformity, valgus deformation
   3) Pistol-grip deformity
   4) Acetabular overgrowth at zenith
   5) Genu valgum or varum
   6) Altered congruity with aging of knees and hips

   B. Generalized heritable disorders, ? biomaterial changes, joint laxity
   a. Multiple epiphyseal dysplasia
   b. Nail-patella syndrome
   c. ? Other such syndromes
6. *Metabolic*
   A. Ochronosis
   B. Chondrocalcinosis—osteoarthritis and mineral deposition interrelations
   C. Gout
   D. Hemochromatosis
7. *Endocrine*
   A. Diabetes mellitus
   B. Acromegaly
8. *Possible Multifactorial Secondary Osteoarthritis— Conditioning Factors (Role for All Still Hypothetical)*
   A. Biomaterial abnormal
   a. Subchondral bone fractures, stiffened bone
   b. ? Altered collagen crosslinking
   ? Altered structure of proteoglycans or glycoproteins in the collagen network to reduce durability
   B. Cellular (chondrocytic) responses abnormal
   a. ? Failure of repair mechanisms to normal wear and microtrauma
   b. Increased matrix degradation
   1) Increased degradative enzyme elaboration
   2) Decreased inhibitors of acid cathepsins B, D, and F or neutral metalloproteoglycanase or collagen
   3) Autolysis at sites initiating:
   Osteoarthritic clefts
   Osteoarthritic progressive changes with cellular coronal proteolysis
   C. Synovial cell injury from microtrauma or cartilage products/reaction to disease
   a. Release of degradative enzymes
   b. Induction of marginal bony proliferative response
   c. Mononuclear cell mediators
   d. Immunologic responses
   D. Somatotypic features
   a. Predominance of endomorphic mesomorphism

teoarthritis versus controls was reported.[123] Excess of growth hormone in acromegaly appears to be responsible for thickened cartilage, marginal bone thickening, and reduced joint mobility, as well as for erosion and splitting of the cartilage secondarily.[124] Secondary joint effusions also appear, probably as a result of the fragmented cartilage. However, the picture in early stages does not seem to mimic the early stages of osteoarthritis. On the other hand, to the extent that the acromegalic arthropathy represents a response to cartilage injury caused by abnormal physical forces, which are in turn generated by overexpansion of the cartilage and poor biomaterial properties, one can consider the response in part a secondary osteoarthritis.

The possible role of estrogens in the etiology of osteoarthritis[125] has been reviewed in Chapter 6. The subject is complicated and provocative with respect to possible therapeutic intervention. The timing of estrogen deprivation with onset of Heberden's and Bouchard's nodes in the genetically defined groups studied by Stecher[126] is probably circumstantial rather than causative. Nevertheless, there are some reports of clinically favorable response of such osteoarthritis to estrogen therapy; the results are not decisive. Relationships to estrogens will probably be further advanced by such studies as those of Rosner and associates on the interplay of estrogens and estrogen antagonists in the production of osteoarthritis.[127]

Diet

The role of diet remains unknown, although considerable studies on aspects of diet have been made in relationship to osteoarthritis.

Diet is a subject charged with emotion, and extremely careful controls are needed to prevent placebo responses from confusing an adequate evaluation. The view that diets high in saturated fat may play a role has never been adequately dealt with, despite studies in mice indicating a severe noxious effect of saturated fat on the microscopic appearance of articular cartilage cells.[128] Other dietary factors such as ingestion of a fungus in food have been suggested as causing osteoarthritis, as described in the syndrome of Kashin-Beck disease.[129] Diets supplemented with ascorbic acid resulted in lessened cartilage injury in a guinea pig osteoarthritic model, as described by Schwartz and colleagues.[130] The low-calorie Oriental diets have been proposed as a reason for the low incidence of osteoarthritis of the hip in Chinese subjects.[131] However, many other factors could have been involved in addition to dietary effect. Accordingly, a role of diet might be only circumstantial.

Metabolic Factors

Recent studies indicated a profound effect of experimental diabetes on proteoglycan synthesis in growth plate cartilages. In our laboratory, the administration of streptozotocin, which caused complete insulin deficiency in rats, was followed by over a 50% reduction in proteoglycan synthesis of articular knee cartilages; similar data have been reported by Caterson and associates.[132] The role of diabetes mellitus in osteoarthritis has been recently reviewed.[133]

Physical Factors

Immobilization of joints followed by exercise that is too intense may constitute a pathogenetic factor leading to the development of osteoarthritis, as studied by Palmoski and coworkers in animal models.[134, 135] At present, a clear-cut relationship has not been defined in humans. Certainly, loss of proteoglycan aggregation and reduced proteoglycan synthesis during immobilization would seem likely conditioning factors that should be considered in the management of patients susceptible to cartilage injury following immobilization of joints for fracture and the like.[135] Overaggressive exercise should be avoided. Finally, diseases in which there is shortening of a limb, such as following tumor removal, for example, may result in shifts of weight bearing that can lead to osteoarthritis of the opposite limb owing to alterations of physical forces in weight bearing.

Excessive Drug Use

The possible impairment of metabolism of cartilage by salicylates and other nonsteroidal drugs is discussed in Chapter 32. Clearly, if chronically suppressed repair responses documented in animal models[136] were also shown to be quantitatively significant in human tissues in vivo, this would be a strong deterrent to their use. Knowledge derived from animal experimentation thus suggests that chronic high-dose administration of oral nonsteroidal anti-inflammatory agents might, under some circumstances, have a noxious conditioning effect that accelerates osteoarthritis. Even stronger would be the contraindication to intra-articular corticosteroids. The subject of local corticosteroids has been well reviewed recently by Gray and associates.[137]

Expanded research has led to a significantly increased understanding of the pathophysiologic responses occuring in osteoarthritis. These observations, in turn, provide the basis for reasonable hypotheses of etiopathogenesis, which can now be tested in more structured fashion. It is obvious from the preceding discussion that these proposed mechanisms are complex and multifaceted. It is hoped that careful (and likely tedious) experimentation to prove or disprove various components of these speculations will lead to better definitions of the etiopathogenesis of this common but complex disorder.

References

1. Magee B: Popper. 7th ed. Glasgow, William Collins Sons and Co., 1978.
2. Peyron JB: Epidemiology of Osteoarthritis. Paris, Ciba-Geigy, 1981.
3. Nuki G (ed.): The Aetiopathogenesis of Osteoarthrosis. Tunbridge Wells, Pitman Medical Publishing Co., 1980.
4. Sokoloff L: The Joints and Synovial Fluid, Vols. I and II. New York, Academic Press, 1980.
5. Maroudas A, Holborow EJ (eds.): Studies in Joint Disease, Vols. I and II. Tunbridge Wells, Pitman Medical Publishing Co., 1980.
6. Inerot S: Studies on cartilage proteoglycans in aging and degenerative joint disease. Doctoral Thesis. Lund University Press, 1983.
7. Howell DS, Talbott JH: Osteoarthritis Symposium. Semin Arthritis Rheum 11(Suppl 1):1, 1981.
8. Blumberg BS: Comments on scientific process in clinical research. Perspect Biol Med 24:15–30, 1980.

9. Gardner DL, Elliott RJ, Armstrong CG, Longmore RB: The relationship between age, thickness, surface structure, compliance and composition of human femoral head articular cartilage. *In* Nuki G (ed.): The Aetiopathogenesis of Osteoarthritis. Tunbridge Wells, Pitman Medical Publishing Co., 1980.

10. Freeman MAR, Meachim G: *In* Freeman MAR: Adult Articular Cartilage. 2nd ed. Tunbridge Wells, Pitman Medical Publishing Co., 1979, pp. 530–531.

11. Harris WH: Idiopathic osteoarthritis of the hip: A twentieth century myth? J Bone Joint Surg 59B:121, 1977.

12. Day WH, Sawson SAV, Freeman MAR: Contact pressures in the loaded human cadaver hip. J Bone Joint Surg 57B:302–313, 1975.

13. Murray RO: The aetiology of primary osteoarthritis of the hip. Br J Radiol 50:81–83, 1965.

14. Radin EL: Mechanical factors in the etiology of osteoarthrosis. *In* Peyron JG (ed.): Epidemiology of Osteoarthritis. Paris, Ciba-Geigy, 1981.

15. Byers PD, Contempomi CA, Farkas TA: A postmortem study of the hip joint: Including the prevalence of the features of the right side. Ann Rheum Dis 29:15–31, 1970.

16. Byers PD, Afoke NYP, Hutton SC: A test of the Freeman hypothesis. *In* Peyron JG (ed.): Epidemiology of Osteoarthritis. Paris, Ciba-Geigy, 1981, pp. 87–89.

17. Altman RD, Meenan RF, Hochberg MC, et al.: An approach to developing criteria for the clinical diagnosis and classification of osteoarthritis. J Rheumatol 10:180–183, 1983.

18. Bullough PG, Goodfellow J, O'Connor J: The relationship between degenerative changes and load-bearing in the human hip. J Bone Joint Surg 55B:746–758, 1973.

19. Urban JPG, Maroudas A, Bayliss MT, Dillon J: Swelling pressures of proteoglycans at the concentrations found in cartilaginous tissues. Biorheology 16:447–464, 1979.

20. Maroudas A: Proteoglycan osmotic pressure and the collagen tension in normal, osteoarthritic human cartilage. Semin Arthritis Rheum 11(Suppl 1):36–39, 1981.

21. Maroudas A, Urban JPG: Swelling pressures of cartilaginous tissues. *In* Maroudas A, Holborow EJ (eds.): Studies in Joint Disease. Tunbridge Wells, Pitman Medical Publishing Co., 1980, pp. 87–116.

22. Hascall VC: Proteoglycans: Structure and function. *In* Ginsberg V (ed.): Biology of Carbohydrates. New York, John Wiley and Sons, 1981.

23. Muir H: Proteoglycans: State of the art. Semin Arthritis Rheum 11(Suppl 1):7–10, 1981.

24. Maroudas A, Venn M: Chemical composition and swelling of normal and osteoarthrotic femoral head cartilage. Ann Rheum Dis 36:399–406, 1977.

25. Kempson GE, Muir H, Swason SAV, Freeman MAR: Correlations between stiffness and the chemical constituents of cartilage on the human femoral head. Biochim Biophys Acta 215:70–77, 1970.

26. Harris ED Jr, Parker HG, Radin EL, Krane SM: Effects of proteolytic enzymes on structural and mechanical properties of cartilage. Arthritis Rheum 15:497–503, 1972.

27. Mankin HG, Thrasher AZ: Water content and binding in normal and osteoarthritic human cartilage. J Bone Joint Surg 57A:76–80, 1975.

28. Mow VC, Myers ER, Roth V, Lalik P: Implications for collagen-proteoglycan interactions from cartilage stress relaxation behavior in isometric tension. Semin Arthritis Rheum 11(Suppl 1):41–43, 1981.

29. Myers ER, Mow VC: Biomechanics of Cartilage and Response to Biochemical Stimuli. *In* Hall BK (ed.): Cartilage. New York, Academic Press, 1982.

30. Meachim G: Cartilage degeneration in the Liverpool population. *In* Peyron JG (ed.): Epidemiology of Osteoarthritis. Paris, Ciba-Geigy, 1981.

31. Meachim G, Bentley G: Horizontal splitting in patellar articular cartilage. Arthritis Rheum 21:669–674, 1978.

32. Maroudas A, Venn MF: Biochemical and physicochemical studies on osteoarthrotic cartilage from the human femoral head. *In* Nuki G (ed.): The Aetiopathogenesis of Osteoarthrosis. Tunbridge Wells, Pitman Medical Publishing Co., 1980, pp. 37–46.

33. Altman RD, Tenenbaum J, Pardo V, et al.: Morphological changes and swelling properties of osteoarthritic dog cartilage. Semin Arthritis Rheum 11(Suppl 1):39–40, 1981.

34. Poole AR, Pidoux I, Reiner A, Rosenberg LC: The ultrastructural organization of proteoglycan monomer and link protein in articular cartilage. Semin Arthritis Rheum 11(Suppl 1):26–28, 1981.

35. Fujimoto D, Moriguchi T, Ishida T, Hayashi H: The structure of pyridinoline, a collagen crosslink. Biochem Biophys Res Commun 84:52–57,.1978.

36. Eyre DR, Oguchi H: The hydroxypyridinium crosslinks of skeletal collagens: Their measurement, properties and a proposed pathway of formation. Biochem Biophys Res Commun 92:403–410, 1980.

37. Eyre DR, Grynpas MD, Shapiro FD, Creasman CM: Mature crosslink formation and molecular packing in articular cartilage collagen. Semin Arthritis Rheum 11(Suppl 1):46–47, 1981.

38. Rosenberg L: Personal communication, 1981.

39. Hewitt AT, Kleinman K, Pennypacker JP, Martin GR: Identification of an adhesion factor for chondrocytes. Proc Natl Acad Sci USA 77:385–388, 1980.

40. Paulsson M, Heinegård D: Matrix proteins bound to associatively prepared protcoglycans from bovine cartilage. Biochem J 183:539–545, 1979.

41. Mejer LE, Noble NL: Hydroxyproline-containing structural glycopeptide fractions from subacute inflammation connective tissue. Connect Tissue Res 4:91–100, 1976.

42. Weightman B: In vitro fatigue testing of articular cartilage. Ann Rheum Dis 34(Suppl 2):108–110, 1975.

43. Kempson GE: Mechanical properties of articular cartilage and their relationship to matrix degradation of age. Biochem J 183:111–113, 1979.

44. Zannoni VG, Malawista SE, LaDu BN: Studies on ochronosis. II. Studies on benzoquinoneacetic acid, a probable intermediate in the connective tissue pigmentation of alcaptonuria. Arthritis Rheum 5:547–556, 1962.

45. Scott JE, Heatley F, Moorcroft D, Olavesen AH: Secondary structures of hyaluronate and chondroitin sulfates. Biochem J 199:829–832, 1981.

46. Mankin HJ, Baron PA: The effect of aging on protein synthesis in articular cartilage of rabbits. Lab Invest 14:658–664, 1965.

47. Mankin HG, Dorfman H, Lippiello L, Zarins A: Biochemical and metabolic abnormalities in articular cartilage from osteoarthritic human hips. II. Correlation of morphology with biochemical and

metabolic data. J Bone Joint Surg 53A:523–537, 1971.

48. Mankin HG, Johnson ME, Lippiello L: Biochemical and metabolic abnormalities in articular cartilage from osteoarthritic human hips. III. Distribution and metabolism of amino sugar containing macromolecules. J Bone Joint Surg 63A:131–134, 1981.

49. Mankin HJ, Lippiello L: Biochemical and metabolic abnormalities in articular cartilage from osteoarthritic human hips. J Bone Joint Surg 52A:424–434, 1970.

50. Sutro CJ: Experimental production of a rapid-type of OA in rabbits—Carborundum granules as the intra-articular irritant. Bull Hosp Joint Dis 23:20–26, 1962.

51. Quintero M, Mitrovic D, Stankovic A, et al.: Quantitative study of the cells in human femoral condylar articular cartilage: Senescence and osteoarthritis. Abstract #0748. XVth International Congress of Rheumatology. Paris, June 1981.

52. Dingle JT: Role of catabolin and arthritic damage. Semin Arthritis Rheum 11(Suppl 1):82–83, 1981.

53. Phadke KD, Lawrence M, Nanda S: Synthesis of collagenase and neutral proteases by articular chondrocytes: Stimulation by a macrophage derived factor. Biochem Biophys Res Comm 85:490–496, 1978.

54. Ridge SC, Oronsky AL, Kerwar SS: Induction of the synthesis of latent collagenase and latent neutral protease in chondrocytes by a factor synthesized by activated macrophages Arthritis Rheum 23:448–454, 1980.

55. Dayer JM, Russel RG, Krane SM: Collagenase production by rheumatoid synovial cells: Stimulation by a human lymphocyte factor. Science 195:181–183, 1977.

56. Stockwell RA: Biology of Cartilage Cells. Cambridge, Cambridge University Press, 1979.

57. Barrett AJ, Saklatvala J: Proteinases in joint disease. In Kelley WN, Harris ED Jr, Ruddy S, Sledge CB (eds.): Textbook of Rheumatology, Vol. 1. Philadelphia, WB Saunders Company, 1981, pp. 195–206.

58. Maroudas A: Metabolism of cartilaginous tissues. In Maroudas A, Holborow EJ (eds): Studies in Joint Disease. Tunbridge Wells, Pitman Medical Publishing Co., 1980, pp. 159–186.

59. Mankin HJ, Johnson ME, Lippiello L: Biochemical and metabolic abnormalities in articular cartilage from osteoarthritic human hips. III. Distribution and metabolism of aminosugar containing macromolecules. J Bone Joint Surg 63A:131–139, 1981.

60. Sapolsky AI, Keiser H, Howell DS, Woessner JF: Metalloproteases of human articular cartilage that digest cartilage proteoglycan at neutral and acid pH. J Clin Invest 58:1030–1041, 1976.

61. Ehrlich MG, Armstrong A, Mankin HJ: Isolation and partial purification and characterization of growth plate neutral proteoglycanase. Trans Orthop Res Soc 6:109, 1981.

62. Bayliss MT, Ali SY: Studies on cathepsin B in human articular cartilage. Biochem J 171:149–154, 1978.

63. Bayliss MT, Venn M: Chemistry of human articular cartilage. In Maroudas A, Holborow EJ (eds.): Studies in Joint Disease. Tunbridge Wells, Pitman Medical Publishing Co., 1980, pp. 2–58.

64. Sandy JD, Brown HG, Lowther DA: Degradation of proteoglycan in articular cartilage. Biochim Biophys Acta 543:536–544, 1978.

65. Greenwald RA, Moy WW: Effect of oxygen-derived free radicals on hyaluronic acid. Arthritis Rheum 23:455–463, 1980.

66. Sapolsky AI, Howell DS: Further characterization of a neutral metalloprotease isolated from human articular cartilage. Arthritis Rheum 25:981–988, 1982.

67. Sapolsky AI, Malemud CJ, Norby DP, et al.: Neutral proteinases from articular chondrocytes in culture. 2. Metal-dependent latent neutral proteoglycanase, and inhibitory activity. Biochim Biophys Acta 658:138–147, 1981.

68. Roughley PJ, Murphy G, Barrett AJ: Proteinase inhibitors of bovine nasal cartilage. Biochem J 169:721–724, 1978.

69. Morales T, Kuettner KE, Howell DS, Woessner JF Jr: Characterization of the metalloproteinase inhibitor produced by bovine articular chondrocyte cultures. Biochim Biophys Acta 760:221–229, 1983.

70. Ali SY, Bayliss MT: Enzymic changes in human osteoarthrotic cartilage. In Ali SY, Elves Mw, Leaback DL (eds.): Normal and Osteoarthrotic Articular Cartilage. London, Institute of Orthopaedics Publications, 1974, pp. 189–205.

71. Ehrlich MG, Mankin HJ, Jones H, et al.: Collagenase and collagenase inhibitors in osteoarthritic and normal human cartilage. J Clin Invest 59:226–233, 1977.

72. Ehrlich MG, House PA, Vigliani G, Mankin HJ: Corrleation between articular cartilage collagenase activity and osteoarthritis. Arthritis Rheum 21:761–766, 1978.

73. Woessner JF, Pelletier JP, Martel-Pelletier J, et al.: Direct measurement of cartilage collagenolytic activity in human osteoarthritis. Semin Arthritis Rheum 11(Suppl 1):58–59, 1981.

74. Bennett GA, Waine H, Bauer W: Changes in the Knee Joint at Various Ages: With Particular Reference to the Nature and Development of Degenerative Joint Disease. New York, Commonwealth Fund, 1942.

75. Gilbertson EMM: Development of periarticular osteophytes in experimentally induced OA in the dog. Ann Rheum Dis 34:12–25, 1975.

76. Chrisman D: Biochemical aspects of degenerative joint disease. Clin Orthop Rel Res 64:77–86, 1969.

77. Lust G, Beilman WT, Dueland DJ, Farrell PW: Intraarticular volume and hip joint instability in dogs with hip dysplasia. J Bone Joint Surg 62A:576–583, 1980.

78. Arnoldi CC, Reinmann I: The pathomechanism of human coxarthrosis. Acta Orthop Scand Suppl 181, 1979.

79. McCarty DJ, Halverson PB, Carrera GF, et al.: "Milwaukee shoulder"—association of microspheroids containing hydroxyapatite crystals, active collagenase, and neutral protease with rotator cuff defects. I. Clinical aspects. Arthritis Rheum 24:464–473, 1981.

80. Dayer J-M, Breard J, Chess L, Krane SM: Participation of monocyte-macrophages and lymphocytes in the production of a factor that stimulates collagenase and prostaglandin release by rheumatoid synovial cells. J Clin Invest 64:1386–1392, 1979.

81. Herman JH, Mowery CS, Koo KK, Dennis MV: Lymphokines: Potential role in the immunopathogenesis of osteoarthritis. Semin Arthritis Rheum 11(Suppl 1):104–107, 1981.

82. Herman JH, Musgrave DS, Dennis MV: Phytomitogen-induced, lymphokine-mediated cartilage

proteoglycan degradation. Arthritis Rheum 20:922–932, 1977.

83. Herman JH, Nutman TB, Nozoe M, et al.: Lymphokine-mediated suppression of chondrocyte glycosaminoglycan and protein synthesis. Arthritis Rheum 24:824–834, 1981.

84. Herman JH, Herzig EB, Crissman JD, et al.: Idiopathic chondrolysis—an immunopathologic study. J Rheumatol 7:694–705, 1980.

85. Glant T, Csonger J, Szucs T: Immunopathologic role of proteoglycan antigens in rheumatoid joint disease. Scand J Immunol 11:247–252, 1980.

86. Gertzbein SD, Tait JH, Devlin SR: The stimulation of lymphocytes by nucleus pulposus in patients with degenerative disc disease of the lumbar spine. Clin Orthop 123:149–154, 1977.

87. Cooke TD, Bennett E, Wright L, Wyllie J: Relationships of immune deposits in osteoarthritic (OA) cartilage to disease site, pattern and synovial reaction. In Peyron JG (ed.): Epidemiology of Osteoarthritis. Paris, Ciba-Geigy, 1981.

88. Howell DS: Diseases due to the deposition of calcium pyrophosphate and hydroxyapatite. In Kelley WN, Harris ED Jr, Ruddy S, Sledge CB (eds.): Textbook of Rheumatology. Philadelphia, W.B. Saunders Company, 1981, pp. 1438–1456.

89. Cheung HS, Halverson PB, McCarty DJ: Chondrocytes release collagenase and lysosomal enzymes after phagocytosis of hydroxyapatite (HA) or calcium pyrophosphate dihydrate (CPPD) crystals. Abstract #0854. XVth International Congress of Rheumatology. Paris, June 1981.

90. Dieppe PA, Crocker P, Huskisson EC, et al.: Apatite deposition disease: A new arthropathy. Lancet 1:266–269, 1976.

91. Schumacher HR, Tse R, Reginato A, et al.: Hydroxyapatite-like crystals in synovial fluid cell vacuoles: A suspected new cause for crystal-induced arthritis. Arthritis Rheum 19:821, 1976.

92. Schumacher HR, Smolyo AP, Tse RL, Maurer K: Arthritis associated with apatite crystals. Ann Intern Med 87:411–416, 1977.

93. Dieppe A: Crystal-induced arthropathies and osteoarthritis. In Dick WC, Buchanan WW (eds.): Recent Advances in Rheumatology. II. Tunbridge Wells, Pitman Medical Publishing Co., 1981.

94. Wilkins E, Dieppe PA, Maddison P, Eveson G: Chondrocalcinosis and osteoarthritis in the elderly. Abstract #832. Rev Rhum XVth International Congress of Rheumatology, Paris, June 1981.

95. Menkes CJ, Simon F, Delrieu F, et al.: Destructive arthropathy in chondrocalcinosis articularis. Arthritis Rheum 19:329–348, 1976.

96. McCarty DJ: Calcium pyrophosphate dihydrate crystal deposition disease—1975. Arthritis Rheum 19:275–285, 1976.

97. Gordon G, Villaneuva HR, Schumacher R, et al.: Autopsy study correlating degree of osteoarthritis, articular calcification, and evidence of synovitis. Arthritis Rheum 23:683, 1980.

98. Howell DS, et al.: Unpublished observations.

99. Bjelle A: Personal communication, 1981.

100. Bullough P: Personal communication, 1981.

101. Lane LB, Villacin A, Bullough PG: A study of endochondral ossification in the adult—a mechanism for continuous joint remodeling. J Bone Joint Surg 57A: 576, 1975.

102. Ali SY: Matrix vesicles and apatite nodules in arthritic cartilage. In Gardner DL (ed.): Diseases of Connective Tissue. London, BMA House, 1978, p. 211.

103. Lemperg R, Boquist L, Rosenquist J: Intracartilaginous defects in adult sheep. Virchows Arch [Pathol Anat] 354:1–16, 1971.

104. Reginato A, Schumacher HR: Experimental hydroxyapatite articular calcification. (Abstract.) Arthritis Rheum 21:585, 1978.

105. Yosipovitch Z, Glimcher MJ: Chondrocalcinosis in rabbits. Isr J Med Sci 7:503–540, 1971.

106. Moskowitz RW, Davis W, Sammarco J, et al.: Experimentally induced corticosteroid arthropathy. Arthritis Rheum 13:236–243, 1970.

107. Howell DS, Pita JC: Calcification of growth plate cartilage with special reference to studies on micropuncture fluids. Clin Orthop 118:208–229, 1976.

108. Howell DS, Woessner JF Jr: Enzymes in articular cartilage. In Maroudas A, Holborow EJ (eds.): Studies in Joint Disease. Tunbridge Wells, Pitman Medical Publishing Co., 1980.

109. Howell DS, Muniz O, Pita JC, Enis JE: Extrusion of pyrophosphate into extracellular media by osteoarthritic cartilage incubates. J Clin Invest 56:1473–1480, 1975.

110. Tenenbaum J, Muniz O, Schumacher HR, et al.: Comparison of phosphohydrolase activities from articular cartilage in calcium pyrophosphate deposition disease and in primary OA. Arthritis Rheum 24:492–500, 1981.

111. Pritzker KPH, Cheng P, Omar SA, Nyburg SC: Calcium pyrophosphate crystal formation in model hydrogels. II. Hyaline articular cartilage as a gel. J Rheumatol 8:451–455, 1981.

112. Cheng P, Pritzker KPH, Adams ME, et al.: Calcium pyrophosphate crystal formation in aqueous solutions. J Rheumatol 7:610–616, 1980.

113. Pritzker KPH: Crystal-associated arthropathies: What's new in old joints. J Am Geriatr Soc 28:439–445, 1980.

114. Kellgren JH, Moore R: Generalized factors in generalized osteoarthrosis. Ann Rheum Dis 22:237–255, 1963.

115. Stewart IM, Marks JS, Hardinge K: Generalized osteoarthrosis and hip disease. In Peyron JG (ed.): Epidemiology of Osteoarthritis. Paris, Ciba-Geigy, 1981, pp. 193–197.

116. Crain DC: Interphalangeal osteoarthritis. JAMA 175:1049–1053, 1961.

117. Ehrlich GE: Inflammatory osteoarthritis. I. The clinical syndrome. J Chronic Dis 25:317–328, 1972.

118. Ehrlich GE: Inflammatory osteoarthritis. II. The superimposition of rheumatoid arthritis. J Chronic Dis 25:635–643, 1972.

119. Wright V: Biomechanical factors in the development of osteoarthrosis: epidemiological studies. In Peyron JG (ed.): Epidemiology of Osteoarthritis. Paris, Ciba-Geigy, 1981, pp. 140–146.

120. Scott D, Bird H, Wright V: Joint laxity leading to osteoarthrosis. Rheumatol Rehabil 18:167–169, 1979.

121. Dieppe P: Calcium phosphate crystal deposition and clinical subsets of osteoarhtiritis. In Peyron JG (ed.): Epidemiology of Osteoarthritis. Paris, Ciba-Geigy, 1981.

122. Bird HA, Tribe CR, Bacon PA: Joint hypermobility leading to osteoarthrosis and chondrocalcinosis. Ann Rheum Dis 37:203–211, 1978.

123. Dequeker J, Burssens A, Creytens G, et al.: Front Horm Res 3:116, 1975.

124. Bluestone R: Arthropathies associated with endocrine disorders. In Kelley WN, Harris ED Jr, Ruddy S, Slege CB (eds.): Textbook of Rheuma-

tology. Philadelphia, W.B. Saunders Company, 1981, pp. 1622–1637.

125. Moskowitz RW: Clinical and laboratory findings in osteoarthritis. *In* McCarty DJ (ed.): Arthritis and Allied Conditions. Philadelphia, Lea & Febiger, 1979.

126. Stecher RM: Heberden oration: Heberden's nodes; clinical description of osteoarthritis of finger joints. Ann Rheum Dis 14:1–10, 1955.

127. Rosner IA, Malemud CJ, Goldberg VM, Papay RS, Moskowitz RW: Pathologic and metabolic responses of experimental osteoarthritis to estradiol and an estradiol antagonist. Clin Orthop 171:280–286, 1982.

128. Silberberg M, Silberberg R, Orcutt B: Modifying effect of linoleic acid on articular aging and osteoarthrosis in lard-fed mice. Gerontologia 11:179–187, 1965.

129. Nesterov AI: The clinical course of Kashin-Beck disease. Arthritis Rheum 7:29–40, 1964.

130. Schwartz ER, Leveille CR, Stevens JW, Won HO: Proteoglycan structure and metabolism in normal and osteoarthritic cartilage of guinea pigs. Arthritis Rheum 24:1528–1539, 1981.

131. Lee P, Rooney PJ, Sturrock RD, et al.: The etiology and pathogenesis of osteoarthritis: A review. Semin Arthritis Rheum 3:189–218, 1974.

132. Caterson B, Baker JB, Christner JE, et al.: Diabetes and osteoarthritis Ala J Med Sci 17:292–299, 1980.

133. Waine H, Nevinny D, Rosenthal J, Joffe IB: Association of osteoarthritis and diabetes mellitus. Tufts Folia Med 7:13–19, 1961.

134. Palmoski MJ, Colyer RA, Brandt KD: Joint motion in the absence of normal loading does not maintain normal articular cartilage. Arthritis Rheum 23:325–334, 1980.

135. Palmoski MJ, Brandt KD: Running inhibits the reversal of atrophic changes in canine knee cartilage after removal of a leg cast. Arthritis Rheum 24:1329–1337, 1981.

136. Palmoski MJ, Colyer RA, Brandt KD: Marked suppression by salicylate of the augmented proteoglycan synthesis in osteoarthritic cartilage. Arthritis Rheum 23:83–91, 1980.

137. Gray RG, Gottlieb NL: Intra-articular corticosteroids: An updated assessment. Clin Orthop 177:235–263, 1983.

GENERAL ASPECTS OF DIAGNOSIS

Roland W. Moskowitz, M.D.
Section Editor

SECTION
2

8

Osteoarthritis—Symptoms and Signs

Roland W. Moskowitz, M.D.

Although pathologic evidence of degenerative changes in joints has been demonstrated to occur as early as the second decade of life, symptoms due to primary osteoarthritis are relatively uncommon before 40 years of age.[1] The frequency and severity of symptoms due to the primary form of the disease increase progressively with age, so that osteoarthritis is a major cause of symptomatic arthritis presenting in persons in the middle to older age groups.[2, 3] The presence of severe osteoarthritis in younger persons should suggest the presence of secondary underlying etiologic factors such as chronic occupationally related trauma, preceding joint disorders such as congenital abnormalities of the hip, old fractures, avascular necrosis, past infection, and neuropathic or metabolic disorders.[4, 5]

This chapter provides an overview of general symptomatology and physical findings of osteoarthritis as it affects various joints of the body. Differences in clinical presentation and ongoing manifestations are noted, based on differences in disease stage and severity and involvement of particular joints. The pathophysiology of these manifestations is identified. Further details of the clinical signs and symptoms of osteoarthritis are provided in later chapters that address this disease entity as it involves various specific joints of the body.

Joints most frequently involved by primary osteoarthritis include the distal and proximal interphalangeal joints of the fingers, first carpometacarpal joints of the hands, hips, knees, first metatarsophalangeal joints, and cervical and lower lumbar vertebrae. The metacarpo-phalangeal joints, wrists, elbows, and shoulders are almost always spared in primary osteoarthritis. In most patients, joint involvement is limited to one or only a few joints. In some forms of the disease, however, such as primary generalized osteoarthritis, symptomatic involvement of a number of joints, including the hands, knees, hips, metatarsophalangeal joints, and spine, may be noted. Involvement of multiple joints may suggest systemic forms of arthritis; the differential diagnosis from early forms of inflammatory connective tissue disease may be difficult at times. Systemic manifestations such as *generalized* morning stiffness, fever, anorexia, weight loss, and fatigue are not associated with osteoarthritis and should provide a clue to other forms of connective tissue disease being present in any individual patient.

The lack of correlation between joint symptomatology and the extent or degree of pathologic or roentgenologic change may be striking. Although degenerative changes in weight-bearing joints have been described in 90% of persons under age 40 studied at autopsy,[1] there is a notable lack of related clinical symptoms in the majority of these patients. Lack of association between morning stiffness and roentgenographic evidence of osteoarthritis has been described; only about 30% of persons with roentgenographic evidence of degenerative joint disease complain of pain at the relevant sites.[6] Despite these findings, however, other studies have demonstrated a general relationship between roentgenographic findings and clinical symptoms.[2, 7] Lawrence,

Bremner, and Bier,[2] for example, showed that the presence of osteoarthritis on roentgenographic examination was associated with a definite predisposition for related symptoms to develop, except for correlations performed on the lumbar apophyseal joints. Similarly, Gresham and Rathey[7] reported a positive correlation between clinical symptoms and roentgenographic evidence of degenerative joint disease of the knee. These apparent disparities in reports of the relationship between joint symptoms and roentgenologic abnormalities may represent differences in roentgenographic definitions of the disease. For example, both osteophytes and structural cartilage loss have long been considered characteristic roentgenographic and pathologic manifestations of degenerative joint disease. Long-term studies of the hip and knee, however, suggest that the presence of osteophytes does not imply later development of other structural changes of osteoarthritis such as joint space narrowing, subchondral bone cysts, and eburnation.[8-10] Accordingly, correlation of symptoms with osteophytes alone may provide different parallels between clinical findings and objective roentgenographic and pathologic manifestations as compared with similar studies that correlate symptoms and structural cartilage loss.

The clinical manifestations of osteoarthritis, either peripheral or spinal, may be continuous or intermittent. Disease progression is not invariable, and not all patients inevitably deteriorate.[11, 12] Stabilization of disease findings and joint space recovery have been described.

SYMPTOMS

In most cases, the clinical presentation of degenerative joint disease has an insidious onset. Symptoms (Table 8–1) depend on a number of variables, including which specific joints are involved, the duration and severity of changes, and the tolerance of the patient to

Table 8–1. SYMPTOMS CHARACTERISTIC OF OSTEOARTHRITIS

Pain
   Deep, aching, poorly localized
   Early, pain with use; later, pain at rest
Stiffness
   Localized to involved joints
   Rarely exceeds 15 to 30 minutes' duration
   Related to weather change
Crepitus, crackling
Limitation of joint motion
Giving way of weight-bearing joints

symptoms. The cardinal symptom of the disease is *pain*. It is usually described as deep and aching in character and tends to be poorly localized. Typically, pain at first occurs after joint use and is relieved by rest. With disease progression, minimal motion may induce pain, and pain at rest eventually ensues. In severe advanced cases, the pain not infrequently awakens the patient during sleep owing to loss of protective joint splinting that limits painful motion during the waking hours.

The pathogenesis of the pain is usually multifactorial. Cartilage itself is aneural and is therefore insensitive to pain. Consequently, the pain in osteoarthritis evolves from noncartilaginous intra-articular and periarticular structures. Intra-articular sources of pain include periosteal elevation associated with marginal bone proliferation, pressure on exposed subchondral bone, trabecular microfractures, degenerative involvement of intra-articular ligaments, distention of the joint capsule, and pinching or abrasion of synovial villi. Secondary inflammatory synovitis undoubtedly plays a significant role in the pathogenesis of pain in many patients with this disease. Gross and histologic evidence of inflammation is frequently observed in patients coming to surgery for treatment of their osteoarthritic disorder (see Figure 4–7). It has been demonstrated that cartilage and chondroitin sulfate are capable of generating kinin-like substances that act as mediators of inflammation.[13] Further studies have demonstrated induction of inflammatory synovitis following intra-articular injection of autologous cartilage into dog knees.[14] It is suggested that phagocytic ingestion of these cartilage fragments by synovial macrophages leads to release of lysosomal enzymes and resultant inflammatory reaction. In studies with experimental models of osteoarthritis, moderate to severe synovitis was induced in osteoarthritic knees exposed to treadmill running.[15] Deposits of crystals of calcium pyrophosphate[16, 17] or calcium apatite,[18, 19] seen more frequently in patients with degenerative joint disease, likely play a significant role in acute, subacute, and chronic inflammatory reactions seen in patients with osteoarthritis.

Restriction of venous drainage with subsequent vascular congestion of bone has been suggested as a primary etiology of pain associated with degenerative joint disease, particularly in patients with osteoarthritis of the hip.[20] Prostaglandins released from synovial tissues and chondrocytes contribute further to the overall pain response.[21] Involvement of periarticular tissues such as tendons and fascia that are richly supplied with sensory nerves is a further source of pain in these patients. Spasm of muscles around the joint or pressure on contiguous nerves, seen most frequently in osteoarthritis involving the spine, may lead to more pain than involvement of intra-articular structures. Some forms of osteoarthritis, such as erosive inflammatory osteoarthritis, which primarily involves the distal and proximal interphalangeal joints of the hands, are characteristically associated with a prominent inflammatory response.[22-25]

Joint *stiffness* is localized to involved joints and of short duration in contrast to the more prolonged, generalized stiffness seen in rheumatoid arthritis and other forms of inflammatory connective tissue disease. Rarely does it last more than 15 to 30 minutes. When present, it is most notable upon awakening in the morning and after inactivity during the day. Pain and stiffness, as with other forms of arthritis, are characteristically related to changes in weather. In the presence of severe, advanced disease, the patient may complain of a feeling of *crepitus* or *crackling* as the joint is moved. With disease progression, the patient may note and complain of *limitation of joint motion*. Involvement of weight-bearing joints leads to a history of abrupt giving way of weight-bearing joints with use.

SIGNS

Signs of joint involvement by osteoarthritis (Table 8–2) are once again variable and depend on disease severity and stage and specific joint involvement. In early stages, *tenderness* on palpation may be absent. When present, it may be localized to widely separated areas of the joint. In patients in whom synovitis is a prominent manifestation of the disease, tenderness over the joint is likely to be more diffuse. *Pain on passive motion* may be a prominent finding even though local tenderness is absent. *Crepitus* or *crunching* of the joint may be palpated and at times heard; patients may not spontaneously complain of this manifestation when their history is being taken. Crepitus appears to result from cartilage loss and joint surface irregularity. *Joint enlargement* is due primarily to proliferative changes in cartilage or bone with osteophyte formation. Later, secondary synovitis contributes to joint swelling. Significant joint effusions are uncommon; they are most likely to occur in patients with an acute flare following trauma, or in association with crystal deposi-

Table 8–2. SIGNS OF OSTEOARTHRITIS

Tenderness on palpation
  May involve widely separated areas of the joint
Pain on passive motion
Crepitus, crunching on joint motion
Joint enlargement—due to
  Cartilage and bone proliferative spur formation, or
  Synovitis with acute flares or after prolonged disease
Limitation of motion—due to
  Joint surface incongruity
  Muscle spasm and contracture
  Mechanical block (osteophytes, loose bodies)
Deformity, subluxation (seen late)—due to
  Cartilage loss
  Subchondral bone collapse
  Bone cysts
  Bony overgrowth
  Muscle atrophy
  Rarely, ankylosis

tion disease. *Limitation of motion* is observed as a result of joint surface incongruity, muscle spasm and contractures, capsular contracture, and mechanical block due to osteophytes or loose bodies. Both *deformity* and *subluxation* are seen in late stages of the disease owing to cartilage loss, collapse of subchondral bone, formation of bone cysts, and gross bony overgrowth (Fig. 8–1). When present, *muscle atrophy* is associated with severe disease of long progression. Complete joint immobilization due to fibrous or bony ankylosis is rare.

FINDINGS IN SPECIFIC JOINTS

The disease manifestations outlined above will often vary in presentation, depending on the specific joint involved. In patients with osteoarthritis of the distal interphalangeal joints (Heberden's nodes) and proximal interphalangeal joints (Bouchard's nodes) of the hands, osteophyte formation at the dorsolateral and medial aspects of the joints is prominent (Fig. 8–2). Flexion and lateral deviations of the distal phalanx are common. It should be noted that lateral deviation is an extremely uncommon manifestation of arthritis of the interphalangeal joints in other forms of arthritis. In some patients, Heberden's nodes develop with little or no pain over a period of many years. In other patients, osteoarthritic involvement of these joints is associated with a marked inflammatory response. Many patients complain of paresthesias and loss of dexterity. Small gelatinous cysts that appear on the dorsal aspects of the distal interphalangeal joints may be relatively asymptomatic and may be of concern to the patient mainly because of their cosmetic effects. In other

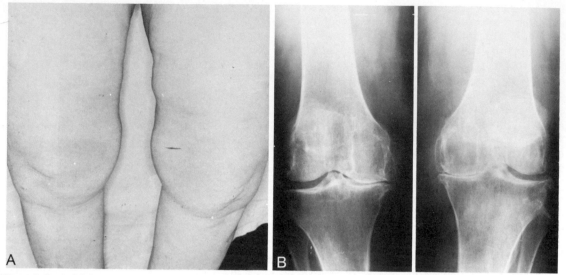

Figure 8–1. *A,* Bilateral genu varum (bowleg deformity) due to osteoarthritis. *B,* Roentgenogram of right and left knees. The genu varum seen clinically is related to marked cartilage loss with narrowed joint spaces at the medial femorotibial compartments of both knees. Osteophyte formation, which is most marked at the distal aspect of the medial femoral condyle, is also seen.

patients, these cysts become painful and inflamed and lead to significant disability (see Figure 11–1). Progressive lateral deviation of the interphalangeal joints leads to a snake-like configuration of the hands. Metacarpophalangeal joint involvement occurs but is rare.

Involvement of the first carpometacarpal joint is associated with localized pain and tenderness at the base of the thumb; symptoms may suggest a stenosing tenosynovitis at the medial aspect of the wrist (de Quervain's disease). The joint may have a squared appearance (shelf sign). Motion is often limited and painful. These changes occur frequently in association with involvement of the distal and proximal interphalangeal joints but may be present for a long period as an isolated finding.

Symptoms and signs include pain in the wrist and base of the thumb, radial and volar swelling, and tenderness over the navicular bone.

Degenerative involvement of the first metatarsophalangeal joint is usually insidious in onset, with very slow progression of swelling and associated pain. Not infrequently, inflammation of the bursa at the medial aspect of the joint secondary to trauma leads to an associated acute increase in swelling and pain in this area. The joint is irregular in contour and may be tender on palpation.

Involvement of the knee with osteoarthritis (see Figure 8–1) is associated with characteristic symptoms and signs of osteoarthritis. The patient complains of pain on motion, considerably relieved by rest. Stiffness is present after

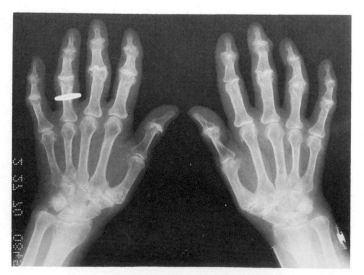

Figure 8–2. Joint space narrowing, osteophyte formation, and mild subchondral erosions are observed involving the distal interphalangeal joints (Heberden's nodes) and proximal interphalangeal joints (Bouchard's nodes) in this patient with osteoarthritis of the hands.

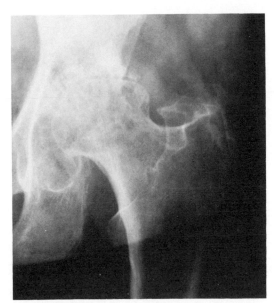

Figure 8–3. Roentgenogram of the left hip. Osteoarthritic changes are characterized by joint space narrowing, osteophyte formation, and subchondral cyst formation. Limitation of motion was observed on physical examination, and a limp was prominent on ambulation.

prolonged inactivity; crepitus is not uncommon. Tenderness may be localized to various aspects of the joint, and pain can be induced by passive or active motion. Osteophytes may be palpated as irregular hard enlargements. Synovitis and joint effusions are more likely to occur with involvement of this joint than elsewhere. Limitation of active or passive joint motion may occur. Quadriceps muscle atrophy is seen with late severe disease. Joint instability and subluxation are particularly associated with disproportionate involvement of the medial or lateral knee compartments. Abnormalities in joint biomechanics and instability are aggravated by laxity of collateral ligaments.

The common presenting manifestations of degenerative joint disease of the hip (Fig. 8–3) are an insidious onset of pain followed by a characteristic limp. Pain of true hip origin is usually felt at the outer aspect of the hip, in the groin, or along the inner aspect of the thigh. It should be noted that hip pain may be referred to the buttocks or sciatic region and is often referred along branches of the obturator nerve down to the knee. In some patients, referred knee pain is so severe that its true origin in the hip is overlooked. Stiffness is common, particularly in the morning and after joint inactivity. Examination will often reveal limitation of motion even early. A notable disparity between joint range of motion and roentgenographic findings is not uncommon. The leg is most characteristically held in exter-

nal rotation, with the hip flexed and abducted. The patient walks with an awkward shuffling gait, and functional shortening of the extremity may be apparent. Limitation of hip motion leads to difficulty in sitting or rising from a sitting position.

Pain and stiffness are characteristic manifestations of spinal osteoarthritis. In addition, radicular pain plays a prominent role in the patient's complaints. Local pain due to osteoarthritis of the spine appears to originate in paraspinal ligaments, joint capsules, and periosteum. Pain is not uncommonly referred along dermatomes related to the primary local lesion. Experimental investigations have demonstrated such pain referral following injections of saline solution into soft tissue structures in and about spinal articulations. Compression of nerve roots due to joint space narrowing or osteophyte formation leads to classic radicular pain. Nerve root impingement may result from spurs that compromise the foraminal space (Fig. 8–4), from prolapse of a degenerative disk, or from foraminal narrowing as a result of apophyseal joint subluxation. Radicular pain and paresthesias, and reflex and motor changes in the distribution of the involved roots are noted. Neurologic complications of this type are seen most often in the

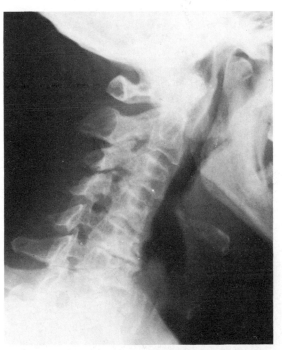

Figure 8–4. Roentgenogram of the cervical spine, oblique view. Cervical spondylosis is characterized by narrowing of multiple disk spaces and osteophyte formation; involvement of apophyseal joints is associated with spur formation and marked foraminal space narrowing at multiple levels.

cervical spine area owing to the relatively small spinal canal and intervertebral foramina as compared with other areas of the spine. Thoracic involvement is less common; radicular pain due to degenerative joint disease must be differentiated from pain due to other disorders such as neoplasms. Nerve root involvement in the lumbosacral area is associated with low back pain, sensorimotor changes on examination, and reflex abnormalities.

Dermatomal pain is generally deep, dull, and ill-defined. Patients often find it difficult to describe this symptom, and it is of little help in determining the level of spine involvement. Nerve root compression, on the other hand, produces symptoms that are much better localized with respect to symptomatic complaints and objective neurologic findings.

Further neurologic symptoms may be associated with osteoarthritis of the spine, particularly in the cervical area, if large posterior spurs or protruded disks compress the spinal cord. Symptoms result from direct cord compression or by compression of the anterior spinal artery. Compromise of the vertebral arteries as these vessels course upward through foramina to the brain may lead to a spectrum of clinical signs and symptoms that simulate basilar artery insufficiency. Dizziness, vertigo, and headaches are common complaints. Visual symptoms include blurring of vision, diplopia, and field defects. The disparity noted earlier between clinical and roentgenographic manifestations of osteoarthritis is particularly likely to be observed in the spine. Roentgenographic evidence of osteoarthritis may be extensive but bear little relationship to the patient's symptoms. On the other hand, severe symptoms may result with only mild anatomic abnormalities if such changes are located in particularly critical areas.

As noted earlier, this chapter is intended to provide a brief overview of symptoms and signs associated with osteoarthritis. Detailed expanded descriptions of clinical joint manifestations are provided in ensuing chapters targeted to specific areas of joint involvement.

References

1. Lowman EW: Osteoarthritis. JAMA 157:487–488, 1955.
2. Lawrence JS, Bremner JM, Bier F: Osteoarthrosis. Prevalence in the population and relationship between symptoms and x-ray changes. Ann Rheum Dis 25:1–24, 1966.
3. Roberts J, Burch TA: US Public Health Serv. Publ. No. 1000, Series 11, No. 15, 1966.
4. Harris WH: Idiopathic osteoarthritis of the hip; a twentieth century myth? J Bone Joint Surg 59B:121, 1977.
5. Solomon L: Patterns of osteoarthritis of the hip. J Bone Joint Surg 58B:176–183, 1976.
6. Cobb S, Merchant WR, Rubin T: The relation of symptoms to osteoarthritis. J Chronic Dis 5:197–204, 1957.
7. Gresham GE, Rathey UK: Osteoarthritis in knees of aged persons; relationship between roentgenographic and clinical manifestations. JAMA 233:168–170, 1975.
8. Danielsson LG, Hernborg J: Morbidity and mortality of osteoarthritis of the knee (gonarthrosis) in Malmö, Sweden. Clin Orthop 69:224–226, 1970.
9. Danielsson LG, Hernborg J: Clinical and roentgenologic study of knee joints with osteophytes. Clin Orthop 69:302–312, 1970.
10. Hernborg JS, Nilsson BE: The natural course of untreated osteoarthritis of the knee. Clin Orthop 123:130–137, 1977.
11. Seifert MH, Whiteside CG, Savage O: A 5-year followup of fifty cases of idiopathic osteoarthritis of the hip. Ann Rheum Dis 28:325–326, 1969.
12. Perry GH, Smith MJG, Whiteside CG: Spontaneous recovery of the joint space in degenerative hip disease. Ann Rheum Dis 31:440–448, 1972.
13. Moskowitz RW, Schwartz HJ, Michel B, Ratnoff OD, Astrup T: Generation of kinin-like agents by chondroitin sulfate, and human articular cartilage: Possible pathophysiologic implications. J Lab Clin Med 76:790–798, 1970.
14. Chrisman OD, Fessel JM, Southwick WO: Experimental production of synovitis and marginal articular exostoses in the knee joints of dogs. Yale J Biol Med 37:409–412, 1965.
15. Moskowitz RW, Goldberg VM, Berman L: Synovitis as a manifestation of degenerative joint disease: An experimental study. (Abstract.) Arthritis Rheum 19:813, 1976.
16. Moskowitz RW, Garcia F: Chondrocalcinosis articularis (pseudogout syndrome). Arch Intern Med 132:87–91, 1973.
17. McCarty DJ: Calcium pyrophosphate dihydrate crystal deposition disease: Nomenclature and diagnostic criteria. (Editorial.) Ann Intern Med 87:241–242, 1977.
18. Dieppe PA, Crocker P, Huskisson EC, Willoughby DA: Apatite deposition disease. A new arthropathy. Lancet 1:266–269, 1976.
19. Schumacher HR, Smolyo AO, Tse RI, Maurer K: Arthritis associated with apatite crystals. Ann Intern Med 87:411–416, 1977.
20. Phillips RS: Phlebography in osteoarthritis of the hip. J Bone Joint Surg 48B:280–288, 1966.
21. Ferreira SH: Prostaglandins, aspirin-like drugs and analgesia. Nature [New Biol] 240:200–203, 1972.
22. Crain DC: Interphalangeal osteoarthritis; characterized by painful, inflammatory episodes resulting in deformity of the proximal and distal articulations. JAMA 175:1049–1053, 1961.
23. Peter JB, Pearson CM, Marmor L: Erosive osteoarthritis of the hands. Arthritis Rheum 9:365–388, 1966.
24. Ehrlich GE: Osteoarthritis beginning with inflammation; definitions and correlations. JAMA 232:157–159, 1975.
25. Utsinger PD, Resnick D, Shapiro RF, Weisner KB: Roentgenologic, immunologic, and therapeutic study of erosive (inflammatory) osteoarthritis. Arch Intern Med 138:693–697, 1978.

9

Roentgenologic Diagnosis

Alex Norman, M.D.

Osteoarthritis (OA) is a disorder of advancing years and the most common form of arthritis. Nine out of ten people will show some degenerative changes in their weight-bearing joints by the time they reach 40 years of age.[1] OA is often painful and disabling and can be severe and crippling, particularly when it affects the hips and knees.

Osteoarthritis affects both large and small diarthrodial joints. The hip and knee are essentially the most symptomatic, although the severity of symptoms may not correlate with the degree of joint involvement. Traditionally, the disease is described as occurring in two stages: First, there is loss of articular cartilage; and second, reparative responses take place in adjacent bone and cartilage in an attempt to remodel the joint.[2-4] Some authorities believe that remodeling at the osteochondral junction occurs simultaneously with cartilage degeneration.[3]

Radin postulates that the first manifestation of osteoarthritis is stiffening of the subchondral bone, which results in greater stress on the overlying articular surface and eventually joint cartilage deterioration. His concepts are supported by animal studies that show that impulsive peak loading on the weight-bearing area causes microfracturing of the trabeculae. Subsequently, fracture healing stiffens the subchondral bone, subjecting the overlying cartilage to increased stress and breakdown.[5, 6] Pogrund and associates pointed out that if the bone is osteoporotic, it has greater resilience and the joint cartilage is spared.[7] This is why osteoarthritis and osteoporosis are so rarely found together.[7]

ETIOLOGY

Although the physical stress of "wear and tear" is the time-honored explanation for the etiology of osteoarthritis, physical stress alone is not the cause. The specific alterations that occur when a joint undergoes degeneration are by no means clearly understood. Many factors, e.g., biomechanical, biochemical, metabolic, enzymatic, genetic, immunologic, and inflammatory, play a role in priming the cartilage[5, 6, 8-13] for injury (see Chapter 7). Significant stress on concentric joint surfaces rarely induces cartilage breakdown. Excess load on incongruous surfaces, however, will trigger cartilage degeneration.

PRIMARY AND SECONDARY OSTEOARTHRITIS

The disease is classified as primary or "idiopathic" when no precipitating cause is apparent; it is classified as secondary when there is a related or pre-existing condition that may have laid the groundwork for its development.[14, 15] The incidence of osteoarthritis in each group is uncertain. In one series of 327 cases of OA of the hip, about 8% of the patients were diagnosed as having primary disease.[16] In several other series, however, the majority of cases were classified as primary.[17]

In an attempt to eliminate some of the confusion, Danielsson[18] set up strict criteria for the roentgenologic diagnosis of primary coxarthritis. He insisted that the roentgenograms show joint space narrowing and structural changes in the bone; the presence of osteophytes alone, he felt, was insufficient. Strict adherence to these criteria indicates an incidence of primary osteoarthritis of 3.4% in patients over 55 years of age and 10% in patients over 85.[18]

Murray[14] assessed the roentgenograms of 200 cases diagnosed as primary OA and concluded that only 70 (35%) were truly idiopathic. The anatomic changes in the other 130 patients were the result of pre-existing asymptomatic disease such as "forme fruste congenital dislocation of the hip" or of a "tilt" deformity, a residuum of adolescent epiphysiolysis. His findings suggest that as more is learned about degenerative joint disease and the conditions that predispose to it, the number of cases classified as primary osteoarthritis will dwindle and secondary OA will assume greater importance.

Conditions associated with secondary osteoarthritis include osteonecrosis, trauma, congenital hip disease, epiphysiolysis, neuropathic disorders, ochronosis, and inflammatory disease[15, 19] (see Chapter 14). In both primary and secondary osteoarthritis, the joint most commonly affected is the hip.[15] Our experience suggests that the four disorders most frequently underlying OA of the hip are osteonecrosis (30%); "burnt-out" inflammatory arthritis (i.e., rheumatoid arthritis and ankylosing spondylitis) (28%); congenital dislocation of the hip (26%); and epiphysiolysis (9%) (Table 9–1).

At a 1961 symposium on population studies related to chronic rheumatic disorders, an attempt was made to establish clinical criteria for defining patterns of OA, but without success.[20] For this reason, it was decided that degenerative arthritis should be graded solely on the basis of roentgenographic data.

The pathogenesis of OA of the hip suggests that subgroupings based on patterns of migration of the femur are most effective in showing the degenerative course of the disease. The pattern of hip displacement is recognized by the initial site of joint narrowing. Lequesne[21] categorized osteoarthritic hips into four groups: superior, superolateral, superomedial, and internal. Hermodsson[22] observed that the type and severity of the osteoarthritis are affected by the center-edge (CE) angle of Wiberg (an angle that defines the acetabular coverage of the femoral head [see Figure 15–1A]). If the outer margin of the acetabulum is less well developed, the CE angle will be proportionately smaller, and the more likely it will be that the load-bearing segment will shift to the superolateral part of the joint. Osteoarthritic joints frequently have subnormal CE angles. Migration of the femoral head is predominantly proximal or superolateral. In contrast, inflammatory joints have normal CE angles and tend to move in an axial or medial direction.[22]

Resnick[23, 24] observed three basic patterns of hip translocation in his series: superior, medial, and axial. Macys and associates[25] categorized the patterns of displacement as superior (which was subdivided into superolateral, lateral, and superior), intermediate, and medial (after Lequesne[21]).

In a study of 67 osteoarthritic hips, Gofton[26] found the most common displacement of the femur to be superior and the least common to be medial (superomedial—15%, medial—13%). Bilateral hip disease occurred most often in the hips that migrated medially (78%). He noted that it was rare for patients with progressive unilateral OA to develop bilateral hip disease after 11 years.[22, 24, 26, 27]

Gofton's statistics are at variance with those of Macys and associates,[25] who found bilateral hip disease in 78% of the patients with superior and lateral hip displacement in their series.[25] Perhaps it was in an attempt to resolve such uncertainties that Solomon[28] proposed a new classification characterized by three forms of pathology: (1) failure of essentially normal cartilage subjected to abnormal or incongruous loading for long periods; (2) damage of defective cartilage failing under normal conditions of loading; and (3) breakup of cartilage due to defective subchondral bone.[28]

ROENTGENOLOGIC CHARACTERISTICS OF OSTEOARTHRITIS

The first roentgenologic manifestation of OA is joint space narrowing. It reflects the

Table 9–1. THE FREQUENCY OF PRE-EXISTING CONDITIONS UNDERLYING SECONDARY OSTEOARTHRITIS OF THE HIP IN AN ANATOMIC STUDY OF 69 PATIENTS

Condition	Number and Percentage of Patients
Osteonecrosis	21/69 (30%)
Inflammatory arthritis	19/69 (28%)
Rheumatoid arthritis	14/69 (20%)
Ankylosing spondylitis	5/69 (7%)
Congenital dislocation of the hip	18/69 (26%)
Subcapital femoral epiphysiolysis	9/69 (9%)
Miscellaneous	7/69 (7%)

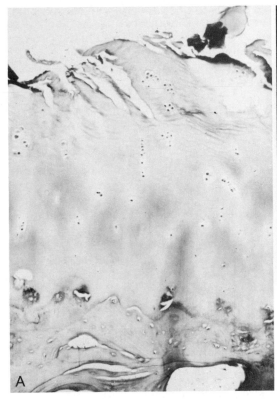

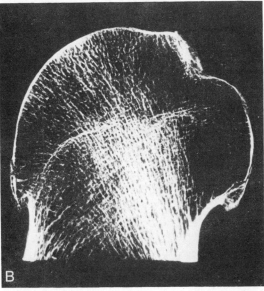

Figure 9–1. *A*, Limited fibrillation of the articular cartilage ($\times$ 125) in a patient with joint senescence. *B*, Note the small osteophytes at the margin of the head on the roentgenogram of the anatomic specimen.

thinning of the articular cartilage. However, joint space narrowing per se need not herald the onset of osteoarthritis, because it is also a phenomenon of aging.[15, 29]

Based on their findings, Byers and colleagues[29] postulated that two types of joint changes occur in the hip: (1) a commonly occurring type with limited progression that is age-related and does not lead to exposure of the subchondral bone or to a joint deformity; and (2) a less frequent form that is unrelated to aging and is progressive. The two types appear to be independent of one another. Only the second is regarded as true osteoarthritis.

The nature of the changes that take place in the senescent and the osteoarthritic joint is similar. Both show a loss of articular surface and production of osteophytes. Where they differ is in the magnitude of the involvement. Aging is characterized by limited deterioration of the cartilage and no restriction of joint function.[29] Fibrillation of the articular surface is generally mild, and osteophytes are small (Fig. 9–1). Occasionally, a senescent joint may almost imperceptibly turn into an osteoarthritic one, but this is rare.[15] OA, on the other hand, is characterized by asymmetric progressive narrowing of the joint cavity, prominent osteophytes, eburnation of the subchondral bone, and pseudocyst formation.[4, 15, 24, 25, 30]

It is often difficult to distinguish roentgenologically between the osteoarthritic and the senescent hip, and sometimes the normal hip as well. The following discussion may be helpful.

In the normal hip, the articular surfaces of the femur and the acetabulum are congruent. At least two thirds of the femoral head is contained by the acetabulum. The articular

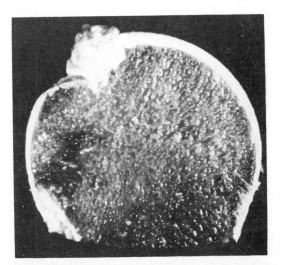

Figure 9–2. The thickest joint cartilage in this femoral head is at the weight-bearing segment lateral to the fovea centralis.

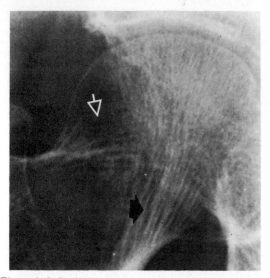

Figure 9–3. Basically, two primary systems of trabeculation are seen in the femoral head: a cone of compressive trabeculae (solid arrow), and the tensile system of trabeculae radiating like a fan from the lateral cortex to the medial side of the femoral head (open arrow). Between the two is Ward's triangle, a segment of minimal stress.

cartilage measures approximately 4 mm in thickness over the weight-bearing segment and tapers to 1 to 2 mm at the periphery (Fig. 9–2). Older adults may have thicker articular cartilage than young adults. Remodeling of the subchondral plate is also a more active process in the elderly patient.[31, 32]

The architecture of the proximal end of the femur is determined by the magnitude of the forces acting on the hip. A cone of compressive trabeculae extends from the load-bearing surface of the hip inferiorly to the medial cortex of the femoral neck.[33] The tensile trabeculae arise from the lateral cortex and traverse the neck to the medial articular surface in a fan-like pattern. Between these two is Ward's triangle, a zone of minimal pressure[33] (Fig. 9–3).

Early-Stage Joint Destruction

The first sign of joint destruction is fibrillation and fissuring of the cartilage in the zone of high pressure. The loss of cartilage accounts for the narrowing of the articulation and the pattern of migration of the femur.[22, 25, 26] A loss of the full thickness of the articular surface of the femoral head and acetabulum can mean a 4- to 5-mm joint narrowing.[25] With further destruction of the joint, the subchondral bone becomes eroded and eburnated, and shards of articular cartilage and bone are deposited in

the joint cavity and work their way into the synovium. The collapse of the femoral head and the erosion of the acetabulum can lead to further displacement, which may amount to 5 to 9 mm and not infrequently to as much as 1 or 2 cm.

Early-Stage Joint Repair

Osteophytes typically characterize OA and are often the most prominent roentgenographic feature of the disease. The exostosis is the reparative response to joint destruction. The etiology is unclear, but the pathology is well understood.[3, 4, 15, 16, 24, 25, 32, 34, 35]

Osteophytes are of two types: peripheral osteophytes, which arise at the chondro-osseous junction of the femoral head and neck and at the sites of capsular attachments; and surface osteophytes, also referred to as "surface bumps" or, occasionally, as central osteophytes, which develop at the perimeter of the pressure zones.[24] Osteophytes do not develop in the weight-bearing area because this segment is subjected to overwhelming stress and constant mechanical abrasion.[30]

Osteophytogenesis has been described as a biomechanical attempt to develop a more favorable distribution of load across the joint. When the surface area is increased by the apposition of new bone, the load per unit segment is diminished. This has a sparing effect on the joint.[36, 37] Ideally, joint remodeling can reach a stage of "incongruous congruity," at which point the arthritis may be slowed or even arrested.

Pathogenetically, osteophytes develop by one of two basic mechanisms: endochondral ossification or intramembranous bone formation. Peripheral osteophytes develop by intramembranous ossification. They parasitize the blood supply from the subsynovial tissue, articular capsule, and ligaments,[4] and grow into nonrestricted areas of the joint cavity, extending into the inferior and medial portions of the joint.

Surface osteophytes also arise in low-pressure areas. They develop by endochondral ossification, which resembles the maturation of the cartilaginous growth plate, and commonly form around the fovea and enlarge along the medial articular surface of the femur. Surface osteophytes ordinarily are not visible roentgenographically or to the naked eye.

During the progressive stage of OA, both types of osteophytes continue to enlarge and eventually coalesce into large exostoses that

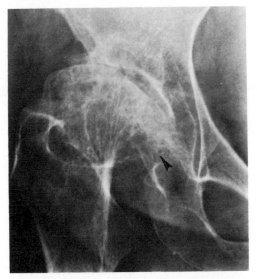

Figure 9–4. Superolateral displacement of the hip by a huge osteophyte extending into the joint (arrow). The excrescence from the acetabulum is not visualized.

Bone formation in the articular capsule and at ligamentous insertions is an example of intramembranous ossification. These changes occur frequently not only about the hip but also are common at the interphalangeal joints (distal interphalangeal joint, proximal interphalangeal joint). Martel and associates noted that these excrescences resembled wing-like expansions of the bone and called them the "seagull sign."[39]

Late-Stage Joint Destruction

Destruction continues in the high-pressure segment unless corrective measures are taken. The limitation of joint motion caused by muscle spasm, capsular scarring, and deformity places an additional load on a particular segment of the joint already weakened by subchondral vascular invasion and thinning of the articular surface. The femoral head, weakened by hyperemia and osteoclastic resorption, deforms under the crushing load.[4, 24] Microfractures develop in the subchondral zone initially, and later deeper in the head. Ultimately, the femoral head collapses, and the articular surfaces become even more incongruous, further aggravating the condition (Fig. 9–6). The femoral head becomes eburnated by the combination of increased pressure and friction.[4] Microfractures are more numerous, and osteonecrosis and pseudocysts develop where the subchondral bone is exposed.

The roentgenologic detection of osteonecrosis in OA is difficult because the lesions are usually microfocal in size and are often concealed in the densely sclerotic head. Distinguishing dead from viable bone in such a setting is almost impossible. For that reason, it is difficult to assess how frequently osteo-

tend to ring the femoral head and neck juncture. Surface osteophytes give the head a lumpy and irregular contour.[15] They are usually small, whereas peripheral osteophytes are frequently large and develop into areas where they are least constrained.[38] Similar changes occur on the inferoposterior wall of the acetabulum. These apposing excrescences mechanically displace the femur from the joint (Fig. 9–4). Some joints suffer major destruction without evidence of repair. In these cases, the joint cavity is clear and there is no hindrance to the destructive erosion of the joint, the deepening of the acetabular cavity, and the medial or axial migration of the femur (Fig. 9–5). More often, however, the growth of osteophytes parallels the extent of the destruction of the joint.

Figure 9–5. Axial migration of the right hip. The femur protrudes deep into the joint beyond the ischial-pelvic line. Compare with the normal left hip.

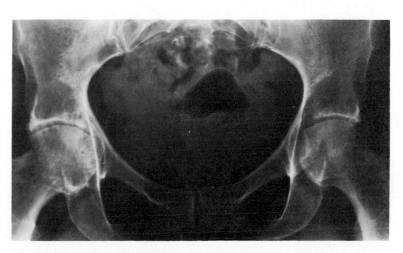

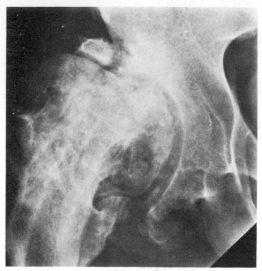

Figure 9–6. The acetabular surface collapsed in late stage OA, and the hip is further displaced from the acetabulum. Fragmentation of the outer border of the acetabulum is seen.

necrosis occurs in late-stage disease. Some researchers believe superficial bone necrosis is common.[4, 25] Others report that microscopic foci of osteonecrosis are always present but that they found sizable necrosis deep in the femur in only 14% of the surgical specimens examined in their series.[16] After excluding patients who had been treated with corticosteroids or who had alcoholic arthropathies, Solomon[28] found osteonecrosis in only 5% of those in his series.

Degenerative "Cysts"

Degenerative "cysts" are a roentgenographic hallmark of osteoarthritis, although the same lesions are seen in other arthritic disorders as well. The term "cyst" is a poor one for these lesions because a cyst is a distinct histopathologic entity. Sokoloff[38] prefers to call them "pseudocysts." Others use terms such as "geodes"[40] or "synovial cysts" (even though they are not limited by synovium). I prefer to call these lesions "cyst-like," which is roentgenologically descriptive and more accurate morphologically.

These cyst-like lesions tend to be small, circular or piriform in shape, and confined to a subarticular conical area of sclerotic bone within the segment of high pressure (Fig. 9–7).[4, 15, 24, 25, 28, 38, 40] Larger ones sometimes develop deeper in the femoral head and acetabulum (Fig. 9–8).[15] The size range is approximately 2 to 20 mm.[24] Whatever their size, however, these lesions are almost exclusively found in the line of load bearing. Harrison and associates[4] reported that every osteoarthritic femoral head removed at surgery contained "cysts." Others found these formations in fewer than half their patients with OA.[25]

A communicating channel from the neck of the lesion to the joint cavity can be identified in some, but not all, cases.[40] Landells[41] speculates that all these "cysts" are open to the joint cavity at one stage of development.

Not all radiolucencies on the surface of the joint are necessarily degenerative "cysts." More often, they are solid foci of fibrous or cartilaginous metaplasia (Fig. 9–9). Indeed, the surfaces of anatomic specimens are frequently punctuated by plugs of fibrocartilaginous nodules or fronds of fibrous tissue.

The etiology of these lesions continues to be debated.[15, 24, 38, 40, 41] Most investigators suggest a trophic or destructive cause, e.g., synovial

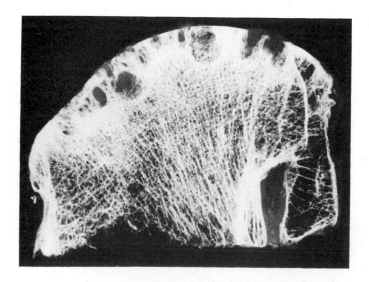

Figure 9–7. A specimen roentgenogram showing small, subarticular degenerative pseudocysts. These are circular or piriform in shape, and at least three communicate with the joint surface. The cysts are confined to the segment of high pressure within the zone of sclerosis.

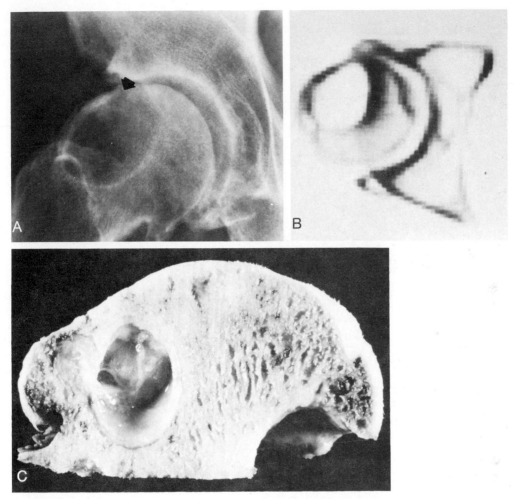

Figure 9–8. *A,* Giant cysts may extend deep into the femoral head. This 37-year-old man had a precocious onset of osteoarthritis. A pathologic fracture occurred in the superior aspect of the cyst (arrow). *B,* The cyst is well circumscribed by a zone of sclerosis, as noted on the computed tomogram. Note the anterior displacement of the femoral head. *C,* This specimen photograph of an osteoarthritic femoral head shows a large intracapital mucoid "pseudocyst" remote from the articular surface. This should not be confused with an intraosseous ganglion, which occurs in normal joints.

Figure 9–9. Roentgenographically, these lesions were mistaken for degenerative "cysts." Morphologically, they were solid foci of cartilage and fibrous metaplasia undergoing cyst formation.

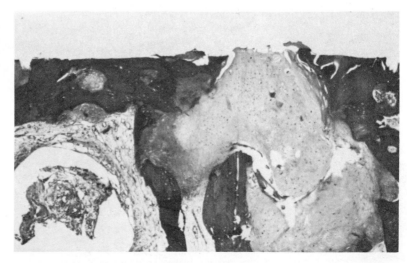

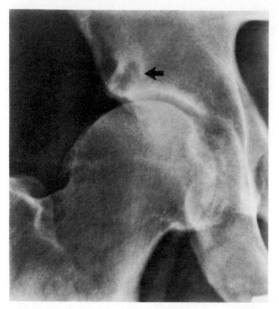

Figure 9–10. Eggers' cyst (arrow) evolving at the classic site in the acetabulum.

fluid intrusion or a bony contusion.[41, 42] Eggers and coworkers[43] contend that the lesions often occur in the acetabulum prior to their formation in the femur or to roentgenographic evidence of arthritis (Fig. 9–10). They suggest that they are secondary to hypervascularity of marrow spaces and bone resorption. Later, fibrous and cartilage marrow metaplasia occurs, and eventually these foci become encysted.

Late-Stage Joint Repair

The vascularity of the subarticular bone is decreased in late-stage OA. Reparative proc-esses become increasingly apparent, and subchondral bone sclerosis is roentgenographically evident in almost every case. Bone sclerosis accompanies the attrition of the articular cartilage and denotes the site of concentrated stress.[25, 34] Occasionally, advanced subchondral sclerosis (thickening of trabecular bone) may be present with little loss of joint cartilage; on the other hand, there may be complete narrowing of the joint with only a minor increase in bone density.[34]

Batra and Charnley[44] observed "eburnation and vertical collapse in the pressure zone" of the femoral head removed at surgery. They detected significant amounts of osteoid in the bone where the stress was greatest and considered it a sign of active osteogenesis and heightened reparative response to degenerative changes occurring in the joint.

Continued pressure on the bone results in increased eburnation and a highly compact polished articular surface. The normal fatty and hemopoietic marrow is replaced by cellular fibrous marrow in which bone trabeculae may form.[4, 15] Trias[45] confirmed by animal experiments that continuous stress on rabbit knees for greater than 12 days results in sclerosis, fibrosis, and cartilage metaplasia. Whitish to gray cartilage nodules of macroscopic or microscopic size project above the articular surface and to a depth of as much as 1 cm in the bone.[15] These cartilaginous foci may calcify and mature to bone or may undergo mucoid and cystic degeneration.[15] For the most part, the late sequelae in the high-pressure zone proceed as follows: (1) cartilage thinning; (2) further abrasion and exposure of the articular cortex; (3) subsurface sclerosis; (4) fibrous and cartilage marrow metaplasia; and (5) partial or complete encystment without vestige of the original tissue. The pathogenesis of OA is summarized in Table 9–2. An 8-year study of

Table 9–2. PATHOGENESIS OF OSTEOARTHRITIS

	Destruction (Weight-Bearing Area)	Repair (Non–Weight-Bearing Area)
Early-stage OA	Fibrillation of cartilage Erosion (minimal)	Osteophytes 　"Surface bumps" 　Marginal "Buttressing" of the femoral neck
Intermediate-stage OA	Erosion and exposure of the bone Focal osteonecrosis Pseudocysts 　Small to large	Sclerosis Osteophytes enlarge and coalesce, and 　the femoral head migrates Fibrous and cartilage marrow 　metaplasia "Buttressing"
Late-stage OA	Progression Collapse and deformity of the 　femoral head	Progression 　Spontaneous subsidence (rare) 　Resurfacing of joint (fibrocartilage)

the evolution of osteoarthritis illustrates the points made above (Fig. 9–11).

Spontaneous improvement of osteoarthritis is known to occur but seldom. With a redistribution of forces about the hip, cysts in the acetabulum and femoral head may heal,[4] the fibrous marrow may revert to fatty tissue,[15] and there is tendency for the eburnated bone to become resurfaced with fibrocartilage.[4, 25] Usually, this takes place after surgery (osteotomy or cup arthroplasty).[46]

Perry and colleagues[47] reported spontaneous joint space recovery and stabilization of 14 hips in the natural course of osteoarthritis. Roentgenographic evidence of restoration of the joint cavity correlated with an improve-

ment in clinical well-being and a reduction of the need for analgesic medication in these patients; hip motion remained restricted, however. After a 10-year prospective study, Perry and coworkers concluded, as did Storey and Landells,[46] that when hip stabilization was achieved as the result of the development of large (retaining) osteophytes, clinical complaints subsided and structural and roentgenographic findings of OA regressed.

Cortical Buttressing

Thickening of the medial cortex of the femoral neck is often present in osteoarthritis (Fig. 9–12), although some researchers found it in

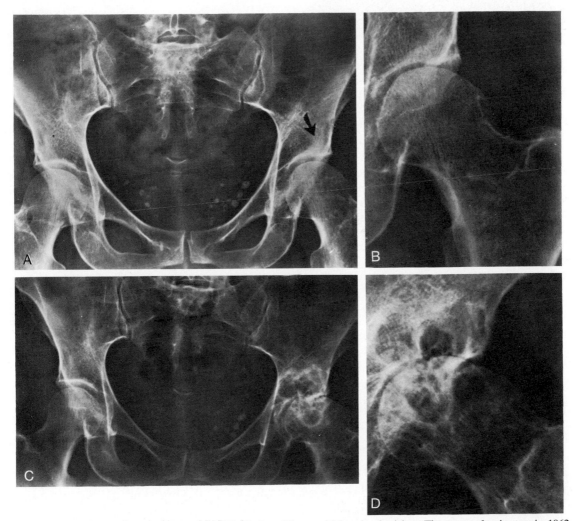

Figure 9–11. A, The evolution of OA of the left hip in a 58-year-old female physician. The onset of pain was in 1962. This first roentgenogram was taken in 1964. Although both joint spaces appear to be of normal width, there is sclerosis in the left acetabulum (arrow) as a response to excessive stress. *B*, (1967) Narrowing of the superior aspect of the joint space; early osteophyte formation at the lateral margin of the head and a buttressing of the medial cortex. The hip has migrated laterally (mild). *C*, (1969) Further joint narrowing; lateral migration of the hip; progressive enlargement of the marginal osteophyte. Subarticular pseudocysts are present in the load-bearing segments of the acetabulum and femoral head. Note that the right hip remains unaffected. *D*, (1970) Late-stage OA with collapse of the femoral head and continued enlargement of degenerative cysts in the acetabulum and femur. The joint space is destroyed.

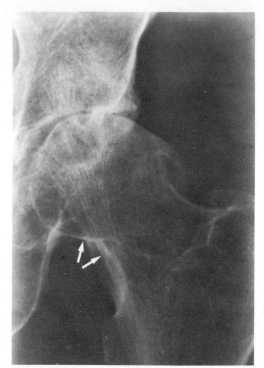

Figure 9–12. Buttressing of the medial cortex is a response to stress along the femoral neck.

only 7% of the patients in their series.[17] Secondary forces acting on the medial aspect of the femoral neck have been implicated as a cause of periosteal new bone response. This buttressing can be seen in early-onset OA. The cortex thickens in response to the concentrated stresses along the femoral neck, and if periosteal new bone is formed quickly, the cortex looks lamellated and shredded. Martel and Braunstein believe buttressing is due to the healing of microfractures.[39] An alternative theory is offered by Lloyd-Roberts, who suggests that a contracted scarred capsule produces traction upon the periosteum that evokes an irritative periostitis.[48]

Buttressing of the cortex is not limited to the hips. It can occur in the shoulders and at extra-articular sites such as the supracondylar portion of the femur.[49]

Other Joint Sites

Originally OA was thought to involve only a single joint or to be limited locally to related articulations. It is now known that it can be a generalized disorder. When it is, the distribution resembles that of rheumatoid arthritis.[50] No joint is spared from degenerative structural changes, but the weight-bearing articulations tend to suffer the greatest deterioration and advanced disease. Certain weight-bearing joints, such as the hip, knee, and first metatarsophalangeal joint, are affected more than others.[51]

In a study of 100 consecutive cases of osteoarthritis, the hands (66%) and knees (61%) were the most common sites of involvement, with the hip being involved less frequently (48%)[50]; involvement of the spine (ankylosing vertebral hyperostosis) occurred in 44% of the cases. In comparison with rheumatoid arthritis, OA most often affects two to five joint sites; rheumatoid arthritis generally involves six to ten joints.

We recently evaluated the extent and distribution of osteoarthritis in a series of patients with OA of the hip by radionuclide imaging and roentgenograms of the scintigraphically "hot" areas. Degenerative disease of the spine (facet joints and spondylosis deformans) was present in almost every instance (92%), and in decreasing frequency, the disease was found in the hands (66%), knees (58%), and feet (42%), predominantly in the great toe and first metatarsophalangeal joint. As a result, a convincing argument can be made for a type of OA characterized by widespread joint disease other than the condition described by Kellgren and Moore in 1952[52] as primary generalized OA (PGOA).

Roentgenographic surveys are regularly performed in a rheumatologic work-up to establish the extent of joint involvement. However, radionuclide imaging is far more efficient and has the additional advantage of exposing the patient to a lower burden of radiation. The radionuclides commonly used are technetium-99m (^{99m}Tc) polyphosphate and ^{99m}Tc methyl diphosphonate. The latter is preferred because it has a high target background ratio. These radiopharmaceutical agents seek out the sites of enchondral ossification, which roughly parallel the location of the alkaline phosphatase activity. Macroautoradiographs have shown that the target sites of these materials are those areas where osteogenesis is occurring, mainly in the osteophyte, cyst wall, and weight-bearing areas.

Scintimetry is more sensitive than roentgenography in detecting affected arthritic joints. If the scan can be quantified, it can also be useful in assessing the effectiveness of therapy.[53] When clinical and laboratory evidence of arthritis is lacking in a patient with known polyarthralgia, a ^{99m}Tc-diphosphonate scan can be helpful in establishing the diagnosis if it reveals significant uptake at the symptomatic joint (Fig. 9–13). A positive bone scan, however, is a nonspecific test because it measures only physiologic blood flow and osteogenesis.[53–56] Clinical experience and laboratory data are still necessary for an exact diagnosis.

OSTEOARTHRITIS OF THE KNEE

OA of the knee is likely to be symptomatic and disabling.[15, 24, 50] The knee is a complex hinged joint with three major compartments: medial tibiofemoral, lateral tibiofemoral, and patellofemoral. Interposed between the condyles are the menisci—anatomic spacers that increase the contact area between the condylar joint surfaces and protect the articular cartilage from excessive wear and tear.[57, 58] The joint surface beyond the coverage of the menisci is the first to undergo degeneration.[59]

Fairbank[60] called attention to the preponderance of osteoarthritis in the postmeniscectomy knee years after surgery. Johnson and colleagues[61] confirmed this finding in their re-

view of the late results of meniscectomy. They speculated that the menisci spare the knee from both physiologic and biomechanical damage. Once osteoarthritis intervenes, however, as Fukubayashi and Kurosawa[58] point out, the meniscus no longer effectively reduces the pressure across the joint, and a degenerated or torn meniscus may expose the articular surface to further damage.

The morphologic alterations that take place in the degenerative knee are the same as those that occur in the hip. Bennett and associates[59] report that the pathogenesis of OA of the knee joint begins in the articular surface. If weight-bearing continues on an impaired joint, abnormalities develop not only in the cartilage but also in the subchondral bone, meniscus, and synovium. In a typical case, degeneration will advance until the surface cartilage is ulcerated and the underlying bone exposed. Marginal repair (osteophyte formation) occurs (Fig. 9–14). The marrow spaces below the eburnated bone are filled with fibrous and cartilaginous tissue. Subsequently, pseudocysts develop, and

Figure 9–13. This patient had polyarthralgia. Roentgenograms confirmed OA of the left hip and cervical spine. Other sites of arthritis are seen on this radionuclide scan, e.g., acromioclavicular joints and lumbar spine (mild).

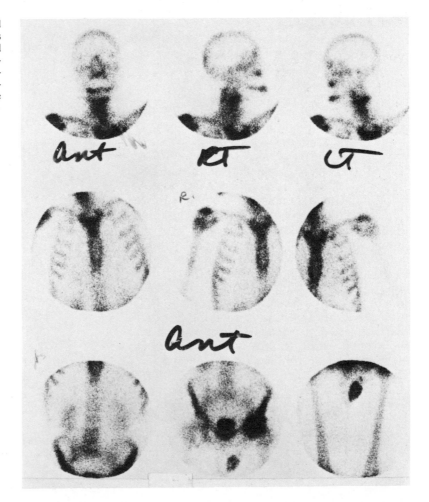

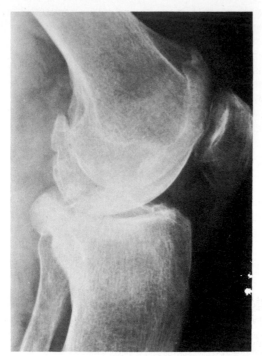

Figure 9–14. Note the marginal osteophyte repair at the posterior extremes of the opposing femoral and tibial condyles.

detritic fragments loosen from the joint surface and are discharged into the cavity. Shards of bone and cartilage are imbedded in the synovium, resulting in a "detritic synovitis."

Attrition of the menisci may parallel the deterioration of the articular surface. The free edge of the meniscus becomes wavy and frayed, and the semilunar cartilage calcifies (chondrocalcinosis), particularly in the elderly.

An appropriate roentgenographic assessment of the knee should include multiple views covering all joint compartments. The conventional frontal and lateral roentgenograms will not ordinarily show the full extent of pathology.[24] A tunnel view is often needed in order to visualize the posterior surface of the femoral condyles.[62] Frequently, a change in the direction of the central beam will show joint bodies, osteochondritis dissecans, erosions of the articular surface, and osteophytes not noticed on the frontal view. Routine lateral and axial views are ideal for examining the patellofemoral joint.

Thomas and associates[63] emphasized the need for careful preoperative assessment of the joint and evaluated the importance of roentgenographic and clinical study versus bone scintimetry, arthrography, and arthroscopy. Clearly, bone imaging is the easiest way to detect an involved joint, but it gives no indication of any anatomic changes that may have occurred. Thomas and coworkers did not consider roentgenograms showing the effects of weight bearing essential to their study, but other studies have demonstrated that roentgenograms in load bearing disclosed joint narrowing when non–weight-bearing films were normal.[63, 64]

Standing views of the knee are invaluable when measuring varus or valgus deformities. The static view is often the decisive film for planning the osteotomy.[64] Maquet[57] stresses that roentgenograms taken with the patient standing can be used for accurate assessment of the knee under load. Displacement of the weight-bearing line from the normal axis of gravity will lead eventually to ipsilateral narrowing of the joint space, sclerosis of the tibial condyle, and, later, changes in the apposing femoral surface (Fig. 9–15).

Bicompartmental (medial tibiofemoral and patellofemoral disease) is a more common pattern of involvement than tricompartmental disease. Even when all compartments are affected, however, the symmetric joint diminution noted in inflammatory arthritis rarely occurs.

A loss of articular surface accounts for the narrowing of the joint cavity. Roentgenograms taken with the patient erect are more effective than conventional ones in detecting the presence of minimal joint degeneration.

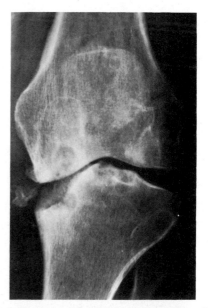

Figure 9–15. Weight-bearing film showed the collapse of the medial joint compartment and accentuated the varus angle of the knee and the fragmentation of the tibial trabecular surface.

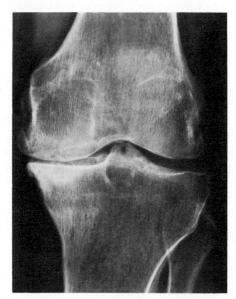

Figure 9–16. The wedge of sclerotic bone in the medial tibial condyle identifies the primary reaction to stress across the medial compartment of the knee.

Focal subchondral sclerosis is often the secondary finding after joint cavity narrowing. A triangular wedge of sclerosis sharply delineates the segment of increased stress and load (Fig. 9–16). Later, changes develop in the femoral condyle. Detritic pseudocysts are not as common a development in the knee as they are in the hip, and when they do occur, they are small and often obscured by the bony sclerosis.[22] Occasionally, a large subarticular cyst appears remote from the line of stress; how-

ever, weight-bearing studies show that the cyst lies under the pressure zone. Osteophytes are always marginal to the segment of weight bearing and are more pronounced when the joint narrowing is advanced. Prominence and broadening of the tibial spines are still other manifestations of osteophyte formation.

A "vacuum sign" may be seen in advanced cases of OA, usually in the medial joint compartment. The vacuum phenomenon disappears on weight bearing.

Patellofemoral arthritis is as common as medial tibiofemoral compartment disease. Subchondral patellar sclerosis underscores the area of concentrated stress. Because patellofemoral incongruence is a key factor in the development of osteoarthritis, it is important to determine patellar subluxation roentgenographically. This is best accomplished by an axial "skyline" view. The Merchant projection[65] is most valuable for demonstrating this change, but when patellar subluxation is advanced, any of the axial projections will disclose the pathology.[65–68]

Erosion or "scooping out" of the anterior femoral cortex proximal to the condyles is not unusual in advanced osteoarthritis (Fig. 9–17). Debris may collect in the soft tissue filling the defect (Fig. 9–18). Occasionally, tibiofemoral arthritis may be absent or minimal. An abnormal quadriceps pull when the knee is in extension has been proposed as the mechanism for this lesion. Because women tend to have greater extension of their knee joints than men do, Alexander[69] speculates that this may explain why seven of his eight patients were

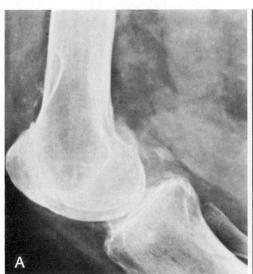
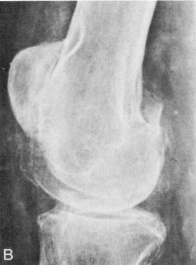

Figure 9–17. *A*, Note the "scooped-out" defect in the femur proximal to the condyles. *B*, When this woman extends her knee, the patella falls into the defect.

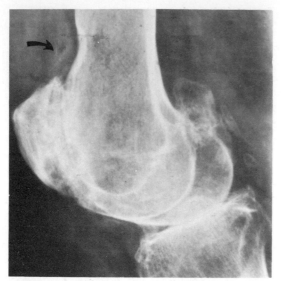

Figure 9–18. Detritic material may collect in the granulation tissue filling the defect (arrow).

women. None had patella alta or an unusually long patella ligament.

Degenerative changes in the patella at the insertion of the quadriceps tendon are common and present as early as adolescence, although they are most pronounced after the fifth decade of life. This lesion should not be confused with patellofemoral osteoarthritis, and there is no correlation between the clinical symptoms of the two disorders. The more advanced the stage of degenerative patellar changes, the more prominent are the vertical ridges and the long excrescences projecting from the upper pole of the patella. An axial view of a patella so affected can simulate dentate structures, which is why Greenspan and associates[70] called such changes the "tooth sign" of patellar degenerative disease.

OSTEOARTHRITIS OF THE SHOULDER

Osteoarthritis of the shoulder is similar in pattern to OA of the hip. The articular surface of the glenoid is the more severely involved side of the joint, perhaps because stresses are concentrated on a smaller joint surface area than that of the humeral head.[71] Nevertheless, the largest osteophytes are seen at the inferior margin of the humeral head (Fig. 9–19). The disorder is usually secondary to osteonecrosis, inflammatory arthritis, trauma, or a metabolic bone disease such as gout or ochronosis.[72] Although it is not rare in older adults, it is seldom clinically significant. A small percent-

age of patients will have severe pain and limitation of motion and may eventually require surgery.

OSTEOARTHRITIS AND OSTEONECROSIS

Osteoarthritis and osteonecrosis are related to each other in two different ways. Segmental osteonecrosis is observed in most femoral heads removed because of advanced osteoarthritis.[4, 25, 28] The necrotic foci of bone and marrow are of microscopic size and are rarely apparent on the roentgenogram. Osteonecrosis is almost always present in the pressure zone, which surmounts the fibrous or pseudocystic region.

Osteonecrosis complicated by secondary osteoarthritis, on the other hand, is a different condition both roentgenographically and anatomically. Although the symptoms may be similar, the necrotic zone is larger and continuous and extends deeper into the bone. Ahuja and Bullough[73] emphasize that the reactive zone of granulation tissue in osteonecrosis far exceeds that found in osteoarthritic joints.

Mankin and collaborators[74] confirm that even in severe cases of osteonecrosis with long-standing symptomatic hip disease, there are limited changes of OA, despite femoral head collapse and joint incongruity. In several in-

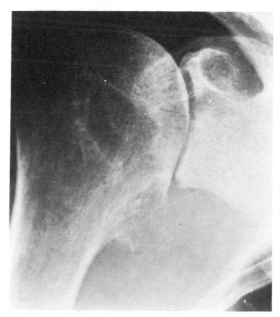

Figure 9–19. This athletic female has a painful frozen shoulder. The opposing joint surfaces are eroded, and a large osteophyte projects from the inferior aspect of the humeral head.

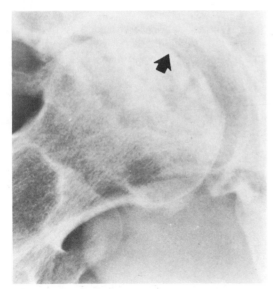

Figure 9–20. An advanced case of osteonecrosis of the hip with secondary OA. The joint space is well preserved for this stage of disease. The "radiolucent crescent" (arrow) is the hallmark of osteonecrosis.

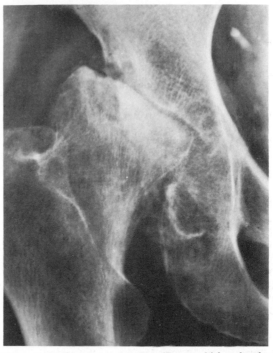

Figure 9–21. Roentgenogram in a 67-year-old female who, after having a smoldering osteoarthritis for 3.5 years, experienced acute pain in the hip that was disabling. The sudden destructive coxarthrosis with very little repair is characteristic of "Postel's" arthropathy.

stances in which cortisone or trauma induced osteonecrosis, the cartilage overlying the necrotic bone was histologically, biochemically, and metabolically normal. Contrary to roentgenographic observations in primary OA of the hip, these patients had less joint space narrowing and smaller osteophytes (Fig. 9–20).

SPECIAL FORM OF OSTEOARTHRITIS: POSTEL'S "DESTRUCTIVE COXARTHROPATHY"

This rapidly destructive degenerative arthritis of the hip was first reported by Postel and Kerboull in 1970.[75] In a matter of weeks, a traditionally slowly progressive osteoarthritis of the hip is converted into a rapidly aggressive disease that could completely destroy the joint in 6 to 10 months. The pain in the hip was typically disabling and unrelenting in 40 of the 44 patients described in their series. In 32 patients, the major portion of the femoral head had disappeared. In many cases, the severity of the changes in the acetabulum equaled that of those in the femoral head. The acetabulum became concentrically enlarged, and a small femoral head stump floated within it. Occurring with equal frequency was the destruction of the roof of the iliac acetabulum and subluxation of the hip. Dissolution of the acetabular

floor was extensive in only five patients (Fig. 9–21).

Features unique to this swift, destructive form of arthritis are the absence of degenerative pseudocysts and the lack of osteophyte formation. The speed of the process inhibits any effort at repair. At pressure sites, however, the articular surfaces are eburnated. In 1979, Jacqueline[76] described a rapidly destructive coxarthrosis in 20 hips that was similar to the sudden massive bone resorption reported by Postel and Kerboull 9 years earlier. These cases were also distinguished by a lack of reparative response.

The roentgenographic characteristics of Postel's destructive coxarthropathy are quite similar to the changes noted by Norman and associates[77] in the "acute disorganizing form of neuropathic arthropathy" (Fig. 9–22). Other differential considerations include the severe generalized joint destruction that occurs in juvenile rheumatoid arthritis and the subacute septic joint. The exclusion of pyogenic hip is of singular importance, for the only option open to the surgeon treating a case of Postel's coxarthropathy is total hip arthroplasty. If occult sepsis is overlooked, the result of the surgery could be catastrophic.

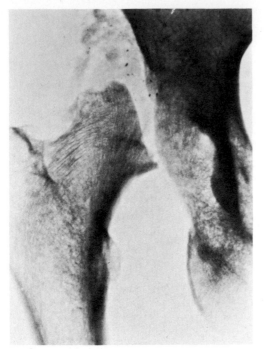

Figure 9–22. Note the striking resemblance of Postel's osteoarthritis to this case of acute neuropathy.

NEUROPATHIC ARTHROPATHY

Neuropathic arthropathy is an acute or chronic destructive arthritis and the most severe manifestation of degenerative joint disease. The resemblance to osteoarthritis is striking. In the advanced stages of the disease, the joint cartilage is destroyed, subchondral sclerosis is pronounced, and marginal osteophytes may form; the last are frequently fragmented, and shards of cartilage and bone debris are discharged into the joint space. Chronic synovitis, which thickens the synovium and capsule, is classically seen morphologically.

Neuroarthropathy and osteoarthritis differ only in the degree of the reaction.[78, 79] Patients with neuropathic arthritis lack the protective sense of pain, and minor injury may trigger severe disorganization and discombobulation of the articulation.

In his treatise on "the arthropathy of the ataxic patient," Charcot limited his commentaries to the neuropathic arthropathy of tabes dorsalis. No other underlying neurologic disorder was considered. Hence, the eponym "Charcot joint" may best be reserved for the specific type of neuroarthropathy and not the condition secondary to other neurologic disorders.

Despite the variety of conditions implicated in the evolution of a neuropathic joint, trauma and impaired sensation are the primary precipitating factors. Charcot stated that the ataxic patient with tabes dorsalis will be less likely to develop a neuropathic joint if confined to bed. Neuropathies rarely occur in patients with spasticity. The increased muscle tone splints the joint and protects it from injury.[80] Eloesser[81] showed the importance of trauma as a cause of neuropathic joint complication in cats. He induced an acute neuropathic joint by first sectioning the posterior roots to the hind limbs of three cats; after an interval of several weeks, the femoral condyles were seared by thermocautery. The "sudden response of an anesthetic joint to the acute trauma of the operation" resulted in an acute Charcot joint in all of the animals.[81] Despite the accumulated evidence favoring trauma as a precipitating factor, some investigators still question whether injury can induce a neuropathic joint in less than 6 weeks. Brower and Allman suggest that perhaps a neurovascular mechanism is the underlying basis.[82]

Neuroarthropathy is a complication of a variety of neurologic disorders, most frequently tabes dorsalis, diabetes mellitus, and syringomyelia.[77, 80] With the increasing number of patients with diabetes in the United States, diabetes ranks a close second to tabes dorsalis as an etiologic factor.[77] Jordan was the first to bring attention to the effect of diabetes on the nervous system and reported spine changes in diabetic patients akin to those recognized in neurosyphilis.[83, 84]

In young patients (children) with neuroarthropathy, congenital insensitivity or indifference to pain, spina bifida, or meningomyelocele are the most likely underlying neurologic disorders recognized. Recently, steroids and nonsteroidal anti-inflammatory agents have been implicated.

Statistically, 85% of neuropathic joints are in the lower extremity. The knee is affected almost as frequently as the total of all other joint sites.[80] In diabetic patients, there is a greater predilection for the joints of the foot and ankle. Patients with syringomyelia and leprosy are more commonly affected in the upper extremities (80%). As many as 25% of patients with syringomyelia develop joint complication. Despite the high percentage of neuropathic changes in patients with syringomyelia, tabes dorsalis and diabetes mellitus are still the more common underlying neurologic disorders.

The spine is involved in approximately 5% to 10% of patients with neuropathy, but as this rarely causes symptoms, the diagnosis is often overlooked unless a roentgenogram is taken of that area. Multiple joint involvement in tabetic neuropathies is not uncommon (40%). Fitzgerald[85] reported a 17-year-old patient with an atypical presentation of congenital indifference to pain who had as many as six neuropathic joints and seven neuropathic fractures.

Fractures play an initiating role in the majority of patients. Charcot mentioned that spontaneous fractures in tabes dorsalis were not uncommon. Fractures may involve the articular surface or the shaft of the bone. Whereas simple traumatic injuries often produce oblique or spiral fractures, the neuropathic fracture tends to be transverse.[80] Metaphyseal infractions are common in youngsters, particularly in the patient with congenital insensitivity to pain.

The early sign characterizing a neuropathic joint is an effusion, which is often massive and persistent. The fluid may be straw-colored or may be hemorrhagic when there is repeated trauma to the joint.[80] Joint capsule distention and a lack of sensibility lead to abnormal stresses of the articulation, stretching of the ligaments, and subluxation.[86] Unsuspected trauma to the articular surfaces results in joint destruction, early onset of a detritic synovitis, thickening of the capsule, and soft tissue swelling (Fig. 9–23).

Although many features of a neuropathic joint are indistinguishable from OA, the detritic joint changes and the reparative responses in the neuropathic arthropathy occur at an earlier stage.

Johnson[78] emphasized that fractures probably trigger the onset of disease. In addition, spontaneous fractures in diabetes mellitus have been heralded as the cause of joint derangement.[83, 87, 88]

Disorganization after minor injury or unrecognized trauma of the joint may occur in 1 to 15 months.[87] The speed with which a neuroarthropathy evolves led Norman and colleagues[77] to classify the arthropathy as "acute and chronic" disease. If the joint disorganization evolves in less than 2 months, it is regarded as an acute neuroarthropathy; all others are considered chronic (Fig. 9–24).

Massive resorption at the end of the bone has been noted about the hip, shoulder and ankle joints. The roentgenographic features are dramatic. Some contend that the pathologic findings are secondary to neurovascular alterations, with increased blood flow to bone and striking osteoclastic resorption.[82] Johnson regards the process as secondary to neuro-

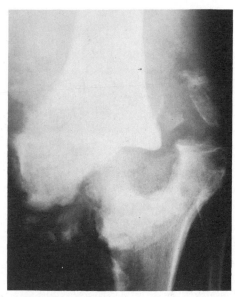

Figure 9–23. The hallmarks of a neuropathic joint are massive effusion and swelling, articular destruction and debris, and instability.

pathic fractures.[78] The fibrovascular invasion is the initial stage of fracture repair. There is resorption of the debris and increased vascularity, which further weakens the bone and exposes it to a greater risk of injury.

As the neuroarthropathy progresses, the reparative responses become more pronounced. The subchondral bone is more sclerotic, and bony debris is dispersed into the soft tissue. Fragmentation of the articular margins, dia-

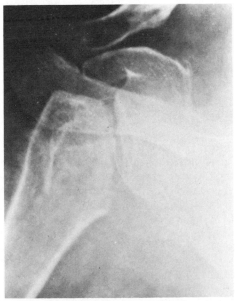

Figure 9–24. Joint destruction occurred in this patient within 7 weeks.

physeal fractures, and subperiosteal new bone formation are the consequences of abnormal stress on the joint in an ataxic patient. Osteophytes become more prominent than those recognized in OA, but often they are fragmented by the chronic forces on the joint margin.

Later, in the more florid stage of the arthritis, there is a greater disorganization of the joint and more pronounced subluxation and dislocation (malalignment). Bony debris in soft tissue may become more pronounced. It can penetrate the capsule and extend into the adjacent muscle groups tracking for some distance away from the joint. Some densities have the appearance of rice bodies.[89] Subsequently, intra-articular and soft tissue debris may be pulverized into bone "dust" and phagocytized by macrophages (Fig. 9–25). At one point, the process stabilizes and comes to a halt. Sclerosis of the bone extends for a distance into the diaphysis; periosteal new bone is pronounced; and marginal osteophytes may grow to massive size. The latter processes widen the bone.

Complications of chronic soft tissue infection are a common source of trouble in leprosy, diabetes mellitus, and tabes dorsalis. "Insensitivity ulcerations" over bony prominences, particularly about the foot, may be a source of the problem. As a consequence, secondary soft tissue and joint infection may produce absorption of the metatarsals and phalangeal heads, giving the appearance of "pencil-sharp" ends of the bone.[86]

SPONDYLOSIS DEFORMANS

Degenerative spine disease is an all-encompassing term often denoting osteoarthritis. It is the most common arthritic condition of the vertebral column and can be present as early as 40 years of age, but more often it occurs in the older adult group. It affects almost all individuals over 60 years of age.[15]

Spondylosis deformans is the more common term for this condition. The disorder is characterized by osteophytes beginning at the anterior margins of the vertebrae near the insertion of the annulus fibrosus. The osteophytes enlarge and frequently coalesce with an exostosis arising from the apposing vertebral surface.[15, 24]

Initially, the disk space is normal; later, it degenerates and narrows. Osteophytes at the posterior aspect of the vertebrae are more common in the cervical region and occur less commonly in the lumbar and thoracic segments.[90]

Spondylosis deformans is decidedly a male disease and is related to occupation. Patients, including women, who do heavy physical labor, have more extensive involvement of the spine. Jaffe[15] quotes a study by Gantenberg[91] that showed a high incidence of spondylosis in miners, a lower incidence in factory workers, and the least incidence in sedentary workers.

Although degenerative spine disease may be asymptomatic, symptoms may develop as the disease progresses. At first, there is mild aching and stiffness of the back. Subsequently, more acute and chronic back complaints develop. These episodes may be punctuated by bouts of radiculitis.

Degenerative disease of the synovial apophyseal joints is the only true manifestation of spinal osteoarthritis. Schmorl and Junghauns[92] observed a dissociation of anatomic findings between spondylosis and true spinal arthritis (spondylarthritis). In one of their series, the spines with extensive spondylosis had only minor involvement of the apophyseal joints (OA); whereas in the second group with significant osteoarthritis of the synovial joints, only a few had changes of spondylosis. One assumes that because both conditions are manifestations of aging and degeneration, the two would run a parallel course. This is not necessarily so, however.

Degenerative spine disease may be a manifestation of a generalized osteoarthritis. Huskisson and colleagues[50] reported that in a survey of 100 patients with osteoarthritis, 44% had roentgenologic features of degenerative spine disease. In our study of patients more than 50 years of age, spondylarthritis was present in 92% of individuals with OA of the hip.

The early changes of spondylosis deformans affect the anterolateral margin of the vertebrae where the annulus fibrosus inserts. Tearing of the fibers weakens the annulus. The restraints on the nucleus pulposus are lost, and the disk protrudes forward. Further stress will lift the anterior longitudinal ligament from the vertebral body, and a buttress of periosteal new bone fills in the area of separation. The osteophytes enlarge in a horizontal direction and curve to bridge the intervertebral disk space (Fig. 9–26).

Macnab[93] describes a "traction spur" that is short and horizontal and arises approximately 1 to 3 mm above the vertebral margin. This exostosis is a reaction to spinal instability. Disk degeneration further aggravates the instability,

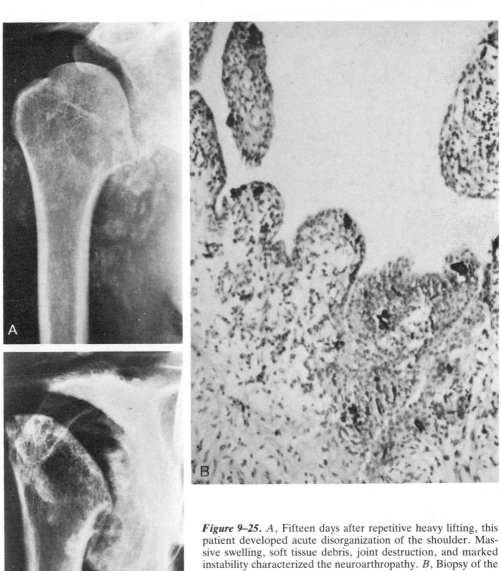

Figure 9–25. *A*, Fifteen days after repetitive heavy lifting, this patient developed acute disorganization of the shoulder. Massive swelling, soft tissue debris, joint destruction, and marked instability characterized the neuroarthropathy. *B*, Biopsy of the synovium showed a detritic synovitis diagnostic of a neuropathic joint. *C*, Three years later, the debris and swelling are resorbed (late-stage findings). Note the disappearance of the humeral head and atrophy of bone.

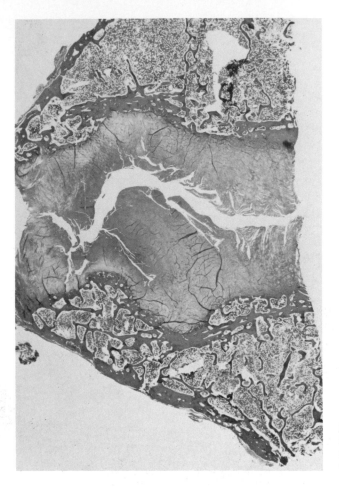

Figure 9–26. Photomicrograph of two large opposing vertebral osteophytes. The lateral course of the osteophyte before bridging the interspace is typical of spondylosis.

and the "spur" increases in size. If fusion or immobilization of the unstable segment occurs, the "traction spur" will remodel and disappear.

Osteophytes arising from the posterior margin of the vertebrae occur less frequently. Anatomically, the posterior longitudinal ligament is firmly anchored to the disk and the edge of the vertebral bodies. It does not strip from the bone as readily as its anterior counterpart. The posterior osteophytes are "claw-like" and small; these can be differentiated from the "traction spur" of instability.

See Chapters 26 to 28 for a complete discussion of spondylarthritis.

SPINAL ENTHESOPATHIES

The enthesopathies are conditions that affect the paraspinal and extra-axial ligamentous structures and tendons in the body. When these structures suffer attrition and degeneration, they customarily become ossified. In the spine, the anatomic sites that are affected are (1) the anterior longitudinal ligament (ALL); (2) the posterior longitudinal ligament (PLL); and (3) the vertebral arch ligaments (VAL) (intraspinous, supraspinous, intratransverse, ligamentum flavum).

There are three syndromes associated with paraspinal ligamentous ossification, and each will be discussed in detail. The most common enthesopathy is ossification of the anterior longitudinal ligament (OALL), more frequently called Forestier's disease or ankylosing hyperostosis (AH). A diffuse idiopathic form called diffuse idiopathic skeletal hyperostosis (DISH) is the extra-axial manifestation of the disorder (see Chapter 13).

Ossification of the posterior longitudinal ligament (OPLL) is a disease primarily of the Japanese. However, like Forestier's disease, there can also be an extra-axial involvement.

The third and rarest of the group is ossification of the vertebral arch ligaments (OVAL). There is no prior reference in the literature to this conditon. Like the other syndromes, it is a noninflammatory degenerative spondylosis and is also punctuated by the DISH syndrome.

Forestier's Disease, or Ankylosing Hyperostosis (AH)

Forestier and collaborators[94] described the entity of ankylosing spine disease that is distinctive from ankylosing spondylitis and osteoarthritis. In their initial report in 1950, all patients were males between 50 and 75 years of age. Since then, the condition has been recognized in females.

Clinically, the patients have moderate stiffness of the back and a limited amount of pain. Posture is generally unaffected; however, an occasional patient may have kyphosis.[94]

Forestier's disease is a common clinical entity with an occurrence as high as 6% to 12% in any unselected autopsy series.[95, 96] The etiology is still open to speculation.

A flowing ossification along the anterior surface of the vertebrae extends across the disk spaces in a distinctive fashion. The thoracic spine is always affected; to a lesser extent, the lumbar and cervical regions of the spine are involved.[97] In their studies, Forestier and Rotes-Querol alluded to other sites of ossification such as supraspinatus ligaments and thickening of the iliac crest.[97]

The roentgenographic features of ankylosing hyperostosis are variable. At the onset, ossification of the spinal ligaments is delicate (1 to 2 mm); subsequently, the osteophytes may be as broad as 20 mm. A layer of lamellated reactive new-bone is deposited in apposition to the anterior cortex of the vertebra but is separated from it by a narrow clear zone. The longitudinal ligament can easily be stripped from the bony mass (Fig. 9–27). As the condition becomes more pronounced, thick hyperostotic, lumpy masses flow in a continuous fashion along the anterior surface of the spine (Figs. 9–27 and 9–28). In the thoracic region, the protuberances are primarily on the right; in the lumbar and cervical regions, the osteophytes extend from both sides of the vertebra. Broad "candle-flame–like" exostoses grow upward from the vertebra across the disk.[95, 97] The disk is of normal height (Figs. 9–28 and 9–29). Only infrequently is there a loss of disk height (10%) or a vacuum phenomenon.[95, 98] Harris and coworkers,[99] like Forestier, estab-

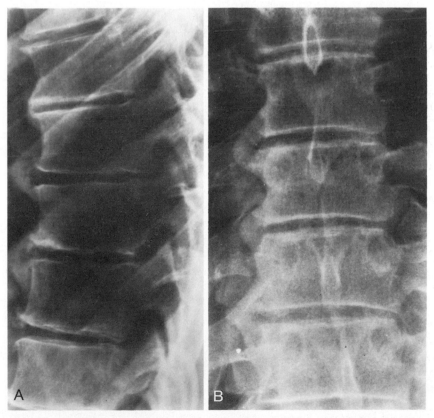

Figure 9–27. *A,* Early onset of thoracic ankylosing hyperostosis with small osteophytes arising from the anterior cortex of the vertebra away from the vertebral margin. Although a few disks appear slightly narrow, they are still intact. *B,* The affinity for the right side of the thoracic spine is clear.

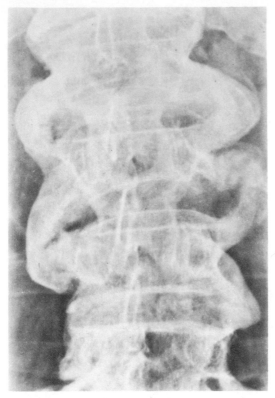

Figure 9–28. Forestier's disease with large lumbar osteophytes approaching a breadth of 20 mm. The disk spaces are of normal height.

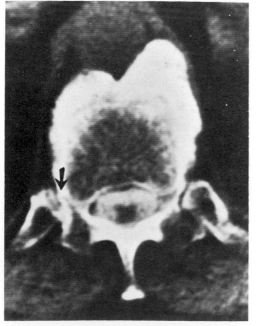

Figure 9–29. Computed tomogram of a thoracic vertebra showing large lumpy ossification of the anterior longitudinal ligament. The aorta sits between the peaks of these exostoses. Ossification of the costovertebral joint is noticed on the left (arrow).

lished the following criteria for AH: There are hyperostotic excrescences along the anterior vertebral aspect of the spine that bridge at least two to four interspaces; the sacroiliac joints must be normal; and there is no associated spine disease to explain the bony ankylosis.

In a study of 20 autopsies, Vernon-Roberts and associates[95] described large endesmophytes (syndesmophytes) bridging the disk space and causing ankylosis. In many macerated specimens, there were narrow clefts of disk material or fibrous tissue separating the bridging osteophytes. In addition, the articular capsule of the apophyseal and costovertebral joints were ossified, and short segments of calcification of the ligamentum flavum and the supraspinous ligaments were seen. These findings illustrate an overlap of Forestier's disease (primary enthesopathy) and, to a minor extent, posterior vertebral arch ossification. Two of Forestier's patients had large bony outgrowths from the ventral surface of the cervical spine with anterior block fusion and remodeling of several segments. This anatomic change may be associated with dysphagia (Fig. 9–30).

When there is an ossifying diasthesis at extraspinal locations in Forestier's disease, the entity is called diffuse idiopathic skeletal hyperostosis (DISH) (see Chapter 13). The incidence of DISH is variable (60% to 100%).[98, 99] The condition was popularized by Utsinger and collaborators[96] and by Resnick and associates.[98]

The favored sites of involvement are the following:

Pelvis. Calcification and ossification occur near the capsule of the hip joints and ligamentous attachments to the iliac crest and at the iliotransverse process. "Whiskering" of the ischial tuberosities, ossification of the sacrotuberous ligament, and ossification of the pubic symphysis are common. The absence of sacroiliitis distinguishes AH from the inflammatory spondylarthitides (ankylosing spondylitis, Reiter's disease, and psoriatic arthritis).

Foot. Other sites of involvement are in the foot. Ossification at the insertion of the tendo Achillis and plantar aponeurosis to the heel is common. In a large series, 76% of the patients had ossification at the dorsal aspect of the talus; the medial aspect of the scaphoid; and the base of the fifth metatarsal.

Elbow. Ossification of the triceps insertion to the olecranon is a usual finding.

Knee. Ossification within the quadriceps and infrapatellar ligaments also occurs frequently.

Skull. Ossification can be found in the ligamentum nuchae.

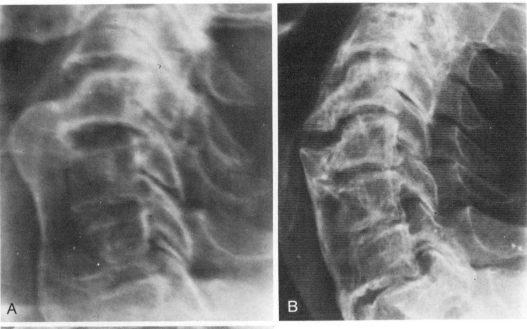

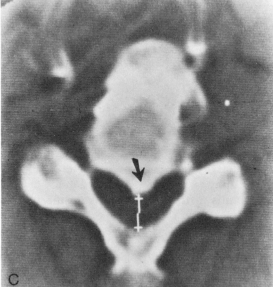

Figure 9–30. *A*, Anterior block fusion of the cervical vertebra similar to Forestier's cases. The block fusion leads to remodeling and resorption of the anterior cortex of the involved segments. Despite extensive cervical fusion, disk space height is normal. *B*, A 76-year-old man with dysphagia secondary to cervical ankylosing vertebral hyperostosis (AVH). This is one of the few cases with degenerative disk narrowing and a faint vacuum sign at C5 to C6. *C*, A correlative computed tomogram through the mid-cervical spine shows posterior longitudinal ligamentous ossification (arrow) and significant narrowing of the spinal canal.

The association of ankylosing hyperostosis and ossification of the posterior longitudinal ligament can have an incidence as high as 50%. However, the extent of posterior longitudinal ligament calcification is not nearly as striking as that in primary OPLL.

Ossification of the Posterior Longitudinal Ligament (OPLL)

Although this condition is an established entity among Japanese, the first paper on OPLL, by Key, appeared in 1839 in the Guy's Hospital Report.[100]

The Japanese Ministry of Public Health and Welfare[101] became aware of the seriousness of this situation after Onji and colleagues[102] published a review of 18 cases of OPLL and cervical myelopathy. A rapid increase in the number of patients with neurologic signs prompted the establishment of a committee to investigate the epidemiology of the disease. Data on 2142 patients were collected in a pilot study that began in 1975. Currently, there are 4000 patients with OPLL in Japan.

In a random series of necropsies, 20% of the patients over 60 years of age had OPLL. Like AH, ossification of the posterior longitudinal ligament is a disease with a male predominance (2:1). The peak incidence is in the seventh decade of life. There is speculation that OPLL is an endemic disease in Japan. The etiology remains obscure. Environmental and genetic factors have been implicated. However, further investigation is necessary to clarify the cause of the condition.

Eighty-five per cent of patients admitted to hospitals with this disorder are symptomatic. They complain of neck pain, dysesthesia, pain and motor dysfunction in the upper and lower extremities, and bladder problems that develop insidiously. Acute signs of tetraparesis can develop after minor injury.

The incidence of OPLL in a asymptomatic adult population, as identified by roentgenograms, is approximately 2%. Very few cases occur outside Japan. Occasional reports are recorded in Caucasians and blacks.[101, 103]

The roentgenographic presentation of OPLL may be (1) segmental, (2) continuous, (3) mixed, or (4) circumscribed foci of ossification. Segmental ossification is the most common presentation and occurs in 39% of patients.[101] The bony masses may be linear or lumpy and can cross several disk spaces, sometimes extending from the upper cervical spine to the thoracic region (Fig. 9–31). A routine lateral roentgenogram may not always show ligamentous ossification. In such instances, if the diagnosis is suspected, tomography and computed tomography are useful, particularly if the lesions are asymptomatic. The features of OPLL are more common in the neck than in the thoracic and lumbar regions of the spine. However, in the latter locations, OPLL may cause more serious disability than in the neck (Fig. 9–32). In many patients, however, the disease is asymptomatic and subclinical throughout life.

Animal experimentation has shown that the spinal canal can be narrowed gradually to 70% of its dimension before neurologic complaints evolve. In humans, however, cervical myelopathy is likely to occur when the sagittal diameter of the spine is reduced to 60% of normal.[104]

In 23.9% of Japanese with OPLL, there is an associated ankylosing hyperostosis. Ono and coworkers[105] studied 166 patients and confirmed the relationship between the two conditions; they speculated that an etiologic kinship exists between OPLL and AH. They suggested that some "hyperostotic diasthesis" may play a role in the pathogenesis of these conditions.

Clinically, posterior ligament ossification is more serious than Forestier's disease. One case of spinal cord compression with neurologic changes was reported in a 68-year-old male with the classic features of ankylosing hyperostosis and DISH. He had suffered weakness in the right leg for 10 years. Two weeks prior to admission, he developed a spastic gait. Complex tomography, CT scanning, and metrizamide myelography demonstrated compression of the cervical cord. Whereas the association of DISH and ossification of the posterior vertebral ligament has been described, the occurrence of neurologic changes in AH has not been substantiated.[95, 96, 98, 99, 101, 106, 107] Alenghat and associates and Becker and colleagues[107, 108] warn that neurologic findings in ankylosing hyperostosis should prompt a search for associated OPLL and cord compression.

Minor cord impingement by calcified ligamentous masses responds to conservative management in 70% of patients. If treatment fails, posterior decompression can be effective.[101]

Metabolic data in the Japanese population show that 12.4% of patients with OPLL have clinically verified diabetes. Although not firmly documented, there may be a relationship between diabetes mellitus and all the enthesopathies.

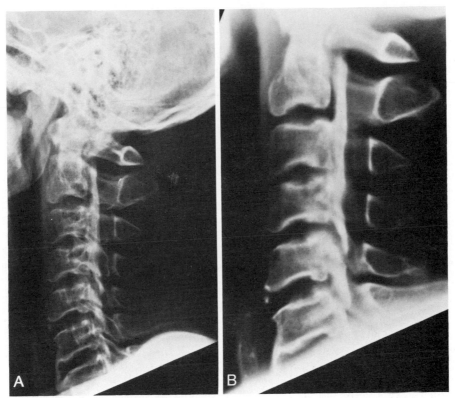

Figure 9–31. *A,* A long continuous lesion of OPLL extending from C2 to C4 and a circumscribed lesion bridging C5 to C6. *B,* Lateral tomography better defines the lesion. (Courtesy of Dr. William Fielding.)

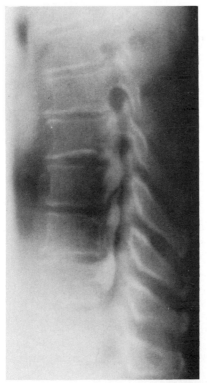

Figure 9–32. A long mixed segment of OPLL in the thoracic region significantly compromised the spinal canal.

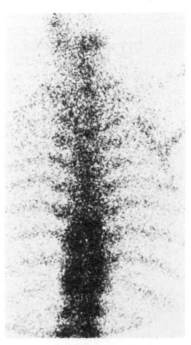

Figure 9–33. Intense uptake of radiopharmaceuticals in the heavily ossified portion of the lumbar spine.

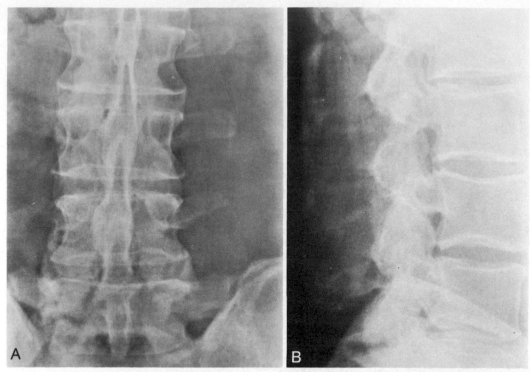

Figure 9–34. A and *B*, Views of the lumbar spine show a massive bony fusion of the posterior arches of the vertebrae. The anteroposterior view identifies the interspinous ossification (simulating railroad tracks); the lateral projection illustrates the extensive posterior ossification and the bony encroachment on the spinal canal. Note the maintained disk height.

Ossification of the Vertebral Arch Ligaments (OVAL)

Ossification limited to the ligaments of the vertebral arch (ligamenta flava, interspinale, supraspinale, and intertransversarium) is an enthesopathy for which no clinical reference could be found in the literature. It is the rarest of the spinal ligamentous syndromes, and manifests some features of AH, OPLL, and the full-blown picture of diffuse idiopathic skeletal hyperostosis. Forestier and associates,[94] Alenghat and coworkers,[107] and others[96, 104, 106] mention focal ossification in the ligamentum flavum and supraspinous ligaments in their cases of AH. However, these findings were in no measure as extensive as the findings in our case of ossification of the vertebral arch ligaments (OVAL).

The condition that we call OVAL was identified in a 40-year-old Hispanic male who complained of progressive stiffness of his back and increased pain, as well as heel pain and limited motion of his spine, shoulders, and hips. A study of the histocompatibility antigens (HLA) was made. There were no markers to suggest a spondylarthropathy or ossifying diaphysis in this patient.

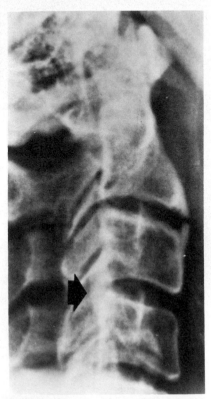

Figure 9–35. A small focal segment of ankylosing hyperostosis at C2 to C3 and a circumscribed lesion at C3 to C4 of OPLL (arrow).

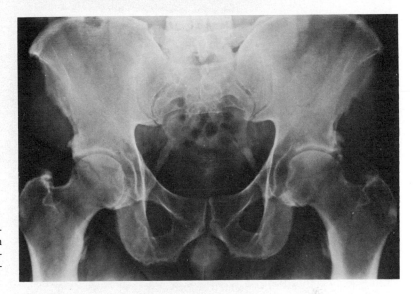

Figure 9–36. Lumpy, tendinous, ligamentous and capsular ossification is seen about the hip and the sacrotuberous and iliolumbar ligaments.

Scintimetry with ^{99m}Tc methyldiphosphonate showed avid uptake in the lumbar region from the first to fifth vertebral segments. This was the site of intense ossification of the vertebral arch ligaments (Fig. 9–33).

A uniform sheet of ossification in the ligaments of the posterior vertebral elements and capsule of the facet joints was demonstrated (Fig. 9–34). The massive bony fusion encroached on the spinal canal and produced a spinal stenosis in this patient.

Other sites of spine involvement appeared to overlap those seen in AH and OPLL. In the cervical spine, there was a small ventral circumscribed segment of ossification in the anterior longitudinal ligament and a lesion of similar size in the posterior longitudinal ligament at C3 to C4 (Fig. 9–35).

The extraspinal components were as prominent as those recognized in AH and OPLL. There was ossification of the musculocapsular attachments about the hip joint. Fluffy and bumpy bony ligamentous irregularities involved the iliolumbar and sacrotuberous ligaments. Other sites of ossification in the pelvis were at the tendinous insertions to the lesser and greater trochanters and the lateral pelvic margin from anterior superior to inferior spine; there was also a "whiskering" of the ischial tuberosities. These findings are consistent in this entire group of enthesopathies (Fig. 9–36). Ossification of ligaments and tendons about the feet, knees, and elbows was also noted.

Computed tomography delineated the fluffy ossification of the capsule about the zygoapophyseal joints and the intraspinal extension of the bony masses that arose in the ligamentum flavum. The synovium-lined apophyseal joints were spared. The computed tomographic scans showed ossification of the tendons and ligaments of the foot with sparing of the subtalar joint, similar to changes at other anatomic sites.

Although initially it was difficult to categorize these lesions into a single entity, it was soon apparent that the pathology (ligamentous ossification) was confined to the posterior spinal elements. For this reason, the name ossification of the vertebral arch ligaments (OVAL) was considered to be appropriate.

Although the etiology remains obscure, the findings suggest an anatomic interrelationship among Forestier's disease (OALL), ossification of the posterior longitudinal ligament (OPLL), and OVAL. They share several features, particularly DISH.

References

1. Lowman EW: Osteoarthritis. JAMA 157:487–488, 1955.
2. Moskowitz RW: Experimental models of degenerative joint disease. Semin Arthritis Rheum 1:95–116, 1972.
3. Ilardi CF, Sokoloff L: The pathology of osteoarthritis: Ten strategic questions for pharmacologic management. Semin Arthritis Rheum 11:3–6, 1981.
4. Harrison MHM, Schajowicz F, Trueta J: Osteoarthritis of the hip: A study of the nature and evolution of the disease. J Bone Joint Surg 35B:598–626, 1953.
5. Radin EL: The physiology and degeneration of joints. Semin Arthritis Rheum 2:245–257, 1973.
6. Radin EL, Parker HG, Pugh JW, Steinberg RS, et al.: Response of joints to impact loading. 3. Relationship between trabecular microfractures and cartilage degeneration. J Biomech 6:51–57, 1973.

7. Pogrund H, Rutenberg M, Makin M, et al.: Osteoarthritis of the hip joint and osteoporosis: A radiological study in a random population sample in Jerusalem. Clin Orthop 164:130–135, 1982.

8. Barrett AJ: Which proteinases degrade cartilage matrix? Semin Arthritis Rheum 11:52–56, 1981.

9. Lippiello L: Prostaglandins and articular cartilage metabolism: Does prostaglandin perturbation perpetuate cartilage destruction? Semin Arthritis Rheum 11:87–91, 1981.

10. Cooke TD: Immune deposits in osteoarthritic cartilage—their relationships to synovitis and disease site and pattern. Semin Arthritis Rheum 11:109–110, 1981.

11. Peyron J: Inflammation in osteoarthritis (OA): Review of its role in clinical picture, disease progress, subsets, and pathophysiology. Semin Arthritis Rheum 11:115–116, 1981.

12. Schumacher HR, Gordon G, Paul H, et al.: Osteoarthritis, crystal deposition and inflammation. Semin. Arthritis Rheum 11:116–119, 1981.

13. Bollet AJ: An essay on the biology of osteoarthritis. Semin Arthritis Rheum 12:152–163, 1982.

14. Murray RO: The aetiology of primary osteoarthritis of the hip. Br J Radiol 38:810–824, 1965.

15. Jaffe HL: Metabolic, Degenerative and Inflammatory Diseases of Bones and Joints. Philadelphia, Lea & Febiger, 1972, p. 735.

16. Meachim G, Whitehouse GH, Pedley RB, et al.: An investigation of radiological, clinical, and pathological correlations in osteoarthrosis of the hip. Clin Radiol 31:565–574, 1980.

17. Hughes GRV: Osteoarthritis. Age Ageing 8:1–8, 1979.

18. Danielsson L: Incidence and osteoarthritis of the hip (coxarthrosis). Clin Orthop 45:67–72, 1966.

19. Moskowitz RW: Clinical and laboratory findings in osteoarthritis. In McCarty DJ (ed.): Arthritis and Allied Conditions. 9th ed. Philadelphia, Lea & Febiger, 1979, p. 1161.

20. Kellgren JH: Diagnostic criteria for population studies. Bull Rheum Dis 13:291–292, 1962.

21. Lequesne M: Coxarthrose. In Encyclopédie Médico-Chirurgicale. Tome Os-Articulations. Paris, Éditions Techniques, 1958.

22. Hermodsson I: Roentgen appearances of arthritis of the hip. Acta Radiol [Diag] (Stockh) 12:865–881, 1972.

23. Resnick D: Patterns of migration of the femoral head in osteoarthritis of the hip. Roentgenographic-pathologic correlation and comparison with rheumatoid arthritis. Am J Roentgenol 124:62–74, 1975.

24. Resnick D, Niwayama G: Degenerative joint diseases. In Diagnosis of Bone and Joint Disorders, Vol 2. Philadelphia, W.B. Saunders Company, 1981, pp. 1322–1332.

25. Macys JR, Bullough PG, Wilson PD Jr: Coxarthrosis: A study of the natural history based on a correlation of clinical, radiographic, and pathologic findings. Semin Arthritis Rheum 10:66–80, 1980.

26. Gofton JP: Studies in osteoarthritis of the hip. 1. Classification. Can Med J 104:679–683, 1971.

27. Danielsson LG: Incidence and prognosis of coxarthrosis. Acta Orthop Scand [Suppl] 66:1–114, 1964.

28. Solomon L: Patterns of osteoarthritis of the hip. J Bone Joint Surg 58B:176–183, 1976.

29. Byers PD, Contepomi CA, Farkas TA: A post mortem study of the hip joint including the prevalence of the features of the right side. Ann Rheum Dis 29:15–31, 1970.

30. Meachim G, Hardinge K, Williams DR: Methods for correlating pathological and radiological findings in osteoarthritis of the hip. Br J Radiol 45:670–676, 1972.

31. Lane LB, Bullough PG: Age-related changes in the thickness of the calcified zone and the number of tidemarks in adult human articular cartilage. J Bone Joint Surg 62B:372–375, 1980.

32. Gardner DL: General pathology of the peripheral joints: In Sokoloff L (ed.): The Joints and Synovial Fluid, Vol. II. New York, Academic Press, 1980, pp. 384–396.

33. Pauwels F: Biomechanics of the Normal and Diseased Hip: Theoretical Foundation, Technique and Results of Treatment—An Atlas. Berlin, Heidelberg, and New York, Springer-Verlag, 1976, p. 18.

34. Cameron HU, Fornasier VL: Fine detail radiography of the femoral head in osteoarthritis. J Rheumatol 6:178–184, 1979.

35. Gilbertson EM: Development of periarticular osteophytes in experimentally induced osteoarthritis in the dog. Ann Rheum Dis 34:12–25, 1975.

36. Johnson LC: Joint remodeling as the basis for osteoarthritis. J Am Vet Med Assoc 141:1237–1241, 1962.

37. Cuccurullo GDG, Croce F: Macroscopic and microscopic aspects of osteophytes in advanced osteoarthritis of the hip. Ital J Orthop Traumatol 6:117–122, 1980.

38. Sokoloff L: The Biology of Degenerative Joint Disease. Chicago, University of Chicago Press, 1969, pp. 5–23.

39. Martel W, Braunstein EM: The diagnostic value of buttressing of the femoral neck. Arthritis Rheum 21:161–164, 1978.

40. Resnick D, Niwayama G, Coutts RD: Subchondral cysts (geodes) in arthritic disorders: Pathologic and radiographic appearance of the hip joint. Am J Roentgenol 128:799–806, 1977.

41. Landells JW: The bone cysts of osteoarthritis. J Bone Joint Surg 35B:643–649, 1953.

42. Rhaney K, Lamb DW: The cysts of osteoarthritis of the hip. A radiological and pathological study. J Bone Joint Surg 37B:663–675, 1955.

43. Eggers GWN, Evans EB, Blumel VA, et al.: Cystic changes in the iliac acetabulum. J Bone Joint Surg 45A: 669–686, 1963.

44. Batra HC, Charnley J: Existence and incidence of osteoid in osteoarthritic femoral heads. J Bone Joint Surg 51B:366–371, 1969.

45. Trias A: Effect of persistent pressure on the articular cartilage. J Bone Joint Surg 43B:376–386, 1961.

46. Storey GO, Landells JW: Restoration of the femoral head after collapse in osteoarthrosis. Ann Rheum Dis 30:406–412, 1971.

47. Perry GH, Smith MJG, Whiteside CG: Spontaneous recovery of the joint space in degenerative hip disease. Ann Rheum Dis 31:440–448, 1972.

48. Lloyd-Roberts GC: The role of capsular changes in osteoarthritis of the hip joint. J Bone Joint Surg 35B:627–642, 1953.

49. Norman A, Baker ND: Spontaneous osteonecrosis of the knee and medial meniscal tears. Radiology 129:653–656, 1978.

50. Huskisson EC, Dieppe PA, Tucker AK, et al.: Another look at osteoarthritis. Ann Rheum Dis 38:423–428, 1979.

51. Trueta J: Studies on the etiopathology of osteoarthritis of the hip. Clin Orthop 31:7–17, 1963.
52. Kellgren JH, Moore R: Generalized osteoarthritis and Heberden's nodes. Br Med J 1:181–187, 1952.
53. Hoffer PB, Genant HK: Radionuclide joint imaging. Semin Nucl Med 6:121–137, 1976.
54. Christensen SB, Arnoldi CC: Distribution of 99mTc-phosphate compounds in osteoarthritic femoral heads. J Bone Joint Surg 62:90–96, 1980.
55. Siegel BA, Donovan RL, Alderson PO, et al.: Skeletal uptake of 99mTc-diphosphonate in relation to local bone blood flow. Radiology 120:121–123, 1976.
56. Genant HK, Bautovich GJ, Singh M, et al.: Bone-seeking radionuclides: An in vivo study of factors affecting skeletal uptake. Radiology 113:373–382, 1974.
57. Maquet PCJ: Biomechanics of the Knee, With Application to Pathogenesis and Surgical Treatment of Osteoarthritis. Berlin, Heidelberg, and New York, Springer-Verlag, 1976, pp. 71–121.
58. Fukubayashi T, Kurosawa H: The contact area and pressure distribution pattern of the knee. Acta Orthop Scand 51:871–879, 1980.
59. Bennett GA, Waine H, Bauer W: Changes in the Knee Joint at Various Ages With Particular Reference to the Nature and Development of Degenerative Joint Disease. New York, The Commonwealth Fund, The New York Academy of Medicine, 1942, pp. 42–63.
60. Fairbank TJ: Knee joint changes after meniscectomy. J Bone Joint Surg 30B:664–670, 1948.
61. Johnson RJ, Kettelkamp DB, Clark W, Leaverton P: Factors affecting late results after meniscectomy. J Bone Joint Surg 56A:719–729, 1974.
62. Resnick D, Vint V: The "tunnel" view in assessment of cartilage loss in osteoarthritis of the knee. Radiology 137:547–548, 1980.
63. Thomas RH, Resnick D, Alazraki NP, et al.: Compartmental evaluation of osteoarthritis of the knee. A comparative study of available diagnostic modalities. Radiology 116:585–594, 1975.
64. Leach RE, Gregg T, Siber FJ: Weight-bearing radiography in osteoarthritis of the knee. Radiology 97:265–268, 1970.
65. Merchant AC, Mercer RL, Jacobsen RH, Cool CR: Roentgenographic analysis of patellofemoral congruence. J Bone Joint Surg 56A:1391–1396, 1974.
66. Maquet P: Mechanics and osteoarthritis of the patellofemoral joint. Clin Orthop 144:70–73, 1979.
67. Clark KC: Positioning in Radiography. 8th ed. London, Heinemann Medical Books, 1964, pp. 113–114.
68. Hughston JC: Subluxation of the patella. J Bone Joint Surg 50A: 1003–1026, 1968.
69. Alexander C: Erosion of the femoral shaft due to patellofemoral osteoarthritis. Clin Radiol 11:110–113, 1960.
70. Greenspan A, Norman A, Tchang FK: "Tooth" sign in patellar degenerative disease. J Bone Joint Surg 59A:483–485, 1977.
71. Neer CS II: Degenerative lesions of the proximal humeral articular surface. Clin Orthop 20:116–125, 1961.
72. Neer CS II: Replacement arthroplasty for glenohumeral osteoarthritis. J Bone Joint Surg 56A:1–13, 1974.
73. Ahuja SC, Bullough PG: Osteonecrosis of the knee: A clinicopathological study in twenty-eight patients. J Bone Joint Surg 60A:191–197, 1978.
74. Mankin HJ, Thrasher AZ, Hall D: Biochemical and metabolic characteristics of articular cartilage from osteonecrotic human femoral heads. J Bone Joint Surg 59A:724–728, 1977.
75. Postel M, Kerboull M: Total prosthetic replacement in rapidly destructive arthrosis of the hip joint. Clin Orthop 72:138–144, 1970.
76. Jacqueline F: Résorptions osseuses massives et brusques au cours des coxarthroses destructrives rapides. Rev Rhum 46:619–627, 1979.
77. Norman A, Robbins H, Milgram JE: The acute neuropathic arthropathy—a rapid severely disorganizing form of arthritis. Radiology 90:1159–1164, 1968.
78. Johnson JTH: Neuropathic fractures and joint injuries. J Bone Joint Surg 49A:1–30, 1967.
79. King EJS: On some aspects of the pathology of hypertrophic Charcot's joints. Br J Surg 78:113, 1930.
80. Bruckner FE, Howell A: Neuropathic joints. Semin Arthritis Rheum 2:47–69, 1972.
81. Eloesser L: On the nature of neuropathic affections of the joints. Ann Surg 66:201–207, 1917.
82. Brower AC, Allman RM: Pathogenesis of the neuropathic joint: Neurotraumatic vs. neurovascular. Radiology 139:349–354, 1981.
83. Jordan WR: Neuritic manifestations in diabetes mellitus. Arch Intern Med 57:307, 1936.
84. Jordan WR: The effect of diabetes on the nervous system. South Med J 36:45–49, 1943.
85. Fitzgerald JAW: Neuropathic arthropathy secondary to atypical congenital indifference to pain. Proc R Soc Med 61:663–664, 1968.
86. Norman A: Neuropathic Arthropathy. Categorical Course on the Skeletal System. American College of Radiology, 1976, pp. 96–99.
87. El-Khoury GY, Kathol MH: Neuropathic fractures in patients with diabetes mellitus. Radiology 134:313–316, 1980.
88. Kristiansen B: Ankle and foot fractures in diabetics provoking neuropathic joint changes. Acta Orthop Scand 51:975–979, 1980.
89. Harrison RB: Charcot's joint: Two new observations. Am J Roentgenol 128:807–809, 1977.
90. Oppenheimer A: Calcification and ossification of vertebral ligaments (spondylosis ossificans ligamentosa): Roentgen study of pathogenesis and clinical significance. Radiology 38:160–173, 1942.
91. Gantenberg R: Zur Klinischen Bedeutung deformierender prozesse der Wirbelsaüle. Fortschr Geb. Rontgenstrahlen 42:740, 1930.
92. Schmorl G, Junghauns H: The Human Spine in Health and Diseases. New York, Grune and Stratton, 1971, p. 185.
93. Macnab I: The traction spur—an indicator of segmental instability. J Bone Joint Surg 53A:663–670, 1971.
94. Forestier J, Jacqueline F, Rotes-Querol J: Ankylosing Spondylitis—Clinical Considerations. Roentgenology, Pathologic Anatomy, Treatment. Springfield, Illinois, Charles C Thomas, 1956, pp. 231–233.
95. Vernon-Roberts B, Pirie CJ, Trenwith V: Pathology of the dorsal spine in akylosing hyperostosis. Ann Rheum Dis 33:281–288, 1974.
96. Utsinger PD, Resnick D, Shapiro R: Diffuse skeletal abnormalities in Forestier disease. Arch Intern Med 136:763–768, 1976.
97. Forestier J, Rotes-Querol J: Senile ankylosing hy-

perostosis of the spine. Ann Rheum Dis 9:321–330, 1950.

98. Resnick D, Shaul SR, Robins JM: Diffuse idiopathic skeletal hyperostosis (DISH): Forestier's disease with extraspinal manifestations. Radiology 115:513–524, 1975.

99. Harris J, Carter AR, Glick EN, Storey GO: Ankylosing hyperostosis. Clinical and radiological features. Ann Rheum Dis 33:210–215, 1974.

100. Key CA: On paraplegia depending on disease of the ligaments of the spine. Guys Hosp Rep 3:17, 1939.

101. The Investigation Committee on OPLL of the Japanese Ministry of Public Health and Welfare: The ossification of the posterior longitudinal ligament of the spine (OPLL). J Jpn Orthop Assoc 55:425–440, 1981.

102. Onji Y, Akiyama H, Shimomura Y, et al.: Posterior paravertebral ossification causing cervical myelopathy. A report of eighteen cases. J Boint Joint Surg 49A:1314, 1967.

103. Hyman RA, Merten CW, Liebeskind AL, et al.: Computed tomography in ossification of the pos-

terior longitudinal ligament. Neurology 13:227–228, 1979.

104. Sakou T, Atsuhiro M, Tomimura K, et al.: Ossification of the posterior longitudinal ligament of the cervical spine: Subtotal vertebrectomy as a treatment. Clin Orthop 140:58–65, 1979.

105. Ono K, Ota H, Tadak K, et al.: Ossified posterior longitudinal ligament, a clinicopathologic study. Spine 2:126–138, 1977.

106. Resnick D, Guerra J Jr, Robinson CA, Vint VC: Association of diffuse idiopathic skeletal hyperostosis (DISH) and calcification and ossification of the posterior longitudinal ligament. Am J Roentgenol 131:1049–1053, 1978.

107. Alenghat JP, Hallett M, Kido DK: Spinal cord compression in diffuse idiopathic skeletal hyperostosis. Radiology 142:119–120, 1982.

108. Becker DH, Conely FK, Anderson ME: Quadriplegia associated with narrow cervical canal, ligamentous calcification and ankylosing hyperostosis. Surg Neurol 11:17–19, 1979.

10

Laboratory Findings in Osteoarthritis

Roy D. Altman, M.D.
Robert G. Gray, M.D.

Osteoarthritis (OA) is characterized by a constellation of clinical, roentgenologic, and synovial fluid (SF) findings. There are, however, no pathognomonic laboratory abnormalities: Conventional tests of blood and urine generally are remarkable for their normality; synovianalysis yields abnormal but nonspecific results. Nevertheless, tests of body fluids (i.e., blood, urine, and synovial fluid) serve to exclude other arthritides and may identify those metabolic disorders associated with secondary OA. Other diagnostic modalities, including synovial membrane biopsy, radionuclide bone scanning, interosseous phlebography, and thermography, exert a more limited and selective role in the evaluation of osteoarthritis. This chapter presents the results of clinically applicable and certain investigational laboratory studies that may aid in the diagnosis of primary and secondary osteoarthritis.

BLOOD

Cellular Constituents

The cellular components of blood are normal quantitatively and morphologically in uncomplicated primary OA. Leukocytosis rarely, if ever, occurs, even during exacerbations of the disease. The platelet count, as a nonspecific marker of "inflammation," may rise slightly during generalized flares but still remains within the normal range.

Erythrocyte Sedimentation Rate

The erythrocyte sedimentation rate (ESR) frequently is normal. Nevertheless, modest elevations in the ESR and, to a lesser extent, other acute-phase reactants[1, 2] may be observed transiently during clinical flare-ups and more persistently in patients with generalized polyarticular osteoarthritis. Kellgren and Moore[1] observed the ESR to be less than 20 mm/hour in 59%, between 20 and 40 mm/hour in 34%, and more than 40 mm/hour in 7% of 112 patients with generalized OA. The mean ESR was 19 mm/hour, in contrast with a mean value of 11 mm/hour in 20 patients with monarticular osteoarthritis. In the latter group, the ESR was invariably less than 20 mm/hour. Marked ESR elevations (more than 50 mm/hour) should engender suspicion of an unrelated, coexistent inflammatory or neoplastic disease.

Serum Chemistry

Glucose. Osteoarthritis does not impair glucose tolerance; however, diabetes mellitus may accelerate the osteoarthritic process.[3] Thus, screening tests for hyperglycemia are indicated in OA patients with early onset or inordinately severe joint disease. Hyperglycemia is commonly noted in patients with the degenerative arthritis associated with hemochromatosis and acromegaly.

Calcium, Phosphorus, and Alkaline Phos-

Table 10–1. LABORATORY ASSESSMENT OF DISORDERS ASSOCIATED WITH OR CAUSING
AN OSTEOARTHRITIS-LIKE ARTHROPATHY

Disorder	Laboratory Studies
Calcium pyrophosphate dihydrate Crystal deposition disease (CaPPD) }	Synovial fluid: positively birefringent, rhomboid-shaped crystals; roentgenograms: chondrocalcinosis
CaPPD induced by hyperparathyroidism }	*Suggestive:* ↑ serum Ca, AP; ↓ serum P *Definitive:* ↑ serum parathyroid hormone
Acromegaly	*Suggestive:* ↑ serum P and blood glucose *Definitive:* ↑ fasting plasma growth hormone
Hemochromatosis	*Suggestive:* ↑ blood glucose; serum iron > 150 μg/dl and > 75% saturation of iron-binding capacity *Definitive:* tissue (liver, synovium) iron deposition
Ochronosis	*Suggestive:* darkening of urine on standing; pigmented shards in synovial fluid ("ground pepper" sign) *Definitive:* ↑ serum and urine homogentisic acid
Wilson's disease	One or more of the following: serum copper < 80 μg/dl; serum ceruloplasmin < 20 mg/dl; urine copper > 100 μg/24 hr; liver copper > 250 μg/gm dry weight

↑ = increased; ↓ = decreased; Ca = calcium; AP = alkaline phosphatase; P = phosphorus

phatase. Routine biochemical assessment of bone metabolism is unrevealing in primary OA. When osteoarthritic joint changes are associated with calcium pyrophosphate dihydrate crystal deposition ("pseudo-osteoarthritis," McCarty Types C and D[4]) (Table 10–1), underlying primary hyperparathyroidism may be disclosed in a minority of patients by elevation of serum ionizable calcium, depression of serum phosphorus, hyperchloremic acidosis, a chloride/phosphorus ratio greater than 32, and, more specifically, by an increase in serum radioimmunoassay parathyroid hormone.

Plasma growth hormone is normal in primary OA. However, in one study,[5] radioimmunoassay growth hormone levels were significantly elevated in menopausal women with OA compared with those in a control group. Rarely, elevation of serum phosphorus in a patient with an OA-like arthropathy may suggest growth hormone hypersecretion. Acromegaly, however, usually is clinically obvious prior to the development of symptomatic joint disease.

An increase in serum alkaline phosphatase, occasionally to an extraordinary degree, and enhanced urinary hydroxyproline excretion are laboratory hallmarks of Paget's disease of bone. Bone deformation and replacement of normal subchondral bone with structurally weaker, fibrous pagetic bone may mediate joint incongruity and secondary OA of large joints (i.e., hip, knee, and shoulder).[6] In such instances, it may be difficult to distinguish pain of pagetic origin from that due to OA. Normalization of serum alkaline phosphatase and urinary hydroxyproline following antipagetic suppressive therapy suggests that persistent pain is due to osteoarthritis and may be ameliorated by nonsteroidal anti-inflammatory agents. Unfortunately, in an occasional patient, recalcitrant bone or "joint" pain proves to be due to sarcomatous degeneration of a pagetic lesion.

Ferrokinetics

Serum ferrokinetics are normal in uncomplicated primary OA. Occasionally, reduction in serum iron is associated with elevation of serum iron-binding capacity and ferritin levels, signaling iron deficiency from chronic blood loss. Although bleeding may be due to erosive gastritis or peptic ulcer disease induced by nonsteroidal anti-inflammatory agents, other considerations (e.g., gastrointestinal and uterine neoplasia) must be excluded. If serum ferrokinetic studies fail to distinguish clearly between impaired iron utilization and iron deficiency, bone marrow assessment of iron stores may be necessary. In the degenerative arthropathy associated with hemochromatosis, serum iron is markedly increased (more than 150 μg/dl) and serum iron-binding capacity is heavily saturated (75% to 100%).

Copper Metabolic Studies

Serum copper and ceruloplasmin are normal in primary OA. An OA-like arthropathy may be a feature of Wilson's disease, a disorder characterized by aberrant copper metabolism and deficient serum ceruloplasmin (see Table 10–1). Infrequently, the arthropathy may precede other manifestations of the disease. Therefore, the development of hepatic dysfunction, personality change, or abnormalities of basal ganglionic function (e.g., tremor, rigidity, and incoordination) should provoke a careful slit-lamp examination for Kayser-Fleischer rings and laboratory and histologic evaluation of copper metabolism. Suggestive laboratory abnormalities include renal tubular acidosis with proteinuria, hyposthenuria, aminoaciduria, glycosuria, and hyperuricosuria with or without hypouricemia. A normocytic or slightly macrocytic anemia, reticulocytosis, and depressed serum haptoglobin indicate an associated hemolytic anemia.

When the pattern, distribution, age of onset, ancillary laboratory findings, or roentgenologic characteristics of a degenerative arthropathy are atypical for primary OA, a primary metabolic disorder should be suspected. Specific chemical or histologic investigation (see Table 10–1) should be guided by suggestive clinical features and screening laboratory studies.

Immunologic Studies

Thus far, studies of the immune system have failed to identify clearly aberrant cellular or humoral immunity in the pathogenesis of OA.

Cellular. Sensitization to proteoglycan antigens was demonstrated in 9 of 22 patients with OA by the lymphocytotoxin production test[7] but in only 1 of 14 patients by the lymphocyte transformation test.[8] It remains unclear whether this cellular immune response contributes to joint damage or merely reflects the incidental unmasking of proteoglycan antigenic sites during cartilage breakdown.

Humoral. The prevalence of serum rheumatoid factor in OA parallels that observed in the general population. Inasmuch as rheumatoid seropositivity increases in frequency with advancing age, low-titer serum rheumatoid factor may be anticipated in 5% to 20% or more of patients with OA.[9, 10] Circulating immune complexes are not observed.[11]

Antinuclear antibodies (ANA) are not associated with OA. Low-titer ANA may infrequently be encountered in patients with OA, as in a similarly aged healthy population without OA.[12, 13]

Antiproteoglycan antibodies, detected by passive hemagglutination, have been noted in the serum of patients with severe OA as well as severe rheumatoid arthritis.[14] This finding seems more likely to be an epiphenomenon of joint destruction than to be of etiologic significance.

Complement. Serum total hemolytic complement and various complement components are normal. In one study,[15] the ninth component of complement was elevated twofold in patients with OA compared with controls; similar elevations were observed in rheumatoid arthritis and nonrenal systemic lupus erythematosus.

URINE

Routine and special studies of urine are normal in primary OA. Urinary calcium and phosphorus levels vary widely, depending largely on dietary intake. Urinary hydroxyproline is also normal, usually in the range of 14 to 38 mg/24 hours for the age group most commonly afflicted with OA. Urinary estrogen and gonadotrophin excretion is similar in postmenopausal women with and without osteoarthritis.[16]

Urinary abnormalities may be noted in patients with certain forms of secondary osteoarthritis. When OA is secondary to juxtaposed *Paget's disease,* augmented urinary hydroxyproline excretion is expected. In the degenerative joint disease of *ochronosis,* alkaline urine may darken on standing. The ability of ochronotic urine to reduce alkaline copper solutions accounts for a false-positive Benedict's test for glycosuria. Confirmation requires specific enzymatic assay of urine (or serum) for homogentisic acid. Renal tubular acidosis is frequently associated with the degenerative arthropathy of *Wilson's disease* and may produce hyposthenuria, glycosuria, aminoaciduria, proteinuria, and hyperuricosuria.

SYNOVIAL FLUID

Synovial fluid in primary OA is generally considered "noninflammatory" (Ropes and Bauer classification Type I[17]). However, increased volume of joint fluid, frequent decrease in viscosity, a mild but significant pleo-

Table 10–2. SYNOVIAL FLUID FINDINGS IN NORMAL AND PRIMARY OSTEOARTHRITIC JOINTS

	Normal (17 Patients)	OA (17 Patients)	OA*
Number of fluid specimens	29	27	113
Appearance	Yellow, clear	Yellow, clear	Yellow, clear (occasionally faintly turbid)
Mucin clot	Good	Good	Good
Mean total WBC count (cells/mm³)	63	720	951
Range	13–180	20–3600	98–6310
Percent polymorphonuclear	< 25	< 25	< 28
Mean total protein (gm/dl)	1.7†	3.1‡	3.1
Range	1.1–2.1†	1.3–4.9‡	1.0–4.2
Viscosity	Normal	Normal–decreased	Normal–decreased

*Unpublished data (RG Gray)
†Ten synovial fluid specimens
‡Sixteen synovial fluid specimens

cytosis, and modest elevation of synovial fluid protein all indicate a mildly inflammatory synovitis (Table 10–2).

Volume

In OA, the volume of synovial fluid in the knee may vary from normal (0.5 to 1.5 ml)[17] to greater than 100 ml. Generally, smaller effusions may be evident in other affected joints. Inexplicably, minimal cartilage loss roentgenographically may be associated with large effusions, and conversely, severe osteoarthritis roentgenographically may elicit only minimal or no synovial effusion.

Appearance

The fluid usually appears pale yellow but infrequently may be blood-tinged or frankly bloody. Such episodes of joint bleeding occur notably in affected glenohumeral and unstable knee joints and often in association with an acutely painful exacerbation, trivial trauma, or increased activity. Hemarthrosis probably reflects "pinching" of synovium between contiguous osteophytes or irregular joint surfaces or, less frequently, a microfracture of subchondral or osteophytic bone. The sanguineous nature of the fluid is evident throughout arthrocentesis, and the fluid subsequently fails to clot. In contrast, bloody fluid resulting from traumatic aspiration technique clears during the course of withdrawal, or alternatively, blood is seen to enter the syringe and mix with initially yellow fluid at the termination of joint aspiration.

In primary OA, shed cartilage fragments are visible as floating white specks and particles. In the degenerative arthritis associated with ochronosis, pigmented shards of cartilage may assume the appearance of "ground pepper" in joint fluid.[18]

Clarity

Synovial fluid is generally nonsanguineous and clear but occasionally appears very faintly turbid.

Viscosity

Viscosity is dependent on a protein–hyaluronic acid complex in synovial fluid; the hyaluronate complex consists of an unbranched glycosaminoglycan macromolecule with a molecular weight of approximately two million daltons, composed in turn of polymerized disaccharide dimers of glucuronic acid–glucosamine coiled into a spherical or ellipsoidal conformation. This conformation allows the structure to occupy a solvent domain considerably larger than the volume of the polymer chain. Hyaluronate depolymerization or synovial membrane secretion of a poorly polymerized hyaluronate or a hyaluronate complex with altered conformation results in diminished viscosity.

In OA, viscosity parallels clinical evidence of inflammation: Fluid from "cool" joints usually has a normal viscosity and produces a "string" sign (Fig. 10–1). Markedly poor viscosity, in which the fluid drops like water from the syringe, is uncommon and may reflect

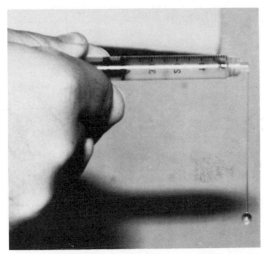

Figure 10–1. High viscosity allows the synovial fluid to "string" when dropped from a syringe.

coexistent pseudogout or another inflammatory arthritis. Conversely, extremely thick, viscous fluid should suggest osteochondromatosis or hypothyroidism.[17, 19] Pseudomucinous synovial cysts, found over the dorsum of osteoarthritic distal interphalangeal joints, contain pale, gelatinous fluid similar to that observed in ganglia.

Mucin

The precipitation of the protein salt of hyaluronic acid after acidification of joint fluid is the basis of the mucin clot test. An aliquot of synovial fluid is added to a beaker containing a four times greater volume of 2% acetic acid and mixed with a glass rod. The resulting mucin clot (hyaluronate-protein) reflects the degree of polymerization of hyaluronic acid. In OA, a tight, ropy mass is formed (graded good), whereas in rheumatoid arthritis and other inflammatory arthritides, the mass shows friable edges (graded poor). The mucin clot is almost invariably good in OA, even when viscosity is significantly diminished.

If it is uncertain that synovial fluid has been aspirated, mucin clot formation and metachromatic staining are capable of detecting as little as 0.5 µl of SF.[20]

Microscopy

Leukocytes. Synovial fluid in OA may be relatively acellular, but a mild increase in the white blood cell count (1000 to 3500 cells/mm³) often indicates a mildly inflammatory synovitis. Synovial pleocytosis in excess of 5000 cells/mm³ is uncommon (see Table 10–2). The majority of leukocytes are lymphocytes (see Table 10–2), predominantly T cells.[21]

Cytoplasmic Inclusions. Leukocytes containing refractile intracytoplasmic inclusions may be noted by phase-contrast microscopy but are sparse in comparison with the numerous "ragocytes"[22] of rheumatoid arthritis and other inflammatory arthritides. These spherical inclusions, measuring 0.5 to 2.0 µ in diameter, do not contain the immunoglobulin–anti-immunoglobulin complexes of rheumatoid synovial fluid and appear to be composed largely of triglycerides (Fig. 10–2).[23]

Figure 10–2. Wet mount microscopic preparation of synovial fluid in OA may demonstrate cells containing many inclusions, composed mostly of triglycerides.

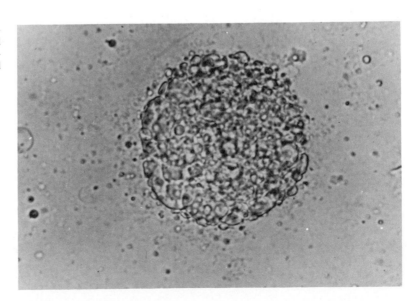

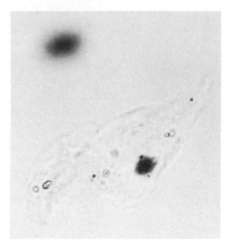

Figure 10–3. Wet mount microscopic preparation of synovial fluid in OA may reveal synovial lining cells. Better cellular definition would necessitate fixation and Wright staining.

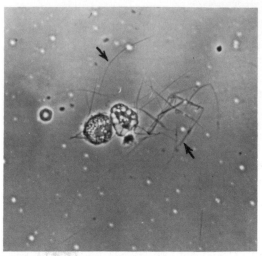

Figure 10–4. Wet mount microscopic preparation of synovial fluid in OA may demonstrate occasional polymorphonuclear leukocytes and fibrils of fibrin or collagen fibers (arrows). These are thin and should not be confused with crystals. (Phase contrast microscopy.)

Synovial Lining Cells. Large exfoliated mononuclear synovial lining cells, measuring 20 to 40 μm in length, may be seen singly (Fig. 10–3) or in sheets[24, 25] and are best identified with Wright's stain. The nucleus, which often has prominent nucleoli, is eccentric and encompasses less than half the cell volume. These cells may be distinguished from macrophages by their smaller nuclei and by lack of staining with Sudan black.[26]

Cartilage Fragments and Bone Cells. The most distinctive microscopic feature of osteoarthritic synovial fluid is the occasional presence of multinucleated cells, probably osteoclasts. These cells appear singly or, more often, in sheets or clusters.[24, 25] Cartilage fragments may contain mononuclear chondrocytes. These chondrocytes may be normal in appearance but often display varying degrees of degeneration and fail to stain properly for proteoglycans, e.g., with safranin O. In ochronotic degenerative arthritis, sloughed cartilage fragments exhibit a golden (ochre) hue.[18]

Fibrils. Wet mount microscopy often shows thin, faintly positively birefringent "fibrin" strands that are morphologically indistinguishable from sloughed collagen fibers (Fig. 10–4).[27] The collagen fiber of osteoarthritic synovial fluid appears to be Type II, derived from articular hyaline cartilage.[28]

Crystals. Calcium hydroxyapatite crystals have been implicated in flares of OA and may be detected by electron microscopy.[29, 30] Occasionally, clumps of hydroxyapatite crystals appear as nonrefringent amorphous globular matter on routine wet mount microscopy.[29] A semiquantitative technique employing ^{14}C-labeled etidronate disodium binding has detected crystals, which seem to be hydroxyapatite, in osteoarthritic joint fluid.[31] A strong correlation was noted between crystal presence and roentgenologic evidence of cartilage loss. Recently, electron microscopy has identified synovial fluid microspherules containing hydroxyapatite crystals, active collagenase, and neutral protease in patients with glenohumeral osteoarthritis and rotator cuff defects ("Milwaukee shoulder" syndrome).[32]

Cholesterol crystals may be observed in the joint fluid of patients with chronic rheumatoid synovitis. More recently, cholesterol crystals were identified by light microscopy in synovial fluids of four patients with recurrent osteoarthritic knee effusions.[33] Synovial fluid white blood cell counts varied from 125 to 3100 cells/mm³. The cholesterol crystals showed a large (10 to 80 μm) notched plate configuration in all fluids and also occasionally appeared as irregular rod- and needle-shaped (1 to 5 μm) structures; in three fluids, identification was confirmed by x-ray diffraction or ultrastructural studies. Previous experiments have established that cholesterol crystals may exert a mild phlogistic effect,[34–36] and thus, these crystals may contribute to the synovitis of OA.

Weakly positively birefringent, rhomboid-shaped calcium pyrophosphate dihydrate crystals may be noted in the fluid of joints affected with the pseudo-osteoarthritis associated with calcium pyrophosphate crystal deposition.[37]

Electrolytes

The synovial fluid is largely an ultrafiltrate of plasma, and concentrations of sodium, potassium, chloride, and bicarbonate approximate those found in serum.

Sugars

The glucose of osteoarthritic synovial fluid parallels serum values. In the fasting state, SF glucose is usually within 5 to 10 mg/dl of serum levels. Marked depression of glucose to less than one third to one half of serum values, as usually occurs in septic arthritis and rarely ensues in rheumatoid and crystal-induced arthritides, is not observed in OA.[17] SF levels of sulfated sugars such as chondroitin sulfate are elevated in osteoarthritis.[38]

Lipids

Few studies of lipid levels in normal or pathologic synovial fluids are available. Normal joint fluid contains minute quantities of cholesterol and phospholipids but lacks triglycerides.[39] Chung and associates[40] detected considerable amounts of cholesterol, phospholipids, and triglycerides in osteoarthritic synovial fluid. The mean cholesterol/phospholipid ratio (1:21) resembled that of a lipoprotein fraction of density of over 1.063. Synovial fluid findings were similar in OA and rheumatoid arthritis and differed from normal serum levels.

Early studies noted a relative increase in short-chain fatty acids in osteoarthritic joint fluid.[41] However, Kim and Cohen,[42] using gas-liquid chromatographic analysis, found a fatty acid composition similar to that in serum. The total fatty acids present in synovial fluid were approximately a third of the amount detected in matching sera. Palmitic, oleic, and linoleic acids represented nearly 80% of the total fatty acids, with myristic, palmitoleic, stearic, and arachidonic acids constituting minor components. Findings were similar in synovial fluid in OA and rheumatoid arthritis. No correlation was noted between joint fluid fatty acid concentration and leukocyte count, and fatty acid analysis failed to differentiate between inflammatory and noninflammatory effusions.

There is one short-chain fatty acid, succinic acid, that is not usually present in synovial fluid. Its presence, as detected by gas-liquid chromatography, suggests septic arthritis and can be used in that differential diagnosis.[43] Although septic joint fluids are not usually confused with those of osteoarthritis, occasional infections, particularly those with *Neisseria gonorrhoeae*, make this a useful test of synovial fluid.

Synovial fluid lipoprotein values, assessed by analytic ultracentrifugation, have been studied in a single patient with OA.[44] Total synovial fluid lipoprotein was 19% of serum level. Class I low-density lipoprotein was absent. Classes II and III lipoprotein concentrations were similar to matched serum values (6.7% versus 5.7% and 5.6% versus 3.7%, respectively); Class IV lipoprotein concentration was slightly decreased (44.7% versus 52.7%). Class V lipoprotein components V_a and V_b were increased and decreased, respectively.

Oxygen Tension and pH

Studies of synovial fluid oxygen tension and pH have, in part, elucidated the pathophysiology of joint disease, although these determinations currently have little clinical applicability. Lund-Olesen[45] noted that the mean oxygen tension in 13 osteoarthritic knee joints was 43 mm Hg (range: 20 to 71 mm Hg), significantly lower than the mean oxygen tension in traumatic effusions (63 mm Hg; range: 42 to 87 mm Hg) ($p < 0.01$), and higher than values in rheumatoid effusions (27 mm Hg; range: 0 to 91 mm Hg) ($p < 0.01$). Values for PCO_2 appeared to correlate with those for PO_2. Richman and coworkers[46] observed that effusions greater than 50 ml were invariably associated with reduction of synovial fluid PO_2 below 50 mm Hg, and they postulated that high intra-articular pressure resulting from sizable effusions may shunt blood from the synovium by collapsing subsynovial capillaries. Synovial fluid pH paralleled that in serum until joint fluid PO_2 decreased below 45 mm Hg; at that point, further reductions in PO_2 were associated with proportional reductions in pH.

Superoxide radical O_2^-, which is capable of degrading cartilage proteoglycans and collagen in vitro[47] and of reducing hyaluronate viscosity,[48] is detectable in osteoarthritic synovial fluid.[49]

Enzymes

Lactic Dehydrogenase. Synovial fluid lactic dehydrogenase, especially fractions 3 and 4, is slightly increased in OA, correlating with the white blood cell count; levels are considerably lower than those observed in rheumatoid arthritis.[50]

Lysosomal Enzymes. The concentrations of a variety of lysosomal enzymes, including acid phosphatase, glycosidase, β-glucuronidase, and *N*-acetylglucosaminidase, are elevated in the synovial fluid[27, 51–54] and extracts of synovial membrane[55] in OA. Enzyme activity is in direct relation to synovial fluid pleocytosis and is less than that noted in joint fluid in rheumatoid arthritis. These enzymes may play a role in the degradation of articular glycosaminoglycans.[55]

Lysozyme. Synovial fluid lysozyme, derived from leukocytic lysosomes and nonlysosomal cartilage matrix, is elevated in OA.[56] Lysozyme activity appears to reflect both synovial inflammation and cartilage degradation.

Collagenase. Free and latent collagenase has been detected in osteoarthritic synovial fluid.[57, 58]

Neuroregulatory Enzymes. Dopamine-β-hydroxylase mediates the conversion of dopamine to norepinephrine and is released from sympathetic neuron synaptic vesicles. The enzyme was detected in normal synovial fluid and, in significantly higher concentrations, in osteoarthritic joint fluid.[59] Conceivably, dopamine-β-hydroxylase may influence the secretory function of articular cells.

Hyaluronidase. The synovial fluid in osteoarthritis contains small amounts of plasma filtrated hyaluronidase with a molecular weight of 60,000 daltons.[60] The concentration of the enzyme correlates with SF white blood cell counts and the presence of synovial debris.[61]

Proteins

The total protein concentration of osteoarthritic synovial fluid is slightly elevated (see Table 10–2). The relative concentrations of various protein moieties (IgG, IgM, IgA, transferrin, and α_2-macroglobulin) parallel normal serum values.[62, 63] Others have observed a higher ratio of synovial fluid/serum concentration for nonimmunoglobulin proteins, haptoglobin, α_2-macroglobulin, orosomucoid, transferrin, and ceruloplasmin in osteoarthritic joints compared with normal joints.[64–66] The enhanced concentrations correlated with the molecular weight of the particular protein. No correlation could be found between increased protein concentration and the degree of synovial inflammation noted on biopsy. However, the highest ratios were observed when histologic changes suggested an early "proliferative" phase with synovial edema and large numbers of dilated venules and capillaries rather than late "fibrous" synovial scarring.[65]

Type II collagen, which is characteristic of hyaline articular cartilage, was recently observed in two of six osteoarthritic effusions. The presence of sufficient collagen to be detected correlated with decreased roentgenographic joint space and SF pH.[28]

Clotting Factors

Normal synovial fluid lacks fibrinogen and contains only trace amounts of plasminogen. Both fibrinogen and plasminogen are detectable in osteoarthritic joint fluid but in lower concentrations than observed in traumatic and inflammatory arthritides.[67]

Copper

Synovial fluid copper (measured by atomic absorption spectrophotometry) and ceruloplasmin (measured by single radial immunodiffusion) levels were significantly lower in primary OA compared with rheumatoid arthritis.[66, 68] Mean synovial fluid copper concentration was approximately one half of serum concentration in normal controls.

Immunologic Studies

Cellular. Lymphokines have been noted occasionally in osteoarthritic fluid. Stastny and associates[69] detected migration inhibitory activity in 20% of 15 osteoarthritic joint fluid specimens, a frequency considerably less than that observed in specimens from rheumatoid arthritis (73% of 22 fluid specimens). The presence of this soluble mediator of cellular immunity possibly reflects an autoimmune response to osteoarthritic joint debris.

Humoral. Significant titers of synovial fluid antinuclear antibody are absent.[70] Other autoantibodies may be detectable in joint fluid when simultaneously present in the serum.[71]

Antithyroid antibodies were found in the synovial fluid of three of six patients with OA who lacked serum antibodies,[72] suggesting the possibility that these immunoglobulins were produced by the synovium.

Immune complexes (immunoglobulins and

complement) have been detected in the synovial membranes and hyaline articular cartilage of osteoarthritic joints but have not been reported as yet in synovial fluid.[73]

Complement. Synovial fluid complement levels are not depressed in OA, in contrast to reported findings in rheumatoid arthritis.[74, 75] None of 12 osteoarthritic synovial fluid specimens showed joint fluid total hemolytic complement less than 10% of mean normal serum values.[76] No relationship was found among synovial fluid complement activity, clinical activity, protein concentration, and leukocyte count.

Cryoprecipitates may be detected in osteoarthritic synovial fluid,[77] but in contrast to RA, they do not contain IgM, infrequently contain IgG, and seem largely composed of nonspecific, cold-insoluble proteins.

Bone and Cartilage Metabolic Studies

Hydroxyproline. Small-fragment, dialyzable hydroxyproline is increased in osteoarthritic synovial fluid, presumably reflecting accelerated collagen metabolism; nondialyzable hydroxyproline is normal.[78]

Inorganic Pyrophosphate. Synovial fluid inorganic pyrophosphate is increased in osteoarthritis[79, 80] as well as in calcium pyrophosphate crystal deposition disease when compared with normal fluids or serum. The degree of elevation seems to correlate with the roentgenographic severity of the joint disease.

SYNOVIAL HISTOLOGIC EXAMINATION

Synovial histologic examination in primary osteoarthritis reveals nonspecific changes of chronic, mild inflammation.[81–83] Closed needle or open biopsy of the synovium is seldom necessary. However, in selected cases, synovial biopsy may serve to exclude other arthritides or to confirm the presence of the degenerative arthropathies associated with ochronosis or hemochromatosis.

Primary Osteoarthritis

In early cases, the synovium may appear normal. Generally, however, focal hyperemia and edema are evident. Not infrequently, villous hypertrophy is noted, although usually not to the degree observed in rheumatoid arthritis. Light microscopy reveals proliferation of synovial lining cells, with scattered collections of lymphocytes and plasma cells. Venules and arterioles may be dilated, with extravasation of red blood cells. Iron may be noted within occasional macrophages of the synovial intima and in both macrophages and the stroma of subintimal and deeper synovial layers.[84] Fragments of calcified and uncalcified cartilage are frequently embedded in the synovium, and synovial lining cells may ingest cartilage debris (Fig. 10–5).[81] In more advanced cases, considerable fibrosis may be evident.

Electron-microscopic studies[82] have demonstrated ultrastructural abnormalities in syno-

Figure 10–5. Synovial biopsy demonstrates mild synovial proliferation with a degenerating cartilage fragment engulfed by the synovium (arrows).

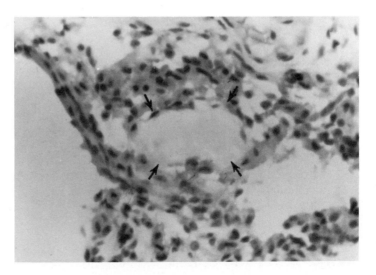

vial lining cells, including (1) increased rough endoplasmic reticulum with dilated cisternae, (2) decreased number and size of Golgi apparatus and smooth-walled cytoplasmic vesicles, and (3) an increased number of lysosomes.

Ochronosis

A pathognomonic feature is the presence of darkly pigmented (ochre) shards of cartilage, embedded with homogentisic acid–derived polymer, within the synovium.[85] Contiguous macrophages may also contain pigmented granules. Other changes are similar to those observed in primary OA.

Hemochromatosis

Hemosiderin is observed within synovial lining cells and, to a lesser extent, in subsynovial tissues. In contrast to osteoarthritis, rheumatoid arthritis, hemophilia, and pigmented villonodular synovitis, the most intense iron deposition is in the superficial synovial layer.[86]

BONE AND JOINT SCANNING

Joint imaging with radionuclide tracer agents may supplement physical examination and plain roentgenograms in assessing the extent and severity of OA.[87]

Pertechnetate joint scans depend on an increased permeability and/or enhanced blood pool of the inflamed synovium. When OA is associated with a mild inflammatory synovitis, increased uptake with ^{99m}Tc pertechnetate will be evident; when the disease is early or advanced and without local inflammatory signs, the joint scan often appears normal.[88] Increased synovial blood flow may be detected by obtaining views of the joints within the first 15 minutes following radionuclide injection.[89]

Enhanced joint uptake of ^{99m}Tc phosphate or phosphonate agents partly reflects increased soft tissue perfusion, and the degree of inflammatory synovitis correlates with the degree of scanning nuclide localization. However, these agents also preferentially chemabsorb to hydroxyapatite crystals, particularly newly formed crystals present in remodeling bone. Consequently, intense uptake is noted in areas of subchondral sclerosis or cyst formation, with variably increased uptake present at all stages of OA.[89, 90] OA with moderate synovitis is often associated with nuclide localization to the synovium, the synovial fluid, subchondral bone, and, occasionally, even the entire extremity as a result of increased extremity blood flow (Fig. 10–6). Spinal osteophytes may also accumulate the nuclide.[91] In the preoperative assessment of OA of the knee, scanning may help in documenting unicompartmental disease.[92]

INTRAOSSEOUS PHLEBOGRAPHY AND PRESSURE MEASUREMENTS

In symptomatic osteoarthritis of the hip and knee, intraosseous phlebography shows impaired drainage from the juxta-articular bone marrow.[93, 94] The normal extraosseous venous route is visualized poorly, if at all; rather, contrast material drains through descending intramedullary channels to the trochanteric region and, subsequently, down the femoral shaft. Venous stasis and engorgement are generally associated with intramedullary hypertension. Arnoldi and associates[93] observed that

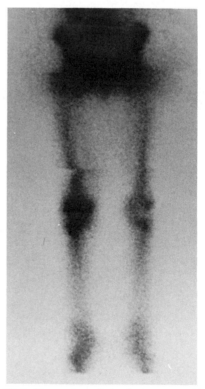

Figure 10–6. Bone scan of the lower extremities of a patient with OA demonstrates intense localization of the nuclide to the right knee synovium, distal femur, and proximal tibia. The left knee demonstrates some increased localization of the nuclide to the lateral compartment.

hip pain at rest was invariably accompanied by intraosseous pressure in the femoral neck greater than 40 mm Hg. Femoral osteotomy, which causes an immediate decrease in the intramedullary pressure of the proximal femur,[95] produces a dramatic amelioration of rest pain.

Intraosseous phlebography requires general or spinal anesthesia, carries a small risk of bone marrow infection, and is not employed routinely in the assessment of osteoarthritis of the hip. However, phlebography and intraosseous pressure measurements, in conjunction with bone scanning, may be useful in evaluating patients who have hip pain at rest without roentgenologic abnormalities (intraosseous engorgement–hypertension syndrome) and in the early diagnosis of ischemic necrosis.

THERMOGRAPHY

Thermography provides a pictorial image of surface temperature, based on the detection of infrared emissions from the skin. Normal joints appear cool, with no discernible difference in temperature from contiguous skin regions. In osteoarthritis, findings may be normal as well, although osteoarthritic joints with concomitant synovitis may appear warmer than adjacent skin. In cases of erosive osteoarthritis, increased joint temperature may be indistinguishable from rheumatoid disease and other inflammatory arthritides.[96, 97] The technique appears to add little to findings evident on physical examination.

References

1. Kellgren JH, Moore R: Generalized osteoarthritis and Heberden's nodes. Br Med J 1:181–187, 1952.
2. Denko CW, Gabriel P: Serum proteins—transferrin, ceruloplasmin, albumin, α1-acid glycoprotein, α1-antitrypsin—in rheumatic disorders. J Rheumatol 6:664–672, 1974.
3. Waine H, Nivinny D, Rosenthal J, et al.: Association of osteoarthritis and diabetes mellitus. Tufts Folia Med 7:13–17, 1961.
4. McCarty D: Calcium pyrophosphate deposition disease: Pseudogout, articular chondrocalcinosis. *In* Arthritis and Allied Conditions, Philadelphia, Lea and Febiger, 1979, p. 1285.
5. Franchimont P, Denis F: Détermination du taux de la somatotrophine et des gonadotrophines dans des cas d'arthrose apparaissant lors de la ménopause. J Belge Rhum Med Phys 23:59–64, 1968.
6. Altman RD, Collins B: Musculoskeletal manifestations of Paget's disease of bone. Arthritis Rheum 23:1121–1127, 1980.
7. Herman JH, Houk JL, Dennis MV: Cartilage antigen dependent lymphotoxin release: Immunopathological significance in articular destructive disorders. Ann Rheum Dis 33:446–452, 1974.
8. Herman JH, Wiltse DW, Dennis MV: Immunopathologic significance of cartilage antigenic components in rheumatoid arthritis. Arthritis Rheum 16:287–297, 1973.
9. Mikkelson WM, Dodge HJ, Duff IF, et al.: Estimates of the prevalence of rheumatic disease in the population of Tecumseh, Michigan, 1950–60. J Chronic Dis 20:351–369, 1967.
10. Bennett PH, Wood PHN (eds.): Population Studies of the Rheumatic Diseases. Amsterdam, Excerpta Medica, 1968.
11. Lambert PH, Casali P: Immune complexes and the rheumatic diseases. Clin Rheum Dis 4:617–642, 1978.
12. Cammarata RJ, Rodnan GP, Fennell RH Jr, et al.: Serologic reactions and serum protein concentrations in the aged. (Abstract.) Arthritis Rheum 7:297, 1964.
13. Robitaille P, Zvaifler J, Tan EM: Antinuclear antibodies and nuclear antigens in rheumatoid synovial fluids. Clin Immunol Immunopathol 1:385–397, 1973.
14. Herman JH, Carpenter BA: Immunobiology of cartilage. Semin Arthritis Rheum 5:1–40, 1975.
15. Ruddy S, Everson LK, Schur PH, et al.: Hemolytic assay of the ninth complement component: Elevation and depletion in rheumatic diseases. J Exp Med 134:2595–2755, 1974.
16. Rogers FB, Lansbury J: Urinary gonadotrophin excretion in osteoarthritis. Am J Med Sci 232:419–420, 1956.
17. Ropes MW, Bauer W: Synovial Fluid Changes in Joint Disease. Cambridge, Massachusetts, Harvard University Press, 1953.
18. Hunter T, Gordon DA, Ogrylo MA: The ground pepper sign of synovial fluid: A new diagnostic feature of ochronosis. J Rheumatol 1:45–53, 1974.
19. Dorwart BB, Schumacher HR: Joint effusions, chondrocalcinosis, and other rheumatic manifestations in hypothyroidism. A clinicopathologic study. Am J Med 59:780–789, 1975.
20. Goldenberg DL, Brandt KD, Cohen AS: Rapid, simple detection of trace amounts of synovial fluid. Arthritis Rheum 16:487–490, 1973.
21. van de Putte LBA, Meijer CJLM, Lafeber GJM, et al.: Lymphocytes in rheumatoid and nonrheumatoid synovial fluids. Ann Rheum Dis 35:451–455, 1976.
22. Hollander JL, McCarty DJ, Rawson AJ: The "RA cell," "ragocyte," or "inclusion body cell." Bull Rheum Dis 16:382–385, 1965.
23. Hersko C, Michaeli D, Shibolet S, et al.: The nature of refractile inclusions in leukocytes of synovial effusions. Isr J Med Sci 6:838–846, 1967.
24. Naib ZM: Cytology of synovial fluids. Acta Cytol 17:299–309, 1973.
25. Broderick PA, Corvese N, Pierik MG, et al.: Exfoliative cytology interpretation of synovial fluid in joint disease. J Bone Joint Surg 58A:396–399, 1976.
26. Shehan HL, Storey GW: Improved method of staining leukocyte granules with Sudan black. Br J Pathol Bacteriol 59:336–337, 1947.
27. Kitridou R, McCarty DJ, Prockop DJ, et al.: Identification of collagen in synovial fluid. Arthritis Rheum 12:580–588, 1969.
28. Cheung HS, Ryan LM, Kozin F, et al.: Identification

of collagen subtypes in synovial fluid sediments from arthritic patients. Am J Med 68:73–79, 1980.

29. Dieppe PA, Huskisson EC, Crocker P, et al.: Apatite deposition disease. A new arthropathy. Lancet 1:266–270, 1976.

30. Schumacher HR Jr: Pathogenesis of crystal-induced synovitis. Clin Rheum Dis 3:105–131, 1977.

31. Halverson PB, McCarty DJ: Identification of hydroxyapatite crystals in synovial fluid. Arthritis Rheum 22:389–395, 1979.

32. McCarty DJ, Halverson PB, Carrera GF, et al.: "Milwaukee shoulder"—association of microspheroids containing hydroxyapatite crystals, active collagenase and neutral protease with rotator cuff defects. II. Synovial fluid studies. Arthritis Rheum 24:474–483, 1981.

33. Fam AG, Pritzker KPH, Cheng P-T, et al.: Cholesterol crystals in osteoarthritic joint effusions. J Rheumatol 8:273–280, 1981.

34. Zuckner J, Uddin J, Ganter GE, et al.: Cholesterol crystals in synovial fluid. Ann Intern Med 60:436–446, 1964.

35. Bland JH, Gierthy JF, Suhre ED: Cholesterol in connective tissue of joints. Scand J Rheumatol 3:199–203, 1974.

36. Pritzker KPH, Fam AG, Omar SA, et al.: Experimental cholesterol crystal arthropathy. J Rheumatol 8:281–290, 1981.

37. McCarty DJ: Calcium pyrophosphate dihydrate crystal deposition disease—1975. Arthritis Rheum 19:275–285, 1976.

38. Sweet MBE: An ultracentrifugal analysis of synovial fluid. S Afr Med J 45:1205, 1971.

39. Bole GG: Synovial fluid lipids in normal individuals and patients with rheumatoid arthritis. Arthritis Rheum 5:589–601, 1962.

40. Chung AC, Shanahan JR, Brown EM Jr: Synovial fluid lipids in rheumatoid and osteoarthritis. Arthritis Rheum 5:176–183, 1962.

41. Sugiyama Y, Ono S: Fatty acid metabolism in the synovial fluid in the patients with rheumatoid arthritis and osteoarthritis. Arch Jpn Chir 35:1020–1025, 1966.

42. Kim IC, Cohen AS: Synovial fluid fatty acid composition in patients with rheumatoid arthritis, gout and degenerative joint disease. Proc Soc Exp Biol Med 123:77–80, 1966.

43. Borenstein DG, Gibbs C, Jacobs RP: Synovial fluid (SF) analysis by gas-liquid chromatography (GLC): Succinic acid (SA) and lactic acid (LA) as markers for septic arthritis. (Abstract.) Arthritis Rheum 24:590, 1981.

44. Small DM, Cohen AS, Schmid K: Lipoproteins of synovial fluid as studied by analytical ultracentrifugation. J Clin Invest 43:2070–2079, 1964.

45. Lund-Olesen K: Oxygen tension in synovial fluids. Arthritis Rheum 13:769–776, 1970.

46. Richman AI, Su EY, Ho G Jr: Reciprocal relationship of synovial fluid volume and oxygen tension. Arthritis Rheum 24:701–705, 1981.

47. Greenwald RA, Moy WW, Lazarus D: Degradation of cartilage proteoglycans and collagen by superoxide radical. (Abstract.) Arthritis Rheum 19:799, 1976.

48. Greenwald RA, Moy WW: Effect of oxygen-derived free radicals on hyaluronic acid. Arthritis Rheum 23:448–454, 1980.

49. Lunec J, Halloran P, White AG, et al.: Free radical oxidation (peroxidation) products in serum and synovial fluid in rheumatoid arthritis. J Rheumatol 8:233–245, 1981.

50. Veys EM, Wieme RJ: Lactate dehydrogenase in synovial fluid diagnostic evaluation of total activity and isoenzyme patterns. Ann Rheum Dis 27:569–576, 1968.

51. Yoshinari G: Acid phosphatase activity in synovial fluid. Arch Jpn Chir 35:1010–1019, 1966.

52. Jasani MK, Katori M, Lewis GP: Intracellular enzymes and kinin enzymes in synovial fluid in joint diseases. Origin and relation to disease category. Ann Rheum Dis 28:497–512, 1969.

53. Stephens RW, Ghosh P, Taylor TKF, et al.: The origins and relative distribution of polysaccharidases in rheumatoid and osteoarthritic fluids. J Rheumatol 2:393–400, 1975.

54. Veys EM, Gabriel P, Decrans L, et al.: N-acetyl-β-D-glucosaminidase activity in synovial fluid. Rheumatol Rehabil 14:50–56, 1975.

55. Kar NC, Cracchiolo A III, Mirra J, et al.: Acid, neutral, and alkaline hydrolases in arthritic synovium. J Clin Pathol 65:220–228, 1976.

56. Bennett RM, Skosey JL: Lactoferrin and lysozyme levels in synovial fluid: Differential indices of articular inflammation and degradation. Arthritis Rheum 20:84–90, 1977.

57. Abe S, Shinmel M, Nagai Y: Synovial collagenase and joint diseases: The significance of latent collagenase with special reference to rheumatoid arthritis. J Biochem 73:1007–1011, 1973.

58. Peltonen L: Collagenase in synovial fluid. Scand J Rheumatol 7:49–54, 1978.

59. Sanchez-Martin M, Garcia AG: Dopamine beta-hydroxylase in human synovial fluid. Experientia 33:650–652, 1977.

60. Stephens RW, Ghosh P, Taylor TKF: The characterization and function of the polysaccharidases of human synovial fluid in rheumatoid and osteoarthritis. Biochim Biophys Acta 399:101–112, 1975.

61. Palmer DG: Total leukocyte enumeration in pathologic synovial fluids. Am J Clin Pathol 49:812–814, 1968.

62. Panush RS, Bianco NE, Schur PH: Serum and synovial fluid IgG, IgA and IgM antigammaglobulins in rheumatoid arthritis. Arthritis Rheum 14:737–747, 1971.

63. Veys EM: Comparative investigation of protein concentration in serum and synovial fluid. Scand J Rheumatol 3:1–12, 1974.

64. Nettelbladt E, Sundblad L, Jonsson E: Permeability of the synovial membrane to proteins. Acta Rheum Scand 9:28–32, 1963.

65. Reinmann I, Arnoldi CC, Nielsen OS: Permeability of synovial membrane to plasma proteins in human coxarthrosis: Relation to molecular size and histologic changes. Clin Orthop 147:296–300, 1980.

66. Scudder PR, McMurray W, White AG, et al.: Synovial fluid copper and related variables in rheumatoid and degenerative arthritis. Ann Rheum Dis 37:71–72, 1978.

67. Anderson RB, Gormsen J: Fibrin dissolution in synovial fluid. Acta Rheum Scand 16:319–333, 1970.

68. White AG, Scudder P, Dormandy TL, et al.: Copper: An index of erosive activity. Rheumatol Rehabil 17:3–5, 1978.

69. Stastny, P, Rosenthal M, Andreis M, et al.: Lymphokines in the rheumatoid joint. Arthritis Rheum 18:237–243, 1975.

70. MacSween RNM, Dalakos TK, Jasani MK, et al.:

Antinuclear factors in synovial fluids. Lancet 1:312–314, 1967.

71. Wordsworth P, Ebringer R, Jones D, et al.: Thyroid antibodies in synovial effusions. Lancet 1:660, 1980.

72. Blake DR, McGregor AM, Stansfield E, et al.: Antithyroid-antibody activity in the synovial fluid of patients with various arthritides. Lancet 2:224–226, 1979.

73. Cooke TDV, Bennett EL, Ohno O: Identification of immunoglobulin and complement components in articular collagenous tissues of patients with idiopathic osteoarthritis. *In* Nuki G (ed.): The Aetiopathogenesis of Osteoarthritis. Tunbridge Wells, Pitman Medical Publishing Co., 1980, pp. 144–154.

74. Ruddy S, Fearon DT, Austin KF: Depressed synovial fluid levels of properdin and properdin factor B in patients with rheumatoid arthritis. Arthritis Rheum 18:289–295, 1975.

75. Perrin LH, Nydegger UE, Zublev RH, et al.: Correlation between levels of breakdown products of C3, C4 and properdin factor B in synovial fluid from patients with rheumatoid arthritis. Arthritis Rheum 20:647–656, 1977.

76. Sheppeard H, Lea DJ, Ward DJ: Synovial fluid total hemolytic complement activity in rheumatic diseases: A reappraisal. J Rheumatol 8:390–397, 1981.

77. Ludivido CL, Myers AR: Survey of synovial fluid cryoprecipitates. Ann Rheum Dis 39:253–259, 1979.

78. Manicourt D, Rao VH, Orloff S: Serum and synovial fluid hydroxyproline fractions in microcrystalline arthritis and osteoarthritis. Scan J Rheumatol 8:193–198, 1979.

79. Altman RD, Muniz OE, Pita JC, et al.: Articular chondrocalcinosis: Microanalysis of pyrophosphate (PPi) in synovial fluid and plasma. Arthritis Rheum 16:171–178, 1973.

80. Camerlain M, McCarty DJ, Silcox DC, et al.: Inorganic pyrophosphate pool size and turnover rate in arthritic joints. J Clin Invest 55:1373–1381, 1975.

81. Lloyd-Roberts GC: Osteoarthritis of the hip; study of clinical pathology. J Bone Joint Surg 37B:8–47, 1955.

82. Roy S: Ultrastructure of synovial membrane in osteoarthritis. Ann Rheum Dis 26:517–527, 1967.

83. Arnoldi CC, Reimann I, Bretlau P: The synovial membrane in human coxarthrosis: Light and electron microscopic studies. Clin Orthop 148:213–220, 1980.

84. Darrell JO-H, Fornaiser VL: Synovial iron deposition in osteoarthritis and rheumatoid arthritis. J Rheumatol 7:30–36, 1980.

85. Schumacher HR, Holdsworth DE: Ochronotic arthropathy. I. Clinicopathologic studies. Semin Arthritis Rheum 6:207–246, 1977.

86. Schumacher HR: Ultrastructural characteristics of the synovial membrane in idiopathic haemochromatosis. Ann Rheum Dis 31:465–473, 1972.

87. Hoffer PB, Genant HK: Radionuclide joint imaging. Semin Nucl Med 6:121–137, 1976.

88. Maccardi DJ, Polcyn RC, Collins PA: 99mTechnetium/scintiphotography in arthritis. II. Its specificity and clinical and roentgenographic correlations in rheumatoid arthritis. Arthritis Rheum 13:21–32, 1970.

89. Koorji AH, Altman RD: Qualitative evaluation of bone-joint function. (Abstract.) Society of Nuclear Medicine, Anaheim, California, June 1978.

90. Bekerman C, Genant HK, Hoffer PP, et al.: Bone and joint scanning of the hand: A definition of normal and a comparison of sensitivity using 99m-Tc-diphosphonate. Radiology 118:653–659, 1975.

91. Snable RD, McDaniel MM, Morton ME: Unilateral osteophytes simulating metastatic lesions on bone scan. Clin Nucl Med 3:116, 1978.

92. Thomas RH, Resnick D, Alazraki MP, et al.: Compartmental evaluation of osteoarthritis of the knee; a comparative study of available diagnostic modalities. Radiology 116:585–594, 1975.

93. Arnoldi CC, Linderholm H, Müssbichler H: Venous engorgement and intraosseous hypertension in osteoarthritis of the hip. J Bone Joint Surg 54B:409–421, 1972.

94. Arnoldi CC, Djurhuus JC, Heerfordt J, et al.: Intraosseous phlebography, intraosseous pressure measurements and 99mTC-polyphosphate scintigraphy in patients with various painful conditions in the hip and knee. Acta Orthop Scand 521:19–28, 1980.

95. Arnoldi CC, Lemperg RK, Linderholm H: Immediate effect of osteotomy on intramedullary pressure in the femoral head and neck in patients with degenerative osteoarthritis. Acta Orthop Scand 42:454–455, 1971.

96. Haberman JD, Ehrlich GE, Levenson C: Thermography in rheumatic diseases. Arch Phys Med Rehabil 49:187–192, 1968.

97. Cosh JA, Ring EFJ: Thermography and rheumatology. Rheumatol Phys Med 10:342–348, 1970.

11

Erosive Inflammatory and Primary Generalized Osteoarthritis

George E. Ehrlich, M.D.

Osteoarthritis is generally thought of as a lesion of a single joint. The common exception may well be Heberden's nodes, benign bony enlargements of distal interphalangeal joints that predominate in women, develop in men only later in life, and appear to have a strong genetic predisposition.[1] However, a polyarticular pattern of development of osteoarthritis can also be recognized.

William Heberden had asked "what those little hard knobs (were), about the size of a pea, which are frequently seen upon the fingers, a little below the top, near the joint. They have no connection with gout, being found in persons who never had it; they continue for life, and being hardly ever attended with pain, are disposed to become sores, are rather unsightly than inconvenient, though they must be some little hindrance to the free use of the fingers."[2] Only 3 years after Heberden was unable to answer his own question, Haygarth proposed that a polyarticular form of osteoarthritis must exist.[3] In 1857, Adams described such a presentation in some detail,[4] and in 1926, Cecil and Archer, attempting a classification of arthritis in general, included nodose deformities of distal and proximal interphalangeal joints among the noninfectious degenerative forms of arthritis.[5]

Still, in general, the nodose deformities of the hands were thought to be relatively pain-less, more unsightly than distressing, rarely painful, and occurring predominantly without associated involvement of other joints. That was the position taken by Stecher in his article on Heberden's nodes, in which he posited strong hereditary association—mendelian dominant in women, recessive in men.[1] Even then, however, several observations led to further clinical and epidemiologic studies: In many patients, evidence of osteoarthritis existed at joints other than those of the hands, and signs of inflammation, especially pain and stiffness, attended osteoarthritis of finger joints and some of these other joints in a considerable proportion of patients. Kellgren and Moore published a concept of primary generalized osteoarthritis (osteoarthrosis) that attempted to link the various sites of osteoarthritis occurring together with Heberden's nodes into a single syndrome.[6] They described primary generalized osteoarthritis as a disorder predominantly of middle-aged women in a ratio of at least 10:1 over men. The mean age of onset was 52 years. They suggested that the mendelian dominant trait in women indeed characterized the affliction of the distal interphalangeal joints of the fingers, but they thought that a secondary hereditary factor might be responsible for encouraging the rest of the syndrome. Kellgren and coworkers later elaborated on this concept and accepted the view that reces-

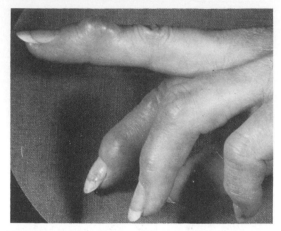

Figure 11–1. Synovial (mucoid) cyst. These lesions generally appear on the dorsal aspect of the distal interphalangeal joint or just proximal to it. Resembling ganglia, they contain gelatinous material and may be extremely inflammatory and painful. Not infrequently, they precede the appearance of the Herberden's node itself.

sive hereditary factors best explained the lower incidence of this disorder in men.[7]

In primary generalized osteoarthritis, the onset was sometimes abrupt, attended by inflammation, so that infection or gout could even have been suspected in some of the patients. There was often an associated thick gelatinous fluid in the tissues overlying the joint, even if no major inflammatory changes had occurred. This presentation anticipated the later description of the "mucoid cyst" (Fig. 11–1) thought to be characteristic of some presentations of erosive osteoarthritis.[8] A serial symmetric involvement of finger joints could be observed, with no apparent relation to trauma or mechanical factors. In fact, Stecher's discovery of a pair of identical twins with mirror-image symmetry of their Heberden's nodes was thought to confirm the nontraumatic nature of this lesion.[9] In the patients who had primary generalized osteoarthritis, periodic attacks of pain intensified at night with a burning characteristic, and despite the prolonged nature of the disorder, rarely did crippling occur in any of the joints. There was no influence upon the general health. The erythrocyte sedimentation rate remained normal or only slightly elevated, and the then newly described rheumatoid factor tests were repeatedly recorded as negative. Few of the patients originally reported by Kellgren and Moore appeared to have had joint effusions. In a subsequent patient who fit the same description, Swezey described a relatively acellular

fluid with otherwise fairly normal characteristics.[10]

In studying the full syndrome, Kellgren and coworkers pointed to the first carpometacarpal articulation as commonly involved in patients who had nodal distal interphalangeal involvement.[6, 11] Proximal interphalangeal joints were frequently involved, but not as often as the distal joints, as were the apophyseal joints of the spine and the sacroiliac joints. The disorder was later separated into nodal and non-nodal forms. The nodal forms included the disorder in all those patients who had nodose deformities in their fingers as well as other articular manifestations, and the non-nodal forms were characterized by osteoarthritic involvement of more than five joints, but not in the fingers, at least at first. It was believed that the nodal forms were the ones that were strongly predisposed to by heredity, whereas the non-nodal forms followed inflammation.[6, 12] Rheumatoid arthritis was specifically cited as one potential precursor of non-nodal polyarticular osteoarthritis.[6, 12]

This concept is still controversial. Noninflammatory polyarticular degeneration is thought by many simply to be osteoarthritis in many joints,[13, 14] and erosive change associated with inflammation is thought to be a separate syndrome.[15, 16] What unites all the concepts of polyarticular osteoarthritis is that on histologic examination, the classic changes of osteoarthritis are found in the various joints, even if the presentations differ and if the generalized forms appear at times both to have inflammatory antecedents and to emerge with inflammatory signs and symptoms of a secondary nature.[17]

Dissociation of generalized osteoarthritis into two syndromes, the primary generalized osteoarthritis attended by little pain and the erosive inflammatory osteoarthritis attended by considerable resemblance to other inflammatory polyarticular disorders, was heralded by a description of 23 patients by Crain.[18] His patients had involvement of finger joints by what appeared to be osteoarthritis. In six of his patients, no joints other than those of the fingers were involved. In 15 patients, the distal interphalangeal joints were involved first, but in the other 8, the proximal interphalangeal joints manifested involvement initially. Concomitant development chiefly involved the spine, as in Kellgren's series; in 12 patients, the cervical spine was involved and in 3, the lumbar spine. There was rare involvement of other joints. Crain named the syndrome interphalangeal osteoarthritis. He recognized a polyarticular onset, but the lack of involvement of the hips and knees and assorted other joints, by now included in Kellgren's concept, segregated the syndrome from the more generalized form. Because of an apparent lack of provocation, the appellation "primary" was given to Crain's syndrome as well. This specifically denied the possibility that vocational and avocational uses of the joints could have resulted in the pattern of development. Crain also disclaimed the eponym Bouchard's nodes that was often attached to the nodes developing at proximal interphalangeal joints (Bouchard's nodes are thought to be the equivalent of Heberden's nodes, occurring one row closer to the hand), as he pointed out that Bouchard's patients were younger (around 20 years old) with flexion deformities of their fingers and that they were said to have had gastric dilatation as an associated feature. However, Crain's pleas seem to have fallen on deaf ears, as most contemporary clinicians use the term Bouchard's nodes to refer to nodose deformities of proximal interphalangeal joints in interphalangeal osteoarthritis.

A proportion of patients who have prominent interphalangeal osteoarthritis develop erosive changes in the finger joints. The term erosive osteoarthritis was thus chosen to emphasize the juxta-articular erosions simulating "those of rheumatoid arthritis in patients who do not have classical or definite rheumatoid arthritis by any of the usual criteria."[15] Although the clinical syndrome here is quite distinctive, the label emphasized the roentgenologic features. Later recognition that the onset in these cases was usually abrupt and accompanied by the cardinal signs of inflam-

mation led to the introduction of the term inflammatory osteoarthritis,[19] now commonly modified to erosive inflammatory osteoarthritis in various contemporary descriptions. Although inflammation signaled the development of this syndrome, it might have produced only the features that brought the syndrome to the attention of the patient and the physician. Because bony enlargements were already present and roentgenographic evidence of osteoarthritis already existed, one can assume that, even here, inflammation was a secondary phenomenon and not immediately causative. Thus, there still may not be adequate justification for separating erosive inflammatory osteoarthritis from primary generalized osteoarthritis, and both terms might be describing a continuum of polyarticular osteoarthritic events to which many factors contribute.

EROSIVE INFLAMMATORY OSTEOARTHRITIS (EOA)

An abrupt onset of pain, swelling, redness, warmth, and limited function of interphalangeal joints of the hands characterize the clinical recognition of this syndrome.[15] Nodose deformities involve the distal interphalangeal joints of the fingers in a symmetric fashion in almost all the patients (Fig. 11–2). The distal interphalangeal joints of the second and third fingers are more commonly involved than those of the fourth and fifth fingers, and the interphalangeal joint of the thumb is involved about as often as the distal interphalangeal joint of the second finger.[19] The skin over the enlarging joint is often quite red (Fig. 11–2), and besides the pain that is complained of,

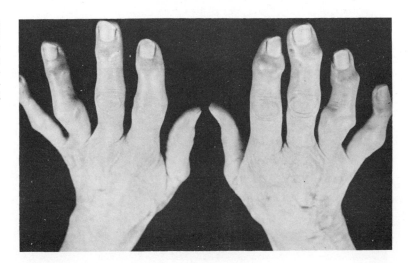

Figure 11–2. Erosive osteoarthritis with involvement of the distal and proximal interphalangeal joints. Bony enlargements due to spur formation are associated with a moderately severe inflammatory reaction, more severe in the distal interphalangeal joints in this patient.

tenderness can be elicited by examining these joints.[19] The distal interphalangeal joints will often be held in slight flexion, and complete extension may be difficult or impossible. Proximal interphalangeal joints are also involved (Fig. 11–2) but only about two-thirds as often as the distal interphalangeal joints. Again, symmetric involvement is the rule. There is a slight tendency toward asymmetry at both the distal and the proximal interphalangeal joints in the slight preponderance of involvement of the dominant hand. This suggests that additional factors of use play a role in predilection for the specific joints, but in general, the symmetry would deny the probability that traumatic factors are responsible for this syndrome. Flexion deformity of the proximal interphalangeal joints is quite common, and in some patients in whom the distal interphalangeal joints are not initially involved, the presentation suggests the collar-button deformity commonly ascribed to rheumatoid arthritis.[19]

Ankylosis of interphalangeal joints may also occur.[20] In erosive inflammatory osteoarthritis, this ankylosis may be an unfavorable prognostic sign. In one series, almost all the patients who had developed ankylosis as part of the osteoarthritic syndrome were later found among those who developed a supervening rheumatoid arthritis.[21]

The metacarpophalangeal joints are rarely involved by the syndrome, but they are by no means spared in all patients. The metacarpophalangeal joints of the thumbs and, less commonly, those of the second fingers will sometimes develop nodose deformities. The third, fourth, and fifth metacarpophalangeal joints are rarely the seat of erosive inflammatory osteoarthritis.[18]

The first carpometacarpal joint is involved in at least one third of the patients (Fig. 11–3).[18] This is an incongruous joint to begin with, and some explain the incongruity by claiming that the first metacarpal is missing from the human hand and that what we call the metacarpal is actually the proximal phalanx of the first finger. The disappearance of the metacarpal and the resultant incongruity of the carpometacarpal joint permit rotation of the thumb and led to opposition and the prehensile grasp that has made so much difference in hand use for man compared with animals. There is a price to be paid for this development, however, and it is the propensity of this joint to develop osteoarthritic changes. Such changes occur in an isolated fashion, of course, as a result of various types of trauma, but they also occur in this joint as part of the syndrome of erosive inflammatory osteoarthritis in a proportion of patients.[6, 18] Osteoarthritis of this joint is called rhizarthrosis in the European literature.[22] Symmetric involvement of these joints is not as common as symmetric involvement of distal interphalangeal joints (approximately 75%) but may be more common than symmetric involvement of proximal interphalangeal joints.[18] The adjacent trapezioscaphoid joint may also be involved in a number of instances. Osteoarthritis between the carpus and the radius or at the distal radioulnar joint or at other carpometacarpal joints is so rare as to be noteworthy if it occurs.

Similar involvement is also seen in the toes, but far less commonly. Perhaps the protection

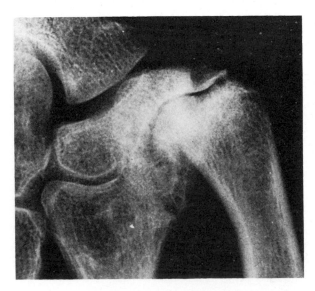

Figure 11–3. Roentgenogram of the first carpometacarpal joint. Osteoarthritis had led to cartilage loss with joint space narrowing, marked subchondral sclerosis, osteophyte formation and subchondral cysts.

of the feet by shoes and the different uses to which toes are put compared with fingers offer some explanation of this difference.[23] The first metatarsophalangeal joint, or bunion joint, however, is commonly involved, perhaps by a separate mechanism, and here, the wearing of shoes may predispose to the development of the lesion, as it is uncommon in barefoot peoples.[24]

On careful examination, most of these patients will be seen to have osteoarthritic lesions of the hips, knees, and cervical spine, although not necessarily with erosive changes or the same degree of symptomatic involvement.[25] In the fingers, morning stiffness is common, although of relatively short duration (minutes, contrasted with an hour or more in active rheumatoid arthritis), localized (the hands but not usually the generalized stiffness seen in rheumatoid disease), and easily worked out (movement of the hands or immersion in warm water generally succeeds in removing the stiffness quickly). Still, it is described by patients and, unless carefully analyzed, can lead to the erroneous impression that one is dealing with rheumatoid arthritis.[26]

As stated, the signs of inflammation are prominent at the time the syndrome is presented to the physician. However, considerable changes have often already occurred in the affected joints, so that this need not necessarily be the onset of the disease but merely the onset of clinically apparent or distressing disease. The disease is predominant in women; at the time of greatest distress, they are usually at or just beyond menopause, between the ages of 45 and 55 years. Later onset is seen in women whose menopausal transition is treated with estrogenic hormones, and in these women, the acute symptoms seem to follow the cessation of hormone administration.[19] Earlier occurrence will be found in women with strong familial predisposition who undergo surgical menopause prematurely.[19] Strong family predisposition exists. Men can develop the syndrome, but in later years as a rule, perhaps in the sixth decade or beyond.

The physical examination of the patient confirms the presentation and distribution of this polyarticular form of osteoarthritis. Side-to-side instability is common in afflicted finger joints and sometimes also in joints remote from the hands, such as the knees when they appear to be afflicted. Careful statistical analysis, however, cannot relate involvement of remote joints to the syndrome in the hands, even though both occur simultaneously in the same people.[19] Coincidence seems to play a

role here, and in the case of the knees and hips, the relationship results more from increasing age than it does from concomitant finger involvement.

Although many of the patients are heavy, obesity does not appear to play a role in initiation of the syndrome, although it will aggravate pains in weight-bearing joints without necessarily being responsible for those pains.[11] None of these patients have rheumatoid arthritis by the usual criteria, although most develop the gnarled fingers with deviation of specific phalanges in both radial and ulnar directions as a result of the disorder. The residual deformities are attended by chronic low-grade pain and often some instability, but the acute inflammation that was manifested at presentation seems to be self-limited. Joint effusions are uncommon, and muscle atrophy rarely complicates the picture. Demineralization adjacent to joints does not occur as it does in rheumatoid arthritis.

On roentgenograms, narrowing of the joint space (cartilage space) is seen and is usually irregular, with erosions at the joint margins and also within the articulating surface (Fig. 11–4).[8] The deviation of the specific phalanx in juxtaposition with these erosions is in the lateral or medial direction. Bony ankylosis can

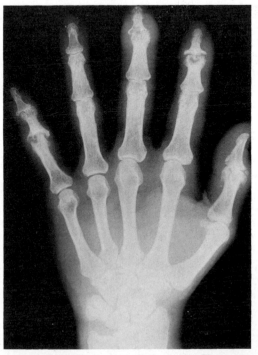

Figure 11–4. Roentgenogram of the hand. Changes seen in this patient with erosive osteoarthritis are characterized by severe bony erosions, cartilage loss, and osteophyte formation.

be detected in some instances.[18, 19] No periosteal new bone formation develops, but subchondral sclerosis, osteophytes, and altered shape of bone ends are characteristic.[26] At times, the erosions are so mutilating as to suggest psoriatic arthropathy.[27, 28] In one case reported by Schumacher, similar changes followed frostbite in one hand and were not reflected in the contralateral hand.[29] In this case, the syndrome presumably did not fall into the category of primary osteoarthritis. Dramatic erosive changes can involve large joints such as the hips and knees as well.[25, 30]

In several studies, histologic evidence of inflammation was gleaned from biopsies or operations on the joints.[17, 19, 31] In most instances, the synovium resembled that in rheumatoid arthritis more closely than it did that considered characteristic of osteoarthritis. However, palisading and fibrinoid necrosis were not seen.[17] Increased local vascularity in the synovium was accompanied by some areas of cellular aggregation. Some of the cartilage and synovium from erosive osteoarthritis examined by Cooke and coworkers contained deposits of immune complexes, as demonstrated by immunofluorescence.[32, 33] Other studies have suggested a role for immune mechanisms in erosive osteoarthritis. Synovial fluid and synovial specimens from patients with EOA had increased numbers of Ia^+ T lymphocytes, similar to that seen in specimens from patients with rheumatoid arthritis.[34] The expression of Ia antigens in both patients with EOA and those with rheumatoid arthritis was in the OKT8 T-lymphocyte subset. These findings, not seen in patients with OA of other types, suggested that EOA represented a subset of patients with osteoarthritis. Singleton and colleagues noted evidence of sicca syndrome in 17 of 22 patients with EOA.[35] Serum gamma globulins were diffusely elevated, and thyroid antibodies were common.

Clinical laboratory tests are singularly unhelpful in making this diagnosis.[25] No abnormalities attend erosive osteoarthritis other than a modest elevation of the erythrocyte sedimentation rate. However, a proportion of these patients appears to be at risk of developing later onset of something that closely resembles rheumatoid arthritis and that seems to have its inception in the upper extremities.[21] This second syndrome, evolving after a period during which the hands have become relatively asymptomatic but still bear the stigmata of the earlier erosive osteoarthritis, develops in about 15% of such patients. In these instances, the erythrocyte sedimentation rate becomes quite rapid, as would be expected in rheumatoid arthritis, and rheumatoid factor emerges in the majority of such patients. Histologic examination of tissues from joints obtained at surgery in these patients reveals evidence that the disorder is clearly rheumatoid in nature, with the classic changes having developed. Soft tissue involvement usually points to the supervention of rheumatoid arthritis, because in osteoarthritis soft tissues are not involved.

GENERALIZED OSTEOARTHRITIS

This concept encompasses a wider range of manifestations. Many of the manifestations of erosive inflammatory osteoarthritis described above would qualify for inclusion in this syndrome, but in other patients the onset is slow and insidious and they never experience acute inflammatory symptoms and signs. Gradual development of nodose deformities in the fingers is the rule, and it is occasionally punctuated by episodes of acute pain. Again, individuals between the ages of 40 to 60 years are most at risk, with a few cases occurring earlier in life and some later, and women are affected far more often than men. Besides distal and proximal interphalangeal joints, the first carpometacarpal joint again is frequently involved, with squaring of the thenar eminence as another presenting sign.[6]

Besides the hands, the hips, knees, and spine are also commonly involved in this generalized syndrome.[6, 11] Although some have claimed that hip and hand involvement are linked,[6, 36] others assert that there is no connection,[19, 25] and both sides can marshal data to support their viewpoints. If the presentations are segregated by sex, however, a relationship between hip and knee osteoarthritis and nodal hand involvement does appear to be present in men, but not in women.[37] Because nodal osteoarthritis is present in more than 60% of women over the age of 55 years, it would be expected that in those with hip involvement, the chances are 2:1 that nodal involvement of the fingers would also be present.[38] Thus, mechanical overload is added to degenerative and inflammatory features and to poor bone response as being among the causes of osteoarthritic development in these various joints.[37]

Roentgenologic changes in the various joints involved are similar to those seen at any single joint that manifests osteoarthritic changes, i.e., narrowing of the joint space, marginal osteophytes, cysts adjacent to joints, and geodes (enlarging cavernous cysts within the bone adjacent to the joint, usually in the subchondral area). The original descriptions also stressed certain features on roentgenograms that differed from the usual pattern of isolated multifocal osteoarthritis: enormous enlargements of articular facets, spinous processes, and neural arches were seen, often tending to approach each other as "kissing spines" (or osteophytes) (Fig. 11–5).[36] The osteophytes at the knees were described as resembling molten wax, and the sharply pointed osteophytes generally seen in osteoarthritis were notably absent. Some resemblance to ankylosing changes of diffuse idiopathic skeletal hyperostosis (DISH) could be inferred,[39] and indeed, on axial roentgenograms, it is sometimes difficult to tell which of these syndromes the specific film is depicting. However, as the concept of primary generalized osteoarthritis per se is receding, such careful differentiation may be unnecessary.

In some instances of generalized osteoarthritis, chondrocalcinosis can be found.[40–43] One family suffered from a familial form of chondrocalcinosis due to apatite crystal depo-

sition, with symptoms indistinguishable from those ascribed to generalized osteoarthritis alone.[44] Morning stiffness occurred in the afflicted joints, with involvement of the small joints of the hand and the dorsolumbar spine and periarthritic involvement of the shoulder predominating. Other studies have implicated calcium pyrophosphate dihydrate in the development of symptoms in osteoarthritis.[45–47] A proportion of patients who had symptomatic deposition of this substance had generalized osteoarthritis and deposited crystals of this material in osteoarthritic joints. Shedding of crystals and of cartilaginous debris[48] could account for some of the secondary changes. However, although diagnostic confusion between calcium pyrophosphate dihydrate deposition disease and generalized or erosive inflammatory osteoarthritis can exist because many of the same joints are involved, these syndromes can be segregated from each other.

Differential diagnosis is complicated by concurrent developments in patients who have polyarticular osteoarthritis. Periarthritis and other afflictions of the shoulder are common in the appropriate age group and when seen together with stiffness-producing interphalangeal arthritis and perhaps coincidental involvement of other large joints may simulate the picture of rheumatoid arthritis.[25, 49] Similarly, polymyalgia rheumatica may present with painful shoulder afflictions in patients who have benign Heberden's nodes, the latter being very common.[50] Again, a generalized syndrome may be supposed, and if scintiscans show apparent involvement of the shoulder joints in these patients, as has been claimed,[51] a resemblance to rheumatoid arthritis as it presents in older age groups[52] obviously also exists. In fact, rheumatoid arthritis intrudes as the major differential diagnosis in most instances.[53, 54] Carpal tunnel syndrome is common in all forms of interphalangeal osteoarthritis, and thus, the syndrome needs differentiation from diabetes mellitus and para-amyloid deposition secondary to multiple myeloma coincidentally occurring in someone who has developed ubiquitous Heberden's nodes. In other words, almost any joint disorder afflicting especially women but also men in the older age groups needs to be ruled out, because the majority of those Buchanan and Park call "elderly folk" will also have osteoarthritic interphalangeal changes of different origin.[55] Finally, the interphalangeal osteoarthritis secondary to vocational trauma might lead to an erroneous diagnosis if one is not aware

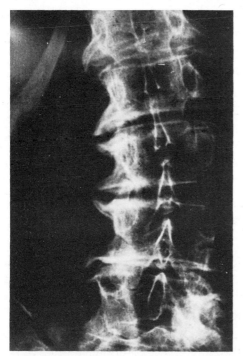

Figure 11–5. Anteroposterior roentgenogram of the lumbar spine. Florid osteophyte formation, disk space narrowing, and sclerosis of articular facets are seen in this patient in whom there was evidence of severe diffuse osteoarthritis in numerous peripheral joints as well.

of the specific distribution of lesions that some tasks will promote.[56]

It is clear that the concept of primary generalized osteoarthritis is undergoing an evolutionary change. Wood has pointed out, "With the advent of disease, one may be confronted with the complexity of multilocus involvement. A simple dichotomization, such as can be applied to single organs or organs that function as a single unit, is not possible."[57] He suggests that osteoarthritis will be interpreted differently by epidemiologists, pathologists, roentgenologists, and clinicians. This explains some of the confusion in terminology—the various descriptions of phenomena come from different sources. The plea by Wood to remember that the musculoskeletal system exists only for the anatomist and not for the clinician seems to have some validity, as the supposition that some disease afflicts the cartilage even in generalized osteoarthritis does not explain the sparing of so much cartilage and the involvement of so little. Thus, the term generalized osteoarthritis merely fuels the controversy of whether osteoarthritis is a disease or whether it is a process that accompanies other disorders, including, perhaps, aging. In the instance of the subset in which inflammation is a clinical feature, some argument could be made that it represents an interface between ordinary osteoarthritis, a balance between degeneration and repair, and inflammatory polyarthritis, such as may be represented by rheumatoid disease.[58]

PROGNOSIS

If one regards generalized osteoarthritis as distinct from erosive inflammatory osteoarthritis, the outlook is quite good. Although nodose deformities tend to occur in finger joints, on the whole, motion is not seriously compromised in the majority of joints, and pain and stiffness tend to be relatively episodic, with considerable pain-free intervals. Longitudinal ridging and concavity of nails may develop because of impingement of large Heberden's nodes on the nail matrix,[59] although successful anti-inflammatory treatment can counter this phenomenon. However, erosive inflammatory osteoarthritis has already been distinguished as a destructive process in the finger joints. Marked limitation of function of the hands tends to result, and further episodes of acute inflammation are likely to punctuate the future course, being responsible at least for consid-

erable discomfort. As noted earlier, about 15% of patients who have erosive inflammatory osteoarthritis are likely to develop a syndrome indistinguishable from rheumatoid arthritis of old-age onset.[21, 60] The prognosis appears to be better in this group than in a younger age group with rheumatoid arthritis.[21, 52] This may be related to the fact that patients in the older age group tend to already be under medical care for previous osteoarthritis and other concurrent illnesses; thus, treatment is initiated earlier.

Since the advent of the low-friction arthroplasty, surgical correction of some of the problems at major joints has become feasible; unfortunately, surgery of finger joints is still in relatively early stages, and in osteoarthritis, it is performed relatively infrequently, with the exception of replacement of the scaphoid by a silicon-rubber prosthetic implant. Progressive destruction of large joints occasionally continues[61]; surgical correction is now eminently feasible.

TREATMENT

The response to anti-inflammatory therapy has been sufficiently gratifying to permit recommendation of treatment with anti-inflammatory drugs and intra-articular corticosteroids when pain and other symptoms of inflammation are present.[25, 62–64] Although analgesic compounds alone will reduce some of the pain, the attendant signs and symptoms of inflammation yield to anti-inflammatory treatment, and this must be recommended. Aspirin is still widely used, but some of the findings by Palmoski, Coyer, and Brandt[65] that suggest that aspirin interferes with the regeneration of cartilage through blockage of proteoglycan repair may be relevant. To a lesser extent, some other nonsteroidal anti-inflammatory compounds also seem to prevent proper repair in this test system, both in vitro and in vivo, but other compounds do not. In particular, indole derivatives seem to react favorably in this test system.[66] However, there appears to be little justification for administration of these compounds during periods of relative absence of pain. Even low-grade pain can often be accepted by patients if they understand that it is not premonitory of a crippling disease; therefore, the prolonged use of any anti-inflammatory medication is to be discouraged. Intra-articular corticosteroid treatments can help the individual highly inflamed joint by reducing the distressing inflammatory signs and symptoms and promoting function, but the same caution that guides such therapy in the treatment of single osteoarthritic joints should also prevail here.[25, 64] There is no justification for the administration of oral corticosteroids or for the use of drugs that encourage remissions in rheumatoid arthritis in a generalized or erosive inflammatory osteoarthritic syndrome. Nor can one countenance the intra-articular administration of cytotoxic substances or other compounds used for synoviorthesis, the chemical equivalent of synovectomy.

A properly constructed program of physical and occupational therapy can help much more. Occupational therapy generally deals with fine movements and is therefore appropriate to treat the hands and to teach joint conservation. The muscle toning and administration of moist heat, perhaps in the form of paraffin dip baths, generally become the responsibility of the department of physical therapy. Many patients can be helped by the overnight wearing of two-way nylon and spandex gloves,[67] which can be purchased at most glove counters (but usually not in pharmacies or surgical supply stores). Surgical correction has already been alluded to as an ultimate recourse.

CONCLUSIONS

The various multilocal osteoarthritic syndromes discussed should be regarded as intermediates between unicameral osteoarthritis, as it is generally conceived, and the inflammatory arthritides. Inflammation is a direct result of the syndrome and is secondary, but it may be remotely causative if one accepts that inflammation attends trauma and that trauma remote in time has set the process into motion that ultimately develops into osteoarthritis. In generalized osteoarthritis, there clearly has to be more than this, as it is necessary to explain the sex predilection, familial clustering, and racial characteristics (generalized osteoarthritis, particularly of the nodal variety, is almost never seen in African blacks, and non-nodal osteoarthritis is seen more commonly in male than in female African blacks, in contradistinction to the distribution in whites). The relationship of generalized osteoarthritis to concomitant disorders, such as hypertension or hyperuricemia,[38] may well be fortuitous, but it does suggest the possibility that some as yet unidentified genetic factors play a major role. No studies successfully linking any HLA abnor-

malities with generalized osteoarthritis have yet been published. Even though it is unlikely, given the presenting syndrome, mechanical pathogenesis still has its advocates, suggesting that the nodose deformities derive from thickening of extensor tendons[14] and that the subchondral microfractures described by Radin[68] might well play an additional role. Those who advocate this view point to the undoubted fact that generalized osteoarthritis is not really generalized but has a predilection for distal and proximal interphalangeal joints, the first carpometacarpals, specific segments in the neck and back, the hips, knees, and first metatarsophalangeal joint and that other joints are not involved. Others would argue that the wrists and ankles are so rarely afflicted because of a diffusion of forces through mosaic joints that fit bones together much like the parts of a jigsaw puzzle and that the elbows and shoulders are rarely the seat of osteoarthritis because they do not often bear weight. When they become weight-bearing, as in patients who need to use assistive devices because of lower extremity afflictions, they become involved more commonly.

Biomechanical explanations emphasize not only crystal induction but also similarities to specific metabolic disorders accompanied by osteoarthritis, such as alkaptonuric ochronosis, hemochromatosis, acromegaly, and congenital disorders of connective tissue.[69] In this construct, proteoglycans, collagen, water content and binding, and a host of other factors induced by inflammation, such as release of various enzymes and the positioning of immune factors, play a role. Tissue pathologists cannot distinguish osteoarthritic cartilage of unicameral osteoarthritis from that of generalized osteoarthritis, however. Epidemiologic studies have been unable to confirm that generalized osteoarthritis exists as an entity.[70, 71] Nevertheless, it is seen often enough that an articular index has been devised for assessment of osteoarthritis so that the effect of various drugs on this disorder can be measured.[72] Most thoughtful investigators believe that the syndrome is only a final common pathway of a number of different disorders and that our methods of discovery are still too crude to distinguish among these processes.

References

1. Stecher RM: Heberden's nodes. A clinical description of osteoarthritis in the finger joint. Ann Rheum Dis 14:1–10, 1955.

2. Heberden W: Commentaries on History and Cure of Diseases. London, T. Payne, 1802, pp. 148–149.
3. Haygarth J: Clinical History of Diseases. London, Gadell and Davies, 1805.
4. Adams R: A Treatise on Rheumatic Gout. London, Churchill, 1857.
5. Cecil RL, Archer BH: Classification and treatment of chronic arthritis. JAMA 87:741–746, 1926.
6. Kellgren JH, Moore R: Generalized osteoarthritis and Heberden's nodes. Br Med J 1:181–187, 1952.
7. Kellgren JH, Lawrence JS, Bier F: Genetic factors in generalized osteoarthrosis. Ann Rheum Dis 22:237–255, 1963.
8. Kidd KL, Peter JB: Erosive osteoarthritis. Radiology 86:640–647, 1966.
9. Stecher RM: Heberden's nodes: Concordant osteoarthritis of fingers in identical twins. Acta Genet Med (Roma) 3, 4:84–91, 1954–55.
10. Swezey RL: Primary generalized osteoarthritis. Case report with knee joint fluid analysis. JAMA 192:147–148, 1965.
11. Kellgren JH, Lawrence JS: Osteo-arthrosis and disk degeneration in an urban population. Ann Rheum Dis 17:388–397, 1958.
12. Francon F: Extensive form of hypertrophic arthritis. Rheumatology 6:17–19, 1950.
13. Rasker JL, Davis P, Bacon PA: Seronegative chronic polyarthritis: Clinical and serological correlates. Ann Rheum Dis 39:550–553, 1980.
14. Solomon L: OA, local and generalized—a uniform disease? J Rheumatol 10(Suppl 9):13–15, 1983.
15. Peter JB, Pearson CM, Marmor L: Erosive osteoarthritis of the hands. Arthritis Rheum 9:365–388, 1966.
16. Peyron J: Inflammation in osteoarthritis (OA): Review of its role in clinical picture, disease progress, subsets, and pathophysiology. Semin Arthritis Rheum 11(Suppl 1):115–116, 1981.
17. Gardner DL, Oates K, O'Connor P, Orford CR: The microscopic heterogeneity of osteoarthrosis. J Rheumatol 10(Suppl 9):9–10, 1983.
18. Crain DC: Interphalangeal osteoarthritis characterized by painful, inflammatory episodes, resulting in deformity of the proximal and distal articulations. JAMA 175:1949–1953, 1961.
19. Ehrlich GE: Inflammatory osteoarthritis. I. The clinical syndrome. J Chronic Dis 25:317–328, 1972.
20. McEwen C: Osteoarthritis of the fingers with ankylosis. Arthritis Rheum 11:734–743, 1968.
21. Ehrlich GE: Inflammatory osteoarthritis. II. The superimposition of rheumatoid arthritis. J Chronic Dis 25:635–643, 1972.
22. Balboso B, Cirillo R, Malara B: La rizartrosi del pollice. Rheumatilismo 20:195–208, 1968.
23. Ehrlich GE: Pathogenesis and treatment of osteoarthritis. Compr Ther 5:36–40, 1978.
24. Solomon L, Beighton P, Lawrence JS: Rheumatic disorders in the South African Negro. II. Osteoarthrosis. S Afr Med J 49:1737–1740, 1975.
25. Utsinger P, Resnick D, Shapiro RF, et al.: Roentgenologic, immunologic, and therapeutic study of erosive (inflammatory) osteoarthritis. Arch Intern Med 128:683–697, 1978.
26. Ehrlich GE: Osteoarthritis beginning with inflammation. Definitions and correlations. JAMA 232:157–159, 1975.
27. Goldie I: Erosive osteoarthritis of the distal finger joints. Acta Orthop Scand 43:469–478, 1972.
28. Swezey RL, Alexander SJ: Erosive osteoarthritis and the main en lorgnette deformity. Arch Intern Med 128:269–272, 1971.
29. Schumacher HR: Unilateral osteoarthritis of the hand. JAMA 191:180–181, 1981.
30. Keats TE, Johnstone WH, O'Brien WM: Large joint destruction in erosive osteoarthritis. Skeletal Radiol 6:267–269, 1981.
31. Waxman BA, Sledge GB: Correlations of histochemical, histologic and biochemical evaluation of human synovium with clinical activity. Arthritis Rheum 16:376–382, 1973.
32. Cooke TD, Hurd ER, Jasin HE, et al.: Identification of immunoglobulins and complement in rheumatoid articular collagenous tissues. Arthritis Rheum 18:541–551, 1975.
33. Ohno O, Cooke TD: Electron microscopic morphology of immunoglobulin aggregates and their interaction in rheumatoid articular collagenous tissues. Arthritis Rheum 21:516–517, 1978.
34. Utsinger PD, Fite FL: Immunologic evidence for inflammation (I) in osteoarthritis (OA): high percentage of Ia$^+$ T lymphocytes (L) in the synovial fluid (SF) and synovium (S) of patients with erosive osteoarthritis (EOA). Arthritis Rheum 25:S44, 1982.
35. Singleton PT, Cervantes AG, McKoy J: Sicca complex and erosive osteoarthritis: Immunologic implications of a new osteoarthritis subset. Arthritis Rheum 25:S33, 1982.
36. Kellgren JH, Lawrence JS: Radiological assessment of osteo-arthrosis. Ann Rheum Dis 16:494–502, 1957.
37. Solomon L, Schnitzler CM, Browett JP: Osteoarthritis of the hip: The patient behind the disease. Ann Rheum Dis 41:118–125, 1982.
38. Lawrence JS: Generalized osteo-arthrosis in a population sample. J Epidemiol 90:381–389, 1969.
39. Resnick D, Shapiro RF, Wiesner KB, et al.: Diffuse idiopathic skeletal hyperostosis (DISH) (ankylosing hyperostosis of Forestier and Rotes-Querol). Semin Arthritis Rheum 7:153–189, 1978.
40. Doyle EV, Huskisson EC, Willoughby DA: A histological study of inflammation in osteoarthritis: The role of calcium phosphate crystal deposition. Ann Rheum Dis 28:192, 1979.
41. Dieppe PA, Doyle DV, Huskisson EC, et al.: Mixed crystal deposition disease in osteoarthritis. Br Med J 1:150–152, 1978.
42. Schmidt KL, Leber HW, Schütterle G: Arthropathie bei primärer Oxalose—Kristallsynovitis oder Osteopathie? Dtsch Med Wochenschr 106:19–22, 1981.
43. Schumacher HR, Gordon G, Paul H, et al.: Osteoarthritis, crystal deposition, and inflammation. Semin Arthritis Rheum 11(Suppl):116–119, 1981.
44. Marcos JC, de Banyacar MA, Garcia-Morteo O, et al.: Idiopathic familial chondrocalcinosis due to apatite crystal deposition. Am J Med 71:557–564, 1981.
45. Utsinger PD, Resnick D, Zvaifler NJ: Wrist arthropathy in calcium pyrophosphate dihydrate deposition disease. Arthritis Rheum 18:485–491, 1975.
46. Dieppe PA, Alexander GJM, Jones HE, et al.: Pyrophosphate arthropathy: A clinical and radiological study of 105 cases. Ann Rheum Dis 41:371–376, 1982.
47. Alexander GM, Dieppe PA, Doherty M, et al.: Pyrophosphate arthropathy: A study of metabolic as-

sociations and laboratory data. Ann Rheum Dis 41:377–381, 1982.

48. Chrisman OD, Ladenbauer-Bellis IN, Fulkerson JP: The osteoarthritic cascade in associated drug actions. Semin Arthritis Rheum 11(Suppl 1):145, 1981.

49. Waxman J: Menopausal osteoarthritis and bursitis. Clin Res 23:25A, 1975.

50. Ehrlich GE: Polymyalgia rheumatica. JAMA 240:57–58, 1978.

51. O'Duffy JD, Wahner HW, Hunder GG: Joint imaging in polymyalgia rheumatica. Mayo Clin Proc 51:519–524, 1976.

52. Ehrlich GE, Katz WA, Cohen SH: Rheumatoid arthritis in the aged. Geriatrics 25:103–113, 1970.

53. Boni A: Die progredient chronische polyarthritis. *In* Schoen R, Boni A, Miehlke R (eds.): Klinik der Rheumatischen Erkrankungen. Berlin, Springer, 1970, p. 156.

54. Bland JH, Brown EW: Seronegative and seropositive rheumatoid arthritis. Clinical, radiological, and biochemical differences. Ann Intern Med 60:88–94, 1964.

55. Buchanan WW, Park WM: Primary generalized osteoarthritis: Definition and uniformity. J Rheumatol 10(Suppl 9):4–6, 1983.

56. Hadler NM, Gillings DB, Imbus HR, et al.: Hand structure and function in an industrial setting. Influence of three patterns of stereotyped repetitive usage. Arthritis Rheum 21:210–220, 1978.

57. Wood PHN: Rheumatic complaints. Br Med Bull 27:82–88, 1971.

58. Ehrlich GE: Osteoarthritis. Arch Intern Med 138:688–689, 1978.

59. Alarcón-Segovia D, Vega-Ortiz JM: Heberden's nodes' nails. J Rheumatol 8:509–511, 1981.

60. Ehrlich GE: Osteoarthritis before, during, and after rheumatoid arthritis. Semin Arthritis Rheum 11(Suppl 1):123–124, 1981.

61. Edelman J, Owen ET: Acute progressive osteoarthropathy of large joints: Report of three cases. J Rheumatol 8:482–485, 1981.

62. Bollet AJ: Analgesic and anti-inflammatory drugs in the therapy of osteoarthritis. Semin Arthritis Rheum 11(Suppl 1):130–132, 1981.

63. Ehrlich GE: Brief review of rheumatic diseases and their response to drug therapy. *In* Paulus HE, Ehrlich GE, Lindenlaub E (eds.): Controversies in the Clinical Evaluation of Analgesic/Anti-Inflammatory/Antirheumatic Drugs. Stuttgart, F. K. Schattauer, 1980.

64. Dieppe PA, Sathapatayavongs D, Jones HE, et al.: Intra-articular steroids in osteoarthritis. Rheumatol Rehabil 19:212–217, 1980.

65. Palmoski MJ, Coyer RA, Brandt KD: Marked suppression by salicylate of the augmented proteoglycan synthesis in osteoarthritic cartilage. Arthritis Rheum 23:83–91, 1980.

66. Brandt KD, Palmoski M: Effects of nonsteroidal anti-inflammatory drugs on proteoglycan metabolism in articular cartilage. Semin Arthritis Rheum 11(Suppl 1):133–134, 1981.

67. Ehrlich GE, Di Piero AM: Stretch gloves: Nocturnal use to ameliorate morning stiffness in arthritic hands. Arch Phys Med Rehabil 52:479–480, 1971.

68. Radin EL: Aetiology of osteoarthrosis. Clin Rheum Dis 2:509–522, 1976.

69. Mankin HJ: Speculation regarding the biochemical pathogenesis of generalized osteoarthritis. J Rheumatol 10(Suppl 9):7–8, 1983.

70. O'Brien WM, Clemett AR, Acheson RM: Symptoms and patterns of osteoarthrosis in the hand in the New Haven survey of joint disease. *In* Bennet PH, Wood PHN (eds.): Population Studies in the Rheumatic Diseases. Amsterdam, Excerpta Medica, 1968, pp. 398–406.

71. Acheson RM, Chan YK, Clemett AR: New Haven survey of joint diseases. XII. Distribution and symptoms of osteoarthrosis in the hands with reference to handedness. Ann Rheum Dis 29:275–286, 1970.

72. Doyle DV, Dieppe PA, Scott J, et al.: An articular index for the assessment of osteoarthritis. Ann Rheum Dis 40:75–78, 1981.

12

Chondromalacia Patellae

David S. Hungerford, M.D.
Dennis W. Lennox, M.D.

The term chondromalacia patellae was first used by Koenig in 1924, although, according to Karlson, it had been in use in Aleman's clinic since 1917.[1] Aleman inserted the word "post-traumatica" in his classic publication in 1927, after which the term came to be widely used in the Scandinavian literature and subsequently in the English literature.[2] During this time, the term had specific meaning and signified a softening and splitting of the articular cartilage on the undersurface of the patella following injury. The traumatic nature of the lesion was universally accepted, as was the specific pathologic entity that was encountered at surgery. The seeds of confusion were sown by Owre with the publication of his doctoral thesis, in which he used the same term to describe a pathologic lesion on the undersurface of the patella in cadavers.[3] Owre's work was the first to point out the widespread and nearly universal changes of fissuring and softening that occurred with increasing frequency with age and could not necessarily be related to either injury or disease.

In 1941, Wiberg defined the main contact patterns of the patellofemoral joints as well as the principal anatomic variations that bear his name.[4] Although he felt that these anatomic variations might be related to patellofemoral disorders, particularly chondromalacia patellae, he was unable to demonstrate a relationship in his investigations. In 1944, Hirsch related the loss of mucopolysaccharides in the ground substance in articular cartilage to a change in its physical characteristics.[5] He hypothesized that this was the result of faulty cartilage nutrition, which led to softening and finally to fissure formation. The seeds sown by Owre came to fruition with the widespread use of the term "chondromalacia patellae" to mean a clinical entity signifying ill-defined anterior knee pain that was probably referable to the patellofemoral joint.[6] A myriad of clinical papers that did not include demonstration of the state of the patellar articular cartilage began to appear, culminating in the paper by Darracott and Vernon-Roberts describing the bony changes in "chondromalacia patellae," in which the majority of the patients had no articular cartilage lesion.[7] Thus, in the space of 50 years, a term that had a precise clinical and anatomic meaning had come to represent an ill-defined clinical entity obviously encompassing a multitude of clinical disorders, with the only common characteristic being anterior knee pain.

Goodfellow and associates suggested that the term "patellofemoral arthralgia" replace the clinical term chondromalacia patellae, although their use of the forbidden term in the title of their publication indicates the extent to which this terminology has become ingrained in clinical usage.[8] Medical practice is replete with imprecise terms, some more impressive than others. The term "internal derangement of the knee" has become much less frequently used as numerous specific disorders of the knee have become more clearly defined and more easily diagnosed. The use of that term also implies the need for further diagnostic investigation, and the clinician would seldom be satisfied to carry such a diagnosis indefinitely. However, for "chondromalacia patellae," the dilemma persists because both Aleman and Owre have defined valid concepts using the same terminology. It is certain that softening and fibrillation of patellar articular cartilage in the absence of clinical symptoms are widespread in an occidental population. It is also clear that deep fissuring associated with crepitus, swelling, and pain can occur following injury or recurrent patellar instability. Finally, anterior knee pain can exist in the absence of any articular cartilage abnormality.

Although we think that the term chondromalacia patellae would best be replaced by the term patellofemoral arthralgia, I have little hope that this will actually be accomplished. If the term would be used in the sense of internal derangement or fever of unknown origin (FUO), we would have little quarrel with its continued use. The user would then recognize the need for further investigation in order to more precisely define the origin of symptoms.

It is beyond the scope of this chapter to detail the processes by which articular cartilage fibrillates and softens; rather it will deal with delineating some of the known clinical syndromes that are manifested as anterior knee pain. There is no evidence to suggest that patellar articular cartilage is fundamentally different from articular cartilage in any diarthrodial joint. It is the thickest cartilage in the body, and the proteoglycan content has been demonstrated to be considerably lower than that in other cartilage, for example, the thinner cartilage covering the femoral head.[9] Because the patellofemoral joint is more incongruent than most diarthrodial articulations, it is likely that this reduced proteoglycan concentration and the attendant increased compliance allow the joint to achieve a larger contact area than it would with stiffer articular cartilage.

THE DIAGNOSTIC PROCESS

When a patient presents with anterior knee pain, a logical sequential utilization of available information-gathering techniques, rather than employment of the umbrella or, as some would say, "wastebasket" term of chondromalacia patellae, can aid significantly in establishing a specific diagnosis.

Clinical History

A history of anterior knee trauma is common in patients complaining of anterior knee pain. A significant injury may even have occurred in the relatively distant past, such as a fall on the flexed knee or a dashboard injury. If the patellar articular cartilage has been damaged, it may take many months or even years before its degeneration leads to symptoms. In addition, anterior knee trauma may lead to the development of post-traumatic reflex sympathetic dystrophy, which can be misinterpreted or missed. This will be covered in more detail later. Twisting injuries may also have resulted in damage to the extensor mechanism, so that even the positive diagnosis of a torn collateral ligament or meniscus would not rule out patellofemoral disease.

Anterior knee pain after prolonged sitting is one peculiar feature of patellofemoral disorders. Patients frequently give a history of aching pain after 45 to 60 minutes of sitting with the knee flexed at 90 degrees that subsides after moving about. Difficulty ascending and particularly descending stairs is also more common with patellofemoral disorders than with tibiofemoral pathology. The common symptom of "giving way" has been classically attributed to ligamentous instability or meniscal tear, but it may also be common with patellofemoral pathology.

Physical Examination

Examination of the knee must include a careful examination of the extensor apparatus. This begins with observing the patient rising from a chair. The use of the hands or excessive bending forward to bring the center of gravity more anteriorly is a positive indication of a painful knee. Because nonspecific anterior knee pain may be a common complaint in malingering and hysteria, additional confirmation of knee disability should be sought by observing patients when they are not aware that they are being observed.

The next step is to carefully examine the gait. Patellar abnormalities occur more frequently in patients with femoral anteversion and external tibial torsion. Observation of the gait may reveal the so-called "squinting knee cap," which is common with excessive femoral anteversion. With the patient supine on the examining table and the quadriceps mechanism relaxed, the Q angle should be measured. This is the angle made by the intersection of two lines, one connecting the center of the patella and the tibial tubercle, and the other connecting the center of the patella and the anterosuperior iliac spine along the line of the rectus femoris tendon. It should not measure more than 15 degrees. The presence of an abnormal Q angle is not necessarily associated with symptoms, however.

The quadriceps mechanism should be measured 6 and 10 inches above the tibial tubercle on both sides. Significant patellofemoral disorders are almost always associated with some quadriceps atrophy.

With the patella between the thumb and index finger and the quadriceps mechanism relaxed, the patella should be subluxated medially (Fig. 12–1A) and laterally (Fig. 12–1B). This excursion, referred to as the "play" of the patella, varies considerably from individual to individual but should be symmetric. Marked reduction in this patellar play is a frequent finding in reflex sympathetic dystrophy. Lateral patellar subluxation may be associated with the apprehension sign, in which the patient involuntarily contracts the quadriceps or otherwise restricts the examiner from performing further lateral subluxation. During this lateral subluxation, the lateral retinaculum should be palpated to search for any constricting bands.

Finally, starting with the leg in full extension, the patient should be requested to actively flex and then extend the knee while the examiner observes the tracking of the patella. Normally, the patella begins by being slightly lateral to the trochlear groove. As flexion occurs, the patella proceeds medially into the depth of the trochlear groove and, with flexion beyond 90 degrees, moves slightly laterally. This then describes a gentle "C" open laterally. During this action of flexion and extension, the patella should be palpated for crepitus. It should also be noted whether any crepitus is painful or asymptomatic.

Other chapters deal more completely with the total physical examination of the knee, but in the difficult patient in whom a diagnosis is not obvious, much more attention to detail than is customary must be directed to the extensor apparatus.

Roentgenographic Examination

We continue to see many patients referred for a second opinion who have not had a proper roentgenologic examination of the patellofemoral joint. Good-quality axial roentgenograms with the knee in 30, 60, and 90 degrees of flexion are essential to define the state of the patellofemoral articulation (Fig. 12–2). Anteroposterior and lateral roentgenograms of the knee provide relatively little information about the condition of the patellofemoral joint. Similarly, a poor roentgenographic examination of the patellofemoral joint itself is not helpful. In order to be useful,

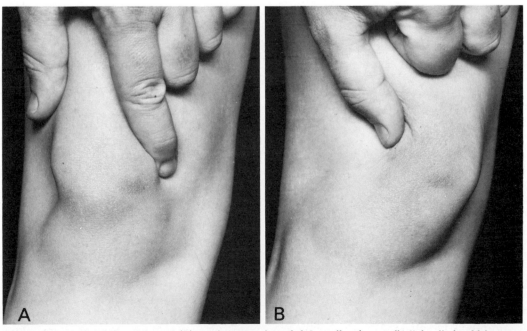

Figure 12–1. The medial (A) and lateral (B) passive excursion of the patella, the patella "play," should be compared with the asymptomatic side in all patients with anterior knee complaints.

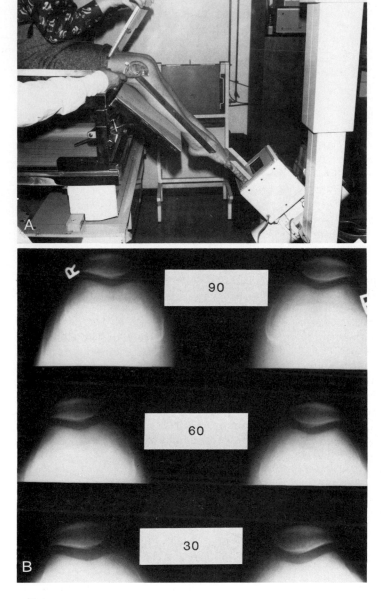

Figure 12–2. *A,* The x-ray technique of Ficat and Philippe maintains the beam parallel to the joint line and perpendicular to the x-ray cassette. *B,* Axial views in 30, 60, and 90 degrees of knee flexion show the full functional contact range of the patellofemoral articulation. (From Ficat P, Hungerford, DS: Disorders of the Patello-Femoral Joint. Baltimore, Williams and Wilkins, 1977.)

the x-ray beam must be perpendicular to the plate and parallel to the joint line. The technique described by Ficat and Philippe[10] is extremely useful, and such roentgenograms should be a part of at least the first roentgenologic examination of any patient with a knee complaint.

Arthrography

An arthrogram is generally performed when the diagnosis is in some doubt. Although it is a minimally invasive procedure, it is expensive

and exposes the patient to a significant amount of ionizing radiation. Therefore, the maximal amount of information should be gained; this includes axial views of the patellofemoral joint with the contrast material in place. Ficat and Philippe have routinely done this with single-contrast arthrography and have found identifiable disorders of patellar articular cartilage in 66% of patients with knee arthrography, compared with meniscal disorders in 13% of patients.[10] However, if double-contrast arthrography is performed, inflation of the joint with air may actually cause patellar subluxation not seen on the plain films. This would therefore be an artifact of the technique and not indicative of patellar subluxation. The subluxation itself, however, might be helpful in that the patella would be separated from the trochlea, and thus, defects in the patellar articular cartilage could be even more readily visible.

Diagnostic Arthroscopy

Diagnostic arthroscopy, particularly under local anesthesia on an outpatient basis, is extremely helpful in delineating various disorders of the knee. The menisci can usually be visualized in their entirety, and the undersurface of the patella can be well seen. There are, however, some pitfalls that must be recognized. The knee is insufflated with saline solution, and because the lateral retinacular structures are tighter than the medial retinaculum, this almost always leads to some lateral drift of the patella. We do not believe that the diagnosis of patellar subluxation should be made arthroscopically with the knee full of saline solution. It should be made on the basis of physical examination and appropriate standard roentgenograms. In addition, articular cartilage surface fibrillation and even deep cartilage fibrillation appear much more significant through the magnification of the arthroscope than they do to the naked eye at arthrotomy. Furthermore, we know from autopsy studies that most occidental adults over the age of 30 will have some fibrillation or fissure formation in their patellar articular cartilage, and we also know that in the vast majority of these patients it will be asymptomatic. Therefore, the mere presence of cartilage fibrillation does not identify the abnormality as the cause of the anterior knee pain.

DIFFERENTIAL DIAGNOSES

There are many specific causes of anterior knee pain, and an attempt at a specific diagnosis should always be made.

Bursitis

The prepatellar bursa, which is subcutaneous, can usually be easily identified when it is inflamed and the source of symptoms. However, the retropatellar tendon bursa, which is not so obvious, can also be the source of anterior knee pain. This bursa, which is situated proximal to the tibial tubercle and between the patellar tendon and the anterior tibia, can be palpated through the patellar tendon when the quadriceps is relaxed. When the quadriceps is tense, tension is transmitted to the patellar tendon and the bursa is protected from the examining finger. It is particularly useful to search for this area of tenderness in a patient with pain following a patellectomy, because the patella normally holds the patellar tendon away from the proximal tibia. The absence of the patella allows the patellar tendon to come into contact with the proximal tibia when the knee is flexed.

Although situated on the medial aspect of the tibial metaphysis, the pes anserinus bursa, when symptomatic, is frequently referenced as the source of diffuse anterior and anteriomedial pain. Symptoms are often confused with those of a meniscal lesion because of the medial localization, but abnormalities in the bursa can also be misdiagnosed as a patellofemoral disorder. This bursa should also be specifically palpated during an examination of the knee.

Plica Synovialis

There are at least two *normal* plicae in the knee, which are more or less prominent. The suprapatellar plica is a remnant of the septum that separates the embryonic suprapatellar bursa from the knee cavity. This septum rarely remains intact to completely separate the bursa from the knee. Its remnant may be vestigial or prominent, but because of its position, 1.5 to 2 cm proximal to the patella, it rarely causes symptoms. The medial plica is a synovial pleat running from the medial side of the suprapatellar plica to the ala of the fat pad. Owing to trauma or chronic irritation, it may hypertrophy and cause a snapping sensation with knee flexion and extension. Perhaps the main significance of the plicae are that they can be an obstacle to the easy manipulation of the arthroscope from one compartment to the other. Although hypertrophied plicae can certainly cause anterior knee symptoms, it is unlikely that they are the culprit as frequently as is claimed by many arthroscopists.

Apophysitis

Both the tibial tubercle and the distal pole of the patella are the site of apophysitis in adolescents and may lead to the complaint of anterior knee pain. Physical examination will demonstrate point tenderness at these sites, and the roentgenogram will generally show separation of the apophysis from the main bone. Tibial tubercle apophysitis is referred to as Osgood-Schlatter disease, and the apophysitis at the distal pole of the patella is termed Sinding-Larsen-Johansson disease. Both of these are self-limiting conditions, and the symptoms generally resolve when growth is complete. It is important not to mistake the symptoms for a more serious disorder.

It is also not uncommon to see tendinitis in both of these areas in active and sports-minded adults. Quick stop-and-go sports such as racquetball and squash are more likely to produce these symptoms, which presumably originate from minor separation of tendon fibers from the bony attachments. This disruption accompanied by point tenderness is most likely to occur at the distal pole of the patella, but unless specifically sought by digital palpation with the quadriceps relaxed, it is easily missed.

Malalignment

The patellofemoral joint is probably the joint most frequently afflicted by malalignment syndromes. Dysplasia of both the patella and the patellofemoral groove (trochlea) leads to a disruption in the normal balance of forces around the patellofemoral joint. Rotational malalignments of the femur and tibia may also lead to an increase in the Q angle, which increases the tendency of the patella to subluxate laterally. Finally, injury may produce atrophy of the vastus medialis, which causes a shift of the resultant vector in a more valgus direction, thereby functionally increasing the Q angle. The diagnosis can be suspected by a history of recurrent giving way, particularly with rotational movements of the knee (turning and cutting), and at physical examination by the apprehension sign. In most instances, the 30-degree axial view will show either frank subluxation of the patella or a patellar tilt (Fig. 12–3).

Merchant and coworkers[11] have developed

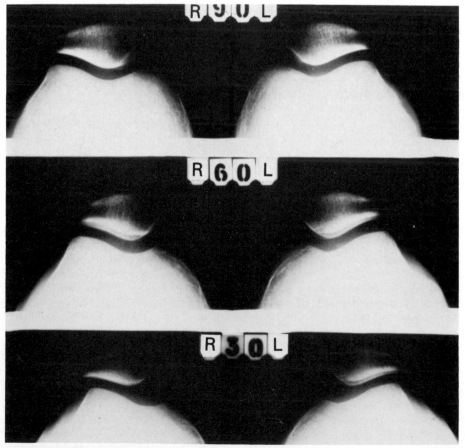

Figure 12–3. This axial view in 30 degrees of knee flexion shows significant lateral subluxation of both patellae but perfect recentering at 60 and 90 degrees of flexion. (From Ficat P, Hungerford DS: Disorders of the Patello-Femoral Joint. Baltimore, Williams and Wilkins, 1977.)

a technique for measuring the roentgenograms to show minimal degrees of subluxation, and Laurin and colleagues[12] have a method for showing minimal degrees of tilt. In most instances, the subluxation will have reduced by 60 to 90 degrees of flexion, but occasionally patients will be seen in whom the patella is subluxated in all flexion views. These patients are less likely to have symptoms of giving way and are more likely to have symptoms of pain. The stable malalignments, i.e., those that maintain malalignment throughout the full range of movement, are much more likely to undergo rapid degeneration of the articular cartilage because of a significantly reduced weight-bearing area.

Post-Traumatic Chondromalacia

Before 1936, the term chondromalacia patellae was limited to this particular clinical entity. The history includes a significant blow to the anterior knee, such as a dashboard injury; a significant fall, with landing occurring directly on the flexed knee; an athletic injury in which the knee cap was forcefully struck; or a patellar fracture. After the initial sequelae

Figure 12–4. A and B, Routine axial views in a patient with post-traumatic painful retropatellar crepitus show no abnormality. C and D, Axial views with contrast material demonstrate cartilage erosion. E, Surgical findings demonstrate massive deep fissuring of the central portion of the patella articular cartilage. (From Ficat P, Hungerford DS: Disorders of the Patello-Femoral Joint. Baltimore, Williams and Wilkins, 1977.)

of the injury have passed, there is usually a relatively or completely asymptomatic period, after which crepitus, recurrent effusion, and anterior knee pain return. The physical examination shows significant retropatellar crepitus associated with pain, and an effusion. Patellar facet tenderness may also be present but is not mandatory for diagnosis.

The roentgenograms are often completely within normal limits, although in good-quality films, a mild reduction in joint-line thickness can usually be detected without evidence of subluxation. Any subluxation that may be present is simply secondary to lateral drift of the patella due to loss of cartilage substance. The gross pathologic findings at surgery are usually much more extensive than would be expected from the plain roentgenograms (Fig. 12–4).

The Excessive Lateral Pressure Syndrome

Ficat and Hungerford have defined a syndrome that is based on a systematic, careful roentgenographic evaluation of patients with anterior knee pain.[13] It is likely that the exces-

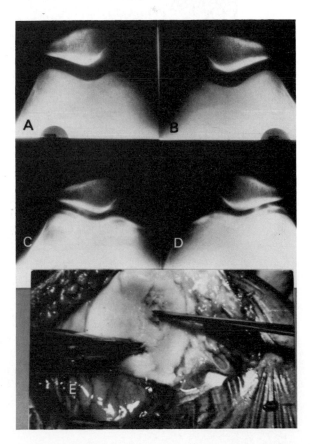

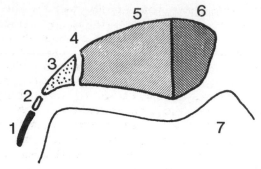

Figure 12–5. Evidence of excessive lateral tethering can be identified on good quality axial patellofemoral radiographs (1 = fibrosis of lateral retinaculum; 2 = calcification of lateral retinaculum; 3 = lateral osteophyte; 4 = bipartite patella; 5 = lateral facet hyperplasia; 6 = medial compartment hypoplasia; 7 = medial compartment hypoplasia). (Redrawn from Ficat P, Hungerford DS: Disorders of the Patello-Femoral Joint. Baltimore, Williams and Wilkins, 1977.)

sive lateral pressure syndrome (ELPS) represents the first stage of a continuum of malalignment syndromes in which the malalignment is first seen as an imbalance in the forces applied to the anterior knee. Evidence of this imbalance is seen in two areas. In the first instance, there is roentgenographic evidence of excessive lateral tethering (Fig. 12–5). This is seen in increased density in the soft tissue of the lateral retinaculum in the skyline view, calcification in the lateral retinaculum, traction osteophytes on the lateral side of the joint, or even stress fractures along the lateral facet.

The other evidence of excessive lateral pressure is seen in the skyline views of the patellofemoral joint in the form of increased subchondral sclerosis, altered orientation of the trabecular stress pattern, medial facet osteoporosis, lateral facet predominance, and lateral trochlear hypoplasia (Fig. 12–6).

Pauwels has shown that trabecular bone, responding as described by Wolfe's law, can literally be read like a photoelastic model.[14] Therefore, a critical examination of the stress patterns in the subchondral plate and the trabecular bone can afford great insight into the forces to which the patellofemoral joint is subjected. The delineation of the excessive lateral pressure syndrome as a clinical roentgenologic entity is therefore useful in detecting the application of abnormal force patterns before such patterns are manifested by the mechanical destruction of the tissues making up the joint.

Reflex Sympathetic Dystrophy

It has not been common to think of reflex sympathetic dystrophy (RSD) as affecting an isolated intermediate joint. However, over the past several years, we have seen nearly 50 patients who presented with symptoms of cutaneous hypersensitivity, sensitivity to cold, and marked osteoporosis limited to the knee. These symptoms responded to sympathetic block and, when necessary, sympathectomy. More subtle forms of this syndrome may also play a role in lesser degrees of anterior knee pain. Moreover, if the diagnosis is not included as a part of the differential diagnosis, even the more flamboyant forms of this condition will be missed, as evidenced by the fact that the majority of patients presenting to our clinic with this syndrome have undergone multiple fruitless surgical procedures. In our experience, reflex sympathetic dystrophy of the knee has always followed an injury. In that sense, it is a complication of an injury that may have produced other derangements as well. Therefore, the positive identification of other pathology—such as a torn ligament or meniscus or post-traumatic chondromalacia patellae—does not necessarily exclude the diagnosis of RSD. Because surgical intervention in the face of RSD will almost inevitably fail, it is important to rule out this condition in any patient who is considered a surgical candidate for other reasons.

A strong suspicion of RSD can be established by the clinical history alone. No other conditions around the knee are characterized by cutaneous hypersensitivity. The patient who

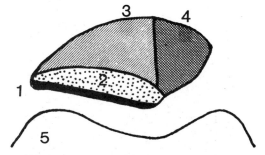

Figure 12–6. Evidence of excessive lateral pressure can be read into the form of the joint and the quality and orientation of the trabecular and subchondral bone (1 = thickening of subchondral plate; 2 = increased density of lateral facet cancellous bone; 3 = lateralization of trabeculae; 4 = medial facet osteoporosis; 5 = hypoplasia of the lateral condyle). (Redrawn from Ficat P, Hungerford DS: Disorders of the Patello-Femoral Joint. Baltimore, Williams and Wilkins, 1977.)

reacts almost hysterically to even the gentlest knee examination may be suffering from RSD rather than hysteria. The anterior aspect of the knee is frequently noticeably colder than that of the opposite knee, particularly if the temperature in the examining room is not above 70°F. This temperature differential can be documented and quantitated on a thermogram, which is an extremely useful diagnostic aid. Although all cases give a history of significant hypersensitivity to cold, this history must be sought by direct questioning and only seldom is volunteered by the patient. Although the pain associated with RSD is similar to anterior knee pain of other etiologies, it is usually more intense, more disabling, and less frequently associated with activity. Night pain is almost exclusively limited to RSD, and some patients will report an irritation of the anterior knee by the bedclothes at night, often leading to unique solutions of avoiding this discomfort.

The diagnostic suspicion can be further enhanced by good-quality axial patellofemoral roentgenograms in which both patellae appear. Although osteoporosis of the patella (Fig. 12–7) is not pathognomonic of RSD, the severe microcystic changes found in the more advanced cases of RSD are seldom seen in other conditions. Likewise, the bone scan in RSD is nonspecific, and increased uptake may be seen with a variety of conditions about the knee,

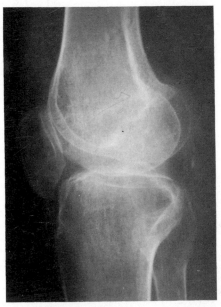

Figure 12–7. The patella shows marked osteoporosis. Although not pathognomonic of RSD, this finding is strong evidence of the condition, particularly in a suggestive clinical setting.

including disuse osteoporosis, fracture, infection, and tumor. However, in RSD, the uptake is particularly intense and is often limited to the anterior aspect of the knee. The sine qua non in establishing the diagnosis is the response to a sympathetic block. Dramatic reduction in symptoms can be expected during the effect of the sympathetic block, and the area that was cool on the preblock thermogram can be shown on a postblock thermogram to have undergone the greatest vasodilation and increased warmth (Fig. 12–8).

PATHOLOGY

As mentioned previously, there is nothing to indicate that patellar articular cartilage is different from other cartilage in the body. However, the particular anatomy of the patellofemoral joint and the thickness of the cartilage, together with the accessibility of the patellofemoral joint to direct visualization either at arthrotomy or at arthroscopy, have led to a better documentation of the earliest stages of patellar articular cartilage degeneration. Patellar articular cartilage is subject to surface fibrillation in the areas of habitual noncontact, similar to changes found in other joints.[15] This particularly affects the odd facet because this area does not make contact until after 90 to 100 degrees of flexion. This area on the medial margin of the medial facet almost never undergoes progressive full-thickness cartilage loss, and the mild softening and surface fibrillation that are frequently seen at arthrotomy must not be mistaken for the more significant lesions in the weight-bearing area of the patella.

The first lesion of patellar articular cartilage is the blister lesion, in which the mid-layer fibers in the C2 region of articular cartilage (Fig. 12–9) have ruptured, allowing the proteoglycans to swell though increased water absorption. The ruptured C2 fibers allow the C1 layer to tent into the typical blister lesion. It is not common to find such a beautiful example as shown in Figure 12–10. Usually, the C1 layer has already ruptured, and the fissures in the articular cartilage can be seen extending deep within the cartilage substance (Fig. 12–11). Once the intrinsic fabric of the cartilage structure has ruptured, much of the mechanical characteristics of articular cartilage has been lost. Under continued use, the fragments shed into the joint and may provoke a synovitis, although this is usually mild. Further

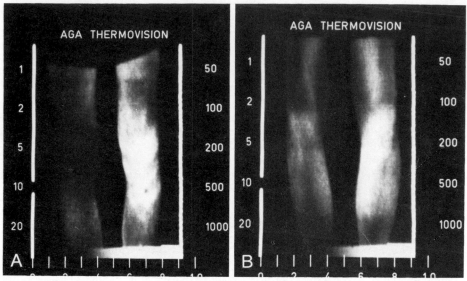

Figure 12–8. *A,* The preblock thermogram shows significant reduction of temperature over the anterior knee on the symptomatic right side. *B,* After a lumbar sympathetic block, the area of previously decreased temperature shows dramatic vasodilation.

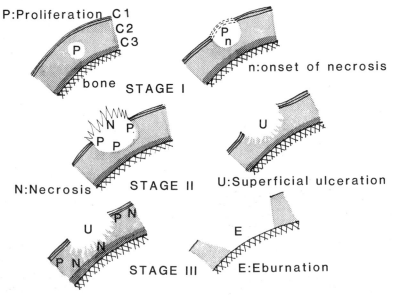

Figure 12–9. The schematic representation of the pathway of patellar articular cartilage degeneration (C1, C2, and C3 represent superficial, mid, and deep cartilage layers, respectively). (Redrawn from Ficat P, Hungerford, DS: Disorders of the Patello-Femoral Joint. Baltimore, Williams and Wilkins, 1977.)

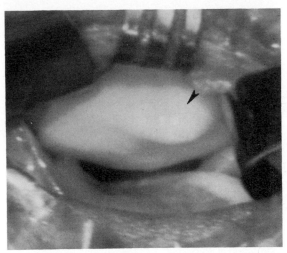

Figure 12–10. "Blister" lesion at the medial margin of the medial facet.

loss of cartilage substance leads to erosive changes, which eventually progress to full-thickness cartilage loss and subchondral sclerosis. Osteoarthrosis of the patellofemoral joint in this stage is indistinguishable from that in other diarthrodial joints. The sequence of events is schematically diagrammed in Figure 12–9. From autopsy studies, it is certain that this sequence can span several decades and, in many individuals, will never pass the area of fibrillated fissured articular cartilage, which produces no symptoms.

TREATMENT

First and foremost must be a determined attempt to establish a specific diagnosis. The concept that chondromalacia patellae is a single disease entity must be rejected. The term should be regarded in much the same way as the nephrologist regards the term nephrotic

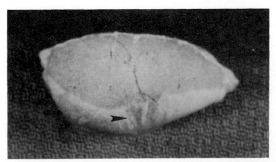

Figure 12–11. Cross section of a patella showing fissure formation extending to calcified cartilage (arrow).

syndrome. The malacic change that occurs in the patellar articular cartilage is simply the final common pathway through which the articular cartilage in the patella degenerates. The specific condition effecting the malacic change must be sought and, if possible, corrected.

It must also be recognized that the origin of the symptoms is unclear. Some have thought that the symptoms emanate from synovial irritation due to the cartilage debris. However, at arthroscopy, the synovium is seldom more than mildly inflamed, and a significant effusion is more uncommon. It is likely that the symptoms come from subchondral bone to which forces are abnormally transferred through articular cartilage that has an altered mechanical state.

Conservative Management

In spite of this deficiency in our understanding of the mechanisms of joint pain, a number of empiric conservative modalities have been recommended that are successful in relieving symptoms in most instances. DeHaven and associates[16] reported an overall success rate of 82% in controlling symptoms through a treatment program consisting of (1) an anti-inflammatory agent (usually aspirin); (2) a progressive resistance exercise program of isometric quadriceps and isotonic hamstring exercises; (3) a graduated running program; and (4) a maintenance program consisting of activities as tolerated, continuation of the progressive resistance exercises 2 to 3 days a week, and patellar braces and shoe orthoses where indicated. Most authors reporting on surgical management of anterior knee pain report a high percentage of success with similar conservative management programs, restricting surgery to those patients who fail to have symptomatic relief after having completed an extensive period of conservative management.

The exact mechanism by which quadriceps rehabilitation produces symptomatic relief of anterior knee pain is not specifically understood, but it must be remembered that the final common vector of quadriceps pull is a function of the balance between its four heads. Specifically, vastus medialis atrophy could lead to a valgus orientation of the quadriceps vector, which would result in improper tracking of the patella. This might be below the level that could be detected roentgenologically. Rehabilitation would then serve the same function as surgically reorienting this vector.

Lateral Patellar Release

This procedure has become increasingly popular, and the overall results have been reported as good.[17] It is currently frequently being done as an arthroscopic procedure in the belief that it at least does no harm. However, overzealous lateral release can lead to an imbalance in the quadriceps mechanism in the opposite direction, and in one recent case, medial dislocation occurred following an extensive lateral release (Fig. 12–12). As with any surgical procedure, it should be performed only in those cases for which there is a specific indication, i.e., ELPS or one of the malalignment syndromes.

Patellar Shaving

There has been a general dissatisfaction with shaving fibrillated patellar articular cartilage via open arthrotomy. However, the widespread use of arthroscopy and particularly motorized shaving equipment has led to the common practice of debridement of cartilage debris from the undersurface of the patella. Patients frequently report reduction in their symptoms following such procedures, although some report similar improvement from arthroscopy and joint lavage alone. The advisability of shaving fibrillated articular cartilage surface can be determined only after longer-term follow-up than has been currently reported. However, what is known about the metabolism and healing of articular cartilage would suggest that such procedures could be expected to offer only temporary relief at best.

Chondrectomy

Ficat and associates have reported good results in severe cases of patellar articular cartilage degeneration utilizing a procedure that consists of removal of the articular cartilage with vertical borders and removal of the subchondral plate in its entirety.[18] This was termed spongialization because the cancellous bone, or spongiosa, was exposed. This concept is an extension of the Pridie procedure, in which the sclerotic subchondral plate was perforated in order to facilitate recovering of the joint surface with fibrocartilage.[19] This procedure requires a very long rehabilitation period to allow the defect first to fill with granulation tissue and then to undergo metaplasia to fibrocartilage and should be reserved for cases in which significant disability exists.

Proximal Realignment

Insall, Bullough, and Burstein have described a technique for realigning the pull of the quadriceps through a proximal imbrication and have reported good results.[20] We have no personal experience with this technique.

Distal Realignment

The results of the Hauser procedure have been discouraging when followed for long periods.[21] However, overzealous medial and distal transfer of the tibial tubercle can probably account for at least some of the failures. Medial displacement of the tibial tubercle by the method described by Hauser results in a posterior displacement of the tibial tubercle that exerts an adverse biomechanical effect that results in increased patellofemoral compression. The procedure as described by Trillat and associates[22] and attributed to Elmsly does not result in posterior displacement, and the results to date have been very satisfactory.

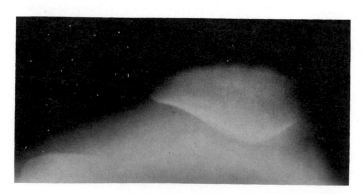

Figure 12–12. Medial dislocation of the patella following overzealous lateral release.

Tibial Tubercle Elevation

Both Maquet[23] and Bandi and Brennwald[24] have reported in large series the relief of anterior knee pain in patients with significant cartilage lesions or even cartilage and bone lesions by osteotomizing the tibial tubercle and elevating it with a bone block. This procedure can also be combined with a medial displacement of the tibial tubercle if necessary. The procedure improves the biomechanics of the patellofemoral joint and reduces the patellofemoral compression load. It also has a role in improving strength in a knee following patellectomy.

SUMMARY

The patellofemoral joint is the site of a wide variety of conditions that have a similar clinical presentation—that of anterior knee pain. In the past, the identification of anterior knee pain has led to a diagnosis of "chondromalacia patellae," which is about as meaningful as the term "internal derangement of the knee." The term "chondromalacia patellae" should be restricted to a description of the pathologic changes on the undersurface of the patella that are the result of a number of specific underlying conditions. The symptom of anterior knee pain in a given individual should lead to a rigorous search for a specific underlying cause. Only then can the appropriate treatment be instituted.

References

1. Karlson S: Chondromalacia patellae. Acta Chir Scand 83:347–381, 1940.
2. Aleman O: Chondromalacia post-traumatica patellae. Acta Chir Scand 63:194–199, 1928.
3. Owre AA: Chondromalacia patellae. Acta Chir Scand (Suppl)77:41, 1936.
4. Wiberg G: Roentgenographic and anatomic studies on the femoropatellar joint. Acta Orthop Scand 12:319–410, 1941.
5. Hirsch C: A contribution to the pathogenesis of chondromalacia of the patella. A physical, histologic and chemical study. Acta Chir Scand 90 (Suppl):83, 1944.
6. Robinson AR, Darracott J: Chondromalacia patellae. A survey conducted at the Army Medical Rehabilitation Unit, Chester. Ann Phys Med 10:286–290, 1970.
7. Darracott J, Vernon-Roberts B: The bone changes in "chondromalacia patellae." Rheumatol Phys Med 11:175–179, 1971.
8. Goodfellow JW, Hungerford DS, Woods C: Patellofemoral mechanics and pathology. II. Chondromalacia patellae. J Bone Joint Surg 58B:291–299, 1976.
9. Ficat C, Maroudas A: Cartilage of the patella. Ann Rheum Dis 34:515–519, 1975.
10. Ficat RP, Philippe J: Contrast Arthrography of the Synovial Joints. New York, Masson Inc., 1981.
11. Merchant A, Mercer R, Jacobsen R, Cool CR: Roentgenographic analysis of patello-femoral congruence. J Bone Joint Surg 56A:1391–1396, 1974.
12. Laurin CA, Levesque MP, Dussault R, et al.: The abnormal lateral patello-femoral angle: A diagnostic roentgenographic sign of recurrent subluxation. J Bone Joint Surg 60A:55–60, 1978.
13. Ficat P, Hungerford DS: Disorders of the Patello-Femoral Joint. Baltimore, Williams and Wilkins, 1977.
14. Pauwels F: Biomechanics of the Locomotor Apparatus. New York, Springer-Verlag, 1980.
15. Goodfellow JW, Bullough P: The pattern of aging of the articular cartilage of the elbow joint. J Bone Joint Surg 49B:175–181, 1967.
16. DeHaven KE, Dolan WA, Mayer PJ: Chondromalacia patellae in athletes. Am J Sports Med 7:1–5, 1979.
17. Merchant A, Mercer R: Lateral release of the patella. A preliminary report. Clin Orthop Rel Res 103:40–45, 1974.
18. Ficat RP, Ficat C, Gedron P, Toussaint JB: Spongialization—a new treatment for diseased patellae. Clin Orthop Rel Res 144:74–83, 1979.
19. Pridie KH: A method of resurfacing osteoarthritic knee joints. J Bone Joint Surg 41B:618, 1959.
20. Insall J, Bullough PG, Burstein AM: Proximal "tube" realignment of the patella for chondromalacia patellae. Clin Orthop Rel Res 144:63–69, 1979.
21. Crosby EB, Insall J: Recurrent dislocation of the patella. J Bone Joint Surg 58A:9–13, 1976.
22. Trillat A, Dejour H, Coutette A: Diagnostic et traitement des subluxations récidivantes de la rotule. Rev Chir Orthop 50:813–824, 1964.
23. Maquet PGJ: Biomechanics of the Knee with Application to the Pathogenesis and the Surgical Treatment of Osteoarthritis. New York, Springer-Verlag, 1976.
24. Bandi W, Brennwald J: The significance of femoropatellar pressure in the pathogenesis and treatment of chondromalacia patellae and femoro-patellar arthrosis. *In* The Knee Joint. New York, American Elsevier Publishers, Inc., 1974.

13

Diffuse Idiopathic Skeletal Hyperostosis (DISH, Ankylosing Hyperostosis)

Peter D. Utsinger, M.D.

Diffuse idiopathic skeletal hyperostosis (DISH) is a common skeletal disease of unknown etiology seen in middle-aged and elderly patients. The principal manifestations of DISH are ligamentous calcification and ossification of the anterolateral aspect of the spinal column, sometimes leading to bony ankylosis (Figs. 13–1 and 13–2). DISH also frequently involves the peripheral skeletal system, where ligamentous calcification and osteophyte and spur formation are seen (Figs. 13–3 and 13–4). DISH has been described in various forms for at least 50 years; it is one of the curiosities of modern rheumatology that such a common illness should have received so little attention. It is only recently that more extensive work has been done, leading to the establishment of diagnostic criteria, a description of the primary clinical features, and the delineation of the extensive roentgenographic abnormalities. In addition, insights into hypotheses of pathogenic and etiologic mechanisms can now be developed.

HISTORICAL ASPECTS

Patients who have clinical features consistent with DISH have been described in the literature, primarily in anecdotal form, for decades (Table 13–1). In 1938, Meyer and Forster[1] described a patient with hyperostosis and calcification on the right side of the thoracic spine and named the entity "moniliform hyperostosis." In 1942, Oppenheimer[2] described 282 elderly patients with calcification of vertebral ligaments; he called the condition "spondylitis ossificans ligamentosa." Eighteen of these patients had abnormalities of the spine unaccompanied by changes of typical spondylosis deformans. Ossification was found predominantly in the thoracic spine, involving the anterior longitudinal ligament. He theorized that the calcification was secondary to immobilization of the spine causing undifferentiated connective tissue to ossify. A similar condition was described by Lacapère[3] in 1949, which he called "melorheostosis of the spine." In 1950, Forestier and Rotes-Querol[4] were the first to systematically study the abnormalities that collectively they called "senile ankylosing hyperostosis." This paper, a classic in clinical rheumatology, was based on a study of nine patients and two cadavers. The patients described moderately severe spinal stiffness, sometimes associated with "lumbago" or sciatica. Attention was called to the characteristic roentgenographic findings in the patients, and the authors hypothesized that "internal secretions" of the prostate, traveling via anastomoses of venous and lymphatic channels between the prostate and the vertebral column, might be of pathogenetic importance. These authors and others further defined the condition over the next 20 years.[5, 6] In 1975 and 1976, Resnick, Utsinger, and coworkers emphasized the frequency of extraskeletal manifestations of the condition,[7, 8] and Resnick suggested the name DISH, a term that is currently widely accepted.

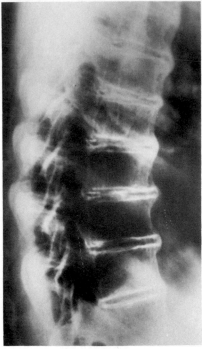

Figure 13–1. Flowing ossification along the anterior aspect of the mid-thoracic spine has resulted in a bumpy vertebral contour. The apophyseal joints are normal.

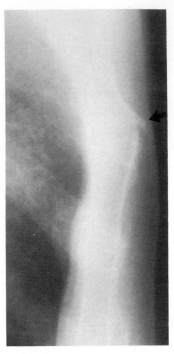

Figure 13–3. Anterior osseous excrescences at the manubriosternal joint (arrow).

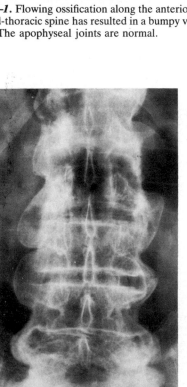

Figure 13–2. Extensive osteophytosis is apparent involving the right and left aspects of the lumbar spine. The osseous bridges have resulted in complete bony ankylosis across multiple intervertebral disk spaces.

DIAGNOSTIC CRITERIA

Criteria for the diagnosis of DISH have not been uniform. For epidemiologic purposes, we have found it convenient to use the following diagnostic criteria for DISH:

1. Continuous calcification and ossification along the anterolateral aspect of at least four contiguous vertebral bodies.

2. Essentially normal disk space height in the involved areas.

3. Absence of apophyseal joint ankylosis.

4. Absence of erosions, sclerosis, or fusion of the sacroiliac joints.

5. Continuous calcification and ossification along the anterolateral aspect of at least two contiguous vertebral bodies.

6. Calcaneal, olecranon, or patellar spurs.

7. Enthesis ossification. (Enthesis = site of muscular or tendinous attachment to bone.)

8. Thoracic spine stiffness and pain with relative preservation of spinal motion and without fibromyositic pressure points in an adult older than 50 years of age.

9. Palpable, discrete spurs around the patella, elbow, or heel or a hard mass within tendons.

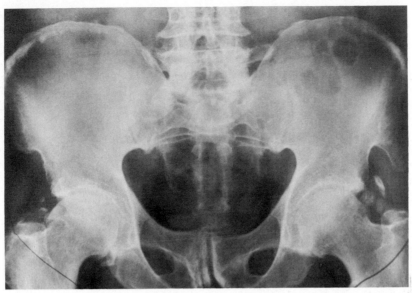

Figure 13–4. Eburnation and sclerosis involving large segments of the iliac crest, para-articular bone formation about the hips, bridging of the superior aspect of the symphysis pubis, and osteophytes developing across the inferior aspect of both sacroiliac joints.

Categories of DISH according to criteria (criteria 2 to 4 must be present in all categories) are as follows:

   A. Definite: 1
   B. Probable: 5, 6, 7, 8, 9
   C. Possible: (i) 5 and two of 6 to 9
           (ii) 6, 7, 8, 9

Definite criteria are highly specific at the expense of being insensitive. However, for epidemiologic purposes, they are quite useful. Probable criteria identify a set of patients who statistically are more likely to have DISH than another isolated rheumatic disease or group of rheumatic diseases. Possible criteria identify a set of patients who may be in the early stages of DISH. We believe that high specificity is a function of the duration of DISH. Credence for this concept comes from analysis of the ages of patients divided into these categories: Category A (definite DISH): 200 patients, mean age 63; Category B (probable DISH): 63 patients, mean age 60; Category C (possible DISH): 22 patients, mean age 56.

We have seen 18 patients in whom characteristic clinical and roentgenographic extra-axial features of DISH were unaccompanied by axial skeleton involvement; four of these have developed typical axial skeleton changes. Consequently, we feel that physicians may entertain a tentative diagnosis of DISH (Category Cii) even in the absence of any spinal abnormalities.

CLINICAL FEATURES

A large-scale population study will be needed to define with certainty the incidence of symptoms in subjects with DISH. Such a study is important because DISH is very common. A recent study in Finland involved following 6167 persons over age 29 for 6 years. The incidence of DISH was 0.7/100 patient years in males and 0.4/100 patient years in females over age 30.[9]

DISH has a marked male predominance, with clinical and autopsy studies showing an approximate 2:1 male-to-female ratio[5, 6, 10] (Table 13–2). In our group of 200 patients, 71% were males.[11] There is a strong suggestion that

Table 13–1. SOME OF THE MORE WIDELY USED SYNONYMS FOR DISH AND APPROXIMATE DATE OF INTRODUCTION

Moniliform hyperostosis, 1938
Spondylitis ossificans ligamentosa, 1942
Senile ankylosing hyperostosis of the spine, 1950
Ankylosing hyperostosis of Forestier and Rotes-Querol, 1952
Physiologic vertebral ligamentous calcification, 1955
Hyperostotic spondylosis, 1965
Ankylosing vertebral hyperostosis, 1969
Ankylosing hyperostosis, 1967
Hyperostosis of the spine, 1971
Diffuse idopathic skeletal hyperostosis, 1975

Table 13–2. AGE, SEX AND RACE CHARACTERISTICS IN FIVE GROUPS OF PATIENTS WITH DISH

| | Number of Patients | Age (years) | | Sex | | Race | | | | | |
| | | Mean | Range | Male | Female | Patients | | | Referral Population | | |
						Black	White	Other	Black	White	Other
Forestier and Lagier[6]	245	85%	> 50	65%	35%	?	?	?	?	?	?
Harris et al.[5]	34	67	47–83	17	17	?	?	?	?	?	?
Utsinger[11]	200	63	44–98	143	57	28	172	0	41	57	2
Resnick et al.[10]	21	66	49–80	21	0	1	20	0	30%	?	?
Shapiro[10]	24	65	51–81	16	8	0	24	0	10%	?	?

DISH affects whites more than blacks (Table 13–2).

Most clinical knowledge of DISH comes from studies[5-8] in which the patients are a unique subset because they were referred to rheumatologists. Our group of 200 patients with definite DISH,[11] from whom most of our experience has been culled, is also a skewed group, because they represent primarily hospitalized patients or patients referred to a rheumatology practice. As might be expected, the majority of patients described in the aforementioned studies have musculoskeletal symptoms.

Symptoms. An overwhelming number of our 200 patients (84%) have symptomatic disease (Tables 13–3 and 13–4). The hallmark and most striking clinical finding is stiffness, primarily in the thoracic spine. This stiffness is usually bimodal, being most marked in the morning, with recrudescence in the late evening after a reasonably stiffness-free day. Stiffness is precipitated by three events: inactivity, cold, and wet weather. Unfortunately, most patients also have pain. This pain is usually mild and involves primarily the thoracic spine; it rarely radiates. It is of interest that some patients describe thoracic pain years before roentgenographic documentation of definite DISH. Occasional patients describe spinal pain in the absence of any roentgenographic abnormality of the spine but in the presence of typical extra-axial roentgenographic changes (Category Cii).

In our series, 38% of the patients had peripheral joint and bone problems. The major areas of involvement were the heel, elbow, knee, and shoulder. Pain was worsened by both use and prolonged rest of the involved area. An important complaint in 56 patients was heel pain; indeed, in 11 patients it was the chief complaint. Fifty patients had elbow pain, and in 20 it was the chief complaint. Forty-two patients had knee or shoulder pain, and in seven it was the chief complaint. Pain in these peripheral sites was uniformly associated with roentgenographic abnormalities, typically spur formation or periostitis ("whiskering") (Fig. 13–5).

Table 13–3. SYMPTOMS IN 200 PATIENTS WITH DISH

	Percentage Involved
1. Spine	
A. Stiffness	84
Morning stiffness	83
Thoracic	80
Lumbar and/or cervical	32
Evening stiffness	36
Aggravated by sitting and inactivity	48
Aggravated by cold weather	42
Aggravated by wet weather	38
B. Pain	72
Thoracic	68
Lumbar and/or cervical	52
C. Dysphagia	14
2. Peripheral joints	
Pain	38
Swelling, heat, or redness	9
3. Bone pain	
Heel	28
Elbow	25
Shoulder	19
Knee	19
4. Neurologic symptoms	4

Table 13–4. PRIMARY CLINICAL CLUES TO THE PRESENCE OF DISH

1. Generalized tenderness at peripheral entheses.
2. Recurrent Achilles tendinitis.
3. Recurrent shoulder "bursitis."
4. Recurrent lateral or medial epicondylitis.
5. Palpable bony spurs (calcaneus, olecranon, patella).
6. Soft tissue mass adherent to quadriceps, patella, or Achilles tendon.
7. Dysphagia.
8. Restricted loss of motion following joint surgery, primarily total joint replacement.

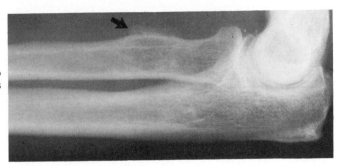

Figure 13–5. Ossification is apparent adjacent to the radial tuberosity (arrow). There is hyperostosis at the ulnar attachment of the triceps.

Dysphagia is commonly found.[8, 12–14] In our series, 28 patients were afflicted, and it was the major and presenting complaint in 19. The dysphagia is due to compression of the esophagus by cervical osteophytes (Fig. 13–6); compression sometimes is severe enough to make eating solid food a strenuous chore.

Neurologic abnormalities occasionally occur in DISH. These reflect a myelopathy, secondary to either posterior osteophyte formation or posterior longitudinal ligament calcification.[15, 16] Symptoms are most commonly paresthesias, but motor disturbances can also be found. Urinary and rectal incontinence and sexual dysfunction are rare.

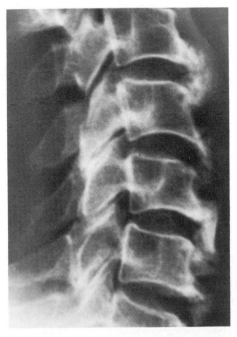

Figure 13–6. Osseous excrescences on the anterior aspect of multiple cervical vertebral bodies. The intervertebral disk spaces are preserved, and there is minor narrowing of the apophyseal joints.

Physical Signs. In the majority of studies, physical examination of the axial skeleton has been reported to be essentially normal, with two exceptions: slight loss of full flexion and extension and a decrease in lumbar lordosis. However, a study[10] in which particular attention was paid to recording range of motion demonstrated a decrease in both thoracolumbar and cervical range of motion in 48% and 55% of patients, respectively. Mildly decreased thoracic cage movement was also noted. In our series, the patients' spinal range of motion was compared with that in 50 age- and sex-matched controls with normal or minimally abnormal spine roentgenograms. Although spine motion appeared to be decreased on initial examination, after exercise and spinal massage only 9% of patients had significantly impaired motion, primarily a decrease in thoracolumbar motion.

In our series, spinal tenderness was noted frequently, with a 90% incidence in the thoracolumbar spine and a 60% incidence in the cervical spine. The characteristic location of fibromyositic "tender points" and postpressure cutaneous erythema was lacking.[17] Fifty-six of our patients had heel tenderness, 20 had palpable spurs, and all had calcaneal spurs on roentgenogram. Likewise, all 50 patients with elbow pain had olecranon spurs; in 46 patients, a bony mass was palpable. A palpable nodular mass is occasionally appreciated in the area of the infrapatellar and quadriceps tendons, Achilles tendon, medial and lateral collateral ligaments of the elbow, and the subdeltoid bursa of the shoulder. Decreased range of motion is often seen in the peripheral skeleton, but motion commonly increases after "limbering up."

Laboratory Aspects. Hyperglycemia is the best-defined laboratory abnormality in patients with DISH. In most studies,[5, 6, 8, 10, 11] the incidence of abnormal glucose tolerance tests is about 22%, and the incidence of overt diabetes is about 9%, a prevalence about twice that in an age-, sex-, and weight-matched population. In one recent study,[18] the incidence of diabetes mellitus was 40%. Laboratory studies that have been investigated extensively and are seemingly normal include complete blood count; erythrocyte sedimentation rate; calcium, phosphorus, alkaline phosphatase, and uric acid levels; VDRL; serum protein electrophoresis; serum immunoelectrophoresis; antinuclear antibody; and rheumatoid factor. Serum growth hormone and somatomedin and parathyroid hormone levels[11, 19] have been consistently normal. We have measured serum fluoride levels in 78 patients; in addition, we measured their water, food, and air fluoride levels at home and at work.[11, 20] No abnormalities have been detected.

Special Clinical Problems. Resnick and associates discussed three patients with DISH who developed heterotopic calcification as a consequence of total hip replacement.[21] This complication is similar to the "re-ankylosis" commonly encountered after total hip replacement in patients with ankylosing spondylitis.[22] None of these patients with DISH had predisposing factors for this complication (e.g., infection or history of multiple surgical procedures). The authors postulated that the same pathogenetic mechanisms underlying DISH may have been responsible for the extensive postsurgical ossification. We have seen this same complication after total hip arthroplasty in four patients with DISH. However, because the incidence of postsurgical heterotopic ossification varies from 5% to 53% in different series,[21] the small number of patients with DISH described with this complication makes it difficult to reach a meaningful conclusion about causality.

Resnick and colleagues reported eight patients who had coexistent rheumatoid arthritis and DISH.[23] These patients had unusual clinical features, including an increased frequency of flexion contractures and decreased joint range of motion of the elbows, wrists, ankles, and knees. Roentgenograms demonstrated features atypical for rheumatoid arthritis: lack of osteoporosis, sclerosis and proliferation around erosions, osteophytes in association with erosions, and ankylosis of joints, including carpal, tarsal, carpometacarpal and tarsometatarsal articulations. A reasonable speculation is that an attempt to heal the injuries due to rheumatoid arthritis resulted in an increased proliferation of bone owing to the coexistent abnormality of DISH.

Coexistent Diseases. In our group of 200 patients, 41% were obese, defined as being more than 15 pounds over the recommended weight for sex, age, body habitus, and height. In a sex- and age-matched hospitalized population without DISH, only 18% were obese. Ten per cent of the patients with DISH had diabetes mellitus, which required treatment, and another 16% had asymptomatic hyperglycemia. Although a hospitalized population is certainly not an ideal control group, the incidence of diabetes and asymptomatic hyperglycemia in age-, sex-, and weight-matched controls was only 9%. Hypertension was found in 22% of the patients with DISH, compared with 16% in the control group. An increased incidence of obesity, diabetes, and hypertension in patients with DISH has been found in other studies,[5, 8, 9, 24–26] suggesting that endocrine and metabolic factors may play a role.

Because there is no cogent reason for DISH protecting one from other rheumatic diseases, the clinician must also be alerted to the development (superimposition) of a new rheumatic disease in patients presenting with joint complaints. Indeed, DISH does coexist frequently with rheumatoid arthritis, erosive osteoarthritis, gout and calcium pyrophosphate dihydrate deposition disease but not in a higher incidence than that in the population at large.

TREATMENT

There is only symptomatic therapy for DISH; it is unknown whether any treatment alters the natural history of the disease. Patients should be reassured that the disease is comparatively benign and does not resemble potentially crippling forms of spinal arthritis. In most patients, spinal stiffness is ameliorated with a physical therapy program emphasizing the application of wet heat, ultrasound, peripheral joint range of motion exercises, and back extension exercises. We encourage swimming programs on a thrice-weekly basis. Many patients have more mobility while receiving nonsteroidal anti-inflammatory agents. We commonly use analgesic drugs such as acetaminophen to decrease pain in the spine. Obese patients are encouraged to lose weight. Pain in the peripheral skeleton usually responds to nonsteroidal anti-inflammatory drugs and analgesics. Pain from spurs can be relieved with injections of lidocaine with or without steroids. If pain continues to be troublesome, we use orthoses to diminish pressure on heel spurs and foam-rubber "donuts" to encase knee or elbow spurs. If spur-induced pain is not helped by these measures, the spur may be removed. We have seen one patient with massive heterotopic ossification around the elbow after an olecranon spur was removed; this patient's experience may be a caveat. Patients with dysphagia due to osteophytes are first instructed to chew food thoroughly; if dysphagia continues, they are encouraged to eat soft foods. In the uncommon situation in which this is unsuccessful, surgical removal of the osteophytes generally relieves symptoms. Before dysphagia is attributed to DISH, all patients should undergo a careful evaluation for esophageal carcinoma. Laminectomy helps the majority of patients disabled by a myelopathy due to posterior osteophytes.[11, 17]

ETIOLOGY AND PATHOGENESIS: AREAS OF INVESTIGATION

The etiology and pathogenesis of DISH are unknown. Research has focused on possible genetic, metabolic-endocrine, and toxic factors. Because of the striking association of ankylosing spondylitis with HLA-B27, we and others studied small numbers of patients, looking at alleles of the HLA-B locus. Discrepant results have been found. In an original report, 16 of 47 patients with DISH were HLA-B27–positive,[20] and in our new group of 200 patients, 21 were HLA-B27–positive.[11] However, other studies[27–29] have shown no increase in this allele or have shown an increase in other antigens such as HLA-B5,[28] HLA-B8,[27] and HLA-A11.[29] Extensive studies of the Pima Indians have shown a prevalence of DISH of 50%, with an 18% frequency of HLA-B27.[30] However, no significant association was seen between any A or B locus antigens when Pima Indians with DISH were compared with age-matched controls. Several points are worth considering when viewing these contradictory findings. First, patients culled from a practice-hospital setting may be more likely to have a coexistent disease, and that disease may be present in linkage disequilibrium with a B or A locus antigen. Second, there may be genetic differences in susceptibility to DISH; the Pima Indians may differ from the Caucasians (the putative predisposing gene may be different in both groups but may be in linkage disequilibrium with the same alleles). Third, the striking fact about HLA-disease associations is that most diseases are associated with alleles of the HLA-D locus. There is a real possibility that certain HLA-A and HLA-B locus antigens exist in a common linkage disequilibrium with a D locus antigen, with which there is a much stronger genetic association, analogous to the situation seen in multiple sclerosis. In other words, it is possible that described associations are due to a linked gene in linkage disequilibrium with the measured genes. Clearly, studies similar to the epidemiologic one described by Spagnole and coworkers[30] need to be done; in particular, D locus typing should be performed.

Metabolic factors may play a role in DISH, because field studies[9] excluding so-called Berkson's fallacies[31] have shown a higher than expected incidence of both diabetes mellitus and obesity.[32]

The relationship between diabetes mellitus and DISH may provide seminal insight. It is interesting that the Pima Indians, in whom DISH is so prevalent, also have an increased incidence of diabetes.[32] There may be an increased incidence of DISH in diabetic patients.[33] Diabetes is mysteriously associated with several rheumatic conditions in which there is proliferation of fibrous tissue:[33, 34] (1) periarthritis, which commonly leads to limitation of joint motion; (2) flexor tenosynovitis, which commonly leads to trigger finger and de Quervain's disease; (3) shoulder-hand syndrome, which may eventually cause extensive shoulder or hip contractures; and (4) Dupuytren's contracture. In addition, a group of juvenile diabetics has been described who have short stature, thickened skin on the back of the hands, and flexion contractures of the proximal interphalangeal joints. The increased risk of microvascular disease in diabetic children with limited joint mobility has also been described recently.[35] The inciting factor or factors that cause rheumatic problems in the diabetic are unclear, and it has been suggested that microvascular disease per se is not the culprit.[33] Interestingly, as previously discussed, Pima Indians have a 50% incidence of glucose intolerance and a 50% incidence of DISH. Pima Indians would be an ideal population in which to study the association of diabetes and DISH.

Attempts to link the excessive bone growth of DISH with abnormalities in growth hormone or somatomedin levels have not been successful.[11, 19] However, recent work by Littlejohn and coworkers[19] shows a significantly higher serum insulin level after glucose challenge in patients with DISH. This suggests that higher than physiologic concentrations of insulin may influence bone growth or that abnormal insulin kinetics may influence bone growth. Obesity, even in the absence of glucose intolerance, is also associated with abnormalities of insulin metabolism. This may explain the increased incidence of obesity in patients with DISH.

There are other areas of investigation worth pursuing. It has been known for years that cats that are given large doses of vitamin A develop extensive bony proliferation.[36] However, some investigators have felt that the roentgenographic changes in these cats, even their extensive cervical spondylosis, do not resemble DISH.[10] In addition, chronic vitamin A poisoning in humans leads to periosteal reaction or deformity of long bones but not to the axial skeletal changes of DISH.[37, 38] Now, however, Abiteboul and associates[39] have presented evidence that patients with DISH have increased serum vitamin A levels, possibly related to accelerated transformation of beta carotene. Because no long-term study of hypervitaminosis A in human adults is available,[38, 40] this work of Abiteboul and colleagues is of great interest. Of special note is the recent observation that patients receiving high doses of the synthetic vitamin A derivative 13-cis-retinoic acid were observed to develop an ossification disorder resembling DISH.[41]

Environmental toxins can cause microvascular abnormalities, and some toxins directly affect bone metabolism. Fluorosis is associated with marked osteophytosis of the spine, spinal ligament ossification, and calcification of paraarticular ligaments and tendons.[42] Although, in a recent limited report 5 patients with DISH syndrome were noted to have elevated plasma and urine fluoride levels,[43] abnormal levels of fluoride have not been noted in a single patient of ours with DISH.[8, 11]

With the growing interest in DISH and its establishment as a discrete disease entity distinct from spondylosis deformans,[23] clearer insights into its etiology and pathogenesis will almost certainly be forthcoming soon.

References

1. Meyer M, Forster E: Considérations pathogéniques sur l'hyperostose moniliforme du flanc droit de la colonne dorsale. Rev Rhum 5:286–293, 1938.
2. Oppenheimer A: Calcification and ossification of vertebral ligaments (spondylitis ossificans ligamentosa). Roentgen study of pathogenesis and clinical significance. Radiology 38:160–164, 1942.
3. Lacapère A: Étude de L'ostéophytose vertébrale. Acta Physiother Rheum Belg 4:145–158, 1948.
4. Forestier J, Rotes-Querol J: Senile ankylosing hyperostosis of the spine. Ann Rheum Dis 9:321–330, 1950.
5. Harris J, Carter A, Glick E, Storey G: Ankylosing hyperostosis: Clinical and radiological features. Ann Rheum Dis 33:210–215, 1974.
6. Forestier J, Lagier R: Ankylosing hyperostosis of the spine. Clin Orthop 74:65–83, 1971.
7. Resnick D, Shaul S, Robins J: Diffuse idiopathic hyperostosis (DISH): Forestier's disease with extraspinal manifestations. Radiology 115:513–524, 1975.
8. Utsinger PD, Resnick D, Shapiro R: Diffuse skeletal abnormalities in Forestier disease. Arch Intern Med 136:763–768, 1976.
9. Julkunen H, Knekt D, Aromaa A: Diffuse idiopathic skeletal hyperostosis in relation to spondylosis deformans in Finnish population. (Abstract.) Rev Rhum 0984, 1981.
10. Resnick D, Shapiro RD, Wiesner KB: Diffuse idiopathic skeletal hyperostosis (DISH) (ankylosing hyperostosis of Forestier and Rotes-Querol). Semin Arthritis Rheum 7:153–187, 1978.
11. Utsinger PD: A clinical and laboratory analysis of 200 patients with DISH. Clin Exp Rheumatol (in press).
12. Meeks L, Renshaw T: Vertebral osteophytosis and dysphagia. J Bone Joint Surg 55A:197–201, 1973.
13. Carlson M, Stauffer R, Payne W: Ankylosing vertebral hyperostosis causing dysphagia. Arch Surg 109:567–570, 1974.
14. Prince D, Luna R, Cohn M, Sibiston W: Osteophyte-induced dysphagia. JAMA 234:77–78, 1975.
15. Resnick D, Guerra J, Robinson C, Vint V: Association of diffuse idiopathic skeletal hyperostosis (DISH) and calcification and ossification of the posterior longitudinal ligament. Am J Roentgenol 131:1049–1053, 1978.
16. Gibson T, Shumacher R: Ankylosing hyperostosis with cervical spinal cord compression. Rheumatol Rehabil 15:67–70, 1976.
17. Yunus M, Masi AT, Calabro JJ: Primary fibromyalgia (fibrositis): Clinical study of 50 patients with matched controls. Semin Arthritis Rheum 11:151–171, 1981.
18. Robbes-Ruy E, Rojo-Mejia A, Harrison-Garcin Calderon J, Discoya-Arbanil J: Diffuse idiopathic skeletal hyperostosis: Clinical and radiological manifestations in 50 patients. Arthritis Rheum 25:101, 1982.
19. Littlejohn GO, Herington AC, Smythe HA: Studies into various growth factors in diffuse idiopathic skeletal hyperostosis (DISH) (Forestier's disease). (Abstract.) Rev Rhum 0987, 1981.
20. Shapiro R, Utsinger PD, Wiesner KB: The association of HLA-B27 with Forestier's disease (vertebral ankylosing hyperostosis). J Rheumatol 3:4–8, 1976.
21. Resnick D, Linovitz R, Feingold M: Post-operative heterotopic ossification in patients with ankylosing hyperostosis of the spine (Forestier's disease). J Rheumatol 3:313–320, 1976.
22. Resnick D, Dwosh IL, Goergen TA, et al.: Clinical and radiographic "re-ankylosis" following hip surgery in ankylosing spondylitis. Am J Roentgenol 126:1181–1188, 1976.
23. Resnick D, Curd J, Shapiro RF, et al.: Modified radiographic abnormalities of rheumatoid arthritis in patients with diffuse idiopathic skeletal hyperostosis. Arthritis Rheum 21:1–7, 1978.
24. Julkunen H, Heinonen O, Kalevi P: Hyperostosis of

the spine in an adult population: Its relation to hyperglycemia and obesity. Ann Rheum Dis 30:605–612, 1971.

25. Hajkova K, Streda A, Skrha F: Hyperostotic spondylosis and diabetes mellitus. Ann Rheum Dis 24:536–543, 1965.

26. Bywaters EGL, Doyle FH, Oakley N: Senile hyperostotic ankylosing spondylosis in diabetes mellitus. Arthritis Rheum 9:495–501, 1966.

27. Rosenthal M, Bahous I, Miller W: Increased frequency of HLA-B8 in hyperostotic spondylitis. J Rheumatol 4:94–96, 1977.

28. Ercilla MG, Brancos MA, Breysse Y, et al.: HLA antigens in Forestier's disease, ankylosing spondylitis and polyarthrosis of the hands. J Rheumatol 4(Suppl):89–93, 1977.

29. Brigode M, Francois R: Histocompatibility antigens in vertebral ankylosing hyperostosis. J Rheumatol 4:429–434, 1977.

30. Spagnole A, Bennett P, Terasaki P: Vertebral ankylosing hyperostosis (Forestier's disease) and HLA antigens in Pima Indians. Arthritis Rheum 21:467–472, 1978.

31. Berkson J: Limitations of the analysis of fourfold table analysis to hospital data. Biometrics Bull 2:47–53, 1946.

32. Felig P, et al.: Endocrinology and Metabolism. New York, McGraw-Hill, 1981, p. 816.

33. Füebl H, Seidl O, Goebel FD: Spondylosis hyperostotica and medial calcification of arteries in diabetes mellitus—a related disorder. (Abstract.) Rev Rhum 0985, 1981.

34. Bland J, Frymoyer J, Newberg A, et al.: Rheumatic syndromes in endocrine disease. Semin Arthritis Rheum 9:23–65, 1979.

35. Rosenbloom A, et al.: Limited joint mobility in childhood diabetes mellitus indicates increased risk for microvascular disease. N Engl J Med 305:191–194, 1981.

36. Seawright AA, English PB, Gartner RJW: Hypervitaminosis A and hyperostosis of the cat. Nature 206:1171–1172, 1965.

37. Rothman PE, Leon EE: Hyper-vitaminosis A: Report of two cases in infants. Radiology 51:368–374, 1940.

38. Ruby LK, Mital MA: Skeletal deformities following chronic hypervitaminosis A: A case report. J Bone Joint Surg 56A:1283–1287, 1974.

39. Abiteboul M, Mazieres B, Laffont F, et al.: Hyperostose vertébral ankylosante et métabolisme de la vitamine A. Rev Rhum 0989, 1981.

41. Pittsley RA, Yoder FW: Retinoid hyperostosis. N Engl J Med 308:1012–1025, 1983.

42. Gerber A, Raab A, Sobel A: Vitamin A poisoning in adults. Am J Med 5:729–745, 1954.

42. Singh A, Dass R, et al.: Skeletal changes in endemic fluorosis. J Bone Joint Surg 44B:806–814, 1962.

43. Mills DM, Taves DR, Pal DP, Bartholomew BA: Association of diffuse idiopathic spinal hyperostosis and fluorosis. Arthritis Rheum 26(Suppl):511, 1983.

14

Secondary Osteoarthritis

H. Ralph Schumacher, Jr., M.D.

Osteoarthritis (OA) in increasing percentages of patients can now be classified as "secondary" on the basis that an identifiable congenital, traumatic, or systemic disease appears to explain the degenerative changes in the articular cartilage. All diseases considered in this chapter have clinical, roentgenologic, and pathologic features in common with "idiopathic" osteoarthritis to varying degrees. However, there are also unique features that suggest each underlying cause. These distinguishing features will be emphasized along with brief descriptions of each disease process. Although osteoarthritic changes associated with these underlying diseases will be emphasized, other musculoskeletal symptoms produced by these diseases that may be confused with osteoarthritic manifestations will also be described. The systemic diseases causing arthritis receive major emphasis because (a) in some patients the osteoarthritis may be an early or even initial clue to a potentially dangerous and treatable systemic disease; (b) these secondary osteoarthritides may have specific therapies in contrast to the largely symptomatic treatment used in most osteoarthritides; and (c) the mechanisms identified in these examples of secondary osteoarthritis may provide helpful clues to mechanisms in "idiopathic" disease.

Specific treatments for or related to underlying diseases are discussed in this chapter. Unless otherwise noted, symptomatic and general therapy is as described in Section 3 (Chapters 17 to 20) for general management of osteoarthritis.

SYSTEMIC METABOLIC DISEASES

Hemochromatosis

Hemochromatosis is a chronic disease characterized by excess iron deposition and fibrosis in a variety of tissues. Although it can result from chronic excess iron ingestion, multiple transfusions with or without hemolysis, or alcoholic cirrhosis of the liver, it is most often idiopathic. Idiopathic cases may be familial, with association with HLA-A3 and HLA-B14. This is not a rare disease; its estimated incidence is about 1:500. Frequent manifestations are hepatomegaly and cirrhosis, increased skin pigmentation (in large part due to increased melanin), diabetes, other endocrine deficiency, and cardiomyopathy. Iron overload usually requires many years to develop, so that most patients have onset of symptoms between the ages of 40 and 60 years. Hemochromatosis is uncommon in premenopausal women, presumably because of menstrual blood loss. The largest iron deposits are in the liver, and biopsy is frequently done here for diagnosis. Elevation of serum iron with nearly complete saturation of iron-binding capacity or elevated serum ferritin can help suggest the diagnosis. Liver function abnormalities are often minimal, even with advanced hepatic deposition of iron.

Osteoarthritis-like changes in hemochromatosis were first described in 1964[1] but have since been recognized to occur in 20% to 50% of patients.[2] Onset of the arthritis has varied from 26 to 70 years of age but is most common

235

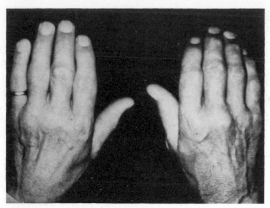

Figure 14–1. Bony osteoarthritis–like enlargement of some of the distal interphalangeal, proximal interphalangeal, and metacarpophalangeal joints in hemochromatosis.

in the 50's. Arthritis generally coincides closely with the onset of other manifestations of hemochromatosis but may antedate other findings and be the first clue to the disease.[3, 4]

The hands, knees, and hips are most commonly involved, although virtually any joint, including those in the feet,[5] can be affected. Helpful in diagnosis is the characteristic involvement of metacarpophalangeal (MCP) joints as well as proximal interphalangeal (PIP) and distal interphalangeal (DIP) joints with a firm, bony, and often only mildly tender enlargement that is different from rheumatoid arthritis (Fig. 14–1). Involvement of the second and third metacarpophalangeal joints is particularly characteristic. Involvement of the metacarpophalangeal joints, of course, is not typically seen in idiopathic OA, although it can occasionally be seen in patients with erosive inflammatory osteoarthritis and primary generalized osteoarthritis and, more often, in association with calcium pyrophosphate deposition disease. Joints are stiff and become limited in motion, but morning stiffness is not prominent.

Joint effusions have been "noninflammatory" with leukocyte counts less than 2000/ mm^3, except when studied during the infrequent attacks of associated pseudogout. Cells are predominantly mononuclear; these cells occasionally have been noted to contain iron on staining with Prussian blue.[6] Measurements of iron levels in synovial fluid are comparable to serum levels.

Synovial tissue shows a striking deposition of iron that is most prominent in the synovial lining cells and, as seen by electron microscopy, is actually greatest in the Type B or synthetic cells.[7] By light microscopy, the iron is golden-colored and may be missed unless specifically looked for. Other synovial changes are only mild lining cell proliferation, fibrosis, and scattered chronic inflammatory cells. Although few cases have been studied, iron is also demonstrable in the chondrocytes of articular cartilage and at the line of ossification. There are degenerative changes in cartilage.[8] All cartilages studied to date by electron microscopy have also shown either apatite or calcium pyrophosphate dihydrate (CPPD) crystals, which may be important in pathogenesis.[8]

Roentgenographic studies show the characteristic joint distribution noted previously that often includes metacarpophalangeal joints. There is joint space narrowing and irregularity, subchondral sclerosis, and often large cystic erosions, bony proliferation, and even subluxation (Fig. 14–2). In up to 60% of patients, chondrocalcinosis and periarticular soft tissue calcification are seen. Aside from the distribution and frequency of calcifications, the involvement at the hips and other sites seems indistinguishable from idiopathic OA.

Musculoskeletal manifestations other than osteoarthritis are also seen. As noted earlier, pseudogout attacks can occur from CPPD crystals. Apatite may also be involved in some crystal-induced arthritis. Osteopenia is seen and may be related to the cirrhosis or to androgen or other endocrine deficiency.

Mechanisms involved in the arthritis are not established, although there are intriguing possibilities.[9] Iron deposition in the chondrocytes could alter the proteoglycan, collagen, or enzymes released by these cells, leading to the degenerative change in the matrix. Iron could bind directly to some proteoglycans and alter their function, as it has been shown to do in vitro. Iron in vitro also inhibits the enzyme pyrophosphatase and could thus contribute to the deposition of CPPD crystals. Because the iron and calcium crystal depositions are not spatially related, iron would appear to favor calcification in some indirect way, or alternatively, the calcifications may be due to unrelated mechanisms or related inherited factors. Although cartilage appears to be primarily involved in the OA, the synovium also has heavy deposits of iron, and altered enzymes from the synovium might contribute to the process. Synovial siderosis might alter the clearance of factors involved in calcification.[10]

Hemochromatosis can be treated and many systemic features reversed or prevented by removal of excess iron with intensive and con-

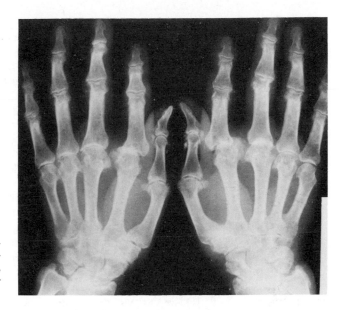

Figure 14–2. Roentgenogram of the hands in hemochromatosis showing joint space narrowing, subluxations, subchondral cysts, periarticular sclerosis, spurs, and soft tissue calcifications, all most prominent at the metacarpophalangeal joints.

tinued phlebotomies or with the chelating agent desferrioxamine. Once established, joint disease has not been reversed, and in fact, some patients have had their first joint symptoms or exacerbations of arthritis after phlebotomy. Episodes of acute crystal-induced arthritis should be watched for and can be treated with nonsteroidal anti-inflammatory agents. Prosthetic hip and knee replacements have been successfully performed for chronic changes. Etiologies for the iron deposition should be sought, and families should be studied for early case detection and prophylactic phlebotomies.

Wilson's Disease (Hepatolenticular Degeneration)

This is an uncommon familial disease characterized by the Kayser-Fleischer ring, consisting of brown pigment at the corneal margin, cirrhosis, and basal ganglion degeneration leading to tremor, rigidity, or other neurologic problems. Many patients also develop renal tubular acidosis. The onset of symptoms occurs between the ages of 4 and 50 years. A disorder of copper metabolism can be demonstrated by an increase in urinary excretion of copper and a general decrease of the serum copper-binding protein, ceruloplasmin. Copper concentration is increased in liver, brain, and other tissues.

Arthropathy is rare in children but occurs in up to 50% of adults.[9, 11, 12] The osteoarthritis may be asymptomatic despite positive roentgenographic findings or may be markedly symptomatic with worsening on activity. More commonly involved joints have been the wrists, elbows, shoulders, hips, and knees and, occasionally, the fingers. The early age of onset and the prominent involvement of the wrists in many patients suggest a difference from primary osteoarthritis.[9, 11–13]

Joint effusions are usually small and consist of clear, viscous fluid. Leukocyte counts have been approximately 200 to 300/mm³, with predominantly mononuclear cells. Crystals have not been identified. Synovial biopsies have shown mild lining cell hyperplasia and few chronic inflammatory cells.[9, 12, 14] Cartilage and subchondral bone biopsies have not been reported.

Roentgenographic joint findings have included subchondral bone fragmentation and sclerosis, cortical irregularity, cartilage space narrowing, periarticular cysts, vertebral wedging,[9, 11, 12] osteochondritis dissecans,[15] and severe chondromalacia patellae.[12] Periarticular calcifications are common. Some calcifications have been thought to represent bone fragments or chondrocalcinosis, but these have not been examined pathologically.

Mechanisms for this osteoarthritis-like arthropathy have not been defined. No correlation has been found between total disease severity, spasticity or tremor, osteopenia, or liver or renal disease and the arthritis. Studies are still needed to ascertain whether copper is deposited in the cartilage or subchondral bone. Experimental studies of only short-term copper loading have not produced an arthropathy. Although the nature of the joint calcifications is not yet known, it should be mentioned that McCarty and Pepe[16] showed that cupric (as well as ferrous) ions could inhibit pyrophosphatase in vitro, suggesting a possible cause for deposition of CPPD crystals.

Wilson's disease is associated with osteopenia in 25% to 50% of different series. It is usually asymptomatic but can be painful in the presence of pathologic fractures. Some of the bony demineralization results from definite rickets or osteomalacia attributed to the renal tubular disease. Joint hypermobility occurred in 9 of 32 patients in one series.[15]

This is a treatable disease; penicillamine appears to be the most effective chelating agent for mobilizing copper from the tissues. Treatment is continued for life. Although neurologic improvement is often reported, there is no evidence that the established arthropathy has been helped; in fact, some penicillamine-treated patients have subsequently developed the osteoarthritis. Whether very early diagnosis and treatment can prevent the arthritis is not yet known. Family members should always be checked to try to establish an early diagnosis. Remember that penicillamine seems occasionally to produce polymyositis, lupus, inflammatory polyarthritis,[15] or other immunologic syndromes.

Ochronosis

Ochronosis is the result of a hereditary deficiency of a liver enzyme, homogentisic acid oxidase.[9, 17, 18] Lack of this enzyme allows accumulation of homogentisic acid, which, when excreted in large amounts, imparts a dark-brown or black color to the urine. This is termed "alkaptonuria." Freshly passed urine usually appears normal but darkens with standing or with alkalinization. This inherited defect is felt to be transmitted as a simple autosomal recessive gene.

Ochronosis occurs when polymers of homogentisic acid become deposited in connective tissue. The exact mechanisms of affinity of homogentisic acid for connective tissue are not known. Deposition is reversible until the homogentisic acid is polymerized. It is proposed that benzoquinone acetic acid may be an intermediate compound involved in the pigment formation and binding.[17] Ochronotic pigment is black when viewed grossly in masses in tissues; when seen in thin histologic sections under the light microscope, it is ochre or golden yellow in color.

Alkaptonuria is often detectable during infancy and youth by black staining of diapers or underwear. By the fourth decade, ochronotic pigment becomes detectable as a blue-black hue to the external ear cartilage or tympanic membrane, scleral pigmentation, or malar and other cutaneous darkening. Pigment deposits in the mitral and aortic valves can deform the leaflets and cusps, producing murmurs in 15% to 20% of patients. Calcified prostatic calculi containing ochronotic pigment occur in a large percentage of men with ochronosis.

Deposition of the pigment in intervertebral disks and in articular cartilages leads to degenerative disk disease and peripheral arthropathy. The majority of patients over 30 years of age develop spondylosis, which may present with low back stiffness and aching or, in about 15%, herniation of a lumbar nucleus pulposus. Involvement of the dorsal and cervical spine occurs only later. Symptoms may be minimal despite prominent roentgenographic changes.

Peripheral arthropathy generally occurs later and is milder than the spondylosis. The knees, shoulders, and hips are most commonly involved.[19] In peripheral joints, symptoms may antedate detected roentgenographic changes. As with other forms of OA, symptoms are predominantly pain, crepitation, limited motion, and stiffness. Hip and knee flexion contractures can develop.

Joint effusions occur in about 50% of involved knees. Synovial fluid is clear, viscous, and yellow. Occasionally, dark specks of ochronotic cartilage can be seen floating in the fluid.[20, 21] Leukocyte counts are generally in the "noninflammatory" range, with counts from 112 to 700/mm^3; in one large series, mononuclear cells were predominant. Joint fluids have been described with CPPD crystals without inflammatory reaction or with acute attacks of pseudogout superimposed on the degenerative arthropathy.[22] Although small amounts of homogentisic acid occur in joint fluid, the amount is insufficient to cause darkening with alkalinization.[19]

The earliest roentgenographic changes suggestive of ochronosis are calcification and even ossification in the lumbar intervertebral disks. Hydroxyapatite has been identified as the calcium salt in the disks. Although typical of ochronosis, disk calcification (Fig. 14–3) is not diagnostic, as it has also been seen with CPPD deposition disease, hemochromatosis, chronic respiratory paralytic poliomyelitis, ankylosing spondylitis, acromegaly, amyloidosis, tuber-

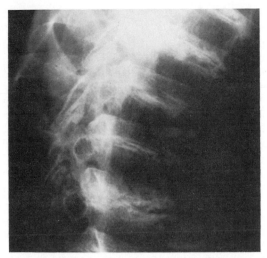

Figure 14–3. Intervertebral disk ossification in ochronosis.

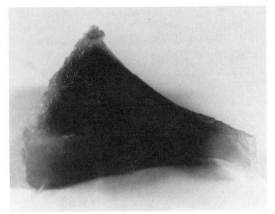

Figure 14–4. Blackening of the knee meniscus in ochronosis.

culosis, and trauma or without any identifiable systemic disease. The calcification in ochronosis is followed later by disk space narrowing; osteophytes tend to be small but may bridge occasional vertebrae. The sacroiliac joints can show narrowing but do not fuse; typical syndesmophytes like those found in ankylosing spondylitis are not seen.

On roentgenograms, peripheral joints do not differ from those in other forms of OA except in the distribution. Ochronosis tends to involve the larger joints and spare or only mildly involve the hands and feet. Protrusio acetabuli has been reported in one case.[19] Loose bodies occur in some peripheral joints.[19] Chondrocalcinosis may be seen. As in the spine, the osteophytes tend to be small.

Ochronotic pigment deposition is initially in the deeper and midzone cartilage but eventually produces grossly visible diffuse blackening of cartilage (Fig. 14–4). This cartilage is so friable that it progressively erodes, with fragments breaking loose into synovial fluid. Pigmented shards become embedded in synovial membrane (Fig. 14–5). Ochronotic pigment can be seen by light and electron microscopy to be associated with collagen fibers of cartilage but not with synovial collagen.[19] Cartilage collagen and associated substances appear to be primary sites of the pigment deposition.[23] Ochronotic pigment is probably secondarily phagocytized by chondrocytes and synovial cells. Because chondrocytes show some degenerative changes in virtually all cases studied by electron microscopy, they may also be affected in some way early in the disease.[19]

What it is about cartilage matrix that attracts the ochronotic pigment is not definitely known. The presence of Type II collagen and glycosaminoglycans different from those seen in synovium is a possible explanation.[19] Whatever the factors, the matrix ochronotic pigment and the cellular changes result in a dramatically friable cartilage that predictably degenerates in early middle age. Joint loose bodies appear to arise from osteochondrometaplasia around the ochronotic shards embedded in synovium.[19]

No satisfactory treatment for the enzymatic defect has yet been developed. Unfortunately, a diet low in phenylalanine and tyrosine precursors has been too unpalatable to demonstrate if it might have any long-term clinical benefit, although urinary homogentisic acid levels can be decreased with it.[9, 19] High doses of ascorbic acid, although not decreasing total urinary homogentisic acid, have been reported

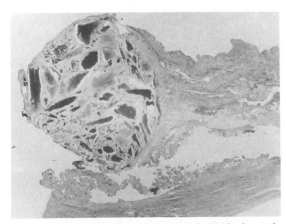

Figure 14–5. Golden-brown pigmented shards from the friable cartilage embedded in synovium in ochronosis.

to inhibit binding to connective tissue in experimental alkaptonuria of rats.[24] Corrective orthopedic measures have been effective, without any special problems.[25]

Gaucher's Disease

Gaucher's disease is an inherited metabolic disease characterized by the accumulation of glucocerebroside in distinctive Gaucher cells, most prominently in the liver, spleen, and bone. The glucocerebroside deposits occur because of a deficiency of the enzyme glucocerebrosidase.[26] The disease is more common in, but not restricted to, people of Ashkenazi Jewish background. Clinical severity can vary widely. Different clinical types with different prognoses have been defined.[27] Some individuals are disabled by age 30, whereas others live relatively symptom-free lives to old age.[28] Common findings in adults are splenomegaly, hepatomegaly, anemia and thrombocytopenia (due to hypersplenism and, occasionally, marrow replacement), pingueculae, and bone marrow expansion causing such findings as the Erlenmeyer-flask appearance of the distal femur. Neurologic problems are more common in children. The age of onset and severity tend to correlate with the degree of glucocerebrosidase deficiency.[26]

Definitive diagnosis can be made by bone marrow or other biopsies or by biochemical study of leukocytes. Gaucher cells are large reticuloendothelial cells with profuse "wrinkled," pale-pink cytoplasm on hematoxylin-eosin staining and with one or more small nuclei. Electron microscopy shows that the cytoplasm of these cells is occupied by membrane-bounded inclusions filled with tubular structures typical of glucocerebroside. Acid phosphatase is demonstrable in some vacuoles within the tubules. Gaucher cells are also rich in ferritin. Chemical analysis also shows iron and other components in the vacuoles.[26] Gaucher-like cells are not diagnostic of Gaucher's disease, as they have also been seen in thalassemia[29] and chronic myelogenous leukemia.[30] Much of the material in the cells in all these conditions appears to be derived from phagocytized erythrocytes.

Elevated serum levels of acid phosphatase are observed and may be helpful in suggesting a diagnosis of Gaucher's disease. Increased angiotensin-converting enzyme[31] and relative Factor IX deficiency have been reported.

The degenerative arthritis in Gaucher's disease follows marrow infiltration, aseptic necrosis[32] or pathologic fracture,[33] with resulting joint distortion. It is most common in the hip but has also been seen in the shoulders and knees.[32] Joint space narrowing is secondary.

Synovial fluid has rarely been examined. In one patient with pathologic fractures of tibial plateaus, joint fluid was clear yellow and contained 600 white blood cells, 7050 red blood cells, and no crystals under polarized light.[33] Actual infiltration of Gaucher cells into cartilage has not been noted.

In addition to aseptic necrosis, roentgenographic changes of the skeleton include demineralization and cortical thinning due to the medullary expansion, foci of sclerosis, and pathologic fractures. Epiphyseal and diaphyseal areas of long bones are prominently involved. Shafts of long bones may be widened with the infiltrative process, as is most typically described in the distal femur.

Musculoskeletal symptoms are not all due to the OA but also appear to result from pathologic fractures, episodic periostitis (often with fever) that may be difficult to distinguish from osteomyelitis,[32, 34, 35] and deep, aching bone pain.[36] Many bone lesions detected roentgenographically are asymptomatic.[32] Amyloidosis[37] has been noted in two reports in association with Gaucher's disease and might offer a secondary cause for musculoskeletal problems.

Reconstructive joint surgery,[34] including total hip replacements, has been successful, but hemorrhage has been an important complication. Increased postoperative infections have been reported.[35] Replacement of the deficient enzyme has been performed experimentally.[36] Enzyme replacement or other theoretic treatments such as replacement of genetic material, extracorporeal degradation of the glucocerebroside, stimulation of residual endogenous enzyme, or alteration of other normal related enzymes have been considered[26] and may be clinically possible in the future.

Hemoglobinopathies

Sickle Cell Disease

This is by far the most common hemoglobinopathy associated with musculoskeletal manifestations.[38] Homozygous sickle cell disease is an inherited disease most common in blacks and caused by a substitution of valine for glutamic acid as the sixth amino acid in the beta chain of hemoglobin. This results in sickling of erythrocytes, which presumably occludes small vessels, causing the painful crises and bone lesions.[39] Other manifestations described include hemolytic anemia, renal involvement with hyposthenuria, leg ulcers, hyporegenerative crises, increased infections, especially with salmonella, and a variety of rheumatic or bone and joint problems.

Diagnosis is generally made by identification of sickled cells in vitro by use of reducing agents such as metabisulfite or by hemoglobin electrophoresis. Hemoglobin S composes 76% to 100% of hemoglobin in homozygous sickle cell disease.

Aseptic necrosis appears to be the basis for any OA seen in these patients.[38] As with other causes of aseptic necrosis, homozygous sickle cell disease, sickle cell–hemoglobin C disease, and sickle cell–thalassemia can lead to osteoarthritis as a result of the incongruity of the joint space and loss of normal bony support for the articular cartilage. This is most common at the hip but can also involve the spine, knee, shoulder (Fig. 14–6), and, occasionally, other joints.

In addition to aseptic necrosis, roentgenographic changes in sickle cell disease can include coarse trabeculae with hair-on-end appearance in the skull, osteopenia, vertebral indentations, medullary infarctions, and periosteal elevation. Aseptic necrosis has been reported in sickle cell trait but does not seem to be more common than in the general population.[40]

Other bone and joint problems in sickle cell disease that are clearly more typical than OA for this disease include infarction of bone away from joints, hyperuricemia and occasional gout,[41] the "hand-foot syndrome" in young children, osteomyelitis and rare septic arthritis, and acute joint effusions, usually, but not always, with low leukocyte counts.[38, 42] An element of synovitis for which there is no clear explanation[43] can damage cartilage and contribute to the later development of OA.

Total hip and knee arthroplasties[38, 44] have been done and have been highly successful. Preoperative transfusions have been used to decrease the chances of sickling during surgery. Tourniquets should be avoided to reduce anoxia and stasis, which contribute to thrombosis. Good hydration and efforts during anesthesia to avoid any hypoxia and acidosis are also warranted.[44]

Thalassemia

Beta-thalassemia describes a group of inherited disorders of hemoglobin synthesis resulting in a relative decrease in beta chains. Alpha chains of hemoglobin accumulate, producing unstable hemoglobin, Heinz bodies, and hypochromic microcytic erythrocytes. Early erythrocyte death results in marrow expansion and splenomegaly. Levels of hemoglobin F or A_2 are elevated.

Frequent transfusions are required and often lead to secondary iron overload. Thalassemia major with severe anemia often leads to death in the second to third decades. Milder thalassemia minor may be asymptomatic and may not require therapy.

Osteoarthritis has been described as developing prematurely in both thalassemia major and minor. Weight-bearing joints (including the ankles) have been predominantly involved, with the wrists and elbows also being af-

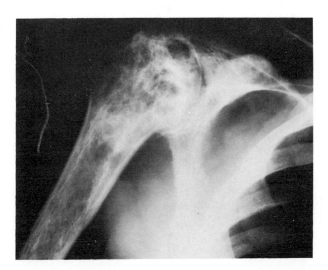

Figure 14–6. Severe marrow infarctions at the shoulder with associated OA in sickle cell disease.

fected.[45, 46] The speculation is that marrow hyperplasia may weaken the subchondral bone and allow microfractures that then alter the normal support required by the articular cartilage.[47, 48] Osteomalacia has been confirmed in the areas of microfractures.[48] Multiple transfusions and iron overload might contribute to osteoarthropathy in some patients, as is described in hemochromatosis,[49] but early OA has also been described without iron overload.[47] Juxta-articular osteopenia may be seen on roentgenograms. Osteonecrosis has been reported, but whether it is increased in incidence has not been established.[46, 50] Widened medullary spaces with thin cortices, coarse trabeculations, and microfractures are seen in bone with marrow expansion. When studied, synovial fluid has been "noninflammatory."

Dull, aching pain, especially at the ankles, has been described after strenuous exercise.[48] Because the cartilage space in the roentgenograms was normal, the pain was attributed to the periarticular bone involvement.[48]

No specific treatment is available for the osteoarthritis due to thalassemia.

Ehlers-Danlos Syndrome and Other Joint Hypermobility

The Ehlers-Danlos syndrome consists of a group of heritable disorders of connective tissue[51] with features that include hypermobility of joints (Fig. 14–7), hyperextensible skin, poor wound healing, bruising, and cigarette paper scars. Even extreme degrees of body contortion are possible, as in the "India rubber man" of old-time side shows at circuses. At least seven different types of Ehlers-Danlos syndrome have been identified, with clinical differences, different inheritance, and, in some cases, identified biochemical defects.

The most serious type of Ehlers-Danlos syndrome is the Type IV vascular or ecchymotic type; patients with this form of the syndrome rarely survive past 20 years of age. A deficiency of Type III collagen has been identified. Type III Ehlers-Danlos syndrome with benign hypermobility is inherited as an autosomal dominant trait and is one of the types in which secondary OA can become prominent. The biochemical defect is not known. Type I has large, irregular collagen fibers by electron microscopy. It is also inherited as an autosomal dominant trait and has been associated with premature OA.[52]

Quantification of the degree of hypermobility has been described.[53] A typical collapsing skeletal structure on the initial handshake may be a clue.

The development of OA seems to be directly related to the severity of hypermobility and the frequency and degree of trauma to which any given joint is exposed.[54] Osteoarthritis associated with Ehlers-Danlos syndrome has been reported in the hands, knees, ankles, and shoulders. It often appears before the age of 40 years. Beighton[54] reported finding no cases of OA of the hip.

Synovial effusions studied have had few cells. Synovial biopsies have shown no distinctive changes by light microscopy.[55] Pathologic studies of articular cartilage have not been reported. Abnormal bone morphology has been suggested.[56] Roentgenograms of joints have no unique features, and subluxations, when correctable, may not be appreciated on films.

Mechanisms of production of the osteoarthritis are suspected to include abnormal cartilage wear due to excessive motion and inadequate protection from trauma. Whether structural abnormalities related to abnormal collagen also occur in capsule and cartilage is not yet known. Studies based on pressure-volume relationships in the knee during distention showed no definite evidence of altered collagen functional properties.[57]

In addition to osteoarthritis, joints may be involved by dislocations, instability, noninflammatory effusions, and spinal deformities (kyphoscoliosis).[55, 58] Other potentially confusing and complicating problems include increased muscle cramps and spasm; peripheral circulatory disease, especially in Type IV Ehlers-Danlos syndrome; congenital abnormalities of bones; and periarticular hemorrhage.

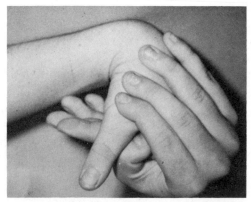

Figure 14–7. Joint hypermobility in Ehlers-Danlos syndrome.

Treatment in symptomatic patients should include educational efforts to help avoid activities that hyperextend joints. Swimming can be used to strengthen muscles to try to aid joint support. Hypermobility is not always a disadvantage, as it may have aided Paganini in his violin virtuosity![59] One study showed no correlation between knee laxity and the frequency of injuries in football players,[60] although others have postulated a relationship. Surgery may be made difficult by unpredictable increased bleeding and poor wound healing.

Isolated joint hypermobility without Ehlers-Danlos syndrome also seems to be associated with an increased incidence of OA and, in one study,[61] also with chondrocalcinosis. These were not prospective studies, so that the exact reasons for such relationships are not clear.[62] Scott and associates[62] found more OA in patients with mild idiopathic joint hypermobility than in age-matched controls. The neck, thumb, and knee have been involved with OA before 30 years of age.[53] It should be noted that in one recent study, no correlation could be found between "benign hypermobility" and arthritis or arthralgias.[63] Recurrent subluxation of the patella can lead to patellofemoral osteoarthritis, but Crosby and Insall actually found that OA was more common in their series after attempted surgical realignment to prevent dislocation.[64]

Other causes of hypermobility that have been described include Larsen's syndrome[58] (a congenital condition characterized by depressed bridge of the nose and other altered facial features), acromegaly, Marfan's syndrome, Jaccoud's arthropathy after rheumatic fever or in systemic lupus erythematosus, hereditary osteo-onychodysplasia, progressive arthro-ophthalmopathy, Wilson's disease, and Noonan's syndrome.[65]

ENDOCRINE DISEASES

Acromegaly

A growth hormone–secreting tumor of the anterior pituitary in adults leads to slowly progressive overgrowth of soft tissue, bone, and cartilage. Because linear growth is not possible at this time, enlargement is prominent in the acral parts, with gradually increasing size of the hands and feet as well as the nose and mandible. There is typical coarsening of features. Patients with acromegaly often have increased sweating and moist, thick skin. Mild glucose intolerance occurs in 50% of patients because hyperexcretion of growth hormone causes insulin resistance. The pituitary tumor may also produce symptoms such as headaches and visual problems. Other pituitary functions may be altered. Diagnosis is based on clinical findings together with laboratory confirmation by demonstration of elevated serum growth hormone levels, suppression of growth hormone after glucose ingestion, and abnormal increased release of growth hormone in response to thyrotropin-releasing hormone. The severity of acromegaly does not correlate directly with growth hormone levels, probably at least partly because growth hormone effects are mediated indirectly through somatomedins produced in the liver.[66]

Peripheral and spinal osteoarthritis is common in acromegaly. Peripheral joint symptoms occur in about 60% of acromegalic individuals.[67, 68] The joints most commonly involved have been the knees, hips, shoulders, elbows, and, occasionally, ankles. Although the hands have soft tissue swelling, widened distal phalanx bone tufts, and carpal tunnel syndrome, they have little osteoarthritis. Hip and knee involvement has been disabling in severe acromegaly. Crepitus is very common. There may be small or, rarely, large effusions and apparent synovial thickening, but acute inflammation has not been reported.

Backache occurs frequently, but back motion (as well as peripheral joint motion) is often normal or increased. This is tentatively attributed to the thickened disks and cartilages plus laxity of acromegalic ligaments.[69] A kyphotic posture is common.

Synovial effusions have been "noninflammatory," as in other osteoarthritides. Fluids with high leukocyte counts have been seen in our series only in patients who also have rheumatoid arthritis or gout.[70] Synovial biopsies have shown only mild villous proliferation, focal increased lining cells, and increased vascularity.[70]

The early increased cartilage thickness producing wide "joint spaces" on roentgenograms can be seen at various joints. Later, joint space narrowing, osteophytes, and subchondral sclerosis occur. Chondrocalcinosis, capsular calcification,[67] and osteochondromas have occasionally been seen. Remodeling of phalanges can produce thickening of the shaft at the tendon and capsular attachments, but thin metacarpal shafts have also been seen, possibly owing to remodeling. In the spine, large anterior osteophytes and ossification in widened disks and in ligaments can be seen. Vertebral bodies often develop anteroposterior elongation.[69]

Mechanisms involved in the secondary osteoarthritis appear to include dramatic cartilage overgrowth that produces joint incongruity and abnormal wear. Whether abnormal cartilage composition also contributes to degeneration is not known. Hypermobility might also contribute to cartilage abuse. Hypermobility was severe in seven patients studied by Kellgren and coworkers, with actual subluxations in two.[69] Chondrocalcinosis seen on roentgenograms[71] and apatite crystals seen so far mainly in synovial biopsies[70] might also contribute to osteoarthritis by either local mechanical effects in the cartilage or low-grade inflammation. Histologic studies of articular cartilage show hyperplasia and hypertrophy of the columnar and basal zones of chondrocytes. Superficial fibrillation and erosion of cartilage at weight-bearing sites occur with time.[67] Marginal osteophyte formation is often excessive.

As noted previously, musculoskeletal symptoms in acromegaly are due not only to osteoarthritis but also may be due to carpal tunnel syndrome, hypermobility, and possibly other related endocrine deficiencies.

Acromegaly can be treated by surgical resection of small adenomas or pituitary irradiation. There is no suggestion that this alters established osteoarthritis, although associated conditions due to overgrowth of soft tissue, such as the carpal tunnel syndrome, are dramatically relieved.

When needed, surgery such as total hip arthroplasty has been successful, with the firm trabecular bone of acromegaly appearing to tolerate the prosthesis well.[67] Careful evaluation of other endocrine values is essential before surgery. Adrenal insufficiency secondary to hypopituitarism, for example, may require steroid supplementation.

Hypothyroidism

Only fairly severe hypothyroidism with detectable clinical features such as cold intolerance, weight gain, lethargy, and constipation has been definitely associated with arthropathy. In addition to low serum T_3 and T_4 levels, reported cases have highly elevated TSH, suggesting that they are due to primary thyroid disease rather than pituitary insufficiency.

Osteoarthritis has been described in association with hypothyroidism,[72] but whether it is definitely increased over the expected frequency in the population is not known. Chondrocalcinosis and CPPD deposition do occur and could explain some OA.[73]

Roentgenograms may or may not show chondrocalcinosis, even if CPPD crystals are found in the synovial fluid. Some patients have a very destructive OA.[72]

Other manifestations of hypothyroidism cause musculoskeletal symptoms that can be confused with OA. These include carpal tunnel syndrome, viscous joint effusions, myalgias, myopathy, secondary gout, flexor tenosynovitis, and fibrositis. Serum creatine phosphokinase may be elevated and may cause confusion with polymyositis.

There is no evidence that treating hypothyroidism alters any associated OA, but thyroid hormone replacement may relieve some of the associated symptoms. One should be aware that patients with CPPD crystals but no inflammatory reaction can and do develop acute pseudogout with thyroid hormone therapy.[7]

Hyperparathyroidism

Increased levels of parathyroid hormone, whether primary or secondary, can produce a wide variety of rheumatic problems in addition to the classic features of osteitis fibrosa cystica. Other systemic manifestations include peptic ulcer disease, nephrolithiasis, symptoms due to hypercalcemia, pancreatitis, or a variety of other less common problems. Serum calcium levels are usually elevated at some time; hyperparathyroidism can be confirmed by elevated parathyroid hormone levels. Serum uric acid may be increased.

Osteoarthritis has been described complicating hyperparathyroidism,[74] and two major mechanisms have been postulated. These are (1) cartilage damage from the mechanical or inflammatory effects of the frequently associated CPPD crystal deposition (chondrocalcinosis has been reported in up to 25% of patients with primary hyperparathyroidism[75]); and (2) subchondral bone erosion due to the resorptive effects of parathormone, leading to subchondral bone change and secondary collapse of articular cartilage. This has been seen most often at the distal interphalangeal, proximal interphalangeal, metacarpophalangeal, and wrist joints.[74] Parathormone increases collagenase activity, which also contributes to tendon ruptures and avulsions.[76] The resulting instability might be a factor in some OA.

Roentgenograms classically show subperiosteal bone resorption along the middle phalanges or elsewhere and cystic or sclerotic changes in bone and may show typical chondrocalcinosis.[77]

Synovial effusions may contain CPPD crystals, and these sometimes are accompanied by elevated leukocyte counts. Because of the impaired urate clearance, urate crystals can also be present. Concomitant occurrence of synovial fluid urates and CPPD should suggest a search for hyperparathyroidism.[78]

Other musculoskeletal problems[79] seen in hyperparathyroidism include gout related to impaired renal clearance of urate, a proximal neuromyopathy, fatigue that is probably partially due to hypercalcemia, and ischemic problems due to intravascular calcification in secondary hyperparathyroidism. Parathyroidectomy does not consistently alter the chondrocalcinosis, and, in fact, attacks of pseudogout can occur postoperatively coincident with the fall in serum calcium.[77, 80, 81] Bone resorption can be reversed, and systemic features such as the neuromyopathy and fatigue should resolve, although established OA will not.

Diabetes Mellitus

Although diabetes has been mentioned as a possible cause of osteoarthritis,[82] known mechanisms through which OA may develop seem to be limited so far to the neuropathic joints complicating diabetes. These are discussed separately under Charcot joints.

Diabetes does have other effects on the musculoskeletal system that can confuse or complicate the management of OA. These include distal neuropathy, a proximal muscle weakness probably due to neuropathy and termed diabetic amyotrophy, adhesive capsulitis at the shoulders, phalangeal flexion contractures[83] with or without Dupuytren's contracture, septic joints, and osteolysis.

Aspirin has a mild hypoglycemic effect that occasionally needs to be considered in patient management. Use of intra-articular steroids for therapy of OA should be used cautiously in light of their known systemic absorption and ability to cause temporary control problems in severe diabetes.

BONE DYSPLASIAS

Multiple Epiphyseal Dysplasia (MED)

This familial disease of unknown cause produces fragmentation and irregularity of epiphyses of many bones. Patients tend to have short stature with relatively short extremities and stubby fingers. The severity of involvement is highly variable, as is the number of epiphyses involved. Most patients are not dwarfs, and, in fact, the first clue to this disease may be the premature osteoarthritis. For purposes of differentiation from spondyloepiphyseal dysplasia, the spine is uninvolved or only mildly involved, although the cause of neither syndrome is known. There is almost certainly considerable heterogeneity in the cases now called MED. Some cases with mild spinal disease in the Mseleni area in South Africa have tentatively been included with MED.[84]

Routine laboratory studies are normal. Other predictable systemic features have not been identified. It appears that the inheritance is most likely autosomal dominant.[85] Only approximately 100 cases have been reported in the United States, but this figure may represent underdiagnosis.

Osteoarthritis develops typically in affected families any time from the early teens to about 30 years of age. The joints most prominently involved have been the hips, followed by the knees, ankles, shoulders, and elbows.[85–87] Mild joint pain on motion often antedates diagnosable OA. Most reported cases have been mild, with little interference with normal activities. Short hands and limited hip motion have been the most common physical findings. Flexion deformities and hypermobility have been reported.[88] Gait may be waddling.

Hip roentgenograms initially show fragmentation of epiphyses, then flattening and irregularity of the femoral heads, with later secondary osteoarthritis. Ossification centers may be late in appearing. Roentgenographic changes in the hip are similar to those in Legg-Calvé-Perthes disease. Roentgenographic changes are milder in the arms, possibly because of less weight bearing. Epiphyseal abnormalities heal after puberty, leaving only the irregularities and later osteoarthritis.

Other frequent changes have been irregularity of the tibial surfaces at the knee joints, sloping of the tibiotalar joints (with the distal tibia sloping downward from lateral to medial), talar sclerosis and irregularity, and flattening of the metatarsal heads. Knee roentgenograms can show the appearance of osteochondritis dissecans.[89] In a series of six cases from France that included both multiple epiphyseal dysplasia and spondyloepiphyseal dysplasia, osteochondromas and chondrocalcinosis were shown in three cases, with bouts of clinically detected inflammation.[90]

Mechanisms involve alteration of epiphyses, with resulting irregularity of the shape of bone ends leading to secondary osteoarthritis. Epiphyseal cartilage has been examined histologically in only two cases,[91] with decreased chondrocytes identified. More morphologic and biochemical study is needed. Recently, some preliminary study of sternal cartilage has been done in mice with chondrodysplasia as a model of epiphyseal dysplasia. Proteoglycans appeared normal, but there may be abnormal collagen monomer assembly.[92]

Genetic counseling can be useful in reassuring unaffected family members that their children should not be involved. In families with mild disease, prognosis is good.[85] It is not known whether early protection or osteotomy might slow progression of the hip osteoarthritis, but this merits consideration. Non–weight-bearing exercises such as swimming are encouraged to maintain joint range of motion and muscle strength for stability. Because hypothyroidism in children can cause similar epiphyseal changes and delayed bone age, this treatable disease should be considered in the differential diagnosis.

Spondyloephiphyseal Dysplasia (SED)

Familial syndromes that are characterized by short stature and retarded ossification of the vertebral bodies, pelvis, and extremities and that are evident at birth have been identified by Spranger and Langer[93] and Maroteux and associates.[94] In affected infants, the face may be flat, with the eyes widely spaced, the neck short, and the thorax barrel-shaped.

Skeletal shortening is due primarily to impaired growth of the spine and proximal extremities, not the hands and feet. Myopia and retinal detachments can occur (as in arthro-ophthalmopathy). Mild ("tarda") forms may lack the extraskeletal features.[94–97] Inheritance of the congenital form is autosomal dominant. The "tarda" form presenting as early OA is apparently an X-linked recessive trait seen only in males.[95, 96] Published cases considered to be SED may be of diverse causes with different patterns of inheritance. This syndrome must be distinguished from Morquio's syndrome; SED does not have the corneal clouding, keratosulfaturia, hand involvement, and other features seen in the otherwise similar Morquio's syndrome.

Osteoarthritis may be the presenting symptom of "tarda" or mild forms that cause premature OA in young adults, with the spinal changes recognized only in retrospect. The hip is the most involved joint, with stiffness and a waddling gait being manifestations. Two brothers with SED and severe metacarpophalangeal joint involvement and without beta-2 globulin have been reported.[98]

Roentgenograms in infancy show delayed or absent ossification centers. Vertebral bodies are flattened with ossification defects. Vertebrae may appear pear-shaped. In childhood, dorsal kyphosis and lumbar lordosis become greatly exaggerated. Ossification in femoral heads and necks continues slowly; epiphyses are deformed, with the femoral heads always involved but other sites of involvement varying. In adults, the vertebral bodies of the thoracic spine show more typical flattening (platyspondyly) and wedging than those of the lumbar spine. The acetabulum is small, and the femoral heads are distorted with coxa vara deformity. Joint space narrowing, subchondral sclerosis, cysts, and osteophytes develop in young adults at the hips and occasionally have also been described at the knees.

The mechanism for OA of the hip seems to be the severe distortion of the femoral heads. Pathologic study of cartilage in infants dying shortly after birth showed PAS-positive, diastase-resistant inclusions in chondrocytes. By electron microscopy, these inclusions were shown to be due to granular material in greatly dilated, rough endoplasmic reticulum.[99] A biochemical defect has not yet been identified.

Treatment with hip arthroplasty has been reported.

Osteo-onychodystrophy (Nail-Patella Syndrome)

This rare, autosomal dominant condition is manifested by nail dysplasia; skeletal deformities, including iliac horns; dislocated radial heads with elbow deformity; and hypoplasia or aplasia of the patellae.[100–102] Renal disease varying from asymptomatic proteinuria to renal failure can occur.[103] A glomerular basement membrane lesion is postulated.

Premature degenerative arthritis has been reported primarily at the elbows and knees, with variable ages of onset.

Diagnostic roentgenographic changes include dysplasia of the iliac wings, with bony horns arising posteriorly from the ilium in most patients. These horns are present in infancy and may be palpable. The patella may be absent or hypoplastic.

Laxity of fingers with correctable swan-neck deformities has been described.[100] The patella may subluxate with such hypermobility, possibly contributing to degenerative arthritis in addition to the malalignments that may occur at the elbows. Renal osteodystrophy has complicated at least one case and has also contributed to the bone and joint problems.[103] No primary pathologic abnormalities of cartilage or bone have been defined.

Other congenital syndromes reported less commonly can potentially be confused with the nail-patella syndrome. For example, onychodysplasia has also been seen with short stature, short middle phalanges, fused fifth toes, broad nose, wide mouth, and mild intellectual impairment.[102] Onychodysplasia with deafness and finger-like thumbs can also occur.[104]

Observation for and management of any progressive renal disease is important.

Progressive Hereditary Arthro-ophthalmopathy (Stickler's Syndrome)

A familial syndrome of myopia, often leading to retinal detachment, and an early onset of an arthropathy with features of osteoarthritis was described by Stickler and coworkers in 1960.[105] Inheritance is thought to be autosomal dominant. A still unknown defect of eye and bone or joint tissues is postulated. Other associated congenital anomalies occasionally described have been cleft palate, micrognathia, and hearing loss.[106]

Afflicted individuals are reportedly recognized at birth by bony enlargement of the ankles, knees, wrists, and other joints. Pain and stiffness of involved joints during and after use begin during childhood. Progression varies. Some patients have had unexplained bouts of acute inflammation. Crepitus and locking have developed in knees in which OA is often detectable by the time the patient reaches 20 years of age. Other joints prominently involved have been the elbows, hips, shoulders, spine, and fingers (metacarpophalangeal joints but not distal interphalangeal joints). Mild hypermobility has been described without other features of Ehlers-Danlos syndrome. Hips may subluxate, and severe degenerative arthritis can evolve.

Two synovial biopsies have been performed; some intimal thickening of medium-sized artery walls was found in one biopsy specimen but no inflammation or other abnormalities.

Synovial fluids have not been studied. Serum biochemical abnormalities are not known. Popkin and Palomeno[106] described increased urinary hydroxyproline excretion in six patients.

Roentgenograms show irregular epiphyses with abnormal modeling of ends of bones that antedates joint space narrowing as detected on routine films. Joint spaces may initially even be abnormally wide, as has been described with acromegaly. Ossified loose bodies have been seen in established disease. Wedge-shaped vertebrae were observed in some patients.

Mechanisms are not established. Cartilage, bone, or loose bodies have not been studied histologically or biochemically. The primary defect leading to arthritis is proposed to be abnormal epiphyseal bone development.

Recognition of the serious potential for blindness as well as early osteoarthritis should influence career choices when possible. Close ophthalmologic supervision may allow prompt treatment of retinal detachment.

Other Diseases Involving Epiphyses

The previous syndromes emphasize that congenital problems distorting epiphyses do seem to account for some cases of premature osteoarthritis.

Other uncommon familial syndromes to be considered include the following:

1. In *the trichorhinophalangeal syndrome*,[107, 108] hair is sparse and fine; the nose is bulbous; and dwarfism occurs in some patients. Problems are mostly cosmetic, except in the more severe (Type II) form, in which microcephaly and retardation may occur. This appears to be inherited as an autosomal dominant trait. Bony enlargement, OA, and clinodactyly of the proximal interphalangeal joints are prominent. The hips may also be involved. The proximal epiphyses of the middle phalanges are cone-shaped on roentgenograms. The fingers are often short because the epiphyses fuse prematurely.

2. The chondrodystrophy known as *the Kniest* or *"Swiss cheese cartilage" syndrome*[109] is associated with dwarfism, kyphoscoliosis, flat rounded facies, and multiple enlarged joints with limited motion (most prominent at the proximal interphalangeal joints). Neurosensory hearing loss, ptosis, and myopia have been reported. Roentgenograms have shown irregular epiphyses, narrow joint spaces, irregular vertebrae, and wide metaphyses.

Histologic studies of cartilage show matrix holes reminiscent of Swiss cheese. Electron microscopy has revealed dilated, rough endoplasmic reticulum in chondrocytes.

3. *An unnamed autosomal dominant familial disease with fragmentation restricted to digital epiphyses* that causes short, knobby digits with osteoarthritic changes beginning before puberty has been described.[110] Limitation to the hands and occasionally the feet caused the authors to tentatively separate this from other epiphyseal dysplasias.

4. *Thiemann's disease*[111, 112] has been associated with progressive enlargement of the proximal interphalangeal joints and premature OA of the fingers, with some cases probably due to epiphyseal dysplasia. Roentgenograms show flattening and irregularity of the basal epiphyses of the middle phalanx at onset. This may resolve completely or may progress to OA. One or more fingers can be involved, with onset occurring before puberty. Autosomal dominant inheritance is described. Necrosis of an epiphysis has been shown on a single biopsy.

5. In *Ellis–van Creveld syndrome (chondroectodermal dysplasia),* there are defects in tissues of both mesodermal and ectodermal origin, with shortened tubular bones, polydactylism, dysplastic teeth, hair, and nails, and congenital heart disease. Inheritance appears to be autosomal recessive. Deformity of phalangeal epiphyses has been noted.[113]

6. *Chondrodysplasia punctata (Conradi's disease)*[114, 115] begins in infancy with punctate calcifications of epiphyses and is followed by epiphyseal dysplasia with asymmetric shortening of different bones, leading to secondary OA. There may be joint contractures. The severity of reported cases varies widely.

7. In *Turner's syndrome,* there may be epiphyseal abnormalities at the knees and elbow joints.[115]

8. In *Maffucci's syndrome,* which is characterized by multiple cavernous hemangiomas and phlebectasia, there is also asymmetric alteration of epiphyses without obvious relation to the hemangiomas.

9. Recently, a patient was described who had *premature osteoarthritis and cartilage dysplasia associated with massive accumulation of lipids in chondrocytes.*[116] Hip pain began when the patient was 12 years old, and severe OA of the hip required arthroplasties by age 23. Roentgenograms showed severe deformation of femoral heads, but whether primary changes were in epiphyses or just in articular cartilage was not clear. Other joints also had mild OA.

Light microscopy of articular cartilage showed chondrocytes with many large vacuoles containing material that was positive on PAS and Sudan staining. Electron microscopy revealed granular and lamellar material in similar vacuoles.

10. *Kashin-Beck disease,*[117] recognized in Russia and Manchuria, affects epiphyses of growing children and causes skeletal shortening and premature osteoarthritis. The hands are prominently involved. Limited studies have suggested a variety of possible etiologic mechanisms such as contamination of grain with a fungus, or iron excess.

Epiphyseal injuries in childhood can cause growth disturbances and later OA.[118]

A number of other bone dysplasias have not been listed as causes of osteoarthritis. Some are not consistent with survival into adult life. Metaphyseal dysplasias such as "cartilage-hair hypoplasia"[119] cause dwarfism and deformity but apparently, by sparing epiphyses, do not distort joints and cause early OA. Further observations of older patients with these dysplasias are needed. Most mucopolysaccharidoses are often associated with stiff joints and carpal tunnel syndrome but apparently not with early OA. In Morquio's syndrome, with its dramatic platyspondyly, early OA may occasionally evolve from the misshapen peripheral epiphyses, as with SED, with which it can be confused.

More details about epiphyseal and other bone dysplasias are reviewed by Spranger and coworkers.[114]

CALCIUM CRYSTAL DEPOSITION DISEASES

Calcium Pyrophosphate Deposition Disease

Deposition of calcium pyrophosphate dihydrate (CPPD) crystals, which is virtually confined to joints and bursae, can have various overlapping or separate presentations.[120–122] The crystals can be phagocytized by synovial fluid cells[120, 123] and can be associated with acute or chronic gout-like arthritis. Chronic forms may closely mimic joint involvement in rheumatoid arthritis. CPPD can be present in asymptomatic form in articular cartilage and can then be detected only by roentgenogram or histologic examination. Such "chondrocalcinosis" was described in 1957 by Zitnan and Sitaj[124]; the synovial fluid crystals and their apparent role in inflammation were discovered by McCarty and Hollander in 1961.[125] CPPD crystals are also commonly found in many osteoarthritic joint fluids, where they are sometimes, but not invariably, associated with appreciable inflammation.[126, 127]

Calcium pyrophosphate deposition is most often idiopathic, although it clearly increases with age and has been identified in familial clusters in Czechoslovakia,[128] Chile,[129] and elsewhere. The mode(s) of inheritance is not clear. CPPD crystals have been identified in 3.2% to 6.8% of cadavers and have been suspected roentgenographically in 2.2% to 4.6% of subjects in their 60's and in as many as 27% of a group of elderly people with a mean age of 83 years.[120, 130] CPPD deposition has also been described to be increased in association with a number of important, largely metabolic diseases, including hyperparathyroidism, hemochromatosis, hypothyroidism, hypophosphatasia, hypomagnesemia, and possibly also amyloidosis, ochronosis, acromegaly, and Wilson's disease.

CPPD crystals are identified in tissue or synovial fluid as rod- or rhomboid-shaped crystals that are usually 3 to 15 μ in length. With compensated polarized light, they have weakly positive or absent birefringence. Light-microscopic morphologic and birefringence characteristics are highly suggestive of CPPD crystals but are not pathognomonic, because other rod-like, positively birefringent crystals, including depot steroids, some calcium oxalate,[131] and calcium hydrogen phosphate dihydrate,[132, 133] also can occasionally be seen in joint effusions. Lithium heparin used in test tubes as an anticoagulant may also yield crystals that resemble CPPD.[134]

Crystals can be concentrated and prepared for x-ray diffraction study as described by Kohn and coworkers.[135] If specimens have adequate numbers of crystals, this is definitive.

Electron-microscopic examination for crystals can be done with standard glutaraldehyde or other fixation, as done for routine transmission electron microscopy, as the CPPD crystals are minimally soluble in the water-based solutions used. CPPD crystals are electron-dense and foamy after exposure to the electron beam (Fig.14–8). Urate and some other crystals that would be included in the differential diagnosis, however, are dissolved. CPPD crystals are hard and can be dislodged from sections, causing them to be missed. A rapid technique allowing transmission electron-microscopic processing for examination in less than 4 hours[136] may prove useful in prompt diagnosis of problem cases. Small CPPD crystals can be missed by light microscopy and found by electron microscopy.

Drops of crystal-containing synovial fluid can also be dried on Formvar-coated grids or processed for scanning electron microscopy for rapid identification of the presence of crystals. With all these electron-microscopic techniques, crystals can then be further characterized either by electron diffraction[132] or electron probe elemental analysis. The latter can confirm a Ca:P ratio of approximately 1:1, as is seen with CPPD.[132, 137]

CPPD crystals can be identified in the midzone of involved articular cartilage (Fig.14–9) and in tophus-like deposits in synovial biopsy specimens.[133, 138] The only required precaution is to avoid decalcification, which might be done by error if the specimen is submitted with fragments of bone. Serum calcium and phosphorus levels are usually normal, except in hyperparathyroidism.

The osteoarthritis that occurs with CPPD deposition appears to be of at least two patterns:

1. Obvious CPPD deposition antedates significant OA. As cartilage degenerates, OA with joint distribution typical of that of CPPD deposition disease develops, i.e., prominent involvement of the knees, wrists, and second and third metacarpophalangeal joints.

2. The second pattern is osteoarthritis, either idiopathic or related to some other primary cause, in which CPPD crystal deposition develops late in the disease. This is presumably a result of cartilage and other damage, as is also seen in chronic rheumatoid arthritis, gout, and other joint diseases. It is speculated that a cartilage matrix change in these various situations favors CPPD precipitation. Adequate sequential studies have not been done to fully establish this suggested sequence. In an ongoing study in our laboratory, about 60% of OA synovial fluids have contained either CPPD or apatite crystals.

Synovial fluids in chronic OA with CPPD crystals are typically still "noninflammatory" with predominantly mononuclear cells. Only during attacks of crystal-induced arthritis do leukocyte counts rise.

Roentgenographic findings include the typical linear calcification in articular cartilages and menisci. Visible calcification, however, may disappear with loss of cartilage or may rarely be seen only as punctate deposits spread throughout the joint. Other CPPD deposits may be too small to be detected by roentgenography. Joint space narrowing, subchondral sclerosis, and cysts in joints typically involved

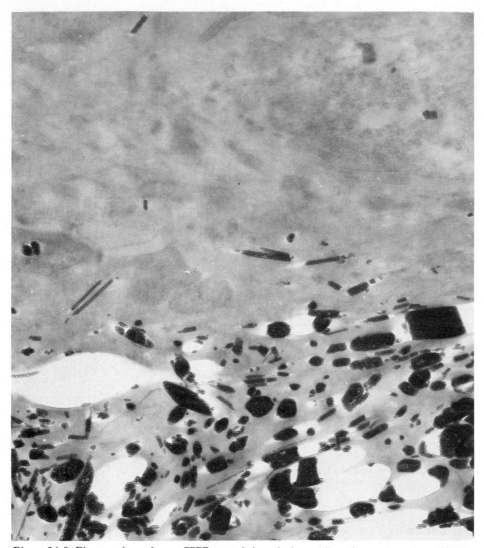

Figure 14–8. Electron-dense foamy CPPD crystals in articular cartilage (approximately ×18,000).

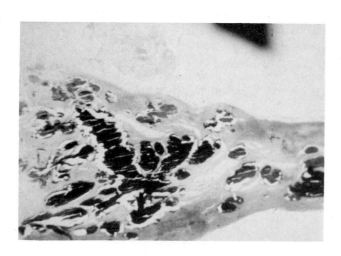

Figure 14–9. Von Kossa staining of CPPD crystals most profuse in the midzone of a knee meniscus.

in CPPD deposition disease should also suggest this diagnosis. Osteophyte formation is variable and inconstant. Occasional joints show severe destruction mimicking Charcot joints even without neurologic disease. Rarely, bony fusion may occur.

Mechanisms of the production of osteoarthritis with CPPD deposition may include mechanical effects of the crystals in the cartilage or acute and/or chronic inflammation induced by the crystals with release of enzymes destructive to cartilage. An element of inflammation has been documented in naturally occurring[126, 127] and experimental OA.[139] Crystals are one possible factor contributing to this, although recent studies in our laboratory do not show any clear correlation between the severity of synovial fluid inflammatory cell response and the presence of crystals.

Many joint fluids, including those of idiopathic osteoarthritis, have been reported to have higher than normal concentrations of pyrophosphate,[140, 141] but whether this is followed by increased precipitation of CPPD crystals is not known.

Treatment of inflammatory episodes with nonsteroidal anti-inflammatory drugs will usually control such bouts. Colchicine may also be effective, especially if administered intravenously. In patients with repeated episodes of inflammation, daily low-dose prophylactic administration of nonsteroidal agents can help control symptoms. There is no evidence that this has any beneficial effect on the cartilage degeneration.

Massive numbers of crystals can be aspirated with at least theoretic advantage to the joint involved, but no methods to deplete CPPD crystals, comparable to the use of allopurinol or probenecid in gout, are available. Associated metabolic disease should be sought and treated when possible.

Apatite Crystal Deposition Disease

Hydroxyapatite, $Ca_5OH(PO_4)_3H_2O_2$, has been recognized to be involved in the acute soft tissue syndromes of calcific tendinitis, bursitis, and periarthritis[142, 143] and the subcutaneous calcifications in scleroderma and dermatomyositis. Although suspected[144] and shown[145] to be present in some articular cartilages, a role for apatite in joint disease was not strongly considered until reports in the 1970's by Dieppe and colleagues[146] and Schumacher and coworkers.[137, 147] Clumps of apatite

crystals can be phagocytized in vivo or in vitro[148] and can induce inflammation when injected into the knee joints of dogs.[137] As with CPPD or urate crystals, they can be present without appearing to cause symptoms or can be associated with acute transient or chronic erosive arthritis.[149] Intra-articular apatite crystals have been seen in collagen-vascular disease,[150] renal failure being treated with dialysis, hypothyroidism, hemochromatosis, CPPD deposition disease, and osteoarthritis,[137] as will be discussed below. Crystals have also been seen without any evident underlying cause,[137] suggesting still incompletely explained systemic factors in their deposition. Trauma is clearly an inadequate explanation for the multifocal deposits. Knee effusions have been studied most often, but there are no good data as to the frequency of involvement of various joints, the ages of individuals affected, and the epidemiologic patterns.

Clumps of apatite crystals are not birefringent and thus are not more readily detected with compensated polarized light. Clumps appear as glossy, homogeneous, and round or angular chunks measuring 1 to 15 μ in diameter. Clumps stain strongly with alizarin red or von Kossa stains. X-ray diffraction can be diagnostic if sufficient numbers of crystals are present. Smaller numbers of crystals can be identified by electron microscopy as tiny needles measuring 75 to 250 Å in diameter (Fig. 14–10). Electron probe elemental analysis shows a Ca:P ratio of approximately 1.7:1.[137, 149] This can be done with either transmission or scanning electron microscopy.

Osteoarthritis with identifiable apatite crystals has to date shown no features different from any other OA except that the presence of apatite correlates with roentgenographic evidence of more severe OA. Whether this is a result or a cause of the OA is not known. Nevertheless, 9 of 34 osteoarthritic joint fluid specimens studied by Huskisson and associates[127] had apparent apatite by scanning electron microscopy, whereas we have found apatite by alizarin red staining and transmission electron microscopy in approximately 50% of the first 100 osteoarthritic joint fluid samples we have studied.[126] Virtually every fluid specimen with CPPD crystals also contains apatite.

Synovial effusions in most OA associated with apatite have been noninflammatory, although occasional elevated leukocyte counts and inflammatory infiltrates or proliferative changes in synovium can be seen. These seem

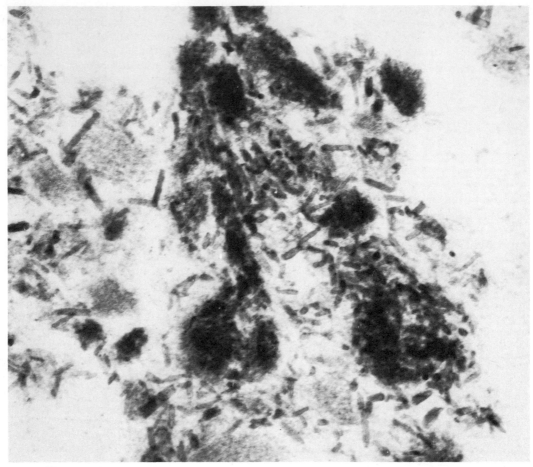

Figure 14–10. Needle-shaped apatite crystals at ×90,000 magnification by electron microscopy.

to correlate with the severity of OA as well as with the presence of crystals,[126] so that the role of the crystals versus other factors in the development of inflammation has not been established.

Apatite clumps can be demonstrated in synovium in OA[126, 127] and, most intriguingly, can be found in articular cartilage by electron microscopy[126, 151] much more often than had been appreciated by light microscopy or roentgenography (Fig. 14–11). Quantitation of crystal frequency and amount in different joints, ages, and patterns of OA is still needed. Basophilia and von Kossa staining in calcified areas can be an important clue to the presence of crystals.[151] Ali has emphasized that the initial apatite deposition is in matrix vesicles, although this is not clearly true in all studies.[152]

Roentgenograms in OA quite commonly show small periarticular calcifications that have previously been little appreciated but can now

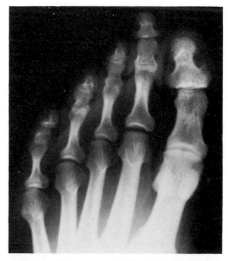

Figure 14–11. Mild osteoarthritis with joint space narrowing and sclerosis at the first metatarsophalangeal joint. Acute inflammation that was proved to be due to apatite crystals developed at this joint.

be shown to correlate with both the severity of OA and the presence of apatite.[126, 127]

Severe degenerative changes of the shoulder in association with apatite-containing particles have recently been described by McCarty and colleagues and termed "Milwaukee shoulder."[153, 154] Patients presented with painful shoulders with decreased mobility or stability. Roentgenographic evidence of a complete tear of the fibrous rotator cuff was present in seven of eight shoulder joints; there were also degenerative changes of the humeral head or glenoid of the scapula and of the acromioclavicular joint and calcification of the tendinous rotator cuff. All synovial fluid samples showed apatite crystals and, in addition, collagenase and neutral protease activity. It was suggested that enzymatic release of hydroxyapatite crystals from the synovium and endocytosis by synovial macrophage-like cells, with subsequent crystal-stimulated release of collagenase and neutral protease into the joint fluid, were components of the pathogenic cycle of this entity. The origin of apatite in such severely destroyed joints is not established; much of it may be from bony debris.

As noted previously, mechanisms relating apatite to low-grade inflammation and OA are still under study. One possibility is that other materials in the fluid or coating the apatite clumps may influence their inflammatory potential. Apatite may also be contributing to OA by its physical presence in the cartilage, as was also suggested with CPPD. Naturally occurring[155] and experimental[156] apatite deposition in rabbit articular cartilage has been documented and should allow study of any of its effects on cartilage with further aging.

As yet, there are no recommended alterations in the routine treatment program for OA that can be predicated on the presence of apatite crystals in synovial fluid. Nonsteroidal anti-inflammatory agents do appear to be more effective, however, when there is a strong inflammatory component.

OTHER SYSTEMIC DISEASES

Neuropathic Arthropathy (Charcot Joints)

Neuropathy due to various causes can be complicated by an arthropathy that has elements of unusually severe osteoarthritis. The neuropathy may vary from mild loss of sensation of pain or proprioception to a severe neurologic problem, including anesthesia.[157] Since an early description by Charcot in 1868, diseases that have been associated with neuropathic joints include diabetes mellitus,[158] syringomyelia, meningomyelocele, syphilis with tabes dorsalis, leprosy, congenital insensitivity to pain,[159] amyloidosis,[160] and hereditary sensory neuropathies.[161] Other less common causes of neurologic dysfunction have also been described with Charcot joints.[157, 162, 163] Sites of involvement tend to vary among diseases and are discussed below.

The arthropathy clinically presents with swelling that may be massive, crepitus from the typically severe destruction of cartilage and bone, instability, palpable loose bodies, and, later, large osteophytes. Some pain may be present and is worse on use. When present, pain tends to be much less than would be expected from the appearance of the joint. Effusions are often intermittent and may be associated with erythema.

Synovial effusions are generally non-inflammatory or hemorrhagic. Cells in the fluid have been mostly mononuclear. In occasional patients with associated calcium pyrophosphate deposition, higher leukocyte counts and more neutrophils are seen.

Synovial biopsies show cartilaginous and bony debris ground deeply into the membrane along with hemosiderin and metaplastic bone formation.[164, 165] Pannus-like synovial proliferation has been described.[166] Mild to moderate infiltration of chronic inflammatory cells has been noted without specific relationship to calcified areas.[167] Histologic examination of cartilage has shown the sequence of changes seen in other OA.[168] Bone has been described as histologically normal except for the fractures.[169]

In tabes dorsalis, the knees are most prominently involved, with hip, ankle, foot, and spine disease also seen in some patients. About 10% of patients with tabes develop arthropathy. In syringomyelia, about 25% of afflicted individuals develop Charcot joints, which in this disease occur most often in the shoulder (Fig. 14–12). Other sites of involvement, in order of frequency, are the elbow, wrist, and cervical spine.

In diabetes mellitus, about 5% of patients with chronic disease and neuropathy develop neuropathic arthropathy in the feet. The tarsal and tarsometatarsal joints are commonly involved (Fig. 14–13). Osteolysis in the phalanges may accompany disease there. Other sites are affected much less often.

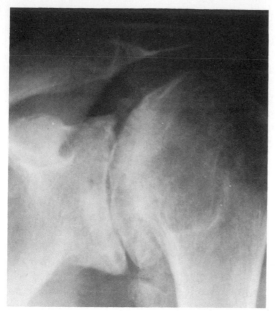

Figure 14–12. Charcot shoulder in syringomyclia. Note fragmentation, sclerosis, osteophytes, and joint space narrowing.

Roentgenograms initially show only soft tissue swelling, but this is soon followed by subluxation and changes seen with any osteoarthritis. Differentiating features may include enormous and bizarre osteophytes, transverse fractures, osteolysis, prominent osseous fragments, or calcifications. The diagnosis should often be suspected on clinical grounds before the more advanced distinctive changes appear. Chondrocalcinosis has been seen, but it is not clear if this is merely a result of the cartilage degeneration or whether a more destructive arthritis results when the neurologic deficit is added to a pre-existing calcium pyrophosphate deposition.[170, 171]

Mechanisms involved almost certainly include repeated joint abuse because of loss of normal pain and proprioceptive protection. Experimental studies have supported this; protection of denervated animal limbs from trauma has been reported to prevent fractures and other changes.[169] Microvascular disease has been thought to be a possible contributing factor in diabetics.

Treatment should include any efforts possible to slow or halt the various associated neurologic diseases. Protection from trauma is more critically important than in most primary osteoarthritides. Splinting, braces, special shoes, and canes are often helpful. Aspiration of large joint effusions can help prevent the stretching of supporting structures. Successful surgical fusions of very unstable joints have been performed, but some difficulties have been encountered in obtaining a fusion, especially if complete, long-duration immobilization is not achieved. Complete removal of the proliferated synovium and detritus, excision of an adequate amount of the damaged bone, and internal fixation seem to improve the chances for success of the fusion.[168]

Charcot joints may become secondarily infected, and this needs to be watched for and treated. Joint replacements have rarely been used and are generally contraindicated. In one instance, limited success at one hip was complicated by poor healing and by recurrent dislocations.[172] Fractures of fragments other than small ones require internal fixation. Osteotomy may provide some help by aligning severely subluxated knees.

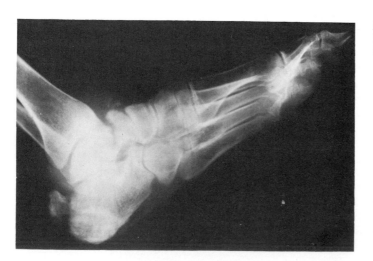

Figure 14–13. Charcot foot in diabetes mellitus. Note fracturing, calcifications, and intertarsal narrowing.

Paget's Disease (Osteitis Deformans)

Paget's disease is a skeletal disorder of unknown cause characterized by thickened trabeculae with disorganized osteoid seams. Both new bone formation and absorption are increased, leading to softening and enlargement of bones and bowing of the long bones. Other well-demarcated areas of bone are normal. Commonly involved sites include the tibiae, clavicles, femurs, pelvis, sternum, skull, and spine. Blood flow is increased in the lesions, occasionally leading to bruits and even high-output heart failure. Serum alkaline phosphatase is increased. Hydroxyproline released from sites of bone resorption is excreted, giving elevated urinary levels. Bone biopsy is needed only occasionally when the diagnosis is unclear. The disease is frequently asymptomatic.

Disease of the hip joint with features of osteoarthritis, i.e., pain on use and limited motion, can result from distortion of the femoral heads or acetabulum due to the underlying bone disease. Altman found OA of the hips in 30% of patients with Paget's disease.[173] The knee was involved in 11% of the patients. OA can develop in other joints, including even the first metatarsophalangeal joint, owing to distortion of the joint by adjacent pagetic bone involvement. Asymptomatic Paget's disease in one leg may lead to painful osteoarthritis on the opposite side as a result of leg-length discrepancy. Juxta-articular bony enlargement is sometimes evident.

Lumbar spine pain is very common[173] and in many patients is associated with straightening of the low back and some hip and knee flexion. Back pain has complex factors related to posture, some pagetic involvement, and secondary or unrelated OA. Synovial fluid examinations or synovial biopsies have not been reported in the studies reviewed.

Roentgenograms of areas involved with Paget's disease show mottled increase in bone density, coarse trabeculae, and incomplete fractures, as well as a variety of deformities due to the bone softening. Protrusio acetabuli with adjacent osteophytes can develop from the pressure of the femoral head into the soft acetabulum.[174] Joint space narrowing occurs. It has been suggested[175] that this is at least partially due to accelerated endochondral ossification and replacement of the deeper layers of cartilage by pagetic bone. Pagetic changes have been seen in the spinal ossifications of ankylosing hyperostosis.[173]

Mechanisms for the osteoarthritis include distortion of joint configuration by the abnormal bone, leading to abnormal wear, alteration in the properties of subchondral bone, and altered biomechanics from bowing and leg-length discrepancies.[173]

Pain obviously also arises from bone itself more often than from the joint disease, and this must be differentiated. Any dramatic increase in pain or swelling should suggest consideration of fracture or osteogenic sarcoma, which has an increased incidence in pagetic bone. Some patients have had overproduction of uric acid and associated gouty arthritis. CPPD deposition disease has also been reported,[176] but the frequency of neither this nor gout is convincingly increased over that in the nonpagetic population.[173]

Treatment of Paget's disease can include the use of aspirin or other nonsteroidal anti-inflammatory agents that seem to help both bone pain and the pain of the secondary osteoarthritis. Salmon calcitonin, 50 to 100 mrc units/day given parenterally, is useful for the bone disease in severe cases, but neutralizing antibodies may develop. Sodium etidronate, 5 mg/kg/day for up to 6 months, may decrease pain and lower alkaline phosphatase levels. Mithramycin has also been used in refractory disease.

Total joint replacements have been performed successfully in joints with pagetic bone involvement,[177] and osteotomies can be used to correct bowing deformities. Treatment with calcitonin or etidronate before any surgery may decrease the hypervascularity and limit the potential for bleeding at operation.

Osteopetrosis

Only about 200 cases of this rare disease have been reported.[178–182] It is characterized by generalized skeletal osteosclerosis, hard but fragile bone leading to easy fracture, and obliteration of the marrow cavity.

Patients with the severe "congenital" autosomal recessive form have not survived past 20 years of age; a milder autosomal dominant form also occurs. The disease mechanism involves defective absorption of calcified cartilage, with the persistence of primitive bone. Bone biopsies show increased trabecular bone that blends with the cortex, and cartilage cores within trabeculae. Varying appearances of osteoclasts have been described. Serum calcium and phosphorus levels are usually normal, but the alkaline phosphatase level is often increased. Renal tubular acidosis has been associated with osteopetrosis in several cases[183] and may actually have ameliorated the osteosclerosis.

Bone marrow encroachment can cause anemia, thrombocytopenia, leukopenia, and extramedullary hematopoiesis. Cranial nerve compression at foramina can occur. Infections may be increased and include osteomyelitis in the abnormal bone.

Osteoarthritis has been noted especially at the hips.[178–180] Factors that may be involved include loss of the normal shock-absorbing qualities for cartilage with this hard bone, subchondral fractures weakening support for the initially normal cartilage, and, in a few of the reported cases, malalignment problems from deformities or aseptic necrosis resulting from femoral neck fractures.[178]

Roentgenograms of bones[181, 182] show diffuse, extreme laminar cortical thickening with a chalky appearance, loss of normal trabeculations, and varying degrees of obliteration of the marrow cavity. Margins of the cortex usually remain sharp, not fuzzy as in metastatic tumor. A "shaft within a shaft" appearance can be seen in long bones. Other causes of relatively diffuse, dense sclerotic bone that should be differentiated include fluorosis,[184] sickle cell disease, Paget's disease, hyperparathyroidism, lymphoma, multiple myeloma,[185] mastocytosis, polyvinylpyrrolidone toxicity,[186] heavy metal poisoning, sarcoidosis, renal osteodystrophy,[187] and myelofibrosis. At least some of these conditions have also been associated with bone necrosis, fractures, and secondary OA.

Although there have been some difficulties in surgery on this brittle bone, successful total hip replacement surgery has been performed.[178, 179] The basic defect in osteopetrosis may include defective osteoclast activity. Osteoclast replacement by marrow transplantation has recently been reported to reverse abnormal pathologic and clinical findings in one infant.[188]

Osteoarthritis Following Miscellaneous Systemic Diseases With Other Initial Mechanisms of Joint Damage

Inflammatory or proliferative joint diseases of many kinds involving synovium can produce cartilage damage that leads to progressively severe osteoarthritis that can persist with or without continued activity of the inflammatory disease. Some examples are rheumatoid arthritis, septic arthritis, gout, seronegative spondyloarthropathies, and hemophilia. Release of destructive enzymes from inflammatory and proliferative cells is a major factor in the cartilage degeneration. In gout, crystals can also become deposited in cartilage and adjacent bone and can destroy cartilage.

Treatment directed effectively at early control of the synovial involvement and systemic features of these diseases can prevent the later OA.

Obesity

The role of obesity in osteoarthritis remains incompletely defined, but it is probably of some significance. The conflicting epidemiologic studies have been reviewed by Lee and associates.[82] Some studies have used only roentgenograms to diagnose OA, which may obviously include many cases of no clinical significance.

Sebo and coworkers[189] studied 664 individuals and found a strong correlation between Grade 2 OA of the knees and first metatarsophalangeal joints and obesity. There was even some correlation between obesity and OA of the distal interphalangeal joints of the fingers, suggesting that not all the association was due to the direct effect of the weight. They suggested that thigh obesity caused varus deformity of the knee that contributed to the knee OA.

Saville and Dickson[190] and Sebo and colleagues[189] found no correlation between weight and OA of the hip, but others have reported the incidence of OA of the hip to be increased in obese patients in population studies.[191] One study[192] claimed no obvious increased incidence of OA in 25 extremely obese patients. This group included patients only up to 54 years of age. It was considered a possibility that these people may have been so obese that they were very inactive and not representative. Six of them did have torn knee menisci requiring surgery.

Some roentgenographic surveys have not found increased evidence of OA with obesity.[193, 194] It is possible that OA of weight-bearing joints is only more symptomatic with obesity. The apparent increased OA in non–weight-bearing joints of obese patients[82, 189, 195, 196] has suggested the possibility that dietary factors (or some other systemic factor linked with

with obesity) might damage cartilage cells or matrix. The Silberbergs[197] produced increased OA in mice given lard-enriched diets; Sokoloff and coworkers could not show any worsening of OA in mice given dietary supplements of vegetable fats or lard.[198]

Treatment of obesity may help reduce the symptoms of osteoarthritis by decreasing strain on supporting structures, by allowing more normal gait and activity, possibly by decreasing abnormal stress on the joint, and by making needed surgery easier. Because proof of the role of obesity in OA is lacking, we should not be judgmental about our obese patients and should use all standard measures for treatment, as for nonobese patients.

Frostbite

Severe cold injury, generally with actual frostbite recalled as occurring prior to closure of epiphyses, has resulted in premature osteoarthritis of the hands.[199–202] The soft tissue changes appropriately evoke the greatest concern at the time of frostbite, as there are usually no identifiable joint symptoms at the time of injury. Joint pain begins months to years later, is often worse in the winter, and is initially associated with few objective findings.[200]

Osteoarthritic involvement is usually identified in the distal and proximal interphalangeal joints. In addition to bony enlargement, stiffness, and crepitus, shortening of the distal phalanges is common and can be a suggestive clue. The age of onset of symptomatic OA has varied from less than 10 years to over 40 years. Unilateral involvement (Fig. 14–14) has been seen after unilateral frostbite.[199] Biopsies or joint aspirations have not been studied.

Roentgenographic studies in children shortly after severe frostbite show destruction of epiphyses. In milder cases and older subjects, the first roentgenographic changes of periarticular bone cysts in hands (or feet) do not occur until after 5 to 12 months. There may be some periosteal new bone formation. Later roentgenograms show osteoarthritis, with shortening of the fingers sometimes the clue differentiating this entity from idiopathic OA.

Possible mechanisms involved include vascular impairment and direct injury to cartilage in response to cold. Widespread vascular occlusion can be shown after cold injury in rabbits.[203] Freezing of a localized area of articular hyaline cartilage induced minimal degenerative changes at 6 months.[204] When animals were studied at 12 months, however, progressive degenerative changes were observed.[205] Peripheral nerve damage can also occur with cold and can complicate symptoms and care.

No specific treatment is available once destruction of the epiphyseal area has occurred. It is not clear whether sympathectomy or other measures to improve blood flow to the bone at the time of frostbite will prevent the later sequelae,[206] although there is some support for this. Rarely, patients with severe deformity due to both the OA and the overlying skin changes may benefit from reconstructive surgery.[207]

Other Mechanical and Local Factors That Appear Important in Localized Osteoarthritis

Jackhammer or pneumatic tool operators with repetitive vibration–type stress on their upper extremities have been described to develop osteoarthritis of the wrists, elbows, and shoulders.[208, 209]

Cotton workers appear to develop more osteoarthritis of the hands, whereas coal workers have more knee involvement.[210] Even repetitive jobs generally considered to be atraumatic influence localization of symptoms, although they do not often cause objective OA. For example, Hadler[211] found more wrist arthritis in textile workers in certain mills who did winding, whereas there were osteoarthritic changes in the second and third metacarpophalangeal joints but no wrist problems in workers in the same mills who did precision gripping.

Severe trauma or distortion of articular structures such as tearing or removal of menisci or severance of anterior cruciate ligaments can produce OA experimentally,[212] and at least some such trauma may be involved in localized OA that occurs in humans after acute or chronic joint injury. Athletes such as American football players[213] (knees), soccer players[214] (ankles, knees, and feet), and baseball pitchers[82] (shoulders and elbows) seem to develop localized OA related to the trauma of their sports. Lee and associates[82] have also reviewed other examples.

In contrast, veteran parachutists do not seem to have any increased osteoarthritis of the knees, ankles, or back.[215] In patients with below-the-knee amputations, more OA of the knee was found on the opposite side than on

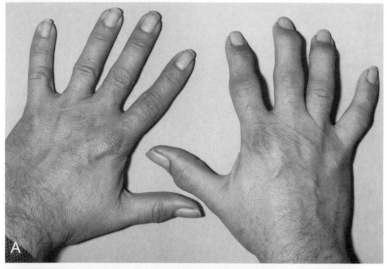

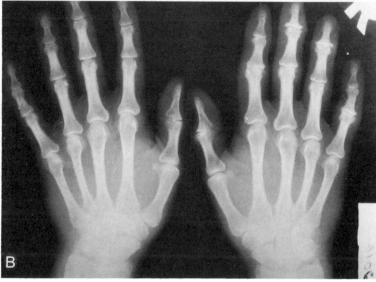

Figure 14–14. *A* and *B*, Unilateral osteoarthritis occurring after frostbite. Roentgenographic study corroborated the severe osteoarthritic changes seen clinically to involve the distal and proximal interphalangeal joints of the right hand.

the amputated side.[216] This difference could be explained either by a diminution in the expected amount of OA on the stress-protected amputated side or by an increase in OA on the intact side exposed to greater stress in walking.

Whether jogging may cause accelerated OA is not known. Former championship runners in Finland did not have an increased incidence of OA of the hip.[217] The authors of the report suggest that proper physiologic running and walking might actually help cartilage nutrition. In untrained individuals, running may have different effects. Prolonged joint immobilization has been shown to contribute to cartilage degeneration.[218, 219] Further studies on knees as well as hips are needed. Studies of sheep walking on concrete showed more cartilage

fibrillation and decreased cartilage hexosamine compared with control animals walking on softer surfaces.[220]

Inequality of leg lengths, or varus and valgus deformities at the knee, have long been felt to contribute to altered concentrations of forces on joints and accelerated OA on the side of the knee exposed to the greatest pressure.[221] Abnormally positioned or shaped joint surfaces have been associated with OA of the hips[222] attributed to congenital deformities such as congenital hip dysplasia, Legg-Calvé-Perthes disease, and slipped femoral capital epiphysis.

Avascular (aseptic) necrosis of the femoral head due to various causes, some of which are discussed elsewhere, can also lead to localized OA in the hip by altering its configuration and shock-absorbing properties.[223] Some causes for aseptic necrosis include fracture of the femoral neck, high-dose adrenocorticosteroid therapy, caisson disease, vasculitis, pancreatic disease, alcoholism, sickle cell disease, and Gaucher's disease.

Intra-articular injections such as the "chemical synovectomies" performed with osmium tetroxide or nitrogen mustard produce some definite surface and midzone cartilage necrosis[224] that may lead to OA in injected joints. Intra-articular injections of depot adrenocorticosteroids may also accelerate osteoarthritic changes by several possible mechanisms, including relief of pain that reduces normal protection from excessive use, catabolic effects on cartilage, and induction of a mild crystal-induced inflammation.[225–227]

Therapeutic implications of the role of localizing factors in the pathogenesis of osteoarthritis vary from changes in occupation or other activities in an attempt to decrease joint abuse to surgical procedures. Osteotomy, for example, can alter the location of stress on joints and is used in some centers to try to prevent progression of early OA due to alignment or mechanical problems.[228]

References

1. Schumacher HR: Hemochromatosis and arthritis. Arthritis Rheum 7:41–50, 1964.
2. Hamilton E, Williams R, Barlow KA, et al.: Idiopathic hemochromatosis. Q J Med 145:171–182, 1968.
3. Gordon DA, Clarke PV, Ogryzlo MA: The chondrocalcific arthropathy of iron overload. Arch Intern Med 134:21–26, 1974.
4. M'seffar A, Fornasier VL, Fox IM: Arthropathy as the major clinical indicator of occult iron storage disease. JAMA 238:1825–1828, 1977.
5. Budiman-Mak E, Weitzner R, Lertratanakul Y: Arthropathy of hemochromatosis. Arthritis Rheum 20:1430–1432, 1977.
6. Kra SJ, Hollingsworth JW, Finch SC: Arthritis with synovial iron deposition in a patient with hemochromatosis. N Engl J Med 272:1268–1271, 1965.
7. Schumacher HR: Ultrastructural characteristics of the synovial membrane in idiopathic haemochromatosis. Ann Rheum Dis 31:465–473, 1972.
8. Schumacher HR: Articular cartilage in the degenerative arthropathy of hemochromatosis. Arthritis Rheum 25:1460–1468, 1982.
9. Schumacher HR: Ochronosis, hemochromatosis and Wilson's disease. In McCarty DJ (ed.): Arthritis and Allied Conditions. Philadelphia, Lea & Febiger, 1979, pp. 1262–1275.
10. McCarty DJ, Palmer DW, Garancis JC: Clearance of calcium pyrophosphate dihydrate crystals in vivo. III. Effects of synovial hemosiderosis. Arthritis Rheum 24:706–710, 1981.
11. Finby N, Bearn AG: Roentgenographic abnormalities of the skeletal system in Wilson's disease (hepatolenticular degeneration). Am J Roentgenol 79:603–611, 1958.
12. Feller E, Schumacher HR: Osteoarticular changes in Wilson's disease. Arthritis Rheum 15:259–266, 1972.
13. Askoy M, Camili N, Dilsen G, et al.: Osteoarticular pains and changes in Wilson's disease. A radiological study in 14 patients in 9 Turkish families. Acta Hepato-Gastroenterol 22:164–170, 1975.
14. Kaklamanis P, Spengos M: Osteoarticular changes and synovial biopsy findings in Wilson's disease. Ann Rheum Dis 32:422–427, 1973.
15. Golding DN, Walshe JM: Arthropathy of Wilson's disease. Ann Rheum Dis 36:99–111, 1977.
16. McCarty DJ, Pepe PF: Erythrocyte neutral inorganic pyrophosphatase in pseudogout. J Lab Clin Med 79:277–284, 1972.
17. Zannoni VG, Malawista SE, LaDu BN: Studies on ochronosis. Arthritis Rheum 5:547–556, 1962.
18. LaDu BN, Zannoni VG, Laster L, et al.: The nature of the defect in tyrosine metabolism in alcaptonuria. J Biol Chem 230:251–260, 1958.
19. Schumacher HR, Holdsworth DE: Ochronotic arthropathy. I. Clinicopathologic studies. Semin Arthritis Rheum 6:207–246, 1977.
20. Hunter T, Gordon DA, Ogryzlo MA: The ground pepper sign of synovial fluid. A new diagnostic feature of ochronosis. J Rheumatol 1:45–53, 1974.
21. Reginato AJ, Schumacher HR, Martinez VA: Ochronotic arthropathy with calcium pyrophosphate crystal deposition. A light and electron microscopic study. Arthritis Rheum 16:705–714, 1973.
22. Rynes RI, Sosman JL, Holdsworth DE: Pseudogout in ochronosis. Report of a case. Arthritis Rheum 18:21–25, 1975.
23. O'Brien WM, LaDu BN, Bunim JJ: Biochemical, pathologic and clinical aspects of alcaptonuria, ochronosis and ochronotic arthropathy. Review of world literature (1584 1962). Am J Med 34:813–838, 1963.
24. Lustberg TD, Schulman JD, Seegmiller JE: Decreased binding of ^{14}C-homogentisic acid induced by ascorbic acid in connective tissues of rats with experimental alcaptonuria. Nature 228:770–771, 1970.
25. Detenbeck LC, Young HH, Underdahl LO: Ochronotic arthropathy. Arch Surg 100:215–219, 1970.
26. Peters SP, Lee RE, Glew RH: Gaucher's disease. A review. Medicine 56:425–442, 1977.
27. Lee RE: The pathology of Gaucher disease. In Gaucher Disease: A Century of Delineation and Research. New York, A. R. Liss, Inc., 1982, pp. 177–217.
28. Beutler E: Gaucher's disease in an asymptomatic 72-year-old. JAMA 237:2529–2530, 1977.
29. Zaino EC, Rossi MB, Pham TD, et al.: Gaucher's cells in thalassemia. Blood 38:457–562, 1971.
30. Kattlove HE, Williams JC, Gaynor E, et al.: Gaucher cells in chronic myelocytic leukemia: An acquired abnormality. Blood 33:379–390, 1969.
31. Silverstein E, Pertschuk LP, Friedland J: Immunofluorescent detection of angiotensin-converting enzyme (ACE) in Gaucher cells. Am J Med 69:408–410, 1980.
32. Silverstein MN, Kelly PJ: Osteoarticular manifestations of Gaucher's disease. Am J Med Sci 253:85–92, 1967.

33. Seinsheimer F, Mankin HJ: Acute bilateral symmetrical pathologic fractures of the lateral tibial plateaus in a patient with Gaucher's disease. Arthritis Rheum 20:1550–1555, 1977.

34. Goldblatt J, Jacks S, Beighton P: The orthopedic aspects of Gaucher's disease. Clin Orthop 137:208–214, 1978.

35. Amstutz HC, Carey EJ: Skeletal manifestations and treatment of Gaucher's disease. J Bone Joint Surg 48A:670–701, 1966.

36. Brady RO, Pentchev PG, Gal AE, et al.: Replacement therapy for inherited enzyme deficiency. Use of purified glucocerebrosidase in Gaucher's disease. N Engl J Med 291:989–993, 1974.

37. Hanash SM, Rucknagel DL, Heidelberger KP, et al.: Primary amyloidosis associated with Gaucher's disease. Ann Intern Med 89:639–641, 1978.

38. Schumacher HR: Rheumatological manifestations of sickle cell disease and other hereditary hemoglobinopathies. Clin Rheum Dis 1:37–52, 1975.

39. Alavi A, Schumacher HR, Dorwart B, et al.: Bone marrow scan evaluation of arthropathy in sickle cell disorders. Arch Intern Med 136:436–440, 1976.

40. Dorwart BB, Goldberg MA, Schumacher HR, et al.: Absence of increased frequency of bone and joint disease with hemoglobin AS and AC [letter]. Ann Intern Med 86:66–67, 1977.

41. Rothschild BM, Sienknecht CW, Kaplan SB, et al.: Sickle cell disease associated with uric acid deposition disease. Ann Rheum Dis 39:392–395, 1980.

42. Espinoza LR, Spilberg I, Osterland CK: Joint manifestations of sickle cell disease. Medicine 53:295–305, 1974.

43. Schumacher HR, Dorwart BB, Bond J, et al.: Chronic synovitis with early cartilage destruction in sickle cell disease. Ann Rheum Dis 36:413–419, 1977.

44. Habermann ET, Grayzel AI: Bilateral total knee replacement in a patient with sickle cell disease. Clin Orthop 100:211–215, 1974.

45. Schlumpf U, Gerber N, Bünzli H, et al.: Arthritiden bei Thalassemia minor. Schweiz Med Wochenschr 107:1156–1162, 1977.

46. Abourizk NN, Nasr FW, Frayha RA: Aseptic necrosis in thalassemia minor. Arthritis Rheum 20:1147, 1977.

47. Dorwart BB, Schumacher HR: Arthritis in β-thalassemia trait: Clinical and pathological features. Ann Rheum Dis 40:185–189, 1981.

48. Gratwick G, Bullough PG, Bohne WHO, et al.: Thalassemic arthropathy. Ann Intern Med 88:494–501, 1978.

49. Sella EJ, Goodman AH: Arthropathy secondary to transfusion hemochromatosis. J Bone Joint Surg 55A:1077–1081, 1973.

50. Schlumpf U: Thalassemia minor and aseptic necrosis. A coincidence. Arthritis Rheum 21:280, 1978.

51. Jimenez SA, Lally EV: Disorders of collagen structure and metabolism. Bull Rheum Dis 30:1016–1022, 1980.

52. Beighton P, Horan F: Orthopaedic aspects of the Ehlers-Danlos syndrome. J Bone Joint Surg 51B:444–453, 1969.

53. Kirk JA, Ansell BM, Bywaters EGL: Hypermobility syndrome. Musculoskeletal complaints associated with generalized joint hypermobility. Ann Rheum Dis 26:419–425, 1967.

54. Beighton P: Articular manifestations of the Ehlers-Danlos syndrome. Semin Arthritis Rheum 1:246–261, 1971.

55. Schumacher HR: Musculoskeletal manifestations of the Ehlers-Danlos syndrome. A clinicopathologic study. (Abstract.) Arthritis Rheum 8:467–468, 1965.

56. Julkenen H, Rokkanen P, Jounela A: Bone changes in Ehlers-Danlos syndrome. Ann. Med Int Fenn 56:55–59, 1967.

57. Steer G, Jayson MIV, Dixon AStJ, et al.: Joint capsule collagen. Analysis by the study of intra-articular pressure during joint distention. Measurements in the knees of control subjects and patients with rheumatoid arthritis and Ehlers-Danlos syndrome. Ann Rheum Dis 30:481–486, 1971.

58. Robertson FW, Kozlowski K, Middleton RW: Larsen's syndrome. Clin Pediatr 14:53–60, 1975.

59. Smith RD, Worthington JW: Paganini: The riddle and connective tissue. JAMA 199:820–824, 1967.

60. Kalenak A, Morehouse CA: Knee stability and knee ligament injuries. JAMA 234:1143–1145, 1975.

61. Bird HA, Tribe CR, Bacon PA: Joint hypermobility leading to osteoarthritis and chondrocalcinosis. Ann Rheum Dis 37:203–211, 1978.

62. Scott D, Bird HA, Wright V: Joint hypermobility in osteoarthritis. (Abstract.) Ann Rheum Dis 38:495, 1979.

63. Jessee EF: The benign hypermobile joint syndrome. Arthritis Rheum 23:1053–1056, 1980.

64. Crosby EB, Insall J: Recurrent dislocation of the patella. Relation of treatment to osteoarthritis. J Bone Joint Surg 58A:9–13, 1976.

65. Boulton MR, Rugh DM, Mattioli LF, et al.: The Noonan syndrome: A family study. Ann Intern Med 80:626–629, 1974.

66. Golde DW, Herschman HR, Lusis AJ, et al.: Growth factors. Ann Intern Med 92:650–652, 1980.

67. Bluestone R, Bywaters EGL, Hartog M, et al.: Acromegalic arthropathy. Ann Rheum Dis 30:243–258, 1971.

68. Detenbeck LC, Tressler HA, O'Duffy JD, et al.: Peripheral joint manifestations of acromegaly. Clin Orthop 91:119–127, 1973.

69. Kellgren JH, Ball J, Tutton GK: The articular and other limb changes of acromegaly. Q J Med 21:405–424, 1952.

70. Weinberger A, Schumacher HR: Unpublished observations, 1981.

71. Lamotte M, Segresta JM, Krassine G: Arthrite microcristalline calcique (pseudogout) chez un acromégale. Sem Hop Paris 42:2420–2424, 1966.

72. Bland JH, Frymoyer JW: Rheumatic syndromes of myxedema. N Engl J Med 282:1171–1174, 1970.

73. Dorwart BB, Schumacher HR: Joint effusions, chondrocalcinosis and other rheumatic manifestations in hypothyroidism. Am J Med 59:780–790, 1975.

74. Bywaters EGL, Dixon AStJ, Scott JT: Joint lesions in hyperparathyroidism. Ann Rheum Dis 22:171–185, 1963.

75. Hamilton EBD: Diseases associated with CPPD deposition disease. Arthritis Rheum 19:353–357, 1976.

76. Preston FS, Adicoff A: Hyperparathyroidism with avulsion of 3 major tendons. N Engl J Med 266:968–971, 1962.

77. Pritchard MH, Jessop JD: Chondrocalcinosis in primary hyperparathyroidism. Influence of age, metabolic bone disease and parathyroidectomy. Ann Rheum Dis 36:146–151, 1977.

78. Grahame R, Sutor DJ, Mitchener MB: Crystal deposition in hyperparathyroidism. Ann Rheum Dis 30:597–604, 1971.

79. Lipson RL, Williams LE: The "connective tissue

disorder" of hyperparathyroidism. Arthritis Rheum 11:198–205, 1971.

80. O'Duffy JD: Pseudogout syndrome in hospital patients. JAMA 226:42–44, 1973.

81. Rynes R, Merzig EG: Calcium pyrophosphate crystal deposition disease and hyperparathyroidism. A controlled, prospective study. J Rheumatol 5:460–468, 1978.

82. Lee P, Rooney PJ, Sturrock RD, et al.: The etiology and pathogenesis of osteoarthritis. A review. Semin Arthritis Rheum 3:189–218, 1974.

83. Rosenbloom AL, Silverstein JH, Lezotte DC, et al.: Limited joint mobility in childhood diabetes mellitus indicates increased risk for microvascular disease. N Engl J Med 305:191–194, 1981.

84. Lockitch G, Fellingham SA, Elphinstone CD: Mseleni joint disease: A radiological study of 2 affected families. S Afr Med J 47:2366–2376, 1973.

85. Gibson T, Highton J: Multiple epiphyseal dysplasia: A family study. Rheumatol Rehabil 18:239–242, 1979.

86. Weinberg H, Frankel M, Makin M, et al.: Familial epiphyseal dysplasia of the lower limbs. J Bone Joint Surg 42B:313–332, 1960.

87. Patrone NA, Kredich DW, Aylsworth AS: Multiple epiphyseal dysplasia and arthritis. (Abstract.) Clin Res 31:654A, 1983.

88. Kaufman EE, Coventry MB: Multiple epiphyseal dysplasia in a mother and son. Mayo Clin Proc 38:115–124, 1963.

89. Mena HR, Pearson EO: Multiple epiphyseal dysplasia: A family case report. JAMA 236:2629–2633, 1976.

90. Kahn MF, Corvol MT, Jurmand SH: Le rhumatisme chondrodysplasique. Sem Hop Paris 46:1938–1953, 1970.

91. Anderson CE, Crane JT, Harper HA, et al.: Morquio's disease and dysplasia epiphysealis multiplex. A study of epiphyseal cartilage in 7 cases. J Bone Joint Surg 44A:295–306, 1962.

92. Monson CB, Seegmiller RE: Ultrastructural studies of cartilage matrix in mice homozygous for chondrodysplasia. J Bone Joint Surg 63A:637–644, 1981.

93. Spranger JW, Langer LO: Spondyloepiphyseal dysplasia congenita. Radiology 94:313–322, 1970.

94. Maroteaux P, Lamy M, Bernard J: La dysplasie spondyloépiphysaire tardive: Description clinique et radiologique. Presse Med 65:1205–1208, 1957.

95. Levy RN, Moseley J, Stiffert RS: Premature arthritis as manifestation of epiphyseal dysplasia. NY State Med J 66:1917–1920, 1966.

96. Weinfeld A, Ross MW, Sarasohn SH: Spondyloepiphyseal dysplasia tarda. A cause of premature osteoarthritis. Am J Roentgenol 101:851–859, 1967.

97. Langer LO: Spondyloepiphyseal dysplasia tarda. Hereditary chondrodysplasia with characteristic vertebral configuration in the adult. Radiology 92:833–839, 1964.

98. Martin JR, MacEwan DW, Blais JA, et al.: Platyspondyly, polyarticular osteoarthritis and absent beta-2-globulin in two brothers. Arthritis Rheum 13:53–67, 1970.

99. Yang SS, Chen H, Williams P, et al.: Spondyloepiphyseal dysplasia congenita—a comparative study of chondrocyte inclusions. Arch Pathol Lab Med 104:208–211, 1980.

100. Carbonara P, Alpert M: Hereditary osteo-onychodysplasia. Am J Med Sci 248:139–151, 1964.

101. Eisenberg K, Potter DE, Bovill EG: Osteoonychodystrophy with nephropathy and renal osteodystrophy. J Bone Joint Surg 54A:1301–1305, 1972.

102. Senior G: Impaired growth and onychodysplasia. Am J Dis Child 122:7–9, 1971.

103. Verdich J: Nail-patella syndrome associated with renal failure requiring transplantation. Acta Derm Venereol (Stockh) 60:440–443, 1981.

104. Nevin NC, Thomas PS, Calvert J, et al.: Deafness, onychoosteodystrophy, mental retardation (DOOR) syndrome. Am J Med Genet 13:325–332, 1982.

105. Stickler GB, Belau PG, Farrell FJ, et al.: Hereditary progressive arthroophthalmopathy. Mayo Clin Proc 40:433–455, 1965.

106. Popkin JS, Palomeno RC: Stickler's syndrome (hereditary progressive arthro-ophthalmopathy). Can Med Assoc J 111:1071–1076, 1974.

107. Cottin S, LeGall G, Lorgeas JM: Le syndrome trichorhinophalangien. À propos de quatre observations familiales. Rev Rhum 47:169–173, 1980.

108. Giedion A, Burdea M, Fruchter H, et al.: Autosomal-dominant transmission of the tricho-rhino-phalangeal syndrome. Helv Paediatr Acta 28:249–259, 1973.

109. Frayha R, Melhem R, Idriss H: The Kniest (Swiss cheese cartilage) syndrome. Arthritis Rheum 22:286–289, 1979.

110. Allison AC, Blumberg BS: Familial osteoarthropathy of the fingers. J Bone Joint Surg 40B:538–545, 1958.

111. Rubinstein HM: Thiemann's disease. Arthritis Rheum 18:357–360, 1975.

112. Melo-Gomes JA, Melo-Gomes E, Viana-Quieros M: Thiemann's disease. J Rheumatol 8:462–467, 1981.

113. Behar A, Rachmilewitz E: Ellis-van Creveld syndrome. Arch Intern Med 113:606–611, 1964.

114. Spranger JW, Langer LO, Wiedemann HR: Bone Dysplasias. An Atlas of Constitutional Disorders of Skeletal Development. Philadelphia, W. B. Saunders Company, 1974, p. 369.

115. Spranger JW, Optitz JM, Bidder U: Heterogencity of chondrodysplasia punctata. Humangenetik 11:190–212, 1971.

116. Stanescu R, Stanescu V, Maroteaux P, et al.: Constitutional articular cartilage dysplasia with accumulation of complex lipids in chondrocytes and precocious arthrosis. Arthritis Rheum 24:965–988, 1981.

117. Nesterov AI: The clinical course of Kashin-Beck disease. Arthritis Rheum 7:228–240, 1964.

118. Specht EE: Epiphyseal injuries in childhood. Am Fam Physician 10:101–109, 1974.

119. McKusick VA, Eldridge R, Hosteller JA, et al.: Dwarfism in the Amish. II. Cartilage-hair-hypoplasia. Bull Johns Hopkins Hosp 116:285–326, 1965.

120. McCarty DJ: Calcium pyrophosphate deposition disease—a current appraisal of the problem. *In* Holt PJL (ed.): Current Topics in Connective Tissue Disease. Edinburgh, Churchill Livingstone, 1975, pp. 181–197.

121. Schumacher HR: Gout and Pseudogout. Garden City, New York, Medical Examination Publishing Co., 1978, pp. 53–73.

122. Moskowitz RW, Garcia F: Chondrocalcinosis articularis (pseudogout syndrome). Arch Intern Med 132:87–91, 1973.

123. Schumacher HR: Pathogenesis of crystal-induced synovitis. Clin Rheum Dis 3:105–131, 1977.

124. Zitnan D, Sitaj S: Calcifications multiples du cartilage articulaire. 9th International Congress sur les Maladies Rhumatismales 2:291, 1957.

125. McCarty DJ, Hollander JL: Identification of urate crystals in gouty synovial fluid. Ann Intern Med 54:452–460, 1961.

126. Schumacher HR, Gordon G, Paul H, et al.: Osteoarthritis, crystal deposition and inflammation. Semin Arthritis Rheum 11:116–119, 1981.

127. Huskisson EC, Dieppe PA, Tucker AK, et al.: Another look at osteoarthritis. Ann Rheum Dis 38:423–428, 1979.

128. Zitnan D, Sitaj S: Natural course of articular chondrocalcinosis. Arthritis Rheum 19:363–390, 1976.

129. Reginato AJ, Schiapachasse V, Zmijewski CM, et al.: HLA antigens in chondrocalcinosis and ankylosing chondrocalcinosis. Arthritis Rheum 22:928–932, 1979.

130. Ellman MH, Levin B: Chondrocalcinosis in elderly persons. Arthritis Rheum 18:43–47, 1975.

131. Hoffman GS, Schumacher HR, Paul H, et al.: Calcium oxalate crystal associated arthritis in chronic renal failure. (Abstract.) Arthritis Rheum 24:573, 1981.

132. Moskowitz RW, Harris BK, Schwartz A, et al.: Chronic synovitis as a manifestation of calcium crystal deposition disease. Arthritis Rheum 14:109–116, 1971.

133. Gaucher A, Faure G, Netter P, et al.: Identification des cristaux observés dans les arthropathies destructices de la chondrocalcinose. Rev Rhum 44:407–414, 1977.

134. Tanphaiachit RK, Spilberg I, Hahn BH: Lithium heparin crystals simulating CPPD crystals. Arthritis Rheum 19:966–968, 1976.

135. Kohn NN, Hughes RE, McCarty DJ, et al.: The significance of calcium pyrophosphate crystals in synovial fluid of arthritic patients: The pseudogout syndrome. II. Identification of crystals. Ann Intern Med 56:738–745, 1962.

136. Cherian PV, Schumacher HR: Diagnostic potential of rapid electron microscopic analysis of joint effusions. Arthritis Rheum 25:98–100, 1982.

137. Schumacher HR, Somlyo AP, Tse RL, et al.: Arthritis associated with apatite crystals. Ann Intern Med 87:411–416, 1977.

138. Reginato AJ, Schumacher HR, Martinez V: The articular cartilage in familial chondrocalcinosis. Arthritis Rheum 17:977–992, 1974.

139. Moskowitz RW, Goldberg VM, Berman L: Synovitis as a manifestation of degenerative joint disease. An experimental study. (Abstract.) Arthritis Rheum 19:813, 1976.

140. Silcox DC, McCarty DJ: Elevated inorganic pyrophosphate concentrations in synovial fluids in osteoarthritis and pseudogout. J Lab Clin Med 83:518–531, 1974.

141. Howell DS, Muniz O, Pita JC, et al.: Extrusion of pyrophosphate in extracellular media by osteoarthritis cartilage incubates. J Clin Invest 56:1473–1480, 1975.

142. Pinals RS, Short CL: Calcified periarthritis involving multiple sites. Arthritis Rheum 7:359–367, 1964.

143. McCarty DJ, Gatter RA: Recurrent acute inflammation associated with focal apatite crystal deposition. Arthritis Rheum 9:804–819, 1966.

144. Bennet GA, Waine H, Bauer W: Changes in the Knee Joint at Various Ages. New York, The Commonwealth Fund, 1942, p. 97.

145. McCarty DJ, Hogan JM, Gatter RA, et al.: Studies on pathological calcification in human cartilage. I. Prevalence and types of crystal deposits in the menisci of 215 cadavers. J Bone Joint Surg 48A:209–235, 1966.

146. Dieppe PA, Crocker P, Huskisson EC, et al.: Apatite deposition disease. A new arthropathy. Lancet 1:266–269, 1976.

147. Schumacher HR, Tse R, Reginato AJ, et al.: Hydroxyapatite-like crystals in the synovial fluid cell vacuoles: A suspected new cause for crystal-induced arthritis. (Abstract.) Arthritis Rheum 19:821, 1976.

148. Maurer KH, Schumacher HR: Hydroxyapatite phagocytosis by human polymorphonuclear leukocytes. Ann Rheum Dis 38:84–88, 1979.

149. Schumacher HR, Miller JL, Ludivico C, et al.: Erosive arthritis associated with apatite crystal deposition. Arthritis Rheum 24:31–37, 1981.

150. Reginato A, Schumacher HR: Synovial calcification in a patient with collagen-vascular disease: Light and electron microscopic studies. J Rheumatol 4:261–271, 1977.

151. Ali SY: Matrix vesicles and apatite nodules in arthritic cartilage. In Willoughby DA, et al. (eds.): Perspectives in Inflammation. Baltimore, University Park Press, 1977, pp. 211–223.

152. Shitama K: Calcification of aging articular cartilage in man. Acta Orthop Scand 50:613–619, 1979.

153. McCarty DJ, Halverson PB, Carrera GF, et al.: "Milwaukee shoulder"—association of microspheroids containing hydroxyapatite crystals, active collagenase, and neutral protease with rotator cuff defects. I. Clinical aspects. Arthritis Rheum 24:464–473, 1981.

154. Halverson PG, Cheung HS, McCarty DS, et al.: "Milwaukee shoulder"—association of microspheroids containing hydroxyapatite crystals, active collagenase, and neutral protease with rotator cuff defects. II. Synovial fluid studies. Arthritis Rheum 24:474–483, 1981.

155. Yosipovich ZH, Glimcher MJ: Articular chondrocalcinosis, hydroxyapatite deposition disease in adult mature rabbits. J Bone Joint Surg 54A:841–853, 1972.

156. Reginato AJ, Schumacher HR, Brighton CT: Experimental hydroxyapatite articular calcification. (Abstract.) Arthritis Rheum 21:585–586, 1978.

157. Bruckner FE, Howell A: Neuropathic joints. Semin Arthritis Rheum 2:47–69, 1972.

158. Sinha S, Munichoodappa CS, Kozak GP: Neuroarthropathy (Charcot joints) in diabetes mellitus. Clinical study of 101 cases. Medicine 51:191–210, 1972.

159. Abell JM, Hayes JT: Charcot knee due to congenital insensitivity to pain. J Bone Joint Surg 46A:1287–1291, 1964.

160. Peitzman ST, Miller JL, Ortega L, et al.: Charcot arthropathy secondary to amyloid neuropathy. JAMA 235:1345–1347, 1981.

161. Pruzanski W, Baron M, Shupak R: Neuroarthropathy (Charcot's joints) in familial amyloid polyneuropathy. J Rheumatol 8:477–481, 1981.

162. Brucker FE: Double Charcot's disease. Br Med J 2:603–604, 1968.

163. Wolfgang GL: Neurotrophic arthropathy of the shoulder—a complication of progressive adhesive arachnoiditis. Clin Orthop 87:217–220, 1972.

164. Horwitz T: Bone and cartilage debris in the synovial

membrane—its significance in the early diagnosis of neuro-arthropathy. J Bone Joint Surg 30A: 579–588, 1948.

165. Lloyd-Roberts GC: The role of capsular changes in osteoarthritis of the hip joint. J Bone Joint Surg 35B:627–642, 1953.

166. Floyd W, Lovell W, King RE: The neuropathic joint. South Med J 52:563–569, 1959.

167. Beetham WP, Kaye RL, Polley HF: Charcot's joints. Ann Intern Med 58:1002–1012, 1963.

168. Drennan DB, Fahey JJ, Maylahn DJ: Important factors in achieving arthrodesis of the Charcot knee. J Bone Joint Surg 53A:1180–1193, 1971.

169. Johnson JTH: Neuropathic fractures and joint injuries. J Bone Joint Surg 49A:1–30, 1967.

170. Rondier J, Cayla J, Guiraudon C, Le Charpentier Y: Arthropathie tabétique et chondrocalcinose articulaire. Rev Rhum 44:671–674, 1977.

171. Jacobelli S, McCarty DJ: Calcium pyrophosphate dihydrate crystal deposition in neuropathic joints. Ann Intern Med 79:340–347, 1973.

172. Ritter MA, DeRosa P: Total hip arthroplasty in a Charcot joint. A case report with a 6 year follow-up. Orthop Rev 6:51–53, 1977.

173. Altman RD: Musculoskeletal manifestations of Paget's disease of bone. Arthritis Rheum 23:1121–1127, 1980.

174. Machtey I, Rodnan GP, Benedek TG: Paget's disease of the hip joint. Am J Med Sci 251:524–531, 1966.

175. Steinbach HL: Some roentgen features of Paget's disease. Am J Roentgenol 86:950–964, 1961.

176. Doury P, Delahaye RP, Leguay G, et al.: Chondro-calcinose articulaire diffuse et maladie de Paget. Rev Rhum 42:551–554, 1975.

177. Detenbeck LC, Sim FH, Johnson EW: Symptomatic Paget disease of the hip. JAMA 224:213–217, 1973.

178. Cameron HU, Dewar FP: Degenerative osteoarthritis associated with osteopetrosis. Clin Orthop Rel Res 127:148–149, 1977.

179. Janecki CJ, Nelson CL: Osteoarthritis associated with osteopetrosis treated by total hip replacement. Cleve Clin Q 38:169–177, 1971.

180. Jaffe HL: Metabolic, Degenerative, and Inflammatory Diseases of the Bones and Joints. Philadelphia, Lea and Febiger, 1972, p. 492.

181. Griscom NT: Very dense bones in a 57 year old man. JAMA 186:251–253, 1963.

182. Beighton P, Hamersma H, Cremin B: Osteopetrosis in South Africa. S Afr Med J 55:659–665, 1979.

183. Whyte MP, Murphy WA, Fallon MD, et al.: Osteopetrosis, renal tubular acidosis and basal ganglia calcification in 3 sisters. Am J Med 69:64–74, 1980.

184. Klemmer PJ, Hadler NM: Subacute fluorosis. A consequence of abuse of an organo-fluoride anesthetic. Ann Intern Med 89:607–611, 1978.

185. Clarisse PDT, Staple TW: Diffuse bone sclerosis in multiple myeloma. Radiology 99:327–328, 1971.

186. Mazieres B, Durroux R, Jambon E: Densification osseuse et nécrose de la tête fémorale par thesaurismose à la polyvinyl-pyrrolidone. Rev Rhum 47:257–265, 1980.

187. Garver P, Resnick D, Niwayama G: Epiphyseal sclerosis in renal osteodystrophy simulating osteonecrosis. Am J Radiol 136:1239–1241, 1981.

188. Coccia PF, Krivit W, Cervenka J, et al.: Successful bone-marrow transplantation for infantile malignant osteopetrosis. N Engl J Med 302:701–708, 1980.

189. Sebo M, Sitaj S, Schultze P: Obesity in the pathogenesis of osteoarthritis. Program of the VI European Rheumatology Congress. Brighton, England, 1971, p. 36.

190. Saville PD, Dickson J: Age and weight in osteoarthritis of the hip. Arthritis Rheum 11:635–644, 1968.

191. Lawrence JS, Bremner JM, Bier F: Osteoarthritis. Ann Rheum Dis 25:1–24, 1966.

192. Goldin RH, McAdam L, Louie JS, et al.: Clinical and radiological survey of the incidence of osteoarthrosis among obese patients. Ann Rheum Dis 35:349–353, 1976.

193. Danielsson LG: Incidence and prognosis of coxarthrosis. Acta Orthop Scand 66(Suppl):1–114, 1964.

194. Engel A: Osteoarthritis and body measurements: United States 1960–1962. Washington, D.C., PHS Publication 1000 Series II, No. 29, 1968.

195. Silberberg M, Frank EL, Jarret SR, et al.: Aging and osteoarthritis of the human sternoclavicular joint. Am J Pathol 35:851–865, 1959.

196. Acheson RM, Collart AB: New Haven survey of joint diseases. XVII. Relationship between some systemic characteristics and osteoarthrosis in a general population. Ann Rheum Dis 34:379–387, 1975.

197. Silberberg M, Silberberg R: Osteoarthrosis in mice fed diets enriched with animal or vegetable fat. Arch Pathol 70:385–390, 1960.

198. Sokoloff L, Mickelsen O: Dietary fat supplements, body weight and osteoarthritis in DBA/ZJN mice. J Nutr 85:117–121, 1965.

199. Schumacher HR: Unilateral osteoarthritis of the hand. JAMA 191:180–181, 1965.

200. Blair JR, Schatzki R, Orr KD: Sequelae to cold injury in 100 patients. JAMA 63:685–695, 1954.

201. Glick R, Parhami N: Frostbite arthritis. J Rheumatol 6:456–460, 1979.

202. Selke AC: Destruction of phalangeal epiphyses by frostbite. Radiology 93:859–860, 1969.

203. Kulka JP: Cold injury of the skin. The pathogenic role of microcirculatory impairment. Arch Environ Health 11:484–497, 1965.

204. Simon WH, Green WT: Experimental production of cartilage necrosis by cold injury: Failure to cause degenerative joint disease. Am J Pathol 64:145–152, 1971.

205. Simon WH, Richardson S, Herman W, et al.: Long-term effects of chondrocyte death on rabbit articular cartilage in vivo. J Bone Joint Surg 58A:517–526, 1976.

206. Golding MR, Dejong P, Sawyer PN, et al.: Protection from early and late sequelae of frostbite by regional sympathectomy: Mechanism of "cold sensitivity" following frostbite. Surgery 53:303–308, 1963.

207. Bigelow DR, Ritchie GW: The effects of frostbite in childhood. J Bone Joint Surg 45B:122–131, 1963.

208. Schumacher HR, Agudelo C, Labowitz R: Jackhammer arthropathy. J Occup Med 14:563–564, 1972.

209. Hunter DA, McLaughlin AIG, Perry KMA: Clinical effects of use of pneumatic tools. Br J Indust Med 2:10–16, 1945.

210. Kellgren JH, Lawrence JS: Osteoarthritis and disc degeneration in an urban population. Ann Rheum Dis 17:388–396, 1958.

211. Hadler N: Hand structure and function in an industrial setting: Influence of 3 patterns of stereotyped repetitive usage. Arthritis Rheum 21:210–220, 1978.

212. Schwartz E, Greenwald R: Experimental models of osteoarthritis. Bull Rheum Dis 30:1030–1033, 1980.

213. Rall KL, McElroy GL, Keats TE: A study of long term effects of football injury to the knee. Mo Med 61:435–438, 1964.

214. Solonen KA: The joints of the lower extremity of football players. Ann Chir Gynaecol Fenn 55:176–180, 1966.

215. Murray-Leslie CF, Lintott DJ, Wright V: The knees and ankles in sport and veteran military parachutists. Ann Rheum Dis 36:327–331, 1977.

216. Burke MJ, Roman V, Wright V: Bone and joint changes in lower limb amputees. Ann Rheum Dis 37:252–254, 1978.

217. Puranen J, Ala-Ketola L, Peltokallio P, et al.: Running and primary osteoarthritis of the hip. Br Med J 2:424–425, 1975.

218. Enneking WF, Horowitz M: The intraarticular effects of immobilization on the human knee. J Bone Joint Surg 54A:973–985, 1972.

219. Salter RB, Field P: Effects of continuous compression on living articular cartilage: An experimental investigation. J Bone Joint Surg 42A:31–49, 1960.

220. Radin E, Eyre D, Schiller AL: Effect of prolonged walking on concrete on the joints of sheep. Arthritis Rheum 22:649, 1979. (Abstract.)

221. Ory M: Des influences mécaniques dans l'apparition et le développement des manifestations dégénérative du genou. J Belge Rhumatol Med Phys 19:103–120, 1964.

222. Solomon L: Patterns of osteoarthritis of the hip. J Bone Joint Surg 58B:176–183, 1976.

223. Radin EL, Parker HG, Pugh JW: Response of joints to impact loading. III. Relationship between trabecular microfractures and cartilage degeneration. J Biomed 6:51–57, 1973.

224. Mitchell NS, Laurin CA, Shepard N: The effect of osmium tetroxide and nitrogen mustard on normal articular cartilage. J Bone Joint Surg 55B:814–821, 1973.

225. Behrens F, Shepard N, Mitchell NS: Alteration of rabbit articular cartilage by intraarticular injections of glucocorticoids. J Bone Joint Surg 57A:70–76, 1975.

226. Salter RB, Gross A, Hall HJ: Hydrocortisone arthropathy—an experimental investigation. Can Med Assoc J 97:374–377, 1967.

227. Gordon GV, Schumacher HR: Electron microscopic study of depot corticosteroid crystals with clinical studies after intraarticular injection. J Rheumatol 6:7–14, 1979.

228. Adam A, Spence AJ: Intertrochanteric osteotomy for osteoarthrosis of the hip. J Bone Joint Surg 40B:219–226, 1958.

15

The Etiology and Natural Course of Osteoarthritis of the Hip (Coxarthrosis)

S. David Stulberg, M.D.

The hip joint has, in a sense, been the stage on which has been conducted the debate as to whether osteoarthritis (OA) is a unique and distinct disease ("primary" osteoarthritis) or whether it is a pathologic process that occurs as the result of an identifiable associated or antecedent cause ("secondary" osteoarthritis).[1–15] Several clinical conditions are associated with the development of osteoarthritis (see Chapter 14). Reviews of series of patients with osteoarthritis of the hip have identified associated diseases or antecedent abnormalities of the hip in 40% to 90% of the affected hip joints.[5, 16–28] This wide range of frequency results from the fact that investigators have taken their series from different populations and have used a variety of methods for determining the existence of associated or pre-existing abnormalities of the hip.

Pathologic femoral heads, which become available for study following the performance of total hip replacement arthroplasties, have been a valuable source of material for increasing our understanding of osteoarthritis.[29–34] Investigators have examined these specimens in differing ways and have provided information that is helping to identify the role that pre-existing abnormalities of a joint play in the development of osteoarthritis in general, and of OA of the hip in particular. Animal models of hip joint OA are also providing important insights into the way in which abnormalities in hip joint anatomy are associated with the development of osteoarthritis.[35–40]

In this chapter, factors thought to affect the incidence of osteoarthritis of the hip will be examined; the ways in which the incidence and natural course of the disease might be better understood by a more knowledgeable interpretation of the role such factors play will be discussed; and, finally, the extent to which current information allows us to resolve the debate as to whether the entity "primary osteoarthritis of the hip" exists will be considered.

THE EPIDEMIOLOGY OF COXARTHROSIS

Epidemiologic studies of osteoarthritis of the hip have identified a number of factors that affect its varying incidence among different populations.[6, 20, 23, 41–46] Coxarthrosis occurs much more commonly in Caucasians than in southern Chinese,[47, 48] Indians,[49] or South African blacks.[50] Although generalized manifestations of osteoarthritis (e.g., hand and spine involvement) occur with approximately equal frequency in Caucasians and these other racial groups, the incidence of OA of the hip is much higher in the Caucasian population.[47, 48, 51–53] It is not known whether this Caucasian predilection reflects a difference in genetic predisposition to develop coxarthrosis or whether factors such as pre-existing childhood hip diseases, hip joint deformities, variations in body size, or type of daily activities are responsible for this difference in the occurrence of hip disease.[47]

The incidence also varies within racial groups. A number of factors have been cited to explain this fact. Osteoarthritis of the hip is relatively common in Japan and is believed to be related to the prevalence of congenital hip dysplasia. In contrast, Hong Kong Chinese rarely develop osteoarthritis of the hip and have a low incidence of childhood hip disease or other conditions of the hip known to be associated with the subsequent development of osteoarthritis. The low incidence of hip disease in the Hong Kong Chinese has been felt to be related, at least in part, to the fact that Chinese infants are carried on their mothers' backs with their hips abducted. This position discourages the development of hip dysplasia, a childhood hip deformity associated with an increased incidence of osteoarthritis.[47] Asian Indians, in whom the incidence of osteoarthritis of the hips is also low, frequently squat, placing their hips in an abducted and flexed posture, thereby discouraging the development of hip dysplasia.[49, 54] That the position in which a child's hips are placed during infancy can have a significant effect on the incidence of hip dysplasia and the subsequent development of OA is also strongly suggested by the experience of the northern Canadian Indians.[55] The incidence of hip dysplasia was apparently significantly altered when an infant-carrying device that kept the hips extended and adducted (a position favoring the development of hip dysplasia) was replaced with one that placed the hips in flexion and abduction.[56, 57] These studies indicate that developmental abnormalities of the hip represent an important cause of osteoarthritis of the hip in susceptible populations. These studies also imply that the incidence of the adult disease might be reduced by early treatment or prevention of the developmental abnormality.

The presence of developmental abnormalities of the hip also explains, in part, the fact that although the incidence of OA of the hip in men and women is approximately equal, women are more likely to develop severe disease at a younger age.[25] The incidence of congenital hip dysplasia is much higher in women than in men. This hip deformity, present at birth, leads to severe OA of the hip in relatively early adulthood.[10, 25, 26, 58–62] Men are more likely to be affected by hip diseases (e.g., Perthes' disease, slipped capital femoral epiphysis) that occur during later childhood and adolescence and that subsequently lead to the development of OA of the hip at a later time than does hip dysplasia.[10, 63–69]

Many of the epidemiologic studies suggest that mechanical factors play an important, perhaps central, role in the development of OA of the hip. How these factors lead to OA of the hip has been the subject of intense interest and discussion among investigators of osteoarthritis.

MECHANICAL FACTORS AND THE INCIDENCE OF COXARTHROSIS

Mechanical factors may influence the development of OA of the hip through one of two mechanisms: (1) normal forces on an abnormal hip joint configuration, or (2) increased forces on normal joint anatomy. A substantial amount of theoretical, experimental, and clinical evidence supports the first mechanism of mechanically induced OA of the hip.[70, 71] There are fewer data supporting the second mechanism, and those that exist are more circumstantial.

Normal Forces on Abnormal Hip Joint Configurations

The relationship of abnormal hip joint anatomy and OA has been examined with two types of studies: those that trace the natural history of pre-existing childhood hip disease into adulthood, and those that attempt to identify evidence of a pre-existing hip joint abnormality in hips with coxarthrosis.

Congenital hip dysplasia (including congenital dislocation of the hip, acetabular dysplasia, coxa valga, and coxa vara) is the developmental abnormality most commonly associated with the development of OA (Fig. 15–1). Most authors believe that OA will inevitably develop if a hip is dysplastic.[10, 25, 26, 57, 59–62] The age at which significant degenerative joint disease will occur varies and is directly related to the extent of lateral and superior femoral head subluxation, femoral head size (coxa magna), femoral head-neck angulation (coxa valga), femoral head sphericity, acetabular inclination, acetabular depth, and acetabular orientation.[61] The earlier the hip dysplasia is recognized and corrected, the more likely that the onset of significant OA will be delayed.[72, 73] Hip dysplasia is probably the most common cause of OA of the hip in women. Therefore, its early detection and treatment could substantially reduce the incidence, severity, and age of onset of severe OA of the hip.

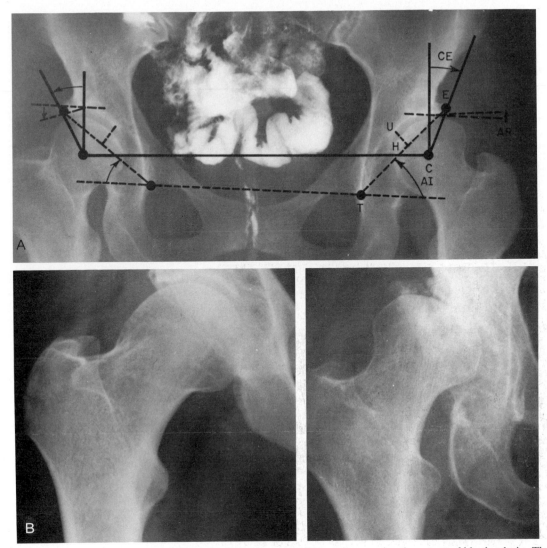

Figure 15–1. *A*, There are numerous methods available for establishing and measuring the extent of hip dysplasia. These measurements include: (1) The acetabular index (AI), which is the angle between the horizontal line connecting the teardrop spaces and the line TE. The AI increases as hip dysplasia becomes more severe. (2) The *center-edge angle* (CE) is the angle between the line that is perpendicular to the horizontal line connecting the centers of the femoral heads and the line from the center of the femoral head to the outer edge of the acetabulum. The CE angle becomes smaller as the dysplasia increases. (3) The acetabular depth is the perpendicular distance, HU, from the line connecting the teardrop and the outer edge of the acetabulum, TE, to the deepest point of the acetabulum. This distance decreases, i.e., the acetabulum becomes shallower, as the dysplasia becomes more severe. (4) The *acetabular roof* angle, AR, measures the lateral inclination of the acetabular roof. The lateral edge of the acetabulum is normally inclined downward. In dysplasia, the acetabular lip may become inclined upward. In this 50-year-old female, the dysplastic left hip has developed secondary osteoarthritis, with narrowing of the superior joint space, subchondral sclerosis, and subchondral cyst formation. *B*, Osteoarthritic changes secondary to congenital hip dysplasia are readily recognizable in this patient who had no history of joint symptoms as a child.

Several acquired childhood hip diseases produce deformities associated with the development of OA in adulthood. These include Perthes' disease, avascular necrosis resulting from a number of systemic diseases (e.g., sickle cell anemia, systemic lupus erythematosus, juvenile rheumatoid arthritis), infection, multiple epiphyseal dysplasia, Morquio's dis-

ease, and the osteochondral dystrophies. These diseases produce hip joint deformities of varying degrees, some of which are very similar to those resulting from congenital hip dysplasia. However, the relationship of deformity to the subsequent development of OA is much less direct in these diseases than it is in hip dysplasia. It has only recently been

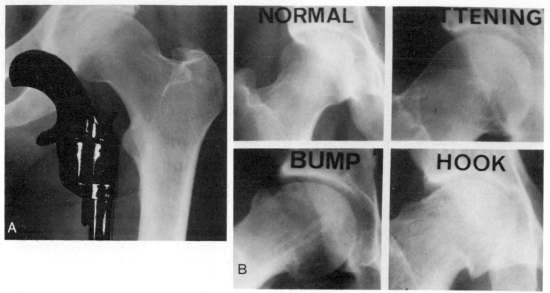

Figure 15–2. *A*, The "pistol-grip" or "tilt" deformity of the femoral head suggests the prior existence of a childhood hip disease, such as a slipped capital femoral epiphysis. *B*, The deformity is characterized by flattening of the superior femoral neck, the presence of a bump on the superior femoral neck, and a prominent hook at the junction of the inferior femoral head and neck. This deformity is frequently associated with the presence of osteoarthritis, especially in males.

appreciated that identical roentgenographic deformities do not necessarily imply similar propensities for the development of coxarthrosis.[10, 63] It is now clear that, contrary to classic mechanical theories of OA, the hip may be able to tolerate for a very long time what appear to be roentgenographically substantial deformities of the joint. Factors other than mechanical ones are important even in hips with abnormal configurations.

Hip deformities can occur without an antecedent history of congenital or acquired hip disease. The "tilt"[7] or "pistol-grip"[10] deformity

(Fig. 15–2) suggests a prior slipped capital femoral epiphysis or Perthes' disease (Fig. 15–3), although a history of these diseases may be lacking. The pistol-grip deformity has been associated with an increased incidence of OA of the hip. Murray and Duncan have suggested that this deformity, which is most common in males, results from participation in athletics during childhood and early adolescence.[8] However, in a long-term follow-up comparative study of Olympic-class marathon runners with age-matched nonathletic controls, Puranen and associates found a decreased incidence of

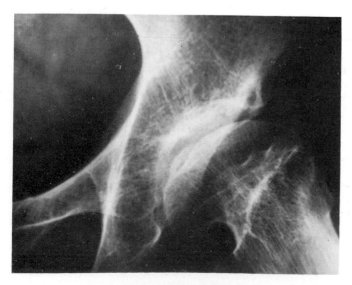

Figure 15–3. In spite of severe deformities of the femoral head and acetabulum, the hip joint of this 65-year-old woman who had Perthes' disease as a child shows very *little* evidence of osteoarthritis. The femoral head is large and mushroom-shaped. The femoral neck is short. A large portion of the femoral head is not covered by the acetabulum, which is itself shallow and steeply inclined. Although both the femoral head and acetabulum are abnormally shaped, they have developed in a nonspherical, congruous way. This congruity appears to have protected the hip joint from the development of arthritis.

the tilt deformity and a decreased incidence of OA of the hip in the marathon runners.[74] The relationship of this deformity to the subsequent development of OA remains intriguing but unclear.[75]

Additional forms of hip joint deformity, including tears of the acetabular labrum[76] and inverted acetabular labrum,[77] have recently been described and their presence implicated in the development of OA. The inverted acetabular labrum is associated with a roentgenographic form of osteoarthritis in which the superior joint space is retained and the medial joint space is narrowed. The primary area of weight bearing within the hip joint is superior, and it is this area that most frequently becomes narrow in osteoarthritis of the hip not associated with inflammatory or metabolic abnormalities. Thus, until the presence of an inverted acetabular labrum and its association with osteoarthritis were noted, there was not a satisfactory biomechanical explanation for this "medial" form of osteoarthritis. It remains, however, to be established whether the inverted labrum plays a significant role in the development of osteoarthritis and whether it alone is the explanation for this roentgenographic form of osteoarthritis.

Increased Forces on Normal Hip Joints

The results of a number of clinical studies have been interpreted to suggest that excessive stresses on normal hip joints will lead to osteoarthritis. For example, it has been observed that the incidence of osteoarthritis in the hip of a limb affected by poliomyelitis is less than that of the contralateral, normal hip.[78] This observation has been interpreted as evidence that the increased stress on the contralateral, normal hip is detrimental and that the reduced stress from paralyzed muscles on the affected leg is beneficial. Although the concept is attractive, the appropriateness of the model to osteoarthritis of the hip in individuals without neuromuscular disease is not clear. It has also been noted that leg-length discrepancies may be associated with an increased incidence of osteoarthritis of the longer leg, the hip being held in adduction and therefore being "uncovered" by the acetabulum. Whether, in fact, this actually occurs in extremities of significantly unequal length has not been established.

Increased body weight alone (without increased activity) has not been shown to be associated with an increased incidence of osteoarthritis of the hip.[79] Athletic activity, especially in muscular young adults, has been implicated in the development of coxarthrosis. Football players, for example, have been observed to have an increased incidence of osteoarthritis of the hip.[80] Whether these findings represent true osteoarthritis or "périarthropathie sportive" (see Chapter 33) is not clear. Moreover, factors other than participation in football (e.g., somatotype) may be influential in the incidence of osteoarthritis of the hip in this group of athletes. Thus, the long-term effects of increased stress, whether from increased weight, increased muscle force, or increased activity on normal hip joints, is uncertain. At the moment, there is *not* strong evidence to suggest that increased forces on a *normal* hip joint will lead to arthritis.

METABOLIC AND SYSTEMIC FACTORS AND THE INCIDENCE OF COXARTHROSIS

Metabolic Factors

Although most epidemiologic data have attributed differences in the incidence of osteoarthritis of the hip among various populations to variations in the occurrence of childhood hip disease that produce abnormal biomechanical stresses on the joint, recent studies have begun to focus attention on the relationship of metabolic abnormalities to the occurrence of osteoarthritis.[41, 81–88] These studies are beginning to support the theory, previously based on experimental investigations,[71] that the capacity of bone to respond to stress may be an important prerequisite for the development of osteoarthritis. These studies have found that the incidence of osteoarthritis of the hip is lowest in groups of patients with osteoporosis. These data have been interpreted to suggest that individuals whose osteoporosis does not respond to measures directed toward correcting this abnormality (e.g., physical activity, diet, and medication) may be less likely to develop osteoarthritis than those individuals whose subchondral bone is capable of responding to these forms of treatment.

Other metabolic diseases (e.g., acromegaly, ochronosis, and hemochromatosis) are associated with an increased incidence of osteoarthritis of the hip. These diseases are also responsible for producing specific abnormalities of articular cartilage metabolism. It is not known how important these mechanisms of cartilage injury are in the production of most forms of osteoarthritis. However, it appears that they play a relatively minor role in the development of osteoarthritis in most individuals with this disease.

Systemic Factors

Although debate continues about the role of inflammation in the development of osteoarthritis, most investigators do not believe that the inflammation often seen in the synovium of osteoarthritic joints is the primary mechanism responsible for the progression of the articular cartilage disease. However, in the past few years, evidence has been accumulating to suggest that the osteoarthritic process may be perpetuated, at least in certain cases, by the presence of immune complexes located within the articular cartilage or by immunologically active inflammatory cells (see Chapter 4).[89-92] These immunologic mechanisms have been associated with the roentgenographic appearance of an arthritic hip characterized by generalized joint space narrowing and protrusio acetabuli, a pattern typically seen in inflammatory diseases. These immunologic abnormalities are also more common in women with multiarticular forms of arthritis, suggesting that this process is a generalized one. Further studies of the role of immune mechanisms in the development of osteoarthritis may provide important and therapeutically useful information about this form of osteoarthritis of the hip.

SUMMARY

In the past few years, particular attention has been directed toward the role that mechanical factors play in the development of osteoarthritis of the hip. Deformities of the hip have been identified that are associated with an increased incidence of arthritis of the hip. Many of these deformities are due to childhood hip diseases. As a result, emphasis is being placed on the detection and treatment of these deformities in early childhood as a means of reducing the incidence of arthritis of the hip. At present, this emphasis appears to be particularly appropriate for dysplasia of the hip. This condition has been shown to be associated with an almost inevitable and often early development of arthritis. It is the most common cause of coxarthrosis in women. When this disorder is discovered in infancy,

treatment may alter its natural course in a significant way. At present, the long-term effects of treating hip dysplasia of late childhood and adolescence are less well defined. Mild forms of acetabular dysplasia, often not diagnosed until adulthood, may progress to osteoarthritis at a slow, unpredictable rate. Thus, the benefits of treatment of dysplasia discovered in adolescence or early adulthood must be carefully weighed against the risks of therapeutic intervention and must be considered with a knowledge of the treatment alternatives that are likely to be available to individuals if or when severe arthritis does occur.

Deformities of the hip that roentgenographically demonstrate incongruity between the femoral head and the acetabulum may be associated with an increased incidence of osteoarthritis. For example, individuals known to have had a slipped femoral capital epiphysis or Perthes' disease are more likely to develop osteoarthritis than those who have not had these diseases. However, the arthritis that occurs after these childhood hip diseases almost always appears relatively late in life. Treatment is directed toward minimizing the deformities produced by these diseases. There is evidence that early recognition and treatment of a slipped capital femoral epiphysis or Perthes' disease do result in a decreased incidence of severe deformity. However, there are as yet few long-term follow-up studies of currently applied treatment programs that would indicate whether or not these programs will be associated with a decreased incidence of arthritis or a delay in its appearance.

There is also no information available about the natural course of those hip deformities, e.g., the "pistol-grip" or "tilt" deformity, that are observed in individuals without a history of childhood hip disease. Therefore, at present, there is no justification for treating these deformities. However, if these deformities are associated with an increased incidence of arthritis and if, as has been shown, they occur quite commonly, directing attention to discovering the metabolic, traumatic, or systemic factors that might be responsible for the appearance of these deformities could lead to a clearer understanding of their relationship to arthritis. It may be that certain deformities biomechanically lead to an unmasking and release of articular cartilage components that are then able to perpetuate the process that leads to arthritis. It may also be that these deformities are associated with an as yet undiscovered concomitant abnormality of one of the components of articular cartilage that predisposes such hips to the development of arthritis. These remain possibilities, perhaps even conjectures, that require further study.

At present, there is no single theory to explain the cause of what has thus far been termed "primary osteoarthritis of the hip." The work in the past decade has called attention to the close relationship that may exist between hip joint deformity and the development of arthritis. It remains to be established by what mechanism these deformities are associated with the development of arthritis. Moreover, it is important to remember that many hips in which osteoarthritis occurs do not have recognizable primary deformities. The mechanism by which the arthritis in these hips occurs may involve immunologic events or metabolic abnormalities currently being studied or may be associated with an as yet undiscovered etiologic factor. Thus, for the time being at least, we shall have to accept the notion that the cause of certain forms of coxarthrosis is still unknown and that, in some cases, the entity "primary osteoarthritis of the hip" still exists.

References

1. Cameron HU, Macnab I: Observations on osteoarthritis of the hip joint. Clin Orthop 108:31–40, 1975.
2. Gofton JP: Studies in osteoarthritis of the hip. I. Classification. Can Med Assoc J 104:679–683, 1971.
3. Gofton JP, Trueman GE: Unilateral idiopathic osteoarthritis of the hip. Can Med Assoc J 97:1129–1132, 1967.
4. Brinckmann P, Frobin W, Hierholzer E: Stress on the articular surface of the hip joint in healthy adults and persons with idiopathic osteoarthrosis of the hip joint. J Biomech 14:149–156, 1981.
5. Lee P, Rooney PJ, Sturrock RD, et al.: The etiology and pathogenesis of osteoarthrosis: A review. Semin Arthritis Rheum 3:189–218, 1974.
6. Hoaglund FT: Osteoarthritis of the hip: Etiologic factors and preventive measures. In Committee on Rheumatoid Arthritis and Allied Diseases, American Academy of Orthopaedic Surgeons: Symposium on Osteoarthritis. St. Louis, C. V. Mosby Co., 1976, pp. 66–79.
7. Murray RO: The aetiology of primary osteoarthritis of the hip. Br J Radiol 38:810–824, 1965.
8. Murray RO, Duncan C: Athletic activity in adolescence as an etiological factor in degenerative hip disease. J Bone Joint Surg 53B:406–419, 1971.
9. Harris WH: Idiopathic osteoarthritis of the hip—a twentieth century myth? J Bone Joint Surg 59B:121, 1977.
10. Stulberg SD, Cordell LD, Harris WH, Ramsey PL, MacEwen GD: Unrecognized childhood hip disease: A major cause of idiopathic osteoarthritis of the hip. In Amstutz HC (ed.): The Hip: Proceedings of the Third Open Scientific Meeting of the Hip Society. St. Louis, C. V. Mosby Co., 1975, pp. 212–228.
11. Elmslie RC: Remarks on aetiological factors in osteoarthritis of the hip joint. Br Med J 1:1, 1933.
12. Trueta J: Studies on the etiopathology of osteoarthritis of the hip. Clin Orthop 31:7–19, 1963.
13. Kellgren JH, Lawrence JS: Radiographic assessment of osteoarthrosis. Ann Rheum Dis 16:494–502, 1957.
14. Harrison MHM, Schajowicz F, Trueta J: Osteoarthritis of the hip: A study of the nature and evolution of the disease. J Bone Joint Surg 35B:598–625, 1953.
15. Trueta J: Osteoarthritis of the hip. Ann R Coll Surg Engl 15:174, 1954.
16. Meachim G, Whitehouse GH, Pedley RB, et al.: An investigation of radiological, clinical and pathological correlations in osteoarthritis of the hip. Clin Radiol 31:565–574, 1980.
17. Macys JR, Bullough PG, Wilson PD Jr: Coxarthrosis: A study of the natural history based on a correlation of clinical, radiographic and pathologic findings. Semin Arthritis Rheum 10:66–80, 1980.
18. Hermodsson I: Roentgen appearance of coxarthrosis. Relation between the anatomy, pathologic changes and roentgen appearance. Acta Orthop Scand 41:169–187, 1970.
19. Danielsson L: Incidence of osteoarthrosis of the hip (coxarthrosis). Clin Orthop 45:67–72, 1966.
20. Kellgren JH, Lawrence JS: Osteoarthrosis of the hip in random population samples. Communicazione al X Congresso della Lega Internazionale contro il Rheumatismo, Rome, 1961.
21. Steven J: Osteoarthritis of the hip: A review with special consideration of the problem of bilateral malum coxae senilis. Clin Orthop 71:152–181, 1970.
22. Danielsson LG: Incidence and prognosis of coxarthrosis. Acta Orthop Scand 66(Suppl):1–114, 1964.
23. Kellgren JH, Lawrence JS: Osteoarthritis as seen in random samples of the population. J Bone Joint Surg 43B:601, 1961.
24. Byers PD, Contepomi CA, Farkas TA: A post mortem study of the hip joint. Ann Rheum Dis 29:15–31, 1970.
25. Stulberg SD, Harris WH: Acetabular dysplasia and development of osteoarthritis of hip. In Harris WH (ed.): The Hip: Proceedings of the Second Open Meeting of the Hip Society. St. Louis, C. V. Mosby Co., 1974, pp. 82–93.
26. Wiberg G: Studies on dysplastic acetabula and congenital subluxations of the hip joint. Acta Chir Scand 83:1, 1939.
27. Murray RO: Degenerative joint disease. Comparative aspects of osteoarthritis of the hip in man. J Small Anim Pract 12:99–100, 1971.
28. Salter RB: Textbook of Disorders and Injuries of the Musculoskeletal System. Baltimore, Williams & Wilkins Co., 1970.
29. Mankin HJ, Lippiello L: Biochemical and metabolic abnormalities in articular cartilage from osteoarthritic human hips. J Bone Joint Surg 52A:424–434, 1970.
30. Mankin HJ, Dorfman H, Lippiello L, et al.: Biochemical and metabolic abnormalities in articular cartilage from osteoarthritic human hips. II. Correlation of morphology with biochemical and metabolic data. J Bone Joint Surg 53A:523–537, 1971.
31. Mankin HJ, Johnson ME, Lippiello L: Biochemical and metabolic abnormalities in articular cartilage from osteoarthritic human hips. III. Distribution

and metabolism of amino sugar-containing macromolecules. J Bone Joint Surg 63A:131–139, 1981.

32. Byers PD, Maroudas A, Oztop F, et al.: Histological and biochemical studies on cartilage from osteoarthritic femoral heads with special reference to surface characteristics. Connect Tissue Res 5:41–49, 1977.

33. Reimann I, Christensen SB: A histochemical study of alkaline and acid phosphatase activity in subchondral bone from osteoarthritic human hips. Clin Orthop 140:85–91, 1979.

34. Reimann I, Mankin HJ, Trahan C: Quantitative histological analyses of articular cartilage and subchondral bone from osteoarthritic and normal human hips. Acta Orthop Scand 48:63–73, 1977.

35. Lust G, Summers BA: Early asymptomatic stage of degenerative joint disease in canine hip joints. Am J Vet Res 42:1849–1855, 1981.

36. Wiltberger H, Lust G: Ultrastructure of canine articular cartilage: Comparison of normal and degenerative (osteoarthritic) hip joints. Am J Vet Res 36:727–740, 1975.

37. Vignon E, Arlot M, Meunier P, et al.: Quantitative histological changes in osteoarthritic hip cartilage. Morphometric analysis of 29 osteoarthritic and 26 normal human femoral heads. Clin Orthop 103:269–278, 1974.

38. Scheck M, Sakovich L: Degenerative joint disease of the canine hip: Experimental production by multiple papain and prednisone injections. Clin Orthop 86:115–120, 1972.

39. Bentley G: Papain-induced degenerative arthritis of the hip in rabbits. J Bone Joint Surg 53B:324–337, 1971.

40. Stulberg SD, Kim YH, Levin JE: An animal model of acetabular dysplasia: A tool for studying the relationship between a developmental joint abnormality and osteoarthritis. Dallas, Texas, Orthopaedic Research Society, February 1978.

41. Solomon L, Schnitzler CM, Browett JP: Osteoarthritis of the hip: The patient behind the disease. Ann Rheum Dis 41:118–125, 1982.

42. Jorring K: Osteoarthritis of the hip. Epidemiology and clinical role. Acta Orthop Scand 51:523–530, 1980.

43. Lawrence JS, Zinn WM: Osteoarthrosis of the hip joint in Switzerland, in the United Kingdom, and in Jamaica, and its relationship to generalized osteoarthrosis. Ann Rheum Dis 29:191, 1970.

44. Lawrence JS, Bremner JM, Bier F: Osteoarthrosis. Prevalence in the population and relationship between symptoms and x-ray changes. Ann Rheum Dis 25:1–24, 1966.

45. Kellgren JH: Osteoarthrosis in patients and populations. Br Med J 2:1–6, 1961.

46. Kellgren JH, Lawrence JS: Osteoarthrosis and disk degeneration in an urban population. Ann Rheum Dis 17:388, 1958.

47. Hoaglund FT, Yau AC, Wong WL: Osteoarthritis of the hip and other joints in southern Chinese in Hong Kong. J Bone Joint Surg 55A:545–557, 1973.

48. Byers PD, Hoaglund FT, Purewal GS, et al.: Articular cartilage changes in Caucasian and Asian hip joints. Ann Rheum Dis 33:157–161, 1974.

49. Mukhopadhaya B, Barooah B: Osteoarthritis of the hip in Indians: An anatomical and clinical study. Indian J Orthop 1:55–62, 1967.

50. Solomon L, Beighton P, Lawrence JS: Rheumatic disorders in the South African Negro. II. Osteoarthrosis. S Afr Med J 49:1737–1740, 1975.

51. Saunders WA, Gleeson JA, Timlin DM, et al.: Degenerative joint disease in the hip and spine. Rheumatol Rehabil 18:137–141, 1979.

52. Yazici H, Saville PD, Salvati EA, et al.: Primary osteoarthrosis of the knee or hip. Prevalence of Heberden nodes in relation to age and sex. JAMA 231:1256–1260, 1976.

53. Roh YS, Dequeker J, Mulier JC: Osteoarthrosis at the hand skeleton in primary osteoarthrosis of the hip and in normal controls. Clin Orthop 90:90–94, 1973.

54. Gunn DR: Don't sit—squat! Clin Orthop 103:104–105, 1974.

55. Ives EJ, Houston CS: Congenital dislocation of the hip in northern Saskatchewan Indians. International Congress Series No. 191. Amsterdam, Excerpta Medica, 1969, p. 69.

56. Salter RB: Etiology, pathogenesis and possible prevention of congenital dislocation of the hip. Can Med Assoc J 98:937–945, 1968.

57. Cooperman DR, Wallensten R, Stulberg SD: The natural history of acetabular dysplasia. Clin Orthop 175:79–85, 1983.

58. Wroblewski BM: Osteoarthritis of the hip secondary to congenital dysplasia. J R Coll Surg Edinb 24:74–78, 1979.

59. Wedge JH, Wasylenko MJ: The natural history of congenital disease of the hip. J Bone Joint Surg 61B:334–338, 1979.

60. Gofton JP: Studies in osteoarthritis of the hip. III. Congenital subluxation and osteoarthritis of the hip. Can Med Assoc J 104:911, 1971.

61. Hart VL: Congenital Dysplasia of the Hip Joint and Sequelae. Springfield, Illinois, Charles C Thomas, 1952.

62. Lloyd-Roberts GC: Osteoarthritis of the hip. A study of the clinical pathology. J Bone Joint Surg 37B:8–47, 1955.

63. Stulberg SD, Cooperman DR, Wallensten R: The natural history of Legg-Calvé-Perthes' disease. J Bone Joint Surg 64A:1095–1108, 1981.

64. Broder H: The late results in Legg-Perthes' disease and factors influencing them. A study of one hundred and two cases. Bull Hosp Joint Dis 14:194–216, 1953.

65. Danielsson LG, Hernborg J: Late results of Perthes' disease. Acta Orthop Scand 36:70–81, 1965.

66. Eaton GO: Long-term results of treatment in coxa plana. A follow-up study of eighty-eight patients. J Bone Joint Surg 49A:1031–1042, 1967.

67. Evans DL: Legg-Calvé-Perthes' disease. A study of late results. J Bone Joint Surg 40B:168–181, 1958.

68. Gower WE, Johnson RC: Legg-Perthes' disease. Long-term follow-up of thirty-six patients. J Bone Joint Surg 53A:759–768, 1971.

69. Ratliff AHC: Perthes' disease. A study of thirty-four hips observed for thirty years. J Bone Joint Surg 49B:102–107, 1967.

70. Arnoldi CC, Reimann I: The pathomechanism of human coxarthrosis. Acta Orthop Scand 181 (Suppl):1–47, 1979.

71. Radin EL, Paul IL, Tolkoff MJ: Subchondral bone changes in patients with early degenerative joint disease. Arthritis Rheum 12:400–405, 1970.

72. Gill AB: The end results in treatment of congenital dislocation of the hip. With an inquiry into factors

that determine the result. J Bone Joint Surg 30A:442, 1948.

73. Muller GM, Seddon HJ: Late results of treatment of congenital dislocation of the hip. J Bone Joint Surg 35B:342, 1953.

74. Puranen J, Ala-Ketola L, Peltokallio P, et al.: Running and primary osteoarthritis of the hip. Br Med J 2:424–425, 1975.

75. Resnick D: The "tilt deformity" of the femoral head in osteoarthritis of the hip: A poor indicator of previous epiphysiolysis. Clin Radiol 27:355–363, 1976.

76. Altenberg AR: Acetabular labrum tears: A cause of hip pain and degenerative arthritis. South Med J 70:174–175, 1977.

77. Harris WH, Bourne RB, Oh I: Intra-articular acetabular labrum: A possible etiological factor in certain cases of osteoarthritis of the hip. J Bone Joint Surg 61A:510–514, 1979.

78. Glyn JH, Sutherland I, Walker GF, Young AC: Low incidence of osteoarthrosis in the hip and knee after anterior poliomyelitis: A late review. Br Med J 2:739–742, 1966.

79. Saville PD, Dickson J: Age and weight in osteoarthritis of the hip. Arthritis Rheum 11:635–644, 1968.

80. Klunder KB, Rud B, Hansen J: Osteoarthritis of the hip and knee joint in retired football players. Acta Orthop Scand 51:925–927, 1980.

81. Pogrund II, Rutenberg M, Makin M, et al.: Osteoarthritis of the hip joint and osteoporosis: A radiological study in a random population sample in Jerusalem. Clin Orthop 164:130–135, 1982.

82. Carlsson A, Nilsson BE, Westlin NE: Bone mass in primary coxarthrosis. Acta Orthop Scand 50:187–189, 1979.

83. Roh YS, Dequeker J, Mulier JC: Cortical bone remodeling and bone mass in primary osteoarthrosis of the hip. Invest Radiol 8:351–354, 1973.

84. Ostrup LT: Fracture of the femoral neck in cases with coxarthrosis on the affected side. Acta Orthop Scand 41:559–564, 1970.

85. Roh YS, Dequeker J, Mulier JC: Bone mass in osteoarthrosis, measured in vivo by photon absorption. J Bone Joint Surg 56A:587–591, 1974.

86. Foss MV, Byers PD: Bone density, osteoarthrosis of the hip, and fracture of the upper end of the femur. Ann Rheum Dis 31:259–264, 1972.

87. Cooperman DR, Wallensten R, Stulberg SD: The consequences of avascular necrosis in congenitally dislocated hips. J Bone Joint Surg 62A:247–258, 1980.

88. Solomon L: Bone density in ageing Caucasian and African populations. Lancet 2:1326–1330, 1979.

89. Cooke TD, Bennett EL, Ohno O: The deposition of immunoglobulins and complement in osteoarthritic cartilage. Int Orthop 4:211–217, 1980.

90. Jasin HE, Cooke TD: The inflammatory role of immune complexes trapped in joint collagenous tissues. Clin Exp Immunol 33:416–424, 1978.

91. Jasin HE, Cooke TD: Persistence of antigen in experimental allergic monoarthritis. In Glynn LE, Schlumberger HD (eds.): Experimental Models of Chronic Inflammatory Diseases. Berlin, Springer, 1977, pp. 28–32.

92. Cooke TD, Hurd ER, Jasin HE, et al.: Identification of immunoglobulins and complement in rheumatoid articular collagenous tissues. Arthritis Rheum 18:541–551, 1975.

16

General Aspects of Differential Diagnosis

Rodney Bluestone, M.B., F.R.C.P.

The diagnostic approach to established or chronic rheumatic disease is a regional one. That is to say, most rheumatic diseases display a typical pattern of distribution throughout the musculoskeletal system. Although any of the common arthropathies may affect one, several, or many of the joints around the body, sooner or later most patients with a well-defined rheumatic disease syndrome display a fairly characteristic pattern of involvement. This concept is crucial to clinical diagnosis, because the distribution of the arthropathy is of itself the most valuable clue available to the clinician. Thus, the history and physical examination of a patient presenting with newly developing or established rheumatic disease must be designed to answer this question. Many of the imaging techniques currently in vogue, including traditional methods such as roentgenography as well as the newer isotope scanning procedures,[1, 2] are all designed to further enhance the clinician's ability to determine the true pattern of distribution of the arthropathy. If the rheumatic disease is well established (of more than 9 to 12 months' duration), the roentgenograms may display some characteristic morphoroentgenographic features that provide further diagnostic clues.[3] Not only is the true pattern of distribution of the arthropathy further disclosed, but also some specific pathologic alterations characteristic of a certain disease process may thereby be inferred.

In certain rheumatic diseases, extra-articular or extraskeletal target organ involvement may be an important component of the disease.[4] This is particularly true in patients with systemic connective tissue diseases such as systemic lupus erythematosus, progressive systemic sclerosis, or vasculitis, for example, as well as in some individuals with rheumatoid arthritis. Thus, the physician must not be content simply to examine the skeleton but must also search for changes in extraskeletal organ systems. Indeed, under some circumstances, the nonarticular manifestations dominate the clinical picture, and their recognition may lead to the diagnosis of a primary rheumatic disease.

The laboratory is often of further diagnostic help in the field of clinical rheumatology.[5] Occasionally, the laboratory test is crucial to the diagnosis, as in crystal-induced arthritis as well as the various infectious syndromes manifesting with joint inflammation. Other laboratory tests help the clinician to assess the extent, severity, and intensity of a well-diagnosed rheumatic disease. Similarly, response to therapy may be reflected in the laboratory parameters.

The clinical diagnosis of osteoarthritis (OA) follows the basic concepts just outlined. In many patients, the clinical manifestations of osteoarthritis are localized to a single joint. In those patients with more generalized primary OA, joint changes are limited to characteristic areas of involvement, which include the distal and proximal interphalangeal joints, first carpometacarpal joints, hips, knees, first metatarsophalangeal joints, and cervical and lumbar spine. Involvement of other joints such as the wrists, elbows, or shoulders by osteoarthritis should suggest a secondary underlying disorder associated with OA (see Chapter 14) or another form of joint disease. Roentgenographic changes are generally confirmatory, especially in the presence of more advanced disease. Systemic extra-articular features are absent. The laboratory profile is negative with respect to systemic inflammation, and antibody studies such as rheumatoid factor or antinuclear antibody are negative.

DIFFERENTIAL DIAGNOSIS

Although the diagnosis of osteoarthritis based on the clinical and laboratory considerations outlined above may be straightforward, the disease is frequently atypical in its presentation and behavior and requires differential diagnostic considerations. Examples of presentations of osteoarthritis that might lead to diagnostic difficulties include the following:

1. Osteoarthritis that occurs in an atypical site outside the characteristic and favored areas for distribution for the disease. As noted, this presentation is likely to be connected with secondary underlying disorders associated with OA.

2. Osteoarthritis associated with a significant inflammatory element. Although clinical evidence of inflammation is generally lacking in most patients with osteoarthritis, inflammation may be more prominent in certain forms of the disease such as erosive inflammatory OA of the hands[6] or in primary generalized OA.[7] Differentiation from systemic forms of arthritis such as rheumatoid arthritis may be difficult at times.

3. Osteoarthritis associated with calcium pyrophosphate deposition disease. Calcium crystal deposition within articular cartilage is often associated with degenerative changes within the cartilaginous substance.[8,9] (See Chapter 14.) Moreover, the degenerative process may be peculiarly brisk and accompanied by inflammatory features that are associated with rapid fragmentation and degeneration of the normal articular surfaces. The appearance of a multifocal arthropathy seen predominantly in the knees, wrists, and shoulders and bearing clinical and roentgenographic features intermediate between primary osteoarthritis and true inflammatory polyarthritis should raise the issue of calcium pyrophosphate deposition joint disease.

4. Osteoarthritis occurring precociously in younger individuals with no strong evidence of mechanical or occupational trauma. Occasionally, patients may present with what seems to be typical osteoarthritis but that is occurring at a much younger age than is usual. In many instances (e.g., in osteoarthritis of the hip), a mechanical abnormality associated with childhood hip disorders may be inferred as the initiating event (see Chapter 15).[10, 11] In other instances, a hereditary disorder with a strong family history may be discerned. Sometimes, however, there appears to be no valid explanation for cartilage destruction to proceed in severe or widespread fashion in a young to middle-aged individual.

5. Postinflammatory osteoarthritis. Chronic or recurrent inflammatory joint disease may completely resolve but may leave damaged joint surfaces in its wake, as may be seen, for example, in patients with rheumatoid arthritis. Once the inflammation has damaged the joint, a progressive secondary osteoarthritis may be inevitable. The clinical picture may then be atypical for primary osteoarthritis because the distribution of joint involvement more faithfully reflects the joint pattern associated with the previous inflammatory joint disease. Moreover, roentgenographic changes resulting from the previous inflammatory process may become combined with and overtaken by osteoarthritic morphoroentgenographic features, leading to a rather atypical roentgenographic appearance.

6. Osteoarthritis associated with metabolic bone disease. In patients with profound metabolic bone disease such as osteoporosis, osteomalacia, or Paget's disease, symptoms may be attributed to age-related findings of OA rather than to the primary bone disorder. Accurate assessment of clinical, roentgenographic, and laboratory findings usually makes the site of origin of the symptoms apparent.

7. Osteoarthritis of the spine presenting with neurologic syndromes. Osteoarthritis that affects the cervical or lumbosacral spine is often associated with symptoms related to nerve root compression. Under such circumstances, for example, the patient may present with upper-extremity radicular pain or lower-extremity sciatica. These symptoms must be differentiated from similar complaints caused by other pathologic processes affecting the spine such as osteoporosis with vertebral collapse, multiple myeloma, or neoplasms. These latter diseases occur primarily in the elderly, in whom some osteoarthritis may also be expected to be present. Caution is necessary to avoid attributing the symptoms to the readily observed OA, especially if changes related to the more serious disorder that is present are in the early stages and less easily detected.

Review of the differential diagnosis of osteoarthritis is best approached by considering specific areas of joint involvement. The major regions within the skeleton that are particularly prone to the primary osteoarthritic process include the middle and lower parts of the cervical spine; the lumbosacral spine; the distal and proximal interphalangeal joints of the hands; the first carpometacarpal joints of the hands; the hips; the knees; and the great toes (first metatarsophalangeal joints). If the osteoarthritic process is confined to one of these regions, specific differential diagnoses must be considered. This differential diagnosis is based on regional considerations and includes a review of the arthropathies that are most likely to affect joints at that specific site. However, if a patient is suffering from atypical osteoarthritis, the more general principles of differential diagnosis applied to rheumatic diseases may apply. Unusual osteoarthritic presentations would therefore call for a full differential diagnostic consideration based on the pattern of distribution of the common rheumatic diseases, extraskeletal manifestations, and appropriate laboratory studies.

DIFFERENTIAL DIAGNOSIS OF REGIONAL OSTEOARTHRITIS

Middle and Lower Cervical Spine

One of the most common pathologic entities afflicting this part of the skeleton is osteoarthritis. However, other pathologic processes may arise at this site and may be manifested as pain in the neck on movement, with or without symptoms and signs of cervical nerve root compression. The potential pathologic conditions in this part of the skeleton include injury, very commonly of a whiplash kind; inflammatory joint disease such as rheumatoid arthritis and ankylosing spondylitis; primary and secondary neoplasms of bone; osteoporosis; neurofibromas of nerve roots manifested as brachial neuralgia; other neurologic conditions primarily affecting nerve roots, such as herpes zoster and trauma to the brachial plexus; and more distal compression syndromes such as the thoracic outlet syndrome.

The fact that so many patients over 40 years of age demonstrate evidence of mild to moderate cervical spondylosis roentgenographically, combined with the fact that many of the conditions outlined above are not uncommon, may make the differential diagnosis of neck pain due to osteoarthritis rather difficult. Indeed, ascribing a patient's symptoms and signs (including signs of nerve root compression) to osteoarthritis of the cervical spine is often a process of exclusion. Moreover, if the neurologic syndrome related to osteoarthritic changes is severe, such as the development of progressive myelopathy, a considerable amount of neurologic investigation is invariably required to exclude other pathologic processes as the cause of the patient's complaints. Nevertheless, most patients over 40 years old with pain in the neck and roentgenographic evidence of significant osteoarthritis affecting the vertebral bodies, intervertebral disks, and apophyseal joints will usually eventually be found to be suffering from primary osteoarthritis of the cervical spine.

Lumbosacral Spine

Osteoarthritis in this region leads to many difficult differential diagnoses. Moreover, as in the cervical spine, the roentgenographic presence of osteoarthritis in this region does not necessarily indicate that the patient's low back pain is due specifically to OA. Among the many other mechanical or pathologic disorders of the lumbosacral spine requiring diagnostic consideration are mechanical low back strain; the various facet joint syndromes, including minor degrees of subluxation; idiopathic or degenerative spondylolisthesis; congenital partial fusions, especially with incomplete sacralization of the fifth lumbar vertebra and pseudoarticulation formation; congenital or acquired scoliosis; and various metabolic and neoplastic disorders of bone that may affect the lumbosacral vertebral structures.

It is important to realize that any of the aforementioned conditions may present in a patient who has already-established osteoarthritis of the lumbosacral spine. It then may become a difficult exercise in clinical and roentgenographic interpretation to elucidate an alternative cause of the patient's symptoms. Moreover, it is not unusual for any of the aforementioned conditions to aggravate or be aggravated by an associated osteoarthritic process within this region of the skeleton, with each component contributing separately to the patient's symptomatic state.

Distal Interphalangeal Joints of the Fingers

Several rheumatic disorders favor this target site within the skeleton. Thus, symptoms or signs located at the distal interphalangeal joints

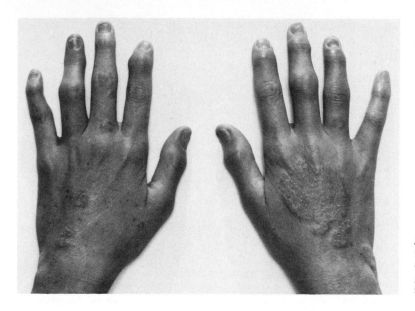

Figure 16–1. Hands of a patient with typical psoriatic arthritis. Swelling of distal and proximal interphalangeal joints is evident. Note extensive nail destruction.

should not automatically be considered due to osteoarthritis. In particular, an inflammatory and destructive arthropathy at this site is well recognized in patients with psoriasis (Fig. 16–1).[12, 13] Pitting of the adjacent fingernail is common (Fig. 16–2), and a psoriatic rash is or becomes obvious. Similar involvement of the distal interphalangeal joints is not uncommonly seen in patients with Reiter's syndrome[14, 15] or in association with the arthritis of chronic ulcerative colitis. Although rheumatoid arthritis usually spares the distal interphalangeal joints, a small proportion of adults with the disease (perhaps 5% of all patients with chronic rheumatoid arthritis) display involvement of this region at one time or another. However, it is not at all uncommon for children suffering from polyarticular juvenile rheumatoid arthritis or acute-onset systemic juvenile rheumatoid arthritis to display artic-

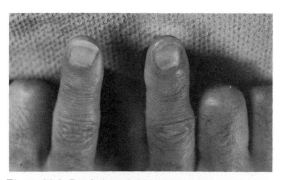

Figure 16–2. Psoriatic arthritis. Pitting of the nail of the right second finger is associated with a chronically inflamed distal interphalangeal joint.

ular inflammation in the regions of their distal interphalangeal joints.

Proximal Interphalangeal Joints of the Fingers

Osteoarthritis quite commonly affects the proximal interphalangeal joints but nearly always in association with more obvious distal interphalangeal joint involvement (Fig. 16–3). Unfortunately, when the disease does affect the proximal joints, there is often an inflammatory component evident and a tendency to develop erosive osteoarthritis. Thus, the differential diagnosis of a primary inflammatory polyarthritis must be considered. In effect, this means the need to consider the possible presence of rheumatoid arthritis as the only other common type of persistent, and potentially destructive, inflammation of all the proximal interphalangeal joints. However, the inflammatory component associated with osteoarthritis at this site is usually transient and often regresses after 6 to 9 months. Moreover, the other bony hypertrophic features characteristic of OA usually become the dominant sign at both the proximal and distal interphalangeal joints, and the absence of more widespread articular inflammation should be evident.

First Carpometacarpal Joint

This joint may be involved in any patient with an inflammatory polyarthritis, so that

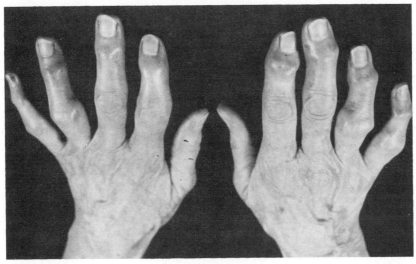

Figure 16–3. Osteoarthritis involves the distal and proximal interphalangeal joints in characteristic distribution.

osteoarthritic pain and swelling in this region must be differentiated from almost any other kind of chronic inflammatory rheumatic disease. Moreover, osteoarthritis at this site may be associated with relative instability of the thumb and a mild articular effusion with synovial distention. Thus, it becomes necessary to screen the patient carefully for signs of a more generalized rheumatic process. In addition, the base of the thumb is a readily traumatized area; acute sprain of the first carpometacarpal joint has to be considered in patients presenting with pain in that region whether or not they show clinical and roentgenographic changes of early osteoarthritis. Tenosynovitis involving the abductor pollicis longus and extensor pollicis brevis tendons at the wrist (De Quervain's tenosynovitis) is common, and symptoms emanating from this area may be difficult to differentiate from osteoarthritic changes of the first carpometacarpal joint.

Hips

Patients with a diverse number of rheumatic diseases may present with pain and limitation of range of motion within a hip joint. Accordingly, in patients who are presumed to have osteoarthritis of the hip, the presence of another arthropathic process must always be considered. In particular, rheumatoid arthritis may begin in a hip joint or the hip may become involved in someone with established rheumatoid arthritis, even at a late stage of the disease. If evidence of rheumatoid disease is already well established in other joints, subsequent involvement of the hip is usually an accurate diagnosis. However, it should not be forgotten that many elderly patients with rheumatoid arthritis may also develop osteoarthritis as a separate pathologic entity. In younger individuals, osteoarthritis must be distinguished from hip disease associated with the seronegative spondyloarthropathies such as ankylosing spondylitis. Although ankylosing spondylitis nearly always presents with back pain as its most prominent feature, large root joint involvement may predominate early in the disease. Osteoarthritis may be seen in younger patients, especially in someone who has had primary hip abnormalities such as congenital hip dysplasia, Legg-Perthes disease, retroversion of the hip, or slipped capital femoral epiphysis, which, even if mild, may lead to secondary osteoarthritis. Pain in the hip with later roentgenographic evidence of development of osteoarthritis may result from avascular necrosis of the femoral head (Fig. 16–4).[16] This may be a difficult diagnosis to approach unless one is suspicious of the process. Very often, the pain of avascular necrosis is out of proportion to any roentgenographic changes; radioisotope scanning often aids in identifying an area of subchondral bone necrosis long before roentgenographic changes are apparent.

Other causes of hip disease to be considered in the differential diagnosis are pigmented villonodular synovitis[17, 18] and synovial chondromatosis. Both of these entities may be subtle in their presentation, and establishment of the

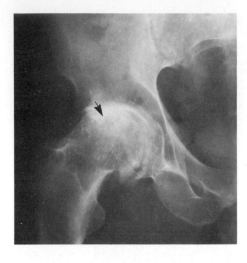

Figure 16–4. Avascular necrosis of the hip. An area of relative radiolucency (arrow) is surrounded by a rim of increased bone density.

diagnosis may be difficult. Pigmented villonodular synovitis, with characteristics of both an inflammatory process and a benign neoplasm, is characterized by specific histologic features that include multinucleated giant cells, hemosiderosis, and distended synovial cells laden with lipid deposits. Recurrent hemorrhage into the joint is common and accounts for the presence of grossly bloody or xanthochromic synovial fluid. Although plain roentgenograms that demonstrate large cystic erosions of bone may suggest the diagnosis, pneumoarthrograms are helpful in demonstrating the lesion, especially if it is small. Synovial chondromatosis is characterized by metaplasia of synovium with replacement of synovial tissue by normal-appearing hyaline cartilage. Ossification with osteochondromatosis follows. Neoplasms of the joint, although relatively uncommon, must also be considered in the differential diagnosis. Finally, inflammatory monarthritis due to *Mycobacterium* tuberculosis or various fungi may be slow in onset and progression and symptoms may mimic those of OA. The diagnosis of an infectious etiology may be readily missed if osteoarthritic changes commonly observed in older age groups are considered the cause of the patient's symptoms without careful clinical evaluation and appropriate observation.

Knee

Osteoarthritis of the knee is always a valid diagnostic consideration in a patient over 50 years of age. Subacute or chronic monarthritis due to other disorders is common, however, and differential diagnosis may be complex.

Mechanical internal joint derangements may result from tearing of one of the menisci or cruciate ligaments. A history of trauma can usually be elicited but may be minor and overlooked. Secondary degenerative joint disease is common. Plica syndrome due to persistent folds or bands of synovial membrane may induce symptoms similar to those associated with osteoarthritis.[19] Pain is increased with activity, and a sensation of clicking or snapping may be noted. Plain roentgenograms are usually normal. Lateral pneumoarthrograms are more definitive. Osteochondritis dissecans most frequently involves the knee and occurs more commonly in children and young adults (Fig. 16–5). The disorder is characterized by separation of a section of cartilage and underlying bone from the larger bone to which it is attached. Secondary OA is a common complication. Idiopathic osteonecrosis of the knee is a form of avascular necrosis.[20] It occurs in older individuals and typically involves the weight-bearing surface of the medial femoral condyle. Pain is typically abrupt in onset. Other diseases that may produce a subacute or chronic arthritis of the knee are avascular necrosis, pigmented villonodular synovitis, and synovial chondromatosis (Fig. 16–6), as described previously in the hip. Similarly, chronic infection with tuberculosis or fungi, as well as primary neoplasms, need to be excluded.

Hypertrophic pulmonary osteoarthropathy is characterized by clubbing of the fingers and toes, periostitis of the ends of the long bones (Fig. 16–7), and synovial swelling of joints. Large joints such as the knees, ankles, and wrists are involved most frequently. An association with neoplasms, particularly of the lungs, is common. Accordingly, this syndrome

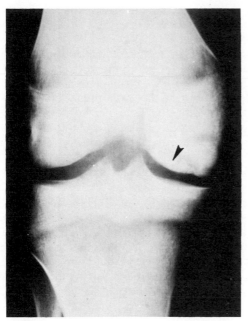

Figure 16–5. Osteochondritis dissecans. Separation of the osteocartilaginous fragment is evident (arrow).

in association with calcium apatite crystal deposition in the knee have been described.[21]

Rarely should there be difficulty in distinguishing rheumatoid arthritis of the knee from osteoarthritis. However, it is not uncommon for rheumatoid disease to begin within the knee joints; when this event is seen in an elderly individual, the consideration of this differential diagnosis becomes pertinent. However, simple osteoarthritis should rarely be associated with a persistent inflammatory reaction within the synovium of the knee that dominates the clinical picture, except when there is associated calcium pyrophosphate deposition and crystal-induced synovitis. In patients with more established rheumatoid arthritis, new involvement of the knee joint usually points to the correct diagnosis once the more generalized pattern of the arthropathy is recognized.

is an important one in the differential diagnosis of OA, which, like neoplasms, affects older individuals.

Because the knee is also a favorite site for calcium pyrophosphate deposition (Fig. 16–8), any patient with OA of the knee may also have acute and chronic episodes of inflammation within the joint. This is one of the few joints in the body, therefore, where the clinical presentation of OA may possess a variable component of active inflammation with the additional signs and symptoms of synovitis. More recently, acute episodes of inflammation

Great Toe (First Metatarsophalangeal Joint)

Osteoarthritis of the great toe is commonly seen, but several pertinent differential diagnoses have to be considered. First, the presence of hallux valgus as part of the degenerative process as opposed to an idiopathic and separate entity must be considered in the presence of the typical deformity. It is often difficult to decide whether the hallux valgus is partially secondary to the osteoarthritis at this site or whether the valgus deformity itself has induced a secondary mechanical osteoarthritis within the great toe. The condition of hallux rigidus may be seen in remarkably young in-

Figure 16–6. Anteroposterior and lateral roentgenograms of the knee showing synovial osteochondromatosis. Multiple rounded calcified masses are readily seen.

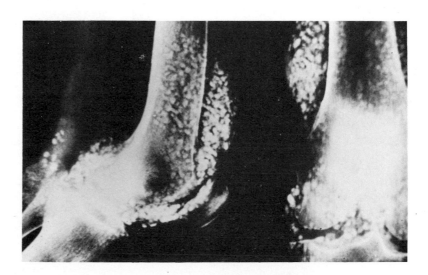

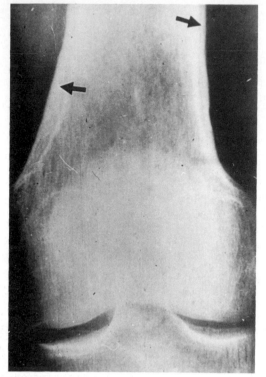

Figure 16–7. Hypertrophic pulmonary osteoarthropathy. Subperiosteal new bone formation (arrows) is prominently seen.

osteophytosis may be surprisingly mild over the dorsal aspect of the joint. Because chronic gout may leave the great toe thickened, enlarged, and somewhat destroyed, this diagnosis needs to be considered in patients with chronic joint deformities in this region (Fig. 16–9). Usually, the history will reveal characteristic episodes of acute gouty arthritis in the past. Aspiration of a relatively asymptomatic gouty great toe may reveal the urate crystals required for the definitive diagnosis.[22] It is rare for osteoarthritis of the toe to be coupled with significant inflammatory findings unless there has been recent trauma to the area or unless there is an associated acute bursitis. Reiter's syndrome or psoriatic arthritis may lead to so much inflammation and destruction of the great toe that the eventual clinical and roentgenologic features may at first simulate severe osteoarthritis. However, the clinical findings suggestive of Reiter's syndrome or psoriasis are usually apparent and together with the roentgenographic picture of an erosive destruction of the joint should quickly dispel any diagnostic difficulties.

DIFFERENTIAL DIAGNOSIS FROM OTHER COMMON RHEUMATIC DISEASE SYNDROMES THAT PRESENT WITH ARTHROPATHY

dividuals, especially those with a history of recurrent trauma to the toe joint (e.g., incorrect kicking posture in soccer). Under these circumstances, all the symptoms and signs of osteoarthritis of the great toe are evident;

As opposed to clinically typical primary osteoarthritis, a greater differential diagnostic problem exists when osteoarthritis appears at unusual sites or when the clinical features, such as a prominent inflammatory component, suggest the possible presence of other disor-

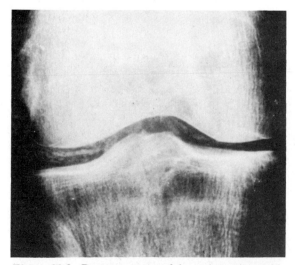

Figure 16–8. Roentgenogram of knee in patient with chondrocalcinosis reveals calcification of the menisci and articular hyaline cartilage with calcium pyrophosphate.

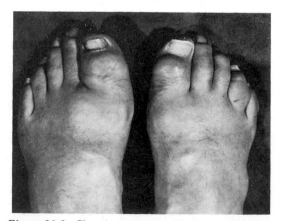

Figure 16–9. Chronic gouty arthropathy of both great toes. Roentgenograms revealed tophaceous joint destruction.

ders. Under these circumstances, it is generally apparent to the clinician that the arthropathy is unlikely to be due to osteoarthritis and is more likely to be due to another rheumatic disease. Thus, the differential diagnosis involves the ability to recognize and diagnose those other common rheumatic disease syndromes that present with arthropathy. Clearly, this involves the entire field of clinical rheumatology, but fortunately, the common rheumatic diseases are rather easily recognized when they appear in their evolved or typical form.

Inflammatory Joint Disease of Nonspecific Etiology

Rheumatoid arthritis is characterized by prominent active synovitis; many small peripheral joints are usually involved in a fairly symmetric fashion. Common extra-articular manifestations include carpal tunnel syndrome, synovitis of the flexor tendon sheath in the hands, subcutaneous rheumatoid nodules, and sicca syndrome. The roentgenographic changes include symmetric loss of joint space, profound periarticular osteopenia, and marginal erosions. Laboratory tests often reveal a low-grade anemia, an elevated erythrocyte sedimentation rate, and the presence of rheumatoid factor.

Ankylosing spondylitis is characterized by inflammation of the axial joints, both cartilaginous and synovial, but predominantly cartilaginous. This is manifested as pain and stiffness in the back and thoracic cage and around the pelvic and shoulder girdles. A common extra-articular manifestation is a history or presence of recurrent acute iritis. Roentgenograms display disruption of the cartilaginous osseous junction, especially in the sacroiliac joints, syndesmophyte formation along the vertebrae of the spine, and, later, prominent ligamentous ossification and bony fusion. Laboratory tests may reveal a mild anemia, an elevated erythrocyte sedimentation rate, elevated serum alkaline phosphatase, and the presence of the tissue antigen HLA-B27.

Patients with psoriatic arthritis usually demonstrate obvious evidence of skin and/or nail psoriasis, although this is not invariably true.[12, 13] Although psoriatic arthropathy may assume one of many forms, about 70% of all patients with this type of joint disease display an intermittent asymmetric oligoarthritis of small and large joints with or without tendon sheath involvement. The roentgenographic changes are similar to those of ankylosing spondylitis but with a more severe involvement of peripheral joints, with a tendency toward joint fusion and periosteal reaction. The laboratory profile is characterized by the absence of rheumatoid factor.

Patients with Reiter's syndrome usually display a lower-limb oligoarthritis that is especially marked within the knees and around the hindfoot.[14, 15] They frequently relate a history of conjunctivitis and iritis. The syndrome is usually most evident in sexually active young men. Other extra-articular features include mucosal and skin lesions, including the skin of the glans penis, palms, and soles (keratoderma blennorrhagicum). The roentgenograms are very similar to those of psoriatic arthritis, revealing a tendency toward early destruction of the joint, followed by bony fusion. Once again, the laboratory profile may simply reflect the presence of inflammation but is typically negative for rheumatoid factor. However, like individuals with ankylosing spondylitis, most patients with Reiter's syndrome are HLA-B27–positive.

Patients with systemic lupus erythematosus often display a symmetric small- and medium-sized joint polyarthritis that is most marked in the joints of the hands, feet, wrists, elbows, and knees. Very soon, the extra-articular tissue involvement dominates the clinical picture, so that the typical polysystem involvement becomes obvious. Despite persistent synovitis, it is unusual to see destructive joint changes in this type of arthritis, although chronic subluxations are well recognized in a minority of patients. The serologic stigmata of the disease are usually evident from the beginning.

Specific Chronic Infective Arthritis

Tuberculous and fungal joint disease may involve any articulation in the body (Fig. 16–10). Symptoms are usually gradual in onset and may simulate joint changes seen in rheumatoid arthritis, the seronegative spondyloarthropathies, and other conditions. A high index of suspicion is frequently required to accurately establish the diagnosis.

Crystal Deposition Diseases

Gout most often affects the great toe and is characterized by repeated episodes of acute inflammation. The disease is also commonly seen, however, in the forefoot and ankle and

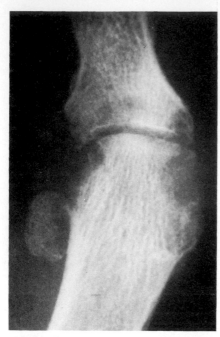

Figure 16–10. Tuberculous infection of the first metatarsophalangeal joint.

around the wrist. There may be signs of chronic arthropathy during the intercritical period, depending especially on the presence of tophaceous deposits. Associated clinical features frequently include obesity, hyperlipidemia, hypertension, and evidence of arteriosclerotic vascular disease. Laboratory findings that are helpful in the diagnosis include previous or current demonstration of urate crystals from an inflamed joint and, usually, an elevated serum urate concentration.

Patients with calcium pyrophosphate deposition arthropathy may develop attacks of acute pseudogout. A differential diagnostic consideration of osteoarthritis occurs when the pyrophosphate deposition disease is more continuous and chronic in its manifestations. Under the latter circumstances, the typical pattern of distribution is in the knees, wrists, and shoulders, usually in an elderly individual. The roentgenograms frequently reveal evidence of chondrocalcinosis. The laboratory profile would be expected to reveal abnormalities only if the chondrocalcinosis is associated with one of the known metabolic endocrine diseases seen in this condition, such as hyperparathyroidism, hemochromatosis, hypophosphatasia, and hypothyroidism. (See Chapter 14.)

References

1. Dick WC: The use of radioisotopes in normal and diseased joints. Semin Arthritis Rheum 1:301–325, 1972.
2. Kirchner PT, Simon MA: Radioisotopic evaluation of skeletal disease. J Bone Joint Surg 63A:673–681, 1981.
3. Resnick D, Niwayama G (eds.): Articular Diseases, Radiographic-Pathologic Correlations. Philadelphia, W. B. Saunders Company, 1981.
4. Bluestone R, Bacon PA (eds.): Extraarticular manifestations of rheumatoid arthritis. Clin Rheum Dis 3:385–406, 1977.
5. Cohen AS: Laboratory Diagnostic Procedures in Rheumatic Diseases. 2nd ed. Boston, Little, Brown & Co., 1975.
6. Ehrlich GE: Osteoarthritis beginning with inflammation. Definitions and correlations. JAMA 232:157–159, 1975.
7. Kellgren JH, Moore R: Generalized osteoarthritis and Heberden's nodes. Br Med J 1:181–187, 1952.
8. Moskowitz RW, Garcia F: Chondrocalcinosis articularis (pseudogout syndrome). Arch Intern Med 132:87–91, 1973.
9. McCarty DJ: Calcium pyrophosphate dihydrate crystal deposition disease—1975. Arthritis Rheum 19:275–285, 1976.
10. Murray RO: The aetiology of primary osteoarthritis of the hip. Br J Radiol 38:810–824, 1965.
11. Solomon L: Patterns of osteoarthritis of the hip. J Bone Joint Surg 58B:176–183, 1976.
12. Moll JMH, Wright V: Psoriatic arthritis. Semin Arthritis Rheum 3:55–78, 1973.
13. Roberts MET, Wright V, Hill AGS, et al.: Psoriatic arthritis: Follow-up study. Ann Rheum Dis 35:206–212, 1976.
14. Ford DK: Reiter's syndrome. Bull Rheum Dis 20:588–591, 1970.
15. Lassus A, Karnoven J: Reactive arthritis, Reiter's disease and psoriatic arthritis. Clin Rheum Dis 3:281, 1977.
16. Ibels LS, et al.: Aseptic necrosis of bone following renal transplantation: Experience in 194 transplant recipients and review of the literature. Medicine 57:25–45, 1978.
17. Smith JH, Pugh DG: Roentgenographic aspects of articular pigmented villonodular synovitis. Am J Roentgenol Radium Ther Nucl Med 87:1146–1156, 1962.
18. Granowitz SP, Mankin HJ: Localized pigmented villonodular synovitis of the knee. J Bone Joint Surg 49A:122–128, 1967.
19. Hardaker WT, Whipple TL, Bassett FH: Diagnosis and treatment of the plica syndrome of the knee. J Bone Joint Surg 62A:221–225, 1980.
20. Rozing PM, Insall J, Bohne WH: Spontaneous osteonecrosis of the knee. J Bone Joint Surg 62A:2–7, 1980.
21. Schumacher HR, et al.: Arthritis associated with apatite crystals. Ann Intern Med 87:411–416, 1977.
22. Agudelo CA, et al.: Definitive diagnosis of gout by identification of urate crystals in asymptomatic metatarsophalangeal joints. Arthritis Rheum 22:559–560, 1979.

GENERAL ASPECTS OF MANAGEMENT

David Howell, M.D.
Section Editor

SECTION

3

17

Rehabilitation in the Management of Patients with Osteoarthritis

Lynn H. Gerber, M. D.
Jeanne E. Hicks, M. D.

The dual purpose of this chapter is to introduce the readers, all those interested in the patient with osteoarthritis (OA), to the discipline of rehabilitation medicine and its methodology as it applies to patients with OA and to outline those treatments the rehabilitation team traditionally uses to help patients maximize their potential for function.

Rehabilitation medicine is that specialty that assists a patient in reaching his maximum potential for function—physically, psychologically, and vocationally. The rehabilitation effort is a composite of input from several disciplines, including rehabilitation medicine, occupational therapy, physical therapy, vocational counseling, social work, and the medical subspecialties of orthopedics and neurology. The rehabilitation team member who is called upon to assist a patient in reaching his goals must initially perform an evaluation that is comprehensive and that can be individually tailored to the needs of the patient with arthritis. This approach must include an assessment of the relationship of the biomechanical deficits as they relate to joint function, as well as the impact of the disease and disability on the patient's independence, self-image, family and job status, and sexual functioning.

Factors pertinent to the patient with osteoarthritis that need to be considered are the stage and extent of the arthritis; the specific joints involved; the influence of the biomechanical alterations on the involved joints and contiguous ones; the pain threshold of the patient; whether the pain is due to the altered biomechanics or inflammation; the current medications used for the osteoarthritic process (i.e., [a] anti-inflammatory agents and [b] pain medication); the patient's life style and how it is altered by the OA; the extent of the patient's understanding of the natural history of OA, and, finally, the patient's medical problems and how they may affect the rehabilitation process.

Rehabilitation intervention addresses three stage-specific issues in the patient with arthritis: prevention, restoration, and maintenance. When the effort of the rehabilitation team is to prevent dysfunction, treatment begins before the development of a disability, and the goal is to lessen the severity of the disability or to shorten its duration. When prevention is not possible, treatments may be designed to restore function, and the goal is to help the patient achieve a significantly better functional level. A treatment plan designed to maintain a particular level of function assumes that the patient will be left with a handicap, perhaps a progressive one, and has as its goal an increase in comfort and a decrease in complications. Despite a well-designed plan, not all patients are able to accept treatment, even though there is an apparent need. Accommodation to the patient's idiosyncrasies on the part of the health care provider is essential; a compromise plan is often better than total rejection of an ideal plan.

Using the aforementioned factors that are

to be considered in evaluating the patient with arthritis, the general types of intervention offered by rehabilitation, and the individual patient's needs, short- and long-term goals can be set. The first goal is to control pain, both acute and chronic. Pain can have adverse effects on motor function by fostering decreased muscle activity, muscle atrophy, and osteopenia, which is often due to decreased muscle tension on bone, decreased joint range of motion, interruption of sleep (e.g., in the fibrositis syndrome), and psychologic stress.

Another major goal is to maintain strength and range of motion and thus preserve functional level and prevent further pain, weakness, and disability. A third goal is energy conservation, which is taught to the patient in order to maximize function and to avoid fatigue of muscle. When muscle becomes fatigued, the joint is improperly supported, and as a result, increasing joint destruction may occur. The fourth goal is to provide supportive measures, either adaptive equipment or some substitutive function to compensate for a lost function on the part of the patient. The rehabilitation professional must prescribe appropriate treatment. Frequently, local measures are used for local problems, when possible, incorporating the use of modalities of heat and cold, orthoses or splints, and adaptive devices.

The fifth goal is to arm the patient with enough information as well as certain behavioral adaptive strategies for coping with his functional level or disability. A good educational program is essential to help the patient adapt or cope with his illness. The purpose of this educational program is to encourage behavioral changes to effect a higher level of independence and satisfaction. The substantive information should be designed to educate the patient about the natural history of the disease and about what resources are available for developing a successful coping strategy.

Although there are really no "hard" data to support the hypothesis that good comprehensive rehabilitation prevents disease progression or deformity, it is hoped that a comprehensive patient management program will promote maximal function and pain control.

PATIENT ASSESSMENTS USED IN REHABILITATION

Evaluation tools used in rehabilitation are designed to answer questions about how much pain and how much change in strength and range of motion the patient has endured, how much financial and emotional impact the arthritic condition has had on the patient, and how the patient is managing his daily activities. The measurements used attempt to be comprehensive, easy to perform, reproducible, informative, and useful in assessing the outcome of treatment. Although effort is focused on the musculoskeletal system, it is the juxtaposition of musculoskeletal performance with the patient's overall function in all aspects of life that is of greatest concern to the rehabilitation team.

Goniometry. Joint movement, called range of motion (ROM), is the standard assessment used to evaluate deformity. Several techniques are currently used to measure the range of motion of peripheral joints, in which well-established notation is described.[1, 2] These techniques are also used for measurement of the range of motion of the axial skeleton.[3, 4]

Muscle Strength Testing. A manual muscle test (MMT) is frequently performed in addition to a joint ROM assessment in the patient with arthritis. This test, which is standardized and quite reliable when done by a trained health professional, identifies weak muscles. In the face of a contracted muscle, or a painful one, strength grades are not very reliable. In most instances, the manual muscle test is performed with the patient trying to overcome the therapist's resistance to the muscle pull. It does not provide a good picture of the patient's "stamina" or ability to perform repetitive or sustained contractions; hence it is not a very good indicator of why a patient "fatigues."

Activities of Daily Living (ADL) Measurements. A number of tests currently in use measure activities of daily living. Some were developed especially for patients with arthritis[5-7]; some have been adapted from general assessments.[8] They do include questions about use of adaptive equipment. The purpose of these tests is to determine how independent the person is in several categories: toileting, grooming, dressing, mobility, and feeding.

Biomechanical Assessments. Recently, with the advent of computers and high-speed video cameras, more quantitative biomechanical measurements of motion have become available. These have provided data on internal joint forces and their relationships to specific activities[9] (such as walking versus jumping) and on the significance of stride length and the impact of the various kinds of ground surfaces one walks or jumps on.[10] Further application of these techniques includes more precise goniometric measurement, which can capture motion on video at more than 100 frames per second. Such analysis can help the physician to determine how much torque or undue flexion or extension there is around a joint during certain movements. Eventually, these observations may lead to clinical management decisions, for it has long been known that the position of a joint during exercise or motion can influence joint compressive force[11]; this compressive force is related to joint stress, which may be causative in abrasion and remodeling of the joint. Biomechanical assessments are not yet routinely available but are gaining wider acceptance because of their application to sports and their potential use in elucidating preventive measures in joint protection.

Psychosocial Measurements. The psychosocial impact of a chronic, often painful illness that can restrict mobility and function is measurable.[12] This is often a critical measurement because it helps identify individual needs of patients and may suggest certain interventions to help improve rehabilitation or adjustment to disease.

Part of this psychosocial evaluation includes several questions pertaining to adult behaviors that reflect self-esteem. This permits us to learn more about where the patient's strengths lie and how to utilize them to achieve a better functional outcome. It identifies those areas in which the arthritis has had the greatest impact and where therapeutic intervention is needed. The areas of assessment include (1) vocational and/or educational activity; (2) recreational/sports activity; (3) interpersonal (family, social, sexual) activity; and (4) spiritual activity.[13]

Pain Assessment. Pain is a commonly reported symptom of patients with arthritis. Measurements of pain intensity are easily and reliably recorded on a visual analogue scale and can be added to the patient's record.[14]

Some investigators have tried to combine several of the aforementioned assessments into a more comprehensive one and have developed disease impact measurement scales.[15–17] Some of these evaluation tools can be used in a repetitive way to evaluate outcome. For example, one can follow change in range of motion, activities of daily living, or self-esteem as a method of determining the success of treatment. As the arthritis progresses or is successfully controlled, the goals and needs of patients may change. These should be reflected in a change in the treatment plan.

A typical rehabilitation reply format is presented in Table 17–1.

Table 17–1. REHABILITATION REPLY FORMAT

I. Biographical Data of Patient
   a. Age
   b. Sex
   c. Patient number
   d. Medical diagnosis
   e. Occupation
   f. Language
II. Medical/Rehabilitation Evaluation
   a. History of present illness, including
     1. Reason for referral
     2. Medications
     3. Other related medical problems
   b. Physical findings related to history of present illness, with inclusion of
     1. Pain assessment
     2. Musculoskeletal and neurologic examination
     3. Gait
     4. Statement about psychologic or cortical function and communication skills
   c. Current functional level and goals
III. Assessment
   a. Key problems(s)—impact on patient's function
   b. Statement of patient's needs and understanding of the impact of the disease on function
IV. Treatment, to Include Outline of Modalities and
   a. Referrals: OT_____, PT_____, Speech_____, Other_____
   b. Education
   c. Precautions
   d. Discharge plan

BIOMECHANICAL PRINCIPLES USED IN REHABILITATION

Implicit in the minds of many physicians and orthopedists is that disability results from impairment. An analysis of the impairment, which incorporates the role of mechanical alteration, may suggest treatments that are more likely to be effective in relieving pain, maximizing function, and minimizing deformity. Activities of daily living often have an impact on impaired joints in ways that may favor disability. Intervention based on data collected from the measurements described earlier may alter the natural history of the disease by changing ways of performing routine or automatic tasks.

We will first discuss the natural history of the deformities and the biomechanical alterations frequently encountered in joints affected by osteoarthritis. (More detail on this subject is presented in Chapter 5.) Although we are not entirely certain of what the initiating events are in osteoarthritis, the end results are often joint space destruction, pain, deformity, and disability. Because we do not know all the variables that predict which patients are at greatest risk for developing severe changes and disability, we utilize the notion of a predictable sequence of events in which intervention can be placed on a rational basis at any point.

Pain is frequently the first reported symptom and is often associated with swelling. In response to this pain, muscles go into spasm, often creating a deforming force. Two events that potentiate osteoarthritic changes are increased load or compressive force on the joint and decreased congruency of the joint, functionally decreasing the articulating surface. The rationale behind this was elegantly demonstrated in Maquet and Pelzer's studies on the knee, in which stress across the joint was reduced by decreasing the force transmitted, distributing the weight over a larger articular surface (i.e., increasing congruency), and reducing any varus or valgus deformity.[18] In other words, reduction of articular pressure and improvement of joint congruity are desirable goals to preserve and protect joints.

It is known that relaxation of muscles about a joint can reduce joint pressure.[19] Conversely, muscles that go into spasm or are severely contracted can increase joint pressure and alter kinematics. When muscle spasm, contracture, or range of motion abnormalities are found, a treatment plan should be formulated to reduce or eliminate them.

Muscles perform an important protective function for joints by maintaining normal alignment. They serve as excellent shock absorbers when they function normally, and they can lengthen under tension.[20] In fact, they are very important in protecting the joint during unexpected impulsive loading.[21] It is this kind of loading that poses a serious threat to joint integrity and may be relevant to the pathogenesis of OA.[22] Preservation of muscle strength may protect joint alignment.

General treatment plans should include methods of reducing pain, preventing and reducing contractures, preserving and restoring range of motion and muscle strength, and reducing joint loads.

Biomechanics as It Applies to the Rehabilitation of Specific Joints

Specific joints that appear to be at risk for developing OA in order of decreasing frequency are the knees, first metatarsophalangeal joints (MTP), distal interphalangeal joints (DIP), carpometacarpal joints (CMC), hips, shoulders, cervical spine, and lumbar spine.

When general treatment principles apply (as listed previously), some issues pertain to specific anatomic loci.

The foot is a common site for OA. Although the metatarsophalangeal joint is most commonly affected, subtalar joints are often involved. A problem of alignment in the foot can be translated to other joints. For example, if the ankle is internally rotated, there is increased stress in the proximal and distal joints; the lateral compartment of the knee is affected, and the fifth metatarsophalangeal joint bears a greater load. There may even be increased external rotation at the hip in order to compensate for the internal rotation at the tibia. Conversely, if the tibia is externally rotated, the first metatarsophalangeal joint and the medial compartment of the knee will receive increased stress. Because the knee and the first metatarsophalangeal joint are at high risk for developing OA and in fact are frequently the sites of presenting symptoms, careful attention to the ankle and attempts to return it to the neutral position for both preventive and restorative care are appropriate.[23]

Adaptations for shoes often alter the mechanics of walking. For example a low, beveled, or cowboy-style heel will decrease the amount of torque at the knee.[24] This may be useful for a patient with arthritis who is suffering from knee pain. On occasion the amount of valgus or varus deformity of the knee can be reduced using a medial or lateral wedge and a flare of the sole of the shoe.[25]

Pain and deformity in the carpometacarpal joint are often seen in OA. Evidence for normal daily activities possibly producing deforming forces in the hand came from investigations by Linscheid.[26] He demonstrated that a 2-kg force applied at the tips of the first and second digits produced six to nine times the force at the carpometacarpal joint. The occupational therapist can recommend techniques to decrease the pinch force at the finger tips in order to decrease the deforming force at the carpometacarpal joint.

A painful hip is a common complaint of the patient with osteoarthritis. This pain may be lessened with removal of weight bearing from the extremity. The most effective way to do this is to use two crutches with partial weight-bearing or toetouching of the affected extremity. This not only distributes the weight to the upper extremities but also reduces the muscle action across the joint, further unloading the hip.

GENERAL INFORMATION ABOUT REHABILITATION TREATMENT

General rehabilitation goals in treating patients with osteoarthritis are (1) to increase function (restorative goal); (2) to maintain current function (maintenance goal); and (3) to prevent dysfunction or preserve normal function (preventive goal).

There are many modalities, adaptive devices, orthoses, exercises, environmental changes, and educational plans that may be therapeutically employed to accomplish both general goals and more specific goals. Specific goals include (1) relief of pain; (2) maintenance of strength and range of motion; (3) preservation of energy; (4) provision of supportive measures; and (5) facilitation of coping with a change in functional status. It is important to reiterate that the effective use of any one treatment method or any combination of methods depends on a thorough analysis of the patient's osteoarthritic problem and the formulation of an individualized comprehensive rehabilitation treatment plan for that particular patient. This plan must be formulated and agreed upon by the patient and the rehabilitation treatment team and should be reasonable and attainable.

Establishing an appropriate program and putting it into action therefore depends on first identifying the main type of rehabilitation goal for which the patient will be striving (i.e., preventive, maintenance, or restorative). In general, patients with restorative goals make the greatest functional gains in a rehabilitation program.

To organize the program, the physician must have sufficient knowledge in three areas: (1) the major factors for consideration regarding the patient's OA (as discussed previously); (2) a specific and practical design to insure success of the program; and (3) a specific treatment armamentarium of modalities, orthoses, aids, and patient education plans and the knowledge of how to apply these to alleviate the particular patient's problem.

The program should be performed at the best time of day for the patient, when pain and stiffness are at the lowest level and when he is not too tired to perform. An analgesic or another modality (e.g., hot packs, or ultrasound) should be used before initiating exercise or gait training, because this may alleviate the patient's pain and allow him to participate more fully in the program.

The patient's tolerance for pain should be assessed, because patients have different levels of tolerance for pain. A therapy program should work within a comfortable range. Patients can accept stretching, range of motion exercises, strengthening exercises, and gait training to a varied degree depending on the severity of pain, their tolerance for it, and their general medical condition. This can be determined by trial and error and by asking the patient to assign a number to quantitate his pain level.

The use of a comfortable position for the patient during treatment is essential. This should be determined, and the range of motion and exercise program should be performed in this position, if possible (e.g., lying down to eliminate gravity or in water for the buoyancy effect). It may be more effective to use a few short sessions rather than one prolonged session to remain within the patient's pain tolerance level and to avoid undue fatigue.

The patient is central in planning the program and is the most important member of the rehabilitation team. He must assist in the goal setting, agree that the goals are realistic, and be motivated to accomplish them.

Informal education should be incorporated with each treatment session. This makes the patient aware of the problems caused by the disease, the outcome of the disease, and the goals of and reasons for treatment. The education process will reassure him, give him confidence, and maximize compliance.

SPECIFIC TREATMENTS OFFERED IN REHABILITATION

The treatment armamentarium used in rehabilitation includes heat, cold, sound, electricity, orthoses, adaptive aids and devices, appropriate exercises, environmental design, and education.

Heat Modalities

Therapeutic heat can be applied using a number of devices and techniques. One must keep in mind the goals of the treatment and choose between vigorous deep heat and gentle superficial heat. Thus, the location, surface area, and depth of the tissue to be treated must be considered in selecting the type of heat therapy.

Superficial Heat. Superficial heat has long been useful in the treatment of musculoskeletal and articular disorders. The following facts are known about it:

The threshold for pain can be raised in man and animals with the application of superficial and deep heat.[27] It produces sedation and analgesia by acting on free nerve endings (both peripheral nerves and gamma fibers of muscle spindles).[28]

The skin penetration of superficial (infrared) heat is rarely more than a few millimeters in depth, so that penetration of heat into the joint is not accomplished.[29]

Heat may effect a change in superficial and intra-articular circulation. Increased intra-articular circulation in osteoarthritis and decreased circulation in rheumatoid arthritis have been reported.[30] The demonstrable increases in peripheral circulation have been used as objective measures of the effect of superficial heating, but their relevance to pain and muscle relaxation has not been determined scientifically.[31]

The application of superficial heat (37°C [98°F]) to extensive areas of body surface can cause an increase in the core body temperature, as well as peripheral vasodilatory effects.[32]

Gentle superficial heat may be produced by various methods (Table 17–2).

Moist heat has been reported to elevate subcutaneous temperature more than dry heat. The general impression is that moist heat is preferable for relieving articular pain, but the significance of this in terms of the mechanism of pain relief or alteration of inflammatory processes in joint disease has not been determined.[33] In the presence of inflammatory articular disease, moist heat is generally more comforting than dry heat, regardless of the mode of application (hot pack or hydrotherapy treatment in a tub, shower, or pool). Both dry and moist heating measures can produce skin temperatures above 44°C (111°F), so that care must be taken to avoid burns (particularly with uneven application over bony prominences).[34]

Hot paraffin wax mixed with mineral oil at temperatures of 47.5° to 52°C (118° to 126°F) can be applied by dipping the hand in a paraffin bath.

The Hubbard tank is a form of hydrotherapy, which is external application of water for therapeutic purposes. This has long been used for treatment of rheumatic conditions. It can provide (1) a generalized form of heat and (2) a generalized form of cooling. Therefore, all the benefits that are derived from heat or cryotherapy accrue. In addition, the buoyancy of water is most useful when minimal stress on joints is desired during range of motion exercises. It can be used when one wishes to resist or assist range of motion. When a patient has muscle weakness caused by myopathy or pain, motion in air is either too difficult or too painful. A whirlpool Hubbard tank or swimming pool can be used for exercise in these cases.

Deep Heat. Deep heat is also useful in treating painful musculoskeletal disorders. It affects the viscoelastic properties of collagen. As tension is applied, stretch is effected, and an increase of the "creep" (the plastic stretch of ligamentous structures placed under tension) occurs.[35] Heat may enhance the efficacy of stretching if applied after its use.

Diathermy (heating through) is effected by the use of short-wave (11.0 meters at 27.33 Hz) or microwave (12.2 cm at 2456 Hz) electromagnetic irradiations or by the conversion to heat of high-frequency sound waves (approximately 1.0 Hz) in body tissues.[36]

Short waves, microwaves, and ultrasound deliver deep heat.

Ultrasound. The depth of penetration of ultrasound is greater than that of shortwave or microwave diathermy. Ultrasound is a well-established deep-heating modality. There is much evidence to demonstrate its ability to heat deep structures, and there is the suggestion that it may have specific application.[37] Only ultrasound can raise the intra-articular temperature of the hip joint.[38] Although not entirely substantiated by a definitive study, ultrasound is used by most clinicians in preference to other types of diathermy in painful periarticular conditions.

Typical energy exposures are 0.5 to 4.0 watts/cm^2 for 5 to 10 minutes. The machine should be adjusted to initially produce a pain-

Table 17–2. METHODS OF HEAT APPLICATION

Conduction (S)	Radiation (S)	Convection (S)	Diathermy (D)
Hubbard tank	Infrared	Sauna	Short waves
Heating pad		Steam room	Microwaves
Water bottle			Ultrasound
Hydrocollator			
Paraffin			Enhances
Decreases pain, stiffness, muscle spasm →			← stretch
Precautions: impaired circulation, sensation			

S = superficial heat
D = deep heat

ful sensation and then adjusted for lower intensity. Clinically, some patients report an exacerbation of pain after ultrasound therapy rather than relief. In the latter situation, lower-energy exposure (≤ 1 watt/cm^2) may be tried.

Ultrasound should be used only in areas of normal sensation. It is reflected rather than concentrated by metal and can be used in the presence of a metallic implant. Ultrasound requires the use of a coupling agent (water or mineral oil) to prevent damping of sound waves in the air.[39] The therapist must keep the ultrasound applicator in constant motion to decrease excess focal heating. Deep heat is contraindicated in patients with local malignancy, those with a bleeding diathesis,[40] and postlaminectomy patients.[39]

The risk of thermal injury with any heat modality is increased with poor circulation, sedation, or sensory impairment. This is particularly true with use of diathermy.[41]

Cold Modalities

Cold is used to decrease pain and may be delivered by ice packs, ice massage, and local spray. Applications of cold decrease skin temperature and muscle temperature, which in the past were considered to be aggravating factors in arthritis and musculoskeletal disease.[42]

Superficial cooling decreases muscle spasm and spasticity,[43] and it has been demonstrated to decrease muscle spindle activity and to raise the threshold of pain.[44] The use of vapo-coolant sprays over areas of painful muscle trigger points has been highly successful.[45] Fluorimethane, which is nonflammable, is preferred over flammable ethyl chloride.[46]

Cold should not be used in patients with Raynaud's phenomenon, cold hypersensitivity, cryoglobulinemia, or paroxysmal cold hemoglobinuria.[47] The abrupt application of cold causes discomfort and produces a stressful response.

In summary, the efficacy of specific superficial heating measures and cooling measures (e.g., ice pack, ice massage) in terms of relief of pain or reduction of inflammation in either rheumatoid arthritis or osteoarthritis has not been fully established.[48] Therefore, decisions about the use of superficial heat or cold for pain relief must be made arbitrarily. Such decisions are based on empirical observations that the pain of acute inflammatory and traumatic disorders is best relieved by cold compresses, whereas subacute to chronic inflammation is best relieved by superficial heat.[49]

On the other hand, deep heat delivered by ultrasound and selectively absorbed by bone is widely accepted for heating joints and periarticular structures.

Other Modalities and Combinations

Electrical stimulation of muscle itself is possible. Muscle spasm around painful joints may be relaxed after intermittent electrically induced contractions.[50] Although no controlled studies have been done to validate this, anecdotal reports indicate there may be decreased pain and muscle spasm.[50] The Microdyne machine employs electrical stimulation and may be used with the joint immersed in water. Clinically, it seems to be effective in decreasing periarticular tissue swelling (particularly of the knees and ankles), pain, and muscle spasm. The Medcosonlator is a machine that combines the use of electrical stimulation and ultrasound.

Transcutaneous Electrical Nerve Stimulation (TENS). The gate control theory provided a rational basis for the use of transcutaneous nerve stimulation techniques for the relief of pain.[51, 52] Essentially, TENS is designed to preferentially stimulate large-diameter cutaneous fibers in an effort to inhibit transmission of painful stimuli to the spinal cord. It is simple, effective in some patients, and safe to use, but it is also expensive.

Acupuncture. This technique has been used for pain relief and as a form of anesthesia and has been applied to manage pain in the patient with arthritis.[53, 54] Its value over placebo for pain relief has been suggested but not clearly established.[55]

Auricular Stimulation. In auricular stimulation, electrical stimulation is used at acupuncture points of the ear. It may effect relief of pain in some individuals. Clinically, it is used for headache and cervical pain.[56]

REHABILITATION TECHNIQUES

Traction

Traction may be utilized to (1) relieve pain; (2) decrease flexion contractures of the arthritic knee and hip[57–59]; and (3) relieve pressure on a compressed nerve root. Great force in excess of that used clinically would be needed to increase vertebral spaces.

Traction has long been used to provide pain relief in cervical disk disease and the resultant radiculopathy. It may be applied in various positions and with different techniques.[60–63] A common method, as described by Swezey,[33] is accomplished with the patient seated. A halter is fitted under the chin and occiput, with the neck in 20 degrees of flexion; the halter is attached to a spreader bar suspended by a rope from an extension arm fitted at the top of a closet door. The traction force is 15 to 25 lbs and maintained for 5 minutes twice daily. Home traction is less desirable than standard traction. Lumbosacral traction has been similarly utilized to decrease pain in patients with discogenic disease.

Massage

Massage is frequently used to relieve pain, stiffness, and spasm and can be delivered by three different techniques: (1) Stroking (effleurage) is used for deep muscle relaxation and produces a soothing effect. (2) In compression (pétrissage), tissues are kneaded to effect muscle relaxation, to mobilize edema, and to stretch adhesions. (3) Percussion (tapotement) can be used in an isolated manner but is time-consuming. The most commonly used techniques, the first and second ones, may be used after application of heat or cold to augment their effects on muscle relaxation and to decrease pain prior to stretching or strengthening exercises.

Injections

Local injections of lidocaine and steroid may be used to relieve pain; injections are done at muscle trigger points or joints. Although some studies have suggested that adding a steroid does not increase efficacy,[64–66] the completeness and duration of response are generally felt to be superior with their use. The use of lidocaine and steroid intra-articularly or in periarticular or myofascial syndromes is well accepted (see Chapter 19). A trial of up to 2 to 3 treatments over a period of 3 to 6 weeks may at times be justified in the face of partial relief or increasing periods of temporary relief.[33]

Exercise

Exercise is used to increase strength, stamina, or range of motion.

There are three different types of muscle contraction, each with a different outcome. *Static or isometric contraction* produces minimal shortening; no joint motion is involved, although maximal tension is generated. This is the type of exercise most frequently prescribed for patients with arthritis.

Isotonic or dynamic contraction may be shortening (concentric) or lengthening (eccentric). Joint motion occurs. It is most suited for patients without inflamed joints because it stresses the joint through its range.

Isokinetic (dynamic) contraction occurs when maximum torque can be developed against a pre-set rate-limiting device. It has very limited use in rheumatic diseases. All of these types of contraction of muscle may facilitate and increase muscle strength and endurance.

There are different general types of exercise: (1) In passive exercise, the muscle is moved by the therapist or an apparatus. There is no active contraction by the patient. (2) Active or active assisted exercise is performed by active contraction of muscle by the patient or with assistance from the therapist. (3) Resistive exercise is accomplished by the active contraction of muscle by the patient against resistance (mechanical or manual). (4) Stretching exercise is performed by active or passive forceful movement.

Stretching Exercises. In general, stretching exercises may be used to prevent contracture, maintain range of motion, or restore range of motion (increase range of motion) by the breaking of capsular adhesions. Exercises must be graded according to the degree of inflammation, the pain present, and the pain tolerance of the patient.

Passive stretching exercises to preserve or increase range of motion should be used particularly in patients with acute inflammation or with mechanical joint derangement in which active exercise should be avoided.[57] Passive range of motion exercises without stretching are used to maintain optimal functional position, decrease edema, stimulate flexion-extension reflexes, and prepare the limb for active exercise(s).

Active assisted stretching can be used to maintain or increase range of motion when the patient's condition is subacute and pain is decreased. The patient may initiate muscle contraction and the therapist or an assistive device aids him. Active stretching is used in the absence of pain or inflammation to maintain range of motion.

Strengthening Exercises. Often, exercise is designed to strengthen muscles. Muscle bulk and strength do not always correlate. A muscle can increase in strength with or without evidence of hypertrophy.[67, 68] High-resistance exercises (e.g., weight lifting) cause white fiber hypertrophy and increase muscle bulk; low-resistance exercises or repetitive endurance exercises (e.g., long-distance running) do not appreciably increase muscle bulk.[69, 70] More important, a muscle strengthened by a specific technique utilizing a specific movement against resistance (isotonic-isokinetic) or static resistance in a fixed position (isometric) will give a maximum response if tested in the precise condition in which it has been trained.[71, 72]

In arthritis, the loss of strength and function in those muscles associated with an arthritic joint occurs often.[73] A muscle can atrophy up to 30% in 1 week.[74] A muscle at complete rest will lose function at a rate of 3% a day.[75]

Forceful muscular contractions increase intra-articular pressures, and repeated forceful contractions have been associated with juxta-articular bone destruction in rheumatoid arthritis.[76] Strengthening exercises that employ repetitive joint motion or that require moving the joint through a full range of motion may increase inflammation and pain and, because of the pain, are unlikely to effect an increase in strength. Thus, isometric (static) exercise is less traumatic. Dynamic (repetitive) exercises are appropriate after articular pain is controlled. These exercises produce general conditioning and enhance endurance in specific muscle groups and often lead to an increase in functional level.[77]

Active resistive exercise often causes an exacerbation of inflammation and therefore increases pain and secondarily decreases range of motion. Resistance given through range increases the strain on periarticular structures and also increases intra-articular pressures, joint temperature,[78] and blood flow. Therefore, such exercises are not recommended for arthritis.

Indications of excess exercise are (1) postexercise pain at 2 or more hours; (2) undue fatigue; (3) increased weakness; (4) decreased range of motion; and (5) joint swelling.

Endurance is the ability of a muscle to continue a particular static or dynamic task.[34] There is controversy as to the extent to which muscle endurance is related to muscle strength. For qualitatively dissimilar tasks, the best training is that task itself.

Management of Specific Joint Problems Seen in Osteoarthritis (Positioning, Stretching, Strengthening)

Hip. The goals of management are to preserve at least 20 to 30 degrees of hip flexion. Osteoarthritis of the hip can be associated with loss of motion in all planes.[33] The abductors and extensors of the hip can become weak, particularly in times of exacerbation of the OA. Hip effusion may cause inhibition of contraction of the gluteus medius.[79] These changes have an adverse affect on the gait cycle. The restrictive motion and the muscle weakness result in loss of function and ability for self-care.

Positioning. The patient should maintain proper hip extension by lying in the prone position for 30 to 40 minutes twice daily.[33] He should not sit with the hip in marked abduction.

Stretching Exercises. Passive stretching exercises to assist in range of motion in extension, flexion, abduction, internal rotation, and external rotation may be done in a pool if the patient has acute pain. Otherwise, exercises can be done on a firm meter board with powder to decrease friction and with use of a foot support that rolls on casters. Prolonged stretching of the hip flexors may be effected in the supine position with a pillow under the affected buttocks and a 10- to 20-lb weight supported by a sling from the knee.

Active stretching exercises to maintain range of motion may be accomplished in the supine position with the legs extended, as follows: (1) Bring the knee to the chest, grasp the front of the knee with the hands, and pull the knee to the chest, keeping the opposite knee extended. Repeat 5 to 10 times with alternate legs. (2) Abduct the extended leg as far away from the midline as possible and then return it to the midline. Repeat 5 to 10 times. (3) With the feet 10 inches apart, rotate the foot as far outward as possible and then inward 5 to 10 times. (4) Stretching may be done in a prone position. Raise the extended leg as high off the mat or floor as possible. Repeat 2 to 4 times daily, depending on the patient's tolerance and the stage of the arthritis. The most functionally important exercises for the hip are extension and abduction.

Strengthening. Isometric exercises can be done with an elastic belt, with emphasis placed on hip abductors and extensors.

Knee. Quadriceps wasting is an early occurrence in OA of the knee. The quadriceps muscle is the guardian of the knee. Quadricep wasting has often been associated with instability, valgus or varus deformity, and knee effusion. Increased volume in the knee joint caused by intra-articular injection has been shown to cause a temporary inhibition of the voluntary contraction of the quadriceps.[79] Active quadriceps contraction in the presence of effusion is inefficient, and wasting may ensue.[79]

In addition, pain and swelling of the knee may lead to restricted range of motion and therefore contractures of the joint capsule and hamstrings. Weakness of the quadriceps follows. If the knee cannot fully extend, it depends on the weakened quadriceps for stability. Therefore, increased mechanical stresses and further joint dysfunction result. Deep knee bends may increase intra-articular pressure and should be avoided.

Positioning. The patient should avoid the use of a pillow under the knee at night; this encourages knee and hip flexion contracture as well as plantar flexion at the ankle. In addition, venous obstruction in the popliteal area may lead to phlebothrombosis.

The most functionally important goal is to maintain extension. More than 10 degrees of flexion contracture results in less than optimal biomechanics. Joint congruity is also affected; hence, weight bearing may unduly stress the joint.

Stretching Exercises. When the patient has acute pain, exercises should be done under water. Active stretching may be accomplished with the patient in the supine position with the legs straight. The patient brings the knee to the chest and then grasps the knee with the hand and flexes it maximally. The exercise is repeated 5 to 10 times two to four times daily, as tolerated.

For strengthening, non–weight-bearing quadriceps exercises should be done daily by patients with OA of the knee. The knee is positioned in slight flexion to minimize pain; an elastic belt is looped over the ankle for resistance. A maximum contracture is held for 6 seconds twice daily.

Ankle and Foot. *Positioning.* A low-heeled shoe should be worn when walking, and loose bed sheets should be used at night to permit near-normal range of motion of the foot.

Stretching Exercises. Stretching exercises to maintain mobility involve active assisted stretching in the following planes of motion: ankle—dorsi/plantar flexion; tarsal bones—foot circling into inversion and eversion; toes—flexion and extension. Repeat 5 to 10 times two to four times daily.

Strengthening. Isometric strengthening for extrinsic foot muscles can be done by pushing or pulling the foot against a beach ball or a loop of an elastic belt for 6 seconds two times daily.[80] Active flexion and extension of the toes may be done on a towel, with the patient flexing and extending the toes to advance the towel toward him.

Neck. Decreased range of motion in the neck may be caused by osteoarthritic bony proliferation, most commonly at the C5–C6 level, or by muscle and ligamentous shortening. The most significant limitation is in extension and lateral rotation. The latter problem alone is amenable to stretching exercises. A simple procedure is for the patient to passively drop the chin on the chest and then rotate the chin first toward one shoulder, then the other, and retract the chin. This technique should be avoided in patients with subluxation or radiculopathy.

Positioning. A soft pillow (not foam) should be used, with the patient assuming a mild flexion position.

Strengthening. Cervical isometrics may be used to preserve or increase strength in patients with chronic neck pain or in patients who have been immobilized in a collar. The therapist turns the patient's head toward one side as far as can be tolerated, and holding both sides of the head, the therapist has the patient push the head against one hand for 6 seconds. Similar pushing against the hand is done with the forehead and occiput. This exercise can be done twice daily.

Lumbosacral Spine. Exercises of the lumbosacral spine should help restore or maintain back mobility and function and develop supporting musculature such as the abdominal muscles. They are done when pain is subsiding and not during the acute phase.

Pelvic tilting and knee-chest exercises stretch the lumbar and gluteal fascia and muscles and strengthen the gluteal and abdominal muscles. The patient lies in a supine position on the floor with the hips and knees flexed and the feet flat on the floor and presses the lower back flat onto the floor (contracting the abdominal and gluteal muscles). The pelvis is then rotated by raising the buttocks with the back remaining flat on the floor; the patient then proceeds with rhythmic pelvic elevation. The pelvic movement is repeated three to five times as a stretch and is held for 6 seconds on the final tilt as an isometric exercise; this utilizes passive back extension to tolerance.

Abdominal isometric exercises minimize intradiskal pressure and assist in pain relief.

They are necessary to maintain muscle tone in patients who wear a corset or brace. The patient lies in the supine position with the knees flexed and the feet flat and back flat. The neck is then flexed, and the arms are extended toward the toes. The position is held for 6 seconds and repeated twice daily.

Pelvic rotation exercises provide a pain-relieving stretch and are good for stretching tight hip external rotators; they are a good preparation for future vigorous activity. They are performed with the patient in the supine position with the knees bent and the feet flat; a foot is placed on the opposite knee, and the knee is lowered. This is repeated five times daily on each side.

Hand. The carpometacarpal joint is a common site of involvement and may be the most symptomatic joint. Radial subluxation and squaring off at the base of the first metacarpal are seen. Pain ensues with repetitive use. In the distal interphalangeal joints, cartilage loss, osteophyte formation, and rupture of the distal attachment of the extensor mechanism may occur, allowing the profundus to pull the distal interphalangeal joints into flexion (mallet deformity).

Positioning. A plastic working splint that holds the thumb in a few degrees of adduction, allowing the pad of the second finger to touch the thumb without the base moving, relieves pain. A mallet deformity can be reduced with a splint to allow adequate pinch with the thumb.

Stretching. Mobilization by passive range of motion exercises at the carpometacarpal, proximal interphalangeal, and distal interphalangeal joints may be tried if long-standing contracture is not present.

Shoulder. Osteoarthritis of the glenohumeral joint is rare, occurring in only about 5% of patients with painful shoulder conditions.[81] When seen, it is usually the result of trauma. Soft tissue problems around this joint such as subacromial bursitis, supraspinatus tendinitis, and bicipital tendinitis occur often after 40 years of age.

Exercises. Stretching is needed because significant contracture can develop in a few weeks. After acute pain is relieved, passive or passive assisted range of motion exercises can be initiated. Exercises may be easier if the patient is in the supine position with the therapist supporting the limb and gravity assisting in flexion. Codman pendulum exercises can then be done. A reciprocal pulley may be used to stretch the shoulder beyond 90 degrees.

Strengthening. Isometric strengthening exercises are geared toward increasing strength in the abductors and internal and external rotators and may be accomplished utilizing a belt or a beach ball.

ORTHOSES AND ASSISTIVE DEVICES

Orthoses and assistive devices for patients with osteoarthritis should be prescribed after an assessment of the stage of their degenerative disease, the altered biomechanics of the joint, and the willingness of the patient to accept the device. In general, orthoses are used to (1) decrease pain by removal of weight bearing from the joint (in acute and chronic situations); (2) decrease motion around a painful joint (acute and chronic situations); (3) provide stability to an unstable joint (chronic situation); and (4) improve patterns of motion (acute and chronic situations). They are also used to achieve restorative or maintenance goals.

The orthotic or assistive device may be needed temporarily to relieve an acute problem (e.g., acute pain and swelling) that will abate in the future, or the orthosis may be a permanent device for a problem that is chronic.

Lower-Extremity Orthoses

The goals of casting or an orthosis for the lower extremity must incorporate the positions of the joints that provide maximum function.

Ankle. The ankle should be in neutral position or, at most, in 10 degrees of plantar flexion, and the subtalar position should allow the foot to be in neutral position and to make full contact with the floor.

A patellar tendon–bearing ankle-foot orthosis (Fig. 17–1) may be used to remove the weight bearing from an ankle with osteoarthritis.[82]

Forefoot. As a rule, a balanced foot will minimize the need for compensatory valgus or varus strain at the knee and external rotation at the hip. The role of the foot is critical to efficient walking. Foot abnormalities that alter the normal role in weight acceptance create imbalances that may produce hypermobility and create painful, inefficient, and, occasionally, unsafe gait patterns.

In the patient with OA, the foot is often uninvolved. When it is affected, the most commonly encountered conditions are hallux valgus, with or without bunion, hallux rigidus and

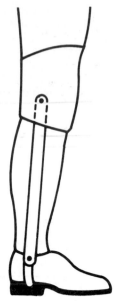

Figure 17–1. Patellar tendon–bearing ankle-foot orthosis. This appliance allows unweighting of the ankle involved with arthritic change.

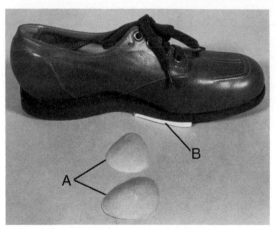

Figure 17–3. Metatarsal pads *(A)* and transverse metatarsal bar *(B)*. Metatarsal pads placed within the shoe or a transverse metatarsal bar affixed to the sole of the shoe allows protection of the metatarsophalangeal joints.

cock-up toes, and some metatarsal head calluses and abrasions on the dorsum of the toes.[83] The first step in management is proper shoe fitting. The forefoot must be wide enough to accommodate the degree of hallux valgus, and the toe-box must be deep enough to permit clearance of the phalanges (Fig. 17–2). As long as critical ankle motion is preserved, the arc of motion is 20 degrees of dorsi/plantar flexion, and the longitudinal arch is intact, the usual modification that needs to be made in the shoe itself in the patient with metatarsalgia is a cushioned sole (neoprene crepe), with a metatarsal pad or external metatarsal bar placed proximal to the metatarsal heads (Fig.

17–3). If there is a painful first metatarsophalangeal joint or hallux rigidus, sufficient mobility at the toe-off portion of the gait cycle may be lacking. Thus, the patient would benefit from a rocker sole or an inserted rocker surface to facilitate toe-off (Fig. 17–4).

Occasionally, shoe modifications may be used to relieve valgus or varus deformity at the knee or to alter the weight-bearing column so that the portion of the hip with the best preservation of cartilage (either medial or lateral) is shifted to do most of the weight bearing. These attempts to realign the whole weight-bearing column are only rarely successful. Some evidence suggests that high heels increase the intra-articular pressure on various joints of the lower extremity.

Leg-length discrepancies of more than 1 cm require leg-length equalization, both because this abnormality produces a compensatory sco-

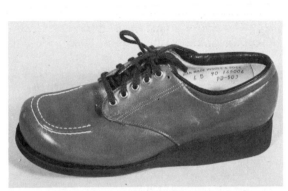

Figure 17–2. Wide toe-box shoe. The forefoot configuration should be wide enough to accommodate any hallux valgus present; the toe-box must also be deep enough to permit clearance of the phalanges.

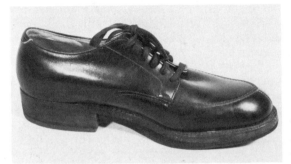

Figure 17–4. Shoe with a rocker sole. Use of a rocker sole or inserted rocker surface facilitates toe-off in patients with limited mobility of the toe joints.

liosis and because one hip may be stressed more than another. This has been called the long-leg syndrome and has been implicated in producing OA of the hip. An external lift of up to 1 cm can be added without having to add some height to the sole; an internal lift of up to 0.5 cm can be added without being concerned about lifting the foot out of the shoe.[83]

Knee. Bracing the knee for pain and instability may be necessary. A Swedish knee cage (Fig. 17–5) or a hinged knee brace (Fig. 17–6) provides some support in limiting extension and may help decrease pain.[84] A long leg brace with a single upright strut or a Lenox Hill brace provides greater medial-lateral stability and alignment of the knee.[85] An ankle-foot orthosis (plastic or metal Klenzak type) may control knee instability by creating either a flexion or extension moment at the knee when plantar flexion or dorsiflexion is blocked at the ankle.[86]

Immobilization of the knee is energy-inefficient and frequently promotes atrophy of the quadriceps, but sometimes it is the only choice short of surgery when there is great instability. Increased stability and normal weight bearing result in less pain and less compensatory joint reaction above and below the affected joint and permit muscles to function to their best mechanical advantage.

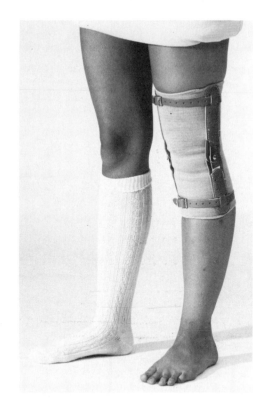

Figure 17–6. Hinged knee brace. Lateral support and limitation of extension may help limit instability and decrease pain.

The influence of heel design must be considered when prescribing braces. A solid ankle-cushioned heel (SACH) made with a medium-density polyurethane center or a beveled hard-rubber heel that makes a 20-degree angle with the floor reduces flexion torque at the knee—a finding of benefit to patients with knee instability.[25]

An elastic bandage may control soft tissue swelling but, strictly speaking, is not an orthosis. Immobilization of the knee acutely during periods of increased pain or inflammation may be useful. This may be done with a posterior splint, which supports the knee in extension, permits some relaxation of the flexor muscles, and promotes a gradual stretch. For a patient with flexion contracture at the knee, serial casting or wedging from the mid thigh to the malleolus may be done. Gains in knee extension are facilitated by either recasting or advancing a turn buckle 1 to 2 degrees daily or by wedging 1 to 2 degrees daily.[87] Only a gradual increase in knee extension must be attempted in order to prevent tearing of the skin or injury to the peroneal nerve.

Hip. No orthoses are used for hip problems.

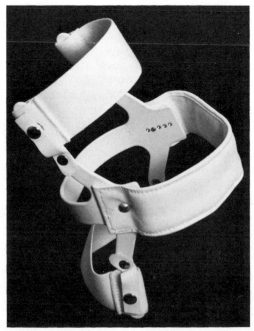

Figure 17–5. Swedish knee cage, which reduces knee pain and instability.

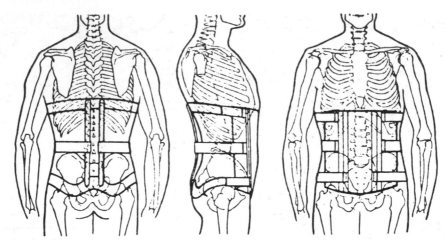

Figure 17–7. Lumbosacral corset. A three-point pressure system limits lordosis and assists abdominal musculature to increase intra-abdominal pressure.

A forearm crutch on the opposite side is used to remove weight bearing from the hip. A toe-touch gait is better than a swing-through gait.[88] Sometimes, two crutches are used, with partial weight bearing on the affected side.

Spine. Although they may potentiate osteoporosis, spinal orthoses may provide significant pain relief for those with pain in the lumbosacral and cervical areas.

Osteoarthritis of the spine is often asymptomatic. When it is symptomatic, this is often attributed to a specific action such as bending or transitional movement, such as getting out of a car, that exceeds the accustomed range of motion. Often, the problem occurs in the elderly in whom there is a reduction of spinal elasticity and motion and/or weakened abdominal musculature.

The orthosis or spinal brace is indicated for symptomatic back pain unresponsive to bed rest and analgesic or anti-inflammatory medication. A spinal brace can limit motion and bending loads by supporting the spine in a semi-erect position and by reinforcing weak muscles.[89] Occasionally, symptoms are attributable to chronic inflammation of the paraspinal soft tissue, the annulus, ligaments, muscles, or synovium of one or more facets. For problems with this etiology, if conservative measures fail, an orthosis may help rest inflamed tissue by immobilization and may reduce lordosis as well as unload the spine and reinforce abdominal muscles.[90]

The orthosis of choice for lumbosacral problems is a lumbosacral corset.[91] This is the most comfortable orthosis, and patient compliance with its use is best. This orthosis (Fig. 17–7) provides a three-point pressure system consisting of posteriorly directed forces from pelvic and thoracic straps and abdominal support and anteriorly directed forces from paraspinal bars and the pelvic and thoracic bands. This system limits lordosis and assists the abdominal musculature to increase intra-abdominal pressure. A lumbosacral cinch acts more like a girdle, providing support for the abdominal musculature without limiting movement.

When the problem is in the thoracic or thoracolumbar area, an orthosis that can restrict movement at that level is indicated. The motion that needs to be controlled is usually flexion-extension. The orthosis for such a condition is similar to the lumbosacral corset, with the addition of axillary straps and extension of the thoracic band. It provides a three-point pressure system with posteriorly directed forces from the axillary and chest straps, pelvic strap, and abdominal corset; anteriorly directed forces are from the posterior uprights at the thoracolumbar area, the pelvic band, and the interscapular bar. Adaptations of these orthoses are available for more or less anterior/posterior control and relief over bony contours. These are custom made by certified orthotists.

The indications for use of a spinal orthosis are for relief of pain, increased function, and stabilization and unloading of the spine. In general, osteoporosis and continued weakening of the abdominal musculature occur with use of orthoses and may even be accelerated. Therefore, activity and carefully prescribed abdominal muscle strengthening are to be encouraged to tolerance; an attempt to discontinue the use of the orthosis at the earliest possible time should be a goal of treatment.

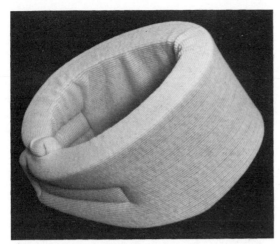

Figure 17–8. Soft cervical collar, which reduces pain related to neck motion and muscle spasm.

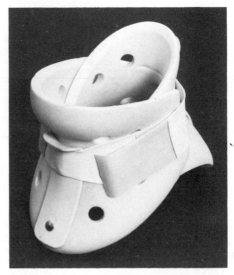

Figure 17–9. Philadelphia collar. This more rigid collar offers more support and limitation of extension for neck arthritis.

The initiation of progressively longer amounts of time out of the brace is one effective way of proceeding, using pain and function as indicators of positive response.

The cervical spine is frequently involved in osteoarthritis, with the C5–C6 level being most commonly affected. A soft cervical collar (Fig. 17–8) is useful in relieving pain, but limits hyperextension only minimally.[92] A Philadelphia collar offers more support and limitation of extension (Fig. 17–9).[93]

Upper-Extremity Orthoses

Upper-extremity orthoses are used when the goals are (1) to relieve pain by limiting joint motion; (2) to improve function or substitute for lost function; and (3) to offer support to joints and possibly slow the rate of deformity. Goals should incorporate principles of preserving positions that assure maximal function: metacarpophalangeal joint—30 to 40 degrees of flexion; proximal interphalangeal joint—35 degrees of flexion; thumb—interphalangeal joint: straight, metacarpophalangeal joint: 20 degrees of flexion and 40 degrees of abduction; wrist—neutral.

Hand. Hand resting splints support the entire hand and wrist but interfere with function. They are best used at night and periodically during the day to support affected joints. They are mainly used to limit contractures and to maintain a joint in a position of maximal function.

Functional wrist splints (Fig. 17–10) stop at the mid-palmar crease and permit phalangeal function; they are useful for wrist inflammation or instability. They prevent flexion at the wrist. A thumb post splint (Fig. 17–11) is useful in patients with a painful carpometacarpal joint. It immobilizes the thumb in a functional, abducted position. Ring splints (Fig. 17–12) are

Figure 17–10. Functional wrist splint. Splinting proximal to the mid-palmar crease permits phalangeal function. This splint is useful for patients with wrist inflammation or instability.

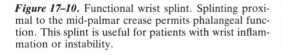
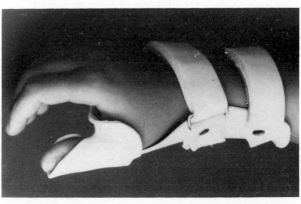

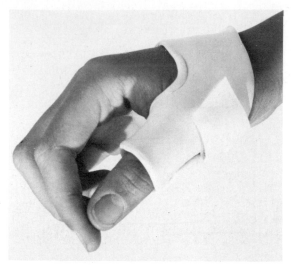

Figure 17–11. Thumb post splint. The thumb is mobilized in a functional, abducted position.

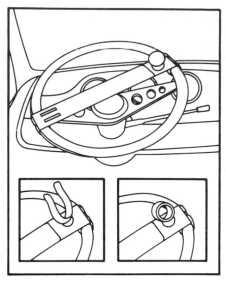

Figure 17–13. Spinner bar. This device, which is attached to the automobile steering wheel, is useful for patients with significant hand problems.

beneficial for severe osteoarthritis of the distal interphalangeal joints with mallet finger.

Adaptive Aids

Adaptive aids are devices that compensate for functional deficits, particularly where there is limited range of motion and pain in joints. They may also be used to overcome some architectural barriers.

Many assistive devices are available today. It is important for the physician to be aware of their existence, so that given the patient's

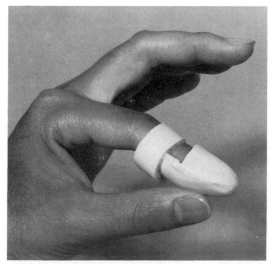

Figure 17–12. Ring splint for mallet finger. This appliance is useful for patients with severe osteoarthritis of the distal interphalangeal joint.

functional level, level of pain, and environmental design problems, he may supply him with the appropriate adaptive devices. The patient must, however, be ready to accept the aid or appliance. Mobility is one of the most important goals for patients with osteoarthritis; the car is the main source of mobility, and hence, the ability to get in and out of it is a critical function. Sliding boards, overhead straps, and automatic seat-height adjustments may help. Use of sideview and rearview mirrors is essential for patients with osteoarthritis of the cerivcal spine. A spinner bar (Fig. 17–13) for the steering wheel is a useful device when the patient has significant hand problems, and a car door opener (Fig. 17–14) and a key ignition piece (Fig. 17–15) are also helpful.

If the problem is ambulation, a gait aid may be needed. When prescribing a gait aid, it should be determined if the functional deficit is in strength, endurance, balance, or pain. If the functional deficit is in strength or endurance, a wheelchair may be needed. A small lightweight one is recommended; there are small motorized types, if necessary, such as the Amigo sporty-type chair (Fig. 17–16). If the problem is one of balance, a cane is usually prescribed first. For more severe problems, a walker may be needed. If balance problems are severe, a wheelchair will be required.

If the problem is joint pain secondary to loss of cartilage, effusion, or synovitis, it is best treated by unloading the joint in question. Weight reduction should also be encouraged

Figure 17–14. This car door opener is useful for patients with limited motion or weakness of grasp.

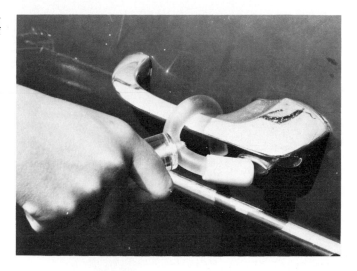

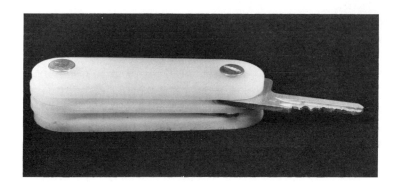

Figure 17–15. Key ignition piece. A built-up attachment allows easier handling and manipulation.

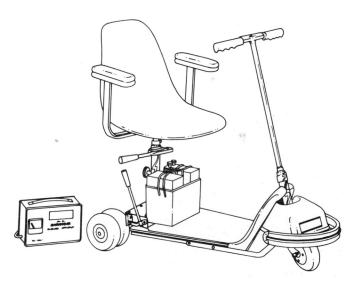

Figure 17–16. Amigo chair. This type of chair has the advantages of being lightweight and motorized for easy use.

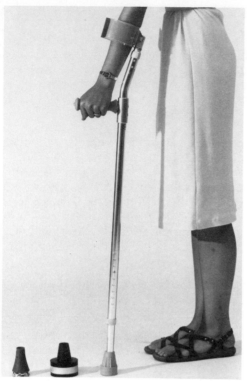

Figure 17–17. Forearm crutch. Crutches are usually utilized in the hand opposite the affected hip or knee. Stresses across the involved joint are considerably reduced.

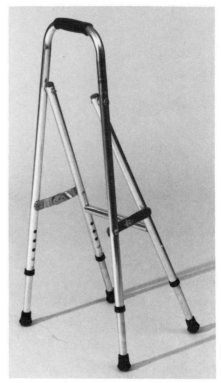

Figure 17–18. Quad cane. This cane is advantageous when balance is a problem in individual patients.

at the same time. A 1-kg weight loss effects a 3- to 4-kg decrease in load across the joint.[94]

Assistive devices to unload the hip or knee are most effectively used on the side opposite the pathologic condition. The use of a forearm or axillary crutch (Fig. 17–17) will reduce by one-half the amount of weight borne by the limb in question.[88] A straight cane is good for balance but is not nearly as efficient in unloading the limb as a crutch is. A quad cane (Fig. 17–18), like a straight cane, is used when balance is a problem.

In rheumatoid arthritis, it is critical that the grip is suited to the hand deformity; platform crutches or a walker is often used. Although this is less important in patients with osteoarthritis, a custom grip may be needed for some patients with severe first metacarpophalangeal, distal interphalangeal, and proximal interphalangeal joint involvement (Fig. 17–19).

Custom hand pieces can be made by making a mold of the patient's grip with the hand placed in a functional position of weight bearing.[95] Forearm rest attachments can be added to wheelchairs as an additional standing aid.[96] Because OA is usually chronic, a permanent and comfortable device should be chosen.

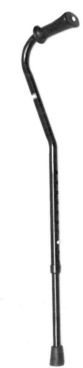

Figure 17–19. Lumex cane. A customized grip allows improved hand grasp for control of cane use.

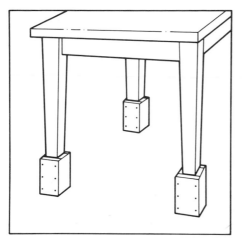

Figure 17–20. Chair blocks. Elevation of the level of the seat provides improved comfort and allows easier push-off to a standing position.

Adaptive Devices for Specific Areas of Transfer. In the patient with OA of the hip with chronic pain and limited motion, transfers from low-level chairs, toilets, and beds are difficult. The upper extremities may be needed for push-off. When there are upper-extremity problems (less common in OA) and lower-extremity muscle atrophy of hip and knee extensors, arising becomes impossible. Elevating the level of the seat to a comfortable height can grant comfort and independence. A 3- or 4-inch block (Fig. 17–20) can be placed under each leg of chairs, tables, and beds. Chairs with seats that can be elevated by motor can be purchased. A clip-on elevated seat can be mounted on the toilet (Fig. 17–21). A free-standing or clamp-on tub seat can make getting in and out of the bathtub easier (Fig. 17–22). Getting in and out of the car may be a significant problem because of a low seat or difficulty in grasping the door or steering wheel. An extra-thick seat cushion to raise the seat can be used, as can a mounted grab bar to increase leverage (Fig. 17–23).

Adaptive and self-care aids include long-handled reachers, shoehorns, elastic shoelaces, sponges, brushes, and toothbrushes (Fig. 17–24). Stirex scissors, button hooks, zipper hooks, toilet paper holders (when grip strength is weak) (Fig. 17–25), and large-handled items (Fig. 17–26) are all helpful devices. Clothing designed with elastic and Velcro may be superior to that with buttons and hooks for patients with OA.

ENVIRONMENTAL DESIGN

Proper adaptation of the environment to maximize function and conserve energy is important. Although elements of normal architectural and environmental design are not barriers to as great an extent in the patient with osteoarthritis as in the patient with rheumatoid arthritis, they should still be addressed with care.

As stated before, the main functional problems in the patient with OA are pain and

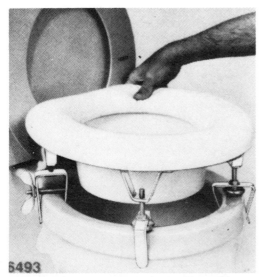

Figure 17–21. A clip-on elevated seat allows easier access to getting on and off the toilet.

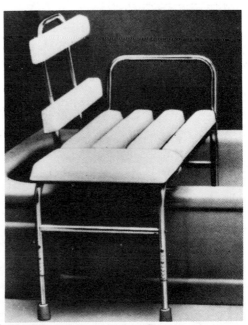

Figure 17–22. Tub seat. This appliance facilitates getting in and out of the bathtub.

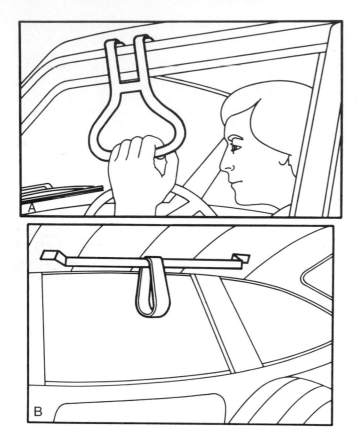

Figure 17–23. Car-mounted grab bars. Externally *(A)* and internally *(B)* mounted grab devices assist the patient in getting in and out of the car.

decreased mobility because of spine, hip and knee involvement. Some problems are encountered in the area of decreased hand function secondary to degeneration of the carpometacarpal joint and proximal and distal interphalangeal joints. The main architectural problems that arise are the following: (1) *Mobility-Ambulation.* Outdoors, going up and down steps, slopes, stairs with deep steps, and high curbs and getting in and out of buses or cars may be difficult to negotiate with OA of the hips and knees. Appropriate placement of

curbs that are dropped and the building of suitable inclines and ramps help. Indoors, thick carpets or certain other surfaces increase friction and are more difficult to walk on. In the bathroom, problems arise if the toilet seat is too low; those without guardrails may prove impossible to use. The bathtub should have nonskid strips or an entire nonskid surface. In the living area, getting in and out of low chairs may be very difficult for the patient with OA of the hip. Doorways should be wide enough to permit wheelchair access. Low cabinets are

Figure 17–24. Long-handled brushes and shoehorn are useful in activities of daily living.

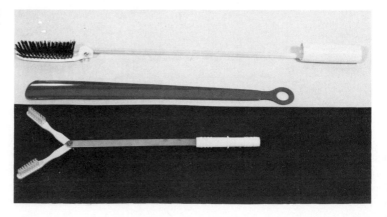

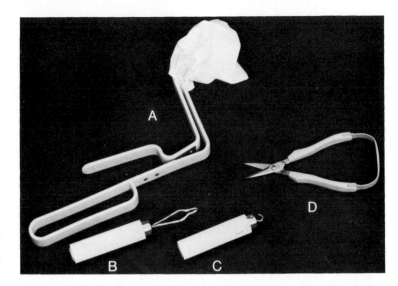

Figure 17–25. Toilet paper holder *(A)*, button hook *(B)*, zipper hook *(C)*, and Stirex scissors *(D)*. Assistive devices are of aid when hand function is compromised, and particularly when grip strength is weak.

often inaccessible, and high ones are difficult to reach; chest-high storage areas and work surfaces are best. (2) *Dexterity*. Opening regular doors or car doors may be difficult for the patient with OA of the carpometacarpal joint. Special door openers are available (Fig. 17–27). For those patients in wheelchairs, proper positioning of door knobs, light switches, and kitchen equipment is necessary. Large-handled items (e.g., pencils and forks) are helpful. Devices to help with the use of spray cans are also available (Fig. 17–28).

EDUCATION

The goals of patient education include reduction of anxiety, increase in cooperation with treatment, and a change in behavior, when appropriate, to assure a better functional outcome. Patient education in the area of osteoarthritis should include a discussion about the natural history of OA and the possible impact this might have on job and leisure activities. The information supplied to the patient should be relevant and cautiously optimistic.

Osteoarthritis is a chronic disease, and although it may affect different joints at various times and have different degrees of severity, there is usually some degree of chronic pain, stiffness, and limitation of motion and, therefore, limitation of function. The element of chronicity must be understood by the patient in a realistic manner. One can then proceed to methods that may (1) relieve pain, (2) preserve motion as much as possible, and (3) adjust the environment to accommodate for functional deficits.

A good liaison must exist between physician

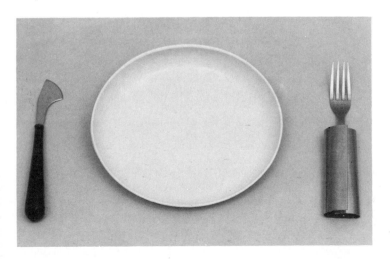

Figure 17–26. Large-handled eating utensils facilitate hand function when osteoarthritic involvement is severe.

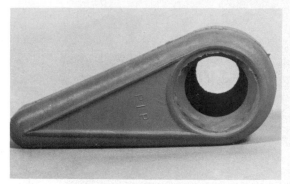

Figure 17–27. This special door opener is useful when hand function is painful or limited.

and patient in discussing these problems. The patient and family must be educated in the disease process itself, what the likely functional deficits will be, and what aids are available to help overcome these limitations. The physician can be of invaluable help if he recognizes the importance of this area, properly guides the patient through the adjustment to his illness and disability, makes the appropriate referrals (i.e., physiatry, physical therapy, occupational therapy, social work, vocational counseling), and helps solve the patient's disease-related problems.

Depending on the joints involved and the extent of involvement, there may be an impact

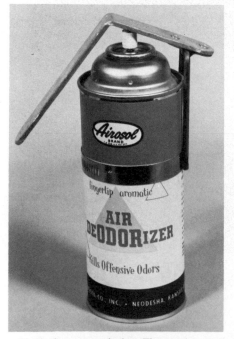

Figure 17–28. Spray can device. The special attachment allows more effective gross hand maneuvering.

of the disease on the life style or vocation of the patient. It is important for the physician to know the patient's general life style, the responsibilities of his work, his relationship to his family, and his premorbid sexual history. Chronic disease does not limit its impact to the patient alone but also affects his family, his work environment, and his psychosexual expression. Therefore, the physician must take a comprehensive approach to the patient in order to be able to assist him in his rehabilitation or adjustment to the chronic disease process.

In general, chronic OA may cause pain, limit mobility, and decrease self-image. These effects can lead to depression, marital discord, and difficulty in job situations. The physician must stress the importance of maintaining one's self-image and life style while utilizing all available means of assistance.

Specific Education

Education about joint function is best done using a simple but informative approach. The patient should be told about how particular joints work biomechanically and which forces alter their normal function. Pointing out a correlation between the stage of the disease and its relationship to function is often helpful.

Joint Protection

Elements in a program for joint protection in patients with OA include avoiding prolonged periods in the same position; minimizing stress on particular joints by promoting good posture; maintaining range of motion, strength, and good joint alignment; reducing pain; unloading the joint when it is very painful; avoiding overuse during acute periods of pain; using appropriate adaptive equipment and splints when necessary; and modifying tasks to decrease joint stress. By applying these concepts, external forces on affected joints can be minimized.[97]

Posture

Good body posture when sitting or standing balances the weight of the head and limbs on the bony framework so that the force of gravity helps maintain joint position. Significant deviation from the correct posture causes muscles to exert more energy to pull against the force of gravity. To perform an activity standing requires 25% more energy than performing the same activity sitting. Ideal posture cannot be maintained unless care is taken to preserve range of motion and strength of muscles around the joints.[97] Particular elements of proper positions for joints are discussed in the section on stretching and strengthening exercises.

Sexual Counseling

One area of major adjustment for the patient with OA is sexuality. Because problems in this area are not always clearly addressed, we wish to do so here.

A comprehensive rehabilitation evaluation should include inquiry into the sexual problems that arise as a result of physical disability. Sexual problems are common in arthritis. Assisting the patient to reachieve normal sexual function is part of a good rehabilitation plan.

Sexual problems in the patient with arthritis arise as a result of (1) mechanical problems associated with decreased range of motion, pain, and stiffness; (2) depression and resultant decreased self-image and interest; (3) drug therapy causing decreased libido; (4) psychosocial problems in the family unit related to the patient's arthritis; and (5) fatigue.

Because there is often more than one contributing factor to the sexual problems of the patient with arthritis,[98] all factors should be evaluated. This evaluation includes an assessment of the patient's mental status, self-image, mood, and current adjustment to his disability; problems existing in the family unit, including a good history from the spouse; and previous sexual history, in order to determine what changes have occurred. A physical examination and documentation of medications used may help to determine other factors influencing sexual activity.

Arthritic involvement of the hips, knees, and lumbar spine may cause mechanical problems that interfere with sexual performance. With regard to arthritis of the hips, 67% of all patients (males—46%; females—81%) with arthritis of the hips have some sexual disability related to their arthritis.[99] Swinburne[100] found that 75% of his patients with rheumatoid arthritis felt it interfered with their sexual life in some way. In both unilateral and bilateral hip disease characterized by pain and stiffness, analgesics and warm baths prior to intercourse

may be helpful. In women with more advanced disease, intercourse in the position with the man on top may become impossible. Intercourse may be achieved if a posterior approach is used by the man. With very severe limitation of motion, either unilateral or bilateral hip replacements may be a requisite for intercourse. After total hip replacement, intercourse should not be resumed at all for 6 weeks postoperatively, and marked hip flexion should be avoided.

Pain, stiffness, or limitation of motion of the knees should not mechanically limit intercourse, but a change in position may be required for more comfort. For patients with back pain, a lateral position for intercourse may be preferable for both the man and the woman. If both OA of the spine and hips exists in the woman, a lateral and posterior approach by the male may be best.

Problems in the joints of the hands and arms are more restrictive for the man than for the woman, and a side-lying position may alleviate this. In both the man and the woman, arthritis in these joints may interfere with the earlier stages of love-making that involve caressing and manual stimulation.

Often, patients with arthritis experience a decrease in self-image, a feeling of helplessness, and, ultimately, depression, which in turn is associated with decreased libido.[101] A comprehensive rehabilitation plan to increase the patient's general functional level, educate him about the disease, and give proper advice in sexual problems, thus greatly improving his self-image, may also increase his suppressed libido. In some cases, an antidepressant such as amitriptyline may be indicated.

Psychosocial Problems

The deformities caused by arthritis may cause decreased self-image. This in turn causes a loss in body image as perceived by both the patient and the spouse. Deformity of the hands is particularly distressing to the woman's body image.[100] Chronic pain may reduce a patient's efforts to make herself more attractive for her partner. The woman who has significant joint deformities is difficult to reassure that she is still physically attractive. The spouse may develop a pathologic fear and horror of the deformity that may be reflected in the marriage. There may also be resistance to making the necessary alterations in sexual techniques.

Chronic arthritis may cause the man to be

unemployed and lose his "head of the household" status, resulting in role-reversal stress. Financial problems may ensue, and ultimately, problems with depression and decreased libido may occur.

It is the physician's obligation to assist the patient in making the required adjustments to the sexual problems arising from disability; the physician should feel comfortable in doing so, making the patient feel at ease. This encourages honest and free communication between the patient and the physician. The physician should not wait for the patient to broach his or her problems in the area of sexuality—most of them would then not be addressed. In taking a holistic viewpoint, as outlined previously, the physician encourages the return of a positive self-image in the patient and fosters a better understanding of his or her disability; a great deal of undue stress that would otherwise potentiate the patient's disabilities is thereby eliminated. This approach can have a significant impact on the patient's acceptance by his or her spouse.

POSTOPERATIVE REHABILITATION

The specific techniques of rehabilitation in the postoperative management of patients who have undergone surgery for OA are not universally agreed upon. Each joint requires a different therapeutic regimen, and frequently, each surgeon practices his own method.[102–104] There is a consensus among orthopedic surgeons that patients who are active in a postoperative rehabilitation program will increase strength, motion, and knowledge about how to protect (and perhaps preserve) the operated joint. Although postoperative hip surgery programs vary, in general the patient is alerted to the potential problems of flexing more than 100 degrees and adducting and internally rotating the operated side. His sitting time is also limited just after surgery. A crutch is frequently used to protect the hip until the muscles (abductors) are strong.

The goals for postoperative management of the knee following arthroplasty or osteotomy are similar to those for postoperative management of the hip. They are to progress to independence in ambulation, to have as near normal a range of motion as possible and as near normal strength as possible, and to achieve independence in daily activity.

Both knee and hip management includes active or active assisted range of motion and isotonic exercises. Education includes full dis-

cussion of precautions, which vary from surgeon to surgeon but usually include some limitation of antigravity sports, including running, basketball, and tennis. A full discussion with the patient about when to alert the physician with respect to concerns about the replaced joint is important both for management of potential mechanical failure and for early recognition and treatment of complications.

Surgery on the foot for patients with OA usually includes treatment of bunion, hallux valgus, and hallux rigidus. The principles include achieving goals of maximal range of motion and comfort. Active assisted range of motion exercises and a splint are used for several weeks after the hallux valgus procedure.

Surgery on the upper extremity usually involves the carpometacarpal joint of the thumb, the proximal interphalangeal joints, and, occasionally, the shoulder. Range of motion exercises and an attempt to increase strength are undertaken by the rehabilitation team. The patient is cautioned about heavy manual labor, which may accelerate subluxation or disruption of the arthroplasty.

APPLICATION OF SPECIFIC INTERVENTIONS AS APPLIED TO THE PROBLEMS OF THE PATIENT WITH ARTHRITIS

In the previous sections, the focus has been on the assessment of problems affecting the patient with arthritis (i.e., pain and stiffness, weakness, loss of range of motion, and functional deficits) and the presentation of a compendium of treatments traditionally used to alleviate these problems. Specific recommendations for control of these difficulties frequently faced by the patient with OA will now be presented.

Specific Recommendations for Control of Pain

Pain is the most common and disabling problem experienced by patients with OA, especially when joints of the lower extremities are involved.[105] Patients learn quickly that positioning may relieve pain, and often, there is a position of greatest comfort; conversely, certain positions may induce pain. For example, flexion and external rotation of the hip and 25 degrees of flexion of the knee lower intra-articular pressure[106] and, hence, are often favored positions. Unfortunately, they are neither the best functional positions nor the most energy-efficient and generally should be discouraged.

Bed rest is often ineffective for control of pain. Pain may increase as the muscles around the joints relax, thus awakening the patient from sleep. This may be due to changes in blood flow.[105] Stiffness is usually increased by immobilization and is often relieved with motion and heat. Pain on motion usually has as its source free nerve endings in the capsule.[105]

Control of pain is often achieved by utilizing a combination of the following: (1) Superficial heat, including warm water; deep heat; or cold. Care must be taken to assess the patient's response to the modality chosen. If heat increases the pain in a particular patient, cold should be tried. (2) A suitable anti-inflammatory medication during the treatment program. (3) Adjustment for altered biomechanics by decreasing the weight-bearing load on an affected joint or shifting the weight to an unaffected joint by use of aids, appliances, or orthoses. (4) Splinting or resting acute joints. (5) Joint conservation techniques to minimize deformity and stress. (6) Relief of muscle spasm, fibrositis, and tendinitis using injection or vapo-coolant spray. (7) Appropriate techniques of massage and transcutaneous electrical nerve stimulation. (8) Techniques to accustom patients to certain levels of pain using relaxation techniques and positioning. All of the techniques can be successful in managing pain in the patient with arthritis.

Specific Recommendations for Maintaining or Increasing Range of Motion

Joint contractures resulting in decreased range of motion involve the joint capsule, synovium, ligaments, and adjacent muscles.[34] Contractures can occur in noninvolved joints as a compensatory mechanism to relieve pain or preserve function. Methods of stretching to increase range of motion in a joint include stretching exercises, traction, serial casting, and progressive splinting. The last three techniques involve prolonged gentle forces to cause a gradual "plastic" stretch.[107] Stretching exercises are best used to preserve range of motion or to increase recently lost range of motion. Patients with long-standing or moderate contractures are best treated by the other three methods.

Exercises to increase range of motion should be designed and performed to cause the least amount of stress to a joint. Often, a bit of longitudinal traction helps to loosen the joint capsule. The goal of maintaining or increasing range of motion cannot be accomplished until pain is adequately controlled. There must be potential for increasing range of motion before applying any stretching techniques. This program is usually advised for the hip, knee, shoulder, and cervical or lumbar spine.

Specific Recommendations for Increasing Strength

In general, patients with arthritis develop decreased muscle bulk and decreased muscle strength around inflamed and/or painful joints. The primary cause of this in OA is disuse, which occurs because of pain and limited joint motion; a vicious circle is set up that results in functional decline.

Before undertaking a strengthening program, care must be taken to decrease pain, relax the patient, and decrease muscle spasm around the joints. Strengthening is not a high priority in the management of OA except for the quadriceps muscle and in postoperative situations (especially for hip abductors, knee flexors or extensors, and shoulder abductors and flexors that have been operated on). Isometric exercises are best tolerated, probably because the joint is least stressed. The fewer the number of joints in need of exercise, the more likely the regimen is to be followed. The program should be clearly understood, and written instructions should be given about which joints are to be exercised and in which position (e.g., supine, side lying), the number of repetitions recommended, whether weights should be used, and how quickly to increase the weight or repetition. We usually start with 5 repetitions and advance to 25 or 30 repetitions, cautioning the patient that if pain occurs, the exercise is stopped and the next day resumed at a lesser intensity and increased as tolerated. The exercises should be done twice daily.

Specific Recommendations About Energy Conservation and Joint Protection

As discussed earlier, energy conservation is that process by which effort is budgeted over time and distributed so that it is adequate to complete a task or a series of tasks. Because osteoarthritis is frequently associated with pain and inflammation, it can cause fatigue. Tense muscles and abnormal body positions are particularly energy-inefficient, and the patient must be made aware of them. Good posture is energy-efficient because the weight of the body is balanced without active muscle contraction. The greater the deviance from this neutral position, the more muscle activity is needed to maintain body position. This requires energy. To perform a task standing requires 25% more energy than performing the same task sitting. When the head is held forward, neck extensors are inappropriately contracting; when the shoulders are shrugged, the levators and trapezius are needlessly contracting.

Correction of these and other posture-related problems is dependent on the patient's awareness of normal posture and education about what environmental changes can be made to reduce one's energy loss. Correct working heights should permit the back to be straight and supported and the shoulders to be relaxed. Work-surface heights should be 2 inches below the elbows. A high-backed chair or a footstool could be added. Furniture can be raised by blocks to the proper height.

Planning one's day maximizes the likelihood of completing the day's activities. We stress the use of an activities analysis. For example, the patient needs to identify those activities that take a long time to do, have caused excessive pain or fatigue, or cannot be done at all. He should then identify deadlines, availability of help, priorities of tasks, and the best time of day to accomplish particular activities. If this can be done, a program of orderly, predictable activity is more likely to be achieved, and appropriate rest periods can be interposed, if necessary. Frequently, conditioning occurs, and stamina can be increased.

Joint protection techniques are designed to reduce external stress on joints in the course of normal daily activity. In addition to avoiding painful activities and maintaining joint range of motion and muscle strength, the following are recommended: wear splints to support, rest, or relieve painful, unstable joints; use the largest joint possible for a job; push or slide heavy objects rather than pull them; avoid strong and constant pressure against the pad of the thumb, as it stresses the carpometacarpal joint; and use a shorter stride length to minimize the amount of stress across the metatarsophalangeal joints and reduce the amount of time spent on one leg. A low heel will permit the quadriceps to relax and will help to decrease stress across the knee joint.

Specific Recommendations to Supply the Patient with Educational Material to Help Cope with His Illness and Its Impact

The purpose of teaching or informing patients about their disease is to influence behavior. An educational program should be designed to help the patient recognize the need for change, develop the skills to execute necessary change, and recognize when change has occurred. We believe that a guided, learner-centered small-group education program is most efficient and successful in developing awareness and problem-solving skills.[108] Such a program should consist of a list of objectives, worksheets and practice assignments designed to present the content of the program, and a self-evaluation of outcome. The process will take time because permanent changes in routine behaviors are only gradually replaced by newly learned behaviors.[109]

References

1. AAOS: Joint Motion: Method of Measuring and Recording. Chicago, American Academy of Orthopedic Surgeons, 1965.
2. Wright V: Conference on measurement of joint movement. Rheumatol Rehabil 18:261, 1979.
3. Dunham WF: Ankylosing spondylitis: Measurement of hip and spinal movements. Br J Phys Med 12:126–129, 1949.
4. Loebl NY: Measurement of spinal posture and range of spinal movement. Ann Phys Med 2:103–110, 1967.
5. Convery FR, Minteer MA, Avriel D, Connett KL: Polyarticular disability: A functional assessment. Arch Phys Med Rehabil 58:494–499, 1977.
6. Ebert DR, Fasching V, Rahlf V, et al.: Repeatability and objectivity of various measurements in rheumatoid arthritis: A comparative study. Arthritis Rheum 19:1278–1286, 1976.
7. Doyle DV, Dieppe PA, Scott J, Huskisson EC: An articular index for the assessment of osteoarthritis. Ann Rheum Dis 40:75–78, 1981.
8. Granger CV, Greer DS: Functional status measurements and medical rehabilitative outcomes. Arch Phys Med Rehabil 57:103–109, 1976.
9. Smith AJ: A study of forces on the body in athletic activities with particular reference to jumping. Thesis. University of Leeds, 1972.
10. McMahon TA, Greene PR: Fast running tracks. Sci Am 239:148–163, 1978.
11. Smidt G: Biomechanical analysis of knee flexion and extension. J Biomech 6:79–92, 1973.

12. Morrow GR, Chiarello RJ, Derogatis LR: A new scale for assessing patients' psychosocial adjustment to medical illness. Psychol Med 8:605–610, 1978.

13. Schain W: Personal communication, 1978.

14. Huskisson EC, Jones J, Scott PJ: Application of visual analogue scales to the measurement of functional capacity. Rheumatol Rehabil 15:185–187, 1976.

15. Meenan RF, Gertman PM, Mason JH: Measuring health status in arthritis: The arthritis impact measurement scales. Arthritis Rheum 23:146–152, 1980.

16. Jette AM: Functional status index: Reliability of a chronic disease evaluation instrument. Arch Phys Med Rehabil 61:395–401, 1980.

17. Fries JF, Spitz P, Kraines RG, Holman HR: Measurement of patient outcome in arthritis. Arthritis Rheum 3:137–145, 1980.

18. Maquet PG, Pelzer GA: Evolution of the maximum stress in osteoarthritis of the knee. J Biomech 10:107–117, 1977.

19. Hill AV: Production and absorption of work by muscle. Science 131:897–903, 1960.

20. Radin E: Mechanical aspects of osteoarthrosis. Bull Rheum Dis 26:862–865, 1975–1976.

21. Watt EGD, Jones JG: Muscular control landing from unexpected falls in man. J Physiol 291:729–737, 1971.

22. Pauwels F: Kurzer liberblick uber die mechanische beanspruchberg des knochen un ibre bedetunf fur die Funktionelle Anpassung. Z Orthop 111:681, 1973.

23. Giannestras N: Foot Disorders: Medical and Surgical Management. 2nd ed. Philadelphia, Lea & Febiger, 1973.

24. Mann RA: Surgical implications of biomechanics of the foot and ankle. Clin Orthop Rel Res 146:111–118, 1980.

25. Wiest DR, Waters RL, Bontrager EL, Quigley MJ: The influence of heel design on a rigid ankle-foot orthosis. Orthotics and Prosthetics 33:3–10, 1979.

26. Linscheid RL: Demonstration of subluxing force at the metacarpotrapezial joint. Clin Orthop Rel Res 123:87–88, 1977.

27. Lehmann JF, Brunner GD, Stow RW: Pain threshold measurement after therapeutic application of ultrasound, microwaves, and infrared. Arch Phys Med Rehabil 39:560–565, 1958.

28. Fischer E, Solomon S: Physiological responses to heat and cold. In Licht S (ed.): Therapeutic Heat and Cold. New Haven, Connecticut, E. Licht, Publisher, 1965, pp. 126–169.

29. Hollander JL, Horvath SM: The influence of physical therapy procedures on the intra-articular temperature of normal and arthritic subjects. Am J Med Sci 218:543–548, 1949.

30. Harris R: The effect of various forms of physical therapy on radiosodium clearance from the normal and arthritic knee joint. Ann Phys Med 7:1–10, 1963.

31. Millard JB: Conductive heating. In Licht S (ed.): Therapeutic Heat and Cold. New Haven, E. Licht, 1958.

32. Davis FA: The hot bath test in the diagnosis of multiple sclerosis. J Mount Sinai Hosp NY 33:280, 1966.

33. Swezey RL: Therapeutic modalities for pain relief. In Arthritis Rational Therapy and Rehabilitation. Philadelphia, W. B. Saunders Company, 1978.

34. Syllabus of the American Academy of Physical Medicine and Rehabilitation. Chicago, 1977, p. A1.

35. Lehmann JF, Masock AJ, Warren CG, Kublanski JN: Effect of therapeutic temperatures on tendon extensibility. Arch Phys Med Rehabil 51:481–487, 1970.

36. Schwan HP, Piersol GM: The absorption of electromagnetic energy in body tissues: Review and critical analysis of physiological and clinical aspects. Am J Phys Med 34:425, 1955.

37. Lehmann JF, DeLateur BJ, Warren CG, et al.: Heating of joint structure by ultrasound. Arch Phys Med 49:28, 1968.

38. Lehmann JF: Diathermy. In Krusen FH, et al.: Handbook of Physical Medicine and Rehabilitation. 2nd ed. Philadelphia, W. B. Saunders Company, 1971, pp. 273–345.

39. Lehmann JF: Diathermy. In Licht S (ed.): Therapeutic Heat and Cold. New Haven, E. Licht, 1958.

40. Lehmann JF, Krusen FH: Biophysical effects of ultrasonic energy on carcinoma and their possible significance. Arch Phys Med Rehabil 36:452–459, 1955.

41. Berger LH: Rehabilitation of patients with rheumatic diseases. In Kelley WN, et al. (eds.): Textbook of Rheumatology. Philadelphia, W. B. Saunders Company, 1981, p. 1855.

42. Knutsson E, Martensson E: Effects of local cooling on monosynaptic reflexes in man. Scand J Rehabil Med 1:126, 1969.

43. Miglietta O: Action of cold on spasticity. Am J Phys Med 52:198–205, 1973.

44. Benson TB, Copp EP: The effects of therapeutic forms of heat and ice on the pain threshold of the normal shoulder. Rheumatol Rehabil 13:101–104, 1974.

45. Travell J: Ethylchloride spray for painful muscle spasm. Arch Phys Med 33:291–298 1952.

46. Mennell JM: Spray and stretch treatment for myofascial pain. Hosp Phys 12:47, 1973.

47. Olson JE, Stravino VP: A review of cryotherapy. Phys Ther 52:840–853, 1972.

48. Clark GR, et al.: Evaluation of physiotherapy in the treatment of osteoarthritis of the knee. Rheumatol Rehabil 13:190–197, 1974.

49. Stillwell GK: Therapeutic heat and cold. In Krusen FH, et al.: Handbook of Physical Medicine and Rehabilitation. 2nd ed. Philadelphia, W. B. Saunders Company, 1971, pp. 259–272.

50. Stillwell GK: Clinical electrical stimulation. In Licht S (ed.): Ultraviolet Radiation. New Haven, Connecticut, E. Licht, Publisher, 1959, pp. 133–139.

51. Wall PD, Cronly-Dillion JR: Pain, itch and vibration. Arch Neurol 2:365–375, 1960.

52. Melzack R, Wall PD: Pain mechanisms: A new theory. Science 150:971–979, 1965.

53. Mann SC, Baragar FD: Preliminary clinical study of acupuncture in rheumatoid arthritis. J Rheumatol 1:126–129, 1974.

54. Gaw AC, Chang LW, Shaw LC: Efficacy of acupuncture on osteoarthritic pain: A controlled double blind study. N Engl J Med 293:375–378, 1975.

55. Moore ME, Bert SN: Acupuncture for chronic shoulder pain: An experimental study with attention to the role of placebo and hypnotic susceptibility. Ann Intern Med 84:381–384, 1976.

56. Toshikatsu K, Masayoshi H: The effects of stimulation of ear acupuncture points on the body's pain threshold. Am J Chin Med 8:241–252, 1979.

57. Kamenetz HL: Massage, manipulation, and traction. *In* Licht S (ed.): Arthritis and Physical Medicine. Baltimore, Waverly Press, 1969, pp. 304, 407–408.

58. Stein H, Dickson RA: Reversed dynamic slings for knee flexion-contractures in the hemophiliac. J Bone Joint Surg 57A:282–283, 1975.

59. Reich RS: The treatment of flexion deformities of the knee as a complication of rheumatoid arthritis. *In* Gasling J, VanSwag H (eds.): Contemporary Rheumatology. Proceedings of 3rd Rheumatology Congress. New York, Elsevier Publishing Co., 1956.

60. Thiske HG: Neck and shoulder pain: Evaluation and conservative management. Med Clin North Am 53:511–524, 1969.

61. Caillet R: Neck and Arm Pain. Philadelphia, F. A. Davis Co., 1964, pp. 79–82.

62. Gurdjian ES, Thomas LM (eds.): Neck Ache and Back Ache. Proceedings of a workshop sponsored by the American Association of Neurological Surgeons in cooperation with the National Institutes of Health, Bethesda, Maryland. Springfield, Illinois, Charles C Thomas, 1970.

63. Swezey RL: Essentials of physical management and rehabilitation in arthritis. Semin Arthritis Rheum 3:349, 1974.

64. Brown BR: Office management of common musculoskeletal pain syndrome. Am Fam Physician 6:92–98, 1972.

65. Bonica JJ: Management of myofascial pain syndromes in general practice. JAMA 164:732–738, 1957.

66. Gorrell RL: Treatment of skeletal pain with procaine injection; an analysis of 295 cases in general practice. Am J Surg 63:102–104, 1944.

67. Wilson CH: Exercise for arthritis. *In* Basmajian JV (ed.): Therapeutic Exercise. 3rd ed. Baltimore, Williams & Wilkins, 1978, p. 528.

68. McQueen IJ: Recent advances in the techniques of progressive resistive exercise. Br Med J 2:1193, 1954.

69. Gordon EE, Kowalski K, Fritts M: Changes in rat muscle fiber with forceful exercise. Arch Phys Med Rehabil 48:296–303, 1967.

70. Hettinger T: Physiology of strength. *In* Thurlwell MH (ed.): Physiology of Strength. Springfield, Illinois, Charles C Thomas, 1961.

71. DeLateur BJ, Lehmann JF, Fordyce WE: A test of the DeLorme axiom. Arch Phys Med 49:245–248, 1968.

72. Osternig LR, Bates BT, James SL: Isokinetic and isometric torque force relationships. Arch Phys Med Rehabil 58:254–257, 1977.

73. Downey JA: The physiatrist in arthritis management. *In* Ehrlich GE (ed.): Rehabilitation Management of Rheumatic Conditions. Baltimore, Williams & Wilkins, 1980, pp. 31–32.

74. Muller EA: Influence of training and inactivity on muscle strength. Arch Phys Med 51:449–462, 1970.

75. Kottke F: The effects of limitation of activity upon the human body. JAMA 196:825–830, 1966.

76. Jayson MI, Rubenstein D, Dixon AS: Intra-articular pressure and rheumatoid geodes (bone "cysts"). Ann Rheum Dis 29:496–502, 1970.

77. DeLateur BJ: Exercise for strength and endurance. *In* Basmajian JV (ed.): Therapeutic Exercise. Baltimore, Williams & Wilkins, 1978, p. 90.

78. Smith RD, Polley HF: Rest therapy for rheumatoid arthritis. Mayo Clin Proc 53:141–145, 1978.

79. Nichols PJR: Osteoarthrosis. *In* Rehabilitation Medicine. London, Butterworth, 1980, Chapter 7.

80. Collut R: Foot and Ankle Pain. Philadelphia, F. A. Davis Co., 1973, p. 57.

81. Melvin JL: Rheumatic Disease: Occupational Therapy and Rehabilitation. Philadephia, F. A. Davis Co., 1977, p. 59.

82. Lehmann JF, Warren GC, Pemberton DR, et al.: Load bearing function of patellar tendon bearing braces of various designs. Arch Phys Med Rehabil 52:366–370, 1971.

83. Gerber LH: Aids and appliances. *In* Wright V (ed.): Arthritis in the Elderly. Edinburgh, Churchill Livingstone, 1983, pp. 256–274.

84. Rubin G, Dixon M, Danisi M: Prescription procedures for knee orthosis and knee foot orthosis. Orthotics and Prosthetics 31:15, 1977.

85. Smith EM, Juvinoll RC, Corell EB, et al.: Bracing the unstable arthritic knee. Arch Phys Med Rehabil 51:22–28, 1970.

86. Lehmann JF, Warren GC: A biomechanical evaluation of knee stability in below knee braces. Arch Phys Med Rehabil 53:134–141, 1970.

87. Larson CB, et al.: Criteria for evaluation of orthopedic measures in the management of deformities of rheumatoid arthritis. Chapter 3. Splinting. Transactions of conference by ARA, ARF, and NIAMDDK, New York, December 8, 1963. Arthritis Rheum 2:585–600, 1964.

88. Blount WP: Don't throw away the cane. J Bone Joint Surg 38A:695–698, 1956.

89. Norten PL, Brown T: The immobilizing efficiency of back braces: The effect on the posture and motion of the lumbo-sacral spine. J Bone Joint Surg 39A:111–138, 1957.

90. Perry J: The use of external support in the treatment of low back pain. J Bone Joint Surg 52A:1440–1442, 1970.

91. Bunch W, Keagy RD: Principles of Orthotic Treatment. St. Louis, C. V. Mosby Co., 1976, pp. 86, 92.

92. Colachis SC Jr, Strohm BA, Ganter EL: Cervical spine motion in normal women: Radiographic study of the effect of cervical collars. Arch Phys Med Rehabil 54:161–169, 1973.

93. Hartman JT, Palumbo F, Hill BJ: Cineradiography of braced normal cervical spine: Comparative study of five commonly used cervical orthoses. Clin. Orthop 109:97–102, 1975.

94. Saunders JV, Inman VT, Eberhart HD: The major determination in normal and pathological gait. J Bone Joint Surg 38A:543–558, 1953.

95. Bruttstrom M, Persson G, Sandgren L: New walking aid for rheumatic patients. Scand J Rehabil Med 6:141–143, 1974.

96. Cascolan D: Forearm rest attachment as an aid to standing. Phys Ther 55:991–992, 1975.

97. Furst G, Gerber L, Smith C: Rehabilitation Through Learning: Energy Conservation and Joint Protection. Bethesda, Maryland, National Institutes of Health, 1982.

98. Katz W: Sexuality in arthritics. *In* Rheumatic Diseases: Diagnosis and Management. Philadelphia, J. B. Lippincott Co., 1977, pp. 1011–1020.

99. Currey HLF: Osteoarthrosis of the hip joint and sexual activity. Ann Rheum Dis 29:488–491, 1970.

100. Swinburn WR (ed.): Sexual counselling for the arthritic. Clin Rheum Dis 2:639–651, 1976.

101. Shinichi Y, Shoji U: Sexual problems of women with

rheumatoid arthritis. Arch Phys Med Rehabil 62:122–123, 1981.

102. Yaslow W, Simeone J, Huestis D: Hip replacement rehabilitation. Arch Phys Med Rehabil 57:275–278, 1976.

103. Charnley J: Low friction arthroplasty of the hip: theory and practice. Berlin, Springer-Verlag, 1979.

104. Sledge C: Introduction to the surgical management of arthritis. *In* Kelley WN, et al. (eds.): Textbook of Rheumatology. Philadelphia, W. B. Saunders Company, 1981.

105. Hoglund F: Clinical manifestations of osteoarthritis. Clin Rheum Dis 2:543, 1976.

106. Favreau JC, Laurin CA: Joint effusions and flexion deformities. Can Med Assoc J 88:575–576, 1963.

107. Warren CG, Lehmann JF, Kublanski JN: Heat and stretch procedures on evaluation using rat tail tendon. Arch Phys Med Rehabil 57:122–126, 1976.

108. Green LW, Kreuter MW, Deeds SG, Partridge KB: Health Education Planning: A Diagnostic Approach. Palo Alto, California, Mayfield Publishing Co., 1980.

109. Swezey RL: Educational theory as a basis for patient education. J Chronic Dis 29:417–422, 1976.

18

Principles of Drug Therapy

John J. Calabro, M.D.

Drug therapy begins with early diagnosis and rests on the appropriate use of supportive measures, but it depends in large measure on patient cooperation. Generally, what the physician seeks to preserve for the patient with osteoarthritis is a life style as close to normal as possible. The principal aim of management is to prevent or to correct disability. Although drugs play an integral role, their use is individualized to the needs of the patient, clearly governed by an understanding of the principles of drug therapy (Table 18–1).

GENERAL PRINCIPLES

Because osteoarthritis is capricious, it is almost impossible to predict early in management which drugs may eventually be needed or what the ultimate prognosis may be. The most promising outlook is generally for the patient who has only minimal involvement from Herberden's nodes, because he or she will suffer less functional impairment than the

patient whose hips and knees are also involved. Moreover, it is always easier to prevent deformity than to restore joint function once it has been lost. Consequently, the comprehensive management of osteoarthritis has both immediate and long-term objectives. One must first relieve the patient's pain and discomfort with drugs and then begin long-range planning for the prevention or correction of deformity.

Patient Education and Motivation

Although patients with osteoarthritis may need the help of specialists in their long-term care, the outcome will depend in large measure on how capable the physician in charge is in educating and motivating the patient. Clearly, management can succeed only with the active participation of the patient. To some patients, a drug regimen augmented by supportive measures such as remedial exercise will appear too simple. Consequently, the excellent results obtainable by these seemingly undramatic measures must be emphasized. The physician needs to explain that for the great majority of patients with osteoarthritis, medical measures alone will help them maintain full and productive lives. Above all, patients should be educated about the nature of their disease and what they can reasonably expect from treatment.[1] They should also be cautioned about modalities that they would be well advised to avoid, considering that Americans spend over a billion dollars yearly on arthritis quackery in their quest for quick and decisive cures.

Initially, of paramount importance are careful counseling and planning of an individualized regimen that the patient is able and willing to adopt as a way of life. This may help to

Table 18–1. PRINCIPLES OF DRUG THERAPY

Patient education
a. Understanding the nature of the disease
b. Understanding the goals of therapy

Special considerations for the elderly

Choice of drug
a. Analgesic versus anti-inflammatory agents
b. Prescribed on demand or on a regular basis
c. Efficacy, tolerance, interaction with other drugs
d. Cost factor
e. Patient compliance

motivate the reluctant patient as well as improve the cooperation of the patient who is only partially motivated. In long-term management, patients need continuous encouragement because they have the difficult task of adapting their lives to the disease. For the majority, a good relationship with the physician is all the psychologic support needed during prolonged treatment. At the outset, however, the physician should be alert to certain patients who may require the added support of a vocational counselor, social worker, or psychiatrist.

The Elderly Patient

The elderly patient often has medical problems other than osteoarthritis, so that the drug prescribed for arthritis may be taken along with a host of additional ones needed for other disorders.[2, 3] Therefore, the risk of adverse reactions and drug interactions rises sharply in such patients. In a typical skilled nursing facility, the number of drugs that the elderly patient receives may range from one to more than 20, with the median number of 6. If patients receive 6 or more drugs, adverse reactions can be expected in 25% of them, as compared with 10% of patients receiving a single drug.[4]

Medication for the elderly should always be determined by the principle of least toxicity, because the pharmacologic action of various agents prescribed may be significantly affected by the altered physiologic state of aging. These alterations include those in metabolism by the liver and kidneys, diminished cardiac output, and alterations in the binding capacity of plasma proteins.[2] Plasma proteins also decrease in the presence of chronic illness, thereby resulting in a higher free-drug concentration than expected. Therefore, in determining the daily dose of a given drug with a high affinity for binding to plasma proteins, one should be certain that the albumin concentration of the patient is normal.

Many patients with osteoarthritis are elderly. Because the major excretion of analgesic and anti-inflammatory drugs is by the kidney, it is imperative to know whether or not the patient's renal reserves are adequate. It is also important to know whether hepatic function is normal. Impairment of liver function will alter the survival of analgesic and anti-inflammatory drugs, because all are primarily cleared or detoxified by the liver. Clearly, before choosing any drug for an elderly patient, each of these factors must be considered.

Choice of Drugs

The basis of any treatment program is the appropriate use of drugs, preferably started as early as possible. By providing symptomatic relief of pain and stiffness, drugs facilitate a more effective program of exercise as well as other supportive measures. Yet, some patients can be effectively managed without drugs. If drug therapy is needed, it is important to determine which drug is to be used, and whether to use a strict analgesic or one that provides anti-inflammatory effects as well. Even with drugs, general supportive measures should also be considered, because these will often decrease or obviate the need for drugs.

Currently, there is no drug that can prevent or reverse the basic pathologic process of osteoarthritis, although several are being investigated from this standpoint.[5, 6] Consequently, drugs are used essentially for their analgesic and anti-inflammatory effects. Analgesic drugs relieve pain and do nothing more. In contrast, the nonsteroidal anti-inflammatory drugs not only reduce pain but also suppress inflammation. Because there is striking evidence of inflammation in many patients with osteoarthritis,[7, 8] both physicians and patients often prefer nonsteroidal anti-inflammatory drugs to pure analgesics.[9]

The choice of drug depends on the needs of the individual patient. Assessment of the problem posed by osteoarthritis is key in this issue. If the problem is primarily mechanical, with little or no inflammatory element, strict analgesics may be adequate. Drugs primarily for pain relief may also be desirable for patients with only mild or intermittent discomfort, particularly when only one or two joints are affected. However, if the problem is largely inflammatory and pain or discomfort is moderate or severe, the anti-inflammatory drugs are usually more beneficial.

The selection of drug will also rely on efficacy, tolerance, and the potential risk of serious toxicity or of interaction with other drugs taken by the patient. In addition to efficacy and tolerance, other factors play a role. Among these are the cost factor and patient compliance. If the latter is a problem, the physician may opt for a drug that needs to be given only once or twice daily in preference to one that must be given three or four times

Table 18–2. ANALGESIC DRUGS USED IN
OSTEOARTHRITIS

Peripherally Acting Drugs	Centrally Acting Drugs
Aspirin in low doses	Propoxyphene
Other salicylates in low doses	Ethoheptazine
Nonsteroidal anti-inflammatory drugs in low doses	Pentazocine
	Codeine
Acetaminophen	Oxycodone

daily. Regardless of the choice, the potential benefits and risks of the drug should be explained with great care to the patient.

ANALGESIC DRUGS

Most analgesic drugs used in osteoarthritis can be grouped into two major classes (Table 18–2).[10] Drugs of the first group act peripherally at the site of pain, perhaps by suppressing mediators of inflammation that are associated with the production of pain. Those of the second group act centrally, either by affecting pain receptors in the brain or by other mechanisms at the level of the spinal cord or other parts of the central nervous system.

Peripherally Acting Drugs

Drugs in this group include all of the nonsteroidal anti-inflammatory agents, including aspirin and other salicylate preparations, as well as acetaminophen. It appears that all nonsteroidal anti-inflammatory drugs are primarily analgesic at low dosages and are anti-inflammatory at higher dosages.[11, 12] Consequently, a number of anti-inflammatory drugs have recently been either approved or marketed as analgesics. These include 300-mg ibuprofen tablets, 200-mg tolmetin sodium tablets, 200-mg fenoprofen calcium capsules, and 275-mg naproxen sodium tablets (Anaprox). As analgesics, each agent can be administered every 4 to 6 hours daily.

There is a wide individual response to analgesic drugs.[13] Therefore, it is important to find the best drug for each patient. Aspirin is widely used in osteoarthritis, particularly when the problem is primarily mechanical with little or no associated inflammatory component. It is usually well tolerated and safe at a dosage of 325 to 650 mg given three or four times daily. Acetaminophen at a comparable dose is equally effective and is also well tolerated.

Consequently, both drugs can be given to patients for prolonged periods, especially because they have been rarely implicated in causing analgesic nephropathy.

Because older persons are more prone to develop aspirin toxicity, dosage increases that raise the total daily dosage above 2.6 gm should be made with caution.[1] If tinnitus or hearing loss ensues, aspirin should be withheld until toxic symptoms resolve, at which time it can be reinstituted at a lower dosage. Administration of aspirin with meals and with food at bedtime or with oral antacids will decrease gastrointestinal side effects. Otherwise, salicylate preparations designed to produce less gastrointestinal distress may be prescribed. These include enteric-coated aspirin, aspirin-antacid mixtures, salicylsalicylic acid, magnesium salicylate, choline salicylate, and choline magnesium trisalicylate.[1] As with aspirin, the total daily dosage of acetaminophen should not exceed 2.6 gm daily. At higher doses, toxic hepatitis may occur, particularly in patients with underlying liver disease.

For patients who cannot tolerate or receive little benefit from either aspirin or acetaminophen, analgesic quantities of a nonsteroidal anti-inflammatory drug can be prescribed. Certain of these, marketed at dosages specifically for analgesia, have already been cited. Nevertheless, any of the others can be used and are equally effective. The analgesic dose of a nonsteroidal anti-inflammatory drug is generally about half of that needed for its anti-inflammatory effect. Finally, a patient with joint pain aggravated by certain activity may need simple analgesics only periodically or on demand, and not on a regular daily basis.

Centrally Acting Drugs

Centrally acting analgesics are primarily narcotics. Therefore, it is wise to avoid the use of these drugs in osteoarthritis because the disorder is usually chronic and addiction can become a major problem. Moreover, they differ from peripherally acting agents by demonstrating a clear plateau in effectiveness despite progressive increases in dosage.[14] Thus, when all pain receptors are saturated by these drugs, no additional analgesic effect is possible.

Propoxyphene hydrochloride, 65 mg, and ethoheptazine citrate, 75 mg, are effective analgesics in this class. Each may be given three or four times daily on a regular or demand basis.[1] Side effects of propoxyphene include sedation, lightheadedness, and gastrointestinal upset. Drug addiction may also develop.[15] Despite the initial claims that propoxyphene carried minimal risks of dependence, there is growing recognition of its addictive potential, with documentation of both psychologic dependence and physical withdrawal symptoms. The most common signs and symptoms of withdrawal from propoxyphene include abnormal vital signs, "goosefleshing," insomnia, hyperactive deep tendon reflexes, nausea, vomiting, agitation, and seizures. Subjective complaints of muscle cramping, dizziness, irritability, and fatigue have also been observed.

Pentazocine, 50 mg orally three or four times daily, is another effective centrally acting analgesic. Although addiction is uncommon with this narcotic, prolonged use is not recommended.[1] The most common side effects of pentazocine include nausea, lightheadedness, and flushing of the skin. Other narcotic preparations, such as codeine or oxycodone, are rarely required in osteoarthritis.

Because most of the centrally acting analgesics are narcotics, each poses special risks, particularly problems of tolerance and addiction. Consequently, narcotic analgesics are rarely used for prolonged periods to control the pain of osteoarthritis. They may be useful, however, for the short-term treatment of acute and severe pain that is superimposed on joint pain that is chronic and mild,[10] as, for example, when a patient with osteoarthritis sustains an acute injury of an already chronically affected joint. Narcotic analgesics may also prove beneficial when radicular pain from severe spinal involvement is a problem. In these instances, the use of a narcotic analgesic for a week or two will reduce the superimposed acute component of severe pain without the risks of tolerance and addiction that can result from prolonged use.

Combinations

Combinations of centrally and peripherally acting drugs are also available.[10] These combinations provide additive effectiveness, so that the analgesia of weak narcotics can be enhanced without increasing the potential for physiologic addiction.[14] The most common of these combinations are propoxyphene, codeine, or ethoheptazine with either aspirin or acetaminophen. Originally, phenacetin or amidopyrine were also used, but renal and bone marrow toxicity have greatly reduced the popularity of these additives.

The use of combinations of peripherally acting drugs, particularly two nonsteroidal anti-inflammatory drugs, has been discouraged because of the hypothetical problem of competition for plasma protein binding sites. Unfortunately, the available data are inadequate to permit guidelines regarding this issue.[14]

Although suppression of pain is a major objective in the treatment of osteoarthritis, it is important to remember that pain plays a protective role in this disease.[14] A neuropathic (Charcot) joint or rapid destruction of a joint can result from the patient's inability to perceive pain.

Local Analgesics

Local application of a liniment, such as methylsalicylate, as a counterirritant may provide hyperemia with its attendant relief of pain. The benefits of liniments are only temporary, as they are with nonmedicinal measures that provide heat.

ANTI-INFLAMMATORY DRUGS

As noted earlier, these drugs provide both analgesic and anti-inflammatory effects. Although the mechanisms of these effects are not entirely understood, all anti-inflammatory drugs have the capacity to inhibit prostaglandin synthesis and/or other mediators of inflammation. There is a wide individual variation in response to these drugs, so that a trial of several may be required.[5]

Rationale for Use

Inflammation of the synovium occurs intermittently during the course of osteoarthritis, especially in large joints such as the knee.[14] During such flares, there is increased swelling and tenderness, often with warmth and signs of effusion in the affected joint. Examination of the synovial fluid will often disclose an increase in protein and cell count, with a shift toward polymorphonuclear cells.[7, 14]

Flares may occur without an explicable reason but frequently result from a fall or a sudden twist of the joint.[14] They may also be a reaction to fragments worn off the surface of the articular cartilage or to associated crystal deposition disease. Flares may also result from injury to the synovium during excessive motion of malaligned joint surfaces. During such epi-

Table 18–3. NONSTEROIDAL ANTI-INFLAMMATORY DRUGS OTHER THAN SALICYLATES USED IN OSTEOARTHRITIS (CHRONOLOGIC LISTING)

Generic Drug (Trade Name)	How Supplied	Daily Dosage Range
Phenylbutazone* (Butazolidin, Azolid)	100-mg tablets	300–400 mg
Oxyphenbutazone* (Tandearil, Oxalid)	100-mg tablets	300–400 mg
Indomethacin (Indocin, Indocin SR)	25-mg capsules, 50-mg capsules, 75-mg sustained-release capsule	75–200 mg
Ibuprofen (Motrin, Rufen)	300-mg tablets, 400-mg tablets, 600-mg tablets	1600–2400 mg
Fenoprofen calcium† (Nalfon)	200-mg pulvules 300-mg capsules, 600-mg scored tablets	2400–3200 mg
Tolmetin sodium (Tolectin)	200-mg scored tablets, 400-mg capsules	1200–2000 mg
Naproxen (Naprosyn)	250-mg scored tablets, 375-mg tablets, 500-mg tablets	500–1000 mg
Sulindac (Clinoril)	150-mg tablets, 200-mg scored tablets	200–400 mg
Meclofenamate sodium (Meclomen)	50-mg capsules, 100-mg capsules	200–400 mg
Piroxicam (Feldene)	10-mg capsules, 20-mg capsules	10–20 mg

*Phenylbutazone and oxyphenbutazone are indicated only for short-term treatment of acute attacks of osteoarthritis of the hips and knees that are not responsive to other treatment.
†Except for fenoprofen calcium, all drugs should be taken with food.

sodes of acute synovitis, anti-inflammatory drugs may be particularly beneficial. The doses usually prescribed are similar to those recommended for patients with rheumatoid arthritis (Table 18–3).

Untoward Drug Effects

Although reactions to drugs are varied, they fall into five major classes (Table 18–4). These include an allergic or hypersensitivity reaction, in which symptoms are related to the patient's abnormal immunologic response to standard doses of drug. The most common clinical man-

Table 18–4. FIVE MAJOR CLASSES OF UNTOWARD DRUG EFFECTS

1. Allergic or hypersensitivity reaction
2. Drug idiosyncrasy
3. Overdose
4. Drug interaction
5. Side effects

ifestation is a mild systemic illness closely resembling serum sickness. It begins a few days after initiation of the drug and usually lasts only a few days or weeks, unless the drug is continued. Rarely is there progression to hypersensitivity vasculitis with severe skin and widespread major organ involvement resulting in a fatal outcome.

The second type of reaction is drug idiosyncrasy, which is characterized by an inordinate response to a normal or less-than-standard dose of a drug. The third untoward drug effect is a fairly predictable response to overdose of a drug. The fourth is drug interaction, in which unpredictable toxicity evolves when another drug is added, the result of rising levels of free drug because of competition for plasma protein binding sites. All anti-inflammatory drugs have this capacity. The fifth type of effect includes adverse reactions or side effects.

The nonsteroidal anti-inflammatory drugs share a common core of potential side effects (Table 18–5). They differ widely, however, in their innate propensity and frequency in in-

Table 18–5. POTENTIAL ADVERSE REACTIONS TO NONSTEROIDAL ANTI-INFLAMMATORY DRUGS

1. Gastrointestinal upset: nausea, vomiting, dyspepsia, diarrhea, constipation
2. Major gastrointestinal bleeding, ulcer, or perforation
3. Toxic hepatitis
4. Skin rash, pruritus, urticaria, alopecia
5. Ocular toxicity: reversible blurring of vision
6. Central nervous system toxicity: headache, tinnitus, drowsiness, dizziness, lightheadedness, agitation, confusion, lethargy, weakness, depression
7. Cardiovascular toxicity: palpitations, arrhythmias
8. Sodium and fluid retention
9. Renal toxicity: diminished function, interstitial nephritis, papillary necrosis, nephrotic syndrome

ducing these and other adverse experiences. Consequently, the choice of drug for the individual patient often rests on tolerance or the potential for serious toxicity.

The most common side effects occur in the gastrointestinal tract. Adverse reactions include nausea with or without vomiting, dyspepsia, including indigestion and heartburn or epigastric pain, abdominal distress or pain, diarrhea, and constipation. Others are anorexia, bloating, flatulence, proctitis, rectal bleeding, ulcerative stomatitis, intestinal ulceration associated with stenosis and obstruction, and the occurrence or aggravation of ulcerative colitis or regional enteritis. Severe toxicity, such as major bleeding, the development or reactivation of peptic ulcer, or gastrointestinal perforation, occur infrequently. All drugs can induce hepatitis and jaundice.

Skin reactions include rash, pruritus, urticaria, petechiae, ecchymoses, alopecia, erythema nodosum, and, rarely, exfoliative dermatitis. Corneal deposits and retinal disturbances, including those of the macula, have been observed with prolonged nonsteroidal anti-inflammatory drug therapy. Blurred vision is a significant symptom that necessitates not only withdrawal of the drug but also a thorough ophthalmologic examination.

Each of these agents may aggravate psychiatric disturbances, epilepsy, and parkinsonism and should therefore be used with considerable caution in patients with these conditions. Headache is a common central nervous system side effect, as is tinnitus. Drugs may also cause drowsiness, dizziness, or lightheadedness; patients should be warned about engaging in activities requiring mental alertness or motor coordination, such as driving a car. Less common central nervous system side effects include agitation, confusion, lethargy, malaise, and depression.

Palpitations occur in less than 1% of patients receiving nonsteroidal anti-inflammatory drugs. Other cardiovascular reactions include arrhythmias, chest pain, hypotension, hypertension, and elevation of the blood urea nitrogen (BUN). Sodium and fluid retention have been observed with each of these drugs but appear to occur more frequently with certain ones, such as phenylbutazone and ibuprofen.

Impaired renal function and more severe renal abnormalities, including interstitial nephritis, papillary necrosis, acute oliguric renal failure, and nephrotic syndrome, have been described with various of these agents.[16–19] The changes can be explained by inhibition of intrarenal prostaglandin synthesis, with resultant fall in renal blood flow. Toxicity is more likely to occur in patients with renal function that is already compromised, because prostaglandin synthesis in these patients is increased on a compensatory basis. Examples of patients at risk include those with hepatic cirrhosis, congestive heart failure, systemic lupus erythematosus (SLE) with renal disease, and diminished plasma volume.

Contraindications and Precautions

The nonsteroidal anti-inflammatory drugs are contraindicated in patients who are allergic to aspirin or who have nasal polyps associated with angioedema or a bronchospastic reaction to aspirin or other nonsteroidal anti-inflammatory agents. Safe conditions for the use of these drugs in children with traumatic or secondary osteoarthritis have not been established except for drugs approved for children under the age of 15 years, such as aspirin, tolmetin sodium, and naproxen. Furthermore, safe conditions have not been established for their prescription in pregnant and nursing women. All drugs should be used with great care in the elderly. All of these agents may mask the usual signs and symptoms of infection.

Proliferation of Drugs

Historically, until 1973, when ibuprofen was marketed, there were only a handful of nonsteroidal anti-inflammatory drugs. These included aspirin, other salicylates, phenylbutazone, oxyphenbutazone, and indomethacin. Since then, there has been a steady proliferation of drugs (Table 18–6). Of these, aspirin is frequently tried first and thus occupies an important place in the drug therapy of osteoarthritis.[1]

Table 18–6. MARKETING YEAR OF NONSTEROIDAL ANTI-INFLAMMATORY DRUGS IN THE UNITED STATES

Drug	Year
Phenylbutazone	1952
Oxyphenbutazone	1961
Indomethacin	1965
Ibuprofen	1974
Fenoprofen calcium	1976
Naproxen	1976
Tolmetin sodium	1976
Sulindac	1978
Meclofenamate sodium	1980
Piroxicam	1982

ASPIRIN AND SALICYLATES

All salicylate preparations are derivatives of salicylic acid and are formed by substitution on the carboxyl group.[20] Acetylsalicylic acid, however, is formed by substitution on the hydroxyl group. Aspirin is the generic name for acetylsalicylic acid in the United States, but in some countries it is still a trade name. The salicylates act by virtue of their salicylic content and by the amount of salicylic anion liberated in the body. The therapeutic usefulness of salicylates in osteoarthritis is well established. The efficacy and safety of these valuable drugs can be enhanced considerably by an understanding of their unique pharmacokinetics.[21]

Pharmacokinetics

After ingestion, salicylates are rapidly absorbed from the stomach. The rate of absorption is influenced by many factors, including gastric emptying time, rate of tablet disintegration, solubility, and concurrent drug therapy. Food also reduces the absorption of aspirin, but the total availability of salicylate is not reduced.[22] There is considerable variation in the rate of absorption of salicylate preparations.[23] Once absorbed, salicylates are distributed throughout all body fluids and are bound to serum albumin. The liver is the primary site of salicylate metabolism, which may account for the elevated levels of serum transaminase found in patients receiving salicylates.[24]

The plasma half-life of aspirin is relatively short, from 10 to 20 minutes, whereas that of salicylates is more prolonged, between 3 and 5 hours.[25] However, when anti-inflammatory quantities of aspirin are given, the biologic half-life is considerably prolonged, from 9 to 16 hours.[23]

Aspirin is excreted principally by the kidney. The urinary excretion of salicylates is largely influenced by the rate of urine flow and the pH of the urine. Therefore, renal excretion is dependent on renal function but is also affected by the concomitant administration of other drugs that compete for proximal tubular transport, such as probenecid and acetazolamide, by the state of acid-base hydration, and by diuretics.[20] Although aspirin has been suspected of inducing analgesic nephropathy, phenacetin is clearly the major cause of this syndrome.[20]

Therapeutic Applications

Aspirin is one of the most widely used drugs in the world.[26] It is readily available in the United States an an over-the-counter medication. However, it has been banned in some countries because of toxicity.

Salicylates are well established as analgesic, antipyretic, and anti-inflammatory agents.[26–28] A single aspirin tablet contains 325 mg, of which approximately 250 mg are salicylate and the remainder the acetyl moiety. By contrast, a single dose of cation salicylate, such as magnesium salicylate (Magan, Mobidin), choline salicylate (Arthropan), choline magnesium trisalicylate (Trilisate), or salicylsalicylic acid (Disalcid) contains 500 mg of salicylate. Consequently, each 500-mg tablet (or teaspoonful) of each of these salicylate preparations is equivalent to 650 mg of aspirin, and each 750-mg tablet is equivalent to almost 1 gm of aspirin. The recommended initial dosage of these salicylates, when used as anti-inflammatory agents, is 3 gm or more. Depending on the tablet size prescribed, this amount can be delivered with two or three tablets given two or three times daily.

A different type of chemical modification of the salicylate molecule is diflunisal (Dolobid), which was the result of an extensive synthesis program and an exhaustive study of some 500 novel salicylic acid derivatives.[29] It has been shown to have analgesic, antipyretic, and anti-inflammatory properties, to be well tolerated, and to have value in the treatment of osteoarthritis.[29–31] Because of its longer duration of action, diflunisal can be given twice daily. The recommended dose is 500 to 1000 mg daily.

In the treatment of osteoarthritis, the dose of aspirin depends on the therapeutic goal. For anti-inflammatory effects, blood levels between 20 and 30 mg/100 ml are usually desired, requiring doses between 3 and 5 gm daily.

Table 18–7. ADVERSE REACTIONS TO AND DRUG INTERACTIONS OF SALICYLATES

Adverse Reactions
  Acute toxicity: respiratory alkalosis and metabolic acidosis
  Chronic toxicity: reversible tinnitus and hearing loss
  Gastrointestinal dyspepsia, bleeding, ulcer, and perforation
  Hepatotoxicity
  Hypersensitivity: acute asthma, hypotension, nasal polyps
  Hemostatic effects

Drug Interactions
  Enhancement of oral anticoagulant, hypoglycemic, uricosuric, and anticonvulsant drug effects
  Potentiation of pancytopenia from methotrexate
  Reduction of plasma salicylate levels by corticosteroids

However, the amount of aspirin required to achieve therapeutic concentrations varies widely, so that the dose must be individualized for each patient. The maximum tolerated dose must be approached slowly, because it may take a week with each dosage change to achieve a new steady-state level.

Toxicity and Drug Interactions

In using prolonged, high doses of aspirin or salicylates, the physician must be constantly on the alert for the earliest signs of toxicity (Table 18–7). Acute salicylate intoxication is manifested as a disturbance of acid-base balance; respiratory alkalosis and metabolic acidosis occur either singly or in combination.[27] The severity of acidosis is greater from poisoning due to chronic aspirin administration than from that due to acute ingestion. Chronic salicylate intoxication produces reversible ototoxicity, with ringing (tinnitus) and hearing loss. When these signs occur, the drug should be stopped for 24 hours, and then resumed at a slightly lower dosage.

Gastrointestinal intolerance is the major cause of salicylate withdrawal. Aspirin is a known gastric irritant, and its effects can range from minor gastric upset and mucosal irritation and erosion to initiation and exacerbation of gastric ulcers, and life-threatening, massive hemorrhage.[26] It is important to note that aspirin-induced gastric lesions and ulcerations are unpredictable and may exist without symptoms or complaints.

When aspirin is taken with food or milk, gastric tolerance is often improved. There is no conclusive evidence that buffered salicylate preparations cause less gastrointestinal bleeding; however, they may result in less dyspepsia in certain patients. Enteric-coated and cation salicylates may be cautiously used in patients with a history of peptic ulcer. As with the administration of all salicylates, serum salicylate levels should be monitored periodically to ensure adequate anti-inflammatory concentrations.

Serious hypersensitivity to aspirin is manifested by asthma and hypotension but is rarely encountered. Minor sensitivity, such as swelling of nasal mucous membranes and nasal polyps, is more common.

The types of hemostatic effects that may occur with salicylate intoxication include decreased prothrombin formation, decreased Factor VII production, increased capillary fragility, decreased platelet adhesiveness, and decreased platelet levels.[27] Measurement of prothrombin time may disclose a small but significant elevation. Despite these changes, clinical manifestations are rarely observed, except in patients with underlying hemorrhagic disorders. Aspirin is also one of several drugs associated with hemolytic anemia due to glucose-6-phosphate dehydrogenase deficiency.[20]

Of the many interactions between salicylates and other drugs, the most important clinically are enhancement of oral anticoagulant, hypoglycemic, uricosuric, and anticonvulsant drug effects by displacing them from protein binding sites. Aspirin, particularly in anti-inflammatory quantities, potentiates the bone marrow toxicity of methotrexate by displacing it from protein binding sites and by decreasing its urinary excretion, thereby resulting in a significant increase in free drug.

In patients maintained on both salicylates and adrenocorticosteroids, caution must be exercised when steroids are tapered and withdrawn.[28] Steroids increase the renal clearance of salicylates. Consequently, their abrupt reduction or withdrawal may precipitate salicylate toxicity.

PHENYLBUTAZONE AND OXYPHENBUTAZONE

Phenylbutazone, like aspirin, has a broad spectrum of clinical application in the rheumatic diseases. Oxyphenbutazone, a hydroxylated metabolite, has similar activity to the parent compound. These drugs should not be considered as simple analgesics and should never be administered casually. Both drugs are closely related chemically and pharmacologically, including adverse effects, to the pyrazolines amidopyrine and antipyrine.

Therapeutic Limitations

Phenylbutazone and oxyphenbutazone have been used for a number of years in the treatment of osteoarthritis. Recently, however, their usage has been restricted to the short-term treatment of acute attacks of osteoarthritis of the hips and knees not responsive to other treatment. Consequently, they are best reserved for short periods of time in controlling acute exacerbations that are unresponsive to salicylates or other anti-inflammatory agents.[1, 32] The recommended dose is 300 to 400 mg daily for 5 to 7 days, followed by gradually decreasing doses for another 7 to 10 days.[1, 32]

Side Effects

The major hazard of phenylbutazone and oxyphenbutazone lies in the development of fatal blood dyscrasias.[33] These are manifested in two major forms. The first is agranulocytosis, which appears to be an idiosyncratic reaction that is not dose-dependent. The second is aplastic anemia, which occurs more often in patients over the age of 55 and more frequently when the drug has been taken for prolonged periods, especially in high doses. Oxyphenbutazone, initially believed to be safer than phenylbutazone, causes twice as many deaths.[33] The reason for this discrepancy is unknown.

As osteoarthritis may require years of medication, notably in the elderly, the following warnings should be considered before prescribing these two drugs. If these drugs are administered on a long-term basis, hematologic studies should be performed at least every other week for 6 weeks, and then monthly. Hematologic toxicity may appear suddenly and is manifested by anemia, leukopenia, thrombocytopenia, and purpura. Any significant change in the total white count, a relative decrease in granulocytes, the appearance of immature forms, a drop in platelet count, or a fall in hematocrit should signal immediate cessation of therapy and a complete hematologic investigation.

With prolonged use, phenylbutazone and oxyphenbutazone carry a high risk of duodenal ulcers and fluid retention.[34] Furthermore, they may be associated with many of the side effects listed in Table 18-5, and they are also listed among the few antirheumatic drugs, the others being intramuscular gold and penicillamine, that can induce a lupus-like syndrome.[35] Reports associating these pyrazoline drugs with leukemia have appeared. However, a cause-and-effect relationship has not been clearly established.

Drug Interactions

Although oxyphenbutazone plasma levels may be increased considerably by anabolic steroids, phenylbutazone levels are not affected.[36] Desipramine and other tricyclic antidepressants, as well as cholestyramine, inhibit the absorption of phenylbutazone and oxyphenbutazone.

The most important interactions occur with coumarin anticoagulants and with anticonvulsants, which are displaced from binding sites, with consequent potentiation of their effects. Phenylbutazone also interacts with sulfonamides, insulin, and oral hypoglycemic drugs, thereby prolonging their half-life.[36] Displacement of plasma protein-bound thyroid hormone by phenylbutazone and oxyphenbutazone may interfere with the interpretation of thyroid function tests.[37]

INDOMETHACIN

Indomethacin became available for clinical trials in November 1961. Its promise derived from its unique pharmacology as a synthetic indole compound with potent analgesic, antipyretic, and anti-inflammatory properties.[38] In 1965, after 4 years of clinical trials in the United States, indomethacin became available for general prescription. By then, a great deal of clinical investigation had supported its effectiveness in the treatment of osteoarthritis.[38-41]

Therapeutic Application

Indomethacin cannot be considered a simple analgesic and should be used only in conditions for which it is recommended. Its anti-inflammatory activity is likely related to its ability to inhibit cyclo-oxygenase, the enzyme that initiates the conversion of arachidonic acid into prostaglandins. In fact, this enzyme inhibition is so powerful that indomethacin has become the standard reference drug for this effect.[38]

Because of indomethacin's potential to cause adverse reactions, particularly at high doses, its use in osteoarthritis should be carefully considered for active disease unresponsive to an adequate trial of aspirin. Indomethacin is especially effective in patients with moderate to severe hip involvement, for which higher than usual doses may be needed.[39–42] Although hip pain may be reduced and mobility may be improved for relatively long periods, underlying progression of disease may be unaffected.[40]

The usual starting dose of indomethacin is 25 mg two or three times daily, which can be gradually increased, if necessary, by 25-mg increments. An adequate response is usually achieved with a total daily dose of 150 mg or less, so that it is rarely necessary to give the maximum dose of 200 mg daily.[38] Increased dosage tends to increase side effects, particularly with doses of 150 to 200 mg daily, usually without a corresponding increase in clinical benefits. As symptoms subside, the dose of indomethacin should be decreased whenever possible so as to maintain the lowest possible effective dose for the individual patient. Indomethacin is currently available as 25- and 50-mg capsules and as a 75-mg sustained-release capsule (see Table 18–3). In some other countries, a 5 mg/ml oral suspension, and both 50-mg and 100-mg suppositories are available.[34] Indomethacin should always be given with food or an antacid to reduce the possibility of gastric irritation. Careful attention to and observation of the patient are essential to the prevention of serious adverse reactions, especially in the aging patient.

Side Effects

The most common side effects are those of the gastrointestinal tract and the central nervous system.[38] Various gastrointestinal adverse reactions occur in 3% to 9% of patients, but serious problems such as peptic ulcer, major hemorrhage, or perforation occur in less than 1%. Migraine-like headaches occur in 10% of patients; these may subside with elimination of the early-morning dose or with reduction of the total daily dosage.[41] Other central nervous system side effects include dizziness, vertigo, somnolence, fatigue, and depression. Somnolence and depression may appear gradually and can thus be easily overlooked. These reactions are cause for withdrawal of indometh-

acin. Indomethacin may mask the usual signs of inflammation and should be used with extra caution in the presence of coexisting infection.[38]

Drug Interactions

Indomethacin does not influence the hypoprothrombinemia produced by anticoagulants.[43] However, patients receiving the latter drugs should be observed closely for alterations in prothrombin time while on indomethacin.[38] Care should also be taken in giving indomethacin to patients receiving probenecid, because plasma levels of indomethacin are likely to increase when both drugs are administered simultaneously.[44] Although the magnitude of this effect is presently uncertain, it does not seem to be appreciable, based on current clinical practice.[37] However, by reduction of renal lithium clearance, indomethacin may produce a clinically relevant elevation of plasma lithium. Consequently, when both drugs are used simultaneously, the patient should be carefully observed for signs of lithium toxicity. Indomethacin can also reduce the natriuretic and antihypertensive effects of furosemide.[45] A patient receiving both drugs should be observed closely to determine if the desired effects of furosemide are obtained. Indomethacin blocks furosemide-induced increase in plasma renin activity. This should be considered when evaluating plasma renin activity in hypertensive patients. Other prostaglandin-inhibiting anti-inflammatory drugs probably produce similar effects.[46] Consequently, hypertensive patients should be given anti-inflammatory agents with caution and should be monitored frequently for inhibition of antihypertensive drug response.

TOLMETIN SODIUM AND SULINDAC

Both of these drugs are chemically related to indomethacin. The essential feature that distinguishes tolmetin sodium from indomethacin is the substitution of a pyrrole ring for the indole nucleus in the hope of eliminating many of the serotonin-like side effects of indomethacin.[26, 47] Sulindac is an indene acetic acid derivative whose pharmacologic effects are mediated through one of its principal metabolites, a sulfide reversibly formed from the parent sulfoxide.[48]

Tolmetin Sodium

This agent has been compared favorably with indomethacin and high doses of aspirin for the treatment of osteoarthritis affecting the knee or the hip.[49] Therapy should be initiated with 1200 mg daily in three or four equally divided doses, preferably including a dose on arising and one at bedtime. Subsequently, the dosage should be titrated to optimal therapeutic effect but not to exceed 2000 mg daily (see Table 18–3).

Gastrointestinal complaints are the adverse effects most often encountered, but these occur at a frequency and intensity generally less than those caused by aspirin.[47] Headache and dizziness are the chief side effects affecting the central nervous system but are less troublesome than those that occur with indomethacin. False-positive tests for proteinuria can result from the use of methods involving acid precipitation in patients receiving tolmetin sodium. Consequently, tests for urinary protein should be performed by other methods such as heat coagulation or the dipstick test.

Acute interstitial nephritis and reversible renal failure have been reported with tolmetin.[50, 51] It differs from the renal papillary necrosis seen with phenacetin because it occurs suddenly after short-term therapy and is reversible on discontinuation of tolmetin. An important clue to this form of nephritis is the presence of eosinophils in the urine.

Sulindac

The discovery of sulindac culminated a prolonged search for a new drug with a potency comparable to that of indomethacin but with improved patient tolerance.[52] Sulindac is well absorbed following oral administration in humans, and its active sulfide metabolite rapidly appears in plasma.[48] Sustained plasma levels of the sulfide metabolite are achieved by extensive plasma binding, absence of renal excretion, enterohepatic circulation, and reversible metabolism. Unlike tolmetin sodium, which has a short half-life of 4.5 to 6 hours, sulindac, by virtue of its active metabolite, has a half-life of 16 hours.

Therapeutically, doses of 100 to 200 mg twice daily are effective in the relief of pain and inflammation in osteoarthritis.[52–56] The daily dosage should not exceed 400 mg (see Table 18–3). Sulindac is particularly effective in the treatment of osteoarthritis of the hip, knee, or cervical spine.[56] At comparable antiinflammatory doses, it is clearly better tolerated than aspirin.[56]

The most frequently reported adverse reactions are those affecting the gastrointestinal tract.[52] These are often mild and occur early in the course of treatment. Peptic ulcer and major gastrointestinal bleeding have been reported only rarely. Occasionally, elevations of liver function tests also occur. Other side effects include dizziness, vertigo, headache, somnolence, insomnia, sweating, asthenia, and tinnitus. Rash, pruritus, stomatitis, and hypersensitivity reactions have occurred infrequently. Rare adverse reactions include pneumonitis,[57] agranulocytosis,[58] and a pernio-like reaction.[59] The last side effect is manifested as painful toes with a condition resembling pernio or chilblains, with swelling, purple discoloration, red papules, and desquamation of the distal skin of the toes. Its resemblance to certain cryophenomena found in connective tissue and vasculitic disorders suggests that some sort of immune mechanism may be operative. The lesions promptly resolve with discontinuation of the drug.

More recently, the administration of sulindac has been reported to cause an unusual set of severe adverse reactions characterized by fever and by skin and visceral organ involvement.[60] The rash may take the form of maculopapular, blistering, and desquamating eruptions. Hepatomegaly, jaundice, and disordered liver function studies are noted. Central nervous system symptoms, along with confusion, pulmonary involvement, and lymphadenopathy, occur in various patients affected. Recurrence of symptoms upon re-exposure to the drug confirmed a causative relationship in several patients. Resolution of symptoms followed drug withdrawal, although death has occurred. The mechanism by which sulindac produces these reactions is unclear.

PROPIONIC ACID DERIVATIVES

These drugs are related chemically to a group of phenylalkanoic acid compounds studied during the early 1960's.[61] Before its withdrawal from the British market, one of these agents, ibufenac, was shown to have antiinflammatory properties. This finding led to a search for safer, equally potent drugs of the same class. Although several of these drugs are available in other countries, only three are available in the United States. These are ibuprofen, introduced in 1974, and fenoprofen calcium and naproxen, both marketed in 1976 (see Table 18–6). Benoxaprofen, released in 1982, was withdrawn from the market because of serious adverse renal, hepatic, and gastrointestinal reactions possibly related to its administration.

Ibuprofen

The clinical efficacy of ibuprofen in the treatment of osteoarthritis is well established.[61–65] It has anti-inflammatory properties similar to those of aspirin, almost milligram for milligram.[61] Early trials of ibuprofen used inadequate anti-inflammatory doses of up to 1200 mg.[66] Subsequent studies, in which daily doses up to 2400 mg were used, finally established its role as an effective anti-inflammatory agent.[67, 68] Consequently, the usual recommended daily dosage of ibuprofen is 1.6 to 2.4 gm. Because of its relatively short half-life of approximately 2 hours, the drug is usually prescribed three or four times daily. However, a preliminary trial showed that ibuprofen proved to be just as effective when administered only twice daily.[69] Whatever the mode of administration, the maximum daily dosage should not exceed 2.4 gm (see Table 18–3).

Fenoprofen

Experience with fenoprofen has established its usefulness in the treatment of patients with osteoarthritis.[70–74] The usual anti-inflammatory starting dose is 600 mg given four times daily. Lower maintenance doses can often be used subsequently.[70] The dosage of fenoprofen given in a single day should not exceed 3.2 gm (see Table 18–3).

Naproxen

Like other propionic acid derivatives, naproxen is well tolerated and rarely causes serious adverse reactions. Unlike ibuprofen and fenoprofen, however, it has a relatively longer biologic half-life, averaging 13 hours, and is therefore ideally suited for twice-daily administration.[75] Much of its success rests on its dosage convenience, thus facilitating good patient compliance. The efficacy of naproxen in the treatment of osteoarthritis is well documented.[75–80] The usual starting dose is 500 to 750 mg/day, and the recommended daily maximum dose is 1000 mg (see Table 18–3).

Toxicity

The propionic acid derivatives are better tolerated than aspirin when the latter is given in anti-inflammatory quantities. Consequently, they are often selected first when aspirin fails or intolerance proves to be a problem in a given patient. Although the propionic acid derivatives are chemically related, lack of effect of any one does not necessarily mean ineffectiveness of any other in an individual patient.[61] Similarly, side effects from one may not occur when another is used in the same patient.

The pattern of side effects from the propionic acid derivatives is similar to that of other nonsteroidal anti-inflammatory drugs (see Table 18–5). Consequently, they are contraindicated in patients with active peptic ulceration. They should be given with caution to patients with any form of bronchospasm and should be avoided in patients who are allergic to aspirin or other nonsteroidal anti-inflammatory drugs. Long-term studies have failed to show any appreciable adverse effects on the liver or bone marrow. As a result, with these nonsteroidal anti-inflammatory drugs there is less need to monitor patients with serial hematologic laboratory studies. Periodic evaluation of the urine and serum creatinine are indicated to detect evidence of functional renal impairment or more severe renal toxic reactions, as described earlier in this chapter.

Gastrointestinal symptoms are the most common adverse reactions observed with most of the propionic acid derivatives.[61, 70, 75] These include nausea, dyspepsia, and vomiting, but major gastrointestinal problems are uncommon. Skin rash is rare.

Drug Interactions

The propionic acid derivatives do not interfere with anticoagulant therapy. They may, however, decrease platelet aggregation and prolong bleeding time. These effects should be considered when bleeding times are determined. The administration of naproxen may result in increased urinary values for 17-ketogenic steroids because of an interaction between the drug and its metabolites with *m*-dinitrobenzene used in this assay. Although

17-hydroxycorticosteroid measurements do not appear to be artificially altered, it is recommended that therapy with naproxen be temporarily discontinued 72 hours before adrenal function tests are performed.

There may be interaction with each of the propionic acid derivatives when used concomitantly with aspirin.[70, 75] For this reason, the use of aspirin with any of these drugs is generally not recommended. The clinical magnitude of this effect is uncertain.

MECLOFENAMATE SODIUM

Meclofenamate is the sodium salt of meclofenamic acid, the only member of the fenamate series to be approved in the United States. Besides inhibiting prostaglandin synthesis, the drug also competes with prostaglandins for binding at the prostaglandin receptor site, a property characteristic of the fenamates. The biologic half-life of meclofenamate is less than 4 hours, so that the drug is usually administered four times daily.

Therapeutic Place

Meclofenamate sodium is effective for the relief of both acute and chronic osteoarthritis.[81-83] However, it is not recommended as the initial drug for treatment because of gastrointestinal side effects, including diarrhea, which is sometimes severe.

The dosage of meclofenamate sodium is 200 to 400 mg daily, administered in three or four equal doses. The smallest dose that provides clinical control should be employed. Consequently, therapy should be initiated at the lower dosage of 200 mg daily and should then be increased as necessary to improve clinical effectiveness, but it should not exceed 400 mg daily (see Table 18–3). Although improvement may be obtained within a few days, 2 or 3 weeks of treatment may be necessary to obtain optimal benefit in some patients. After a satisfactory response has been achieved, a lower dosage may suffice for long-term therapy. To avoid gastrointestinal upset, it is best to administer meclofenamate sodium with meals, milk, or antacids. Mild gastrointestinal complaints may be relieved by reducing the daily dosage. However, for severe diarrhea or other major toxicity, meclofenamate therapy should be terminated.

Precautions and Interactions

Patients receiving meclofenamate sodium should be evaluated periodically to insure that the drug is still necessary and tolerated. They should also be advised that rash, nausea, vomiting, abdominal pain, and diarrhea are common side effects. Patients receiving long-term therapy should have periodic hemoglobin and hematocrit determinations, especially if signs or symptoms of anemia occur. Serum transaminase and alkaline phosphatase levels as well as serum creatinine and BUN levels may occasionally be elevated in patients receiving prolonged therapy.[84]

Meclofenamate sodium enhances the effect of warfarin. It should therefore be avoided in patients receiving warfarin therapy. The additional administration of aspirin with meclofenamate may lower the plasma levels of the latter. This effect does not occur with the concomitant use of propoxyphene or with antacids and meclofenamate.

PIROXICAM

Piroxicam is an oxicam, a new and different antirheumatic agent with a prolonged plasma half-life of 38 hours.[85] Its anti-inflammatory effects are more than likely due to its ability to inhibit the activity of prostaglandin synthetase.[86] With prolonged administration, the presence of multiple drug peaks suggests enterohepatic recycling of piroxicam.

Efficacy

Long-term effectiveness along with ease of administration makes piroxicam acceptable for long-term treatment of osteoarthritis.[80, 86-91] The recommended starting dose is 10 mg given once daily, which can be increased, if necessary, to a maximum dose of 20 mg/day. The advantage of a once-daily dose is that it is especially suitable for patients who are prone to noncompliance.

Adverse Reactions

Gastrointestinal reactions are the most common adverse reactions to piroxicam, being observed in about 20% of patients.[86] These include peptic ulceration (less than 1%) and occasional gastrointestinal bleeding, each of which are clearly dose-related. Consequently, patients should be closely supervised for gastrointestinal side effects, and doses greater than 20 mg daily should not be used (see Table 18–3).

Piroxicam is highly protein-bound and may therefore displace other protein-bound drugs, such as coumarin anticoagulants and nonsteroidal anti-inflammatory drugs. Although the coadministration of aspirin and piroxicam produces changes in the plasma concentrations of either drug, this effect does not appear to be clinically significant.[86] Nevertheless, the dosage of drugs that are highly protein-bound should be carefully monitored when used in conjunction with piroxicam. Changes in laboratory parameters observed during prolonged piroxicam therapy include bleeding time, platelet and white blood cell counts, hemoglobin and hematocrit, and both hepatic and renal function.

OTHER DRUGS USED IN THE TREATMENT OF OSTEOARTHRITIS

In evaluating claims for novel forms of treatment, it must be remembered that osteoarthritis is a disorder of fluctuating signs and symptoms.[33] Moreover, there is no constant correlation between roentgenologic changes and physical signs, few absolute objective measurements of disease progress, and a strong tendency for patients to respond to placebo therapy.

Systemic Adrenocorticosteroids

Although there has been considerable emphasis recently on the inflammatory component of osteoarthritis, long-term systemic corticosteroid therapy has no part to play in its control.[92] When steroids were first introduced, it was believed that their anti-inflammatory properties might also produce appropriate analgesia in osteoarthritis. However, the equivocal results derived from such therapy, the major potential toxicity from their long-term use, and the relatively benign nature of most forms of osteoarthritis contraindicate their general use in this disorder.[1]

Antirheumatic Drugs

The potent antirheumatic drugs available for rheumatoid arthritis and other rheumatic disorders, such as gold, antimalarial agents, penicillamine, and immunosuppressive agents, have no role in the treatment of osteoarthritis.[33]

Other Forms of Drug Therapy

The oral or intravenous administration of procaine is of no benefit in osteoarthritis but can cause serious toxicity. Therapy with vitamins, calcium, thyroid hormone, or estrogens is of no value.

Intramuscular injections of extracts of bovine cartilage (Catrix-S) have been held to be beneficial.[93] However, no controlled studies have yet been reported.[33] The combination of calf cartilage and bone marrow extract (Rumalon) given by intramuscular injection is widely used in Eurpoe[33] but rarely in the United States.[94] Double-blind controlled investigation has shown some benefit in patients with hip involvement, although at the same time highlighting the high placebo response rate that can be obtained in such trials.[95]

References

1. Moskowitz RW: Treatment of osteoarthritis. *In* McCarty DJ (ed.): Arthritis and Allied Conditions. Philadelphia, Lea and Febiger, 1979, pp. 1181–1186.
2. Ouslander JG: Drug therapy in the elderly. Ann Intern Med 95:711–722, 1981.
3. Marchant B: Pharmacokinetic factors influencing variability in human drug response. Scand J Rheumatol [Suppl] 39:5–14, 1981.
4. Williamson J: Adverse reactions to prescribed drugs in the elderly. *In* Crooks J, Stevenson IH (eds.): Drugs and the Elderly. Baltimore, University Park Press, 1979, p. 243.
5. Moskowitz RW, Goldberg VM, Rosner JA, et al.: Specific drug therapy of experimental osteoarthritis. Semin Arthritis Rheum 11:127–129, 1981.
6. Walton ES, Stevens RW, Ghosh P, et al.: Nonsteroidal antiinflammatory drugs (NSAIDs) and articular cartilage integrity. Semin Arthritis Rheum 11:147–149, 1981.
7. Peyron J: Inflammation in osteoarthritis: Review of its role in clinical picture, disease progress, subsets, and pathophysiology. Semin Arthritis Rheum 11:115–116, 1981.
8. Bullough P: Synovial osseous inflammation in osteoarthritis. Semin Arthritis Rheum 11:146, 1981.
9. Huskisson EC: Routine drug treatment of rheumatoid arthritis and other rheumatic diseases. Clin Rheum Dis 5:697–706, 1979.
10. Kantor TG: Analgesics for arthritis. Clin Rheum Dis 6:525–531, 1980.
11. Huskisson EC, Woolf DL, Balme HW, et al.: Four new anti-inflammatory drugs; responses and variations. Br Med J 1:1048–1049, 1976.
12. Huskisson EC: Classification of anti-rheumatic drugs. Clin Rheum Dis 5:353–357, 1979.

13. Hart FD: Osteoarthrosis. *In* Hart FD (ed.): Drug Treatment of the Rheumatic Diseases. Baltimore, University Park Press, 1978, p. 114.

14. Bollet AJ: Analgesic and anti-inflammatory drugs in the therapy of osteoarthritis. Semin Arthritis Rheum 11:130–132, 1981.

15. Collins GB, Kiefer KS: Propoxyphene dependence: An update. Postgrad Med 70:57–61, 1981.

16. Kimberly RP, Plotz PH: Aspirin-induced depression of renal function. N Engl J Med 296:418–424, 1977.

17. Brezin JH, et al.: Reversible renal failure and nephrotic syndrome associated with nonsteroidal anti-inflammatory drugs. N Engl J Med 301:1271, 1979.

18. Walshe JJ, Venutuo RC: Acute oliguric renal failure induced by indomethacin: Possible mechanism. Ann Intern Med 91:47–49, 1979.

19. Wendland ML, Wagoner RD, Holley KE: Renal failure associated with fenoprofen. Mayo Clin Proc 55:103–107, 1980.

20. Buchanan WW, Rooney PJ, Rennie JAN: Aspirin and the salicylates. Clin Rheum Dis 5:499–539, 1979.

21. Levy G: Clinical pharmacokinetics of aspirin. Pediatrics 62:867–872, 1978.

22. Champion MD, Day RO, Graham GG, et al.: Salicylates in rheumatoid arthritis. Clin Rheum Dis 2:245–265, 1975.

23. Paulus HE, Siegel M, Mongan E, et al.: Variations of serum concentrations and half-life of salicylate in patients with rheumatoid arthritis. Arthritis Rheum 14:527–532, 1971.

24. Rich RR, Johnson JS: Salicylate hepatotoxicity in patients with juvenile rheumatoid arthritis. Arthritis Rheum 16:1–9, 1973.

25. Rowland M, Riegelman S: Pharmacokinetics of acetylsalicylic acid and salicylic acid after intravenous administration in man. J Pharm Sci 57:1313–1319, 1968.

26. Roth SH: Salicylates: Revolution versus evolution. *In* Roth SH (ed.): New Directions in Arthritis Therapy. Littleton, Massachusetts, PSG Publishing Co., Inc., 1980, pp. 23–36.

27. Temple AR: Pathophysiology of aspirin overdosage toxicity, with implications for management. Pediatrics 62:873–876, 1978.

28. Klinenberg JR, Miller F: Effect of corticosteroids on blood salicylate concentration. JAMA 194:601–604, 1965.

29. Van Winzum C, Verhaest L: Diflunisal. Clin Rheum Dis 5:707–731, 1979.

30. Andrew A, Rodda B, Verhaest L, et al.:Diflunisal: Six-month experience in osteoarthritis. Br J Clin Pharmacol 4:45S–52S, 1977.

31. Dieppe PA, Huskisson EC: Diflunisal and aspirin. A comparison of efficacy and nephrotoxicity in osteoarthritis. Rheumatol Rehabil 18:53–56, 1979.

32. Robinson WD: Management of degenerative joint disease. *In* Kelley WN, Harris ED Jr, Ruddy S, Sledge CB (eds.): Textbook of Rheumatology. Philadelphia, W.B. Saunders Company, 1981, pp. 1491–1499.

33. Haslock I: Medical treatment of osteoarthritis. Clin Rheum Dis 2:615–625, 1976.

34. Turner R: Aspirin and newer anti-inflammatory agents in rheumatoid arthritis. Am Fam Physician 16:111–115, 1977.

35. Alarcon-Segovia D: Drug-induced systemic lupus erythematosus and related syndromes. Clin Rheum Dis 1:573–582, 1975.

36. Fowler P: Phenylbutazone and indomethacin. Clin Rheum Dis 1:267–283, 1975.

37. Hart FC, Huskisson ED, Ansell BM: Non-steroidal anti-inflammatory analgesics. *In* Hart FE (ed.): Drug Treatment of the Rheumatic Diseases. Baltimore, University Park Press, 1978, pp. 8–43.

38. Rhymer AR, Gengos DC: Indomethacin. Clin Rheum Dis 5:541–552, 1979.

39. Wanka J, Dixon A St J: Treatment of osteoarthritis of the hip with indomethacin. Ann Rheum Dis 23:288–294, 1964.

40. Hodgkinson R, Woolf D: A five year clinical trial of indomethacin in osteoarthritis of the hip. Practitioner 210: 392–396, 1973.

41. Calabro JJ: Long-term reappraisal of indomethacin. Drug Therapy 5:46–60, 1975.

42. Mills JA: Nonsteroidal anti-inflammatory drugs. II. N Engl J Med 290:1002–1005, 1974.

43. Vessel ES, Passananti GT, Johnson AO: Failure of indomethacin and warfarin to interact in normal human volunteers. J Clin Pharmacol 15:486–495, 1975.

44. Brooks PM, Bell MA, Sturrock RD, et al.: The clinical significance of indomethacin-probenecid interaction. Br J Clin Pharmacol 1:287–290, 1974.

45. Brooks PM, Bell MA, Lee P, et al.: The effect of furosemide on indomethacin plasma levels. Br J Clin Pharmacol 1:485–489, 1974.

46. Hansten PD: Furosemide and indomethacin. Drug Interactions Newsletter 1:1–3, 1980.

47. Ehrlich GE: Tolmetin sodium: Meeting the clinical challenge. Clin Rheum Dis 5:481–497, 1979.

48. Kwan KC, Duggan DE: Pharmacokinetics of sulindac. Acta Rhum Belg 1:168–178, 1977.

49. Rau R, Lobsiger M, Gross D: Tolmetin treatment in patients with osteoarthritis of the hip and the knee. Scand J Rheumatol 4:510–512, 1975.

50. Katz SM, Capaldo R, Everts EA, et al.: Tolmetin. Association with reversible renal failure and acute interstitial nephritis. JAMA 246:243–245, 1981.

51. Chatterjee GP: Nephrotic syndrome induced by tolmetin. JAMA 246:1589, 1981.

52. Rhymer AR: Sulindac. Clin Rheum Dis 5:553–568, 1979.

53. Gengos D: Long term experience with sulindac in the treatment of osteoarthritis. Eur J Rheumatol Inflamm 1:51–54, 1978.

54. Bordier PH, Kuntz D: Sulindac: Clinical results of treatment of osteoarthritis. Eur J Rheumatol Inflamm 1:27–30, 1978.

55. Calabro JJ, Andelman SY, Caldwell JR, et al.: A multicenter trial of sulindac in osteoarthritis of the hip. Clin Pharmacol Ther 22:358–363, 1977.

56. Andelman SY: Long-term double-blind comparison of sulindac and aspirin in the treatment of osteoarthritis. *In* Talbott JH (ed.): Clinical Evaluations of Clinoril. New York, McGraw-Hill, 1979, pp. 21–32.

57. Fein M: Sulindac and pneumonitis. Ann Intern Med 95:245, 1981.

58. Romeril KR, Dube DS, Hollings PE: Sulindac-induced agranulocytosis and bone marrow culture. Lancet 2:523, 1981.

59. Reinertsen JL: Unusual pernio-like reaction to sulindac. Arthritis Rheum 24:1215, 1981.

60. Park GD, Spector R, Headstream T, et al.: Serious adverse reactions associated with sulindac. Arch Intern Med 142:1292–1294, 1982.

61. Kantor TG: Diagnosis and treatment: Drugs five years later. Ibuprofen. Ann Intern Med 91:877–882, 1979.

62. Royer GL Jr, Moxley TE, Hearron MS, et al.: A six-month double-blind trial of ibuprofen and indomethacin in osteoarthritis. Curr Ther Res 17:234–248, 1975.

63. Adams SS, Warwich Buckler J: Ibuprofen and flurbiprofen. Clin Rheum Dis 5:359–379, 1979.

64. Brackertz B, Busson M: Comparative trial of sulindac (Clinoril) and ibuprofen (Brufen) in osteoarthrosis. Br J Clin Pract 32:77–80, 1978.

65. Siegmeth W, Sieberer W: A comparison of the short-term effects of ibuprofen and diclofenac in spondylosis. J Int Med Res 6:369–374, 1978.

66. Brooks CD, Schlagel CA, Sekhar NC, et al.: Tolerance and pharmacology of ibuprofen. Curr Ther Res 15:180–190, 1973.

67. Godfrey R, de la Cruz S: Effect of ibuprofen dosage on patient response in rheumatoid arthritis. Arthritis Rheum 18:135–137, 1975.

68. Blechman WJ, Schmid FR, April PA, et al.: Ibuprofen or aspirin in rheumatoid arthritis therapy. JAMA 233:336–340, 1975.

69. Brugueras NE, LeZotte LA: Ibuprofen: A double-blind comparison of twice-a-day therapy with four-times-a-day therapy. Clin Ther 2:13–21, 1978.

70. Ridolfo AS, Nickander R, Mikulaschek WM: Fenoprofen and benoxaprofen. Clin Rheum Dis 5:393–410, 1979.

71. Wojtulewski JA, Hart FD, Huskisson EC: Fenoprofen in treatment of osteoarthrosis of hips and knee. Br Med J 2:475–476, 1974.

72. Brooke JW: Fenoprofen therapy in large-joint osteoarthritis: Double blind comparison with aspirin and long term experience. J Rheumatol 3(Suppl 2):71–75, 1976.

73. Diamond HS: Double-blind crossover study of fenoprofen and aspirin in osteoarthritis. J Rheumatol 3(Suppl 2):67–70, 1976.

74. McMahon FG, Jain A, Onel A: Controlled evaluation of fenoprofen in geriatric patients with osteoarthritis. J Rheumatol 3(Suppl 2):76–82, 1976.

75. Segre EJ: Naproxen. Clin Rheum Dis 5:411–426, 1979.

76. Blechman WJ, Willkens R, Boncaldo GL, et al.: Naproxen in osteoarthritis: Double-blind crossover trial. Ann Rheum Dis 37:80–84, 1978.

77. Clark AK, Barnes CG, Goodman HV, et al.: A double-blind comparison of naproxen against indomethacin in osteoarthrosis. Drug Res 25:302–304, 1975.

78. Melton JW, Lussier A, Ward JR, et al.: Naproxen vs. aspirin in osteoarthritis of the hip and knee. J Rheumatol 5:338–346, 1978.

79. Blechman WJ: Crossover comparison of benoxaprofen and naproxen in osteoarthritis. J Rheumatol 7(Suppl 6):116–124, 1980.

80. Hybbinette CH: Piroxicam and naproxen in the treatment of osteoarthritis. Br J Clin Pract 35:30–34, 1981.

81. Dresner AJ: Multicenter studies with sodium meclofenamate (Meclomen) in the United States and Canada. Curr Ther Res 23:S90–S106, 1978.

82. Schleyer I: European studies of sodium meclofenamate (Meclomen) in the treatment of osteoarthritis. Curr Ther Res 23:S121–S125, 1978.

83. Eberl R: European studies of sodium meclofenamate (Meclomen) in long-term treatment. Curr Ther Res 23:S131–S137, 1978.

84. Preston SN: Safety of sodium meclofenamate (Meclomen). Curr Ther Res 23:S107–S112, 1978.

85. Hobbs DC, Twomey TM: Piroxicam pharmacokinetics in man; aspirin and anatcid interaction studies. J Clin Pharmacol 19:270–281, 1979.

86. Wiseman EH, Boyle JA: Piroxicam (Feldene). Clin Rheum Dis 6:585–613, 1980.

87. Dessain P, Estabrooks TF, Gordon AJ: Piroxicam in the treatment of osteoarthritis; a multicentre study in general practice involving 1218 patients. J Int Med Res 7:335–343, 1979.

88. Telhag H: Safety and efficacy of piroxicam in the treatment of osteoarthrosis. Eur J Rheumatol Inflamm 1:352–355, 1978.

89. Zizic TM, Sutton JD, Stevens MB: Piroxicam and osteoarthritis; a controlled study. Soc Med Int Cong Symp Ser 1:71–82, 1978.

90. Gordon AJ, Estabrooks TF, Dessain P: Treatment of osteoarthrosis with piroxicam in general practice: Long-term follow-up in a multicentre study. J Int Med Res 8:375–381, 1980.

91. Kantor TG: Report. Pharmacology, efficacy, and safety of a new class of anti-inflammatory agents: A review of piroxicam. Am J Med 72:1–90, 1982.

92. Hart FD: Corticosteroid therapy in the rheumatic disorders. Clin Rheum Dis 6:533–543, 1980.

93. Prudden JF, Balassa LL: The biological activity of bovine cartilage preparations. Semin Arthritis Rheum 3:287–321, 1974.

94. Denko CW: Treatment of osteoarthritis with Rumalon R. Arthritis Rheum 21:494–496, 1978.

95. Dixon A St J, Kersley GD, Mercer R, et al.: A double-blind controlled trial of Rumalon in the treatment of painful osteoarthrosis of the hip. Ann Rheum Dis 29:193–194, 1970.

19

Intra-Articular Steroid Therapy

David H. Neustadt, M.D.

Where fluid is exuded . . . we are often puzzled as to the best means of subduing it. Should there be an excess of fluid present, it may be desirable to tap the joint and withdraw the fluid. I have often seen the mere fact of puncture relieve tension and give ease. I find patients once relieved by this means ask for it to be done again and again.[1]

Although joint aspiration with intra-articular therapy is considered a relatively new therapeutic approach the comment above was taken from Bannatyne's textbook[1] on arthritis, published in 1898.

In 1951, hydrocortisone was introduced and popularized for local intra-articular administration. Observations and a vast experience accumulated during the past 33 years have confirmed the value of this compound and other corticosteroid suspensions for combating pain and inflammation when given at the local tissue level.[2-4] Other drugs and preparations, including phenylbutazone, sodium salicylate, and benzyl salicylate in oil, have also been shown to demonstrate anti-inflammatory effects when injected directly into inflamed joints. However, these compounds offer no therapeutic advantage and possess irritating properties when compared with corticosteroids.

INTRA-ARTICULAR STEROIDS IN OSTEOARTHRITIS

Although the value of intra-articular steroids in the treatment of rheumatoid arthritis and other inflammatory arthropathies is undoubted, their use in the therapy of osteoarthritis has been controversial.[5] Early studies suggested the possibility of a Charcot-like arthropathy occurring after multiple corticosteroid injections,[6-8] and studies performed on experimental small animals (i.e., mice, rats, and rabbits) indicated evidence of altered cartilage protein synthesis and damage to the cartilage.[4, 9-13] These reported deleterious effects curbed the initial enthusiasm for intra-articular corticosteroid therapy in osteoarthritis. However, other investigators reported that clinical observations after repeated administration of intra-articular steroids to knees demonstrated no significant evidence of destruction or accelerated deterioration.[14, 15] A detailed study of the effects of steroid injections on monkey joints disclosed no appreciable joint damage, suggesting that primate joints probably respond in a different way from those of mice and rabbits.[16] Thus, most authorities now consider intra-articular corticosteroid therapy in osteoarthritis of considerable value when administered judiciously and when indicated. It is important to emphasize that this form of treatment must always be considered as an adjunct to a conventional management program.

In this chapter there will be descriptions of the indications for intra-articular steroid therapy, the evidence of its efficacy, contraindications and complications, information on dosage and available corticosteroid compounds, and general and regional techniques for joint injection and a summary of data on nonsteroidal intra-articular agents.

RATIONALE

The major objective of intrasynovial therapy in osteoarthritis is to enter the joint space, aspirate any excess fluid, and instill the corticosteroid suspension that provides the most effective relief for the longest period of time.

333

Precise knowledge of the metabolic pathway and fate of corticosteroids within the joint has not been completely elucidated.[4] Some evidence of the injected steroid can be detected in the synovial fluid cells for 48 hours after injection. Prednisolone trimethylacetate has been identified in synovial fluid 14 days after its injection. The rate of absorption and duration of action are related to the solubility of the compound instilled.[17] Triamcinolone hexacetonide is the most insoluble preparation currently available.[2]

An antilymphocytic action is the probable mechanism of steroid benefit on rheumatoid synovial lining. Corticosteroids inhibit prostaglandin synthesis and decrease collagenase and other enzyme activity. The major basis of benefit in osteoarthritis remains somewhat unclear. A recent study suggests that in addition to their anti-inflammatory action, steroids may also reduce synovial vascular permeability.[18]

Systemic "spill-over" with absorption may occur, varying with the size of the dose and the solubility of the preparation injected. A recent study showed that 40 mg of methylprednisolone acetate was sufficient to induce a transient adrenal suppression, as reflected in depressed cortisol levels for up to 7 days.[17] A post-injection rest regimen or partial immobilization of the injected joint probably delays "escape" of the intra-articular steroid and minimizes systemic effects.[19]

INDICATIONS

In any discussion of indications, it is important to emphasize again that intra-articular therapy must be considered an adjunctive measure, and except in treating a regional problem such as traumatic synovitis or olecranon bursitis, it should be thought of simply as a component modality included in a comprehensive management program.

The indications for the use of intra-articular steroids are summarized in Table 19–1. In addition to the goal of introducing a drug into the joint cavity, arthrocentesis permits the aspiration of synovial fluid, which is useful as a diagnostic aid. Examination of the synovial fluid permits an estimation of the presence and degree of inflammation. An experienced observer can usually distinguish rheumatoid from traumatic or osteoarthritic fluid by its gross appearance and viscosity (see Chapter 10). Only a few drops of fluid may suffice to establish the diagnosis of an accompanying crystal synovitis (gout or pseudogout).

Table 19–1. INDICATIONS FOR INTRASYNOVIAL CORTICOSTEROIDS

1. To provide pain relief and suppress the inflammation of synovitis.
2. To provide adjunctive therapy for one or two joints not responsive to other systemic therapy.
3. To facilitate a rehabilitative and physical therapy program or orthopedic corrective procedures.
4. To prevent capsular and ligamentous laxity (large knee effusion).
5. To bring about a "medical synovectomy."
6. To treat patients unresponsive to or intolerant of oral systemic therapy.
7. To treat acute effusions occurring with associated crystal deposition disease.

When conventional therapy, including nonsteroidal anti-inflammatory agents, analgesics, rest, and applications of heat or cold, has failed to control the symptoms adequately and/or prevent disability, local steroid therapy deserves consideration. The presence of a large, tense, or painful effusion is the strongest indication for prompt arthrocentesis, followed by a steroid injection, pending the synovial fluid findings to exclude infection.

Relief of pain with preservation or restoration of joint motion is the major objective of therapy. When one or more joints are resistant to systemic therapy, consideration should be given to intrasynovial injections. Joint injections are often helpful in preventing adhesions and correcting flexion contractures of the knee, especially when given in the hospital in conjunction with traction. In large tense or boggy effusions, the capsule and ligaments may become stretched, and this can be combated effectively with intra-articular therapy. Finally, in long-standing or recurrent effusions of the knee, a so-called "medical synovectomy" can be performed by instilling a relatively large dose (30 to 50 mg) of an insoluble preparation such as triamcinolone hexacetonide, followed by the postinjection rest regimen, which is described in detail in the section on dosage and administration.

CLINICAL EFFICACY

A lack of prospective controlled studies with adequate observations has led to considerable controversy as to the efficacy of intra-articular steroids in the treatment of osteoarthritis. However, the simple fact that a chapter on this form of therapy is included in a textbook limited solely to the topic of osteoarthritis strongly suggests that current medical opinion supports the value of intrasynovial therapy in osteoarthritis.[5]

Numerous authors reported favorably on the use of intra-articular steroids in the treatment of osteoarthritis.[4, 20–24] Balch and associates[14] reported on repeated intrasynovial injections given over a period varying from 4 to 15 years. The minimum number of injections given was 15 during a period of 4 years, with the interval between injections being not less than 4 weeks. Their results strongly supported the conclusion that this was a "very useful" form of treatment.

Although certain controlled trials[25, 26] failed to demonstrate significant efficacy of steroid injections, these studies did not take into consideration such important factors as adequate dosage, the presence or absence of fluid, removal of excess fluid (dilution factor), and the technique of the injection, and most important, there was no attempt to regulate the postinjection physical activity of the patient.

Dieppe and colleagues[27] reported a beneficial response with significantly greater reduction of pain and tenderness than after placebo in a controlled trial in which 20 mg of triamcinolone hexacetonide were injected into 48 osteoarthritic knees. These results were obtained even though injections were made into the infrapatellar pouch and only 5 ml of fluid were aspirated from each knee at the time of the procedure. In another recent report[28] of 42 patients with osteoarthritis in whom triamcinolone hexacetonide, betamethasone acetate, and betamethasone disodium were compared, the results confirmed that intra-articular steroid treatment of osteoarthritis was highly effective. In other studies,[28, 29] including a similar comparative assessment in a group consisting of 19 patients with osteoarthritis of the knee, favorable results were obtained.[29] The duration of effect varied with different preparations and dosage.

These carefully performed randomized double-blind and single-blind studies support the results of Hollander's[2] 30 years of experience with a large number of injections. He reported that in a 10-year follow-up of the first 100 patients who had been given repeated intra-articular steroids in osteoarthritic knees, 59 patients no longer needed injections, 24 continued to require occasional injections, and only 11 did not obtain a worthwile response.[24]

My own experience is similar to that of Hollander and the other authors cited above. Striking relief of pain, frequently coupled with increased motion, occurred in the majority of injected joints.

Finally, the case for the efficacy of intrasynovial corticosteroid injections in osteoarthritis

Table 19–2. RELATIVE CONTRAINDICATIONS

1. Infection (local or systemic)
2. Anticoagulant therapy
3. Hemorrhagic effusions
4. Uncontrolled diabetes mellitus
5. Severe joint destruction and/or deformity
6. Extreme overnutrition

has been given support in an editorial published in the British Medical Journal.[5]

However, the success of short-term beneficial response must be balanced against the all-important duration of effect and any iatrogenic deleterious response.

CONTRAINDICATIONS AND COMPLICATIONS

The place of intra-articular corticosteroids in osteoarthritis remains controversial despite extensive use and reported beneficial response because of reports of the development of steroid-induced (Charcot-like) arthropathy after multiple injections.[6, 8]

Contraindications are relative (benefits versus risk) and are listed in Table 19–2. Local infection or recent serious injury overlying the structure to be injected or the presence of a generalized infection with possible bacteremia is an obvious contraindication to the local instillation of a corticosteroid. In patients with systemic infections, intra-articular therapy might be performed under the "cover" of appropriate antibiotic therapy, if the indication is considered urgent. The risk of provoking serious bleeding in patients receiving anticoagulants must be determined after a review of the patient's general status, including determination of the prothrombin time. Joints of the lower extremities demonstrating considerable underlying damage, such as an unstable knee, should not be injected with corticosteroids unless there is a relatively large inflammatory effusion and the patient will cooperate by adhering to a non–weight-bearing schedule for several weeks after the procedure.

Complications of intra-articular therapy are listed in Table 19–3. Despite some systemic

Table 19–3. COMPLICATIONS OF INTRA-ARTICULAR THERAPY

Infection
Postinjection flare
"Crystal-induced" synovitis
Cutaneous atrophy (local)
"Steroid" arthropathy

"spill-over," physical evidence of hypercortisolism or other steroid undesirable effects rarely occur from intermittent intra-articular therapy. If rounding of the face appears, this would suggest that injections have been administered too frequently.[30] Although the possibility of introducing an accidental infection is the most serious potential complication, review of our extensive experience and that of others discloses that infections occurring as an aftermath of joint injections are extremely rare.[2, 4, 31] We do not use routine prophylactic antibiotics or concur with the recommendation that they should be administered.

Local adverse reactions are minor and reversible. The so-called *"postinjection flare"* is a rare complication that begins shortly after the injection and usually subsides within a few hours, rarely continuing up to 48 to 72 hours. Some investigators consider these reactions to be a true crystal-induced synovitis due to corticosteroid ester crystals.[3, 32] The application of ice to the site and oral analgesics usually control the pain until the reaction abates. In a few instances, the postinjection synovitis has been sufficiently severe to require "re-aspiration" of the joint to obtain relief.

Another infrequent complication is *localized subcutaneous or cutaneous atrophy*.[3, 4] This cosmetic change can be recognized as a thin or depressed area at the site of the injection, sometimes associated with depigmentation. As a rule, the skin appearance will be restored to normal when the crystals of the corticosteroid have been completely absorbed. Rarely, *capsular (periarticular) calcification* at the site of the injection has been noted in roentgenograms taken after treatment. The calcifications usually disappear spontaneously and are not of clinical significance.[19] Careful technique, avoiding the leaking of the steroid suspension from the needle track to the skin surface, will prevent or minimize these problems. A small amount of 1% lidocaine (or the equivalent) or normal saline solution can be utilized to flush the needle used to administer the crystalline suspension before removing the needle.

An occasional patient may complain of increased warmth and flushing of the skin. There may be central nervous system and cardiovascular reactions to local anesthetics if used in combination with the steroid for injection. It has been suggested that the abolition of pain after the introduction of steroids will permit the patient to "overwork" the involved joint, causing additional cartilage and bone deterioration and finally giving rise to a "Charcot-like" or so-called "steroid" arthropathy.[33] In addition, experimental evidence in rabbit joints indicates that frequently repeated injections of corticosteroids may interfere with normal cartilage protein synthesis.[4, 13] As stated earlier, recent studies on primate joints failed to confirm evidence of significant cartilage damage due to repeated administration of intra-articular steroids, suggesting that the steroid effect on primate joints, including human joints, is probably transient.[16]

The potential hazard of "spontaneous" tendon rupture, especially of the Achilles tendon, after local steroid injections has been reported to develop infrequently. Careful administration with infiltrations around and beneath the tendon to prevent forcing any of the preparation into the substance of the tendon will help to prevent the occurrence of this rare complication.[34]

AVAILABLE COMPOUNDS AND CHOICE OF DRUG

Hydrocortisone and a variety of available repository preparations are listed in Table 19–4. All corticosteroids, with the exception of cortisone and prednisone, can produce a significant and prompt anti-inflammatory effect in an inflamed joint. The most soluble corticosteroid suspension is absorbed rapidly and has a short duration of effect. The tertiary-butylacetate (TBA, tebutate) ester prolongs the duration of action owing to decreased solubility, which probably causes its dissociation by enzymes to proceed at a lower rate. Although an occasional patient may obtain greater benefit from one steroid derivative than another, no single steroid agent has demonstrated a convincing margin of superiority with the exception perhaps of triamcinolone hexacetonide.[7, 24, 35] Prednisolone tebutate has the virtues of price advantage and long-time usage. Triamcinolone hexacetonide is the least water-soluble preparation currently available. It is 2.5 times less soluble in water than prednisolone tebutate and usually provides the longest duration of effectiveness. There is minimal systemic "spill-over" with this agent.

DOSAGE AND ADMINISTRATION

The dose of any microcrystalline suspension employed for intrasynovial injection must be arbitrarily selected. Factors that influence the

Table 19–4. INJECTABLE CORTICOSTEROIDS

Repository Preparations	Mg Per Ml	Range of Usual Dosage*
Hydrocortisone tebutate (Hydrocortone-TBA)	50 mg	25–100 mg
Prednisolone tebutate (Hydeltra-TBA)	20 mg	5–40 mg
Betamethasone acetate and disodium phosphate (Celestone Soluspan)	6 mg†	1.5–6 mg
Methylprednisolone acetate (Depo-Medrol‡)	20 mg	4–40 mg
Triamcinolone acetonide (Kenalog-40)	40 mg	5–40 mg
Triamcinolone diacetate (Aristocort Forte)	40 mg	5–40 mg
Triamcinolone hexacetonide (Aristospan)	20 mg	5–40 mg

*Amount will vary depending on the size of the joint to be injected.
†Available as 3 mg of acetate and 3 mg of phosphate.
‡Supplied in 20 mg per ml, and 40 mg per ml, and 80 mg per ml preparations.

dosage and the anticipated results are listed in Table 19–5.

For estimating dosage, a useful guide is as follows: for small joints of the hand and foot, 2.5 to 10 mg of prednisolone tebutate suspension or the equivalent; for medium-sized joints such as the wrist and elbow, 10 to 25 mg; for the knee, ankle, and shoulder, 20 to 50 mg; and for the hip, 25 to 40 mg. Occasionally, it is necessary to give larger amounts to obtain optimal results. For intrabursal therapy, such as for the hip (trochanteric) or the knee (anserine bursa), 15 to 40 mg are usually an adequate dose.

The longer the intervals between injections, the better. I usually recommend a 4-week minimum between intra-articular procedures, and in weight-bearing joints, I prefer an interval of 6 to 12 weeks between injections. Injections should not be repeated on a "regular" routine basis, and rarely should more than two to three injections into a specific weight-bearing joint be repeated per year. Injections into soft-tissue sites of para-articular inflammation may be given on a more frequent basis. After knee injection, I advise the patient to adhere to the following schedule: The patient should remain in bed for 3 to 4 days, with the exception of bathroom privileges and meals; crutches are then prescribed, to be used with "three-point" gait to protect the injected knee for 2 to 4 weeks. A cane may be substituted at times when crutches are inappropriate or uncomfortable. I believe that this postinjection regimen facilitates a sustained improvement and avoids the hazard of "overworking" or abusing the injected joint. An additional benefit is that the inactivity reduces any systemic effect by delaying absorption of the steroid. This program is optimal for achieving maximal therapeutic benefit and reducing possible deleterious effects of joint overuse after injection.

Table 19–6 presents a comparison of groups of rheumatoid knees demonstrating the prolonged duration of relief after the rest regimen. During the past several years, I have hospitalized five patients with osteoarthritis of the knees who had intractable, recurrent synovitis requiring frequent arthrocenteses and repeated intra-articular injections. After the administration of a steroid (usually triamcinolone hexacetonide) and the completion of the strict rest period, these patients obtained complete resolution of effusions for up to a year or longer.

PREPARATION OF SITE

Preparation of the site for injection of a steroid requires rigid adherence to aseptic technique. "Landmarks" are outlined with a skin pencil. The point of entry is then cleansed with pHisoHex (or the equivalent) or Betadine, and alcohol is sponged on the area. Sterile drapes and gloves are not ordinarily considered necessary. Sterile 4-inch × 4-inch gauze pads are useful for drying the area.

Table 19–5. FACTORS THAT INFLUENCE RESPONSE TO INTRA-ARTICULAR INJECTIONS

Size of joints
Volume of synovial fluid
Choice of corticosteroid preparation
Dosage and technique
Severity (and extent) of synovitis
POSTINJECTION ACTIVITY

TECHNIQUES

General Considerations

Arthrocentesis is easily and relatively painlessly performed in a joint that is distended

Table 19–6. SUMMARY OF COMPARATIVE DURATION OF
EFFECT IN SYNOVITIS OF KNEES

Steroid	Number of Patients (Number of Knees)	Duration of Response (Weeks)
Prednisolone tebutate*	50 (58)	1–16 (average: 5.5)
Prednisolone tebutate and prescribed rest	50 (56)	2–30 (average: 9.5)
Triamcinolone hexacetonide† and prescribed rest	47 (50)	3.5–104 (average: 35)
Triamcinolone hexacetonide‡	37 (44)	2.5–50 (average: 21)

*6-Methylprednisolone instilled in 10 knees.
†Intra-articular therapy administered in hospital in 16 patients.
‡Dosage varied from 1.5 to 2 ml of 40 mg/ml preparation.

with fluid or when boggy synovial proliferation is present. For most joints, the usual point of entry is on the extensor surface, avoiding the large nerves and major vessels that are usually present on the flexor surface. Optimal joint positioning should be accomplished to stretch the capsule and separate the joint "ends" to produce maximal enlargement and distraction of the joint or synovial cavity to be penetrated.

A local anesthetic is sometimes desirable, especially when a relatively "dry" joint is being entered or when only a small amount of fluid is present. A small skin wheal made by infiltration with lidocaine or the equivalent or spraying (frosting) the skin with a vapocoolant such as Frigiderm usually provides adequate anesthesia.

Aspiration of as much synovial fluid as possible prior to instillation of the corticosteroid suspension reduces the dilution factor. After the therapeutic agent is injected in large joints, it is advisable to re-aspirate and re-inject several times within the barrel of the syringe (barbotage) to obtain good "mixing" and dispersion of the therapeutic compound throughout the joint and synovial cavity. I often instill a small amount of air just prior to removing the needle to insure adequate diffusion. Finally, gentle manipulation, carrying the joint through its full excursions of motion, facilitates maximal dispersion of the injected medication.

Specific Joints and Adjacent Sites

The joints most frequently considered for corticosteroid injection in osteoarthritis include the knee, the distal and proximal interphalangeal joints, first carpometacarpal joint, and first metatarsophalangeal joint. Less commonly injected joints include the hip and temporomandibular joint. Shoulder joints are rarely involved in primary osteoarthritis but, like the elbow, may develop osteoarthritis on a secondary, underlying basis.

The Knee

The knee joint contains the largest synovial space in the body and is the most commonly aspirated and injected joint. Demonstrable, visible, or palpable effusions often develop, making it the easiest joint to enter and to inject with medication. When a large amount of fluid is present, entry is as simple as puncturing a balloon.

Aspiration of the knee is usually performed with the patient lying on a table with the knee extended as much as possible. The usual site of entry is medially at about the mid-point of the patella or just below the point where a horizontal line tangential to the superior pole of the patella crosses a line paralleling the medial border. The needle (1.5 to 2-inch, 20-gauge) is directed downward or upward, sliding into the joint space beneath the undersurface of the patella (Fig. 19–1). Aspiration of the knee can be facilitated by applying firm pressure with one hand cephalad to the patella over the suprapatellar bursa. If cartilage is touched, the needle is withdrawn slightly and the fluid is aspirated (Fig. 19–2). A similar approach can be used on the lateral side if the maximal fluid bulge is present laterally. The lateral approach is especially convenient if there is a large effusion in the suprapatellar bursa. The point of penetration is just lateral and superior to the patella, and at this point, puncture is often painless. An approach that is used less frequently is the infrapatellar route,

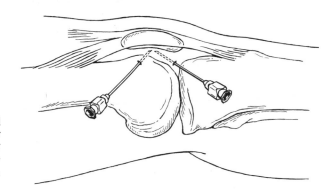

Figure 19–1. Arthrocentesis of the knee joint, medial approach, the usual entry site. (From Steinbrocker O, Neustadt DH: Aspiration and Injection Therapy in Arthritis and Musculoskeletal Disorders: A Handbook on Technique and Management. Hagerstown, Maryland, Harper & Row, 1972.)

which is useful when the knee cannot be fully extended and there is only minimal fluid present. With the knee flexed, the needle is directed either medially or laterally to the inferior patellar tendon and cephalad to the infrapatellar fat pad. It is difficult to obtain fluid with this approach, and there is a slight possibility of injury to the joint surface.

The Knee Region

Although roentgenographic evidence of degenerative changes involving the knee may be present, the "knee" pain and associated disabling symptoms are sometimes due to extra-articular causes. Some of these painful conditions in the knee region, often associated with osteoarthritis, may respond to local injection therapy.

These disorders include bursitides of the knee with involvement of the prepatellar, suprapatellar, and anserine bursae. Other disorders adjacent to the knee that may be responsive to injection therapy include semi-

membranosus tenosynovitis, Pellegrini-Stieda syndrome, painful areas of the collateral ligaments associated with osteoarthritis, and painful points around the edge of the patella associated with patellofemoral osteoarthritis. The differential diagnosis between osteoarthritis of the knee and these disorders is chiefly based on a thorough history and the physical findings.

Prepatellar Bursitis. Prepatellar bursitis ("housemaid's knee"), characterized by swelling and effusion of the superficial bursa overlying the patella, is easily recognized. The chronic bursal reaction commonly occurs from repetitive activity or pressure, such as kneeling on a firm surface ("carpet cutter's knee" and "nun's knee"). Pain is relatively minimal except during direct pressure, and motion is usually preserved. Aspiration, which yields a small amount of clear, serous fluid, is performed, and then 1 to 2 ml of lidocaine and 10 to 20 mg of a prednisolone suspension are instilled. This bursa is not usually a single cavity but a multilocular structure in which

Figure 19–2. Actual arthrocentesis of the knee joint. (From Steinbrocker O, Neustadt DH: Aspiration and Injection Therapy in Arthritis and Musculoskeletal Disorders: A Handbook on Technique and Management. Hagerstown, Maryland, Harper & Row, 1972.)

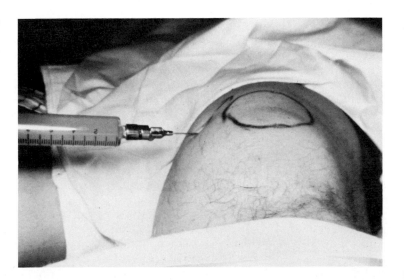

loose areolar tissue separates the walls of the bursa. Thus, in some cases, the procedure may need to be repeated once or a few times to obtain a lasting result. Whenever possible, the activity provoking the bursitis should be eliminated.

Suprapatellar Bursitis. Suprapatellar bursitis is usually associated with synovitis of the knee cavity. Occasionally, the suprapatellar bursa is largely separated developmentally from the synovial cavity. In these cases, effusion is especially prominent at the suprapatellar region.

Anserine Bursitis. Anserine bursitis ("cavalryman's disease") now mainly occurs in obese women with disproportionately heavy thighs in association with osteoarthritis of the knee. The bursa is located at the anteromedial surface of the tibia just below the joint line of the knee, at the site of the insertion of the conjoined tendon of the sartorius, semitendinosus, and gracilis muscles, and superficial to the medial collateral ligament. The entity may simulate or coexist with osteoarthritis of the knee. A relatively abrupt increase in knee pain, localized tenderness with a sensation of fullness in the vicinity of the site of the bursa, or the development of an angular knee deformity should strongly suggest consideration of this often overlooked disorder. Injection of a few ml of lidocaine and approximately 1 to 1.5 ml of a corticosteroid suspension from an anterior or medial approach with a 1.5-inch, 22-gauge needle frequently produces prompt symptomatic relief. The duration of effect is variable and may correlate with the patient's weight-bearing activities.

Semimembranosus Tenosynovitis. Semimembranosus ("popliteal") tenosynovitis is characterized by pain in the posterior or posteromedial aspect of the knee. Localized tenderness over the superoposterior area of the medial condyle of the tibia (the semimembranosus groove) supports the diagnosis. Protective muscle spasm of the medial hamstrings causes a "pseudo-locking" of the knee. This condition is usually superimposed on underlying osteoarthritis, and the onset is relatively sudden. Treatment with local steroid injection to the points of greatest tenderness is frequently beneficial.

Pellegrini-Stieda Syndrome. This syndrome occurs as an aftermath of trauma. Calcification develops in the region of the medial tibial collateral ligament. The major manifestation is progressively impaired knee joint flexion. The diagnosis is made by roentgenographic study disclosing the calcification 3 to 4 weeks after the injury. Early local injections of steroids and/or an anesthetic are the most beneficial form of treatment.

Periarthritis. In periarthritis of the knee, painful areas may be limited to one or two points in the collateral ligaments. In a knee with a valgus (knock-knee) deformity, pain is produced in the medial collateral ligament on forced abduction; similarly, in a varus (bowlegged) knee, pain is felt in the lateral collateral ligament on forced adduction, although this is relatively rare. If tenderness can be accurately localized, an infiltration of lidocaine and approximately 0.5 to 0.75 ml of a steroid preparation directly to the sore points is frequently effective. Postinjection pain is not uncommon for up to 24 hours, and the patient should be duly warned.

Another area where pain may arise in the "unswollen" knee is around the edge of the patella in association with patellofemoral osteoarthritis. Occasionally, one or two localized tender points are detected. Injection of these "pain spots" with 1 ml of lidocaine and 0.5 to 0.75 ml of a steroid suspension may produce significant relief. The injection has to be made under pressure into the actual fibrous tissue attachments of the capsule to the edge of the patella. The use of a relatively short needle (⅞- to 1-inch) will help prevent advancing the needle too far and entering the knee cavity.

The Shoulder

Scapulohumeral Joint. Of the approaches to the shoulder, the anterior route provides the simplest entry. A needle is directed mediodorsally in the groove between the medial aspect of the humeral head at a point just inferior to the tip of the coracoid process (Fig. 19–3*A*). A 1.5- or 2-inch, 20- or 22-gauge needle is advanced into the scapulohumeral interspace; any fluid is aspirated, and 20 to 30 mg of prednisolone suspension is introduced with or without 2 to 3 ml of lidocaine.

The posterior approach is often preferable because it is done out of the patient's line of vision. Internal rotation of the shoulder with adduction of the patient's arm across the chest wall and with the hand resting on the opposite shoulder tends to open up the joint space. The site of needle entry is just below (1 to 2 cm) the posterolateral angle of the posterior aspect of the acromion (Fig. 19–4). A 1.5- or 2-inch, 20- or 22-gauge needle is introduced through a cutaneous wheal to a point within a free space, visualized as the capsule of the scapulohumeral joint. Aspiration, which rarely yields fluid, is performed, and 20 to 30 mg of a steroid preparation is instilled.

Acromioclavicular Joint. Entry is made through a cutaneous lidocaine wheal over the interosseous groove at the point of maximal tenderness (Fig. 19–3B). The joint is relatively superficial, and a ⅞- or 1-inch, 22-gauge needle is adequate. One to 2 ml of lidocaine and 0.75 to 1 mg of a prednisolone suspension are instilled. It is not necessary to advance the needle beyond the proximal margin of the joint surfaces.

Sternoclavicular Joint. Osteoarthritis of the sternoclavicular joint is seldom the cause of much pain. However, in the rare instance that involvement is considered clinically significant, the joint is easily located and injected by sliding a ⅞-inch, 25-gauge needle between the articular surfaces and then 0.25 ml of a steroid suspension is instilled.

The Elbow

The elbow (humeroulnar) joint can usually be readily entered by the posterolateral approach. With the joint incompletely extended and held in a relaxed position, the bulge of any synovial effusion is noted posterolaterally,

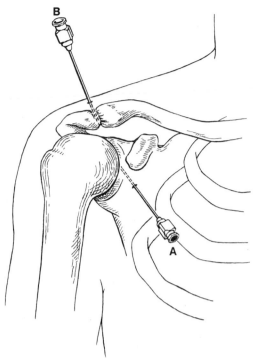

Figure 19–3. A, Arthrocentesis of the scapulohumeral joint, anterior approach. B, Injection of acromioclavicular joint. (From Steinbrocker O, Neustadt DH: Aspiration and Injection Therapy in Arthritis and Musculoskeletal Disorders: A Handbook on Technique and Management. Hagerstown, Maryland, Harper & Row, 1972.)

Figure 19–4. Injection of the shoulder, posterior approach. (From Steinbrocker O, Neustadt DH: Aspiration and Injection Therapy in Arthritis and Musculoskeletal Disorders: A Handbook on Technique and Management. Hagerstown, Maryland, Harper & Row, 1972.)

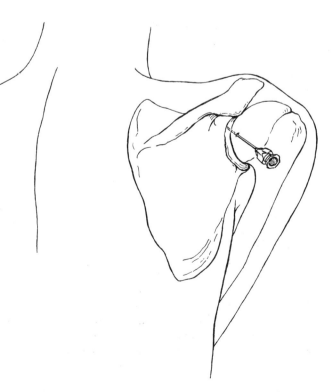

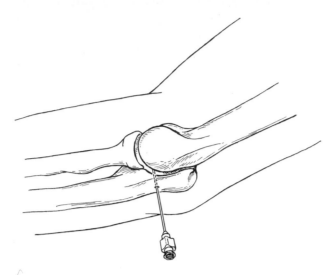

Figure 19–5. Arthrocentesis of the elbow joint. (From Steinbrocker O, Neustadt DH: Aspiration and Injection Therapy in Arthritis and Musculoskeletal Disorders: A Handbook on Technique and Management. Hagerstown, Maryland, Harper & Row, 1972.)

just outside of the olecranon process and inferior to the humeral lateral epicondyle. The needle is introduced at the outer aspect of the olecranon and just below the lateral epicondyle. It is directed medially, proximal to the radial head. The radial head can be easily identified by pronating and supinating the forearm. Aspiration of any fluid is performed, followed by intra-articular injection of 1 to 1.5 ml of a corticosteroid suspension (Fig. 19–5).

Because the elbow region is subject to frequently occurring extra-articular soft tissue forms of pathology such as epicondylitis, it must be kept in mind that the presence of osteoarthritis may not be the source of pain.

Finger and Toe Joints

First Carpometacarpal Joint. The carpometacarpal joint of the thumb is commonly affected with osteoarthritis (thumb base osteoarthritis). With the thumb adducted and held in flexion within the palm, steroid injection is performed from the dorsal side, inserting the needle at the point of maximal tenderness. It is not usually necessary to actually slide the needle between the trapezium (greater multangular) and the base of the thumb metacarpal (Fig. 19–6).

Interphalangeal Joints. Small hand joints are entered on the dorsal surface, utilizing ⅞-inch, 25-gauge needles (Fig. 19–7). The needle is slipped beneath the extensor tendon from either the lateral or the medial side. Aspiration does not usually yield fluid. In small joints, it is necessary to use a gentle teasing technique with the needle, in combination with efforts to distract the joint, but frequently, periarticular injection produces an adequate response, indicating that it is not always necessary to instill

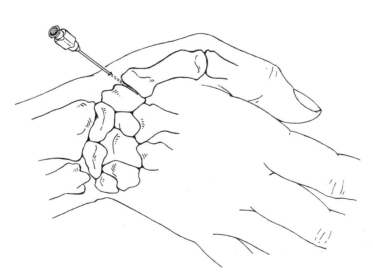

Figure 19–6. Arthrocentesis for the first carpometacarpal joint (thumb base). (From Steinbrocker O, Neustadt DH: Aspiration and Injection Therapy in Arthritis and Musculoskeletal Disorders: A Handbook on Technique and Management. Hagerstown, Maryland, Harper & Row, 1972.)

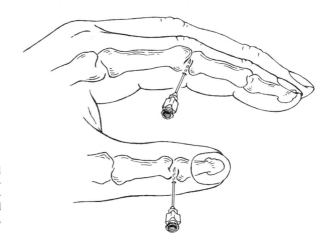

Figure 19–7. Arthrocentesis of the interphalangeal joints. (From Steinbrocker O, Neustadt DH: Aspiration and Injection Therapy in Arthritis and Musculoskeletal Disorders: A Handbook on Technique and Management. Hagerstown, Maryland, Harper & Row, 1972.)

the therapeutic suspension directly into the joint space. Aspiration and steroid injection of distal joints are performed in a fashion similar to those of the proximal joints. Steroids may be injected into toe joints by utilizing traction to facilitate insertion of the needle between the phalangeal joint surfaces.

Injecting a tender, inflamed Heberden's node with a steroid is usually accomplished through a point frozen by spraying Frigiderm; a fine needle, such as a ⅞-inch, 27-gauge one, is used, and any effort to aspirate fluid is avoided. The needle is gently teased through the point of entry into the capsule, depositing the steroid without attempting to enter the tiny joint space. Ready transport of the corticosteroid occurs through inflamed tissue.

Mucous (synovial) cysts associated with He-

berden's nodes at the dorsum of the affected joint can be "unroofed," inspissated fluid can be removed, and a small dose of corticosteroid suspension can be instilled. If the result is not satisfactory after one or two injections, surgical excision should be considered.

Metatarsophalangeal Joints. The metatarsophalangeal joints may be entered through a mediodorsal approach by teasing with 24- or 25-gauge needles. Rarely, a metatarsophalangeal joint is approached from the plantar surface by a subcutaneous entry.

The first metatarsophalangeal joint (bunion joint) may be the site of acute or chronic synovitis. It may be entered through a mediodorsal approach by teasing with a 25-gauge needle. Five to 10 mg of prednisolone suspension may be injected (Fig. 19–8 *A*). Subcuta-

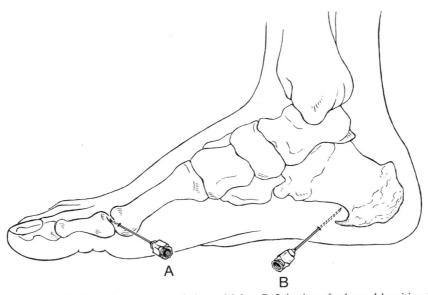

A   B

Figure 19–8. A, Arthrocentesis of the first metatarsophalangeal joint. *B,* Injection of calcaneal bursitis with heel spur. (From Steinbrocker O, Neustadt DH: Aspiration and Injection Therapy in Arthritis and Musculoskeletal Disorders: A Handbook on Technique and Management. Hagerstown, Maryland, Harper & Row, 1972.)

neous entry of the swollen capsule for aspiration and injection, or deposit of the dosage over the joint space is usually sufficient.

Freezing the skin with a vapocoolant (Frigiderm) spray before needling small joints is usually preferred to the injection of lidocaine.

Hip Joint

Although the hip joint is the largest joint in the body, it is usually the most difficult to enter and to aspirate. It has a dense capsule, enclosed by large ligaments and abundant, soft connective tissues. Pathologic joints may have overriding osteophytes, disturbing the anatomic relationship of the femoral head to the acetabulum and making it almost impossible to enter the joint space. Aspiration of fluid, signaling actual entry of the synovial cavity, is uncommon. Injection is performed whether fluid is obtained or not. Accordingly, results are unpredictable, and the duration of relief may be relatively brief. Appropriate roentgenograms and experience help overcome the difficulties of performing the procedure.

The joint may be entered and injected by the anterior or lateral approach. With the anterior method, the patient lies supine, with the extremity straight and slightly rotated externally. A 20-gauge needle, 2.5 to 4 inches long (depending on the patient's size), is used. The entry is made at a point 2 cm below the anterosuperior spine of the ilium and 3 cm lateral to the palpated femoral pulse, approximately at the level of the upper edge of the greater trochanter. The needle is directed at an angle of 60 degrees posteriorly and medially, penetrating the tough capsular ligaments to bone. The needle then is withdrawn slightly,

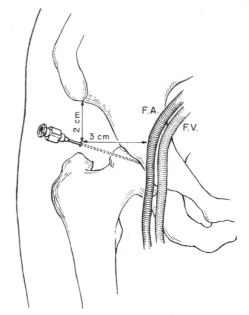

Figure 19–9. Arthrocentesis of the hip joint, anterior approach. (From Steinbrocker O, Neustadt DH: Aspiration and Injection Therapy in Arthritis and Musculoskeletal Disorders: A Handbook on Technique and Management. Hagerstown, Maryland, Harper & Row, 1972.)

and aspiration is attempted. Rarely, fluid is obtained. The joint is then injected (Fig. 19–9).

Injection of the hip joint by the lateral route is simpler only in that the needle follows the line of the femoral neck to the articulation. It is difficult to be sure of the entry through the capsule into the joint space here, too, because only occasionally is fluid aspirated (Fig. 19–10).

The prominence of the greater trochanter of the femur is located by having the patient

Figure 19–10. Arthrocentesis of the hip joint, lateral approach. (From Steinbrocker O, Neustadt DH: Aspiration and Injection Therapy in Arthritis and Musculoskeletal Disorders: A Handbook on Technique and Management. Hagerstown, Maryland, Harper & Row, 1972.)

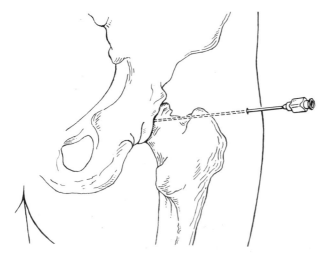

rotate the limb during palpation. With the limb outwardly rotated, a wheal is made just anterior to the greater trochanter. A 3- to 4-inch, 22- or 20-gauge needle is directed medially and is "walked" along the neck of the femur toward a point below the middle of the inguinal ligament to a depth of 2.5 to 3.5 inches, until the joint capsule is reached and penetrated. Aspiration is performed, and the medication is injected through the intact needle after changing syringes.

The femoral (as well as the humeral) head has been an occasional site of osteonecrosis due to repeated, frequent introduction of corticosteroids. Intra-articular injection at this location, as elsewhere, should be repeated at intervals no less than 4 weeks, preferably 6 to 12 weeks, with due consideration for the possibility of so-called "steroid" arthropathy.[33] The popularity of total hip replacement procedures has led to a great reduction in steroid injections of the hip joints.

The Hip Region

Periarticular Pain Points. Localized tender points are found occasionally in the abundant musculature and fibrous tissues in the vicinity of the hip joint and are associated with osteoarthritis of the hip. These secondary sites of irritation may produce the pain and tenderness adjacent to the joint. Injection of the sore joint may prove helpful at one or more circumscribed sites of tenderness. The injections are given deeply with a 2- or 2.5-inch, 20-gauge needle, administering 3 to 4 ml of 1% lidocaine and 0.5 to 1 ml of prednisolone suspension.

Trochanteric Bursa. Involvement of the trochanteric bursa may simulate osteoarthritic hip pain. If the bursa is calcified, it is easily located by roentgenogram. Trochanteric bursitis occurs over or below the greater trochanter, and tenderness is localized over the greater trochanter. Active abduction of the hip when lying on the opposite side typically accentuates the discomfort. Intrabursal injection of 3 to 5 ml of lidocaine and 20 to 40 mg of prednisolone suspension is frequently effective in suppressing the pain.

Temporomandibular Joint

The patient should be in a reclining position with the head facing upward or sitting in a chair with the head supported. The zygomatic arch is palpated, and the tip of the index finger is placed inferior to the arch about 2 cm anterior to the tragus of the ear. When the

patient opens and closes his mouth, the condyle of the ascending ramus is felt. The point of entry lies just inferior to the zygomatic arch and halfway between the tragus and the anterior border of the ascending ramus. The pulsation of the superficial temporal artery is palpated somewhat posterior to this point, near the tragus of the ear, with the patient's mouth closed. A 1- or 1.5-inch, 22-gauge needle is then inserted perpendicular to the surface of the skin. The ramus is near the surface, almost subcutaneous. When bone is touched, 2 or 3 ml of 1% lidocaine solution and 10 mg of a prednisolone suspension are deposited for a periarticular infiltration. Aspiration before injection is advisable.

The procedure may be done intra-articularly after the needle rests on the condyle by having the patient open his mouth. The needle is then slipped from the condyle up 0.15 cm or less into the joint. Aspiration is performed, and the steroid injection is given (Fig. 19–11).

Ankle Joint (Tibiotalar Joint)

Osteoarthritis affecting the ankle joint is relatively rare except as an aftermath of trauma or special occupations such as ballet dancing. Local steroid injections are often ineffective in suppressing osteoarthritic ankle pain.

The ankle joint may be difficult to enter. The usual technique includes holding the foot in slight plantar flexion. The point of entry is

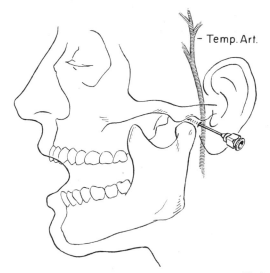

Figure 19–11. Arthrocentesis of the temporomandibular joint. (From Steinbrocker O, Neustadt DH: Aspiration and Injection Therapy in Arthritis and Musculoskeletal Disorders: A Handbook on Technique and Management. Hagerstown, Maryland, Harper & Row, 1972.)

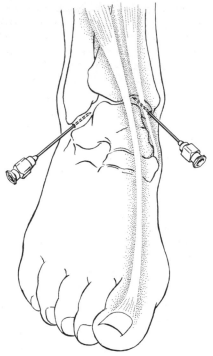

Figure 19–12. Arthrocentesis of the ankle joint, medial and lateral entries. (From Steinbrocker O, Neustadt DH: Aspiration and Injection Therapy in Arthritis and Musculoskeletal Disorders: A Handbook on Technique and Management. Hagerstown, Maryland, Harper & Row, 1972.)

just medial to the extensor hallucis longus tendon. The needle is directed somewhat laterally from a point approximately 1 cm above and 1 cm lateral to the medial malleolus. A slight depression can be felt between the medial malleolus and the extensor hallucis longus tendon. Plantar flexion tends to open up the ankle joint, providing a larger area for injection (Fig. 19–12).

The Foot

Calcaneal Bursitis With Spur. The major condition of the foot associated with osteoarthritis for which steroid injection therapy is suitable is calcaneal bursitis (plantar fasciitis) with painful heel spurs. If orthopedic shoe corrections and aids are ineffective, steroid injection of the painful heel is often beneficial. At the site of maximal tenderness, a 1-inch, 22- to 24-gauge needle is inserted into the plantar surface at 90 degrees, sliding into the space at the mid-point of the calcaneus. The tip of the needle lies in the aponeurosis of the attachment to the os calcis (Fig. 19–8 *B*). One ml of lidocaine and 10 to 20 mg of prednisolone suspension are instilled.

CRYSTAL SYNOVITIS AND OSTEOARTHRITIS

Calcium Pyrophosphate Dihydrate (CPPD) Deposition. The link between osteoarthritis and CPPD is extremely strong. The majority (about 70%) of cases of CPPD are associated with a chronic arthritis identical to osteoarthritis, usually involving the hips and the knees.[36]

In those patients who develop an acute or subacute attack, "pseudogout," arthrocentesis permits diagnostic confirmation and thorough aspiration of synovial fluid; introduction of 1 to 2 ml of a corticosteroid suspension generally suppresses the inflammatory process in the knee. Involved joints other than the knee also respond satisfactorily to intrasynovial therapy.

Hydroxyapatite Crystals and Osteoarthritis. The possible relationship of hydroxyapatite crystal deposition and osteoarthritis was first reported by Dieppe and associates in 1976.[37] The notion that the inflammation may be due to apatite crystals was based on the finding of the crystals in synovial fluid from osteoarthritic patients. Specific diagnosis is made by electron microscopy or x-ray diffraction of crystals. Although clinical recognition of apatite crystals is difficult, when acute or subacute arthritis with an effusion develops, especially in patients on dialysis, it is reasonable to aspirate the contents of the synovial cavity and instill a corticosteroid suspension.

Corticosteroid Postinjection Crystal Synovitis. The rare "postinjection flare" that occurs within a few hours after the administration of a local corticosteroid injection usually subsides spontaneously in several to 24 hours. In some cases, a true crystal-induced synovitis due to microcrystalline corticosteroid ester crystals occurs. If the reaction is severe, a thorough re-aspiration of the joint contents provides prompt relief. Oral administration of analgesics or nonsteroidal anti-inflammatory agents for several days is also beneficial when symptoms are severe.

NONSTEROIDAL INTRA-ARTICULAR THERAPEUTIC AGENTS

Intra-articular injections were performed with a variety of compounds for relief of symptoms long before the advent of corticosteroids. However, none of the preparations available before corticosteroids had dependable or durable effects. Agents that have been injected include lactic acid, phenylbutazone, cytotoxic compounds, sodium salicylate, and aspirin (dissolved in saline solution).[38] Phenylbutazone is beneficial but causes considerable local irritation.[39] In my experience and that of others, nitrogen mustards and thio-tepa produced only minimal benefit and occasionally caused toxic effects with high fever.[40-42]

The terms chemical and radiation (nonsurgical) synovectomy have been introduced to describe the effects of potent agents such as osmic acid and radioisotopes such as gold-198 (^{198}Au) and yttrium-90 (^{90}Y).

Osmic Acid. Failure to produce predictable prolonged local remissions after corticosteroid injections prompted the use of chemical agents such as osmic acid. Osmic acid is an aqueous solution of osmium tetroxide in a 1% or 2% concentration. Intra-articular injection of osmic acid has been used in synovitis of the knee since 1950 in Scandanavia. The drug is relatively widely used in other countries, especially France, and over 4000 injections have been given at the Rheumatism Foundation Hospital in Finland.[43] To my knowledge, osmic acid therapy has not been used in human joints in the United States.

Intra-articular injection of osmic acid produces acute necrosis of the synovial tissue with an intensely painful reaction. When a local anesthetic and corticosteroid are administered in conjunction with the osmic acid, the initial drastic reaction is reduced to a tolerable level. Although this form of therapy has been used chiefly in rheumatoid synovitis, chronic or recurrent synovial effusions with osteoarthritis have been favorably influenced by it. Menkes[44] reported some cases of hemophilic arthropathy with chronic effusion or hemarthrosis that resolved completely after osmic acid therapy. Because concomitant use of a corticosteroid with osmic acid is necessary to combat the local reaction and because in a comparative study the duration of the beneficial effects of triamcinolone hexacetonide alone was similar to the combination, it seems unlikely that osmic acid will ever become a common remedy in the treatment of knee joint synovitis.[45]

Radioisotopes. The use of radioactive gold in the treatment of malignant pleural effusions prompted its trial use in cases of persistent synovial effusions.[46] Despite successful results, the concern with minimizing unwanted radiation led to subsequent studies with ^{90}Yttrium, ^{169}Erbium, and other radioactive isotopes.[47] Satisfactory results have been reported from Europe, including more than 9000 joints treated with radioisotope injections in France.[44]

A double-blind trial comparing yttrium-90 with nonradioactive yttrium for chronic synovitis of the knee failed to demonstrate significant beneficial effect of the radioisotope.[48] In addition, anterior instability developed in a significant number of the knees treated with the radioactive yttrium. The fear of leakage of radioactivity from the joint and the uncertain long-term biologic hazards of radiation has limited this form of therapy in the United States to experimental studies in animals.[49, 50] Some comparative clinical studies indicate that radioisotope therapy is not superior to "long-acting" steroids, including methylprednisolone and triamcinolone hexacetonide.[44, 51, 52]

Hyaluronate Therapy. A new direction in intra-articular therapy in osteoarthritis was initially reported in studies on the effect of exogenous hyaluronic acid in race horses.[53, 54] These equine studies suggested that injections of hyaluronate reversed the synovial fluid molecular matrix changes that occur in osteoarthritis and increased function without any deleterious effect on the cartilage. Preliminary clinical assessment of sodium hyaluronate (Healon) in the treatment of osteoarthritic human knee demonstrated evidence of improvement.[55] A recent trial of the effects of sodium hyaluronate in human knees affected by osteoarthritis utilized sham and saline injections as controls. When the hyaluronate-treated knees were compared with the sham-treated knees, there was improvement in the former, with decreased pain and increased function, without any adverse effects. In a comparison of the effects of hyaluronate compared with saline solution, there was no immediate significant difference, but a reduction of pain and an improvement of flexion occurred after 1 week in the hyaluronate-treated group.[56] Although these studies suggest that intra-articular hyaluronate injections may be of clinical value, further investigation and additional studies, including a comparative evaluation with corticosteroids, are necessary to determine the ultimate usefulness of this substance in synovitis associated with osteoarthritis.

References

1. Bannatyne GA: Rheumatoid Arthritis. 2nd ed. Bristol, John Wright and Co., 1898, pp. 152–153.
2. Hollander JL: Intrasynovial corticosteroid therapy in arthritis. Maryland Med J 19:62–66, 1972.
3. Steinbrocker O, Neustadt DH: Aspiration and Injection Therapy in Arthritis and Musculoskeletal Disorders: A Handbook on Technique and Manage-

ment. Hagerstown, Maryland, Harper and Row, 1972.

4. Gray RG, Tenenbaum J, Gottlieb NL: Local corticosteroid injection treatment in rheumatic disorders. Semin Arthritis Rheum 10:231–254, 1981.

5. Editorial: Intra-articular steroids. Br Med J 1:600–601, 1978.

6. Chandler GN, Jones GT, Wright V, Hartfall LJ: Charcot arthropathy following intra-articular hydrocortisone. Br Med J 1:952–953, 1959.

7. Neustadt DH: Chemistry and Therapy of Collagen Diseases. Springfield, Illinois, Charles C Thomas, 1963, p. 54.

8. Chandler GN, Wright V: Deleterious effect of intra-articular hydrocortisone. Lancet 2:661–663, 1958.

9. Silberberg M, Silberberg R, Hasler M: Fine structure of articular cartilage in mice receiving cortisone acetate. Arch Pathol 82:569–582, 1966.

10. Meyer WL, Kunin AS: Decreased glycolytic enzyme activity in epiphyseal cartilage of cortisone treated rats. Arch Biochem Biophys 129:431–437, 1969.

11. Mankin HJ, Conger KA: The acute effects of intra-articular hydrocortisone on articular cartilage in rabbits. J Bone Joint Surg 48A:1383–1388, 1966.

12. Moskowitz RW, Davis W, Sammarco J, Mast W, Chase SW: Experimentally induced corticosteroid arthropathy. Arthritis Rheum 13:236–243, 1970.

13. Behrens F, Shepherd N, Mitchel N: Alterations of rabbit articular cartilage by intra-articular injection of glucocorticoids. J Bone Joint Surg 57A:1157–1160, 1976.

14. Balch HW, Gibson JMC, El Ghobarey AF, et al.: Repeated corticosteroid injections into knee joints. Rheumatol Rehabil 16:137–140, 1977.

15. Keagy RD, Keim HA: Intra-articular steroid therapy: Repeated use in patients with chronic arthritis. Am J Med Sci 253:45–51, 1967.

16. Gibson T, Burry HC, Poswillo D, et al.: Effect of intra-articular corticosteroid injections in primate cartilage. Ann Rheum Dis 36:74–79, 1976.

17. Armstrong RD, English J, Gibson T, et al.: Serum methylprednisolone levels following intra-articular injections of methylprednisolone acetate. Ann Rheum Dis 40:571–574, 1981.

18. Eymontt MJ, Gordon GV, Schumacher HR, et al.: The effects on synovial permeability and synovial fluid leukocyte counts in symptomatic osteoarthritis after intra-articular corticosteroid administration. J Rheumatol 9:198–203, 1982.

19. McCarty DJ: Treatment of rheumatoid joint inflammation with triamcinolone hexacetonide. Arthritis Rheum 15:157–173, 1972.

20. Bornstein J, Silver M, Neustadt DH, et al.: Intra-articular hydrocortisone acetate in rheumatic disorders. Geriatrics 9:205–210, 1954.

21. Zuchner J, Machek O, Caciolo C, et al.: Intra-articular injections of hydrocortisone, prednisolone and their tertiary-butylacetate derivatives in patients with rheumatoid arthritis and osteoarthritis. J Chronic Dis 8:637–644, 1958.

22. Foreign letters: Hydrocortisone and osteoarthritis. JAMA 170:1451, 1959.

23. Kehr MJ: Comparison of intra-articular cortisone analogues in osteoarthritis of the knee. Ann Rheum Dis 18:325–328, 1959.

24. Hollander JL: Osteoarthritis: Perspectives on treatment. Postgrad Med 68:161–168, 1980.

25. Miller JH, White J, Norton TH: The value of intra-articular injection in osteoarthritis of the knee. J Bone Joint Surg 40A:636–643, 1958.

26. Friedman DM, Moore ME: The efficacy of intraarticular steroids in osteoarthritis: A double-blind study. J Rheumatol 7:850–856, 1980.

27. Dieppe PA, Sathapatayavongs B, Jones HE, et al.: Intra-articular steroids in osteoarthritis. Rheumatol Rehabil 19:212–217, 1980.

28. Valtonen EJ: Clinical comparison of triamcinolone hexacetonide and betamethasone in the treatment of osteoarthrosis of the knee joint. Scand J Rheumatol 41(Suppl):3–7, 1981.

29. Clemmesen S: Triamcinolone hexacetonide in intra-articular and intra-muscular therapy. Acta Rheumatol Scand 17:273–278, 1971.

30. Neustadt DH: Complications of local corticosteroid injection. (Letter to the Editor.) JAMA 246:835–836, 1981.

31. Fitzgerald RH: Intrasynovial injection of steroids: uses and abuses. Mayo Clin Proc 51:655–659, 1976.

32. Gordon GV, Schumacher HR: Electron microscopic study of depo corticosteroid crystals with clinical studies after intra-articular injection. J Rheumatol 6:7–14, 1979.

33. Sweetnam R: Corticosteroid arthropathy and tendon rupture. (Editorial.) J Bone Joint Surg 51B:397–398, 1969.

34. Neustadt DH: Tendon rupture and steroid therapy. (Letter to the Editor.) South Med J 73:271–272, 1980.

35. Bain LS, Balch HW, Wetherly JMR, et al.: Intraarticular triamcinolone hexacetonide: Double-blind comparison with methylprednisolone. Br J Clin Prac 26:559–561, 1972.

36. McCarty DJ: Calcium pyrophosphate dihydrate crystal deposition disease—a current appraisal of the problem. *In* Holt PJL (ed.): Current Topics in Connective Tissue Disease, New York, Longman, Inc., 1975, p. 184.

37. Dieppe PA, Crocker P, Huskisson EC, et al.: Apatite deposition disease. A new arthropathy. Lancet 1:266–269, 1976.

38. Rylance HJ, Chalmers TM, Elton RA: Clinical trials of intra-articular aspirin in rheumatoid arthritis. Lancet 2:1099–1102, 1980.

39. Neustadt DH, Steinbrocker O: Observations of the effects of intra-articular phenylbutazone. J Lab Clin Med 47:284–288, 1956.

40. Henderson ED, Nathan FF: Experience with injection of nitrogen mustard into joints of patients with rheumatoid arthritis. South Med J 62:1455–1458, 1969.

41. Zuckner J, Uddin J, Ramsey RH, et al.: Evaluation of intra-articular thio-tepa in rheumatoid arthritis. Ann Rheum Dis 25:178–183, 1966.

42. Gristina AG, Pace NA, Kantor TG, et al.: Intra-articular thio-tepa compared with depo-medrol and procaine in the treatment of arthritis. J Bone Joint Surg 52A:1603–1610, 1970.

43. Nissila M: Absence of increased frequency of degenerative joint changes after osmic acid injections. Scand J Rheumatol 7:81–84, 1978.

44. Menkes CJ: Is there a place for chemical and radiation synovectomy in rheumatic diseases? Rheumatol Rehabil 18:65–77, 1979.

45. Anttinen J, Oka M: Intra-articular triamcinolone hexacetonide and osmic acid in persistent synovitis of the knee. Scand J Rheumatol 4:125–128, 1975.

46. Makin M, Robin GC: Chronic synovial effusions treated with intra-articular radioactive gold. JAMA 188:725–728, 1964.

47. Ingrand J: Characteristics of the radioisotopes for

intra-articular therapy. Ann Rheum Dis 32 (Suppl):3–9, 1973.

48. Yates DB, Scott JT, Ramsay N: Double blind trial of yttrium 90 for chronic inflammatory synovitis of the knee. Ann Rheum Dis 36:481, 1977.

49. Sledge CB, Noble J, Hnatowich S, et al.: Experimental radiation synovectomy by dyferric hydroxide macroaggregate. Arthritis Rheum 20:1334–1342, 1977.

50. Lee P: The efficacy and safety of radiosynovectomy (Editorial). J Rheumatol 9:165–168, 1982.

51. Ruotsi A, Hypen M, Rekonen A, et al.: Erbium-169 versus triamcinolone hexacetonide in the treatment of rheumatoid finger joints. Ann Rheum Dis 38:45–47, 1979.

52. Gumpel JM, Matthews SA, Fisher M: Synoviortheses with erbium-169: A double blind controlled comparison of erbium-169 with corticosteroids. Ann Rheum Dis 38:341–343, 1979.

53. Asheim A, Lindblad G: Intra-articular treatment of arthritis in race horses with sodium hyaluronate. Acta Vet Scand 17(Suppl):379–394, 1976.

54. Auer JA, Fackelman GE, Gingerich DA, et al.: Effect of hyaluronic acid in naturally occurring and experimentally induced osteoarthritis. Am J Vet Res 41:568–574, 1980.

55. Peyron JG, Balazs EA: Preliminary clinical assessment of Na hyaluronate injection in human arthritis joints. Pathol Biol 731–736, 1974.

56. Weiss C, Balazs EA, Stonge R, et al.: Clinical studies of the intraarticular injection of Healon (sodium hyaluronate) in the treatment of osteoarthritis of human knees. Semin Arthritis Rheum 11 (Suppl)1:143–144, 1981.

20

Surgery in Osteoarthritis: General Considerations

Victor M. Goldberg, M.D.

Osteoarthritis (OA) is ubiquitous and is the most common form of joint disease. The treatment for the most part is nonoperative. However, a small number of patients do not respond to the basic medical program, which usually consists of appropriate rest, physical therapy, analgesics, anti-inflammatory medications, and modifications of daily activities. Surgical management may then be helpful in either correcting structural abnormalities or preventing further progression of the disease. The advent of the total joint replacement era has, of course, made surgery a more appealing therapeutic alternative for the patient suffering from the problems of OA. Beneficial results that can be seen after total joint reconstruction must be tempered by the possibility of failure secondary to mechanical and biologic problems. The end result of these complications may be less than optimal function, sometimes in a relatively young and active individual. Because of these possibilities, although total joint replacement may be an attractive surgical procedure, a number of other less invasive surgical procedures should be considered that may improve the symptoms of the disease or retard the progression of the pathology without the necessity of removing extensive bone stock. It is therefore important to re-examine carefully the indications and outcome of surgical procedures such as osteotomy, which still preserve the biologic diarthrodial joint. This chapter will endeavor to give the reader an overview of the indications for surgery and the types of surgical procedures that are presently available, which will be discussed in detail in the sections that follow.

GENERAL INDICATION CONSIDERATIONS

Before considering surgical treatment, the physician must weigh the risks and benefits of each procedure. This is especially important today, considering the larger number of younger, active patients who are developing secondary arthritis after trauma or sports-related injuries. Although there are no absolute indications or contraindications for considering any surgical procedure, certain general concepts are important. For each individual patient, the physician should endeavor to develop a quantitative assessment of parameters of function in order to determine the appropriate therapeutic program. Not only is this an aid in the therapeutic decision process, but it can also be of help in prospective studies evaluating the outcome of different surgical procedures. Figure 20–1 summarizes a scoring system for the evaluation of the knee used at our hospital.[1] Similar protocols may be adapted to the hip or other joints.

Pain is a key factor in the therapeutic decision process and is usually given the most points. If rest pain is present, this poses a major problem for the patient and usually requires narcotics for control. Greater consideration should be given in this circumstance for surgical intervention. Activity-related discomfort is also important and may affect the quality of life. However, many times these symptoms may be treated by nonoperative modalities, although lesser surgical procedures than total joint reconstruction may be of greater use during this stage of the disease.

Date: Examiner: Age: Sex:
                                                                             Height:
                                                                             Weight:

Operation: Knee   R   L   Bilateral   Patient's Record No.

Surgery
Date: Preop: _____ Postop: _____ Length of follow-up _____ Surgeon _____
                   O.A., R.A., post-trauma, post-arthrotomy, sepsis, failed prosthesis
                   other (specify)

1. Pain
   a. None/ignores   44
   b. Slight, occasional, no compromise in
      activity   40
   c. Mild, no effect on ordinary activity,
      pain after unusual activity, uses aspi-
      rin   30
   d. Moderate, tolerable, makes conces-
      sions, occasional codeine   20
   e. Marked, serious limitations   10
   f. Totally disabled   0
2. Function
   a. Gait (walking maximum distance)
      1. Limp:
         None   3
         Slight   2
         Moderate   1
         Serious   0
         Unable to walk   0
      2. Support:
         None   11
         Cane, long walks   7
         Cane, full time   5
         Crutch   4
         2 canes   2
         2 crutches or walker   0
         Unable to walk   0
      3. Distance walked:
         Unlimited   11
         6 blocks   8
         2–3 blocks   5
         Indoors only   2
         Bed and chair   0
   b. Functional activities
      1. Ability to use stairs:
         Ascends and descends normally   6
         Ascends normally, has difficulty
            descending   4
         Uses banister at all times   2
         Unable   0

2. Ability to get out of chair:
   Able with ease   5
   Able with difficulty   3
   Unable   0
3. Ability to sit in car or theater:
   No difficulty   1
   Difficulty   0
3. Absence of deformity
   a. None   2
   b. Varus or valgus, 10°   0
   c. Flexion contracture, 10°   0
4. Range of motion
   Add each segment to arc to determine
      total score. Do not add point if any
      portion of arc is missing.
   Flexion
      0°–15°   2
      15°–45°   2
      45°–90°   2
      90° or greater   1
                                                        ___
      Total motion points
5. Stability
   a. Never locks or gives way   7
   b. Rarely locks or gives way   5
   c. Frequently locks or gives way   0
6. Effusion or hemarthrosis
   a. Never has an effusion   3
   b. Occasionally has an effusion   1
   c. Frequently has an effusion   0
7. Total knee function rating _____
   Compsensation or litigation involved?
   Yes
   No

Figure 20–1. Quantitative knee evaluation form.

Functional considerations are also central in the therapeutic decision process. The distance one walks may be correlated with the anatomic severity of the joint disease. The need for external supports, e.g., canes, is an objective indication of the functional impairment experienced by the patient. The activities of daily living are also important. The ability to climb stairs and get into and out of an automobile or chair should be quantified. One should

inquire about the loss of time from work and the inability to perform necessary household chores, as well as recreational activities. This information gives the physician an estimate of the quality of the patient's daily life and the socioeconomic problems that the person may be experiencing.

Anatomic considerations include the range of joint motion, the presence or absence of extremity deformity, and an estimation of joint stability. This last function is easier to evaluate for the knee joint than for other joints. For example, when considering the hip, because ligaments cannot be examined, indirect techniques, e.g., evaluation of pain and deformity, may be indicative of joint integrity. The degree of motion and/or the extent of deformity is important not only in defining the stage of the disease but also in influencing the choice of the surgical procedure, as will be described in subsequent chapters.

All these data must be integrated into an overall estimation of the patient's present state of joint disease. Additional important considerations in this regard are the age and weight of the individual. For example, total joint arthroplasty has a higher chance of mechanical failure in a young, overweight, active individual, so that other surgical procedures, e.g., arthrodesis, should be considered. By contrast, an elderly patient with a finite life expectancy who may not have severe anatomic or functional limitations but whose activities have had to be significantly modified may be a candidate for total joint replacement.

The ability of the patient to cooperate in any treatment plan is also important in surgical selection. Certain procedures, i.e., debridement or arthroplasties, require greater involvement of the patient during the postoperative rehabilitation period compared with arthrodeses. In addition, the patient's understanding of the disease must be considered, because possible limitations in functional gains from any surgical procedure must be understood by the person. The patient's own perception of what he hopes to obtain as a result of the surgery is central in the decision process. The important question that all too frequently is not asked by the physician is what are the desires of the patient himself. Although each person must be considered individually, information relative to the known outcome of each surgical procedure is important in educating that individual. In some circumstances, an individual may desire a curative procedure that is unrealistic. At other times, cosmetic correction is foremost in the patient's mind. However, the patient may have become well adjusted to the presence of the malposition of the extremity, and if his function is not compromised and the deformity does not constitute an anatomic threat to other joints, the mere presence of malposition may not be a reason for surgery.

Long-term bed-bound or wheelchair-confined patients may desire a return to a community ambulatory status, but there may be extra-articular anatomic factors that militate against this goal. However, the improvement of function to an effective, household ambulatory status may be an attainable goal. These outcomes must be understood clearly by the patient and the physician.

The general medical health of the patient must be considered in evaluating risk factors of surgery. Diseases of the cardiovascular or respiratory system may be severe enough to be a contraindication to general anesthesia and a major surgical procedure. However, many times, regional or spinal anesthesia may be substituted, thereby reducing the morbidity. It is important to realize that many of the patients who are candidates for reconstructive surgery in the treatment of osteoarthritis are elderly and are poor surgical and anesthetic risks. However, chronologic age alone should not be considered a contraindication; rather, the physiologic age of each patient must be considered in the risk-versus-benefit formula. It is important, however, to recognize, stabilize, and correct medical conditions that may exist prior to surgery. Some of the more common conditions include chronic obstructive lung disease, hypertension, angina pectoris or congestive heart failure, peripheral vascular disease, and diabetes mellitus. If there are any factors that predispose to infection, e.g., chronic steroid treatment, these should be considered and modified, if possible.

In addition to the risk-versus-benefit aspect of any treatment, the cost versus benefit of a procedure must also be weighed. Questions that should be asked include the following: Will the surgery enable the patient to become more self-sufficient, or allow the individual to remain independent? If the surgery is successful, can the person continue working, or will surgery allow the patient to return to employment? The answers to these questions must be considered in the overall decision-making process. Of course, care must be taken not to allow the decision of whether to operate to weigh too heavily on socioecomonic considerations.

It should be evident that there are no absolute indications for surgical intervention in osteoarthritis. Many factors must be considered, and no one treatment algorithm is appropriate for any surgical treatment. In the same light, there are no absolute contraindications to surgery in OA, although relative contraindications do exist after the risks and benefits are weighed for each individual. Active infection, overwhelmingly poor medical health, and inadequate anatomic structures, e.g., motor control, or available bone stock are all reasons to reject surgical modalities of treatment. Other factors may increase the chance for a poorer outcome when considering specific operative procedures. For example, patients with morbid obesity or a neuropathic-type joint usually do poorly when arthroplasties are performed, so that suitable alternatives should be substituted, if possible.

Until we gain more knowledge pertaining to the outcome of many of the presently performed operative procedures as well as which risk factors are most important in determining their fate, the decisions of when, upon whom, and which surgical procedure to utilize must be left to sound clinical judgment. Most important, each person must be considered individually, and the pros and cons of the situation must be carefully weighed for that patient.

TYPES OF SURGICAL PROCEDURES

The surgical treatment modalities presently used in OA may be classified into four broad categories: osteotomy, debridement, arthrodesis (fusion), and arthroplasty. There are general principles that have evolved for each procedure that are applicable to its use in any osteoarthritic joint problem.

Osteotomy

The biologic and mechanical factors influencing the pathophysiology of OA have been discussed previously in great detail. One of the advantages of an osteotomy is that it addresses both biologic and mechanical problems without sacrificing the integrity of the joint. If joint malalignment is present, e.g., genu varum of the knee, with resultant abnormal force distribution, an osteotomy to realign the joint toward a normal configuration will correct the destructive pattern. This will redistribute the forces in a way that healthy cartilages on the relatively uninvolved side of the joint will be brought into apposition. In addition, there is some evidence that cutting the bone changes an abnormal vascular pattern toward a normal distribution, suggesting a biologic effect of the operation.[2]

Osteotomy is one of the earlier procedures to be utilized in the surgical management of OA; the knee and the hip joints are the most frequently treated. Although osteotomy is not curative, when patients are carefully selected, long-term good results may be expected with excellent pain relief, improved function, and maintenance of physiologic joint motion and stability.[3–6] It is particularly applicable for the young, active individual when articular cartilage has not been completely destroyed. A functional range of motion must be present before surgery, because many times some motion may be lost after surgery. The knee joint, for example, should have close to 90 degrees of flexion without a fixed flexion contracture greater than 20 degrees for osteotomy to be considered.[3] If a deformity, e.g., genu valgum, is present, it should not be so excessive that correction to physiologic alignment cannot be obtained. Additional important considerations include appropriate motor control of the joint and intrinsic stability. Considerable patient cooperation and understanding are necessary for a successful outcome. The recent use of internal fixation devices may lessen the postoperative need for casts and may enable maintenance of joint motion, which is so important for healthy cartilage. Recently, there have been reports of the use of the combination of osteotomy and debridement in the knee joint, with encouraging early results in difficult, more advanced problems of OA of the knee.[7] This may delay the need for total knee reconstruction in the younger patient.

Debridement

The concept of smoothing irregular joint surfaces and removing loose bodies and inflamed synovium that adds to the destructive process of OA was popularized by Magnuson in 1946 in the knee joint,[8] although in appropriate circumstances the ankle, wrist, and elbow may benefit from this surgical modality. For this procedure to be considered, no extremity malalignment should be present and a functional range of motion is necessary. The results are variable and depend a great deal on the careful selection of a motivated patient. Pain relief can be impressive, but many times, some joint mobility is lost after surgery. Insall reported about 75% good results of knee joint debridement with an average of 6.5 years of follow-up.[9] Frequently, a joint effusion is present for a prolonged period after surgery; however, this gradually subsides. Maximal improvement usually is not seen before 12 months after surgery. The recent addition of continuous passive motion in the postoperative rehabilitation phase may improve the long-term results of debridement, but this awaits further prospective studies.[10] Advances in arthroscopic techniques, with their attendant decrease in morbidity and postoperative recovery time may make debridement an even more attractive approach in early cases.

Arthrodesis (Fusion)

Although this is the era of artificial joint replacement, there is still a place in the surgical management of OA for the use of arthrodesis of joints. In fact, it must be clearly understood by any patient about to undergo total joint replacement of the knee that fusion may be the only reasonable alternative and may be the end result if failure occurs. However, there are specific instances in which arthrodesis may be the primary procedure of choice. Osteoarthritis of the cervical or lumbar spine unresponsive to medical management may require appropriate fusion of the involved segments combined with decompression of the neural elements.[11, 12] Local intercarpal fusions may be extremely helpful in controlling the pain and instability of carpal OA without completely sacrificing wrist motion and function.[13]

If a single lower-extremity joint is involved with OA in a young, heavy, active patient, arthrodesis may be the procedure of choice when the severity of joint destruction precludes use of a lesser procedure. As long as the contiguous joints are mobile, function is usually maintained and long-term pain relief is achieved. However, if OA is present in other joints, e.g., the lumbar spine, hip, or knee, fusion may be relatively contraindicated, and careful consideration should be given to the performance of an appropriate arthroplasty. Anatomic considerations are also important in the decision. For example, deficient bone stock or inadequate motor power may be contraindications to other procedures and may make arthrodesis attractive. If the shoulder joint lacks adequate rotator cuff and deltoid muscle power but has good scapular muscle stabilizers, fusion may be an effective surgical modality in relieving pain and improving upper-extremity function. The use of modern internal fixation devices has made arthrodesis a more successful procedure and less dependent on prolonged cast immobilization.

Arthroplasty

The modern concepts of joint replacement have their origin in the original Smith-Petersen cup arthroplasty, but with the applications of sophisticated engineering principles to orthopedics, great strides in arthroplasty have been made in the last 20 years.[14] Charnley's adaptation of polymethylmethacrylate as a fixation interface between the metallic or plastic implant and the bone created a major impact on the surgical treatment of severe OA.[15]

Arthroplasty is indicated when severe pain and disability are present. Appropriate bone stock and muscle power must be present to technically accomplish the procedure and to expect a satisfactory result. Because the failure of arthroplasty usually results in less than optimal function, lesser surgical procedures should be considered first, if feasible, and the patient should understand and be willing to accept, if necessary, the possible end-stage procedure. Arthroplasty may be of the excisional, partial, or total replacement type. Recently, biologic substitutes have been used to resurface destroyed articular surfaces in the knee joint, with encouraging early results.[16]

Girdlestone described a hip arthroplasty in which the head and neck of the femur were excised and a fibrous pseudarthrosis developed.[17] The results of this procedure as a therapeutic modality are less than optimal, but patients who are candidates for total hip reconstruction must be willing to accept this type of procedure as a possible consequence of the complications of the total joint arthroplasty. Excellent results are rarely seen in the excisional arthroplasty, as most patients continue to complain of some pain, instability, and shortening of the extremity. External supports such as a cane or crutches are usually required for most activities.[18]

Use of the excisional type of arthroplasty with the interposition of local tissue may be of greater use in small joints, e.g., the first carpometacarpal joint[19] or the first metatarsophalangeal joint.[20] Under these circumstances, the malalignment and pain resulting from OA of these joints are corrected, and function is improved. These joints, of course, are not usually subjected to the marked stresses seen in other large upper- and lower-extremity synovial joints.

The cup arthroplasty was the first modern attempt to resurface destroyed articular surfaces.[14] The initial results were encouraging, but unfortunately, the long-term outcome has been inconsistent and too dependent on the technical expertise of the surgeon and on the postoperative rehabilitation program. Although satisfactory results may be expected in only approximately 60% of patients, there are certain clinical situations in which the procedure should still be considered. Young patients with secondary OA after a remote infected joint may benefit from this procedure, but their expectation of the outcome should not be high as far as ultimate function is concerned.[21]

Another type of hemiarthroplasty that has been used in the past with some success is the Austin-Moore or Thompson femoral head replacement. It has been used extensively for treatment of the displaced femoral neck fracture in the elderly, with satisfactory results.[22] Its application to the surgical treatment of OA has been supplanted by the more dependable total replacement. However, in situations in which OA involves only the femoral articular surfaces, e.g., as a secondary manifestation of osteonecrosis, some consideration should be given to its use.[23] A bipolar femoral head replacement in which polymethylmethacrylate is used to fix the implant to bone has been employed in an attempt to prevent the problems of loosening of the prosthesis that may be seen. Early satisfactory results have been reported.[24]

Biologic materials have also been utilized to resurface articular surfaces destroyed by OA. Osteochondral allografts have been primarily used in the knee joint.[16] The experience has been variable, although satisfactory results have been reported when technical problems have been minimized and a single compartment replaced. The widespread applicability of this technique to articular problems in OA awaits improved techniques of cartilage preservation and fixation.

Today, the surgical treatment of advanced OA has primarily centered on total joint reconstruction. There is no doubt that this procedure is one of the most consistent and dependable operative techniques used in orthopedic surgery. The relief of pain and improved function that it affords are almost universal in technically satisfactory procedures. However, great care must be given to prior consideration of other surgical treatment modalities in view of the possible complications (which occur, fortunately, relatively infrequently) and poor outcome if failure does ensue. Although almost every diarthrodial joint has been replaced in the treatment of OA, the hip and knee have been the major foci.[25, 26] As many as 100,000 total hip replacements and 40,000 total knee replacements are performed each year in the United States.[27] Because these procedures were not done with

such frequency until recently, there are only a few reports that relate long-term follow-up, and these relate primarily to the hip.[28, 29] Wear, initially considered to be the major long-term concern, has not been the problem it was anticipated to be. Infection has been significantly controlled by the use of prophylactic antibiotics and special operating room suites that rapidly exchange air in a laminar flow pattern. The data from the long-term studies indicate that the major problem appears to be loosening of the implants.[28, 29] The weak link of the system in this regard is the polymethylmethacrylate and its bond with the bone. Although a true incidence of loosening is difficult to obtain if only roentgenographic criteria are used, Stauffer reports an 11.3% acetabular loosening and a 29.9% femoral loosening in a 10-year follow-up of 231 hip replacements.[28] Although this surely might be an omen of the future, not all of these hips were symptomatic. If one looks only at the clinical results, 90% of the patients had what would be considered a good result. Many of the early failures occurred in young, heavy, active patients. Because of the problems of total joint reconstruction in young patients, alternative procedures that resurface the destroyed articular surfaces but retain a large part of the bony stock (surface replacement arthroplasty) have been developed (Fig. 20–2). Unfortunately, the early results of these surface replacements have not been as good as anticipated.[30] Loosening of the implants and fracture of the femoral neck have been the major reasons for the failures. Additional investigation is continuing to improve this technique.[31]

Because of the concern with long-term loosening of the components of both total hip replacements and total knee replacements, many centers are investigating different means of fixing the implants to the bone. One of the major areas of research has been the use of porous-surface implants to allow bone ingrowth for biologic fixation.[32] Although this appears to be an attractive concept, certain problems remain unsolved. These include the type of alloys that should be used, rates of corrosion of the surface metal, the role of infection, and, most important, the possible stress shielding that can result in atrophy of the surrounding cortical bone. A major technical consideration still to be answered is the problem of implant removal for whatever reason. In addition, the exact design of the components is critical in determining the effect that the prosthetic device will have on bone

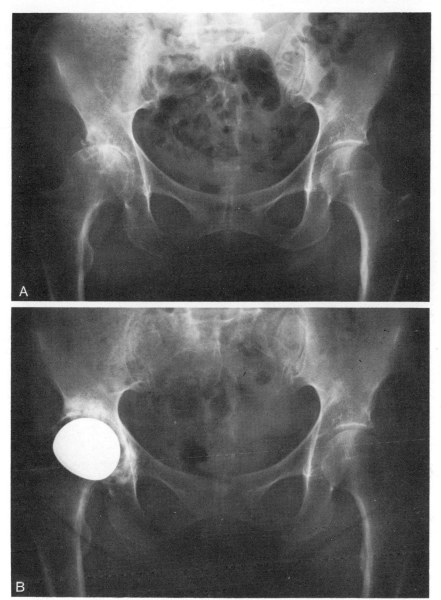

Figure 20–2. *A,* Roentgenogram of the pelvis of an active 51-year-old female demonstrating symptomatically severe primary OA of the right hip. *B,* Roetgenogram of the pelvis of the patient 4 years after a successful surface replacement arthroplasty of the hip.

remodeling. This therefore requires additional careful consideration.

There have been some early clinical reports on the results of sintered titanium fiber composites for replacing bone defects as well as powdered porous-surface cobalt chromium molybdenum (Co-Cr-Mo) implants for hip and knee replacement.[33, 34] These studies are ongoing and should ultimately provide some of the necessary solutions to problems in total joint replacement.

Another new approach to the problem of implant fixation has been the use in the hip of a ceramic articular surface that has an extremely low coefficient of friction.[35] This technique utilizes a ceramic cup in the shape of a cone with large side threads to obtain immediate fixation and to allow bone ingrowth to occur. The femoral implant is a Co-Cr-Mo implant designed so that the geometry results in immediate stability. This implant has been used in Europe for reconstruction in difficult problems of severe OA in young patients, with excellent short-term results (Fig. 20–3). As is evident from this discussion, improved methods of total joint reconstruction will continue

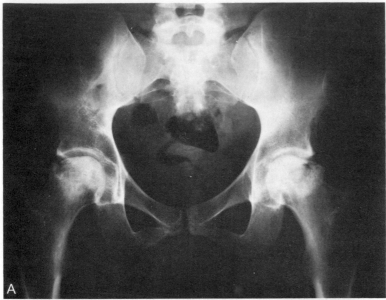

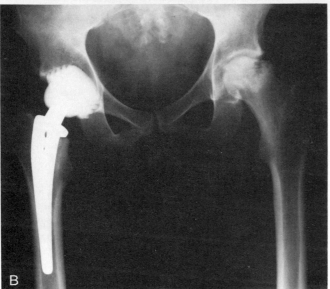

Figure 20–3. *A,* Roentgenogram of the pelvis of a 35-year-old male illustrating idiopathic osteonecrosis of both hips. The right hip was symptomatic and was severely limiting function. *B,* Roentgenogram of the pelvis of this patient 6 months after right ceramic hip replacement.

to evolve as our knowledge of the biologic and mechanical principles of diarthrodial joints increases and our adaptations of engineering advances improve.

CONCLUSIONS

The present state of the art of surgical management of OA offers patients effective methods of alleviating the distressing symptoms of the disease. However, it must be remembered that a vast majority of individuals may obtain adequate relief with judicious nonoperative therapeutic modalities. Prior to surgical intervention, careful consideration should be given to the available surgical alternatives, and great effort should be directed toward educating the patient with regard to the risks and benefits of any procedure. It is hoped that with improved uniform prospective quantitative evaluations of the functional performance of different surgical methods, accurate information to assess the best approach to each patient's needs will become available.

References

1. Goldberg VM, Henderson BT: The Freeman-Swanson ICLH total knee arthroplasty: Complications and problems. J Bone Joint Surg 62A:1338–1344, 1980.
2. Arnoldi CC, Lemperg R, Linderholm H: Immediate effect of osteotomy on the intramedullary pressure in the femoral head and neck in patients with degenerative osteoarthritis. Acta Orthop Scand 42:454–455, 1971.
3. Coventry MB: Osteotomy about the knee for degenerative and rheumatoid arthritis. Indications, operative technique, and results. J Bone Joint Surg 55A:23–48, 1973.
4. Coventry MB: Upper tibial osteotomy for gonarthrosis. The evolution of the operation in the last 18 years and long term results. Orthop Clin North Am 10:191–210, 1979.
5. Insall J, Shoji H, Mayer V: High tibial osteotomy. A five-year evaluation. J Bone Joint Surg 56A:1397–1405, 1974.
6. Hansen FW, Hansen-Leth C, Jensen EG: Intertrochanteric osteotomy with A. O. technique in arthrosis of the hip. Acta Orhop Scand 44:219–229, 1973.
7. MacIntosh DL, Welsh RP: Joint debridement—a complement to high tibial osteotomy in the treatment of degenerative arthritis of the knee. J Bone Joint Surg 59A:1094–1097, 1977.
8. Magnuson PB: Technique of debridement of the knee joint for arthritis. Surg Clin North Am 26:249–266, 1946.
9. Insall JN: Intra-articular surgery for degenerative arthritis of the knee. A report of the work of the late K.H. Pridie. J Bone Joint Surg 49B:211–228, 1967.
10. Coutts RD, Kaita J, Barr R, et al.: The role of continuous passive motion in the postoperative rehabilitation of the total knee patient. Transactions of the 28th Annual Meeting of the Orthopaedic Research Society 7:195, 1982.
11. Paine KWE: Results of decompression for lumbar spinal stenosis. Clin Orthop 115:96–100, 1976.
12. Jacobs G, Krueger EG, Leivy DM: Cervical spondylosis with radiculopathy. Results of anterior diskectomy and interbody fusion. JAMA 211:2135–2139, 1970.
13. Watson HK, Hempton RF: Limited wrist arthrodesis. I. The triscaphoid joint. J Hand Surg 5:320–327, 1980.
14. Smith-Petersen MN: Evolution of mould arthroplasty of the hip joint. J Bone Joint Surg 30B:59–75, 1948.
15. Charnley J: The bonding of prostheses to bone by cement. J Bone Joint Surg 46B:518–529, 1964.
16. Gross AE, Silverstein EA, Falk J, et al.: The allotransplantation of partial joints in the treatment of osteoarthritis of the knee. Clin Orthop 108:7–14, 1975.
17. Girdlestone GR: Acute pyogenic arthritis of the hip: An operation giving free access and effective drainage. Lancet 1:419–424, 1943.
18. Bosquet MMJ, Duncan CP, Mulier JC, Patterson FP: Girdlestone excision arthroplasty of the hip. A review of 49 patients. Orthop Trans 6:336, 1982.
19. Jensen JS: Operative treatment of chronic subluxation of the first carpometacarpal joint. Hand 7:269–271, 1975.
20. Wrighton JD: A ten-year review of Keller's operation. Review of Keller's operation at the Princess Elizabeth Orthopaedic Hospital, Exeter. Clin Orthop 89:207–214, 1972.
21. Hunt DD, Larson CB: Treatment of the residual of hip infections by mold arthroplasty. An end result study of thirty-three hips. J Bone Joint Surg 48A:111–125, 1966.
22. Anderson LD, Hamsa WR, Waring TL: Femoral-head prostheses. A review of three hundred and fifty-six operations and their results. J Bone Joint Surg 46A:1049–1065, 1964.
23. Apley AG, Millner WF, Porter DS: A follow-up study of Moore's arthroplasty in the treatment of osteoarthritis of the hip. J Bone Joint Surg 51B:638–647, 1969.
24. Van Demark RE Jr, Cabanela ME, Henderson ED: The Bateman endoprosthesis: 104 arthroplasties. Orthop Trans 5:507, 1981.
25. Charnley J: The long-term results of low-friction arthroplasty of the hip performed as a primary intervention. J Bone Joint Surg 54B:61–76, 1972.
26. Insall JN, Ranawat CS, Aglietti P, Shine J: A comparison of four models of total knee-replacement prostheses. J Bone Joint Surg 58A:754–765, 1976.
27. Kelsey JL: Epidemiology and Impact. Presented at NIH Consensus Development Conference on Total Hip Joint Replacement, Bethesda, Maryland, March 1–3, 1982. In Total Hip Joint Replacement. Program Abstracts, pp. 23–25. Washington, D.C., U.S. Government Printing Office, 1982, 0–361–132/3806.
28. Stauffer RN: Ten-year follow-up study of total hip replacement. With particular reference to roentgenographic loosening of the components. J Bone Joint Surg 64A:983–990, 1982.
29. Salvati EA, Wilson PD, Jolley MN, et al.: A ten-year follow-up of our first one hundred consecutive Charnley total hip replacements. J Bone Joint Surg 63A:753–767, 1981.
30. Bierbaum BE, Sweet R: Complications of resurfacing arthroplasty. Orthop Clin North Am 13:761–775, 1982.
31. Amstutz HC, Graff-Radford A, Mai LL, Thomas BJ: Surface replacement of the hip with the Tharies system. Two to five year results. J Bone Joint Surg 63A:1069–1077, 1981.
32. Cameron HU, Pilliar RM, MacNab I: The effect of movement on the bonding of porous metal to bone. J Biomed Mater Res 7:301–311, 1973.
33. Andersson GB, Gaechter A, Gallante JO, Rostoker W: Segmental replacement of long bones in baboons using a fiber titanium implant. J Bone Joint Surg 60A:31–40, 1978.
34. Hungerford DS, Krackow KA, Kenna RV: Preliminary experience with the porous anatomic total knee replacement with and without cement. Orthop Trans 6:368, 1982.
35. Mittelmeier H: Selbshaftende Keramik—Metall-Verbund-Endoprothesen. MOB 6:152, 1975.

REGIONAL CONSIDERATIONS
(INCLUDING DIAGNOSIS, DIFFERENTIAL DIAGNOSIS, MEDICAL AND SURGICAL MANAGEMENT, OUTCOMES, AND PROGNOSIS)

Victor M. Goldberg, M.D.
Henry J. Mankin, M.D.
Section Co-Editors

SECTION
4

21

Osteoarthritis of the Hand and Wrist

Richard J. Smith, M.D.

DISTAL INTERPHALANGEAL JOINTS

Primary degenerative osteoarthritis of the distal interphalangeal joints of the fingers (Heberden's nodes) occurs most frequently in women in their fifties or sixties. There is a strong hereditary predisposition to the development of Heberden's nodes. Transmission is usually as an autosomal dominant characteristic.[1–3]

A Heberden's node usually appears gradually, without history of antecedent injury. It is first noted as a painless asymmetric enlargement at the dorsomedial or dorsolateral aspect of the distal joint of one finger. Often, a small nontender cystic swelling just proximal to the fingernail may herald an underlying, asymptomatic osteoarthritic osteophyte.[4] The cyst may reach a diameter of 2 cm and extend proximal to the distal interphalangeal extension crease. The overlying skin is thin, virtually translucent, and may rupture. A viscous, clear fluid with the consistency of currant jelly will escape. This fluid is identical to the contents of a typical ganglion cyst. Osteoarthritic mucous cysts often are not painful, and the patient's chief complaint is likely to be displeasure with the cyst's appearance or with the appearance of the fingernail just distal to it. Often, the pressure of the cyst on the germinal matrix will cause a shallow groove on the dorsum of the nail.

The bony swelling about the distal joint slowly enlarges, and soon the distal joints of the thumb or other fingers are involved. As the swelling becomes larger, the patient notes occasional aching pain in addition to the disfigurement. With advancing osteoarthritis, joint cartilage is lost, osteophytes increase in size, and the supporting terminal tendon of the extensor aponeurosis and the joint ligaments stretch. The distal phalanx subluxates volarly, falls into flexion, and may deviate ulnarly or radially by the forces acting on it in grasp or by the asymmetric enlargement of the joint osteophytes (Fig. 21–1). With deviation, subluxation, and dislocation, there is gross deformity, instability, weakness, and pain. Synovitis contributes to the pain, which is made more severe by activity.

Osteoarthritis of the distal interphalangeal joint may follow a fracture of the base of the distal phalanx. This is most common after a "mallet finger" fracture of the dorsal lip of the base of the distal phalanx that follows an acute flexion injury. In contrast to Heberden's nodes, secondary distal interphalangeal joint osteoarthritis is more likely to occur in younger patients, and the deformity is symmetric. There is uniform bony swelling transversely at the level of the distal interphalangeal joint extension crease. Rarely is more than one finger involved. The lateral roentgenogram will show a beaked dorsal lip of the distal phalanx and a relatively normal articular surface of the middle phalanx. Osteoarthritis of a distal in-

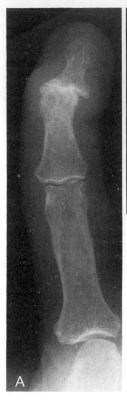

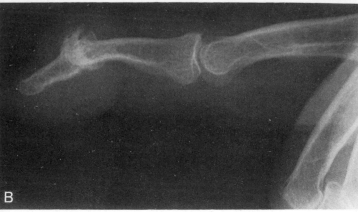

Figure 21–1. Posteroanterior *(A)* and lateral *(B)* views of primary osteoarthritis of the distal interphalangeal joint—"Heberden's node." Osteophytes arise from the dorsum of the base of the distal phalanx and from the head of the middle phalanx. There is an overlying cyst and the joint space is lost. The finger is deviated at the distal interphalangeal joint. Stability and pain relief can be achieved by distal interphalangeal arthrodesis.

terphalangeal joint may also be secondary to a condylar or intercondylar fracture of the distal end of the middle phalanx.

Treatment

For most patients with primary osteoarthritis of the distal interphalangeal joints, treatment is conservative. Small plastic or aluminum-foam splints may be applied to a swollen, tender joint as protection when the patient is engaged in manual activities. Nonsteroidal anti-inflammatory medications are often helpful. There is no reason to use systemic steroids, but local steroid injections intra-articularly or into inflamed para-articular tissues may be beneficial (see Chapter 19).

The osteoarthritic cyst may be improved—or at times even cured—by aspiration. A local anesthetic is injected intradermally with a small-bore needle (26-gauge), and the cyst entered with a larger needle (19-gauge). Often, the cyst fluid will extrude under pressure as soon as the larger needle enters it. Most of the fluid can be expressed from the cyst by digital pressure. Adhesive tape maintains the pressure for several hours.

Unfortunately, the cyst recurs quite fre-

quently after aspiration, with or without use of steroid. If there is a history of repeated infection about the cyst or if its appearance is objectionable to the patient, it may be excised. Because the cyst wall is intimately adherent to the overlying thin skin, many surgeons will excise this skin and replace it with a local rotation flap or skin graft. If there is an osteoarthritic osteophyte beneath the cyst, it too should be removed to lessen the chance of recurrence. After the cyst has been removed, the terminal tendon is retracted and the osteophyte is removed at its base. If the osteophyte protrudes beneath the center of the terminal tendon, the tendon is split longitudinally in order to permit adequate exposure. Postoperatively, the distal interphalangeal joint is splinted in extension for 5 to 7 days. Surgery is usually performed under local infiltration anesthesia using an upper-arm pneumatic tourniquet.

Many patients request removal of a Heberden's node (primary osteoarthritic osteophyte) for aesthetic reasons. If there is no joint space narrowing, subluxation, or instability at the distal interphalangeal joint and if the patient has no complaints of pain, such surgery may be justified. The patient should be warned, however, that the operation will not significantly alter the progress of the disease, and she should anticipate the possibility of further joint changes.

With more advanced changes and functional disability, the joint may be treated by arthroplasty or arthrodesis. Very few surgeons favor arthroplasty, because the joint may remain unstable considering the stresses to which it is subject and the poor quality of the lateral supporting ligaments. Those who favor arthroplasty (I am not among them) will usually use a silicone implant (0 or 00 size), with stems inserted into both the middle and distal phalanges, or hemiarthroplasty using a silicone toe implant. It would appear that arthroplasty is least indicated in the index finger, where normal pinch exerts greater stress on the distal joint.

Arthrodesis is the best way to correct the deformity and instability and to "cure" the pain of primary or secondary osteoarthritis of the distal interphalangeal joint. There is little penalty in arthrodesing the distal joint, as postoperative function is usually excellent. The hand can then be used for manual labor, for fine prehension, and even for typing and playing most musical instruments, provided the more proximal joints are normal. Most patients prefer arthrodesis in a relatively straight position. Our usual elective angle of arthrodesis of the distal interphalangeal joint is 10 degrees for the thumb and 20 degrees for the other fingers. Many other surgeons prefer to fuse the ring and little fingers in greater flexion. We use compression band wiring for most patients requiring arthrodesis of the distal interphalangeal joint.

PROXIMAL INTERPHALANGEAL JOINTS

Osteoarthritis of the proximal interphalangeal joints may be primary (Bouchard's osteoarthritis) or secondary to injury. As with primary osteoarthritis of the distal interphalangeal joint (Heberden's nodes), primary osteoarthritis of the proximal interphalangeal joints is often familial and is more common in women than in men, and its onset is usually in the sixth or seventh decade. Most often, it is associated with primary osteoarthritis of the distal interphalangeal joints.

Primary osteoarthritis of the proximal interphalangeal joint is often painless in its early stages. Although mucous cysts occasionally develop about an osteophyte, they are relatively rare—certainly occurring much less frequently than at the distal joint. The first symptom is likely to be slowly progressive, painless, firm swelling about the condyles of the distal end of the proximal phalanx. Although the joint becomes diffusely enlarged, the swelling is bony hard and not soft and ballotable as in rheumatoid arthritis. Gradually, there is loss of joint motion, and the proximal interphalangeal joint becomes stiff in mild flexion. Although the middle phalanx may deviate as much as 30 to 40 degrees, severe angulatory deformity is *not* typical of the disease. Neither boutonnière deformity nor swan-neck deformity is likely to develop with osteoarthritis, although they are frequently seen in rheumatoid arthritis. The severely affected osteoarthritic joints are more painful with activity. The joints are grossly enlarged with sessile osteophytes. Some joints may be totally ankylosed in about 30 degrees of flexion; others may permit only 20 to 30 degrees of motion. Often, the motion is relatively painless.

Roentgenographic findings may belie the clinical findings. Joint space narrowing and extensive osteophyte formation may suggest a crepitant, swollen, and painful joint. Often, however, clinical signs and symptoms may be scanty. In some cases, loss of motion may be due more to bony impingement of an osteophyte than to cartilage destruction (Fig. 21–2).

Secondary osteoarthritis of the proximal interphalangeal joint is usually the result of intra-articular fracture, fracture-dislocation, or unreduced dislocation. The most frequent causes include avulsion fracture of the volar lip of the middle phalanx, displaced condylar fractures of the proximal phalanx, and compression fractures of the articular cartilage.

Treatment

Early treatment of osteoarthritis of the proximal interphalangeal joint consists of the intermittent use of a resting splint in a position of comfort. Nonsteroidal anti-inflammatory medication may be of help in reducing the pain of an acute flare-up.

For late-stage, disabling osteoarthritis of the proximal interphalangeal joint, operative treatment is of three types: (1) osteophyte excision, (2) arthrodesis, and (3) arthroplasty.

Osteophyte Excision. Excision of osteophytes is rarely indicated for aesthetic purposes. Occasionally, an osteophyte may be painful. If it is large and protrudes prominently beneath the skin, it may press against an adjacent clenched finger when the patient

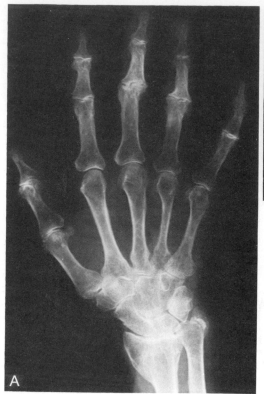

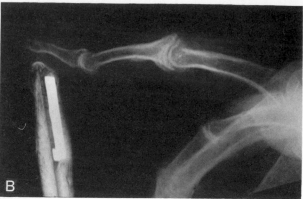

Figure 21–2. *A* and *B,* Roentgenograms showing advanced primary osteoarthritis of the proximal interphalangeal joints of the middle and ring fingers. Despite joint narrowing, sclerosis, and osteophyte formation, the patient had 60 degrees of painless motion at these joints. She sought treatment only because of an unrelated malunion of a Colles' fracture, and she required no treatment for the interphalangeal osteoarthritis.

makes a fist. Under these circumstances, the protuberant osteophyte may be removed at its base. A large volar osteophyte also may limit flexion of the joint because it abuts against the adjacent joint surface. Examination will reveal a bony block to passive joint flexion. Lateral roentgenograms taken in flexion will demonstrate the bone-to-bone contact. The osteophyte is removed through a volar zigzag incision. The flexor tendons are retracted laterally, and the volar plate is separated from the neck of the proximal phalanx proximally to distally. The juncture of the volar plate and the accessory collateral ligament may be repaired (with 5-0 nylon) after the osteophyte is removed. Motion is begun within 1 to 2 days of the operation.

Arthrodesis. If the joint is stable and painless, arthrodesis is not indicated, even with advanced arthritic changes. However, arthrodesis of the proximal interphalangeal joint may be advisable if there is marked deviation of the middle phalanx, joint instability, or disabling pain. Arthrodesis provides a painless and strong but immobile joint. For a manual worker, the strength of grip afforded by arthrodesis of the proximal interphalangeal joint may justify the lack of mobility. Most patients,

however, are at an age at which strength of grip is not as important as dexterity. They would like to be able to handle a pen or a paintbrush, play cards, and use a golf club or tennis racket with comfort. For this reason, in most patients with osteoarthritis, we favor arthroplasty of the proximal interphalangeal joint over arthrodesis.

In those patients for whom arthrodesis is preferred, we will position the joint in mild flexion, with the index and middle fingers at 30 degrees and the ring and little fingers at 45 degrees. The operative technique is similar to that described for arthrodesis of the distal interphalangeal joints.

Arthroplasty. Arthroplasty of the proximal interphalangeal joint may be performed by excising the osteophytes and inserting a fascial interposing membrane or by excising the osteophytes and both articular surfaces of the joint. A silicone or metal-and-ceramic prosthesis is then inserted in the joint space.

After fascial arthroplasty, the range of joint motion usually is about 30 to 40 degrees. Occasionally, exuberant bony overgrowth may cause recurrent ankylosis. However, there are several potential advantages of fascial arthroplasty over implant or prosthetic arthroplasty.

With fascial arthroplasty, less bone is resected, and the operated finger usually remains more normal in length and more stable than after some forms of replacement arthroplasty. In addition, there is no risk of later material failure (implant breakage). Should the arthroplasty prove unsuccessful, secondary arthrodesis may be performed, and the finger remains of acceptable length. Fascial arthroplasty is not indicated unless the joint is well aligned and has limited angulatory deformity. The main goal of the operation is to obtain a strong and painless joint. Joint motion will be limited, however.

Replacement arthroplasty of the proximal interphalangeal joint has been used with varying success for more than 35 years. In the 1950's, hinged metal prostheses were used for traumatized and rheumatoid joints.[5] Although some patients did well, various biomechanical problems plagued the postoperative course.[6] A disturbing number of prostheses unhinged, eroded through the skin and tendons, or sank deep within the shaft of the phalanges. The range of active motion diminished after a few years. The results with silicone and metal-and-ceramic implants have been much better. In the United States, the silicone implants have been most popular. Silicone is relatively nonreactive, and improvements in design and elastomer chemistry have increased the durability and flexibility of the implant.[7] Joints that have undergone an implant arthroplasty are usually painless, and their stability is dependent on soft tissue support. The mean passive assisted range of motion after surgery is about 50 degrees. However, there is a breakage rate of over 20% in 5 years. Implant arthroplasty for osteoarthritis of the proximal interphalangeal joint is indicated chiefly for those patients with pain and stiffness who require good joint mobility, even at the risk of possible loss of stability and strength and ultimate implant fracture.

Secondary osteoarthritis of the proximal interphalangeal joint due to volar-lip avulsion fracture and dorsal subluxation of the middle phalanx may be treated by volar plate arthroplasty if advanced changes have not destroyed the head of the proximal phalanx.[8] At operation, the entire volar side of the proximal interphalangeal joint is exposed. The avulsed fracture fragment is excised from its attachment to the volar plate. The joint is then relocated and held in mild flexion with a Kirschner wire. Reduction is often difficult and may require freeing intra-articular and para-articular adhesions. The volar plate is advanced and sutured into the defect at the base of the middle phalanx, restoring motion and stability.

With painful osteoarthritis of the proximal interphalangeal joint secondary to intra-articular fractures, the surgeon must choose between arthrodesis and arthroplasty. For a young patient with an otherwise normal hand, a fused proximal interphalangeal joint is awkward. Regardless of the position in which the joint is arthrodesed, the finger frequently gets in the way when the patient grasps large or small objects. Machine work is difficult. For this reason, we usually prefer arthroplasty over arthrodesis in the younger patient with only one finger injured. For secondary osteoarthritis of the dominant index finger in a manual worker, stability is more important than mobility. We would probably treat it with fascial arthroplasty. For the nondominant middle or ring fingers of a clerical worker, stability may be augmented by support of the adjacent fingers. Here, silicone arthroplasty would be our choice. In all cases of replacement arthroplasty, the patient is cautioned that there is a chance that the implants may break and that the finger may have to be reoperated on in the years to come. Occasionally, we will pass a Kirschner wire through the proximal interphalangeal joint for a 1- to 2-week trial of "temporary arthrodesis." We will then ask the patient to decide whether hand function with the proximal interphalangeal joints fused is satisfactory. Our decision as to whether to proceed with arthrodesis or arthroplasty will then rest on the patient's evaluation of hand function with a stiffened joint.

METACARPOPHALANGEAL JOINTS

Primary osteoarthritis of the metacarpophalangeal joint of the digits is rare. Most frequently, metacarpophalangeal osteoarthritis is secondary to intra-articular fractures of the head of the metacarpal or the base of the proximal phalanx. In the thumb, secondary metacarpophalangeal osteoarthritis is often the late result of collateral ligament rupture with or without an avulsion fracture of the base of the proximal phalanx. This is known as an acute "gamekeeper's thumb" when the ulnar collateral ligament is involved. In 30% of the cases, with loss of collateral ligament support, the proximal phalanx subluxates volarly and joint congruity is lost.[9] If the ligament is not repaired or reconstructed, secondary osteoarthritic changes may occur. The dorsal lip of the subluxated phalanx compresses the articular cartilage of the metacarpal head, forming a groove. The joint becomes painful and swollen. There is a positive "grind test" (pain and crepitation with compression), and the phalanx can be translocated dorsally or volarly by manipulation.

Treatment

Each of the metacarpophalangeal joints of the fingers lies at the apex of a longitudinal arch of the hand. If any of their joints is ankylosed, the involved finger protrudes from the clenched fist, unable to participate in many types of grasping. For this reason, arthrodesis of the metacarpophalangeal joints of the fingers is rarely advisable. The silicone implants and the metal-and-ceramic prostheses have proved more satisfactory in the metacarpophalangeal joints than in the proximal interphalangeal joints. Metacarpophalangeal joint implants are larger than those of proximal interphalangeal joints, and they are therefore more resistant to lateral and translocational stress fracture. The metacarpophalangeal joints are supported by a relatively strong capsule and are reinforced laterally by the tendons of the interosseous muscles. Each of the metacarpals of the fingers is interconnected by the deep transverse metacarpal ligament. Arthroplasty of the metacarpophalangeal joint of one finger is thus supported by the adjacent portions of the hand.

Although fascial and metal-and-ceramic arthroplasties are favored by some surgeons, we prefer silicone arthroplasty for secondary osteoarthritis of the metacarpophalangeal joint. Should the silicone fracture (20% in 5 years),[10] it may be replaced. Indeed, should the implant fracture after several years, it may be removed, and a functional range of motion with good stability may be maintained by reefing the supporting tendons and ligaments without replacing the silicone.

With secondary osteoarthritis of the thumb metacarpophalangeal joint, however, our preference is usually arthrodesis. Many patients normally have only 20 to 30 degrees of metacarpophalangeal motion. With these patients, the first metacarpal head is usually flat on the lateral roentgenogram. In addition, the thumb metacarpophalangeal joint is subject to repeated lateral stress with pinch and grasp, which are unsupported by adjacent metacarpophalangeal joints. The implant is thus more likely to fracture. If first carpometacarpal (trapeziometacarpal) and thumb interphalangeal joint motions are normal, the function of the thumb with arthrodesis of the metacarpophalangeal joint is excellent. We usually fuse the metacarpophalangeal joint of the thumb in 20 degrees of flexion, 20 degrees of abduction, and 30 degrees of pronation. The compression band wiring technique described for arthrodesis of the distal interphalangeal joint is a preferred method of achieving fusion of the metacarpophalangeal joint.

Should arthroplasty be indicated because of the patient's functional needs and desires, the surgeon should be most conservative with bone resection. He should take care to remove no more of the metacarpal head than is necessary for prosthetic fit. There is an inverse relationship between stability and mobility of silicone arthroplasty, and stability is essential at the metacarpophalangeal joint of the thumb. Although we generally begin protective motion within 1 or 2 days of arthroplasty of the proximal interphalangeal or metacarpophalangeal joint of the other fingers, we will immobilize thumb arthroplasties for 3 weeks in order to encourage firm encapsulation of the implant.

CARPOMETACARPAL JOINTS

Primary osteoarthritis of the second and third carpometacarpal joints has been called "metacarpal boss" or "golfer's boss."[11, 12] An osteophyte will form on either side of the involved joint at the dorsal base of the second or third metacarpal and the distal dorsal lip of the trapezoid or capitate. In some patients, the osteophyte represents growth of an accessory ossicle. The usual history is the gradual onset of a somewhat tender, firm mass at the dorsum of the hand. With manual activity, there may be redness or acute pain at the dorsum of the wrist. This appears to be due to tendinitis of the overlying extensor carpi radialis brevis or extensor carpi radialis longus. Most patients and many doctors may misdiagnose the lump as a ganglionic cyst. All attempts at aspiration are futile. The metacarpal boss usually appears in patients in their twenties and is more frequent in men than in women. It rarely measures more than 0.5 cm in diameter. It is bony hard and lies just proximal to the insertion of the radial wrist extensors and 1 or 2 cm distal to the usual location of a ganglion cyst. The boss is most prominent with the wrist palmar flexed. Lateral roentgenograms will show dorsal lipping at the carpometacarpal joint.

Treatment

Treatment is usually conservative. If the patient develops tendinitis, the area of inflammation may be injected with steroids and local anesthetics. A course of nonsteroidal anti-inflammatory agent (5 days) often is helpful. A canvas cock-up wrist splint will prevent irritation of the radial extensor tendon, and symptoms should soon subside.

If there is persistent pain from a large osteophyte, surgery may be necessary. The radial wrist extensor tendon that lies over the mass is mobilized and retracted. The osteophyte on both sides of the joint is removed and the bone is curetted, so that there are concavities where the osteophytes were. Postoperatively, the wrist should be splinted for 2 to 3 weeks.

Post-traumatic osteoarthritis of the second or third carpometacarpal joint is usually the result of caropmetacarpal dislocation. Because there is normally very little motion at these joints, persistent carpometacarpal pain should be treated by arthrodesis. The joint surfaces are curetted, and cancellous bone chips are inserted.

Post-traumatic osteoarthritis of the fifth metacarpal–hamate joint is more common than that of the adjacent carpometacarpal joints. Fracture of the base of the fifth metacarpal often results in dislocation of the fifth metacarpal shaft at its ulnar basal condyle. The radial condyle remains strongly held to the carpus and the fourth metacarpal base. If the fracture-dislocation is not reduced, painful osteoarthritis often will develop. Because the fifth metacarpal normally has 40 degrees of motion at its base, there will be pain at the ulnar dorsal side of the hand, just distal to the wrist, with grasp. Grip will be weak. Roentgenograms may show malunion of the fifth metacarpal base. Often, tomograms are required to demonstrate the true nature of the problem.

Although some authors have suggested arthroplasty with silicone implants to relieve the pain and preserve metacarpal motion, we have found arthrodesis to be preferable.[13] The fifth metacarpal retains its mobility as compensatory triquetral-hamate motion develops after metacarpal-hamate fusion. We will decorticate the hamate and the fifth metacarpal base, fashion a slot between them, and insert a corticocancellous bone graft from the ilium.

Complete pain relief and excellent function usually result.

The first metacarpal–trapezial joint is a common site of primary osteoarthritis in the hand. As a saddle joint with a concavoconvex articulation, it should permit motion in only two planes, flexion-extension and abduction-adduction. However, rotation also takes place because the joint is loose and somewhat incongruous. The curvature of the metacarpal base is greater than that of the distal articular surface of the trapezium. Strong metacarpocarpal ligaments hold the joint surfaces together. Should these ligaments stretch or weaken, stability is lost. Women in their fifties or sixties are most prone to develop osteoarthritis of this joint. The first metacarpal base subluxates radially and dorsally, the joint space narrows, and a large osteophyte forms at the distal ulnar condyle of the trapezium. Later, with increasing subluxation of the metacarpal base, the first metacarpal shaft angulates into flexion and adduction. Secondary hyperextension of the metacarpophalangeal joint may develop as the proximal phalanx is pushed dorsally when the patient grasps large objects. Over 50% of patients with trapeziometacarpal osteoarthritis also have osteoarthritis between the trapezium and trapezoid or between the trapezium and the scaphoid.

Mild trapeziometacarpal osteoarthritis should be treated with anti-inflammatory medication and splinting.[14] We use a short "C splint," made of plastic and fitted in the first web space. It holds the thumb in opposition and immobilizes the painful trapeziometacarpal joint. It does not immobilize the wrist, the interphalangeal joint of the thumb, or the metacarpophalangeal joint of the index finger. The patient uses the splint intermittently when performing manual activities or at times when the thumb aches or is painful. If pain is disabling, we recommend surgery.

Trapeziometacarpal arthrodesis completely relieves the pain of trapeziometacarpal arthritis.[15, 16] Yet, because many patients with primary trapeziometacarpal osteoarthritis also have intercarpal arthritis, some pain may persist (Fig. 21–3).[17] In addition, with loss of trapeziometacarpal joint mobility, there are many functions of which the thumb is incapable. If the trapeziometacarpal joint is arthrodesed in opposition, the patient will be able to pinch and grasp. However, she will be unable to retract the thumb to the plane of the palm for pushing or supporting flat objects, washing a wall, carrying a tray, or placing the hand in a pocket or narrow space. If the joint

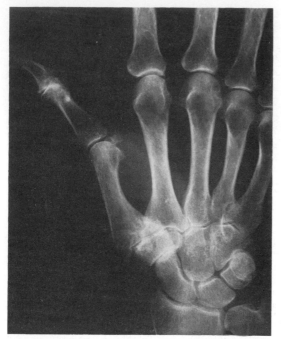

Figure 21–3. Degenerative osteoarthritis of the trapeziometacarpal joint. The first metacarpal is subluxated dorsally and radially. There is a large osteophyte to the ulnar side of the distal articular surface of the trapezium. There is also evidence of advanced osteoarthritis between the proximal articular surface of the trapezium and the distal pole of the scaphoid. Note also the osteoarthritic changes at the interphalangeal joint of the thumb.

is fused in a neutral position, full opposition is lost. Trapeziometacarpal arthrodesis should be considered for a patient who requires strong pinch and only if the osteoarthritis is localized to the trapeziometacarpal joint.[18]

If arthritis is localized to the trapeziometacarpal joint alone, hemiarthroplasty (resurfacing the distal trapezium) or trapeziometacarpal joint replacement with metal and ceramic may relieve pain while maintaining motion and strength of pinch. With pantrapezial arthritis, however, total trapezial resection is usually preferred. The trapezium may then be replaced with a silicone implant.[19] The stem of the implant is inserted into the base of the first metacarpal. The implant rests on the distal pole of the scaphoid. The implant must be seated snugly and stabilized by carefully reconstituting the ligaments that surround it. The techniques of silicone implant arthroplasty after total trapezial resection have advanced as the problems of subluxation have become more evident. Arthroplasty now includes partial resection of the trapezoid, Kirschner-wire fixation of the implant, and transfer of the radial half of the flexor carpi radialis to further stabilize the arthroplasty. Although the mean postoperative pinch strength is about 14 pounds (normal pinch strength is 25 pounds), mobility and pain relief are excellent.

We would agree with many authors who find that fascial arthroplasty after trapezial resection offers equally good results with fewer potential complications than silicone arthroplasty.[20, 21] A rolled-up "pillow" of palmaris longus is placed in the space between the metacarpal and the scaphoid after trapezial resection. The abductor pollicis longus is shortened about 1.5 cm to restore normal metacarpal alignment, and the ligaments surrounding the metacarpal base are firmly closed. The dorsal retinacular ligament is released over the first compartment to prevent the sutured abductor pollicis longus from becoming irritated. Postoperatively, the thumb is splinted in opposition for 3 weeks and then is protected for an additional 3 weeks with a plastic splint. For those patients with primary pantrapezial osteoarthritis who do not require strong pinch and who desire a pain-free mobile joint, resection arthroplasty is a predictable and safe operation (Fig. 21–4).

Secondary osteoarthritis of the trapeziometacarpal joint is usually the result of a Bennett's fracture-dislocation or a comminuted Rolando fracture of the base of the first metacarpal. If the patient is seen many months or years after injury and secondary osteoarthritis has caused pain, weakness, and limited motion, surgery is advised. Unlike primary osteoarthritis of the trapeziometacarpal joint, with post-traumatic osteoarthritis the adjacent joints are usually normal. In these patients, arthrodesis or hemiarthroplasty is preferable to trapeziectomy in order to preserve pinch strength. We prefer to smooth the base of the first metacarpal by subcortical osteotomy, resect the distal third of the trapezium, and then insert a silicone cap to the trapezium (the "Ashworth-Blatt implant").[22] Another alternative is to resect the base of the metacarpal and to replace it with a silicone "great toe" implant.

THE WRIST

Primary osteoarthritis of the radiocarpal joint occurs infrequently. Because the ulnar head is separated from the triquetrum by the triangular ligament, ulnocarpal arthritis is also rare. Radiocarpal and intercarpal osteoarthritis may be secondary to aseptic necrosis of the

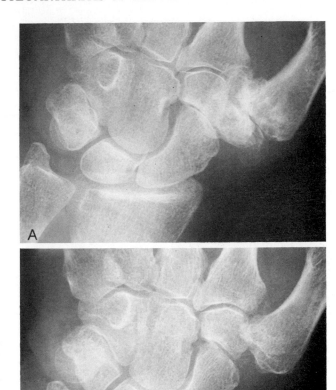

Figure 21–4. A, Advanced osteoarthritic changes of the trapeziometacarpal joint with large osteophyte formation and subluxation of the first metacarpal. *B,* After resection of the trapezium and interposition of palmaris longus tendon between the metacarpal and scaphoid, painless joint motion is restored. (From Smith RJ, Amadio PC: Resection arthroplasty for trapezio-metacarpal osteoarthritis. Strickland JW, Steichen JB (eds.): *In* Difficult Problems in Hand Surgery. St. Louis, C. V. Mosby, 1982.)

lunate (Kienböck's disease) or scaphoid (Preiser's disease) or to fractures and dislocations of the carpal bone or radius. Radioulnar osteoarthritis is usually secondary to fractures of the distal radius or dislocations of the ulnar head.

All cases of lunate necrosis are considered Kienböck's disease. In many cases, a specific history of trauma precedes lunate necrosis.[23, 24] Roentgenograms (particularly lateral tomograms) will show fracture lines in the transverse and frontal planes. The fractures disturb lunate vascularity,[25, 26] and compressive forces cause secondary lunate collapse. In some patients with no history of trauma, lunate ischemia may be caused by vasculitis, as in lupus erythematosus.

There is a high correlation of short ulna ("ulna minus") with Kienböck's disease.[27] This has led some to postulate that in those patients in whom the ulnar head is proximal to the distal articular surface of the radius, the ulnar and radial halves of the lunate may be subject to unequal compressive forces. They reason that this may cause ischemia and collapse of the lunate. This theory has gained wide popularity in recent years. Its proponents, however, have not satisfactorily explained why patients who have undergone ulnar head resection fail to develop Kienböck's disease or why arthrograms of patients with shortening of the ulna usually show perfectly normal support of the lunate by the triangular ligament.

Kienböck's disease is most common in men between 18 and 30 years of age. There is limited wrist motion and pain that is intensified with activity. Examination reveals tenderness and some fullness on deep palpation at the center of the dorsum of the wrist. In early stages, roentgenograms will show only increased radiodensity of the lunate. Often, there is a radiolucent line or cavity on the ulnar side of the lunate at its proximal third. Lateral tomograms showing radiolucent "fracture lines" are almost pathognomonic of the condition. Later, the lunate may collapse. The extent of this collapse may be measured by comparing carpal length (distal capitate to proximal lunate) with the length of the third

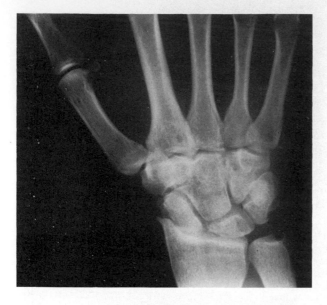

Figure 21–5. Many years following Kienböck's disease, osteoarthritis has developed between the scaphoid and the radius. This is due to proximal migration of the capitate and secondary intercarpal malalignment.

metacarpal (distal to proximal articular cortex) on a posteroanterior roentgenogram of the wrist and hand. Normally, this ratio is 52% to 54%. Any significant decrease in this ratio suggests lunate collapse.[28]

With collapse of the lunate, the capitate migrates proximally and intercarpal malalignment develops (Fig. 21–5). The scaphoid will rotate so that its distal pole faces volarly, and the triquetrum shifts ulnarly. The wrist becomes stiff and painful. If there is more advanced disease, the lunate may be compressed wafer-thin, and severe intercarpal and radiocarpal osteoarthritis develops.

Treatment

There are many methods of treating Kienböck's disease. At an early stage, before lunate collapse and intercarpal shift, some surgeons recommend plaster immobilization of the wrist. Results are disappointing, as compressive forces continue to act on the lunate, which may gradually fragment. Some have suggested lengthening the ulna or shortening the radius in cases of early Kienböck's disease with no carpal collapse.[29, 30] Although they report good clinical results with this treatment, the lunate does not recover normal roentgenographic appearance. Other surgeons have recommended intercarpal arthrodesis.[31] By fusing the capitate to the hamate and to the trapezoid, or the scaphoid to the trapezium and trapezoid, compressive forces on the lunate will be decreased.

It is believed that this will spare the lunate and prevent its collapse. Other methods of treatment include excising the lunate and replacing it with a silicone implant. Recently, there have been attempts to revascularize the lunate by transferring a branch of the ulnar artery or a vascularized bone flap into it.[32]

If the patient is not seen until a late stage, after lunate collapse and intercarpal displacement, equalization of the length of the radius and ulna or capitate-hamate-trapezoid arthrodesis would not correct carpal alignment. Lunate excision without replacement would give relief of pain. However, with continued carpal shift, many patients will develop increasing symptoms of intercarpal osteoarthritis within 3 to 4 years. Lunate excision and silicone replacement are often successful in restoring intercarpal alignment and achieving relief of pain. In time, however, some of these implants may collapse, dislocate, or fragment unless they are supported by intercarpal arthrodesis. If scaphoid rotation has progressed so that the bone lies 90 degrees to the longitudinal axis of the radius, it should be reduced and may be held in its corrected position by scaphoid-trapezoid-trapezial arthrodesis or scaphoid-capitate arthrodesis. Although wrist motion will be limited, a more stable intercarpal alignment may avoid later osteoarthritic changes.

The preferred operation will depend on the patient's age and occupation and the extent of carpal collapse. Arthrodesis would be favored in a younger patient with severe collapse, pain, and limited motion. More conservative measures would be favored in an older patient without collapse. To a large extent, however, the choice of the operation depends on the surgeon's preference and his interpretation of the pathophysiology of the disease.

As a rule, our present plan in patients with an uncollapsed lunate is capitate-hamate-trapezoid arthrodesis without lunate excision. In patients with a collapsed lunate, we realign the scaphoid by fusing it to the trapezoid and trapezium. If arthrograms show good proximal articular cartilage of the lunate, it is not removed. If there is evidence of radiolunate arthritis, the lunate is excised.

Primary aseptic necrosis of the scaphoid (Preiser's disease) is extremely rare. However, aseptic necrosis of the proximal pole of the scaphoid secondary to fracture is relatively common. As the blood supply to the proximal pole of the scaphoid enters from its distal end, a nonunited fracture of the waist or proximal third of the scaphoid will jeopardize its viability. Gradually, the non-united fragment becomes dense and then collapses. Often, compressive forces on the ischemic proximal pole of the scaphoid will cause it to collapse even as the fracture is healing.[33, 34] The scaphoid becomes comma-shaped, with a normal distal pole and a thin, sclerotic proximal pole. Collapse of the proximal pole may permit the capitate to migrate proximally, displacing the lunate and triquetrum ulnarly. Secondary osteoarthritis of the intercarpal and radiocarpal joints will cause gradually increasing pain and stiffness.

The best primary treatment is to secure union of the fractured scaphoid by closed reduction or surgery. If the proximal pole has become necrotic and has collapsed, carpal support should be re-established by scaphoid replacement or intercarpal arthrodesis. The scaphoid implant is preferred if there is joint space narrowing and osteophyte formation at the lateral half of the radius. This is evidence of secondary radioscaphoid osteoarthritis. For persistent nonunion with a collapsed proximal pole, scaphoid implant arthroplasty appears to be indicated as well. With severe intercarpal collapse, we would favor excision of the small proximal scaphoid fragment, scaphoid realignment, and scaphoid-capitate arthrodesis. If carpal collapse and radiocarpal arthritis are advanced, wrist arthroplasty or arthrodesis will most predictably restore function to the hand.

Secondary radioscaphoid osteoarthritis often follows malunion of the displaced scaphoid fracture (Fig. 21–6). Impingement of the fracture callus or fracture fragments on the articular cartilage of the radial styloid may cause localized joint space narrowing and osteophyte formation. There will be pain at the radial side of the joint, intensified by radial deviation of the hand. A local anesthetic infiltrated into the radial side of the wrist will usually relieve the pain. In these cases, radial styloidectomy may result in a painless wrist with normal motion.[35] The radial styloid is removed vertically by osteotomy of the radius where the styloid flare meets the radial shaft. This operation is not indicated if scaphoid replacement arthroplasty

Figure 21–6. Severe radiocarpal arthritis following an ununited scaphoid fracture with necrosis of its proximal pole. Recommended treatment was wrist arthrodesis.

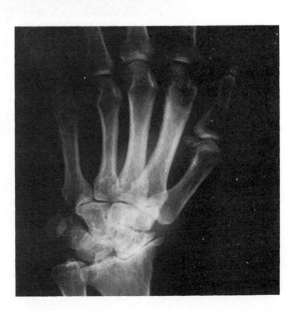

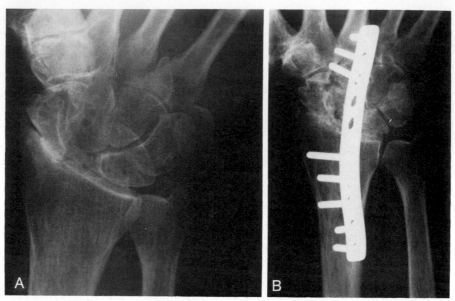

Figure 21–7. *A,* After an unreduced dislocation of the lunate, incongruous radiocarpal joint surfaces led to severe secondary osteoarthritis. *B,* Complete pain relief was achieved with arthrodesis.

is considered, because scaphoid implants are often unstable after styloidectomy.

Secondary radiocarpal osteoarthritis may follow any severe fracture or dislocation about the wrist (Fig. 21–7). Often, symptoms subside with the use of a cock-up wrist splint. If not, arthrodesis (Fig. 21–7B) or arthroplasty must be considered. Frequently, intercarpal arthrodesis may successfully stabilize the carpals while permitting good wrist motion (Fig. 21–8).[36]

Wrist arthrodesis is an effective method of controlling pain and restoring strength to the arthritic wrist.[36, 37] Pronation and supination of the forearm are unaffected, as the radioulnar joint is not involved. Many patients are pleasantly surprised by the versatility of the hand after wrist arthrodesis. They can use the hand for heavy and light grip, for typing, and for many sports. For some patients, it is advisable to immobilize the wrist with a Kirschner wire for 1 or 2 weeks before the operation so that the patient can test hand function prior to making his decision regarding arthrodesis or arthroplasty.

We prefer to fuse the wrist in 20 degrees of dorsiflexion. We align the third metacarpal with radial shaft. The dorsum of the carpus is decorticated. The dorsal cortex of the radius (about 6 cm by 2 cm) is cut with a power saw. Articular cartilage is removed from the intercarpal and radiocarpal joints, and the joints

are filled with cancellous bone from the ilium. The dorsal radial cortex is advanced distally to cover the decorticated carpus and metacarpals and to bridge the wrist joint. It is held in place with screws or with screws and a plate. Cancellous bone is passed about the defect proximal to the sliding graft. When we use the plate, we will immobilize the wrist for only 1 week and then protect it with a volar splint. With screw fixation, we immobilize the wrist with a below-elbow cast for 2 months.

Some patients require wrist motion for their work or hobbies. For example, wrist motion is essential for electricians, who must put their hands around and through small openings, and for most musicians. Arthroplasty will usually provide relatively painless motion, but with some loss of strength and with the risk of material failure.[38, 39] Resection arthroplasty (such as proximal row carpectomy) gives somewhat inconsistent results but has been favored by many. Silicone and metal-and-ceramic arthroplasty will usually permit 50 to 80 degrees of motion. This range is sufficient for most activities of daily living. With improved design in materials, we are confident that wrist implants will soon prove a most satisfactory solution to the problems of the osteoarthritic wrist. For the present, however, their use should be restricted to those who will not use the wrist for heavy manual labor and who require wrist motion for their occupation.

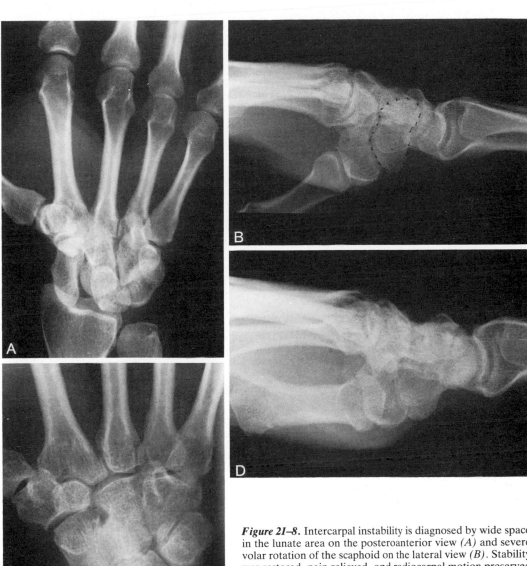

Figure 21–8. Intercarpal instability is diagnosed by wide space in the lunate area on the posteroanterior view *(A)* and severe volar rotation of the scaphoid on the lateral view *(B)*. Stability was restored, pain relieved, and radiocarpal motion preserved by intercarpal arthrodesis of the scaphoid to the capitate and lunate, as shown on the posteroanterior *(C)* and lateral *(D)* views.

References

1. Smith RJ, Broudy AS: Advances in surgery of the rheumatoid hand. Curr Pract Orthop Surg 7:1–35, 1977.
2. Kellgren JH, Lawrence JS, Bier F: Genetic factors in generalized osteoarthrosis. Ann Rheum Dis 22:237–255, 1963.
3. Lawrence JS, Bremmer JM, Bier F: Osteoarthrosis. Ann Rheum Dis 25:1–24, 1966.
4. Eaton RG, Dobranski AI, Littler JW: Marginal osteophyte excision and treatment of mucous cysts. J Bone Joint Surg 55A:570–574, 1973.
5. Brannon EW, Klein G: Experiences with a finger-joint prosthesis. J Bone Joint Surg 41A:87–102, 1959.
6. Ellison MR, Flatt AE, Henard D: Finger joint replacement in the rheumatoid hand. A comparison of 525 implants of varying design and material. J Bone Joint Surg 55A:880, 1973.
7. Swanson AB: Flexible implant arthroplasty for arthritic finger joints. J Bone Joint Surg 54A:435–455, 1972.
8. Eaton RG, Malerich MM: Volar plate arthroplasty of the proximal interphalangeal joint: A review of ten years' experience. J Hand Surg 5:260–268, 1980.
9. Smith RJ: Post-traumatic instability of the metacarpophalangeal joint of the thumb. J Bone Joint Surg 59A:14–21, 1977.
10. Beckenbaugh RD, Dobyns JH, Linscheid RL, Bryan RS: Review and analysis of silicone-rubber metacarpophalangeal implants. J Bone Joint Surg 58A:483–487, 1976.
11. Carter RM: Carpal boss: A commonly overlooked deformity of the carpus. J Bone Joint Surg 23:935–940, 1941.
12. Artz TD, Posch JL: The carpometacarpal boss. J Bone Joint Surg 55A:747–752, 1973.
13. Clendenin MB, Smith RJ: Metacarpo-hamate arthrodesis for post-traumatic arthritis. Orthop Trans 6:168, 1982.
14. Dell PC, Brushart TM, Smith RJ: Treatment of trapeziometacarpal arthritis: Results of resection arthroplasty. J Hand Surg 3:243–249, 1978.
15. Eaton RG, Littler JW: A study of the basal joint of the thumb. The treatment of its disabilities by fusion. J Bone Joint Surg 51A:661–668, 1969.
16. Stark HH, Moore JF, Ashworth CR, Boyes JH: Fusion of the first metacarpotrapezial joint for degenerative arthritis. J Bone Joint Surg 59A:22–26, 1977.
17. Crosby EB, Linscheid RL, Dobyns JH: Scaphotrapezial trapezoidal arthrosis. J Hand Surg 3:223–234, 1978.
18. Weinman DT, Lipscomb PR: Degenerative arthritis of the trapeziometacarpal joint: Arthrodesis or excision? Mayo Clin Proc 42:276, 1967.
19. Swanson AB: Disabling arthritis at the base of the thumb. The treatment by resection of the trapezium and flexible (silicone) implant arthroplasty. J Bone Joint Surg 54A:456–471, 1972.
20. Amadio PC, Millender LH, Smith RJ: Silicone spacer or tendon spacer for trapezium resection arthroplasty—comparison of results. J Hand Surg 7:237–244, 1982.
21. Froimson AI: Tendon arthroplasty of the trapeziometacarpal joint. Clin Orthop 70:191, 1970.
22. Ashworth CR, Blatt G, Chuinard RG, Stark HH: Silicone-rubber interposition arthroplasty of the carpometacarpal joint of the thumb. J Hand Surg 2:345–357, 1977.
23. Mouat TB, Wilkie J, Harding HE: Isolated fracture of the carpal semi-lunar and Kienböck's disease. Br J Surg 19:577, 1932.
24. Beckenbaugh R, Shives T, Dobyns J, Linscheid R: Kienböck's disease: The natural history of Kienböck's disease and consideration of lunate fractures. Clin Orthop 149:98–106, 1980.
25. Taleisnik J, Kelly PJ: The extraosseous and intraosseous blood supply of the scaphoid bone. J Bone Joint Surg 48A:1125–1137, 1966.
26. Gelberman RH, Bauman TD, Menon J, Akeson WH: The vascularity of the lunate bone and Kienböck's disease. J Hand Surg 5:272–278, 1980.
27. Hulton O: Über anatomische variationen der hand gelenkknochen. Acta Radiol 9:1928, 1955.
28. Youm Y, McMurtry RY, Flatt AE, Gillespie TE: Kinematics of the wrist. I. An experimental study of radial-ulnar deviation and flexion extension. J Bone Joint Surg 60A:955–961, 1978.
29. Eiken O, Niechev I: Radial shortening in malacia of the lunate. Scand J Plast Reconstr Surg 14:191, 1980.
30. Lee M: The intraosseous arterial pattern of the carpal lunate bone and its relation to avascular necrosis. Acta Orthop Scand 33:43–55, 1963.
31. Chuinard RG, Zeman SC: Kienböck's disease: An analysis and rationale for treatment by capitate-hamate fusion. (Proceedings.) J Hand Surg 5:290, 1980.
32. Hori Y, Tamai S, Okuda H, et al.: Blood vessel transplantation to bone. J Hand Surg 4:23–33, 1979.
33. Fisk GF: Carpal instability and the fractured scaphoid. Ann R Coll Surg Engl 46:63–76, 1970.
34. Mazet R Jr, Hohl MM: Fractures of the carpal navicular: Analysis of 91 cases and review of the literature. J Bone Joint Surg 45A:82–112, 1963.
35. Barnard L, Stubbins SG: Styloidectomy of the radius in the surgical treatment of non-union of the carpal navicular: A preliminary report. J Bone Joint Surg 30A:98–102, 1948.
36. Watson HK, Hempton RF: Limited wrist arthrodeses. I. The triscaphoid joint. J Hand Surg 5:320–327, 1980.
37. Campbell CJ, Keokaran T: Total and subtotal arthrodesis of the wrist: Inlay technique. J Bone Joint Surg 46A:1520–1533, 1964.
38. Goodman MJ, Millender LH, Nalebuff EA, and Philips CA: Arthroplasty of the rheumatoid wrist with silicone rubber: An early evaluation. J Hand Surg 5:114–121, 1980.
39. Volz RG: The development and implementation of a total wrist joint. J Bone Joint Surg 58A:272, 1976.

22

Osteoarthritis of the Shoulder and Elbow

Alan H. Wilde, M.D.

THE SHOULDER

Osteoarthritis supposedly is rare in the shoulder,[1] but significant numbers of replacements of the glenohumeral joint are now being performed for primary osteoarthritis, including one series of over 100 such replacements.[2] This would suggest that osteoarthritis of the glenohumeral joint is not as rare as the literature might indicate. Anatomic studies of the shoulder joint revealed gross changes of osteoarthritis in approximately 60% of individuals over the age of 15 years in a series of 1000 unselected necropsies.[3]

Osteoarthritis can result from other conditions such as gout, alkaptonuria, septic arthritis, fractures of the head of the humerus, recurrent dislocation of the shoulder, sickle cell disease, lupus erythematosus, Gaucher's disease, idiopathic avascular necrosis of the humeral head, hematologic disorders in which recurrent hemarthroses occur, or a mixed arthritis with an underlying rheumatoid arthritis or juvenile rheumatoid arthritis.[4] Osteoarthritis can also occur as a result of neuropathic conditions such as syringomyelia. Chronic trauma has been implicated as a cause of osteoarthritis in the shoulder, as it has been seen more frequently in bus drivers or pneumatic tool workers.[5]

Shoulder pain is a common complaint in clinical practice. In addition to the impingement syndrome, osteoarthritis attacks the glenohumeral, sternoclavicular, and acromioclavicular joints. Lesions of the rotator cuff and the long head of the biceps will be considered under the discussion of the impingement syndrome. Avascular necrosis of the humeral head and rheumatoid arthritis are not the topic of this book, and the reader is referred to appropriate references elsewhere.[6, 7] In addition, there are a number of extrinsic causes of pain in the shoulder, such as cervical spine lesions, tumors of the apical regions of the chest, gallbladder disease, herpes zoster, cervical rib syndrome, scalenus anticus syndrome, and hyperabduction syndrome.

There are four joints in the shoulder that function in unison: the glenohumeral joint, the sternoclavicular joint, the acromioclavicular joint, and the scapulothoracic joint. The scapulothoracic joint is not a true joint. The glenohumeral, acromioclavicular, and sternoclavicular joints are true joints and can be sites of osteoarthritis. The diagnosis and management of osteoarthritis in each of these joints will be discussed.

Although some studies indicate that 80% of people over 55 years of age will have osteoarthritis, only about 30% complain of symptoms in the joint where osteoarthritis can be demonstrated roentgenographically.[1] One should not attribute shoulder pain to osteoarthritis without first taking a careful history and conducting a careful physical examination. There can be many reasons for shoulder pain, and all of them must be considered in each patient if the proper diagnosis is to be made and the appropriate treatment rendered. The following sections will present the various symptom complexes that may cause shoulder pain and that are intrinsic to the shoulder girdle and its four joints.

Impingement Syndrome

Perhaps the most common reason for shoulder pain is impingement of the rotator cuff. This has also been referred to as the refractory arc syndrome, coracoacromial ligament syndrome, or supraspinatus syndrome. It has been recognized that the rotator cuff can undergo attrition as a result of compression beneath the coracoacromial ligament, a spur on the anteroinferior lip of the acromion, or protruding inferior osteophytes from an osteoarthritic acromioclavicular joint. In the individual patient, any one or a combination of these conditions can be responsible for impingement of the rotator cuff.[7-10] The area of involvement of the rotator cuff is usually the supraspinatus tendon but may also include the anterior portion of the infraspinatus and the long head of the biceps. Rupture of the long head of the biceps can accompany rupture of the rotator cuff.

With elevation of the arm in internal rotation or in the anatomic position of external rotation, the area of likely degeneration of the rotator cuff passes beneath the coracoacromial ligament or the anterior portion of the acromion. When the arm is abducted to about 80 degrees, the rotator cuff comes close to the inferior surface of the acromioclavicular joint. It can easily be seen that the rotator cuff, particularly the supraspinatus tendon, can readily undergo attrition as a result of a repetitive compression by the coracoacromial ligament or by a spur on the anteroinferior surface of the acromion or on the inferior surface of the acromioclavicular joint. Neer has described three grades of impingement lesions: Grade I, edema of the rotator cuff; Grade II, fibrosis; and Grade III, bone reaction and tendon rupture.[2]

Patients with impingement syndrome complain of pain in the shoulder, particularly with elevation of 70 to 120 degrees. If elevation in this range is forced by the physician, there may be pain in the region of the anterior acromion. Night pain is characteristic of a rotator cuff tear. Patients may also complain of crepitus with motion of the shoulder. It is helpful to inject a local anesthetic into the inferior aspect of the acromion as a diagnostic test to see if impingement of the rotator cuff is responsible for the patient's symptoms. Relief of the patient's complaints following injection of the local anesthetic not only confirms the diagnosis but also suggests that surgical correction of the impingement may relieve symptoms.

Treatment. Initial treatment of the impingement syndrome should be conservative. The use of local heat and nonsteroidal anti-inflammatory drugs is standard treatment. Local injections of corticosteroids into the anteroinferior acromial area are commonly given. Repeated, frequent injections of steroids should not be administered, as these in themselves may lead to degeneration of the tendon. A patient who does not respond to conservative treatment after 8 weeks or longer and who demonstrates weakness of abduction should undergo arthrography of the shoulder. If a rotator cuff tear is diagnosed, surgery should be done both to release the impingement and to repair the cuff. If the arthrogram appears normal, surgery is still performed to relieve the impingement.

Surgical treatment of the impingement syndrome is performed by making an incision from the anterior acromion to the coracoid process just inferior to the acromion. The deltoid muscle is split superiorly to inferiorly at the level of the acromioclavicular joint. The muscle-splitting incision should be approximately 3.8 cm in length. It should be no longer than 5 cm; otherwise, the axillary nerve may be injured. The deltoid muscle is freed on either side of the acromioclavicular joint by sharp dissection, leaving a portion of the origin of the deltoid muscle on the bone for later repair. The coracoacromial ligament is exposed and is excised from the acromion and coracoid process. If there is a protruding spur on the inferior surface of the acromion, the Neer acromioplasty is performed as well.[8] This is accomplished by removing a portion of the anteroinferior acromion, measuring 0.9 cm of the inferior acromion at the site of attachment of the coracoacromial ligament. This piece of bone is 2 cm long. The cut surface of the acromion is treated with bone wax to aid in hemostasis and to prevent re-formation of the bone spur. The inferior aspect of the acromioclavicular joint is palpated for bony spurs. If there is osteoarthritis of the acromioclavicular joint and osteophytes protrude inferiorly, the distal 2.5 cm of the clavicle are removed as well. If there is also an osteophyte on the inferior surface of the acromial side of the acromioclavicular joint, this too is removed. Any raw bony surfaces are treated with bone wax. The rotator cuff is inspected for any tears.

By rotation of the humeral head, the rotator cuff can be inspected. This approach allows adequate exposure for rotator cuff repairs, particularly when the distal 2.5 cm of the clavicle have also been removed. If there is a tear of the rotator cuff, the edges are freshened and repaired directly. The repair of the deltoid muscle attachment must be meticulous, because separation of the anterior deltoid muscle from the acromion can result in permanent weakness of elevation of the arm. Postoperatively, pendulum exercises are begun within 3 or 4 days. Assisted external rotation can also be started at this time. The patient can perform assisted total elevation, with the opposite arm helping the operated side until full total elevation can be accomplished. This exercise is done with the patient in the supine position. Active total elevation is delayed for 10 days. When the rotator cuff has been repaired, abduction should not be performed before 6 weeks. Neer reported satisfactory results in 15 of 16 patients with partial tears of the supraspinatus and in 19 of 20 patients with complete tear of the supraspinatus.[8]

"Cuff Tear Arthropathy." A new syndrome called "cuff tear arthropathy" has been described by Neer.[7] Basically, it involves degeneration of the articular cartilage of the humeral head and osteoporosis when there has been a large long-standing rotator cuff tear. This is not like osteoarthritis, in which the rotator cuff is normal, or rheumatoid arthritis, in which the cuff is atrophic and may be penetrated by rheumatoid granulation tissue. Furthermore, in cuff tear arthropathy, the humeral head may ultimately collapse. Treatment is difficult be-

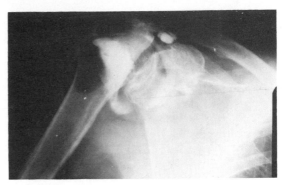

Figure 22–2. Double-contrast arthrogram of the patient shown in Figure 22–1 reveals a massive tear of the rotator cuff.

cause of the massive cuff tear (Figs. 22–1 and 22–2).

Osteoarthritis of the Glenohumeral Joint

Certainly, osteoarthritis of weight-bearing joints such as the hip and the knee occurs more frequently than osteoarthritis of the glenohumeral joint. However, osteoarthritis of the glenohumeral joint is not rare. Now that there is interest in replacement of the glenohumeral joint, this disease is becoming recognized more often.

Anatomic studies of the glenohumeral joint are few. In studies of 96 cadaver shoulder joints by DePalma and associates[11] and of 105 specimens by Neer, similar findings were reported.[12, 13] They found more extensive degenerative changes in the articular surface of the glenoid than in the humeral head. The articular surface of the humeral head was divided into three parts for purposes of reporting: The central area was called the inner circle; the outer area was called the outer circle; and the margin of the articular cartilage was termed the periphery. DePalma found that the most extensive changes in the articular cartilage occurred in the peripheral area. The inner circle demonstrated the fewest changes. Neer has described the typical findings in primary osteoarthritis in the shoulder as found at the time of replacement arthroplasty.[2] Osteophytes were largest at the inferior surface of the humeral head at the head-neck junction. Osteophytes were also found surrounding the periphery of the head and in the bicipital groove. Eburnated bone was commonly found in that part of the humeral head that articulated with the glenoid when the arm was abducted between 60 and 100 degrees. The gle-

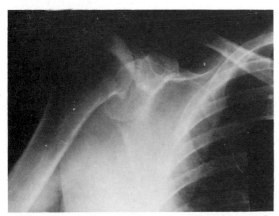

Figure 22–1. Cuff tear arthropathy. Note the superior migration of the humeral head with narrowing of the space between the acromion and the humeral head on the anteroposterior roentgenogram. Note also the osteoarthritis of the shoulder joint as manifested by the osteophyte on the inferomedial aspect of the humeral head.

noid was usually eburnated. Osteophytes were commonly seen at the inferior margin of the glenoid. As in the knee joint, there may be excessive synovial fluid present. At times, the amount of fluid may be so extensive that the subacromial bursa is distended, not unlike a Baker's cyst of the knee.

DePalma felt that degenerative changes in the rotator cuff did not parallel those seen in the articular surfaces of the humeral head and glenoid. He noted a gradual increase in severity of the changes in the articular surface of the humeral head with advancing age, beginning in the third decade. He did find incomplete tears of the rotator cuff, particularly the subscapularis and, more frequently, the supraspinatus and infraspinatus. These tears were on the articular side of the rotator cuff and were not felt to be responsible for symptoms. Neer has confirmed these findings at the time of replacement arthroplasty of the shoulder for osteoarthritis. He stated that tears of the rotator cuff occurred infrequently in primary osteoarthritis.[2] The clinical problem in osteoarthritis of the glenohumeral joint is primarily localized to the articular surfaces. Replacement of the joint surfaces involved should give predictably good results, provided the soft tissues are not unduly disturbed by surgery.

Treatment. The initial treatment of osteoarthritis of the glenohumeral joint is nonsurgical. There are many patients with marginal osteophytes, particularly at the inferior portion of the glenohumeral joint, who have a satisfactory joint space and function well. Nonsteroidal anti-inflammatory drugs and rest during flare-ups of pain are the mainstays of treatment. Intra-articular injections of corticosteroids are useful but should not be repeated more frequently than every 3 to 4 months. Frequent injections may result in degeneration of articular cartilage. When these measures no longer give satisfactory relief from pain and when daily activities such as combing and washing the hair, eating, dressing, and bathing are restricted, surgery of the shoulder should be considered.

Debridement of the shoulder with removal of osteophytes and loose bodies has been tried in the past but without success.[2] Arthrodesis of the shoulder has also been performed for osteoarthritis, but the incidence of pseudarthrosis has been reported to be as high as 40%.[14] Replacement of the shoulder is a more attractive idea and has the prospect of rapid and complete restoration of function. I will describe the approach and technique for the

Neer glenohumeral replacement,[15] as this is the one with which I have experience. The reader is referred to the works of others who also have described shoulder replacements.[16–22]

A new approach to the shoulder, recently described by Neer,[15] preserves both the deltoid muscle and the supraspinatus. As the attachments of the deltoid muscle and supraspinatus are not disturbed, motion of the shoulder can be started early. This has greatly improved the range of motion following replacement of the glenohumeral joint. This approach is accomplished by making an oblique incision from the coracoid process to the insertion of the deltoid muscle (Fig. 22–3). The deltopectoral groove is identified and dissected. The cephalic vein is doubly ligated and excised. The deltoid muscle is dissected from origin to insertion. The clavipectoral fascia is incised, and the coracoacromial ligament is excised. The subscapularis is dissected from the underlying capsule and is released 1 cm from its insertion on the lesser tuberosity. A suture is placed through the proximal end of the subscapularis. The plane between the subscapularis and the capsule is dissected. The capsule is incised superiorly to inferiorly. Usually, it is not necessary to incise the supraspinatus in order to gain exposure. With the shoulder abducted and externally rotated and the deltoid gently retracted, the surgeon can usually gain enough exposure to perform the replacement. Osteophytes, which are commonly found on the inferior surface of the humeral head and joint margins, are removed, so that the junction of the humeral head and neck can be clearly delineated. Only a wafer-thin piece of bone containing the residual articular surface of the

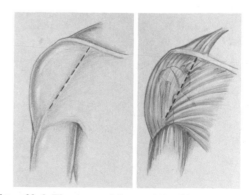

Figure 22–3. The approach for total shoulder replacement. An oblique incision is made from the coracoid process to the insertion of the deltoid muscle. The deltopectoral groove is dissected. The cephalic vein is doubly ligated and excised.

humeral head is removed. This is performed with a power saw. The osteotomy is made in 35 to 40 degrees retroversion. A curved Hohmann retractor is placed beneath the posterior portion of the glenoid. If the long head of the biceps tendon is present, it should be preserved. Any residual articular cartilage on the glenoid is removed with a curette. A slot is cut for the anchoring lug of the glenoid component. This slot is oriented along the long axis of the glenoid. The slot should be started with a small curette and enlarged with a power burr. The intramedullary canal of the glenoid should be located with a curette and enlarged. A trial fit of the glenoid component is made; the component should be supported by bone circumferentially. The glenoid component is removed. The humerus is then maximally externally rotated. The intramedullary canal of the humerus is located with a curette and is enlarged to accommodate the intramedullary stem of the humeral component. The medullary canal of the humerus should be measured from the preoperative roentgenogram. There are three stem sizes for the Neer humeral component—6.5 mm, 9.5 mm, and 12.9 mm. The largest stem size that will fit the humeral canal should be chosen.

There are two prosthetic humeral head sizes, 23 mm and 15 mm (Fig. 22–4). The smaller size should be used when the anatomic humeral head is small or when there is difficulty in closing a defect in the rotator cuff. The larger prosthetic humeral head is used in larger patients and provides a better fulcrum for the rotator cuff.

The glenoid component (Fig. 22–5), which

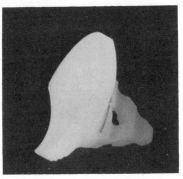

Figure 22–5. The glenoid component for the Neer total shoulder is made of high-density polyethylene. A metal backing on this material is also being used.

is now available, is made of high-density polyethylene, with or without metal backing. Larger metal-backed glenoid components are being tried on an experimental basis. These may be helpful in irreparable rotator cuff lesions.

The surface of the glenoid is further prepared with a water lavage system or water gun to clear the cancellous surfaces of debris. A sponge containing sterile 10 volumes % hydrogen peroxide is packed into the intramedullary canal of the scapula. Hydrogen peroxide aids in hemostasis. The sponge is removed, and methyl methacrylate is injected into the medullary canal of the scapula with a 10-ml syringe, the injecting end of which has been enlarged by removing the inner cylinder of plastic. The glenoid component is inserted and is held firmly until the cement has hardened.

The humeral component is placed into the medullary canal. Usually, bone cement is not necessary because there is sufficient bone present for adequate fixation of the prosthesis but it should be used if fixation is not adequate. The humerus is reinserted into the glenoid, and the range of motion is recorded. The subscapularis is sutured to the remaining tendon on the lesser tuberosity. The rotator interval, i.e., the space between the subscapularis and the supraspinatus, is also sutured. A Hemovac is inserted into the joint. The deltopectoral groove is reconstituted by suturing the deltoid muscle to the pectoralis major muscle. The subcutaneous tissue and skin are repaired. A sling and swath are applied.

Because neither the deltoid muscle nor the supraspinatus cuff has been disturbed in the usual case, active exercises can begin on the day following surgery. We have been following a modified rehabilitation program, described by Hughes and Neer.[23] We start with pendulum

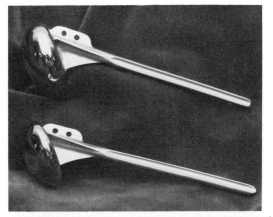

Figure 22–4. The humeral components of the Neer total shoulder replacement. Two humeral head sizes are available—23 mm and 15 mm. There are also three stem sizes—6.5 mm, 9.5 mm, and 12.9 mm.

exercises the day following surgery and continue with range of motion exercises and active assisted exercises as soon as the patient can participate. Abduction and total elevation are encouraged, and active assisted external rotation is allowed within the first 2 weeks. There are at least two formal physical therapy sessions daily while the patient is in the hospital. In addition, the patient is encouraged to perform physical therapy in his room an additional three times a day. Following discharge from the hospital, the patient continues this regimen at home. Patients who live close to the hospital are requested to return for weekly visits to the outpatient physical therapy department. At the 4- to 6-week postoperative visit, the patient is usually ready to engage in resistance exercises and active use of the arm and shoulder for light activities. The use of moist heat and stretching exercises may be advised if there is residual loss of motion. The patient can do this himself by gently stretching the shoulder by holding onto the top of the door and gradually moving the body closer to the door. Exercises should continue for at least 6 months, and longer if there has been significant weakness or stiffness preoperatively. We have recently reported our results with 44 Neer shoulder replacements, 12 of which were performed in patients with osteoarthritis. Relief of pain and improvement in range of motion were gratifying in most cases.[24] Often, the best results from shoulder replacement are in osteoarthritis, because the deltoid muscle and

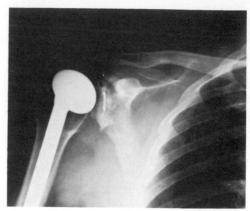

Figure 22–7. Anteroposterior roentgenogram of the right shoulder following Neer total shoulder replacement. Methyl methacrylate has been used to fix the glenoid component but has not been necessary for the humeral component.

the rotator cuff are normal. When the new approach described by Neer is utilized, functional results are superior (Figs. 22–6 to 22–10).

OSTEOARTHRITIS OF THE ACROMIOCLAVICULAR JOINT

In patients with osteoarthritis, involvement of the acromioclavicular joint is common. Waxman found that 70% of patients with a diagnosis of osteoarthritis had clinical involvement of the acromioclavicular joint.[25] In a roentgenographic study, osteophytes at the acromioclavicular joint were found in 39% of patients with osteoarthritis.[26] DePalma has studied 223 sets of acromioclavicular joints and has documented that degenerative changes begin during the second decade and progress

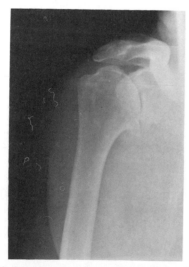

Figure 22–6. Anteroposterior roentgenogram of the right shoulder shows large marginal osteophytes on the inferior aspect of the humeral head and glenoid, with eburnation of the humeral head and glenoid.

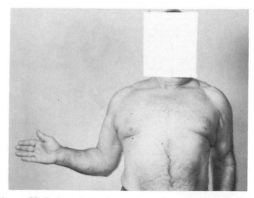

Figure 22–8. Postoperative external rotation of the right shoulder is demonstrated 1½ years following surgery.

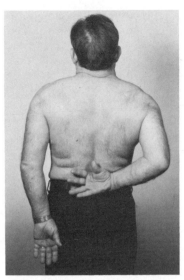

Figure 22–9. Internal rotation of the right shoulder 1½ years following total shoulder replacement.

during the lifetime of the patient.[27] The inferior portion of the joint is in intimate contact with the subacromial bursa and the rotator cuff. The development of osteophytes on the acromioclavicular joint can impinge on the subacromial bursa and produce additional changes in the rotator cuff, leading to rotator cuff tears.

Although the finding of osteoarthritis in the acromioclavicular joint is common roentgenographically and anatomically, these findings may not be associated with clinical symptoms.[27] Furthermore, the degree of roentgenographic

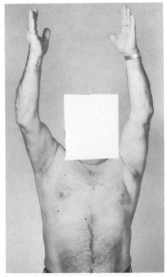

Figure 22–10. Total elevation of both shoulders following right total shoulder replacement.

change may not correlate with the degree of the patient's complaints.[28] Patients with osteoarthritis of the acromioclavicular joint may complain of pain in the shoulder. The pain is likely to be diffuse and not localized to the joint. The pain may be referred to the insertion of the deltoid muscle on the humerus or may be referred down the upper arm but not into the forearm or trapezius area. Patients who have pain in the trapezius region or pain that radiates from the shoulder region into the forearm and hand are more likely to have disease in the cervical spine. The pain is usually aggravated by motion, particularly elevation and abduction. It is likely to be intensified when the arm is used in overhead activities such as washing windows, painting, or hanging draperies.

On inspection, the acromioclavicular joint may be enlarged because of marginal osteophytes. Examination usually reveals local tenderness of the acromioclavicular joint. This is felt to be the most diagnostic single clinical finding in osteoarthritis of the acromioclavicular joint.[28] Clinical tests for disease in the acromioclavicular joint include having the patient adduct the involved shoulder by touching the opposite shoulder. The physician then gently further adducts the humerus. In the presence of osteoarthritis, this maneuver may produce pain in the acromioclavicular joint but not invariably so. A more reliable test is to anesthetize the acromioclavicular joint with a local anesthetic and then have the patient move the shoulder. Relief of symptoms following the injection of a local anesthetic confirms that the acromioclavicular joint is the source of the complaint. However, it should be appreciated that it may be difficult to be certain that the injection has actually been given into the joint, particularly when there may be significant narrowing of the joint space and large marginal osteophytes. Therefore, if a patient with suspected osteoarthritis of this joint does not obtain relief of symptoms after injection of a local anesthetic into the joint, it would be wise to repeat the injection before assuming that the cause of the patient's complaints is arising from another area. In addition to a local anesthetic, a steroid preparation should also be injected into the joint to provide symptomatic relief. Range of motion of the shoulder may be limited, and indeed, an adhesive capsulitis can develop from osteoarthritis of the acromioclavicular joint.

Treatment. Treatment of this condition should be conservative initially. The use of injection of a local anesthetic and steroid into the joint has been mentioned. This should not be repeated more frequently than every 3 or 4 months because of the deleterious effects of steroids on the metabolism of chondrocytes. Local heat and the use of nonsteroidal anti-inflammatory drugs are also prescribed. If conservative treatment fails to provide lasting relief, surgery should be considered.

Excision of the distal 2.5 cm of the clavicle or acromioclavicular arthroplasty is an effective form of treatment.[28–31] As discussed previously, the acromioclavicular joint can be approached through the incision used for the Neer anterior acromioplasty. Acromioclavicular arthroplasty is perhaps performed more frequently with anterior acromioplasty or glenohumeral replacement arthroplasty than as an independent procedure. A 5-cm incision is made over the distal end of the clavicle and acromion obliquely. A transverse incision is made along the distal 3 cm of the clavicle and across the acromioclavicular joint. A round Hohmann retractor is placed superiorly around the clavicle and inferiorly against the coracoclavicular ligaments. The distal 2.5 cm of the clavicle are excised with a power saw. This osteotomy is performed so that more of the clavicle is removed posteriorly than anteriorly and more superiorly than inferiorly. Bone wax is applied to the raw cut surface of the clavicle. More than 2.5 cm of the clavicle should not be removed; otherwise, the coracoclavicular ligaments would be violated. To repair the wound, the capsule is closed and the trapezius muscle is sutured to the deltoid muscle. Postoperatively, the shoulder is immobilized in a sling and swath. Pendulum exercises are begun as soon as the patient can tolerate them. Later, the patient performs range of motion exercises.

OSTEOARTHRITIS OF THE STERNOCLAVICULAR JOINT

It is interesting to note that about twice as much motion occurs at the sternoclavicular joint as at the acromioclavicular joint.[32] For instance, of the total 180 degrees of elevation that is possible in the shoulder, 40 degrees occurs at the sternoclavicular joint and 20 degrees at the acromioclavicular joint. Any condition that would result in incongruity of the sternoclavicular joint can result in restriction of motion of the shoulder joint.

Osteoarthritis of the sternoclavicular joint is surprisingly common when the joint is examined pathologically. The sternoclavicular was involved histologically with changes of osteoarthritis in slightly more than 60% of a series of 1000 unselected autopsies.[3] In a study of 64 sternoclavicular joints obtained at postmortem examination, Sokoloff and Gleason found frequent degenerative changes by the end of the third decade. With advancing age, these changes increased in frequency, and after the fifth decade, a normal-appearing joint was uncommon.[33] These findings were confirmed in a later study of 200 sternoclavicular joints removed at autopsy.[34] Mild changes of osteoarthritis were first observed in 18% of specimens from individuals in the third and fourth decades. The incidence of osteoarthritis increased to 83% during the sixth decade and to 94% during the seventh to ninth decades.

Clinically, primary osteoarthritis of the sternoclavicular joint occurs infrequently. Posttraumatic arthritis of the sternoclavicular joint may be encountered occasionally after fracture or dislocation. Patients are often concerned about the development of swelling about the joint. Symptoms are usually not severe and consist of pain and tenderness in the area. Pain may be increased by abduction and elevation.[35]

Treatment. Reassurance that the enlargement of the joint is the result of osteoarthritis is frequently the only treatment needed. Local heat and nonsteroidal anti-inflammatory drugs may be prescribed in more symptomatic patients. Symptoms are usually not severe enough to require surgery. An arthroplasty of the sternoclavicular joint has been described by Neer for cases that cannot be managed conservatively.[7] The medial 2 cm of the clavicle are resected through a transverse incision over the joint. Dissection is performed carefully around the clavicle to avoid damage to the great vessels lying immediately beneath the clavicle. The resected end of the clavicle is treated with bone wax to aid in hemostasis and to reduce the chances of periosteal new bone formation. The clavicular head of the sternocleidomastoid muscle may be partially released and placed in the defect caused by removal of the medial 2 cm of the clavicle.

THE ELBOW

Osteoarthritis of the elbow is more common than might be suspected. In a study of 1000 unselected postmortem examinations in patients more than 15 years of age, osteoarthritis of the elbow was found in 950 (95%).[3] Goodfellow and Bullough studied the age changes in the elbow joint in 28 postmortem examinations of people aged 18 to 88 years.[36] They consistently found degeneration of articular cartilage in the radial head and mirror changes in the capitellum. The humeroulnar joint was usually spared. They felt that those areas of articular cartilage that did not articulate with cartilage on the opposite side of the joint had undergone chondromalacia. In the radial head, the most severe degenerative changes were found in the posteromedial part of the rim of the radial head. This process begins in the fourth decade and progresses with advancing age until, ultimately, the joint surface is destroyed. In the capitellum, they found ulceration of the posterior crest that divides the capitellum from the trochlea. The humeroulnar joint may reveal grooving of the articular cartilage in the axis of movement, but eburnation is not seen. They stated that the rim of the radial head displays chondromalacia, but it is only the posteromedial portion that impinges on the posterior crest of the capitellum that undergoes degeneration. Furthermore, they felt that the degeneration of the radiohumeral joint was related to its hinge and rotatory movements, whereas the humeroulnar joint uses hinge motion only.

Osteoarthritis may occur secondarily in the elbow from trauma, old infection and hematologic disease in which repeated hemarthroses occur, such as hemophilia, and as a sequela of old, inactive rheumatoid arthritis. Fractures of the radial head that interfere with its normal contour will result in limitation of motion and traumatic arthritis.[31, 37] Chronic trauma, as seen in pneumatic tool workers[5] or foundry workers,[38] has been thought to be responsible for the production of osteoarthritis of the elbow. Osteoarthritis can also occur as a result of osteochondritis dissecans or Panner's disease.[39] The capitellum is the usual site of this condition, but the trochlea may be involved as well. It usually begins in childhood but may cause symptoms in later adult life. The cartilage of the capitellum may degenerate and slough away from the subchrondral bone, forming loose bodies. If the loose bodies are symptomatic, they should be removed.

Trauma may also be responsible for the production of loose bodies, which can result in osteoarthritis if they are allowed to remain in the joint. They should be removed if locking occurs. Synovial osteochondromatosis can also involve the elbow. Indeed, after the knee joint, the elbow is the second most common site.[40]

The elbow can also be the site of neuropathic disease resulting from syringomyelia or tertiary syphilis. The usual treatment is to fit the patient with a hinged elbow brace. Arthrodesis may be considered when pain is severe and cannot be managed by a brace.[39]

Marmor has stated that the most commonly involved portion of the elbow joint in osteoarthritis is the radial head,[31] which can result in limitation of pronation and supination. Ultimately, loss of extension and flexion can also occur as secondary contractures develop. The loss of a few degrees of extension is usually not disabling to a patient, as few activities require full extension of the elbow. Flexion of the elbow is important. It is obviously desirable to have enough flexion of the elbow to enable the patient to place the hand for such activities as eating, dressing, and combing the hair. Pronation and supination are important and enable the patient to place the hand in different positions. For example, pronation is required for writing, and supination is needed for lifting or receiving items into the hand. The patient can compensate somewhat for the loss of pronation and supination by rotation of the shoulder. If both the shoulder and the elbow are restricted in motion, the resultant disability can be severe.

Clinically, the patient with osteoarthritis of the elbow complains of pain and a gradual loss of motion and motor power. There is usually no palpable or visible swelling about the elbow joint. Depending on the amount of pain and stiffness, there will be a proportionate loss in the ability to perform ordinary activities of daily living. It is useful for the surgeon to determine if there is pain only with pronation and supination or with flexion and extension. Often, there is more pain with pronation and supination than with flexion and extension. This differentiation is helpful in determining treatment.

Treatment. Treatment of both types of osteoarthritis of the elbow, primary and secondary, is the same. In the early stages of osteoarthritis, resting the elbow during periods of pain and administration of nonsteroidal anti-inflammatory drugs are sufficient to relieve the symptoms. Intra-articular steroids are useful, especially for episodes of severe pain, but they should not be given more frequently than every 3 to 4 months.

Surgical treatment is required when loose bodies cause locking of the elbow joint; the loose bodies should be removed. In the case of osteoarthritis of the radiohumeral joint that is symptomatic with pronation and supination, resection of the radial head is indicated. In cases of generalized osteoarthritis of the elbow joint, resection of the radial head may also be of value if the pain occurs mainly with pronation and supination and there is little discomfort with flexion and extension. In cases of generalized osteoarthritis, loose bodies and osteophytes should be removed in addition to the radial head. Resection of the radial head may improve pronation and supination and perhaps flexion. Extension of the elbow joint is usually not improved by radial head resection.[31, 41]

There are some who advocate replacement of the radial head with a Silastic prosthesis rather than radial head resection alone.[31, 42] This is an attractive idea, considering that radial shortening and pain at the wrist joint due to subluxation of the distal radioulnar joint have been shown to occur after radial head resection in as many as 50% of patients in one study.[13] Reports as to the usefulness of the Silastic radial head have been mixed, and fractures of the prosthesis have occurred in significant numbers of patients.[44, 45] All the fractures occurred in the older prostheses. None have been reported with the newer high-performance silicone elastomer to date.

Radial head resection alone will not relieve symptoms of patients with severe osteoarthritis of the entire elbow joint. The other alternatives for treatment are arthroplasty and arthrodesis. Traditionally, fascial arthroplasty is done on the elbow. Knight reported long-term results with the Campbell fascial arthroplasty in 45 patients. With an average follow-up of 14 years, the results were good on only 56%. Unsatisfactory results were obtained in 22%.[46]

Total replacement arthroplasty of the elbow has undergone significant change in the last 10 years. Initially, the elbow was replaced by various hinge prostheses, including the Dee, McKee, and GSB prostheses. Unfortunately, these have had a marked number of problems, including a significant incidence of loosening. A hinge prosthesis does not compensate for the torque generated across the elbow joint. This force is transmitted directly to the bone-cement interface and is probably responsible for the prosthetic loosening encountered with the hinge prosthesis.[47–50] Most of the hinge elbow replacements have been performed in patients with rheumatoid arthritis rather than osteoarthritis. Those with osteoarthritis would be expected to place greater demands on an elbow joint, and therefore, problems might occur more frequently.

Newer prostheses have been utilized, such as the nonconstrained capitellocondylar elbow arthroplasty. A recent report listed only one revision for loosening in 69 arthroplasties in patients with rheumatoid arthritis. These results are encouraging enough to suggest that the prosthesis might also be of benefit to patients with osteoarthritis with the possible provision of a radial head prosthesis. Other prostheses are in the developmental stage. At this time, none of the prostheses can be recommended for use in patients with osteoarthritis until more is known of the results.

Arthrodesis of the elbow has been mentioned as a possible mode of treatment. This operation is probably better performed for sepsis such as tuberculosis, for treatment of neurotrophic joints, or perhaps for severe cases of post-traumatic arthritis.

References

1. Bland JH, Stulberg SD: Osteoarthritis: Pathology and Clinical Patterns. In Kelley WN, Harris ED, Ruddy S, Sledge CB (eds.): Textbook of Rheumatology. Philadelphia, W.B. Saunders Company, 1981, pp. 1471–1499.
2. Neer CS II: Replacement arthroplasty for glenohumeral osteoarthritis. J Bone Joint Surg 56A:1–13, 1974.
3. Heine J: Über die Arthritis deformans. Virchows Arch 260:521–663, 1926.
4. Moskowitz RW: Treatment of osteoarthritis. In Hollander JL, McCarty DJ (eds.): Arthritis and Allied Conditions. 8th ed. Philadelphia, Lea and Febiger, 1972, pp. 1054–1067.
5. Lawrence JS: Generalized osteoarthrosis in a population sample. Am J Epidemiol 90:381–389, 1969.
6. Hollander JL, McCarty DJ (eds.): Arthritis and Allied Conditions. 8th ed. Lea and Febiger, Philadelphia, 1972.
7. Neer CS II: Reconstructive surgery and rehabilitation of the shoulder. In Kelley WN, Harris ED, Ruddy S, Sledge CB (eds.): Textbook of Rheumatology. Philadelphia, W.B. Saunders Company, 1981, pp. 1944–1959.
8. Neer CS II: Anterior acromioplasty for the chronic impingement syndrome in the shoulder. J Bone Joint Surg 54A:41–50, 1972.
9. Watson M: The refractory painful arc syndrome. J Bone Joint Surg 60B:544–536, 1978.
10. Pujadas GM: Coraco-acromial ligament syndrome. J Bone Joint Surg 52A:1261–1262, 1970.
11. DePalma AF, White JB, Callery G: Degenerative lesions of the shoulder joint at various age groups which are compatible with good function. Am Acad Orthop Surg Lectures 7:168–180, 1950.
12. Neer C II: Degenerative lesions of the proximal humeral articular surface. Clin Orthop 20:116–124, 1961.
13. Neer CS II, Watson KC, Stanton FJ: Seven year experience in total shoulder replacement. Orthop Trans 5:398, 1981.
14. Barton NJ: Arthrodesis of the shoulder for degenerative conditions. J Bone Joint Surg 54A:1759–1764, 1972.
15. Neer CS II, Cruess RL, Sledge CB, Wilde AH: Total

shoulder replacement. A preliminary report. Orthop Trans 1:244, 1977.

16. Buechel FF, Pappas MJ, DePalma AF: Floating-socket total shoulder replacement: Anatomical, biomechanical and surgical rationale. J Biomed Mater Res 12:89–114, 1978.

17. Fenlin JM Jr: Total glenohumeral joint replacement. Orthop Clin North Am 6:565–583, 1975.

18. Macnab I: Total shoulder replacement—a bipolar glenohumeral prosthesis. J Bone Joint Surg 58B:257, 1977.

19. Post M, Haskell S, Jablon M: Total shoulder replacement with a constrained prosthesis. J Bone Joint Surg 62A:327–335, 1980.

20. Lettin AWF, Scales JT: Total replacement of the shoulder joint (two cases). Proc R Soc Med 65:373–374, 1972.

21. Coughlin MJ, Morris JM, West WF: The semiconstrained total shoulder arthroplasty. J Bone Joint Surg 61A:574–581, 1979.

22. Romano RL, Burgess EM: Total shoulder replacement. J Bone Joint Surg 57A:1033, 1975.

23. Hughes M, Neer CS: Glenohumeral joint replacement and postoperative rehabilitation. Phys Ther 55:850–858, 1975.

24. Wilde AH, Borden LS, Brems JJ: Experience with the Neer total shoulder replacement. Orthop Trans 5:397, 1981.

25. Waxman J: Acromioclavicular disease in rheumatologic practice—the forgotten joint. J Louisiana State Med Soc 129:1–3, 1977.

26. McNair MM, Boyle JA, Buchanan WW, Davidson JK: A clinical and radiological study of rheumatoid arthritis with a note on the findings in osteoarthrosis. I. The shoulder joint. Clin Radiol 20:269–277, 1969.

27. DePalma AJ: Degenerative Changes in the Sternoclavicular and Acromioclavicular Joints in Various Decades. Springfield, Illinois, Charles C Thomas, 1957.

28. Worcester JN, Green DP: Osteoarthritis of the acromioclavicular joint. Clin Orthop 58:69–73, 1968.

29. Gurd FB: The treatment of complete dislocation of the outer end of the clavicle. Ann Surg 113:1094–1098, 1941.

30. Mumford EB: Acromioclavicular dislocation. J Bone Joint Surg 23:799–802, 1941.

31. Marmor L: Surgery of osteoarthritis. Arthritis Rheum 2:117–156, 1972.

32. DePalma AF: Surgery of the Shoulder. Philadelphia, J.B. Lippincott Co., 1973, pp. 125–132.

33. Sokoloff L, Gleason IO: The sternoclavicular articulation in rheumatic diseases. Am J Clin Pathol 24:406–414, 1954.

34. Silberberg M, Frank EL, Jarrett SR, Silberberg R: Aging and osteoarthritis of the human sternoclavicular joint. Am J Pathol 35:851–865, 1959.

35. Bateman JE: The Shoulder and Neck. Philadelphia, W.B. Saunders Company, 1972, p. 289.

36. Goodfellow JW, Bullough PG: The pattern of aging of the articular cartilage of the elbow joint. J Bone Joint Surg 49B:175–181, 1967.

37. Key JA: Treatment of fractures of the head and neck of the radius. J Bone Joint Surg 96:101–104, 1931.

38. Mintz G, Fraga A: Severe osteoarthritis of the elbow in foundry workers. Arch Environ Health 27:78–80, 1973.

39. Smith FM: Surgery of the Elbow. 2nd ed. Philadelphia, W.B. Saunders Company, 1972, pp. 279–295.

40. Spjut IIJ, Dorfman HD, Fechner RE, Ackerman LV: Tumors of Bone and Cartilage. Washington, D.C., Armed Forces Institute of Pathology, Second Series. Fascicle 5, 1971, p. 39.

41. Chrisman OD: Elbow. *In* Milch RA (ed.): Surgery of Arthritis. Baltimore, Williams and Wilkins, 1964, pp. 101–111.

42. Swanson AB, Jaeger SH, LaRochelle D: Comminuted fractures of the radial head. J Bone Joint Surg 63A:1039–1049, 1981.

43. Taylor TKF, O'Connor BT: The effect upon the inferior radio-ulnar joint of excision of the head of the radius in adults. J Bone Joint Surg 46B:83–88, 1964.

44. Morrey BF, Askew L, Chao EY: Silastic prosthetic replacement of the radial head. J Bone Joint Surg 63A:454–458, 1981.

45. Mayhall WST, Tiley FT, Paluska DJ: Fracture of Silastic radial head prosthesis. J Bone Joint Surg 63A:459–460, 1981.

46. Knight RA, Van Zandt IL: Arthroplasty of the elbow, an end result study. J Bone Joint Surg 34A:610–618, 1952.

47. Souter WA: Arthroplasty of the elbow with particular reference to metallic hinge arthroplasty in rheumatoid patients. Orthop Clin North Am 4:395–413, 1973.

48. Dee R: Total replacement of the elbow joint. Orthop Clin North Am 4:415–433, 1973.

49. Inglis AE, Pellicci PM: Total elbow replacement. J Bone Joint Surg 62A:1252–1258, 1980.

50. Morrey BF, Bryan RS, Dobyns JH, Linscheid RL: Total elbow arthroplasty. J Bone Joint Surg 63A:1050–1063, 1981.

23

Osteoarthritis of the Foot and Ankle

Roger A. Mann, M.D.

ANATOMIC AND BIOMECHANICAL CONSIDERATIONS

The foot and ankle joints are subjected to loading forces that exceed the body weight by 15% to 20% during normal walking and by as much as 200% to 250% during running. The dissipation of these forces through these rather small articulations is normally done in an extremely efficient manner. For example, when a 150-lb individual *walks* for 1 mile, about 63 tons of force are dissipated through the foot; when the same 150-lb person *runs* 1 mile, about 110 tons of force are dissipated through the foot. The ability of the foot and ankle to dissipate these forces was probably best stated by Jones when he said that the longitudinal arch composed of the joints of the foot "does not break down, it bends down."[1] This unique characteristic of the bones and joints of the foot and ankle permits them to absorb and dissipate these great forces and at the same time remain asymptomatic.

The foot and ankle cannot be looked upon as isolated entities, but rather must be viewed as a series of interdependent articulations that function in unison in order to absorb the impact of gait and to dissipate its forces, while at the same time providing a stable platform for the body. At the time of initial ground contact, the foot is a flexible structure with the heel in valgus and the longitudinal arch un-

locked, but as it passes through the mid-stance phase toward toe-off, the foot is converted into a rigid lever arm that supports the body weight. A disruption of any one of the joints along this linkage will hamper the dissipation of forces and place increased stress on another joint in this finely balanced mechanism.

During normal gait, dorsiflexion and plantar flexion occur at the ankle joint, as demonstrated in Figure 23–1. If adequate dorsiflexion cannot take place because of osteophyte formation along the anterior aspect of the tibia or the neck of the talus, the patient may experience pain about the anterior aspect of the ankle joint and a decrease in the step length. This will be compensated for in part by some increased motion within the transverse tarsal joint. Lack of ankle plantar flexion due to osteoarthritis rarely will cause any significant gait abnormality.

The motions about the subtalar joint (talocalcaneal joint) are those of inversion and eversion. The main function of the subtalar joint is to transmit the transverse rotation that is occurring in the lower extremity above into the foot below. The subtalar joint axis is aligned approximately 45 degrees to the horizontal, and as a result, it functions similarly to a mitered hinge. In this way, rotation in the tibia above can be transmitted across the ankle joint into the foot below (Fig. 23–2). During normal gait, at the time of initial ground con-

PLANTAR FLEXION-DORSIFLEXION

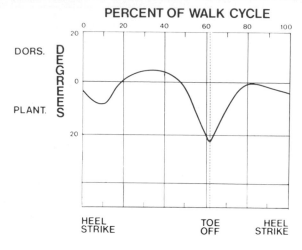

PERCENT OF WALK CYCLE

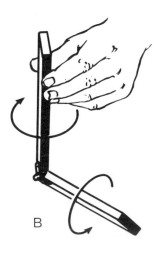

Figure 23–1. A graph depicting ankle dorsiflexion and plantar flexion during walking.

tact, the heel is in valgus or eversion, and at the time of toe-off, the heel is in inversion or varus.[2] The motion in the subtalar joint permits the foot to adapt to a slope or irregular surface during walking. If the function of the subtalar joint is disrupted because of osteoarthritis, it may limit one's ability to ambulate. If the calcaneus can no longer pass into eversion at initial ground contact, the person is more prone to sprain the lateral aspect of the ankle because the line of weight bearing will pass lateral to the calcaneus. Therefore, if the patient steps on an irregular surface, the foot would have a tendency to invert, throwing the person off balance. Conversely, if the patient has lost the ability to invert the subtalar joint, it is compatible with normal gait; however, if the calcaneus becomes too everted, there would be marked flattening of the longitudinal arch, and the patient would tend to roll over

the medial border of his foot, placing a greater stress along this area, increasing the chance of clinical symptoms.

The next functional articulation within the foot as one proceeds distally is the transverse tarsal joint, which consists of the talonavicular and calcaneocuboid joints. The function of this joint system is dependent on normal subtalar joint motion. When the subtalar joint is everted, as at the time of initial ground contact, the transverse tarsal joint is quite flexible, whereas when the subtalar joint is inverted, as in the last half of the stance phase, the transverse tarsal joint is rather rigid (Fig. 23–3).[3] If there is loss of function of either the talonavicular joint or calcaneocuboid joint, the function of both the transverse tarsal joint and subtalar joint is lost. This is due to the interdependence of this joint complex on each joint being functional. If, however, only the subtalar joint is

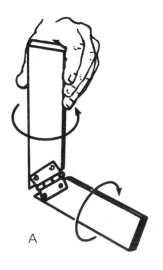

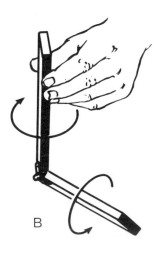

Figure 23–2. Model of the function of the subtalar joint as it translates motion from the tibia above into the calcaneus below. *A,* The action of a mitered hinge demonstrating translation of rotation across a 45-degree hinge is illustrated. This is analogous to the subtalar joint. Inward rotation of the upper stick causes outward rotation of the lower stick, which is analogous to the inward rotation of the tibia producing eversion of the calcaneus. *B,* The concept that outward rotation of the tibia will produce inward rotation of the calcaneus is demonstrated in this figure. (From Mann RA, Inman VT: Biomechanics of the foot and ankle. *In* DuVries HL (ed.): Surgery of the Foot. 2nd ed. St. Louis, C. V. Mosby Company, 1965.)

EVERSION   INVERSION

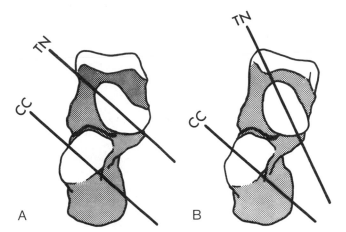

Figure 23–3. Axes of the transverse tarsal joint. *A,* When the calcaneus is in eversion, the conjoint axes between the talonavicular (TN) and the calcaneocuboid (CC) joints are parallel to one another, so that there is increased motion in the transverse tarsal joint. *B,* When the calcaneus is in inversion, the axes are no longer parallel, so that there is decreased motion and increased stability of the transverse tarsal joint.

nonfunctioning, a certain degree of dorsiflexion and plantar flexion can still occur within the transverse tarsal joint. Following an ankle arthrodesis, the limited dorsiflexion and plantar flexion that occur within the foot take place at the transverse tarsal joint.

In a more distal location in the foot are the midtarsal joints, which include the intertarsal joints and the tarsometatarsal joints; these joints are quite rigid, and little or no motion occurs from a functional standpoint. Loss of motion within any of these joints has little or no effect on the function of the foot.

The metatarsophalangeal joints play a vital role in the stability of the longitudinal arch of the foot. This is brought about because the plantar aponeurosis and the intrinsic muscles of the foot, which arise from the calcaneus, insert into the base of the proximal phalanges. As the metatarsophalangeal joints are brought into dorsiflexion in the last half of the stance phase, the proximal phalanx pulls the plantar aponeurosis over the metatarsal heads, thereby raising and stabilizing the longitudinal arch.[4] When this mechanism is disrupted owing to the inability of the metatarsophalangeal joints to dorsiflex, some instability of the foot may result (Fig. 23–4).

GENERAL CLINICAL CONSIDERATIONS

The diagnosis of osteoarthritis of the joints of the foot and ankle usually is not a particularly difficult one to make. It may be difficult to decide, however, whether one is dealing with primary or secondary osteoarthritis, e.g., degenerative arthritis versus traumatic arthritis. From a clinical standpoint, the patient's main complaint is that of pain in the region of the affected joint, which is aggravated by activity and usually diminishes with rest. Not infrequently, the pain is worse when the person first arises and moves around on the extremity, only to improve somewhat after a short period of time. The pain will tend to recur near the end of the day or if increased demands are placed on the extremity. This is frequently associated later in the course of the condition with swelling and increased heat around the affected joint.

The physical findings demonstrate a decrease in the range of motion of the affected joint, often associated with pain and/or crepitus. Not uncommonly, generalized synovial thickening is noted. As the condition progresses, a deformity of the involved joint can often be seen.

The diagnosis is confirmed by obtaining a roentgenogram of the involved area. If necessary, laboratory studies may be indicated to try to specifically define the etiology of the arthritic process. At times, early in the degenerative process, more elaborate studies such as tomograms, computed tomography, and a bone scan may be indicated.

In general, treatment should initially be directed toward relieving the patient's main clinical complaint. Early in the course of the disease process, salicylates or other types of nonsteroidal anti-inflammatory medicine may be all that is required (see Chapter 18). As the process continues, some form of immobilization, in the form of a splint, brace, arch support, and/or shoe modification, may be indicated in order to relieve the symptoms. If

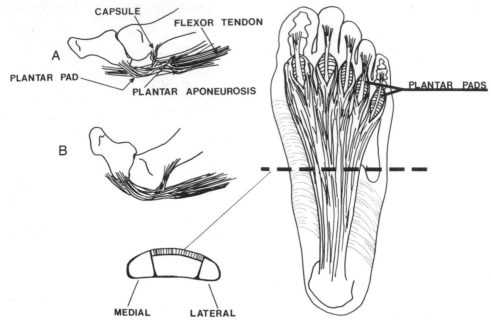

Figure 23–4. The plantar aponeurosis. *A,* The plantar aponeurosis divides as it proceeds distally to allow the flexor tendons to pass through the aponeurosis and combines with the joint capsule to form the plantar pad of the metatarsophalangeal joint. *B,* Dorsiflexion of the toes forces the metatarsal head into plantar flexion and brings the plantar pad over the head of the metatarsal. (From Mann RA, Inman VT: Structure and function. *In* DuVries HL (ed.): Surgery of the Foot. 2nd ed. St. Louis, C. V. Mosby Company, 1965.)

conservative measures are unsuccessful, surgical intervention may be considered.

Now that this general background of the biomechanical aspects of the foot and ankle, diagnosis, physical examination, laboratory evaluation, and conservative treatment of foot and ankle problems has been presented, specific anatomic areas will be discussed.

THE ANKLE JOINT

The main complaint associated with osteoarthritis of the ankle is pain, which is usually well localized to the area of the joint. It is often mild at first but becomes more severe as the joint deterioration increases.

Physical examination will often demonstrate a decrease in the range of motion, particularly in dorsiflexion. As a result of this loss of dorsiflexion, the patient may state that when he walks, his foot is externally rotated more on the affected side than on the uninvolved side. This is a compensatory mechanism to help decrease the dorsiflexion stress on the ankle joint. Not infrequently, there is generalized synovial thickening and increased warmth about the joint.

The diagnosis can usually be confirmed by obtaining a roentgenogram of the ankle joint

(Fig. 23–5). If there are no roentgenographic changes but persistent pain is noted, a bone scan may be of diagnostic benefit.

If degenerative arthritis secondary to trauma is excluded, there are few other entities that mimic primary osteoarthritis of the ankle joint.

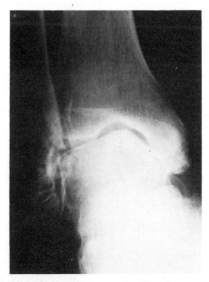

Figure 23–5. Roentgenogram showing degenerative arthritis of the ankle joint. In addition to narrowing and irregularity of the ankle joint, a varus tilt has also occurred, placing increased stress against the lateral side of the ankle.

Occasionally, a nonspecific monarticular synovitis will cause pain about the ankle joint, but this is uncommon. Unrecognized trauma such as an osteochondral or chrondral fracture of the talus should be excluded by tomography or arthroscopy.

Treatment

Conservative Management. The management of osteoarthritis of the ankle joint is essentially based on the patient's symptom complex. Initially, salicylates will be adequate, but as the arthritis progresses, various types of nonsteroidal anti-inflammatory medication may be added to the conservative regimen.

If the patient has rather marked limitation of dorsiflexion, a slight elevation of the heel may be useful. This can be done either by placing a felt pad within the shoe itself or by adding an external elevation to the heel. The use of soft sole material in the heel, e.g., a SACH heel, is helpful because it decreases the impact of initial ground contact.

As the osteoarthritis becomes progressively more symptomatic, it becomes necessary to use some form of orthosis. Initially, the use of a molded leather ankle brace that incorporates a medial and lateral steel stay will help decrease the motion within the ankle joint, although there is still enough "give" in the brace to allow some motion. The only problem that this type of orthosis presents to the patient is that he will often require a mismated pair of shoes because the volume of the brace is such that most people cannot wear regular shoes with it. In order to further increase the stability of the ankle joint, a polypropylene ankle-foot orthosis (AFO) will further restrict ankle joint motion (Fig. 23–6). When such an orthosis is used, the patient should wear a rocker-bottom–type shoe in order to enable him to smoothly roll over his foot. With a rigid ankle, the energy expenditure during walking is increased significantly; a rocker-bottom sole on the shoe greatly facilitates a smoother gait pattern.

There are two other types of braces that may help decrease the stress on the ankle joint: a patellar tendon–bearing orthosis, which helps unload the ankle joint (see Chapter 17), and a double-upright brace with a fixed or restricted ankle and a rocker-bottom shoe. It has been my experience, however, that neither of these braces seems to significantly diminish ankle joint pain and that both are heavier than the polypropylene AFO.

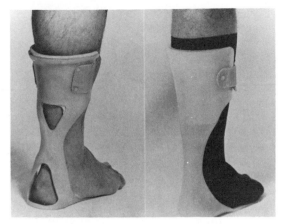

Figure 23–6. An example of a polypropylene ankle-foot orthosis (AFO). This lightweight brace will provide stability to both the ankle and the subtalar joint.

Surgical Management. The overall prognosis for untreated osteoarthritis of the ankle joint is poor because it is a progressive problem. How long the pain can be tolerated, however, is extremely variable from patient to patient. If the patient continues to have significant pain and disability after adequate conservative management, surgical intervention should be considered. The surgical management of osteoarthritis of the ankle consists mainly of performing an arthrodesis of the ankle joint (Fig. 23–7). Once an ankle arthrodesis is achieved in satisfactory alignment, the overall ambulatory capacity of the patient can be significantly improved. Following a successful ankle arthrodesis, most patients can walk with a mild gait abnormality with little or no pain.

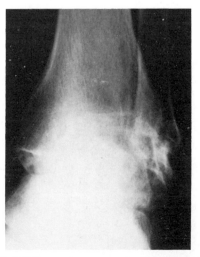

Figure 23–7. This roentgenogram shows an example of an ankle arthrodesis. This is the postoperative roentgenogram of the ankle shown in Figure 23–5.

If only a single joint is involved, i.e., the ankle joint and no joint distal to it, the prognosis is better than if there is involvement of the subtalar or transverse tarsal joint as well. This is mainly because of the interdependence of these joints on one another, because most of the dorsiflexion and plantar flexion that has been lost at the ankle joint is partially compensated for by motion in the subtalar, talonavicular, and calcaneocuboid joints. If these joints are arthritic, the area receiving the added stress will usually cause persistent pain in the patient's foot.

An ankle arthrodesis may be achieved by utilizing the compression technique advocated by Charnley. The fusion rate in the literature varies, but it is usually in the range of 80% to 85%. The most critical factor in performing an ankle arthrodesis is to place the ankle in proper alignment in relation to the tibia. The ideal position is neutral position, insofar as dorsiflexion and plantar flexion are concerned, and in approximately 5 to 7 degrees of valgus. If the ankle is placed into excessive plantar flexion, the patient will have a tendency to vault over the foot and, as a result, will place increased stress on the knee joint and the forefoot. Likewise, the varus-valgus alignment is extremely critical, because if the foot is positioned in a varus position, too much weight will be borne on the lateral aspect of the foot, resulting in pain along the lateral side of the foot and, eventually, a build-up of callus. It will also cause the forefoot to be in a somewhat supinated position, which is a more rigid position and will often result in discomfort in the forefoot with ambulation.

The total ankle replacement should be mentioned for completeness of a discussion of therapy. Most total ankle joints that are currently in use do not provide adequate pain relief, significant improvement in motion, or long-term reliability. The major problem has been loosening of the components in the patient with osteoarthritis, particularly in younger individuals. At present, the main indication for total ankle replacement is in the patient with rheumatoid arthritis with multi-joint involvement. In this group of patients, it usually functions mainly to provide relief of pain, with little or no improvement in ankle joint motion, especially dorsiflexion.

THE SUBTALAR JOINT

The patient with osteoarthritis of the subtalar joint usually presents with the complaint of pain about the hindfoot area. The patient usually will not localize the pain to the subtalar joint specifically but will complain of a diffuse type of pain. At times, subtalar joint pain may be referred and will present as pain localized to a specific area of the hindfoot. This often leads to misdiagnosis of symptoms as being due to a localized area of fasciitis, or possibly tendinitis, rather than arthritis of the subtalar joint. Patients will often note that they can walk fairly comfortably on level ground but that any type of irregular surface will cause a considerable amount of discomfort. They also note a progressive loss of agility. Symptoms are usually aggravated by prolonged activity and diminished by resting the foot.

Physical findings demonstrate restricted motion in the subtalar joint, at times associated with crepitus. The motion is usually associated with pain, especially at the extremes of motion. It is unusual to feel localized warmth or synovitis about the joint. Occasionally, a patient experiences spasms of the peroneal tendons, which results in a peroneal spastic flatfoot. The complete etiopathology of the peroneal spastic flatfoot is not known, except that it is associated with malfunction of the subtalar joint.

The diagnosis is confirmed by a roentgenogram of the subtalar joint, although at times the degenerative changes may not be obvious until the disease process has progressed (Fig. 23–8). If the patient has persistent pain in the subtalar joint region and the roentgenographic findings are persistently negative, a bone scan may be of benefit in demonstrating increased bony activity in this area.

The differential diagnosis includes primary osteoarthritis of the subtalar joint and secondary osteoarthritis related to rheumatoid ar-

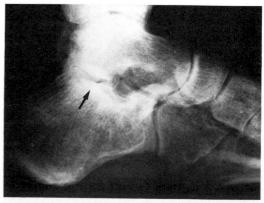

Figure 23–8. A roentgenogram of degenerative arthritis of the subtalar joint. Note the irregularity within the posterior facet (arrow).

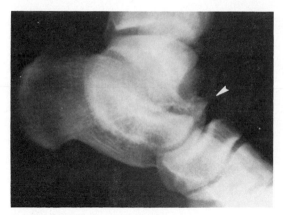

Figure 28–9. Roentgenogram demonstrating a long-standing tarsal coalition. This has resulted in secondary degenerative changes at the talonavicular joint, as demonstrated by the dorsal spurring (arrow) and an abnormal appearance of the subtalar joint.

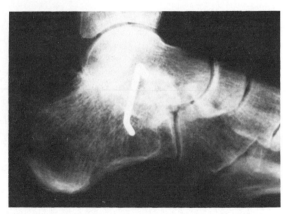

Figure 23–10. Postoperative roentgenogram demonstrating an arthrodesis of the subtalar joint. A staple has been used to maintain fixation following surgery.

thritis or congenital subtalar or tarsal coalition (Fig. 23–9).

Treatment

The initial management of the problem should be symptomatic. Salicylates followed by nonsteroidal anti-inflammatory medications will often be of some benefit early in the management of these cases. As pain increases, however, ambulation becomes increasingly difficult. The use of a broad-heeled shoe will increase the stability of the subtalar joint by presenting more surface to the ground, but either a molded leather ankle brace with medial and lateral steel stays or the polypropylene AFO with a rocker-bottom shoe may eventually be necessary.

After conservative measures no longer provide adequate relief of symptoms, surgical stabilization should be considered. A subtalar arthrodesis can be performed and will usually result in satisfactory relief of symptoms. It should be noted, however, that fusion of the subtalar joint places increased stress on the ankle joint because the transverse rotation that occurs in the lower extremity can no longer pass through the subtalar joint. Therefore, if the patient has concomitant ankle joint problems, a subtalar joint fusion may cause increased ankle joint pain.

A subtalar arthrodesis can be achieved through a lateral approach to the subtalar joint through the sinus tarsi. Usually, this can be accomplished without the addition of a bone graft, but some surgeons prefer to use bone from the iliac crest (Fig. 23–10).

As with an ankle arthrodesis, the position of a subtalar arthrodesis is extremely critical to insure proper placement and function of the foot. It is essential that the subtalar joint be placed in approximately 5 to 7 degrees of valgus to prevent any ankle joint instability. If it is placed into varus, the line of weight bearing will pass lateral to the heel, making the patient susceptible to inversion injuries of the ankle. When the subtalar joint is in a slight degree of valgus, the forefoot is kept flexible, but if the subtalar joint is placed into varus, the forefoot remains rather rigid.

Fusion of the subtalar joint will have an effect on the overall stability of the forefoot because the mechanism by which the transverse tarsal joint is stabilized is no longer functional. Generally, this is not a severe disability.

The question often arises as to whether a subtalar joint fusion alone is sufficient for treating arthritis in this area. It has been my experience that an isolated subtalar joint fusion is usually adequate if there is no associated problem in the talonavicular or calcaneocuboid joint. The greater the mobility that can be maintained in the foot, the better. I have not previously found it necessary to extend a subtalar joint fusion when it has been performed for an isolated subtalar joint problem. Following surgical stabilization of the subtalar joint, the overall functional capacity of patients is quite good. They can often return to many forms of light exercise and usually to their previous occupation, providing it is not one that requires a great deal of agility, such as that of roofer or steel worker.

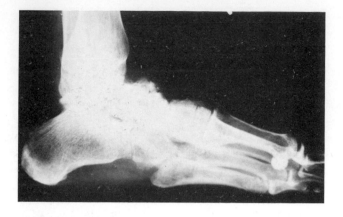

Figure 23–11. Roentgenogram illustrating degenerative arthritis of the talonavicular joint.

THE TALONAVICULAR JOINT

Isolated involvement of the talonavicular joint with osteoarthritis occurs infrequently. The most common types of arthritis are secondary degenerative joint disease following trauma, and rheumatoid arthritis. The patient usually presents with pain that is fairly well localized to the area of the talonavicular joint. The symptom complex is aggravated by activity and diminished with rest. The patient may note progressive loss of height of the longitudinal arch of the involved side.

Physical examination will usually demonstrate localized pain, swelling, and possibly increased heat over the area of the talonavicular joint. Stress of this joint causes increased discomfort. When the patient stands, there may be a sag at the talonavicular joint and, occasionally, a large medial prominence. The diagnosis is confirmed by roentgenographic examination of the joint (Fig. 23–11).

The differential diagnosis includes rupture of the posterior tibial tendon, which also results in a progressive loss of the longitudinal arch.

Treatment

Initial treatment consists of salicylates and nonsteroidal anti-inflammatory medication. These may be supplemented by the use of several types of shoe supports. A molded leather arch support may be adequate, but over a period of time, it may become necessary to use a UCBL type of insert, particularly if there is progressive collapse of the medial longitudinal arch (Fig. 23–12). If conservative measures fail to adequately relieve the patient's symptoms, surgical intervention may be of benefit.

The surgical treatment of choice is an arthrodesis of the talonavicular articulation. This fusion can be performed through either a medial approach or a dorsomedial approach to the joint, following which the joint surfaces are denuded. Occasionally, iliac crest bone may be added. I prefer to stabilize the joint with a staple. Following cast immobilization a firm arthrodesis can usually be achieved in 80% to 90% of patients. Occasionally, a nonunion results, which will require a bone grafting procedure and further immobilization.

When performing a talonavicular arthrodesis, it is important that the forefoot be properly aligned when the fixation device is placed across the joint. If the forefoot is placed in excessive supination, the individual may walk on the lateral border of the foot, causing a moderate amount of discomfort. It is important to place the foot in sufficient pronation at the time of surgery so that it will be flat on the floor.

As mentioned previously, an isolated arthrodesis of the talonavicular joint will eliminate most of the motion in the transverse tarsal and subtalar joints. This will increase stress on the ankle joint, although it is usually not of sufficient magnitude to cause clinical symptoms.

Following a successful talonavicular fusion, most patients can return to a fairly active existence, including light sports, although too much stress may lead to clinical symptoms. At times, the use of a rocker-bottom shoe will improve the patient's gait pattern.

As a general rule, an isolated talonavicular fusion will be adequate for isolated arthritis, but it will fail if other joints in the subtalar complex are involved.

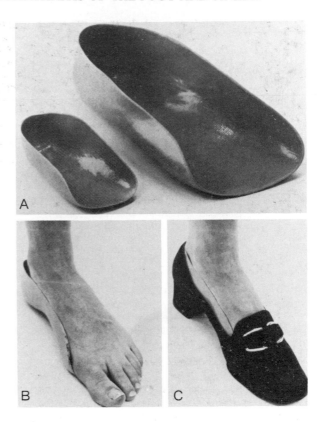

Figure 23–12. UCBL inserts. *A,* Child and adult sizes. *B,* Insert on the foot. *C,* Insert in a shoe.

THE CALCANEOCUBOID JOINT

In my experience, primary osteoarthritis of the calcaneocuboid joint, which makes up the other half of the transverse tarsal joint, has been extremely rare. It almost invariably follows trauma to the subtalar joint.

The management of osteoarthritis of the calcaneocuboid joint is similar to that described for the talonavicular joint. If necessary, arthrodesis of the calcaneocuboid joint can be done with essentially the same functional loss as that encountered with arthrodesis of the talonavicular joint.

THE MIDTARSAL JOINTS

Involvement of the midtarsal or intertarsal joints with osteoarthritis is an extremely unusual occurrence. As pointed out previously, little or no motion occurs within the midtarsal joints, and as a result, even if osteoarthritis were to occur, it would probably have little or no effect on the individual except for possibly an aching feeling within the mid-portion of the foot. There would be essentially no functional loss or deformity. If this condition is encoun-

tered, conservative treatment can be performed, as mentioned earlier, followed by local fusions, if necessary.

THE TARSOMETATARSAL JOINTS

Osteoarthritis of the tarsometatarsal joints usually occurs at the first metatarsocuneiform joint and with decreasing frequency as one moves laterally across the foot. In the early stages, the diagnosis may be difficult to establish owing to the vague nature of the complaint. With time, however, progressive changes are noted in the joints; these are associated with a progressive deformity of the mid-foot region (Fig. 23–13).

With the development of degenerative changes progressive enlargement about the first metatarsocuneiform joint and possibly the second and third metatarsocuneiform joints occurs. This enlargement is usually manifested by dorsal bossing, which makes the wearing of shoes somewhat difficult. As the process progresses, an abduction deformity of the forefoot may develop secondary to the stresses of weight bearing. This progressive abduction of the forefoot leads to a flattening of the longi-

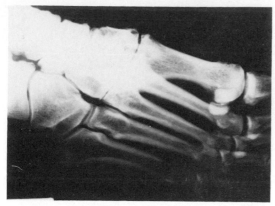

Figure 23–13. A roentgenogram showing degenerative arthritis of the tarsometatarsal joints.

tudinal arch, and a painful callosity may develop along the medial side of the foot.

Physical examination demonstrates tenderness about the involved metatarsocuneiform joints, which is aggravated by stressing the joints. As the degree of deformity increases, the localization of the problem becomes more obvious. The progressive abduction deformity that occurs in the metatarsocuneiform joints becomes quite rigid and cannot be passively corrected. When the patient stands, the abduction deformity of the forefoot is exaggerated.

Not infrequently, osteoarthritis of this area is secondary to prior trauma. The initial trauma may be overlooked by patients, and to the best of their knowledge, they do not remember a significant foot injury. A Charcot foot associated with diabetic neuropathy must also be considered. Almost invariably, however, this neuropathic arthritis is associated with some degree of sensory and/or vibratory loss, which is not observed in the patient with ordinary primary or secondary osteoarthritis.

Treatment

The initial management of the patient with arthritis of the tarsometatarsal joints should be nonoperative. The patient is given a firm arch support to relieve the stress in the area of the metatarsocuneiform joints. This can be quite effective early in the condition. As the foot becomes progressively deformed, however, the ability of the patient to comfortably wear an orthosis diminishes owing to pressure points against the orthotic device. The use of a covering such as Plastazote, which will conform to the medial bony prominence, may be of

benefit to these patients. Along with the orthotic device, the patient should be given a rocker-bottom–type shoe sole, which will allow him to roll over the foot, thereby decreasing some of the stress in the affected area.

Over a period of time, if the deformity progresses, manifested by severe abduction of the forefoot with loss of the longitudinal arch and a large medial bony prominence, surgical intervention should be considered. Surgery consists of stabilization of the involved tarsometatarsal joints, with the first joint being most frequently involved, followed by joints in sequence laterally across the foot. Rarely does the process extend to the fourth and fifth metatarsocuboid joints in primary osteoarthritis. When surgical stabilization is performed, the abduction deformity of the mid-foot should be corrected at the same time. The sites of arthrodesis need to be stabilized with some type of internal fixation, whether it be a staple, screw, or threaded pins. In general, primary bone grafting of these joints is not necessary to obtain a satisfactory fusion; however, if they are being fused in situ, small pieces of bone may be inserted across the joint to effect a satisfactory fusion.

It has been my experience that once the joint deteriorates to the point that a progressive abduction deformity begins, it will continue to progress, resulting in a mid-foot deformity and a painful medial longitudinal arch. As noted previously, as this occurs, conservative management becomes progressively less effective because of pressure points that develop along the medial aspect of the foot, making the use of an orthosis more uncomfortable. Once the patient is caught up in this cycle of progressive deformity and inability to adequately provide support to the mid-foot region with an orthotic device, his ambulatory capacity diminishes to the point that he is eventually housebound. Unfortunately, in some patients, the circulatory status of the foot is poor, so that surgical intervention cannot be performed safely, resulting in a very difficult situation for everyone involved.

THE METATARSOPHALANGEAL JOINTS

Osteoarthritis of the metatarsophalangeal joints usually involves only the first metatarsophalangeal joint. Initially, the patient notes an aching feeling about the joint, usually associated with a certain degree of synovitis and increased warmth. The joint itself progressively enlarges, making usual footwear more

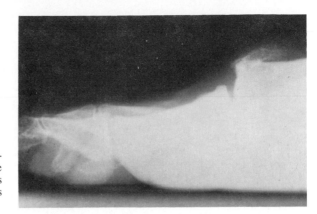

Figure 23–14. Roentgenogram of the metatarsophalangeal joint of the great toe involved with degenerative arthritis producing dorsal spurring. This condition results in a hallux ridigus, because the dorsal spurring blocks normal dorsiflexion of the proximal phalanx.

and more uncomfortable (Fig. 23–14). As this process continues, there is progressive enlargement of the metatarsophalangeal joint region, and range of motion of the joint, particularly dorsiflexion, decreases. These patients usually complain of an inability to walk over their forefoot because of the pain in the area of the dorsal aspect of the metatarsophalangeal joint. Women will also note an inability to comfortably wear high-heeled shoes, again because of pain in the dorsal aspect of the joint.

Although this is an uncomfortable condition for the patient, the ambulatory capacity is not as limited as that with osteoarthritic problems located more proximally in the foot. At times, patients walk with their foot in an increased angle of external rotation to enable them to roll over the medial side of the metatarsophalangeal joint rather than passing directly over the joint, which would cause an increased degree of discomfort.

Physical examination demonstrates a generally thickened metatarsophalangeal joint that is not infrequently associated with dorsal spurring. Occasionally, even a small ulceration can be seen over the area of the spur owing to tight shoes. The range of dorsiflexion is usually diminished considerably when compared with that of the opposite normal foot. Forcing dorsiflexion past the point that the patient can passively achieve usually causes him significant discomfort. The patient often notes that this is the type of discomfort that he experiences during walking.

The roentgenographic findings consist of narrowing of the joint space associated with proliferative new bone and varying degrees of dorsal beaking (Fig. 23–14).

The differential diagnosis of primary osteoarthritis of the first metatarsophalangeal joint includes traumatic arthritis secondary to previous trauma. At times, the findings can be

differentiated only by obtaining a history of trauma to the joint. Gout may cause pain in the first metatarsophalangeal joint but can usually be differentiated from osteoarthritis on the basis of the physical findings and characteristic roentgenographic changes. Occasionally, adolescents will develop osteochondritis dissecans of the first metatarsal head, which results in a symptom complex similar to that seen in hallux rigidus. Osteochondritis dissecans can occur without trauma and can be differentiated from primary osteoarthritis by the characteristic roentgenographic findings seen in osteochondritis (Fig. 23–15). It rarely represents a diagnostic problem with osteoarthritis owing to the younger age of the patients.

Treatment

The initial treatment of osteoarthritis of the first metatarsophalangeal joint consists of con-

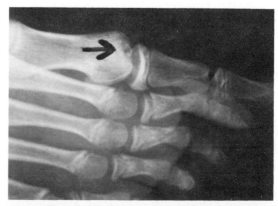

Figure 23–15. An osteochondritic defect in the metatarsal head (arrow) may result in symptoms that resemble hallux rigidus. Roentgenograms reveal changes associated with separation of bone and cartilage from the underlying bone to which it had been attached.

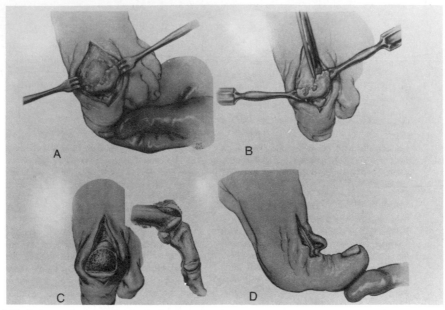

Figure 23–16. Technique of performing a cheilectomy for the treatment of hallux rigidus. *A,* Exposure of the head with the hallux plantar flexed, showing a proliferative bony change. *B,* Removal of excess bone with an osteotome. *C,* Smoothing and rounding of the raw bone surface. *D,* Dorsiflexion of the hallux with normal excursion. (From Mann RA, DuVries HL: Acquired nontraumatic deformities of the Foot. *In* Mann RA (ed.): DuVries' Surgery of the Foot. 4th ed. St. Louis, C. V. Mosby Company, 1978.)

servative management. Prescription of a shoe that has an adequate toe box to prevent excessive pressure is helpful (see Chapter 17). A shoe with a stiff sole or a rocker bottom will help diminish motion at the metatarsophalangeal joint and will decrease joint pain. If the symptoms persist or increase after an adequate trial of conservative management, surgical intervention for this problem may be indicated.

The surgical approach to osteoarthritis of the first metatarsophalangeal joint revolves around four basic procedures. They will be discussed in the order of my personal preference for the procedure. A cheilectomy consists of removing the excessive bone from around the metatarsal head.[5, 6] This removes the impingement to dorsiflexion and has resulted in a satisfactory clinical response in approximately 80% of patients (Fig. 23–16). The patient will usually regain about 40% to 50% of dorsiflexion, which is a sufficient amount to permit ambulation with few or no clinical complaints. The procedure has the advantage that, if necessary, another surgical procedure can be performed if the cheilectomy fails.

My second choice for surgical intervention is an arthrodesis of the first metatarsophalangeal joint. This will assure the patient of a painless joint, but the motion of the joint is lost. From a functional standpoint, this usually does not present a significant handicap to the patient; it is often the treatment of choice if the patient is involved in heavy manual labor. When performing an arthrodesis, the position of the metatarsophalangeal joint should be approximately 15 to 25 degrees of dorsiflexion and approximately 10 degrees of valgus, using the first metatarsal shaft as the reference point. Approximately 30% of patients who have an arthrodesis of the first metatarsophalangeal joint will develop some roentgenographic evidence of degenerative change in the interphalangeal joint, probably secondary to increased stress; this rarely becomes clinically symptomatic. Functionally, these patients can often resume essentially full activities, except for long-distance jogging. At times, however, it is difficult for them to squat because of their inability to dorsiflex the metatarsophalangeal joint.

The third procedure that can be considered is placing a Silastic spacer into the base of the proximal phalanx as well as performing a cheilectomy of the metatarsal head in order to permit adequate dorsiflexion. This procedure may give a satisfactory clinical result, but rarely one that is sufficiently superior to the cheilectomy alone. The problems associated with a prosthesis are a certain degree of soft tissue reaction to the foreign material, which is seen in a select group of patients; a resultant cock-up deformity of the metatarsophalangeal joint due to lack of function of the intrinsic muscles that stabilize the proximal phalanx; and, occasionally, material failure of the prosthesis. In the case of a failure, an arthrodesis may be used to salvage the joint, which results in a shortened but functional great toe.

The fourth and least recommended procedure is the Keller procedure. This is a resection of the proximal third of the proximal phalanx associated with removal of the dorsal spurs. Although this operation provides the patient with a painless first metatarsophalangeal joint, the loss of stability of the joint as a result of the procedure may result in a transfer of pressure to the second metatarsal. The great toe may also develop a cock-up deformity due to the loss of the insertion of the intrinsic muscles into the proximal phalanx. This procedure can be salvaged by performing an arthrodesis, but again, it results in a shortened great toe. Although not my procedure of choice for an active individual, the Keller procedure will give a satisfactory result in a person who is a nondemanding, basically housebound ambulator, because it does relieve the pain associated with the arthritic joint.

The overall prognosis for untreated osteoarthritis of the metatarsophalangeal joint must be guarded, because once the condition begins, it is usually progressive. Unless spontaneous fusion occurs, the joint will become progressively symptomatic. This may result not only in pain but also in sufficient enlargement of the joint, so that it becomes difficult for the patient to obtain shoewear.

THE INTERPHALANGEAL JOINTS

Osteoarthritis of the interphalangeal joints of the toes is manifested by pain either within the proximal or distal interphalangeal joint of the lesser toes or within the interphalangeal joint of the great toe. As the process proceeds, a varying degree of deformity may occur, which is manifested as either a mallet toe or a hammer toe. This deformity may give the patient more clinical symptoms than the actual osteoarthritis of the joint per se. The pain is usually caused by pressure against the dorsal aspect of the proximal interphalangeal joint (hammer toe) or the tip of the toe when a deformity of the distal interphalangeal joint (mallet toe) exists. Because the toes are not really a weight-bearing structure per se, symptoms may not be too bothersome, provided the patient wears a shoe that has a toe box

sufficiently large to keep the pressure off of the involved sites.

In most cases, the diagnosis is not too difficult to make, because patients are usually able to localize the area of their main complaint. The physical findings will demonstrate either a generalized thickening of the involved joint or an actual deformity of either the proximal interphalangeal joint (hammer toe) or the distal interphalangeal joint (mallet toe). In general, these deformities are associated with a loss of motion of the involved joint. The roentgenographic findings will confirm the clinical findings in most cases.

In considering the differential diagnosis, some form of traumatic arthritis may be confused with primary osteoarthritis, but as a rule, the patient will have a positive memory of an injury to the foot. Other types of arthritides such as psoriatic arthritis, Reiter's syndrome, and rheumatoid arthritis may involve these joints (see Chapter 16), but in general, they will be accompanied by characteristic systemic manifestations.

Treatment

The management of deformities of the interphalangeal joints should be conservative. The use of a broad-toed shoe with a large toe box is essential to keep the stress off of the deformed toes. At times, the use of a sandal can be quite useful. The commonly stocked "extra-depth" shoe now places this type of shoewear within the financial reach of most patients.

Along with shoe modifications, various types of felt pads are available to relieve the stress on the involved joints. If this type of conservative management fails, surgical intervention should be considered.

The use of a DuVries-type arthroplasty, in which the distal portion of the proximal phalanx is excised for a hammer toe or the distal portion of the middle phalanx is excised for a mallet toe, provides the clinician with a relatively simple procedure that can be performed under local anesthesia in most outpatient settings.[5] The procedure involves removing an ellipse of skin over the dorsal aspect of the involved joint, releasing the collateral ligaments, and excising the distal portion of the involved bone just proximal to the condyles. This effectively decompresses the involved joint, although it may be necessary at times to cut the flexor digitorum longus tendon to the

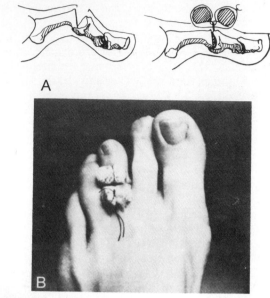

A

B

Figure 23–17. Technique of repair of a hammer toe. *A,* Resection of a wedge of tissue excising the dorsal callosity over the proximal interphalangeal joint and the condyles of the proximal phalanx. A Telfa bolster is made and held in place with a 3–0 silk suture. *B,* The suture is left in place for 1 week, after which it is removed and the toe is taped into proper alignment.

toe. A figure-of-eight suture incorporating a Telfa bolster is utilized to hold the toe in correct alignment until healing begins. The

bolster is removed after 7 days, and the toe is supported with a tape splint (Fig. 23–17). Other procedures may be utilized, such as an arthrodesis, but the previously described procedure is simple, and the results are uniformly good.

The overall prognosis for untreated osteoarthritis of the interphalangeal joints is guarded, because once the deformity begins, it will usually become progressively more severe. As noted earlier, however, it does not involve a weight-bearing structure per se and is certainly not as disabling as some of the other previously mentioned conditions involving the foot and ankle.

References

1. Jones FW: Structure and Function as Seen in the Foot. Baltimore, Williams and Wilkins, 1944.
2. Wright DG, Desai ME, Henderson BS: Action of the subtalar and ankle-joint complex during the stance phase of walking. J Bone Joint Surg 46A:361–382, 1964.
3. Elftman H: The transverse tarsal joint and its control. Clin Orthop 16:41–46, 1960.
4. Hicks HJ: The mechanics of the foot. II. The plantar aponeurosis and the arch. J Anat 88:25, 1954.
5. DuVries HL: Surgery of the Foot. 1st ed. St. Louis, C.V. Mosby, 1959.
6. Mann RA, Coughlin M, DuVries HL: Hallux rigidus. Clin Orthop 142:57, 1979.

24

Osteoarthritis of the Knee

Donald B. Kettelkamp, M.D.
Robert A. Colyer, M.D.

Osteoarthritis or degenerative arthritis of the knee is third in frequency behind that of the spine and hip. Although osteoarthritis of the knee can severely limit the patient's activity, it is better tolerated than osteoarthritis of the hip, primarily because the hip is usually painful at rest, whereas the knee is usually not. Conversely, osteoarthritis of the knee is less satisfactory to treat than osteoarthritis of the hip since the advent of the total hip arthroplasty.

In this chapter, the pathomechanics, clinical presentation, and the nonoperative and operative options available to the physician in the treatment of osteoarthritis of the knee will be discussed.

BIOMECHANICS OF OSTEOARTHRITIS OF THE KNEE

Earlier in this text, the ultrastructural, biochemical, and histologic changes of osteoarthritis were presented. Of all the joints, the knee best illustrates the biomechanical contribution to osteoarthritis and its progression. The primary concept involved at the knee is that of increased stress (force per unit area) and the response of the musculoskeletal system to this stress. An understanding of this concept is imperative in understanding osteoarthritis of the knee and its management.

In most patients with osteoarthritis of the knee, there is no specific known underlying reason for the development of osteoarthritis and the resulting deformity. Obesity and rickets and other growth abnormalities in childhood, including tibial torsion, have variously been implicated in the development of osteoarthritis, but there are not adequate long-term data to substantiate their contribution. Conversely, some preceding problems eventuate in predictable osteoarthritis of the knee. These include knee injury with meniscal tears, meniscectomy, instability secondary to ligamentous disruption, irregularity of the articular surface secondary to tibial plateau and distal femoral fractures, and angular deformity following fractures of the femoral or tibial shaft. All of these produce increased articular surface stress.

When a patient with a normally aligned lower extremity stands on both legs, the line of weight-bearing force goes from the center of the femoral head through the center of the knee and through the center of the ankle.[1] In a patient with genu varum (bowleg deformity), the weight-bearing line falls through the medial side of the knee or medial to the knee. In genu valgum (knock-knee deformity), the weight-bearing line falls through the lateral tibial plateau or lateral to the knee. During normal walking, a force of about three times body weight is transmitted through the knee.[2] The largest portion of this load is borne on the medial side of the knee; however, both plateaus do transmit force.[3] The magnitudes of force are not identical throughout the weight-bearing part of gait on both plateaus.[4] Other activities, such as going up and down stairs, increase the force transmitted through the knee to approximately four to five times body weight.[2]

Loss of the medial meniscus decreases the contact area between the femur and the tibia by approximately 50%.[5, 6] Although the exact percentage of force transmitted by the menisci is not accurately known, the remaining articular surface must transmit all the load after meniscectomy, thus increasing the stress during activity.[7] As a consequence, approximately 85% of patients who have had meniscectomy will show roentgenographic evidence of some degree of osteoarthritis over a long period of time.[8, 9]

Flexion deformity of the knee from whatever cause also increases the force per unit area because the largest area of contact between the tibia, menisci, and femur occurs with the knee in full extension and decreases with flexion.[1, 4, 6, 10] Thus, a fixed flexion deformity results in loads being carried across a smaller surface. This is further compounded by the increased muscle action required by the quadriceps to maintain knee stability in a flexed position (force magnitude increased).

Fracture of the tibial plateau may increase the stress by two modes of action. The first is the initial disruption of the articular cartilage with irregularities of the articular surface, thus creating points of increased stress. The second is the production of either a varus or a valgus deformity if the plateau cannot be reduced and held in a normal anatomic position.

Malunited fractures of the tibial or femoral shaft act in a somewhat different manner. Here, the result of the malalignment is to shift the weight-bearing line to the medial or lateral side of the knee, thus creating an overload on an otherwise normal joint.[1, 3] Over a long period of time, this may result in osteoarthritis of the loaded compartment.

Once an angular deformity is present, one compartment of the knee bears less weight and may eventually bear no weight at all. This means that in varus deformity, all of the load is passing through the medial side of the knee. Because of the ligamentous stays on the lateral side of the knee, the actual force increment is greater than if no deformity existed. Kettelkamp and Chao[3] and Maquet[1] have shown that forces equal to or greater than body weight may occur in one knee with genu varum with the patient standing on both legs. This alteration toward increased loads would be accentuated during the single-limb support phase of gait.

Although the preceding statements would imply that degenerative genu varum is an unremittingly progressive disease, this is not always true for a given patient. Miller and associates[11] studied a group of 48 patients with degenerative genu varum over an average of 6.5 years, with a range of 5 to 11 years. During that period, they found that roentgenographic evidence of progression of osteoarthritis occurred only in 42% of the subjects. Statistical analysis would indicate that progression occurs somewhere between 35% and 65% of the time. Thus, although osteoarthritis may be a steadily progressive disease over extremely long periods of time, it is not predictably progressive for a given patient over a relatively short time interval. Several mechanical factors may enter into this situation. Certainly, one of the most important is the patient's activity level. As a patient's knee becomes more symptomatic, he tends to be less active, thus submitting the joint to decreasing overall stress. Furthermore, adaptive mechanisms in avoiding stairs, using the hands to rise from sitting, using a cane, and avoiding uneven ground may all contribute to delaying the progression of osteoarthritis.

Another biomechanical concept that must be understood is that of mechanical and anatomical axes of the knee (Fig. 24–1). The anatomical axis of the knee is the angle made by the intersection of a line from the center of the knee up the center of the shaft of the femur and a line from the center of the knee down the shaft of the tibia. This angle does not take into account malunions or other abnormalities in the proximal femur, femoral shaft, tibial shaft, foot, or ankle. The mechanical axis is the angle formed by the intersection of a line from the center of the femoral head to the center of the distal femur and a line through the center of the ankle through the center of the proximal tibia. Normally, this angle is 0 degrees. The mechanical axis does take into account abnormalities in the femoral shaft, femoral head, tibial shaft, and ankle. Thus, the mechanical angle must be used in planning any type of reconstructive procedure for osteoarthritis of the knee.

HISTORY AND SYMPTOMS

Pain, usually with activity, is virtually always a presenting complaint of a patient with osteoarthritis of the knee. Associated but less troublesome complaints include stiffness in the morning or after sitting for periods of time and a stiffness that classically tends to improve with activity and then return later in the day.

The history obtained from the patient is helpful in determining the specific problem and the subsequent mode of therapy. The most important item in the history is pain with

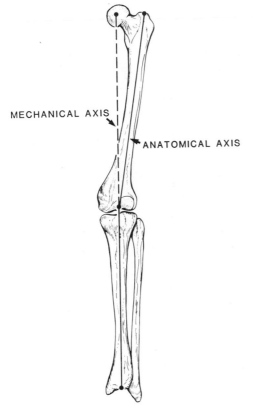

LOWER EXTREMITY
MECHANICAL AXIS
VERSUS
ANATOMICAL AXIS

MECHANICAL AXIS

ANATOMICAL AXIS

Figure 24–1. Lower extremity mechanical axis versus anatomical axis.

activity. The physician needs to know if the patient has pain with all weight bearing, the location of the pain, the distance the patient can walk before the pain becomes limiting, if the patient has pain ascending or descending stairs or sitting down on and rising from a chair, and if rest pain is present. It is important to know the patient's occupation and the relationship of pain to that occupation. Pain that will wake the patient after he has gone to sleep occurs less frequently and usually is not particularly troublesome. Pain may occasionally rouse the sleeping patient when he turns.

Some patients' osteoarthritis will be asymptomatic or virtually so until they have a specific injury, frequently a minor one, or an increase in activity. History of locking, catching, and joint effusion may indicate internal derangement in addition to osteoarthritis. History of an old injury or previous surgery may be useful in determining the initiating cause of the osteoarthritis. Many patients will relate a history

of intermittent difficulty with the knee over a period of years 'that has gradually become worse over the past year or so. They will also sometimes give a history of noting increasing bowing or knock-knee deformity.

Past history of the medications used for the knee, previous exercise programs, and the use of crutches, canes, or other forms of external support should also be obtained. It is important to obtain a history referable to injuries and pain in other areas of both lower extremities, including the hips and feet, and other general medical problems.

CLINICAL EXAMINATION

The knee has one synovial cavity but three articular surfaces (compartments)—patellofemoral, medial femorotibial, and lateral femorotibial. Physical examination of the knee is directed toward demonstrating the location and degree of articular cartilage degeneration.

Gross visual leg alignment is noted with the patient standing. Genu varum (bowleg deformity) or genu valgum (knock-knee deformity) points to a specific pathologic area in the knee joint. Walking with the leg exposed may reveal limping, lateral joint thrust, a shortened stride, and a fixed flexion deformity.

The range of knee motion is measured for future reference. Motion limited by pain should be differentiated from mechanical blocks to motion.

The patellofemoral joint is examined statically and dynamically. The Q angle,[12] measured with the knee extended and the quadriceps relaxed, is formed by the intersection of a line from the tibial tubercle through the center of the patella with a line down the center of the quadriceps and the center of the patella (see Chapter 12). The normal Q angle is 15 degrees or less. An increased Q angle may signify patellar subluxation, which predisposes to increased stress on the lateral patellar facet. A lateral tilt of the patella viewed from above with the knee flexed 90 degrees also indicates patellar subluxation.[13] The patella should ride symmetrically in the intercondylar groove of the femur with flexion and extension. A "J" sign occurs when the patella suddenly moves laterally near full extension and, again, indicates a tight lateral retinaculum and often a high-riding patella (patella alta). Compression of the patella into the femur may reproduce the patient's pain, confirming the location of the osteoarthritis.

Joint effusion, thickened synovium, popliteal cysts, and joint capsule tenderness are indicative of synovial inflammation. Osteophytes are commonly palpable along the joint line of either the tibia or the femur. Their size and location should be noted.

The knee should be stressed to determine if the malalignment in varus or valgus is passively correctible. The correction can be determined clinically and supplemented with a roentgenographic stress film, if necessary. At the point of maximal correction, a firm end point should be present, indicating intact collateral ligaments. The knee is checked for ligamentous stability, including both collateral ligaments and the anterior and posterior cruciate ligaments, and for rotatory instability. Most patients without previous ligamentous injury will have ligamentous stability.

Occasionally, loose bodies can be palpated in the suprapatellar pouch or about the femoral condyle. McMurray's test can be performed in some patients. In those with marked degrees of degenerative arthritis, this particular examination for torn menisci is of limited, if any, value and frequently is uncomfortable; hence, it may usually be omitted. The joint line should be palpated for local areas of tenderness. In degenerative genu varum or genu valgum, it is anticipated that the joint line on the concave side of the deformity will be tender. In the course of this palpation, any bulge along the joint line that might be indicative of a degenerative cyst of the meniscus should be sought.

Because the three major joints of the lower extremity are linked, problems in one can produce abnormal stress in all. Therefore, the knee examination should include examination of the hip, ankle, and foot. The whole pattern of lower-extremity motion should be considered. Determination of distal pulses, the status of the veins, and muscle strength and a neurologic examination should be routine.

ROENTGENOGRAPHIC EXAMINATION

The roentgenographic examination should include an anteroposterior weight-bearing view of the knee. If the mechanical axis is to be determined, a 6-foot standing roentgenogram extending from the femoral head to the ankle must be obtained. The anatomical angle can be measured on either film. From this view, the physician can determine the degree of joint space narrowing (Fig. 24–2), whether or not bone attrition is present, the compartments

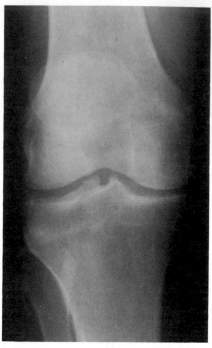

Figure 24–2. Standing anteroposterior roentgenogram demonstrating medial joint space narrowing, subchondral sclerosis of the medial tibial plateau, and a medial femoral osteophyte. This represents the classic roentgenographic appearance of moderate knee osteoarthritis.

that are involved with the osteoarthritis, tibial subluxation, osteonecrosis,[14] and, frequently, the presence of loose bodies (Fig. 24–3). The other roentgenographic views include the lateral, tunnel, and patellar views. We routinely use the Merchant[15] view for the patella. These additional views allow a better examination of the joint for loose bodies, and the patellar view provides information regarding patellofemoral arthritis and patellar subluxation. Stress views are of value in determining the status of the joint space on the convex side. For example, in a knee with a varus deformity, an anteroposterior film is taken with the knee subjected to valgus stress. This view determines the passive correctibility of the joint as well as whether or not the lateral joint space is maintained.

Other diagnostic examinations are sometimes indicated. An arthrogram may be helpful in determining the presence of a meniscal tear and occasionally loose bodies in early, relatively mild degenerative arthritis. Arthroscopy may be of value under similar circumstances and may also ascertain the status of the lateral articular cartilage in genu varum or that of the medial articular cartilage in genu valgum when the stress views are inconclusive.

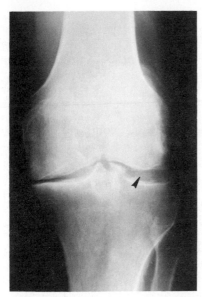

Figure 24–3. Standing anteroposterior roentgenogram demonstrating moderate medial compartment osteoarthritis and a large lateral loose osteocartilaginous body (arrow).

TREATMENT

The treatment of osteoarthritis of the knee varies, depending on the severity of symptoms, the structural abnormalities present, the patient's age, and concomitant medical problems.

Nonoperative Management

Nonoperative management is most suitable for those patients with more than half of the articular joint space present, as demonstrated by the weight-bearing roentgenograms. As noted earlier, osteoarthritis does not always run an unremitting course, and not infrequently, there are periods when symptoms are relatively minor. Some patients who have complete loss of articular cartilage on one half of the knee, with associated bone attrition, are still functioning at a level satisfactory to them without sufficient symptoms to warrant operative intervention. Because of this, each patient must be carefully assessed on an individual basis. Nonoperative management consists of nonsteroidal anti-inflammatory medications, exercises, and rest of the part during the acute episode. Many nonsteroidal anti-inflammatory medications are available to the physician (see Chapter 18). Patients' responses to these medications vary. Usually, if the patient is able to

take salicylates, these are the initial anti-inflammatory agents used. Systemic steroids are not indicated in osteoarthritis. Intra-articular injection of steroids may aid in resolving acute synovial inflammation associated with osteoarthritis; however, this medication changes the biochemical characteristics of the articular cartilage and may lead to additional complications and degenerative changes.

Isometric exercises are used to increase quadriceps and hamstring strength, thus permitting the patient to use muscle control to avoid minor translatory shifts at the knee and to distribute weight bearing better (see Chapter 17). The isometric progressive quadriceps exercises are done with the patient in the supine position with the opposite knee and hip flexed and the foot resting on the bed, floor, or table. The leg to be exercised is in full extension; the quadriceps muscle is tightened; the leg is raised 20 degrees and held for 5 seconds; the leg is then lowered to the table, the muscle is relaxed, and the exercise is repeated. Twenty repetitions are performed twice a day; the patient is permitted to add ankle weights at increments of approximately 1 pound as he becomes able to do 20 repetitions twice a day with ease. Usually, by the time the patient can lift 8 to 10 pounds doing 20 repetitions twice a day, he has regained sufficient quadriceps strength for limited daily activities. Although this exercise is particularly applicable to the arthritic knee because it permits the patient to generate increasing quadriceps tension and yet retain tibiofemoral and patellofemoral forces at a minimum, it does put an additional load on the hip and may aggravate low-back symptoms. Those patients who have osteoarthritis of the hip or symptomatic degenerative changes in the lumbar spine with or without nerve root irritation must modify this exercise. This can be done by supporting the distal thigh so that the knee is flexed about 20 degrees; the exercise is then done through the terminal 20 degrees of extension. This method increases the forces transmitted across the articular surfaces of the knee but markedly decreases the forces at both the hip and the low back. An alternative method is for the patient to do the exercise sitting forward in a chair so that the knee is in an extended position with the hip somewhat flexed; the leg elevation is done only an inch or two from the floor.

The isometric progressive resistance hamstring exercises are done with the patient in the prone position. In this position, the patient flexes the knee 20 degrees, leaving the thigh resting on the table or bed. A program similar to that for the quadriceps, consisting of 20 repetitions of the exercise, with holding for 5 seconds, is used. Again, weights are added at 1-pound increments as the exercises become easy for the patient to perform.

The purpose of both of these exercises is to regain muscle strength while producing minimal transarticular forces. A number of other variations of these exercises are suitable as long as the principle of maintaining low transarticular forces is followed.

Rest of the osteoarthritic knee is indicated when the patient has had an acute flare, frequently secondary to minor trauma or overuse, or has a joint effusion. Depending on the severity of the symptoms, this may require bed rest and immobilization of the knee on a temporary basis. The temporary use of crutches with weight bearing as tolerated is useful until the knee is less painful, the effusion is subsiding, and the patient has had the opportunity to regain muscle strength.

Many patients with osteoarthritis of the knee are overweight or frankly obese. Whether this is an etiologic factor in the development of osteoarthritis or a secondary factor due to reduced activity is not important in treatment. The increased stress on the knee due to the extra weight is the main point. Biomechanically, when bearing weight, the knee receives a compressive force approximately three times body weight. Certain activities can increase the forces even more. Therefore, 1 kg of weight reduction can lead to a joint force reduction of approximately 3 kg. The patient must understand that increased weight leads to increased stress, which is causing the knee pain. A rational weight reduction program must be accomplished over time, as short-term fad diets usually are not long-lasting. The positive feedback of pain reduction is a very powerful incentive for weight loss in these patients.

Flexion deformity is frequently associated with degenerative arthritis of the knee. As noted earlier, a flexion deformity decreases the articular surface contact at the knee, while at the same time requiring increased quadriceps force to stabilize the joint. The net result is increased stress across the knee. The forces involved in flexion deformity markedly increase after 20 to 30 degrees of flexion. Flexion deformity may occur secondary to contracture of the posterior capsule or to intra-articular changes. Frequently, in degenerative genu varum with associated bone attrition, there is

a relative anterior ridge on the tibia, with osteophytes that effectively block extension. It is important to determine whether the flexion deformity is secondary to an internal block or to posterior capsular contracture. Only surgery can improve a flexion deformity secondary to an intra-articular block. Nonoperative management of a capsular contracture should be used initially. Mild degrees of flexion deformity of less than 20 degrees can often be improved by quadriceps setting exercises and passive stretching of the posterior capsule under the patient's control. With less than 20 degrees of contracture, corrective casts are seldom of much benefit. Five to 10 degrees of deformity are acceptable, as the forces generated by this minimal degree of flexion deformity are small and the degree of deformity is well within the normal knee flexion that occurs during the mid-stance phase of walking. Fifteen degrees is probably the maximal acceptable amount and is near the upper limits of normal knee flexion during the stance phase of gait. If the flexion deformity exceeds this, if there is no intra-articular block to extension, and if the deformity is not improved by nonoperative methods, surgical release of the posterior capsule may need to be considered.

Operative Management

The operative procedures that may be applicable to osteoarthritis of the knee include limited joint debridement, procedures for patellofemoral arthritis, proximal tibial or distal femoral osteotomy, unicompartmental joint replacement, total knee arthroplasty, and arthrodesis. Each procedure will be presented separately.

It must be understood throughout the presentation of operative procedures that the procedure being discussed is appropriate for the pathologic condition in the specific knee under consideration and that the patient's symptoms and limitations related to the arthritic knee are of sufficient severity to warrant the risks and convalescence associated with the operative procedure (see Chapter 20).

Debridement

At present, joint debridement in the osteoarthritic knee is limited to intra-articular mechanical derangement that is the primary cause of symptoms in a specific knee. Joint debridement with articular surface drilling of the type described by Magnuson[16] and Pridie[17] has little place in the current management of osteoarthritis of the knee. Abrasion arthroplasty using an arthroscopic approach may have merit, but well-controlled, long-term studies are needed to better define its ultimate role in the treatment of cartilage erosions.

Usually, the knee considered for joint debridement will have more than half of the normal joint space remaining. The situations for which debridement would be considered include the removal of osteocartilaginous loose bodies, the excision of torn menisci, and, occasionally, the removal of osteophytes, either those that are blocking extension or marginal osteophytes on the femur that produce retinacular and patellofemoral symptoms.

Loose bodies characteristically produce intermittent catching episodes or transient locking episodes. Effusion may follow such episodes but frequently does not. Unlike locking secondary to a torn meniscus, the locking secondary to loose bodies can usually be relieved by positional changes or minimal flexion extension motions at the knee. Occasionally, loose bodies can be palpated in the suprapatellar pouch by the patient and the examining physician. Loose bodies are the result of flaked-off articular cartilage that continues to grow, nourished by synovial fluid, and that becomes radiopaque with the deposition of calcium salts. These loose bodies may become attached to the synovium and may obtain a blood supply, with subsequent ossification of the calcified cartilage. In both of these circumstances, loose bodies can be visualized on a standard roentgenogram. Occasionally, there will be symptomatic loose bodies that are still cartilaginous. Arthrography and arthroscopy may be of aid in diagnosing these cartilaginous loose bodies.

Removal of the loose bodies may be performed with either arthroscopic surgery or open arthrotomy, depending on the size, location, and number and whether additional operative procedures are also necessary.

Lesions of the meniscus can occur in the osteoarthritic knee and, in some circumstances, may lead to or aggravate the progression of the osteoarthritis. Usually, in degenerative genu varum or valgum, the meniscus on the concave side is gradually abraded away. Meniscectomy is not indicated in this situation. In early degenerative arthritis, however, menisci may be torn and may present symptoms of internal derangement with intermittent effusion, locking, or catching. A high index of suspicion is necessary to suggest the diagnosis

of a symptomatic torn meniscus in the degenerative knee. Joint line tenderness, a usual finding with a common meniscal tear, is generally also present in degenerative arthritis and, as a result, loses its value as a diagnostic sign. Arthroscopy and arthrography are of considerable aid in establishing the diagnosis of a significant meniscal tear. When a symptomatic longitudinal or flap tear is present, an appropriate partial meniscectomy should be performed. Rarely, a degenerative cyst of the meniscus will be found in a knee that shows evidence of early osteoarthritis. The clinical findings for degenerative cysts are a palpable tender bulge that may vary in size and symptoms with activity. An arthrogram or arthroscopy will be normal unless there is a concomitant tear of the meniscus, which occurs not infrequently. Meniscectomy is the usual treatment for this lesion. Our limited experience with excision of the cyst alone when involvement of the meniscus is not marked and when a tear is not present has not been very satisfactory.

Osteophytes rarely produce sufficient symptoms to justify excision as a primary procedure. On rare occasions, however, large femoral osteophytes will produce sufficient irritation of the synovium to warrant excision when the knee demonstrates relatively little other evidence of tibiofemoral arthritis. Similarly, osteophytes are occasionally seen that pinch the meniscus sufficiently to produce joint line pain and alter the normal mobility of the meniscus. The symptoms may be relieved by osteophyte excision. The raw bed left following osteophyte removal should be covered with bone wax, which tends to decrease the recurrence of the osteophytes.

Osteotomy

Osteotomy of the proximal tibia or, in the knee with a valgus deformity, of the distal femur to realign the extremity and to decrease the stress on a single degenerative compartment has proved to be a useful procedure in the relatively young patient, under age 70, who is active and has unicompartmental osteoarthritis. As a general rule, the patient who is a candidate for osteotomy will have pain with all weight bearing and will be restricted to walking three blocks or less before needing to rest because of discomfort. Night pain is usually absent. Patients with somewhat less restriction of activity (and in an actively working age group) may be candidates for osteotomy, assuming the clinical and roentgenographic findings indicate that the knee is suitable for this procedure.

Ideally, the physical examination would show a varus deformity with good ligamentous stability, no flexion deformity, and active flexion to greater than 100 degrees. Marked ligamentous instability, particularly posterior cruciate instability, flexion deformity of greater than 15 to 20 degrees,[1] and maximal flexion of less than 60 to 70 degrees would militate against proximal tibial osteotomy on the basis of clinical findings. Distal pulses should be present, and the arterial supply to the extremity should be good. Varicose veins and previous phlebitis are not absolute contraindications to osteotomy; however, they greatly increase the risk of phlebitic complications. Previous phlebitis would dictate the use of an anticoagulant postoperatively, but both heparin and warfarin (Coumadin) delay healing of the osteotomy,[18] thus making these patients less satisfactory surgical candidates.

Roentgenographic examination ideally shows degenerative genu varum with loss of the medial joint space. A valgus stress film would demonstrate a good lateral articular surface, and a patellar or Merchant's view would show normal patellofemoral articular surface. Frequently, however, the patellar or Merchant's view shows some evidence of osteoarthritis. Small lateral osteophytes, particularly on the femur, may be present on the lateral side. The stress films, however, still should demonstrate a good lateral joint space.

The reverse findings would be true in a knee with a valgus deformity. Particular attention should be paid to the degree of opening on the medial side, as some knees with valgus deformity will gradually stretch the medial collateral ligament, and if this is excessive, the knee may be unstable after osteotomy. The knee with a valgus deformity is much more likely to show a laterally subluxated patella with patellofemoral arthritis along the lateral facet. This must be corrected at the time of osteotomy if osteotomy is performed for this deformity.

Two other findings on the anteroposterior weight-bearing view must be noted. Frequently, in long-standing degenerative genu varum, there is loss not only of the articular joint space but also of bone from the proximal medial tibia. If the bone loss exceeds 5 mm, one must be certain that the knee is geometrically capable of bearing weight on both plateaus after the osteotomy.[19] The second ab-

normality to be noted is lateral tibial subluxation. In some knees, the tibia will be subluxated laterally, so that the lateral femoral condyle is bearing weight against the intercondylar notch, and even under stress, the tibia does not undergo sufficient correction to permit weight bearing on a good articular surface after osteotomy.[19]

A long, weight-bearing roentgenogram that shows the extremity from the center of the femoral head to the center of the ankle is obtained to determine the mechanical axis and, hence, the amount of correction required (Fig. 24–4). The desired correction varies in the literature. Virtually all authors agree, however, that the correction should produce an anatomic angle of 5 to 12 degrees of valgus. The recommendations of Maquet and associates[10] are correction of a varus deformity to

CORRECTION OF VARUS DEFORMITY WITH
HIGH TIBIAL OSTEOTOMY

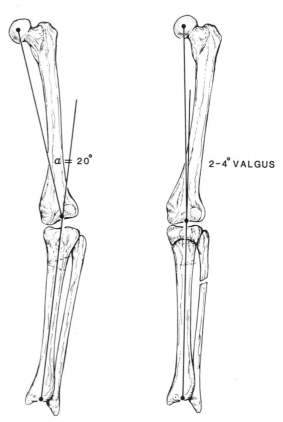

Figure 24–4. High tibial dome osteotomy to correct a 20-degree varus mechanical axis deformity to a 2- to 4-degree valgus mechanical axis position.

a mechanical angle of 2 to 4 degrees of valgus. This roughly equates to 8 to 10 degrees of anatomic valgus. Chao[20] has found that the difference between the anatomic angle and the mechanical angle is 5 degrees ±1 degree. In a valgus deformity, the desired correction is to a mechanical angle of 1 to 3 degrees of varus (Fig. 24–5). This produces a relative varus position based on the normal anatomic position.

There are two basic surgical techniques for correction of a degenerative genu varum. The most widely used is a closing wedge osteotomy (Fig. 24–6).[21–23] In this procedure, a wedge of bone with the base located laterally and the apex located medially is removed from the tibia just proximal to the insertion of the patellar tendon. The fibula may be managed by hollowing the fibular head so that it will collapse with closure of the wedge, with resec-

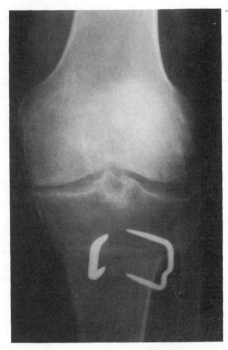

Figure 24–6. Post-valgus closing wedge high tibial osteotomy for medial compartment osteoarthritis and genu varum. The osteotomy is stabilized with two staples.

tion of the fibular head and reattachment of the collateral ligament and biceps tendon, or with osteotomy of the fibula. The wedge is fixed with staples and supported with a cylinder or a long leg cast. Weight bearing is permitted as tolerated by the patient, and the cast is usually required for 6 to 8 weeks. Up to 20 degrees of flexion deformity can be corrected with a closing wedge osteotomy. Although correction of flexion deformity in this manner will result in a shift of the force from the medial plateau toward the lateral plateau, it does not increase the articular surface area back to the amount found in normal extension. A closing wedge osteotomy is most applicable when 15 degrees of correction or less is required. Greater degrees of correction require a larger wedge resection with decreased bone contact for healing.

The second technique of proximal tibial osteotomy for degenerative genu varum is the barrel-vault osteotomy, described by Maquet (Fig. 24–7).[23a] In this technique, 0.5 inch of fibular shaft is removed. The osteotomy is a curved cut through the tibia, proximal to the tibial tubercle. Fixation is with skeletal pins and compression clamps. The distal tibia is moved 1 cm anteriorly, which decreases the patellofemoral joint force. This technique is particularly applicable to the patient with sig-

CORRECTION OF VALGUS DEFORMITY WITH DISTAL FEMORAL OSTEOTOMY

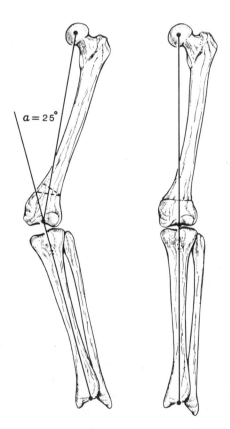

$a = 25°$

PREOPERATIVE   POSTOPERATIVE

Figure 24–5. Distal femoral varus osteotomy to correct a 25-degree valgus mehanical axis deformity to a near-neutral mechanical axis.

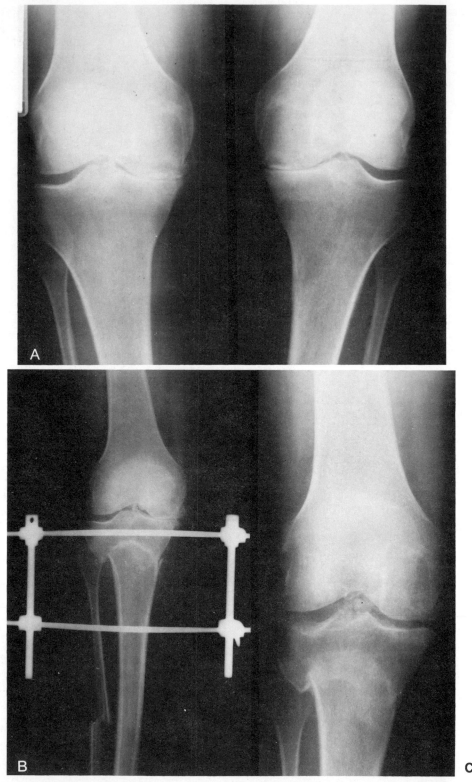

Figure 24–7. *A,* Preoperative standing anteroposterior roentgenogram demonstrating bilateral medial compartment osteoarthritis and genu varum, which is most severe on the right. *B,* Roentgenogram taken soon after high tibial dome osteotomy with fibular osteotomy. The osteotomy is stabilized with an external fixator. *C,* Standing anteroposterior roentgenogram taken approximately 1 year after osteotomy demonstrating an increase in the medial joint space.

nificant patellofemoral arthritis and when more than 15 degrees of correction is required, as the area of bone contact remains high. Flexion deformity cannot be corrected. Pins and compression clamps are used until there is sufficient bone healing, usually 8 weeks. All methods using compression fixation have approximately a 10% risk of pin track infection.[24] A cast is not used with this technique, so that knee flexion and extension can be started soon after surgery. Weight bearing as tolerated, using crutches or a walker, is permitted as soon as the patient is able. With both methods, external support is usually required for 2 to 4 months after removal of the cast or the compression clamps, until healing is complete and the patient has regained motion and muscle strength.

Degenerative genu valgum may be treated by proximal tibial osteotomy with either a closing wedge based medially or a barrel-vault osteotomy if the correction required is 10 degrees or less.[25] In a valgus deformity, correction in the proximal tibia should not produce an obliquity of the proximal articular surface that exceeds 10 degrees. If the required correction produces a joint obliquity of greater than 10 degrees, the osteotomy should be performed at the distal femur (see Fig. 24–5). The distal femoral osteotomy may be fixed internally, or a compression technique may be used.

The risks involved with osteotomy are the same regardless of the site and the technique. The risks include infection at the osteotomy site, infection of the pin tracks with the compression techniques, thrombophlebitis, pulmonary embolus, and peroneal palsy or anterior compartment syndrome.[24, 26] In addition, there is a small risk of nonunion,[27] and correction may be lost or, rarely, excessively increased during the healing process. Arterial damage to the distal leg has been reported.

Results. A satisfactory result (i.e., the patient can maintain his current activities with less discomfort or can increase his activities before discomfort occurs) can be anticipated in 80% of the knees when proximal tibial osteotomy is done for degenerative varum[10, 28] and in about 70% of the knees in which osteotomy, either femoral or tibial, is performed for degenerative genu valgum.[1, 24] The advantage of this procedure is that the patient may resume whatever activities are tolerated by the knee after healing and rehabilitation are complete. Furthermore, if the osteotomy eventually becomes unsatisfactory because of

degenerative changes in the initially unaffected compartment or for other reasons, salvage by total knee replacement has not been jeopardized. The most common cause of unsatisfactory results is undercorrection or loss of correction.[24] This may sometimes be improved by repeat osteotomy. Occasionally, a patient will continue to have symptoms caused by intra-articular pathology such as meniscal tears. Some knees seem to take a period of months to sort of "retrack," and for this reason, the knee that apparently has undergone a successful correction should not be judged a failure sooner than 1 year after osteotomy.

Osteotomy is the procedure of choice for a patient in a younger age group with unicompartmental degenerative arthritis who by desire or necessity must maintain a moderately high activity level on the knee.

Unicompartmental Replacement

Replacement of the involved side of a degenerative genu varum or valgum with tibial and femoral arthroplasty components has been used in unicompartmental arthritis (Fig. 24–8). The results reported for this procedure have been variable.[29–32] The primary problem has been loosening of the tibial component.[29] With longer follow-up, some patients have shown progressive degenerative changes on the unreplaced side of the joint.[29] Unicompartmental arthroplasty, however, is a procedure that may be considered in the elderly patient, particularly when the varus or valgus deformity is passively correctible.[31] On occasion, it may also be considered for a somewhat younger patient who has sufficient bone loss that a total joint replacement would be the only other alternative.

Correction of alignment is mandatory. For this reason, the procedure is most applicable to knees that are already passively correctible. If the procedure is to be used in a knee that is not passively correctible, soft tissue release of the medial collateral ligament and medial structures from the tibia for genu varum and of the iliotibial band and sometimes the lateral collateral ligament and popliteus tendon in genu valgum must be done before the bone cuts are made for insertion of the implant. The primary advantages of unicompartmental replacement are minimal blood loss, perhaps a slightly lower postoperative infection rate, and perhaps a somewhat more rapid convalescence. The operative procedure itself requires nearly as much time as a total joint replace-

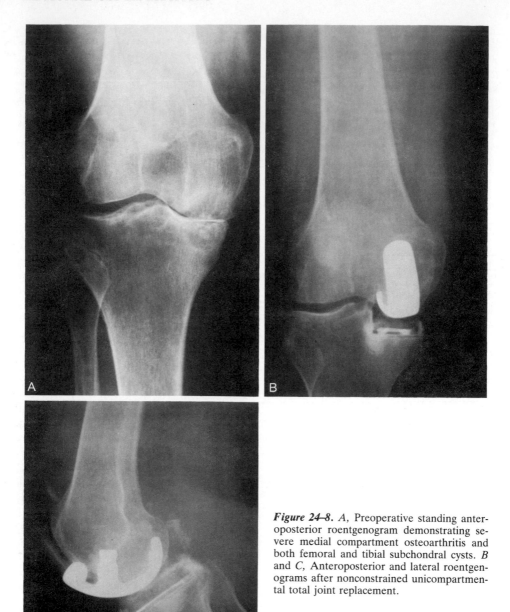

Figure 24–8. *A,* Preoperative standing anteroposterior roentgenogram demonstrating severe medial compartment osteoarthritis and both femoral and tibial subchondral cysts. *B* and *C,* Anteroposterior and lateral roentgenograms after nonconstrained unicompartmental total joint replacement.

ment, and the procedure does not replace or otherwise alter the patellofemoral joint. The primary complication with unicompartmental replacement has been loosening. This may necessitate replacing and recementing the parts, conversion to a total knee arthroplasty, or arthrodesis. Fortunately, conversion to a total knee arthroplasty is not technically difficult. At present, unicompartmental replace-

ment has a limited role in the treatment of osteoarthritis of the knee.

Total Knee Arthroplasty

The advent in 1971 and 1972 of total knee arthroplasty using high-density polyethylene and metal components conformed to the tibia and femur with polymethylmethacrylate represented a major advance in the treatment of the knee with severe osteoarthritis. The primary factors that limit the use of total knee arthroplasty in osteoarthritis are the lack of data on the longevity of the implants, particularly in relation to loosening at the bone-cement interface,[33] and the difficulty in salvage after infection.[34, 35] Total knee arthroplasty is the procedure of choice for osteoarthritis associated with severe deformity, whether it be varus, valgus, or flexion. Usually, these severe deformities are associated with significant bone loss and compound deformities, i.e., varus and flexion deformity with bone loss, and are not amenable to the lesser procedures of debridement, osteotomy, or unicompartmental replacement. A second primary indication is three-compartment osteoarthritis with loss of articular space from both the medial and lateral tibiofemoral compartments. A third primary indication, although one that is weaker than the first two, is the age of the patient. Total knee arthroplasty may be a primary procedure in patients 70 years of age or older because of the shorter convalescence, the expectation of a low loosening rate with the decreased activity of this age group (hence, the longevity of the implant will meet the longevity of the patient), and the better immediate results with total knee arthroplasty than with osteotomy. This procedure does impose activity limitations on a patient. The limitations are particularly referable to most sports, heavy work, prolonged walking on uneven ground, or other situations that produce high forces across the knee.

The primary contraindications to total knee arthroplasty are previous infection in the joint or the immediate surrounding bone; neurotrophic (Charcot) joints; lack of motor control of the extremity, as in paralysis secondary to poliomyelitis; and poor vascularity in the extremity. Known sites of infection such as open sores and infected toenails, bladder infections, and so on must be cleared before performing total knee replacement.

The potential complications associated with total knee arthroplasty are the same as for any other major knee surgery. These include infection, phlebitis, pulmonary embolus, peroneal nerve palsy, and risks associated with anesthesia, transfusion, and antibiotics. Of these, the primary complication, which carries a much worse prognosis than with other knee surgery, is infection. Infection in the presence of a total knee arthroplasty usually requires removal of the implant. Currently, with sensitive gram-positive organisms, there has been a limited experience with replacement of the implant after a course of intravenous antibiotics. The eventual outcome and efficacy of this procedure are yet to be fully realized. The other alternative for gram-positive and for all gram-negative infections is removal of the implant and arthrodesis, which is difficult to achieve. On occasion, above-knee amputations have been required to control infection after total knee arthroplasty.

Four fundamental mechanical types of artificial knee joints are available. The hemiarthroplasties previously mentioned may be used to resurface both the medial and lateral compartments of the knee. This type of implant is truly nonconstrained and depends on the collateral and cruciate ligaments and muscles for knee control. These implants are seldom used today because of the relatively high loosening rate of the tibial component.[36]

The second general type of implant is also frequently classed as nonconstrained and is a posterior cruciate–sparing implant. These implants have a single tibial component with a posterior central cut-out for the posterior cruciate ligament and a single metal femoral component and may be used with a polyethylene patellar button. Intact posterior cruciate and collateral ligaments are required.[37]

The third class of implant is semiconstrained (Fig. 24–9). This implant requires functioning collateral ligaments, but both cruciates are resected and the implant is designed with inherent stability in the anteroposterior direction.[38, 39] Many surgeons prefer this type as their primary implant. Others prefer to use a nonconstrained implant when the posterior cruciate ligament can be retained. At present, there are insufficient data to substantiate a preference for one approach versus the other.

The fourth and last type of implant is totally constrained. This implant has built-in constraints to prevent anterior and posterior shifting and to provide medial and lateral stability in the absence of collateral ligaments.[40-43] The loosening rate is highest with totally constrained implants. For that reason, this type of implant is utilized only when the status of the knee requires the use of an implant with the built-in constraints.

The results observed in multiple reports covering the variety of the implants in the aforementioned categories would indicate acceptable or good results in 85% to 95% of the patients.[37-39, 42] In reports with average follow-ups of 2 years or longer, the loosening rate varies from approximately 5% to 15%, with

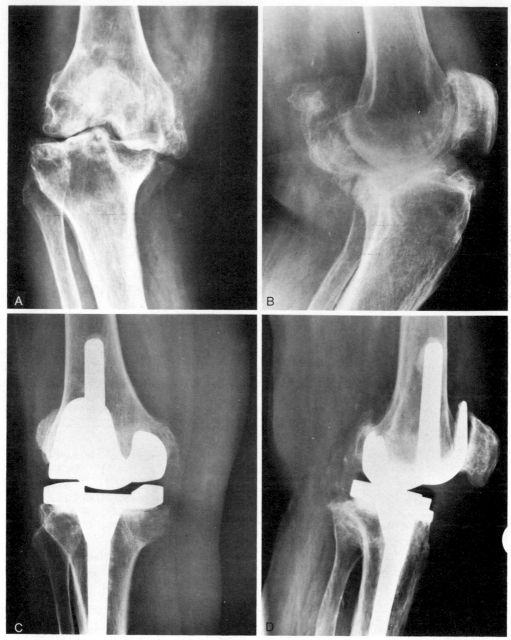

Figure 24–9. Preoperative anteroposterior *(A)* and lateral *(B)* roentgenograms demonstrating severe three-compartment osteoarthritis, genu varum, and bone loss in the medial tibial plateau. *C* and *D,* Roentgenograms taken after implantation of a semiconstrained total joint prosthesis demonstrating good correction of the varus deformity.

the higher loosening rates being in implants of earlier design.[38, 39, 41, 44] The primary question is what will happen to the loosening rate over a longer period of time. Follow-ups of 10 years or longer are not available with the current implants. Some reports indicate that most of the loosening will probably occur within the first 3 years after total knee arthroplasty. Recent investigations have sought alternative methods of fixing the implants to the bone, with early encouraging results (see Chapter 20).

Arthrodesis

Arthrodesis, or fusion, is rarely used for osteoarthritis of the knee. The primary indications for this procedure are a severely limiting osteoarthritis in a knee that has been the site of previous infection (Fig. 24–10), osteoarthritic changes in a Charcot joint, osteoarthritis that is symptomatic in a flail extremity, and severe post-traumatic degenerative arthritis in a young adult whose other lower-extremity joints are normal. The primary disadvantages of arthrodesis are the difficulty in sitting and getting into and out of cars and the additional forces it places on adjacent and contralateral joints.

Procedures for Osteoarthritis of the Patellofemoral Joint

The barrel-vault proximal tibial osteotomy for the patient who has unicompartmental tibiofemoral and patellofemoral arthritis has already been discussed (see Fig. 24–7). Occasionally, however, patients have primarily patellofemoral arthritis with good tibiofemoral articulations. Often, the underlying problem is patellar subluxation or recurrent dislocations.[45] The initial treatment of early patellofemoral arthritis is nonoperative.[46] Isometric quadriceps[47] and hamstring exercises,[48] anti-inflammatory medications, and alteration of activities to avoid those that involve use of the flexed

loaded knee will be sufficient treatment for many patients.

Operative procedures have been used for osteoarthritis of the patella or its earlier stage of chondromalacia with frayed, fibrillated articular cartilage. The older operations include shaving of the articular cartilage and spongiolization (removing the involved cartilage and decorticating the underlying bone so that new fibrocartilage can form).[17, 49] Both of these procedures have given unpredictable results and, hence, have relatively low usage. Arthroscopic shaving has some enthusiastic advocates. Early reports indicate frequent improvement of patients' symptoms. Whether this is from joint washout or primarily from debridement remains an unanswered question. We have, however, seen a number of patients in whom this method has been unsuccessful.

In the patient whose primary problem is patellar subluxation with narrowing of the patellofemoral joint on the lateral facet, a lateral retinacular release followed by quadriceps exercises may provide symptomatic relief for a period of time.[50, 51] Realignment of the extensor mechanism, assuming that there is reasonable articular cartilage remaining, may provide relief in the patient who has patellar subluxa-

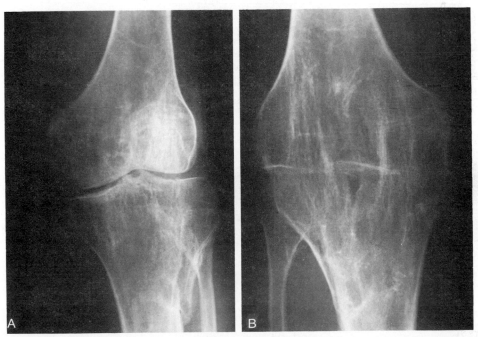

Figure 24–10. *A,* Standing anteroposterior roentgenogram of a relatively young patient several years after an intra-articular tibial fracture complicated by osteomyelitis. Moderate post-traumatic osteoarthritis was debilitating to the patient, and his history of infection precluded total joint implantation. *B,* Roentgenogram taken after arthrodesis of the knee, demonstrating solid union. The patient was able to return to physical employment.

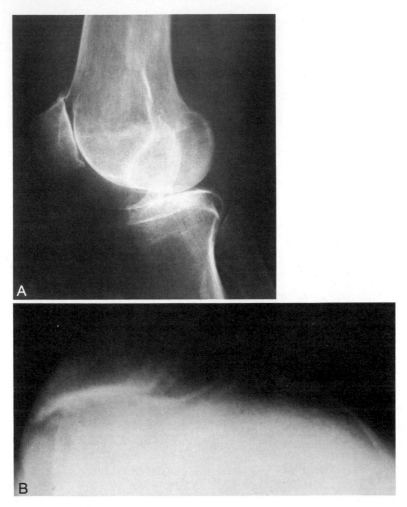

Figure 24–11. *A* and *B,* Lateral and tangential patellar roentgenograms demonstrating patellofemoral osteoarthritis and severe lateral patellar subluxation.

tion or dislocation.[12] Realignment may be a soft tissue proximal realignment, including the lateral release and medial reefing, or this may be combined with realignment of the patellar tendon insertion.[52]

Occasionally, a laterally subluxated patella will show a lateral overhang with primary arthritic involvement at the lateral femoral condylar ridge and the overhanging portion of the patella. Again, lateral release with resection of the patellar overhang may produce an improvement in symptoms.

Tibial tubercleplasty, as described by Maquet[1] and Ferguson,[53] is the most useful of the procedures for the patient who has significant joint space narrowing from patellofemoral arthritis (Fig. 24–11). This procedure consists of splitting the anterior tibial cortex, including the tibial tubercle, so that the tuber-

cle may be elevated 0.5 inch (Fig. 24–12). The elevation is maintained either with local bone from the area of Gerde's tubercle or with bone from the iliac crest. This procedure decreases the load on the patellofemoral joint, while maintaining the mechanical advantage of the extensor mechanism.

The end-stage procedure for severe patellofemoral arthritis is patellectomy. Kaufer,[54, 55] Sutton and associates,[56] and others[57] have demonstrated that loss of the patella decreases the effectiveness of the quadriceps and is frequently associated with knee discomfort, decreased knee flexion during the stance phase of gait, and difficulty in going up and down stairs. Even with these disadvantages, patellectomy can often relieve the symptoms related to severe patellofemoral arthritis sufficiently to permit the patient to return to an increased

ELEVATION OF TIBIAL TUBERCLE FOR
PATELLOFEMORAL OSTEOARTHRITIS

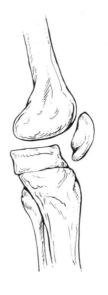 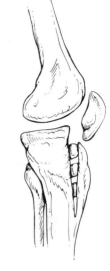

Figure 24–12. Elevation of the tibial tubercle for patellofemoral osteoarthitis.

ASSOCIATED WITH HIGH
TIBIAL OSTEOTOMY

TIBIAL TUBEROPLASTY
ALONE

activity level. Patellectomy remains a useful procedure to a considerably lesser degree than before the development of the tubercleplasty. If quadriceps weakness is a primary problem after patellectomy, the tibial tubercleplasty may be performed in the absence of a patella, thus restoring the mechanical advantage to the extensor mechanism and further lifting the retinacula from the medial and lateral ridges of the femoral condyle.

SUMMARY

The mechanical contributions to osteoarthritis are perhaps best demonstrated and most easily understood at the knee. Osteoarthritis of the knee is no longer always a disease process with which a patient must learn to live. No treatment, however, restores an osteoarthritic knee to normal status. Although osteoarthritis of the knee tends to be progressive, it is not unrelentingly and predictably so for any given knee. Nonoperative management, consisting of exercises, temporary protection, anti-inflammatory medications, and activity alteration, is particularly useful in those knees that still retain some articular cartilage. Local debridement, consisting of the removal of loose bodies, menisci, and, occasionally, osteo-

phytes, may be needed to supplement medical management in knees with early osteoarthritis. Relatively young patients with unicompartmental osteoarthritis may be able to return to increased activity by proximal tibial osteotomy. In the elderly patient with osteoarthritis, total knee arthroplasty and, in selected circumstances, unicompartmental replacement offer the opportunity for an improved life style. Arthrodesis remains a salvage procedure applicable only when other procedures are contraindicated or when ultimate salvage is required. The Maquet or Ferguson tubercleplasty can provide marked improvement in the patient with primarily patellofemoral osteoarthritis.

References

1. Maquet PGJ: Biomechanics of the Knee. New York, Springer-Verlag, 1976.
2. Morrison JB: The Forces Transmitted by the Human Knee Joint. Thesis. University of Strathclyde, Glasgow, Scotland, 1967.
3. Kettelkamp DB, Chao EV: A method of quantitative analysis of medial and lateral compression forces at the knee during standing. Clin Orthop 83:202–213, 1972.
4. Tansey HH III: A Three Dimensional Kinematic and

Force Analysis of the Human Tibio-femoral Joint During Normal Walking. Thesis. Purdue University, West Lafayette, Indiana, 1976.

5. Burke DL, Ahmed AJ, Miller J: A biomechanical study of partial and total medial meniscectomy of the knee. Orthop Trans 2:130, 1978.

6. Kettelkamp DB, Jacobs AW: Tibiofemoral contact area—determinations and implications. J Bone Joint Surg 54A:349–356, 1972.

7. Walker PS, Erdman MJ: The role of the menisci in force transmission across the knee. Clin Orthop 109:184, 1975.

8. Johnson RJ, Kettelkamp DB, Clark W, Leaverton P: Factors affecting late results after meniscectomy. J Bone Joint Surg 56A:719–729, 1974.

9. Jones RE, Smith EC, Reisch JS: Effects of medial meniscectomy in patients older than forty years. J Bone Joint Surg 60A:783–786, 1978.

10. Maquet PGJ, Van de Berg AJ, Simonet JC: Femorotibial weight-bearing areas. J Bone Joint Surg 57A:766–771, 1975.

11. Miller R, Kettelkamp DB, Lauberthal KN, et al.: Quantitative correlations in degenerative arthritis of the knee. J Bone Joint Surg 55A:956–962, 1973.

12. Insall J, Bullough PG, Burstein AH: Proximal "tube" realignment of the patella for chondromalacia patellae. Clin Orthop 144:63–69, 1979.

13. Hughston JC: Subluxation of the patella. J Bone Joint Surg 50A:1003–1026, 1968.

14. Rozing PM, Insall J, Bohne WH: Spontaneous osteonecrosis of the knee. J Bone Joint Surg 62A:1–7, 1980.

15. Merchant AC, Mercer RC, Jacobsen RH, Cool RT: Roentgenographic analysis of patellofemoral congruence. J Bone Joint Surg 56A:1391–1396, 1974.

16. Magnuson PB: Technique of debridement of the knee joint for arthritis. Surg Clin North Am 27:249, 1946.

17. Pridie KH: A method of resurfacing osteoarthritic knee joints. J Bone Joint Surg 41B:618, 1959.

18. Stinchfield FE, Sankaron B, Samilson R: The effect of anticoagulation therapy on bone repair. J Bone Joint Surg 58:537–540, 1976.

19. Kettelkamp DB, Leach RE, Nasca R: Pitfalls of proximal tibial osteotomy. Clin Orthop 106:232–241, 1975.

20. Chao EVS: Biomechanics of high tibial osteotomy. In American Academy of Orthopaedic Surgeons: Symposium on Reconstructive Surgery of the Knee. St. Louis, C. V. Mosby, 1978, pp. 143–160.

21. Coventry MB: Osteotomy of the upper portion of the tibia for degenerative arthritis of the knee. A preliminary report. J Bone Joint Surg 47A:984–990, 1965.

22. Coventry MB: Osteotomy about the knee for degenerative and rheumatoid arthritis. J Bone Joint Surg 55A:23–48, 1973.

23. Kettelkamp DB: Proximal tibial osteotomy. Clin Orthop 103:46, 1974.

23a. Maquet PGJ: Valgus osteotomy for osteoarthritis of the knee. Clin Orthop 120:143–148, 1976.

24. Kettelkamp DB: A review of proximal tibial osteotomy for degenerative arthritis. J Cont Ed Orthop 7:11–19, 1979.

25. Shoji H, Insall J: High tibial osteotomy for osteoarthritis of the knee with valgus deformity. J Bone Joint Surg 55A:963–973, 1973.

26. Shargorodsky FS: Traumatic neuritis of the peroneal nerve complicating the surgical correction of tibia vara. Orthop Traum Protezir (Moscow) 5:32–35, 1969.

27. Tjornstrand B, Hagstedt B, Persson BM: Results of surgical treatment for non-union after high tibial osteotomy in osteoarthritis of the knee. J Bone Joint Surg 60A:973–977, 1978.

28. Vainiopaa S, Laike E, Kirves P, Tiusanen P: Tibial osteotomy for osteoarthritis of the knee—a five to ten year follow up study. J Bone Joint Surg 62A:938–946, 1981.

29. Laskin RS: Unicompartmental tibiofemoral resurfacing arthroplasty. J Bone Joint Surg 60A:182–185, 1978.

30. Marmor L: Marmor modular knee in unicompartmental disease—minimum four year follow up. J Bone Joint Surg 61A:347–353, 1979.

31. Scott RD, Santore RF: Unicondylar unicompartmental replacement for osteoarthritis of the knee. J Bone Joint Surg 62A:536–544, 1981.

32. Skolnick MD, Bryan RJ, Peterson FA: Unicompartmental polycentric knee arthroplasty—description and preliminary results. Clin Orthop 112:208–214, 1975.

33. Ducheyne P, Kagan A, Lacey JA: Failure of total knee arthroplasty due to loosening and deformations of the tibial component. J Bone Joint Surg 60A:384–391, 1978.

34. Broderson MP, Fitzgerald RH Jr, Peterson LFA, et al.: Arthrodesis of the knee following failed total knee arthroplasty. J Bone Joint Surg 61A:181–185, 1979.

35. Hagemann WF, Woods GW, Tullos HJ: Arthrodesis in failed total knee replacement. J Bone Joint Surg 60A:790–794, 1978.

36. Bryan RS, Peterson LFA: Polycentric total knee arthroplasty. Clin Orthop 14S:23–28, 1979.

37. Finerman GAM, Coventry MB, Riley RH, et al.: Anametric total knee arthroplasty. Clin Orthop 145:85–90, 1979.

38. Insall J, Scott WM, Ranawat CS: The total condylar knee prosthesis—a report of 220 cases. J Bone Joint Surg 61A:173–180, 1979.

39. Murray DG, Webster DA: The variable-axis knee prosthesis—two year follow up study. J Bone Joint Surg 62A:687–694, 1981.

40. Hui FC, Fitzgerald RH: Hinged total knee arthroplasty. J Bone Joint Surg 62A:513–519, 1980.

41. Kaufer H, Matthews L: Spherocentric arthroplasty of the knee—clinical experience with an average four year follow up. J Bone Joint Surg 62A:545–559, 1981.

42. Wilson FC, Fajgenbaum DM, Venters GC: Results of knee replacement with Walldius and geometric prostheses—a comparative study. J Bone Joint Surg 52A:197–503, 1980.

43. Bargar WL, Cracchiolo A, Amstutz HC: Results with constrained total knee prosthesis in treating severely disabled patients and patients with failed total knee replacements. J Bone Joint Surg 62A:504–512, 1980.

44. Coventry MB: Two part total knee arthroplasty: Evolution and present status. Clin Orthop 145:29–36, 1979.

45. Ficat RP, Hungerford DS: Disorders of the Patello-Femoral Joint. Baltimore, Williams and Wilkins, 1977.

46. Kettelkamp DB: Current concepts review: Management of patellar malalignment. J Bone Joint Surg 53A:1344–1348, 1981.

47. Lieb FJ, Perry J: Quadriceps function: An electromyographic study under isometric conditions. J Bone Joint Surg 53A:749–758, 1971.

48. Larson RL: Subluxation-dislocation of the patella. *In* Kennedy JC (ed.): The Injured Adolescent Knee. Baltimore, Williams and Wilkins, 1979.

49. Ficat RP, Ficat C, Gedeon P, Toussaint JB: Spongialization: A new treatment for diseased patellae. Clin Orthop 144:74–83, 1979.

50. Ceder LC, Larson RL: Z-plasty lateral retinacular release for the treatment of patellar compression syndrome. Clin Orthop 144:110–113, 1979.

51. Merchant AC, Mercer R: Lateral release of the patella. Clin Orthop 103:40–45, 1974.

52. Hughston JC, Walsh WM: Proximal and distal reconstruction of the extensor mechanism for patellar subluxation. Clin Orthop 144:36–42, 1979.

53. Ferguson AB Jr, Brown TP, Fu FH, Rutkowski R: Relief of patellofemoral contact stress by anterior displacement of the tibial tubercle. J Bone Joint Surg 61A:159–166, 1979.

54. Kaufer H: Mechanical function of the patella. J Bone Joint Surg 53A:1551–1560, 1971.

55. Kaufer H: Patellar biomechanics. Clin Orthop 144:51–54, 1979.

56. Sutton FS, Thompson CH, Lipke J, Kettelkamp DB: Effect of patellectomy on knee function. J Bone Joint Surg 58A:537–540, 1976.

57. Stearer PA, Gradisar IA, Hoyt WA, Chu M: Patellectomy: A clinical study and biomechanical evaluation. Clin Orthop 144:84–90, 1979.

25

Osteoarthritis of the Hip

Harlan C. Amstutz, M.D.
William C. Kim, M.D.

ETIOLOGY

Osteoarthritis of the hip is frequently the result of obvious anatomic defects, congenital or acquired, developmental, traumatic, or metabolic (see Chapters 7, 14, and 15). When there is no known obvious cause, primary osteoarthritis (OA) is diagnosed, although it, too, is probably a collection of disease states (see Chapter 15). Despite the emergence of considerable pertinent information from anatomic and pathophysiologic studies of the hip, the precise etiology is often not well defined. For this reason, treatment continues to be empiric, directed primarily toward palliation rather than prevention and cure. Definition of OA by the traditional pathologic and roentgenographic criteria of joint space narrowing, subchondral sclerosis, cyst formation, and osteophyte formation is useful but incompletely describes the underlying pathogenesis of its many variants. Further studies, including clinical evaluation, roentgenography, gross and microscopic pathologic evaluation of tissues obtained from hips at surgery and autopsy, biochemical assays, and immunologic and biomechanical studies, will lead to a better understanding of the osteoarthritic process. In the following discussion, a model of the natural history of cartilage of the normal hip is developed so that current and future knowledge of the disease state can be incorporated.

NATURAL HISTORY OF ARTICULAR CARTILAGE OF THE HIP

Most of the human specimens for study have been obtained at surgery on end-stage osteoar-

thritic hips with markedly altered topographic landmarks. In addition, other autopsy specimens appear to represent age-related changes without overt clinical manifestations of OA. Findings indicate that with advancing age, there is increasing prevalence of focal fibrillation and erosion of a limited progression (in non–weighting-bearing areas);[1] greater congruence between the femoral head and the acetabulum, perhaps due to attritional wear, remodeling, and change in compliance;[2] less glycosaminoglycan in the areas of erosion; diminished fatigue endurance;[3] more extracellular lipids;[4] and cartilage cellular degeneration in the deeper portions of articular cartilage.[5]

Findings that appear to be independent of aging include normal mean sulfate uptake; total glycosaminoglycan content;[6] and ratio of chondroitin sulfate content and water content.[7] There is evidence that joint remodeling occurs throughout life.[8] These are some of the age-related and independent changes that contrast with findings in OA.

PARAMETERS FOR BIOMECHANICAL HOMEOSTASIS OF THE NORMAL HIP

The articular cartilage and its associated subchondral bone are tissues that are affected by stress (force per unit area).[9, 10] If the applied stress to a chondro-osseous unit of the femoral head exceeds its strength, mechanical failure occurs, possibly from a single excessive peak dynamic stress applied or because of repetitive cyclic loading of lower stress that exceeds the endurance limit. However, the chondro-osseous unit also possesses biologic properties that can respond to the applied stress. Remod-

423

eling occurs in accordance with Wolff's law for bone and Heuter-Volkmann's principle for articular cartilage (the amount of matrix in the articular cartilage is proportional to the stress distributed on it).[9] Hence, a complete expression for homeostasis of the hip, and its chondro-osseous unit in particular, includes biologic as well as mechanical factors.

There is also a less well-defined lower limit of applied stress below which the chondro-osseous unit may become abnormal. Examples that are well recognized in bone include disuse atrophy and stress shielding. Evidence suggests that there may be a similar analogue for articular cartilage,[2, 11, 12] and in addition, it has been shown that motion is important for cell nutritional viability.[2, 13]

Apparently, there is a static and dynamic balance between applied stress and reaction of the chondro-osseous unit to the applied stress mechanically and biologically; as long as the applied stress remains within normal limits, mechanical and biologic changes are reversible.

NATURAL HISTORY OF OSTEOARTHRITIS OF THE HIP

Cameron and MacNab[14] described six different roentgenologic patterns of OA of the hip, dividing them into nonmigratory (concentric, superior, and capital collapse) and migratory (central, downward and medial, upward and lateral) types. Inasmuch as this was not a true natural history study, it is probable that the concentric and central groups, which are the most common types, and the superior and upward lateral groups are representations of the same process at different times.

Recently, reports of inflammatory osteoarthritis have been increasing, particularly with respect to failures after resurfacing procedures.[15–17] This is an inadequately defined entity and may be represented initially by the concentric and central migratory types. Some reports have included the classic forms of juvenile rheumatoid arthritis, adult rheumatoid arthritis, and ankylosing spondylitis in the inflammatory group. However, there appears to be an arthritic condition that is distinct from them and that tends to progress rapidly, associated either with central migration or with superior collapse. In our experience, such cases have a considerably greater inflammatory response, as manifested by synovitis with increased vascularity and osteoporosis. Our observed numbers are less than those reported in other series, and it has been suggested that there may be a relationship to prolonged treatment with indomethacin or other nonsteroidal anti-inflammatory agents. Perhaps the debris produced by the disease causes a synovitis that exacerbates the process through an autoimmune reaction.

In more classic OA, it has been noted that optimal biomechanical homeostasis requires that the applied stress not exceed a certain threshold value beyond which the chondro-osseous unit will fail mechanically and/or biologically, a situation that may cause osteoarthritic changes. At an abnormally low stress, the cells of subchondral bone and perhaps the articular cartilage may not function physiologically. There is evidence to suggest that inadequate stress may predispose to OA of the hip.[2, 11, 12] Evidence then appears to suggest upper and lower limits of normal biomechanical conditions within which osteoarthritic changes do not occur.

Moreover, there appears to be a gray zone outside the limits of normal, where transition between normal and osteoarthritic hip changes occurs that may be time-related. Evidence suggestive of reversibility is based on known ability of injured articular cartilage to undergo mitosis and to synthesize matrix.[18, 19] as well as gross and roentgenographic joint space restoration following proximal femoral osteotomy.[20–22]

SUMMARY OF ETIOLOGIC FACTORS OF OSTEOARTHRITIS OF THE HIP RELATED TO ABNORMAL STRESS

Hip Structure and Material

Etiologic factors related to OA of the hip may stem from abnormally matched force and application to the mechanical and biologic chondro-osseous substrate. High stress may be due to abnormally high force for a given period and area of application, as in a motor vehicle accident, which can cause mechanical failure of the chondro-osseous unit and result in death or physiologic dysfunction of the cells. This is an example of high, single, peak dynamic stress. Such post-traumatic OA is well recognized. Repetitive application of lower peak dynamic force for a given area can result in changes of OA,[23, 24] as will continous application of force or absence of force.[11, 13] In contrast, high stress applied in an oscillatory direction tangential to the surface of the chondro-osseous unit does not appear to produce osteoarthritic changes.[24] Hence, the magnitude and direction of force vector are important variables in the etiology of OA, as is the frequency. In addition, the requirement to stay within upper and lower limits of normal to avoid osteoarthritic changes appears to hold.

Excessive stress can occur if the area is very small, resulting in high concentration. This can occur with trauma, loose bodies, hip dysplasias, slipped capital femoral epiphysis, and Legg-Calvé-Perthes disease. It is believed that a significant number of cases previously diagnosed as primary OA, may be secondary to incongruity of the hip joint (see Chapter 15). Mechanical changes may also occur secondary to inflammatory conditions such as rheumatoid arthritis and septic arthritis, in which there has been irregular destruction of the articular cartilage and subchondral bone.

Osteoporosis is associated with decreased likelihood of osteoarthritic changes, possibly due to increased elasticity and the dampening effect of the subchondral bone (see Chapter 1).[25] Conversely, increased stiffness of subchondral bone, perhaps due to repetitive microfracture with healing, may be associated with OA, as postulated by Pugh and colleagues.[10] Increased stress is then borne by articular cartilage owing to decreased trabecular bone dampening effect.

CLINICAL MANIFESTATIONS

Early Stage

The onset of pain is gradual, often dull or aching, and poorly localized about the hip (thigh, groin, and buttock), or it may radiate to the knee via the anterior branch of the obturator nerve. Initally, the pain is related to activity and subsides with rest. Pain has been attributed to articular cartilage debris resulting in low-grade synovitis, venous congestion within the underlying trabecular bone, and subchondral bone fractures.[26–28]

Physical findings in this early period may include coxalgic (painful) limp, subtle muscle spasm, and decreased internal rotation of the hip. These signs represent compensatory mechanisms to minimize pain. The abductor lurch becomes manifest when the patient bends toward the affected hip, thereby shifting the center of gravity closer to the hip. The lever arm for the center of gravity of the body from the center of the affected head (fulcrum) is thus reduced, which translates into less force applied to the hip. Decreased internal rotation may be due to hip muscle spasm in response to pain or volumetric effect of increased synovial fluid within the hip capsule, which is composed of fibers that twist internally as they proceed from proximal to distal. External rotation of the hip decompresses or unwinds the fibers maximally; this is a more frequently assumed position. Muscle spasm is best detected by rolling the extended hip gently in the rotation arc.

Early roentgenographic changes may not correlate with clinical findings. It should be kept in mind that a considerable number of the general population have roentgenographic evidence of OA but are without symptoms.[28a] Rarely, subtle widening of the medial joint margin may be due to increased joint fluid, but the width of the articular cartilage is generally reduced. Subchondral sclerosis, although of varying prominence, tends to be present. Osteophytes usually appear, possibly as the result of endochondral ossification subsequent to vascular invasion of non–weight-bearing areas.[11]

Intermediate Stage

In intermediate-stage OA, clinically, pain continues as the dominant symptom, becoming exacerbated with weight-bearing activities, which place more stress across the hip joint. Limp and abductor lurch may progress. In addition to limitation of internal rotation, abduction and flexion decrease because of capsular contracture of the hip. Osteophyte formation in the medial inferior region of the hip joint gives the impression of pushing the femoral head laterally and adds to the abduction posture. In addition to narrowing of articular cartilage, cyst formation may be significant, and progressive osteophyte formation confers an abnormal shape to the head and the acetabulum. Pathologically, there is progressive change from focal to general involvement of the femoral head.

Advanced Stage

In advanced-stage OA of the hip, pain is severe, being present at rest and sometimes awakening the patient at night. Frequent use of analgesics is required. Ambulation is restricted to the house, and there is difficulty in sitting for prolonged periods or in climbing stairs. Complaints of leg-length inequality may be more apparent than real because of the posture of the affected limb. The Trendelenburg sign, reflecting abductor weakness, may be present. Significant limitations of flexion, abduction, extension, and internal rotation are noted; there may be evidence of thigh atrophy secondary to relative disuse.

Roentgenographically, the joint space may be obliterated and the femoral head deformed. The direction of migration of the femoral head relative to the acetabulum may vary, depending on a combination of bony and soft tissue changes.

Pathologically, the femoral head shows large patches of denuded bone with eburnation. Cysts may contain fluid similar to synovial fluid but, more often, contain fibrous material; communication with the articular surface frequently occurs and is interpreted to result from subchondral fracture or intrusion of synovial fluid via a cartilaginous defect.

MANAGEMENT

Optimal management of OA of the hip is dependent on many variables including (1) the patient's age, weight, amount of disability, and desired activity level; (2) the stage of the osteoarthritic process; (3) the state of the art and science of treatment modalities available; and (4) the experience, ability, and judgment of the treating physician.

Patient Factors

Because the osteoarthritic process causes disability but is nonfatal, it is particularly important to know how much pain and disability the patient is able and willing to tolerate. Individual variations in pain threshold may be inconsistent with physical findings or the roentgenographic appearance of the hip. The measure of disability is related to the limitation of work and play activity accepted by the patient and bearing on the quality of life. The patient and his disability must be treated rather than isolated clinical or roentgenographic findings.

If the disability is such that treatment needs to be instituted, it is essential that the patient be educated concerning the risk-benefit ratio of a particular treatment modality and the natural history of OA of the hip; management requires full patient understanding and cooperation.

Inasmuch as the pertinent variables in the osteoarthritic process are applied stress to the hip and the mechanical and biologic properties of the hip, the patient's education about this relationship helps to initiate programs that reduce stress. Changes in activity, weight reduction, and the use of supports such as canes or crutches may be necessary.

Influence of the Osteoarthritic Process

Unfortunately, there is no good indicator to prognosticate the speed of disease progression. Roentgenographic changes followed over a time period are helpful; even though such changes may have been slow in the past, there is no guarantee that they will continue at the same rate. Rate of progression does have a bearing on whether management recommendations will remain conservative or surgical. At present, there is no proven method to reverse early osteoarthritic changes. If an interval of reversal occurs after the osteoarthritic process has been initiated, it is usually early in the course of the process.

Nonoperative Treatment

Modes of nonoperative treatment may be divided into those directed at alleviating symptoms and those minimizing progression of the disease.

Medications

Because pain is a dominant symptom, analgesics are an important part of the treatment (see Chapter 18). When inflammation within the hip joint is a significant source of pain, anti-inflammatory drugs are helpful. The choice of analgesic and anti-inflammatory drugs must be based on a thorough understanding of the rationale for use, safe limits of dosage and schedule, possible adverse and allergic reactions, specific indications and contraindications, and interactions with other drugs taken concomitantly. The risk-benefit ratio and use of the safest but most effective drugs must be considered. In practice, empiric trials with one or more drugs may be needed before the patient benefits. Titration of dosage and schedule may be needed. Alleviation of stress across the hip joint may permit the patient to use less potent drugs and to take them less frequently. Patients must be educated to maximize compliance and relief.

Physical Therapy

Warmth can comfort the painful hip joint involved with OA, but because the hip is deep within tissue, application of surface heat is less effective than diathermy and ultrasonic treatments. Appropriate exercises to maintain and regain range of motion should be implemented (see Chapter 17).

In addition to pain, the natural clinical history of the osteoarthritic hip includes progressive deformity, diminished range of motion, and muscle atrophy. The pathophysiology of these changes has been discussed previously. Flexion and adduction deformity can be reduced by lying in a prone position and by placing a pillow between the legs during sleep. Active exercises in abduction, extension, and external rotation also reduce contractures and help to maintain muscle mass. Much of the stress across the hip joint is dissipated by muscles and soft tissues about the hip in addition to subchondral bone; therefore, well-maintained muscle mass and tone may attenuate and dampen the stresses before they reach the articular cartilage.[23, 24]

Rest and Activity

In reviewing current theories on the natural history of OA of the hip and the factors governing it, it is evident that applied stress is a significant, controllable variable. Therefore, treatment modalities that reduce or favorably alter stress across the hip joint appear valid. A large magnitude of stress applied as impact, or impact stresses of lesser magnitude applied repetitively, tends to produce pain and may promote disease progression. Thus, rest and activities that do not involve these types of stress have roles in the treatment of the osteoarthritic hip.

Absolute bed rest is rarely required; occasionally, however, acute inflammation within the hip joint may benefit from several days of bed rest. Such a hip joint must be evaluated for other inflammatory conditions. At times, traction is helpful in reducing undesirable motion in bed and in alleviating muscle spasm.

Activity is usually dictated by the severity of discomfort caused by the involved hip. The patient thus learns to avoid activities that exacerbate symptoms, e.g., jogging (high peak dynamic stress of high frequency) and long walks (low peak dynamic stress of lower frequency). Intervals of rest during ambulation help to alleviate discomfort and permit longer walks. Swimming and bicycling (oscillatory stresses tangential to the articular surface) are better tolerated, because they involve less impact. If the patient has not learned to adjust his own activities and is exceeding his limits, he needs to be educated concerning the principles of adverse activities.

Avoidance of activities of daily living that tend to cause pain because of abnormal stress is possible. Sitting may be better tolerated if the seat is elevated. Maneuvers to decrease stress at the hip when getting into or out of a car can be learned.

Weight Reduction and Assistive Devices

Weight reduction decreases static stress across the hip joint. The total force across the hip joint is equal to the product of the body weight and distance of the center of gravity from the femoral head plus the product of the abductor force required to keep the pelvis level and its distance from the femoral head (Fig. 25–1).[29] If weight is reduced, the total force across the hip joint is diminished. A 1-lb reduction in weight results in a 3-lb reduction of force across the hip joint in simple walking.

Supportive devices can significantly unload the hip joint and improve gait. A cane used in the contralateral hand is an efficient mechanical device.[30] Use of crutches can unload the hip further. As noted, much of the force across the hip joint results from muscular action; accordingly, total lack of weight bearing is associated with increased force across the hip joint because the leg must be held elevated in mid-air.[31] Toe-touch weight bearing sufficient to equal the weight of the leg (one-sixth of the body weight) maximally unloads the hip, and muscle forces are minimized.

Shoes with soft, cushioned soles and heels may dampen forces transmitted during heel-strike and mid-stance and thus help alleviate symptoms.

Surgical Treatment

Basic Considerations

Because conservative or nonoperative measures are only of temporary benefit and because osteoarthritis is usually a progressive disease,

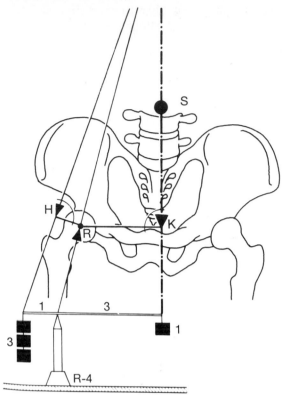

Figure 25–1. The total stress across the hip joint is equal to the product of abduction force and its lever arm (HR) plus the product of body weight (minus the weight of the standing leg) and lever arm (KR).

surgery is often necessary. Operations performed for osteoarthritis of the hips are numerous and ever-changing. The timing and the type of procedure to be performed are related to the degree of disability and the age and medical condition of the patient. Each patient must be individually analyzed, and all alternatives must be considered carefully, keeping in mind the individual's life span and the potential technologic advances. If no effective surgical alternative exists, it is better to continue nonoperative methods. Hip disability causes significant disturbances in the patient's mental health and daily life as well as economic hardship. Appropriate surgical treatment can provide relief and can resolve related problems. It is important to keep in mind the time-dependent nature of osteoarthritis, the needs of the patient, the experience of the surgeon, and the changing refinements in technology. Selection of the optimal procedure must be consistent with these variables in each individual patient.

The feasibility of a surgical procedure is determined by the extent and severity of os-

teoarthritic changes of the hip as assessed by conventional roentgenograms, tomograms, and CAT scans. Osteotomy may be indicated if the weight-bearing area of the hip can be broadened or made more congruent either by proximal femoral osteotomy or by supra-acetabular osteotomy. In prosthetic hip replacement, the optimal size of the implant can be assessed by using a clear template of varying designs superimposed on the diseased hip and corrected for magnification. It is generally desirable to remove diseased bone, to preserve normal bone, and to optimize the biomechanical relationship at the hip and adjacent joints. Arthrodesis is dependent on an adequate amount of bone stock. The Girdlestone procedure, in which the head of the femur is resected, is performed only for sepsis or when there is inadequate bone stock.

The availability of bone stock plays an important role in decision making related to the type of surgical procedure to be considered (Fig. 25–2). If the arthropathy is confined to a focal area of the femoral head, an osteotomy displacing that area away from the weight-bearing zone and moving normal articular cartilage to it is feasible. If the changes are more extensive, involving much of the surface, a hemisurfacing procedure would best fit the pathoanatomy. If the whole head is involved, an entire femoral head replacement may be necessary.

If both the femoral and acetabular sides have related focal changes, an osteotomy may be considered. If the surface of both articular cartilages are involved, a surface type or conventional total hip replacement may be the best solution, especially if the patient is older.

Conventional total hip replacement may follow other more bone-conserving procedures. Total hip replacement performed in the younger patient may be the gateway to a repetitive cycle of loosening and revisions that can lead to a salvage Girdlestone procedure. An osteotomy preserves bone, relying on biologic response, and because of this, it is the most conservative procedure. However, each operation becomes somewhat of a deterrent to the success of future procedures, and therefore, all the "trade-offs" must be carefully evaluated. The durability of any procedure is influenced by the patient, surgeon, procedure, and etiologic factors that can increase or reduce the possibility of failure. Because pain is the primary indication for surgery, complete relief is the goal. Reduction of functional disability is also desirable.

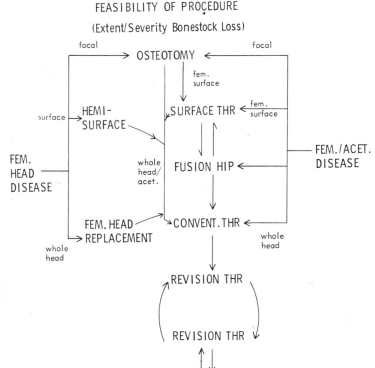

FEASIBILITY OF PROCEDURE

(Extent/Severity Bonestock Loss)

Figure 25–2. This flow diagram summarizes the feasibility of different surgical procedures according to the extent and severity of bonestock loss. Conventional total hip replacement (THR) is the point of convergence that leads into the cycle of revisions.

Virgin cemented total hip replacements have achieved the best overall results. The quality of clinical results of other procedures tends to be poorer and less consistent. Revision total hip replacements have not demonstrated clinical results as satisfactory as those with the primary procedure, and futhermore, good results diminish as the number of revisions increases.[32–35] Conversion of an arthrodesed hip to total hip relacement can alleviate low back pain.[36] The Girdlestone procedure is performed to salvage failures of other procedures.[37]

Indications for the Feasible Procedure

The procedure may be indicated if it has a reasonable chance of attaining the desired balance among clinical result, durability, and complications. Durability is governed by the relationship among stress applied to the hip joint, mechanical resistance of the joint to the applied stress, and the biologic state of the hip tissues. It is influenced by the patient, the surgeon, and etiologic, as well as procedural factors (Fig. 25–3). Etiologic factors are discussed under various procedures.

Patient Factors

The patient's age, weight, activity level, and compliance with postoperative recommendations influence the clinical result and durability of the procedure. In individuals of comparable health and physiologic function, age can predict the stress anticipated and correlates with activity level. Weight and body habitus determine the magnitude of stress. The applied stresses are cumulative of single large forces or lower stress cycles that exceed the endurance limit for the hip procedure.

A judicious rehabilitation program, realistic expectations from the procedure, and an adjustment of priorities favor clinical durability. These variables alter with advancing age, and thus, life expectancy must be taken into account in selecting the procedure.

Surgeon and Procedure Factors

Experience, judgment, and technical ability of the surgeon equally influence the clinical result and durability of the procedure and minimize complications. The surgeon's technical expertise encompasses his experience, his

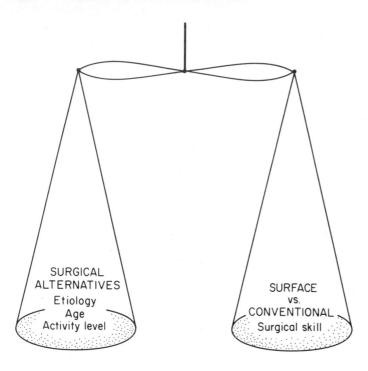

Figure 25–3. Indications for a surgical procedure are based on the patient, surgeon, etiology, and technical factors, which also influence immediate and long-term results.

hospital, and his operating team. Failure to select the appropriate patient for a procedure can doom even the best technically performed surgery. State-of-the-art advances influence the longevity of the procedure, particularly prosthetic hip replacements, which continue to improve. Improved fixation techniques appear to increase the durability of prosthetic hip replacements, and the use of "super alloys" makes stem fracture less common.

Specific Surgical Procedures for Osteoarthritic Hips

The indications and criteria for each procedure for osteoarthritic hips must be related to the risk-benefit ratio and comparison with other procedures. Each clinical situation is unique and cannot be solved by a formula. The specific operative techniques for each procedure are not within the scope of this discussion but can be found in the references at the end of this chapter.

Mold Arthroplasty. Smith-Petersen conceived of interposing a foreign material between raw decorticated surfaces of the femoral head and the acetabulum in order to stimulate the biologic process to form articular cartilage. The initial material, Pyrex glass, was replaced with a more durable cobalt chromium cup. Often, with intermittent passive motion, fibro-

cartilage and, occasionally, hyaline cartilage formed. In 1948, he reported on 90 cups used for osteoarthritis, most of which were pain-free, allowing an active life style.[38] Aufranc emphasized meticulous technique and often needed to revise unsatisfactory results once or twice to produce better results.[39] It was an innovative idea that has contributed significantly to hip surgery in osteoarthritic patients, although its results would not be acceptable by today's standards.

Johnson and Larson reviewed 543 cup arthroplasties followed for periods ranging from 3 to 14 years.[40] Among them, 106 hips in 94 patients were operated on for primary osteoarthritis and were evaluated according to unilateral or bilateral disease; of these, 30% to 40% had pain. All the patients limped; 60% had moderate to severe gait abnormalities sufficient to interfere with daily activities. In 50% of the patients, it took 2 to 3 years to reach a clinical plateau; in 7% there was no clinical improvement; and in 13%, there was deterioration 4 to 12 years postoperatively.

It became generally recognized that cup arthroplasty was a demanding procedure for the patient because rehabilitation was the key to success. According to Blount, the patient must have the "proper emotional background to exercise faithfully until adequate strength and range of motion are established."[20] The arduous and lengthy process required the utmost complicance and determination to adhere to such a protocol. Non–weight-bearing crutch support was recommended for a period of six months. Results were more satisfactory in unilateral disease, especially in cases of post-traumatic osteoarthritis. Unsatisfactory results were often ascribed to aseptic necrosis, but in our view, high stress concentration and motion were the primary causes of failure. Although occasional outstanding results persisted for 10 to 20 years, the quality of pain relief was rarely comparable to that achieved with total joint replacement. However, the decline of cup arthroplasty was mainly due to the far more predictable and rapid results obtained with joint replacement. Today, a cup arthroplasty might be indicated for a young patient, under 40 years of age, with good bone stock, who has the intelligence to understand its benefits and risks and the willingness to accept less-than-perfect results. He must also understand that this would be a time-buying procedure, but one that would require being away from work or school for at least 6 months. In this way, femoral and acetabular bone would be preserved to permit a later conversion to surface or conventional replacement. The potential complications include those associated with anesthesia and hip surgery in general and will be reviewed in the section on total hip replacement. Specific complications include sepsis (low with today's prophylaxis) and erosion of bone stock due to eccentric pressure. Today, very few surgeons have experience with the demanding technique of mold arthroplasty.

Osteotomy. Although the exact mechanism by which osteotomy works to relieve pain is unknown, the biomechanical rationale for osteotomy is improvement in joint congruity and stress distribution (Fig. 25–4). Other reasons cited for pain relief include decompression of increased venous pressure and vascularity.[26] The current concept is mechanically based and may be achieved by using an acetabular osteotomy and other shelving procedures or a proximal femoral varus osteotomy to redirect the head into the acetabular socket. These procedures facilitate alignment of relatively normal cartilage into the weight-bearing area.

The hip force may be reduced by increasing the abductor lever arm with a varus osteotomy, which also decreases muscular forces by relative lengthening of the muscles. Bombelli, however, recommends decreasing the force across the hip joint by moving the center of rotation of the head medially by valgus osteotomy, whereby the capital "drop" osteophyte of Wiberg is moved into apposition with the

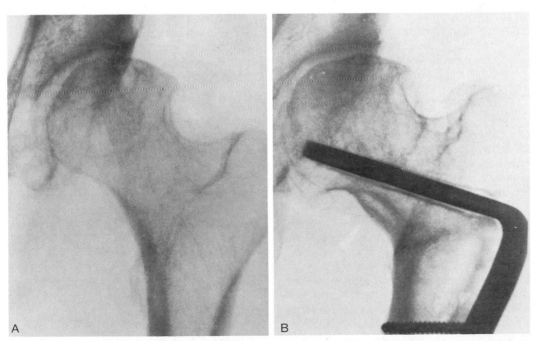

Figure 25–4. Proximal femoral osteotomy is a bone-conserving and time-buying procedure that can be effective in relieving pain and improving the stress distribution at the hip. Joint congruity and stress distribution abnormalities associated with mild osteoarthritis (*A*) are lessened following osteotomy (*B*).

inferomedial "tent" osteophyte.[41] This is particularly applicable to an eccentric-shaped head associated with a slipped capital epiphysis or dysplasia. In contrast to varus osteotomy, which may combine the effects of increased surface area and increased abductor lever arm to reduce stress at the weight-bearing area, valgus osteotomy shortens the abductor lever arm. Its beneficial effect occurs mainly by improving surface area and congruity. An extension osteotomy is useful to compensate for a flexion contracture, and Bombelli frequently combines this with a valgus osteotomy.[41] The surgeon considering an osteotomy that may change the anatomy of the hip must be aware of the effect that such an alteration may have on future surface or total hip replacement. Anterior rotational osteotomy about the axis of the femoral neck, as described by Sugioka, is useful for femoral head osteonecrosis, in which the lesion is usually located in the anterosuperolateral aspect of the head.[42] Because this procedure is not accompanied by marked alteration in the biomechanics or anatomy, later surface replacement is feasible.

There are also implications of hip osteotomy relative to the knee. With varus osteotomy at the hip, the weight-bearing axis is shifted to the medial compartment; the converse holds true for valgus osteotomy at the hip. If there is a pre-existing valgus or varus deformity of the knee, appropriate tailoring of the osteotomy at the hip should be considered. If there is a valgus deformity of the knee, valgus osteotomy at the hip of more than 25 to 30 degrees should be accompanied by lateral displacement of the distal fragment of the femur.[43] Varus osteotomy usually results in a Trendelenburg-type limp, which, although reducing stress across the hip joint, is clinically less than optimal. Therefore, Morscher does not recommend varus osteotomy of more than 15 to 20 degrees except in a completely mobile joint with marked coxa valga, or unless it is combined with distal and lateral transposition of the greater trochanter.[43] In performing osteotomies, preoperative full extension is recommended when doing flexion osteotomy, and adequate preoperative abduction is recommended when doing varus osteotomy.

There are numerous reports citing increased roentgenographic joint space after osteotomies as evidence of healing.[21, 22] However, this apparent increased space may be due to positioning of the joint in relation to roentgenographic projection. Proof of actual joint regeneration remains elusive. The suitability of a patient for an osteotomy is determined by making a "template" of the pathoanatomy of the hip. The femoral head should be placed in various positions to identify optimal congruency by taking roentgenograms in different degrees of abduction and adduction. CAT scans are helpful in delineating specific types of lesions such as those seen in osteonecrosis, with cysts, and in hip dysplasia, which may require bone grafting.

Indications for osteotomy for osteoarthritis vary even among contemporary proponents of these procedures. Morscher[43] reviewed 2251 intertrochanteric osteotomies performed by the Swiss Orthopaedic Association as well as his own 263 cases at the University of Basel. Optimal prognostic factors included age younger than 50 years, minimal obesity, demonstrated mechanical basis for osteoarthritis, white-collar worker, good congruency attainable on functional roentgenograms, and signs of mechanical overload such as local sclerosis, joint space narrowing, and cyst formation. In a recent follow-up of 94 hips with 5 years' follow-up, 45.5% of patients had no pain or only slight pain. One-third achieved a long-lasting excellent result; one-third had a good result; and one-third required total hip replacement. Follow-up of the procedure by roentgenographic evaluation showed that 10% had deteriorated in the first 2 years postoperatively and that 14% had deteriorated at the third or fourth year postoperatively. He believed that intertrochanteric osteotomy permitted a 5-year delay before another surgical procedure was required. Success of the osteotomy was related to good preoperative planning, surgical technique, and a rehabilitation protocol with a period of no weight bearing. Variations in patient acceptance of disability must be taken into account in evaluating the effectiveness of this procedure.

Various types of osteotomies can produce excellent results, but results are less consistent in comparison with total hip replacement. They are less satisfactory and require demanding postoperative rehabilitation, and usually, range of joint motion does not improve. However, intertrochanteric osteotomy is a valuable alternative to prosthetic hip replacement when possible because if successful, it can provide years of improved function in young and active patients. The potential complications from anesthesia for hip osteotomies are comparable to those in other hip procedures. The risk of infection is low, and there is a low incidence of loss of fixation with change in position of the osteotomy, or malunion, and nonunion. In some centers in North America, surgeons are reporting favorable experience with pelvic osteotomies for symptomatic younger patients, who usually have secondary osteoarthritis as a result of hip dysplasia.[44]

Femoral Hemiarthroplasty. Femoral hemiarthroplasty is a practical procedure when the acetabular articular cartilage is normal or only minimally affected by pathologic changes. Traditionally, this has been a stem-type replacement, as proposed by Austin Moore[45] or Thompson.[46] If the entire femoral head is severely involved, with a smooth and intact acetabulum, replacement of the entire head is mandatory; when the procedure is performed for fractures of the neck of the femur and avascular necrosis, good results are generally reported. Anderson and associates reviewed experience with Austin-Moore and Thompson prostheses followed for periods ranging from 12 to 148 months.[47] In patients with recent fractures (less than 3 months), approximately 85% had good or excellent results; in those with avascular necrosis as a result of fractures, about 80% achieved good to excellent results. Femoral head hemiarthroplasty was performed for idiopathic osteonecrosis in six patients whose acetabulum was intact; all had good to excellent results. In marked contrast were the results in patients with osteoarthritis, rheumatoid arthritis, and failed cup arthroplasties, among whom only 40% to 50% had good to excellent results. Salvati and Wilson[48] studied 436 femoral head replacements in 418 patients; 148 were performed for primary or secondary osteoarthritis. In a subgroup with Austin-Moore prostheses, 106 were available for long-term review, at an average of 8 years' follow-up; 19 failures occurred before 5 years (about 20%). The average age at operation was 59 years, and at follow-up, it was 68 years. Of the 30 patients with primary and secondary osteoarthritis, 17 achieved excellent to good results, whereas in 13, results were fair to poor. In eight patients with idiopathic osteonecrosis, all gained good to excellent results. These studies suggest that femoral head replacements when the acetabular cartilage is intact may be expected to be successful in fresh fractures and early idiopathic osteonecrosis. In osteoarthritis involving both sides of the joint, results are poor, and femoral head replacement is not indicated. However, in a young active patient with early acetabular changes secondary to idiopathic osteonecrosis of the femoral head, it may be wise to buy time and preserve bone stock for probable total hip replacement by considering a femoral hemiarthroplasty. The durability of femoral hemiarthroplasty, even with normal acetabular cartilage, depends on many unknown factors, such as the durability of articular cartilage to withstand articulation with a metal sphere whose size match may be less than optimal.

Furthermore, another disadvantage is that often the patient with osteonecrosis is young, and once committed to a stem-type device, any subsequent revision surgery will have to be of the stem type. Recently, we have been performing a hemi-resurfacing with an acrylic-fixed custom THARIES prosthesis for osteonecrosis if a portion of the femoral head is viable. In this situation, both the femoral canal and the acetabulum would be preserved for later reconstruction with advanced technology. The feasibility of this procedure is determined by a CAT scan, and components are custom ordered in millimeter increments, with the appropriate size of the components determined by roentgenogram and then press-fitted at surgery to ensure the best "fit."

Bipolar components are now widely utilized in order to minimize articular cartilage wear by providing a low-friction artificial polyethylene-cobalt/chrome bearing.[49] However, early models were prone to dislocate between the components, and reduction was not possible by closed methods. Newer designs have lessened this tendency, although the efficacy of low wear has not yet been demonstrated.

Arthrodesis. Arthrodesis is rarely performed for osteoarthritis in the United States because of the advantages of joint replacement with its effective pain relief combined with preservation of motion. Advising a patient to undergo a hip fusion can be difficult, and it is even more difficult for the patient to accept. However, there is a clear indication for consideration of this procedure in young active males who are of stout, short stature and otherwise healthy and whose work requires prolonged standing. The procedure may be considered in patients with primary osteoarthritis; it is more applicable to secondary and post-traumatic arthritis of the young. When the hip is fused, the excess strain ordinarily absorbed by a mobile hip must be absorbed by the spine, the contralateral hip, and ipsilateral knee. In time, the strain may produce or accelerate secondary degenerative changes in those joints. It may be feasible to subsequently revise an arthrodesis of the hip to a total hip replacement when the patient is older and activities are less demanding. Today, hip arthrodesis should be performed by intra-articular methods that employ techniques that preserve the normal muscle and skeletal anatomy, so that if a revision to a total hip replacement must be performed, this secondary procedure will be facilitated.

Lipscomb and McCaslin reported on arthrodesis of the hip in 371 patients, 347 of whom were followed for at least a year.[50] Their average age was 36.5 years. The result was a successful fusion at the time of the initial procedure in 78% of cases. Solid fusion was achieved in 84% of the 52 patients with osteoarthritis. These authors recommended a bone graft, internal fixation, and a spica cast, as well as a subtrochanteric osteotomy of the femur, to decrease the lever arm at the hip joint to promote a higher rate of healing. Successful results were reported using rigid internal fixation with a large cobra plate.[51] This technique is applicable only when the abductor muscles can be preserved, leaving a muscle envelope attached to the trochanter to aid a successful revision of the arthrodesis at a later date. In general, some form of internal fixation is advisable. The 155-degree nail-plate combination has been satisfactory. Alternative methods also include screw fixation of the femoral head alone or combined with subtrochanteric osteotomy and the use of a plaster spica cast to insure minimal displacement of the osteotomy. This will permit the use of a stem-type total hip replacement subsequently, if required. Most surgeons recommend arthrodesis in neutral abduction and adduction, 30 to 40 degrees of flexion, and no more than 10 degrees of external rotation.

Conventional Total Hip Replacement. Of all the surgical procedures for osteoarthritic hips, conventional total hip replacement is the most predictable and effective of any procedure so far devised (Fig. 25–5). The resulting pain relief facilitates improved function and range of motion, although early successful results have been tempered by an increasing incidence of loosening, which is now the primary complication. Cupic reported on 409 Charnley low-friction arthroplasties.[52] The revision rate was only 1.5% at an 11.5-year follow-up. However, the average age of his patients at surgery was 68 years, and although many had roentgenographic evidence of loosening, their activity levels were low, permitting relatively symptom-free function. In contrast, Chandler and coworkers reported that of 33 hips operated on in patients who were younger than 30 years old at time of initial surgery,

57% required revision or were potential candidates for revision at the 5-year follow-up.[37] Most of these patients had bone stock deficiencies or technical problems in addition to their youth. Although techniques have improved, even today's replacements are not durable enough for the younger or more active patient.

Risks and potential complications include the rare surgery-related death, sepsis requiring removal of the prosthesis, dislocations, trochanteric problems when the transtrochanteric approach to the hip is used, heterotopic new bone formation, nerve palsy, thrombophlebitis, and pulmonary embolism, as well as blood replacement reactions. The decision to implant a conventional total hip replacement should be guided by the prognostic factors of these variables for any given patient based on etiology, the surgeon's experience, and the available prosthetic design and materials.

Patient Factors. As emphasized earlier, age is a major determinent of mechanical failure of conventional total hip replacements and is related directly to activity level and length of follow-up. Weight is also a risk factor in loosening and in stem fractures. Collis reported four femoral stem fractures (2%) in 200 total hip arthroplasties in patients weighing over 91 kg who were followed for a minimum of 48 months.[53]

Surgeon Factors. The surgeon's knowledge, judgment, experience, and technical ability are important factors with respect to the durability of a conventional total hip replacement. For individual surgeons, there is a "learning curve" that can be accelerated by working in a center focusing on optimizing technique and minimizing complications.

Prosthetic Design and Materials. The material and design of conventional total hip replacement prostheses are significant factors in mechanical failure. Collis has cited metallurgic imperfections in many fractured stems.[53] Corrosion and fatigue failure have been prominent in early stainless-steel prostheses containing a high carbon content and in cobalt-based alloys with casting defects and large grain size. The "super alloys" of today—multiphase, pressed, or forged cobalt and titanium—are stronger, so that fracture of the stem is much less likely than in the past.

Early in the era of total hip replacements, it was feared that the polyethylene socket would wear out; thus far, this has not been a significant problem. Charnley and Halley noted 0.15 mm of wear per year, which decreased after the first 5 years.[54] Beckenbaugh and Ilstrup

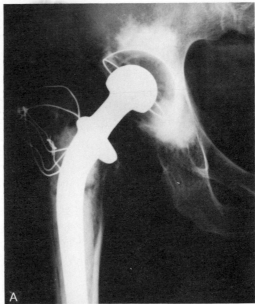

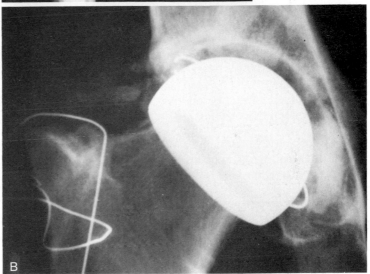

Figure 25–5. Conventional total hip replacement (*A*) is contrasted with surface total hip replacement (*B*). The former has an intramedullary stem for fixation. In the surfacing procedure, the metal cup is seated on a portion of the femoral head.

agree with our own observations that it is difficult to evaluate wear roentgenographically.[55] Rose and colleagues studied wear by an in vitro total joint simulator using cycling equivalent to 2 to 10 years of use of the Charnley-Mueller prosthesis.[56] There were dimensional changes from 0.035 to 0.1 mm per year, but wear accounted for only 1% to 30% of the dimensional changes. Some of the dimensional change appeared to be due to creep or plastic flow. However, there was 0.3 to 10.2 mg of debris particles produced per year. There was a strong correlation of wear to the polymer molecular weight; the higher the mo-

lecular weight, the less wear occurred. Metal-backed acetabular components may diminish this tendency, although it is probably not an important factor in conventional replacement sockets, which are thicker. It may be important in improving stress transfer and "wear" or deformation in thinner-walled surface replacement components.

The design of the femoral stem has evolved as a factor in loosening and stem fracture. Pellicci and associates noted that curved and diamond-shaped stems were prone to loosening.[57] Sharp edges in prostheses cause stress risers in the acrylic cement and have been one of the factors leading to loosening. It is hoped that the current improved technique of inserting larger prosthetic stems in neutral position combined with the full containment of the socket within the acetabulum will improve results. Technique is one of the major determinants of loosening. Technical concepts have been studied experimentally and have been shown to be of paramount importance. The critical techniques of improved cementation include the use of a pulsating lavage and/or mechanical cleansing with a brush, thorough drying of the canal, and the use of a bone plug 1 to 2 cm distal to the stem tip to enhance pressurization and to optimize trabecular intrusion of cement. Bone grafting is important on the acetabular side to provide full coverage for the socket component. The varus position of the femoral stem has been associated with loosening and stem fracture. Trochanteric osteotomy has been emphasized for wide exposure in order to place the femoral component in a valgus position and to optimize fixation. Although trochanteric osteotomy is routinely used by some and is necessary for revision surgery, many surgeons prefer trochanter-sparing approaches. Hypotensive anesthesia, when safely used, has reduced blood loss; less bleeding at the bone-cement interface enhances fixation.

Newer alternative techniques of fixation and design of the implants may decrease the problem of loosening in the future (see Chapter 20).

Etiologic Factors—Anatomic and Pathophysiologic. In primary osteoarthritis, bone stock and vascularity are generally good, and the results after conventional total hip replacements are usually better than in other diseases. In Gaucher's disease, for example, stem loosening may be related to progressive osteoporosis and infiltration of Gaucher cells predisposing to loosening. In congenital hip dysplasia, in which bone stock may be deficient, socket loosening has occurred frequently although bone grafting may minimize this tendency. Chandler and associates reported a higher revision rate in patients who had undergone prior cup arthroplasty.[37] The loss of bone stock in quantity and quality as a result of a prior prosthetic implant or joint replacement can be so extreme that additional reconstructive procedures may be impossible.

Sepsis. Sepsis can jeopardize an otherwise appropriately indicated and well-executed total hip replacement. The prosthesis may have to be removed, leaving the patient with a poorly functioning Girdlestone procedure; on rare occasions, systemic complications may ensue and may endanger the patient's life. The results of the infection depend on host resistance, the virulence and number of organisms, and the efficacy of treatment modalities.

Cupic reported a 4.1% incidence of infection in patients at Wrightington in the initial 409 Charnley total hip replacements.[52] Two cases occurred just after the operation, and 15 developed later, from 1 to 5 years postoperatively. Three cases required Girdlestone procedures. Coventry and associates noted deep infections in 12 hips in a series of 2012 patients at 3 months to 2 years postoperatively.[58] In our experience, risk factors for sepsis include steroid use, debilitation, prior sepsis, prior operation, postoperative urinary tract infection, and hematoma formation.

The diagnosis of an infected total hip replacement can be difficult. Discomfort and pain that never resolved postoperatively raise clinical suspicion of sepsis. The type of infection must be determined, if possible, by aspiration, culturing for both aerobic and anerobic organisms. In addition to characterizing the organism and determining the location of the source of sepsis the presence of osteomyelitis should be established. Bone scans with technetium diphosphonate are helpful, but the use of gallium scans has been disappointing in the differentiation between aseptic and septic loosening. Blood tests, including erythrocyte sedimentation rate and routine blood counts, are sometimes helpful but are not diagnostic.

Superficial infections can be controlled with thorough debridement and antibiotics. Deep infections that are promptly diagnosed may be amenable to debridement if the prosthesis is not loose. Late infections require removal of the prosthesis and debridement. If the organism is a gram-negative one or is a virulent gram-positive one, removal of the prosthesis and open packing are the preferred treatment, with secondary closure. Direct prosthesis exchange should be considered only for organisms of low virulence. Reimplantation after infection with a gram-negative organism has resulted in a high infection recurrence rate. The use of antibiotics combined with laminar airflow and personal isolator systems reduces the incidence of infection after reimplantation. In a multicenter study, Lidwell recently demonstrated the statistical advantage of isolator systems over laminar flow alone.[59]

Relative and absolute contraindications to direct joint exchange include debilitation of the patient, extensive bone loss, established osteomyelitis, previous total hip replacement infected with *Pseudomonas*, and the consideration that the results of the Girdlestone procedure may be acceptable to the patient.

Dislocation. Coventry and coworkers reported a 3% incidence of dislocation in 2012 hips; closed reduction was successful in 76% of the cases.[58] Open reduction was required in 5% of the patients, and revision of the prosthesis was necessary in 13%.[58] Pellicci and colleagues noted that dislocations were due to malposition of acetabular components in 50% of the patients; the risk of dislocation was increased with previous surgery or trochanteric nonunion.[57]

Prevention of dislocation requires correct orientation of the acetabulum and femoral component and the removal of excess bone or cement, which can cause impingement and levering out of the femoral component at extremes of motion. Distal and lateral positioning of the trochanter may assist in reducing the incidence of dislocation.

Nerve Palsy. A 15% incidence of sciatic nerve palsy and a 12% incidence of femoral nerve palsy were reported by Coventry and colleagues.[58] Electromyographic studies showed partial denervation of femoral, sciatic, and obturator nerves of all hips randomly studied subsequent to total hip replacement. In our experience at the University of California at Los Angeles (UCLA) Hospital, there has been a 2% incidence of nerve palsy that is increased in revision total hip replacement. It is believed to be due to retraction at surgery and/or lack of limb support in the lateral decubitus position when the limb is dislocated and placed over the side of the table.

Trochanteric Problems. Total hip replacement requires excellent exposure to optimize fixation and alignment. It can be performed with or without trochanteric osteotomy. The choice is dictated by the trade-offs as perceived by the surgeon. The advantages of trochanteric osteotomy include improved exposure, less injury to the abductor muscles, tightening of muscles, and, theoretically, improved biomechanics associated with transplanting the trochanter distally and laterally. The major disadvantages are nonunion and migration of the trochanter. Durable fixation is dependent on the type and quality of technique.

Total hip arthroplasty without trochanteric osteotomy is said to reduce total blood loss, shorten the operating time, and ease rehabilitation. Its disadvantage is that it provides less than optimal exposure, especially in obese patients and in revision procedures.

The risk factors for avulsion of the trochanter include osteoporosis, previous surgery (especially total hip replacement), a small trochanteric osteotomy, apposition to an acrylic bed rather than to bone, poor wiring technique, and noncompliance on the part of the patient. The use of two vertical wires is recommended in high-risk patients. Occasionally wire mesh and a protracted rehabilitation program are required.

Heterotopic Bone. Coventry and Scanlon reported that radiation therapy administered after operation to those at high risk for ectopic bone prevented massive ectopic bone formation.[60] Patients at risk included those with active ankylosing spondylitis and those with secondary OA after fracture-dislocations of the hip. Radiation-induced sarcoma does not appear to be a hazard with the doses of radiation utilized.

In a multicenter study, Finerman and associates reported that etidronate disodium, a diphosphonate, in a dose of 20 mg/kg/day given for 2 weeks before and for 3 months after surgery lowered the incidence and amount of heterotopic bone in high-risk patients, including those with contralateral ectopic bone from previous surgery, osteoarthritis, old slipped capital femoral epiphysis, and ankylosing spondylitis.[61] This is the current dosage and schedule. The main side effect is diarrhea.

General Complications. Medical complications have been reported in 25% of patients who have undergone total hip replacement.[58] These include myocardial infarction, renal failure, urinary tract infection, cardiac failure, pneumonitis and atelectasis, thrombophlebitis, gastrointestinal disturbance, and death. Careful preoperative medical evaluation and stabilization are important to prevent complications.

Thrombophlebitis and pulmonary embolism are life-threatening conditions. Warfarin sodium has proved to be the most effective preventive agent, but careful regulation of prothrombin time at 1.5 to 2.0 times control is essential to prevent bleeding complications. Aspirin, 600 mg twice a day for males, and dextran are also beneficial, but subcutaneous heparin has not been an effective prophylactic. Dextran has potential problems of fluid overload and anaphylaxis.[62] Once a pulmonary embolism or thrombophlebitis has been documented, intravenous heparin followed by warfarin sodium is recommended.

The risk of hepatitis is decreased significantly by using autologous blood that has been stored several weeks before surgery. Coventry and associates reported a 0.4% mortality rate in the perioperative period.[58] At UCLA Hospital, no deaths have occurred during the immediate postoperative period in more than 2000 cases.

Revision Total Hip Arthroplasty. Pellicci and coworkers reviewed the results of revision total hip arthroplasty in 107 patients who underwent 110 revisions at from 2 to 8.7 years' follow-up.[35] Two deep infections developed, and there were 15 mechanical failures, which required an additional six revisions. It was concluded that the incidence of significant complications was higher than in the original surgery, with doubling of the infection rate. Trochanteric problems occurred in 13% of the patients, three times the usual incidence. Loosening occurred in 5.4%, two to three times more than with the primary surgery, and 8.2% needed reoperation.

Our UCLA Hospital series includes 66 patients who underwent revision of acrylic-fixed conventional total hip replacement for suspected loosening without sepsis. The primary diagnosis included a higher percentage of patients with congenital hip dysplasia and post-traumatic osteoarthritis than in the overall series.[32] The failure rate was lower in patients with rheumatoid arthritis. The average age at revision was 52 years, and there was an equal number of male and female patients. In 51 of the 66 patients, the initial total hip replacement had been performed at another hospital. The average time to the revision surgery was 4 years after the initial surgery, and follow-up averaged 2.1 years. Pain relief, walking ability, and function were less than in the group of patients who had undergone primary replacements, and the flexion arc was also less. Although there have been no fatalities at UCLA Hospital and systemic complications have been no greater, there was a high complication rate due to other causes following the revision. These included a 7.5% incidence of peroneal nerve palsy, seven dislocations (10.6%) (one requiring component change), and one loose acetabular component, and 7.5% of the patients had migration of the trochanter. A high rate of femoral bone fracture (6%) was noted. The majority of patients with dislocations and subluxations had undergone prior surgery. Longer operating time, increased bood loss, and higher complication rates have been universally described in the literature in these cases.[34, 35] There was a high correlation between loosening and bone stock deficiency at UCLA Hospital, with a 9% revision rate over an average of 2 years of follow-up. Roentgenographic analysis revealed 29% femoral and acetabular loosening, defined by 100% lucency around the components and a width of lucency greater than or equal to 2 mm for the acetabular component and greater than or equal to 1 mm for the femoral component. The recent use of bigger stems and special sockets, assuring proper muscular tension and more normal biomechanics, has improved results.

Conversion of Hemiarthroplasty to Conventional Total Hip Replacement. Amstutz and Smith reported on 41 patients who underwent total hip replacement following failed femoral hemiarthroplasty.[63] Although there was notable relief of pain and increased range of motion, three patients required revisions at 55 to 66 months after surgery because of a loosened symptomatic femoral component resulting from failure to remove all of the fibrous membrane at the time of conversion. Five patients had intraoperative fractures of the proximal femur, and an additional 14.6% have had progressive roentgenographic loosening. Improved techniques using wide stems to fill the proximal femur and enhanced cementation have greatly improved the postoperative results.

Conversion of Arthrodesis to Conventional Total Hip Replacement. The indications for conversion of an arthrodesis to a total hip replacement include pain in the hip, knee, or, especially, the low back. Amstutz and Sakai reported effective relief but limited range of motion, depending on duration of ankylosis.[36] Functional results varied. The investigators stressed preoperative assessment of abductors and postoperative rehabilitation of this muscle group, medialization of the acetabulum, and use of a long-neck prosthesis that has a small, straight stem with good inherent stability.

Conversion of the Girdlestone Procedure to Conventional Total Hip Replacement. Although many Girdlestone procedures have been performed because of bone stock deficiency, primarily of the acetabulum, most resection arthroplasties have followed deep infection.[64] In patients with unstable, painful Girdlestone resections, it is possible to use a bone graft for inadequate bone stock and to perform a conventional total hip replacement, although there is increased risk of loosening and sepsis. Pain, instability, and leg-length inequality are improved after the procedure.

Hip Resurfacing. Hip resurfacing offered the hope of improved durability, as well as providing a replacement that would save bone stock for an anticipated revision or, if necessary, conversion to conventional total hip replacement (see Fig. 25–5B). The initial clinical results from other centers were uniformly promising, but unfortunately, these have been followed by reports of a progressive incidence of loosening and neck fracture.

Trentani and Vaccarino recently reported a 46% failure rate in 60 hips followed for 4 to 8 years.[65] The early Eicher (Indiana Conservative Hip)[15] and Freeman (ICLH)[16] series each reported a 45% failure rate with their initial clinical trials that were followed for 2 to 5 years. Even with his subsequent technique and design changes, Freeman noted a 35% failure rate in patients who were an average of 58 years old at operation and who were followed for 3 to 6 years. Although improvements in technique were made with the Indiana Hip, as performed by Capello and Trancik,[15] 27% failed in patients averaging 49 years of age at 3 to 6 years after surgery. Both reported high failure rates in the not-too-well-defined entity known as "inflammatory arthritis."

Wagner has not presented recent detailed statistics of his long-term patients but has reported a failure rate of 29% in inflammatory arthritis and now utilizes a ceramic femoral component exclusively.[17] Recently, Head reported a 30% failure rate due to loosening, fracture, and necrosis in 41 patients followed for 1 to 4 years after using the Wagner prosthesis.[66]

The TARA prosthesis, which has a short, curved stem, is now undergoing clinical trials. This prosthesis is not a true surface replacement because the stem enters the intramedullary canal. Townley has reported a 3.4% failure rate due to loosening in patients who predominantly had osteoarthritis at an average age of 58 years with a relatively short follow-up of only 19 months.[67]

In view of all the statistical bad news and the large number of changes that have been instituted in most reports, it seems appropriate to question the future of resurfacing. We believe most affirmatively that the concept is sound and that the current THARIES resurfacing technique can produce quality and durable results but that age and patient selection are important criteria.

Of the more than 500 THARIES replacements that have been performed at UCLA Hospital, 300 have had a follow-up of 2 to 6.5 years.[68] The first series of 100 patients included 31% with osteoarthritis, 19% with osteonecrosis, 16% with dysplasia, 15% with rheumatoid arthritis and spondylitis, 8% with slipped capital femoral epiphysis, and 11% with miscellaneous other diagnoses. The average age of the patients was 40.7 years, and males predominated. The second and third series of 100 each have progressively more patients with osteoarthritis and fewer with dysplasia and slipped capital femoral epiphysis. The clinical results in terms of pain, walking, function, range of motion, and heterotopic bone formation are not statistically different from those of our conventional replacements. The incidence of sepsis (0.7%), dislocation (0.7%), and systemic complications has been less than in our conventional total hip replacements. There have been two neck fractures. There has been a 1.5% incidence of trochanteric migration, and 2% have required wire removal. The incidence of heterotopic bone and nerve palsy has been comparable to that seen in conventional replacement. Aseptic loosening occurred in 20 (6.6%), including a 10% incidence in the first 100, 8% in the second 100, and 2% in the third 100. The average age of patients whose prostheses loosened was 37 years, with a high incidence in nontraumatic osteonecrosis (17%) and in dysplasias (17.2%). There were no loose prostheses in patients with post-traumatic necrosis or rheumatoid arthritis, and the incidence of loosening was only 1% in patients with osteoarthritis. Poor technique, inadequate case selection, and high activity levels account for most failures. Component, instrumentation, and technical improvements have considerably improved the short-term roentgenographic results. The improved fixation techniques that have evolved include recessing the socket within the acetabular margins to prevent impingement, removal of excess cement, emphasis on full and properly oriented seating of the femoral component in neutral or slight valgus position, and measures to optimize cement interdigitation. Hypotensive anesthesia is used when the patient has no cardiovascular, cerebral, or renal problems in order to decrease bleeding and improve drying of the field. Pressurization techniques are used to achieve optimal cement intrusion, and spacers are utilized to avoid a thin cement layer, which can crack. Timing is important because the acrylic should be used when it is not too viscous. Pulsating lavage removes debris and blood and improves fixation. Spinning the femoral shell in the acetabular component lubricated with blood is done before introduction of the component into the prepared bed in order to detect any abnormal frictional torque. The proper use of THARIES instruments helps to avoid notching of the neck. Protected weight bearing allows the hip tissues to adapt to new material and protects the interface until tissues mature. The lateral extracapsular trochanteric osteotomy approach permits optimal exposure. The trochanteric piece should not be too large, because it could lead to vascular insult of the head and increase the chance of notching the neck.

There are special technical points specific to using this procedure for different diseases. In avascular necrosis, as much necrotic bone should be removed as possible. Surfacing can be done if a third of the volume of the head is maintained. If there is still remaining necrotic bone, it should be drilled with a fine drill to enhance fixation and healing. In acetabular dysplasia, bone grafting may be necessary to assure adequate coverage of the socket. The technique is demanding, with a significant learning curve, but it can produce durable results. The potential causes of complications after resurfacing are similar to those having had high rates with conventional replacement. There is and will continue to be a need to improve long-term interface durability to minimize and, we hope, eliminate loosening. We are encouraged by our experimental results using porous implants to obtain fixation, although we do not believe that the ultimate in materials and technique has been achieved when employing acrylic as the interface material; our currrent protocol includes thicker shells of polyethylene and acrylic. Although metal backing of the socket may help distribute stress, space is at a premium, and sacrifice of additional bone stock to accommodate the increased thickness must be evaluated carefully.

The advantages of surface replacement are considerable: excellent stability, low sepsis, minimal systemic complications, and less blood loss. Especially attractive are the ease of femoral revision and the quality of the available options. We agree that there is concern regarding excessive sacrifice of acetabular bone stock, which has made acetabular revision as difficult as or more difficult than conventional replacement. This problem can be minimized by utilizing the smallest-size femoral component without violating the femoral neck.

There is no doubt that the best time for optimizing fixation is at the initial surgery, when maximal trabecular bone can be exposed by reaming. We do, however, recommend that the hip be protected from excess stress during the postoperative period. The length of protection or the degree to which the surgeon and patient should strive to achieve this goal has not yet been precisely defined.

From our perspective, neither resurfacing nor conventional replacement is recommended for patients younger than 40 years old unless the patient has built-in physical restraint, because lifetime durability cannot be achieved for such patients at this time.

Based on very low dislocation and sepsis rates and easier revision, our own confidence has increased with resurfacing, so that we are applying it to older patients. We believe that resurfacing will become a permanent part of our orthopedic armamentarium. Moreover, it is our opinion that conventional replacement should not be used in youthful patients who have sufficient bone stock to be resurfaced. We believe that time spent in developing facility with use of this procedure is well worth the effort for those who have large numbers of patients with osteoarthritic hips.

Decision-Making Algorithm

The choice of a specific surgical procedure for an osteoarthritic hip in a given patient must be based on adequate information. This information has been processed in the form of prognostic factors bearing on the likelihood of clinical and surgical success, immediate and long-term, and the prognosis for failure and complications. Although the literature review data are pertinent, each patient and clinical setting is unique, and decisions cannot be made with a cookbook formula. The risk-benefit ratio must be defined for each procedure for the patient, based on clinical needs, durability and complications. Then, it is possible to utilize the surgical flow-diagram at the proper entry point, with an awareness of all adverse sequelae (see Fig. 25–2).

References

1. Byers PD, Contemponi CA, Farkas TA: A postmortem study of the hip joint. Ann Rheum Dis 29:15, 1970.
2. Bullough P, Goodfellow J: The relationship between degenerative changes and load-bearing in the human hip. J Bone Joint Surg 55B:746–758, 1973.
3. Weightman B: In vitro fatigue testing of articular cartilage. Ann Rheum Dis 34(Suppl 2):108–110, 1975.

4. Bonner WM, Jonsson H, Malanos C, Bryant M: Changes in the lipids of human articular cartilage with age. Arthritis Rheum 18:461, 1975.
5. Vignon E, Arlot M, Menunler P, Vignon G: Histological changes in osteoarthrotic femoral head cartilage. Ann Rheum Dis 34(Suppl 2):134, 1975.
6. Anderson CE, Ludowieg J, Harper HA, Engleman EP: The composition of the organic component of human articular cartilage. J Bone Joint Surg 46A:1176, 1964.
7. Linn FC, Sokoloff L: Movement and composition of interstitial fluid of cartilage. Arthritis Rheum 8:481, 1965.
8. Johnson LC: Kinetics of osteoarthritis. Lab Invest 8:1223, 1956.
9. Freeman MAR: Adult Articular Cartilage. Tunbridge Wells, Pitman Medical Publishing Co., 1973.
10. Pugh JW, Radin EL, Rose RM: Quantitative studies of human subchondral cancellous bone; its relationship to the state of its overlying cartilage. J Bone Joint Surg 56A:313–321, 1974.
11. Harrison MHM, Schajowicz F, Trueta J: Osteoarthritis of the hip: A study of the nature and evolution of the disease. J Bone Joint Surg 35B:598–626, 1953.
12. Kempson GE, Spivey CJ, Swanson SAV, Freeman MAR: Patterns of cartilage stiffness on normal and degenerative human femoral heads. J Biomech 4:597–609, 1971.
13. Enneking WF, Horowitz M: The intra-articular effects of immobilization on the human knee. J Bone Joint Surg 55A:973, 1972.
14. Cameron HU, Macnab I: Observations on osteoarthritis of the hip joint. Clin Orthop 100:31–40, 1975.
15. Capello WN, Trancik TM: Indiana Conservative Hip: Results, 2–4½ years. AOA Second Annual International Symposium, Boston, May 1981.
16. Freeman MAR: ICLH surface replacement: Frontiers in total hip replacement. AOA Second Annual International Symposium, Boston, May 1981.
17. Wagner H: Cemented surface replacement in the hip joint. AOA Second Annual International Symposium, Boston, May 1981.
18. Mankin HJ, Lippiello L: Biochemical and metabolic abnormalities in articular cartilage from osteoarthritic human hips. J Bone Joint Surg 52A:424–434, 1970.
19. Mankin HJ, Lippiello L: The glycosaminoglycans of normal and arthritic cartilage. J Clin Invest 50:1712–1719, 1971.
20. Blount WP: Osteotomy in the treatment of osteoarthritis of the hip. Clin Orthop 141:28–43, 1979.
21. Harris NH, Kirwan E: The results of osteotomy for early primary osteoarthritis of the hip. J Bone Joint Surg 46B:477–487, 1964.
22. Nissen KI: The arrest of early primary osteoarthritis of the hip by osteotomy. Proc R Soc Med 56:1051–1060, 1963.
23. Radin EL, Paul IL: Does cartilage compliance reduce skeletal impact loads? The relative fore-attenuating properties of articular cartilage, synovial fluid, periarticular soft tissues and bone. Arthritis Rheum 13:139, 1970.
24. Radin EL, Paul IL: Response of joints to impact loading. I. In vitro wear. Arthritis Rheum 14:356, 1971.
25. Smith RW, Rizek J: Epidemiologic studies of osteoporosis in women of Puerto Rico and Southeastern Michigan with special reference to age, race, national origin, and other related or associated findings. Clin Orthop 45:31, 1966.
26. Arnoldi CE, Linderholm H, Mussbichler H: Venous engorgement and intraosseous hypertension in osteoarthritis of the hip. J Bone Joint Surg 54B:409–421, 1972.
27. Lloyd-Roberts GC: The role of capsular changes in osteoarthritis of the hip joint. J Bone Joint Surg 35B:627–642, 1953.
28. Phillips RS, Bulmer JH, Hoyle G, Davies W: Venous drainage in osteoarthritis of the hip. J Bone Joint Surg 49B:301–309, 1967.
28a. Lawrence JS, Bremner JM, Bier F: Osteo-arthrosis: Prevalence in the population and relationship between symptoms and x-ray changes. Ann Rheum Dis 25:1–24, 1966.
29. Denham P-A: Hip mechanics. J Bone Joint Surg 418:550, 1959.
30. Blount WP: Don't throw away the cane. J Bone Joint Surg 38A:695–708, 1956.
31. Pauwels F: Der Schenkelschruch: Ein mechanisches Problem. Stuttgart, Ferdinand Enke, 1953.
32. Amstutz HC, Ma SM, Jinnah RH, Mai L: Revisions of aseptic loose total hip replacements. Unpublished data.
33. Eftekhar NS, Smith DM, Henry JH, Stinchfield FE: Revision arthroplasty using the Charnley low friction arthroplasty technique. Clin Orthop 95:48–59, 1973.
34. Hunter GA, Welsh RP, Cameron JU, Bailey WH: The results of revision of total hip arthroplasty. J Bone Joint Surg 51B:419–421, 1979.
35. Pellicci PM, Wilson PD Jr, Sledge CB, et al.: Results of revision total hip replacement. In The Hip Society: The Hip: Proceedings of the Ninth Open Scientific Meeting of the Hip Society. St. Louis, C.V. Mosby Co., 1981.
36. Amstutz HC, Sakai DN: Total joint replacement of ankylosed hips. Indications, technique and preliminary results. J Bone Joint Surg 57A:619, 1975.
37. Chandler HP, Reineck FT, Wixson RL, McCarthy JC: Total hip replacement in patients younger than thirty years old: A five year follow-up study. J Bone Joint Surg 63A:1426–1434, 1981.
38. Smith-Petersen MN: Evolution of mold arthroplasty of the hip joint. J Bone Joint Surg 30B:59–75, 1948.
39. Aufranc OE: Constructive hip surgery with the Vitallium mold: A report on 1,111 cases of arthroplasty of the hip over a fifteen-year period. J Bone Joint Surg 39A:237–248, 1957.
40. Johnson RC, Larson CB: Results of treatment of hip disorders with cup arthroplasty. J Bone Joint Surg 51A:1461–1479, 1969.
41. Bombelli R: Osteoarthritis of the Hip: Pathogenesis and Consequent Therapy. Berlin, Springer-Verlag, 1976.
42. Sugioka Y: Transtrochanteric anterior rotational osteotomy of the femoral head in the treatment of osteonecrosis affecting the hip: A new osteotomy. Clin Orthop 130:191, 1978.
43. Morscher EW: Intertrochanteric osteotomy in osteoarthritis of the hip. In The Hip Society: The Hip: Proceedings of the Eighth Open Scientific Meeting of the Hip Society. St. Louis, C.V. Mosby Co., 1980.
44. Salter, RB: Innominate osteotomy in the treatment of congenital dislocation and subluxation of the hip. J Bone Joint Surg., 43B:518, 1961.
45. Moore AT: The self-locking metal hip prosthesis. J Bone Joint Surg 39A:811–817, 1957.
46. Thompson FR: Two and a half years experience with a Vitallium intramedullary hip prosthesis. J Bone Joint Surg 36A:489–502, 1954.

47. Anderson LD, Hamson WR, Waring TL: Femoral-head prosthesis: A review of three hundred and fifty-six operations and their results. J Bone Joint Surg 46A:1049–1065, 1964.

48. Salvati EA, Wilson PD Jr: Long-term results of femoral head replacement. J Bone Joint Surg 55A:516–524, 1973.

49. Drinker H, Murray WR: The universal proximal femoral endoprosthesis. J Bone Joint Surg 61A:1167–1174, 1979.

50. Lipscomb PR, McCaslin FE Jr: Arthrodesis of the hip: Review of 371 cases. J Bone Joint Surg 43A:923, 1961.

51. Muller ME, Allgower M, Willenegger H: Manual of Internal Fixation. Berlin, Springer-Verlag, 1970, p. 282.

52. Cupic Z: Long-term follow-up of Charnley arthroplasty of the hip. Clin Orthop 141:28–43, 1979.

53. Collis DK: Femoral stem failure in total hip replacement. J Bone Joint Surg 59A:1022–1041, 1977.

54. Charnley J, Halley DK: Rate of wear in total hip replacement. Clin Orthop 112:170–179, 1975.

55. Beckenbaugh RD, Ilstrup DM: Total hip arthroplasty. A review of three hundred and thirty-three cases with long-term follow-up. J Bone Joint Surg 60A:306–313, 1978.

56. Rose RM, Nusbaum MJ, Schneider II, ct al.: On the true wear rate of ultra-high-molecular-weight polyethylene in the total hip prosthesis. J Bone Joint Surg 62A:537, 1980.

57. Pellicci PM, Salvati EA, Robinson HJ: Mechanical failure in total hip replacement requiring reoperation. J Bone Joint Surg 61A:28–37, 1979.

58. Coventry MB, Beckenbaugh RD, Nolan DR, et al.: 2,012 total hip arthroplasties: A study of postoperative course and early complications. J Bone Joint Surg 56A:273–284, 1974.

59. Lidwell OM: Infections following orthopaedic surgery in conventional and unidirectional air flow operating theaters: The results of a prospective randomized study. Presented at the Scientific Program of the 49th Annual Meeting of AAPS, New Orleans, 1982.

60. Coventry MB, Scanlon PW: The use of radiation to discourage ectopic bone. J Bone Joint Surg 63A:201–208, 1981.

61. Finerman GAM, Krengel WF Jr, Lowell JD, et al.: Role of diphosphonate (EHDP) in the prevention of heterotopic ossification after total hip arthroplasty: A preliminary report. In The Hip Society: The Hip: Proceedings of the Fifth Open Scientific Meeting of the Hip Society. St. Louis, C.V. Mosby Co., 1977, pp. 222–234.

62. Harris WH, Athanasoulis CA, Waltman AC, Salzman EW: High- and low-dose aspirin prophylaxis against venous thromboembolic disease in total hip replacement. J Bone Joint Surg 62A:63–66, 1982.

63. Amstutz HC, Smith RK: Total hip replacement following failed femoral hemiarthroplasty. J Bone Joint Surg 61A:1161–1166, 1979.

64. Girdlestone GR: Discussion on treatment of unilateral osteoarthritis of the hip joint. Proc R Soc Med 38:363, 1945.

65. Trentani C, Vaccarino F: Italian experience: Resurface arthroplasty utilizing the Paltrinieri-Trentani resurface arthroplasty. Eight-year assessment. AOA Second Annual International Symposium, Boston, May 1981.

66. Head WC: Wagner surface replacement arthroplasty of the hip. J Bone Joint Surg 63A:420–427, 1981.

67. Townley CO: Conservative total articular replacement arthroplasty with the fixed femoral cup. Presented at AAOS 48th Annual Meeting, Las Vegas, Nevada, February 1981.

68. Amstutz HC, Kim WC, Thomas BJ, Mai LL: THARIES: 2–6½ year result. In The Hip Society: The Hip: Proceedings of the Eleventh Open Scientific Meeting of the Hip Society. St. Louis, C.V. Mosby Co., 1982. (Unpublished.)

26

Osteoarthritis of the Cervical Spine

Henry H. Bohlman, M.D.

The cause of osteoarthritis (degenerative joint disease) of the cervical spine is not totally understood; however, many factors are probably involved in this life-long process.[1–6] Osteoarthritis of the cervical spine affects all of the major spinal articulations, including the intervertebral disks, the apophyseal joints, the ligamentous connections between the vertebrae, and the vertebral bodies themselves. Some use the term spondylosis to describe degenerative changes that involve the intervertebral disks and vertebral bodies, in contrast to degenerative changes of the apophyseal joints, which are classified as true osteoarthritis because the roentgenologic changes more closely resemble those seen in other diarthrodial joints. Osteophyte spur formation on the vertebral bodies is prominent, most frequently seen at the anterior aspect of the vertebrae. Apophyseal joint involvement characteristically exhibits joint space narrowing, bony sclerosis, and spur formation.

Factors associated with the etiology of osteoarthritis of the spine include aging, trauma, and congenital fractures, as well as biochemical changes. The chondrocytes that are damaged release proteolytic and collagenolytic enzymes that degrade the cartilage matrix. The cartilage breakdown is followed by a repair process with chondrocyte proliferation and, ultimately, osteochondrophyte spur formation in the cervical spine. The pathophysiologic alterations of the intervertebral disk have been studied through various stages of life.[1, 7, 8] Aging of the intervertebral disk results in dehydration and cracking with loss of elasticity of the disk and surrounding ligaments. Fissures occur in the cartilage and plates that ultimately extend into the annulus fibrosus.[7, 9, 10] Once dehydration has occurred, clefts form in the disk. The disk space collapses, producing the narrowing seen on roentgenograms.[11, 12] Narrowing of the disk space then affects the biomechanics of the vertebral segment, producing bulging of the annulus fibrosus anteriorly, posteriorly, and laterally.[13] Cartilage joint surfaces are resorbed, microfractures may occur, and adjacent bony trabeculae become thickened; osteochondrophyte spurs form at the site of ligament insertions to bone. The intervertebral disk may then herniate into the spinal canal through the annulus fibrosus or remain protruding between the posterior longitudinal ligament and the vertebral body.[8] The uncovertebral joints are affected by the degenerative disease process whereby osteophytes grow by the process of enchondral ossification. The apophyseal joints are affected by the same pathologic process that affects other peripheral joints with osteoarthritic disease. Fibrillation of the articular cartilage occurs with loss of joint surface, osteophytes form, and the subchondral bone becomes sclerotic. With progressive osteoarthrosis of the cervical spine, there may be segments of the spine that become more mobile, while others, usually the lower cervical spine, become increasingly stiffer with passage of time.

Early in osteoarthritis of the cervical spine, single segments of the spine may be affected. However, during later decades of life, the fifth, sixth, and seventh cervical segments are frequently involved, producing a less mobile lower cervical spine and a hypermobile upper cervical spine. In addition, it is more common to have zygoapophyseal joints affected in the upper cervical spine between the third, fourth, and fifth cervical levels.

Nerve fibers have been demonstrated in the annulus of the intervertebral disk, in facet joint capsules, and in the longitudinal ligaments of the cervical spine, explaining some sources for pain as a result of degenerative change in the spine.[14, 15] Other authors have pointed out that degenerative change of the cervical spine is very common after 40 years of age and affects at least 70% of individuals over 70 years of age.[4, 11] The end result of the progressive osteoarthritic process includes ankylosis, narrowing of the spinal canal and neural foramina, and, rarely, vertebral artery compression (Fig. 26–1). The roentgenologic appearance of a degenerative cervical spine, however, may not be related to the clinical symptoms.[11] The major complaint of the patient with cervical osteoarthritis may be neck pain, pain in the upper extremities related to compression of involved roots, or motor weakness; all findings may be present.

SYMPTOMS AND SIGNS

The etiology of pain in degenerative disk and joint disease of the cervical spine is less well defined than in the neural compression syndromes secondary to a herniated cervical disk. There is a general misconception that all neck pain originates from neural compression. Any disease that affects the peripheral joints of the musculoskeletal system also may involve the cervical spine to produce pain.[16–19] Basically, the mechanisms that produce neck pain as a result of degenerative osteoarthritis of the cervical spine are direct external compression of the nerve roots or spinal cord, degenerative disk or joint disease itself, intrinsic osseous or ligamentous lesions, and abnormal motion or instability in a segment of the cervical spine. The pain syndrome may be primarily in the cervical spine or may radiate distally to the shoulder and arm as a result of direct neural

compression. Pain may also result from stimulation of deep somatic nerve endings found in the joints and the outer layers of the disk or longitudinal ligaments. Pain originating from the deep somatic nerve endings of the joints, bone, or disk will produce interscapular pain, with aching in the arm or forearm; this is often associated with generalized paresthesias of the hand.[14] Neck pain may be more specific and dermatomal in distribution, following a particular nerve root path. Abnormal motion or compression of the soft tissue structures may stimulate the C nerve fibers, producing a somatic pain syndrome whereby the pain is referred to other sites, such as the shoulder or arm. In addition, bone itself has innervations that travel with the vascular supply; therefore, it can be postulated that abnormal motions or distortion at the osseous structures can produce pain.[20, 21]

Pain from degenerative disk disease may radiate to the occiput, shoulder, interscapular area, and arm (Fig. 26–2). Generally, higher-level cervical spine pathology causes pain radiation into the upper scapular area, whereas lower-level cervical disk disease is more likely to cause pain that radiates distally into the arm. The patient may complain of subjective paresthesias without an absolute dermatomal pattern. Often, the patient will volunteer that lying down and resting the neck relieve the pain from cervical osteoarthritis.

Rarely, pain may be produced as a result of degenerative osteoarthritis of the upper cervical spine involving the atlanto-occipital and atlantoaxial joints. Roentgenologic findings in osteoarthritis of the atlantoaxial joint include narrowing of the joint space with loss of articular cartilage, marginal cortical thickening, and osteophyte formation. Disease involvement may include the lateral atlantoaxial joint, the articulation of the atlas with the odontoid, or mixed findings. Patients complain of occipital pain, shoulder stiffness, and finger paresthesias.

Early in the process of osteoarthritis of the cervical spine, the most common cause of pain is direct neural compression secondary to a laterally herniated degenerate cervical vertebral disk. Ordinarily, cervical disks herniate without previous trauma; the patient may awaken with severe neck and arm pain with associated paresthesias in a specific dermatome. With compression of a nerve root, both sensory and motor abnormalities occur. A less common cause of neck and arm pain is the centrally herniated disk, which may produce

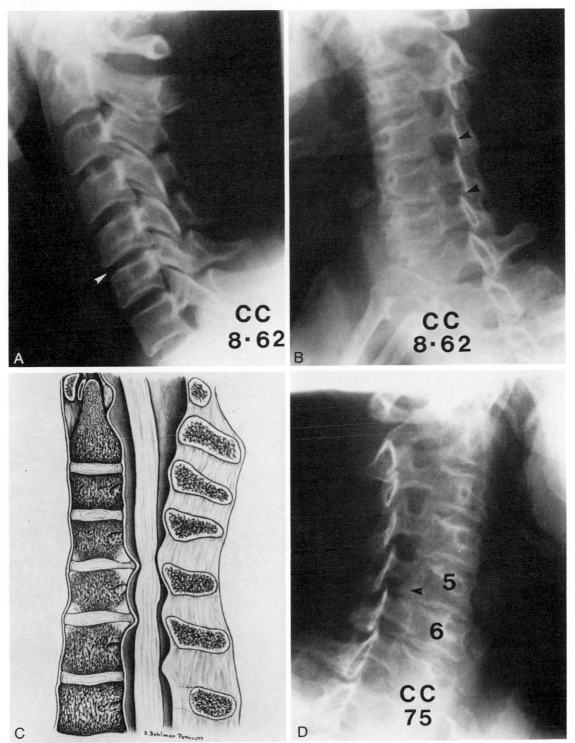

Figure 26–1. *A,* Lateral roentgenogram of a 52-year-old female presenting with neck and left shoulder pain in August 1962. There is minimal disk space narrowing at C5–C6 (arrow). *B,* Note that there is very little foraminal encroachment in the oblique roentgenogram (arrows). *C,* A diagrammatic illustration of a cervical spondylotic spine illustrating a narrow canal, decreased height of the disk spaces, posterior osteophytes, and disk protrusions with a buckled posterior longitudinal ligament and ligamentum flavum. (From Bohlman HH: Cervical spondylosis with moderate to severe myelopathy: A report of seventeen cases treated by Robinson anterior cervical discectomy and fusion. Spine 2:151–162, 1977.) *D,* Oblique roentgenogram revealing a large osteophyte, and osteochondrophyte spur formation in the foramen between the fifth and sixth cervical vertebrae (arrow).

Illustration continued on following page.

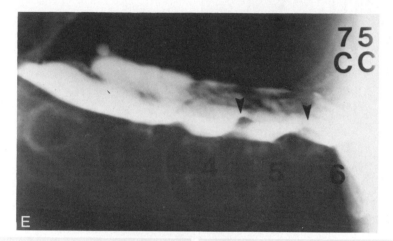

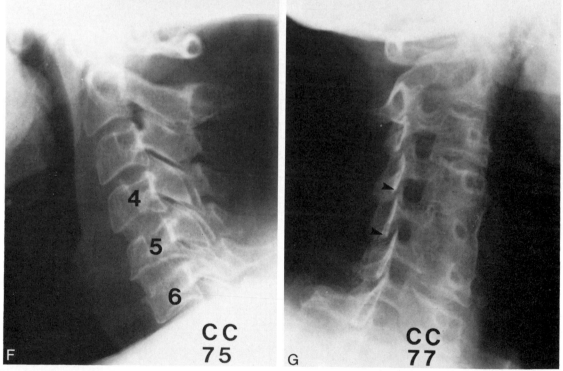

Figure 26–1 *(Continued)*. *E,* Lateral view of the myelogram revealing disk and osteophyte protrusions at C4–C5 and C5–C6 (arrows). *F,* Lateral roentgenogram taken 2 months after Robinson anterior cervical diskectomy and fusions at C4–C5 and C5–C6. Note the distracting bone blocks and the intentional lack of removal of posterior osteophytes. The patient was relieved of her neck and shoulder pain at this point in time. *G,* Oblique roentgenogram 2 years after surgery revealing total resorption of osteophytes in the foramina of C4–C5 and C5–C6 secondary to the normal process of bone remodeling (arrows).

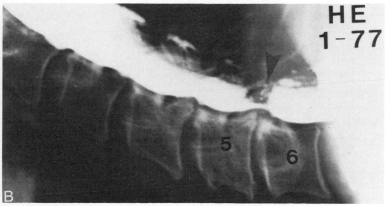

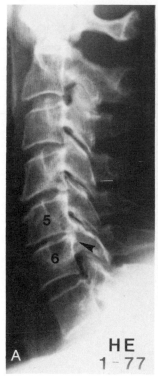

Figure 26–2. *A,* Lateral roentgenogram of a 50-year-old man with cervical spondylosis resulting in neck and right arm pain. Note the narrowing of the C4–C5 and C5–6 disk spaces with posterior osteophyte formation at C5–C6 (arrow). There was no neurologic deficit on examination. *B,* Lateral view of the cervical myelogram revealing anterior indentation of the dye column at C5–C6 (arrow). The patient underwent anterior cervical diskectomy and fusion without removal of osteophytes and was relieved of his neck and arm pain. (From Bohlman HH: Neck pain. *In* Nickel V (ed.): Orthopedic Rehabilitation. New York, Churchill Livingstone, 1982, pp. 467–480.)

anterior spinal cord compression with myelopathy and radiculopathy. A congenitally narrowed cervical spinal canal (13 mm sagittal diameter) is often associated with spinal cord or root compromise in conjunction with a herniated disk.[22–25] In addition, direct neural compression may be aggravated by the pre-existing formation of osteochondrophyte spurs of the cervical spine at the posterolateral joints of Luschka.[23, 26] Soft disk herniations generally occur in the second, third, or fourth decade of life, prior to the onset of severe osteoarthritis. The reason for this is that in younger individuals, the cervical disk has not become totally dehydrated and degenerate; there still is some cartilaginous material that can extrude. In older individuals with more severe osteoarthritis, the disk material is hard and is unable to protrude, and in addition, there is less mobility of the cervical spine. In the patient with a herniated soft cervical disk and mild osteoarthritis, there will generally be very minimal foraminal encroachment by osteochondrophyte spurs, which can be demonstrated on oblique roentgenograms (Fig. 26–3).

Upper motor neuron and other long tract signs may be observed if large posterior spurs or protuded disks compress the spinal cord. Although it is not common, compression of

the anterior spinal cord may result in an anterior cord syndrome. Further compromise of blood supply to the brain may occur if large spurs compress the vertebral arteries as they course upward through foramina to the brain. Symptoms of basilar artery insufficiency may be simulated. Specifically, dizziness, vertigo, and headaches are frequent complaints. Visual symptoms may include blurred vision, diplopia, scotomata, and field defects. Ataxia may be observed in association with nystagmus. Symptoms of vascular compression by cervical osteoarthritis are frequently intermittent, described as attacks by the patient. Loss of leg strength may be abrupt. Postural neck changes that result in compression of vertebral arteries by osteophytes may result in acute exacerbations. Neurologic symptoms must be differentiated from those seen in patients with multiple sclerosis, progressive spinal atrophy, amyotrophic lateral sclerosis, syringomyelia, and spinal cord tumors.

Physical examination of the patient will reveal significant pain with hyperextension of the cervical spine, which produces increased bulging of the herniated disk and further compression of the neural structures. Extension of the neck with lateral rotation may produce a lateral nerve root compression and radicular pain

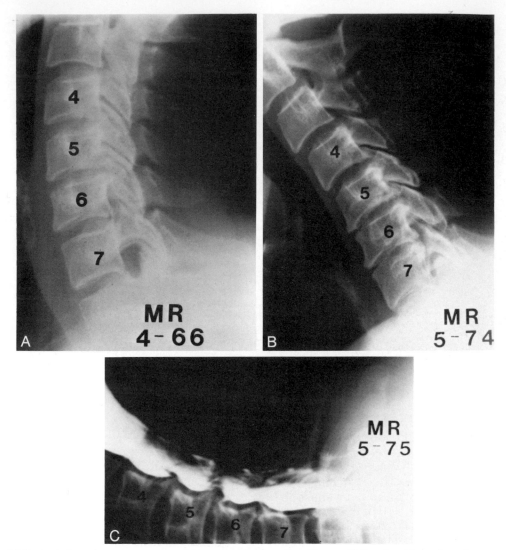

Figure 26–3. *A,* A lateral roentgenogram of the cervical spine of a 40-year-old female with neck and arm pain and radiculopathy presenting in April 1966. Note the slight narrowing at C5–C6 with very slight posterior osteophyte formation. The patient was treated without surgery, with a soft collar and analgesics resolving her symptoms. *B,* Lateral roentgenogram of the same patient 8 years following the initial bout of neck pain, demonstrating progressive narrowing and osteophyte formation at C4–C5, C5–C6, and C6–C7. The radiculopathy had recurred. *C,* Lateral view of the cervical myelogram demonstrating disk protrusions and osteophyte formation, anteriorly indenting the spinal cord at C4–C5, C5–C6, and C6–C7. (From Bohlman HH: Cervical spondylosis with moderate to severe myelopathy: A report of seventeen cases treated by Robinson anterior cervical discectomy and fusion. Spine 2:151–162, 1977.)

Illustration continued on opposite page.

radiating into the shoulder, arm, or fingers with associated paresthesias.[17] Neck limitation may be relatively mild early in the course of the disease; limitation progresses as degenerative changes worsen. Neurologic abnormalities, including diminished or lost reflexes, sensory deficits, and motor weakness, may be observed, depending on the extent and duration of the disease process. The specific location and combination of neurologic findings will depend on the specific nerve root or roots involved.

A complete physical examination is essential in the patient with cervical osteoarthritis and neck pain to rule out other causes of pain as a result of direct neural compression.[17]

TREATMENT

The initial treatment of symptomatic degenerative disk and degenerative joint disease of the cervical spine should be conservative. This includes the use of soft-collar immobilization

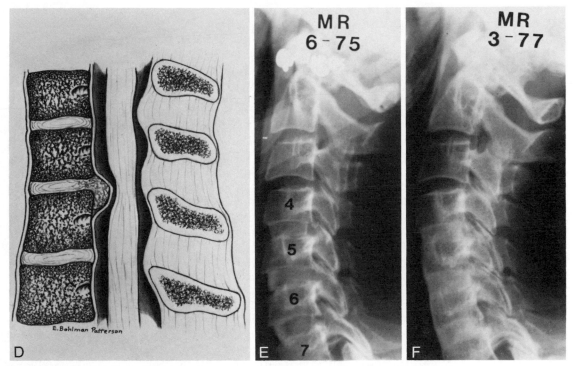

Figure 26–3 (*Continued*). *D,* Illustration demonstrating association of soft disk protrusion and spondylosis with a narrow spinal canal. Cervical disk protrusion is usually anterior to the posterior longitudinal ligament but may be posterior to the vertebral body. (From Bohlman HH: Cervical spondylosis with moderate to severe myelopathy: A report of seventeen cases treated by Robinson anterior cervical discectomy and fusion. Spine 2:151–162, 1977.) *E,* Lateral roentgenogram of the patient 1 month postoperatively revealing the anterior bone blocks at C4–C5, C5–C6, and C6–C7. No attempt was made to remove the posterior osteophytes. *F,* Lateral roentgenogram 2 years after the anterior cervical diskectomy and fusion and 11 years after the initial onset of symptoms, demonstrating resorption of anterior as well as posterior spurs by the process of bone remodeling.

and analgesic and anti-inflammatory medications. Even patients with significant neural compression as manifested by individual muscle weakness and loss of sensation that follows a specific nerve root distribution can resolve their impairment with proper immobilization and the use of these analgesic and anti-inflammatory agents. It is likely that neural compression resolves as the herniated cervical disk is resorbed. Relief of pain and inflammation is associated with decreased associated muscle spasm and improved range of motion. Cervical collars should be properly fitted and are frequently most effective when used with the neck in approximately 15 degrees of flexion. This avoids hyperextension of the cervical spine and aggravation of nerve root compression. Not infrequently, patients tolerate the use of a cervical collar better if the narrow part of the collar is used anteriorly. Cervical traction may be indicated and beneficial. Cervical traction techniques should be taught in the physical therapy office, at which time intermittent trac-

tion may be applied. Cervical traction may be continued in the home with proper instruction. It is important to caution the patient to use cervical traction with the neck in slight forward flexion, once again so as to avoid neck hyperextension and symptom aggravation. Cervical traction may not be well tolerated in older individuals with severe osteoarthritis and marked osteophyte spur formation.

Heat is helpful. Local injections of steroids and lidocaine to associated trigger point areas of pain and spasm may be beneficial at times; several areas may have to be injected. Tranquilizers with muscle-relaxant properties aid in relieving tension and muscle spasm.

In most instances, these modalities of treatment will resolve the pain syndrome. It is our practice to utilize a conservative program for at least 6 to 8 weeks. Although this program does not alter the basic process of disk degeneration and osteochondrophyte spur formation, it frequently provides symptomatic relief and resolution of neurologic findings. Ordinarily, the patient's pain will resolve first, followed by gradual resolution of weakness and, finally, resolution of sensory loss over a period of weeks to months. If the pain syndrome becomes chronic and disabling and the offending vertebral segment can be identified, surgical intervention may become necessary. Significant residual neurologic deficits are a further indication for surgical intervention.[4, 27–29] An anterior cervical diskectomy and fusion performed at the appropriate level are recommended. Prior to surgical intervention, the patient is admitted to the hospital to undergo a diagnostic cervical myelogram to determine the exact level of neural compression. Following surgical intervention, the patient is instructed to wear a rigid cervical orthosis for 6 weeks or until the bone graft is completely healed. We do not recommend cervical diskectomy without fusion, because many of these patients will have continued abnormal motion at the operative segment of the spine; this produces a chronic neck pain syndrome that may later require cervical fusion to resolve the situation.

The purpose of anterior diskectomy and fusion, as described in 1955 by Robinson and Smith,[30] is to remove the offending disk and to stabilize the abnormal motion segment. The ideal patient for an anterior diskectomy and fusion is that individual with a single level of degenerative disk disease and osteoarthritis. At times, extension of the procedure to involve larger numbers of disk spaces may be indicated but results in a higher incidence of pseudoarthrosis and a decreased number of good to excellent results for pain relief and resolution of neurologic deficit.[28, 31]

As the progressive process of cervical osteoarthritis affects older individuals, the cervical spondylosis may produce a myelopathy. Patients who develop cervical cord myelopathy generally have pre-existing congenitally narrow cervical spinal canals that are further compromised by ingrowth of osteochondrophyte spurs. In this situation, the patient may not complain primarily of pain in the cervical spine but may present with an ataxic gait and difficulty walking.[32–34] Physical examination will reveal a limited range of cervical spine motion and aggravation of symptoms with hyperextension of the neck. Neurologically, these patients manifest myelopathy by hyperreflexia, motor weakness of various grades, and sensory loss. Myelopathy is usually associated with radiculopathy, so that there will be a mixture of upper motor neuron as well as lower motor neuron symptoms. It is important to analyze the lateral roentgenogram of the patient with cervical spondylosis and myelopathy to determine the sagittal diameter of the spinal canal, which in this situation is ordinarily less than 13 mm (Fig. 26–4).

The initial treatment of cervical myelopathy should be with cervical-collar immobilization; the spinal cord is in jeopardy, however, and surgical intervention by anterior diskectomy and fusion is usually necessary. Cervical myelography is always performed to determine the number of pathologic levels affecting the spinal cord and nerve roots. The results of Robinson anterior cervical diskectomy and fusion are excellent in patients with moderate to severe myelopathy if they have not progressed to the point where there is loss of position or vibratory sense, or bladder and bowel paralysis.[35] From a technical standpoint, the surgical treatment of cervical spondylosis and myelopathy involves complete anterior removal of the cervical disk; no attempt is made to remove the posterior osteophytes because of the significant risk of iatrogenic spinal cord injury. Laminectomy is associated with a significant risk of paralysis.[36] We believe that it is very important to stabilize the cervical segment with a bone block, which produces immediate rigid immobilization and protects the spinal cord from further damage. Once the bone graft is inserted, there no longer is any posterior cord compression by buckling of the ligamentum flavum, which may be a factor in causing spinal cord compression (Fig. 26–5). Ultimately, the reactive spurs will be resorbed by the normal process of bone remodeling, because motion is stopped at the fused levels.[31, 35, 37]

As previously mentioned, cervical osteoarthritis may produce a pain syndrome secondary to abnormal motion or instability. Long-standing degenerative disk and joint disease results in immobile lower cervical segments and more mobile upper cervical segments with compensatory anterior subluxation (Fig. 26–6). The results are abnormal motion and stretching of the ligamentous structures, which result first in pain and secondarily in nerve root or spinal cord compression and paralysis. Initially, mild cervical subluxations of less than 4 mm can be treated nonoperatively with cervical immobilization and analgesics. If the pain syndrome becomes chronic and disabling, however, and especially if paralysis ensues, operative intervention is necessary to stabilize the segment to relieve pain and paralysis. With compensatory cervical subluxations, it is very important

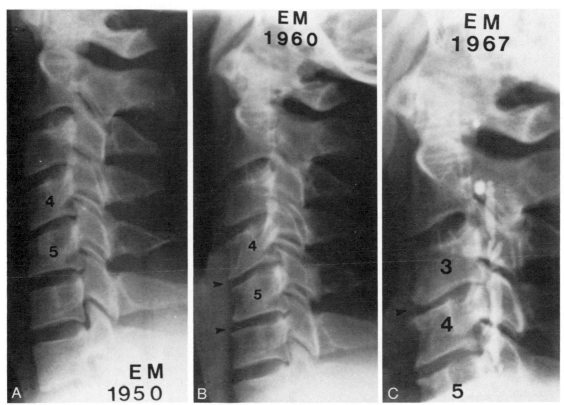

Figure 26–4. A, Lateral roentgenogram of the cervical spine of a 35-year-old physician in 1950, demonstrating mild narrowing of the disk space at C4–C5 (arrow). In addition, there is a congenitally narrow cervical spinal canal. At this stage of cervical spondylosis, there is dehydration of the disk and abnormal mechanics of the affected segment and no osteophytes have formed. *B,* Lateral roentgenogram of the cervical spine of the patient 10 years later at age 45, when he had recurring neck pain as well as arm pain. The illustration demonstrates progressive narrowing of C4–C5 and C5–C6 disk spaces with early osteophyte formation (arrows). *C,* Lateral myelogram of the patient 17 years following onset of the initial symptoms and performed in preparation for surgical intervention. At this point, the patient has progressive disk degeneration and narrowing and osteophyte formation at C3–C4 (arrow) and C4–C5, with cervical radiculomyelopathy.

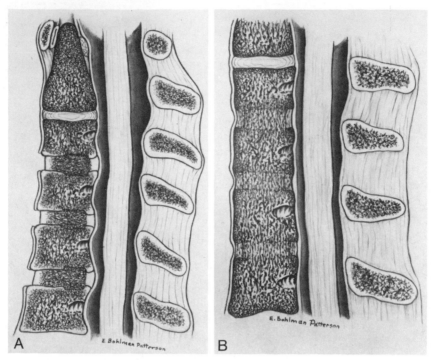

Figure 26–5. *A,* This illustration demonstrates the Robinson anterior diskectomy and bone block insertion at C3–C4, C4–C5, and C5–C6. The entire disk has been removed at each level without violating the posterior longitudinal ligament. Distraction straightens the redundant posterior longitudinal ligament and ligamentum flavum, and immediate stability is achieved. (From Bohlman HH: Cervical spondylosis with mild to severe myelopathy: A report of seventeen cases treated by Robinson anterior cervical discectomy and fusion. Spine 2:151–162, 1977.) *B,* Illustration demonstrating incorporation of the bone graft, loss of osteophytes by normal bone remodeling, and lessened redundance in the ligamentous structures. The pathologic segments have been stabilized. (From Bohlman HH: Cervical spondylosis with mild to severe myelopathy: A report of seventeen cases treated by Robinson anterior cervical discectomy and fusion. Spine 2:151–162, 1977.)

to measure the spinal canal diameter to determine whether it is less than 13 mm and, hence, that spinal cord compression can occur. Serial examinations and roentgenograms of these patients are indicated; treatment with soft-collar immobilization will usually resolve the pain syndrome. As shown by White and Panjabi[38] and others, vertebral body subluxation greater than 3.5 mm anteriorly, translatory displacement of the vertebral bodies, or angulation between two vertebrae greater than 11 degrees at adjacent interspaces indicates pathologic instability. In this situation, arthrodesis is indicated. Usually, anterior cervical diskectomy and fusion by the Robinson technique will be the surgical treatment of choice. Less commonly seen are patients with spondylotic retrolisthesis (Fig. 26–7).

Cervical osteoarthritis, if severe, may affect the upper cervical spine and produce upper cervical pain that radiates to the occiput (Fig. 26–8). Patients may describe clicking and popping on rotation of the neck, which are very

bothersome. Disease in this area of the cervical spine may or may not be associated with previous traumatic episodes. Severe direct blows to the top of the head may produce fractures of the lateral mass of the atlas, damage to the atlantoaxial joint, and osteoarthritis (Fig. 26–9). The etiology of atlantoaxial arthritis involving the odontoid process is unknown. Rarely, the destructive process of osteoarthritis may erode the transverse ligament of the atlas and produce atlantoaxial dislocation, with resultant severe occipital pain with or without paralysis secondary to the spinal cord compression (Fig. 26–10). Physical examination of the patient with atlantoaxial osteoarthritis will ordinarily reveal limitation of motion on neck rotation and pain; atlanto-occipital osteoarthritis produces limitation of flexion and extension. The patient with atlantoaxial dislocation may present with severe upper cervical spine pain; the patient frequently supports the chin in the hands. In general, the treatment of upper cervical osteoarthritis is conservative

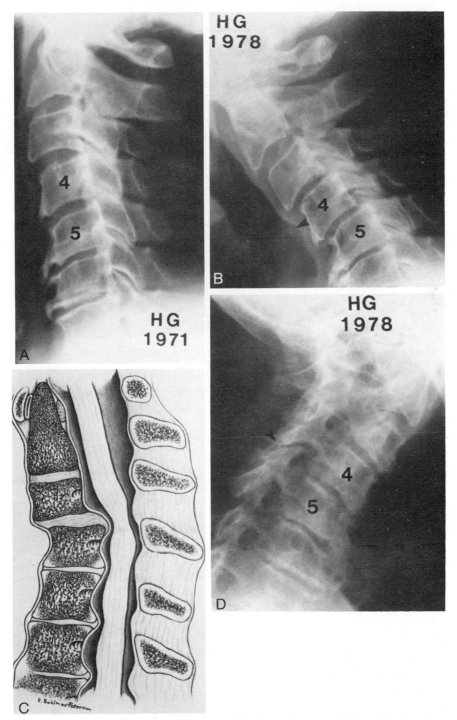

Figure 26–6. *A,* Lateral cervical roentgenogram taken in 1971 of a patient complaining of neck and arm pain without any neurologic deficit. The illustration demonstrates moderately severe cervical spondylosis at C4–C5, C5–C6, and C6–7. *B,* Lateral roentgenogram of the patient 7 years later revealing progression of the cervical spondylosis and compensatory subluxation at C3–C4 and C4–C5 (arrow) above the spontaneously arthrodesed C5–C6 level. The patient was now complaining of severe neck and arm pain. The subluxations are secondary to progression of the disease, involving the facets and producing laxity of the joint capsules posteriorly. *C,* Diagrammatic illustration of compensatory anterior subluxation of the third on fourth cervical vertebrae above the stiff spondylotic segments. The spinal cord compression occurs anteriorly. (From Bohlman HH: Cervical spondylosis with mild to severe myelopathy: A report of seventeen cases treated by Robinson anterior cervical discectomy and fusion. Spine 2:151–162, 1977.) *D,* Oblique roentgenogram of the patient 7 years after the onset of symptoms with subluxation of C4–C5, demonstrating progressive osteoarthritis of the posterior facet joints creating instability and producing neural foramen compromise (arrow).

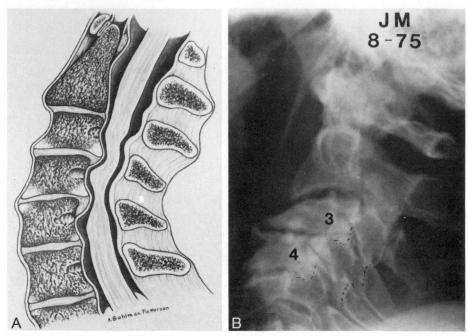

Figure 26–7. *A,* Diagrammatic illustration of retrolisthesis or posterior subluxation that may occur, causing spinal cord compression anteriorly. Although there may be a buckled ligamentum flavum posteriorly, these patients usually present with anterior cord compression syndromes without loss of posterior column functions. (From Bohlman HH: Cervical spondylosis with mild to severe myelopathy: A report of seventeen cases treated by Robinson anterior cervical discectomy and fusion. Spine 2:151–162, 1977.) *B,* Lateral roentgenogram of the cervical spine of a 60-year-old man with severe cervical spondylosis and retrolisthesis of the third and fourth cervical vertebrae.

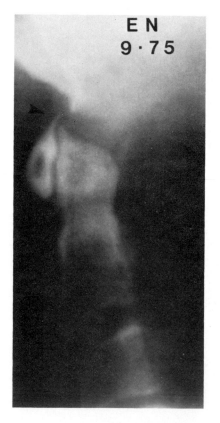

Figure 26–8. Lateral roentgenogram of the cervical-occipital complex demonstrating osteoarthritic change in the atlantoaxial joint. Note the superior spur formation at the anterior arch of the atlas and the tip of the odontoid process (arrow). In addition, there is narrowing of the atlantoaxial joint space, which is a true synovial joint. This patient presented with severe pain and cracking on rotation of the head and neck.

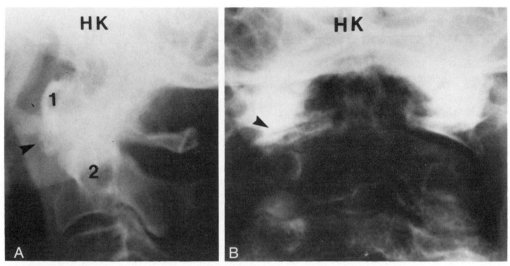

Figure 26–9. *A,* Lateral roentgenogram of the atlantoaxial complex of a 55-year-old man who fell 1 year previously from a one-story window, striking his head and sustaining an injury to the atlantoaxial joint. Note the sclerotic osteoarthritis of the atlantoaxial complex (arrow). The patient complained of severe upper cervical and occipital pain on rotation of the head and the neck. *B,* Open-mouth odontoid view demonstrating total destruction of the lateral atlantoaxial joint with osteoarthritis (arrow).

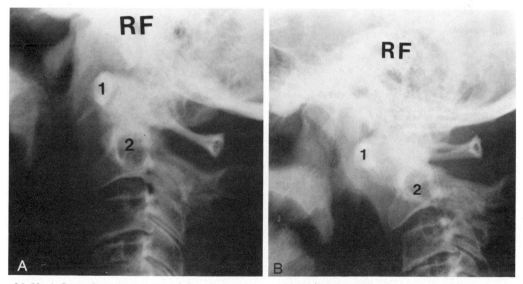

Figure 26–10. *A,* Lateral roentgenogram of the atlantoaxial complex of a patient with known osteoarthritis of the cervical spine. The patient presented complaining of upper cervical and occipital neck pain without paralysis. *B,* Lateral roentgenogram in flexion of the atlantoaxial complex demonstrating a dislocation of C1 on C2 secondary to lysis of the transverse ligament. This process was secondary to osteoarthritis of the atlantoaxial complex.

and consists of soft-collar immobilization, analgesics, and anti-inflammatory agents. These modalities will usually result in relief of the pain syndrome; physical therapy with traction and manipulation are not indicated. On the other hand, the patient with atlantoaxial dislocation requires posterior cervical arthrodesis, because the spinal cord is in jeopardy.

Rare Forms of Osteoarthritis of the Cervical Spine

Adults with athetoid cerebral palsy develop osteoarthritis of the cervical spine. It is likely that this progressively severe disease in these individuals is secondary to the constant abnormal motions of the cervical spine (Fig. 26–11). This, indeed, is an extremely difficult patient to treat when a neck pain syndrome is involved or when there is compromise of the neural elements. Immobilization of the cervical spine is impossible, and one is left with treatment by analgesics or anti-inflammatory agents. Arthrodesis of the cervical spine either anteriorly or posteriorly, although rarely indicated, is difficult to achieve.

Ankylosing hyperostosis of the spine was originally described by Forestier where the characteristic roentgenographic features of the spine included anterior undulating ossification of the cervical spine and cortical hyperostosis (Fig. 26–12) (see Chapters 9 and 13). This variant of cervical osteoarthritis falls into the classification of diffuse idiopathic skeletal hyperostosis or DISH syndrome.[18] Ordinarily, one sees flowing calcification and ossification along the anterior aspect of the contiguous vertebral bodies, with preservation of the intervertebral disk height. In addition, because there is no motion to cause osteochondrophyte spur formation posteriorly, the vertebral foramina are completely clear, as they are in ankylosing spondylitis. It is rare to have pain syndromes as a result of this disease, but occasionally, dysphagia is related to the osteophytosis that occurs posterior to the esophagus (Fig. 26–13).

Although very common in Japan, ossification of the posterior longitudinal ligament of the cervical spine (OPLL) occurs rarely in this country (see Chapter 9). This entity may be associated with DISH.[18] In contrast to DISH, OPLL may produce encroachment on the cer-

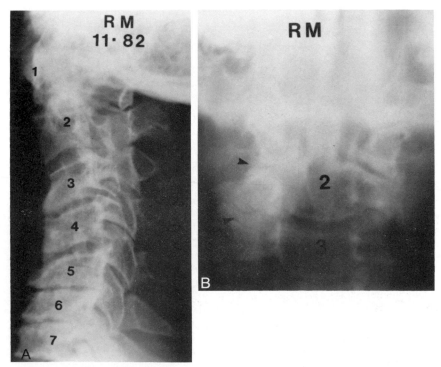

Figure 26–11. *A,* Lateral roentgenogram of the cervical spine demonstrating severe, diffuse osteoarthritis of the cervical spine, including the atlantoaxial complex, in a 50-year-old patient with athetoid cerebral palsy. The patient presented with severe neck, cervical, and occipital pain of 18 months' duration. *B,* Open-mouth odontoid view of the patient demonstrating severe osteoarthritis of the lateral atlantoaxial and C2–C3 joints (arrows).

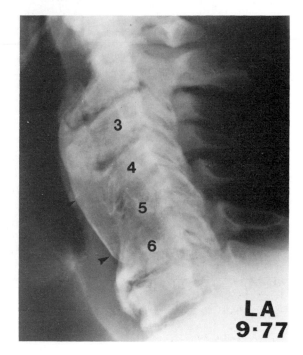

Figure 26–12. Lateral roentgenogram of a patient with long-standing osteoarthritis of the cervical spine and diffuse idiopathic skeletal hyperostosis (DISH). Note the flowing ossification along the anterior borders of the third through sixth vertebral bodies (arrows).

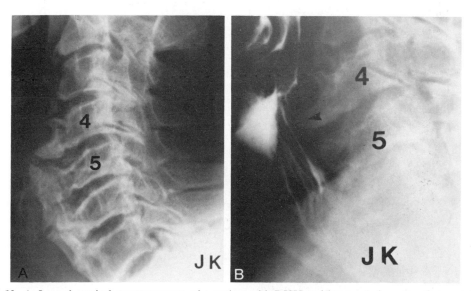

Figure 26–13. *A*, Lateral cervical roentgenogram of a patient with DISH and large anterior osteophytes at the fourth and fifth cervical levels. The patient complained of severe dysphagia. *B*, Lateral roentgenogram demonstrating the barium swallow and marked esophageal impingement by the anterior fourth cervical osteophyte (arrow). This was removed successfully, with relief of the dysphagia.

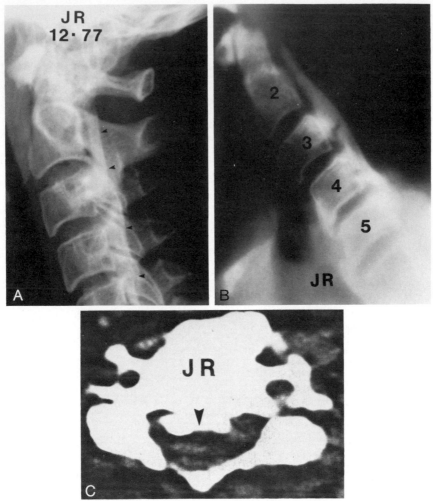

Figure 26–14. *A,* Lateral cervical roentgenogram of a 55-year-old patient presenting with cervical myeloradiculopathy. Note the thickened ossified posterior longitudinal ligament (OPLL) extending from the second through the sixth cervical vertebrae, severely compromising the diameter of the cervical spinal canal (arrows). *B,* Lateral cervical tomograms of the patient further defining the ossified posterior longitudinal ligament and additional osteoarthritis of the atlantoaxial complex. *C,* Cervical computerized axial tomogram demonstrating severe compromise of the cervical spinal canal by the ossified posterior ligament, anterior to the spinal cord (arrow).

vical spinal canal and may result in compression of the spinal cord or nerve root compression. There is no known etiology for OPLL. When neural compression occurs, surgical intervention is necessary to decompress the spinal canal. The roentgenographic appearance of OPLL is diagnostic and consists of a linear band of ossified tissue along the posterior margin of the vertebral bodies. This may involve the entire cervical spine or may be segmental in location (Fig. 26–14).

Osteoarthritis of the cervical spine may become manifest in various degrees of formation, depending on the age of the individual. Pain or neurologic deficit may begin following trauma. Conservative treatment has been outlined previously, and the indications for surgical intervention have been specified. With the aforementioned entities in mind, the physician can proceed with a well-formed plan of treatment, and surgical intervention can be offered where specifically indicated.

References

1. Coventry MB: Anatomy of the intervertebral disc. Clin Orthop Rel Res 67:9–15, 1969.
2. DePalma A, Rothman R: The Intervertebral Disc. Philadelphia, W. B. Saunders Company, 1970.
3. Hadley LA: Anatomico-roentgenographic Studies of

the Spine. 2nd ed. Springfield, Illinois, Charles C Thomas, 1973, p. 447.

4. Kellgren JH, Lawrence JS: Osteoarthritis and disk degeneration in an urban population. Ann Rheum Dis 17:388–397, 1958.

5. Kellgren JH, Lawrence JS, Bier F: Genetic factors in generalized osteoarthrosis. Ann Rheum Dis 22:237–255, 1963.

6. Payne EE, Spillane JD: The cervical spine. An anatomicopathologic study of 70 specimens (using a special technique) with particular reference to the problem of cervical spondylosis. Brain 80:571–596, 1957.

7. Coventry MB, Ghormley RK, Kernohan JW: The intervertebral disc: Its microscopic anatomy and pathology. II. Changes in the intervertebral disc concomitant with age. J Bone Joint Surg 27:233–247, 1945.

8. Friedenberg ZB, Miller WT: Degenerative disc disease of the cervical spine. J Bone Joint Surg 45A:1171–1178, 1963.

9. Compere EL: Origin, anatomy, histology and pathology of the intervertebral disc. In American Academy of Orthopaedic Surgeons: Instructional Course Lectures. Vol. 18. St. Louis, C.V. Mosby, 1961, pp. 15–20.

10. Keyes DC, Compere EL: The normal and pathological physiology of the nucleus pulposus of the intervertebral disc. J Bone Joint Surg 14:897–938, 1932.

11. Lawrence JS, Bremner JM, Bier F: Osteoarthrosis: Prevalence in the population and relationship between symptoms and x-ray changes. Ann Rheum Dis 25:1–24, 1966.

12. Wilkinson M: The morbid anatomy of cervical spondylosis and myelopathy. Brain 83:589–617, 1960.

13. Schmorl G, Junghanns H: The Human Spine in Health and Disease. 2nd ed. Translated by EF Besemann. New York, Grune & Stratton, 1971, p. 138.

14. Cloward RB: The clinical significance of the sinu-vertebral nerve of the cervical spine in relation to the cervical disk syndrome. J Neurol Neurosurg Psychiatry 23:321–326, 1960.

15. Mulligan JH: The innervation of the ligaments attached to the bodies of the vertebrae. J Anat 91:445–465, 1957.

16. Bohlman HH: Neck pain. In Nickel V (ed.): Orthopaedic Rehabilitation. New York, Churchill Livingstone, 1982, pp. 467–480.

17. Bohlman HH: The neck. In D'Ambrosia RD (ed.): Musculoskeletal Disorders: Regional Examination and Differential Diagnosis. Philadelphia, J. B. Lippincott, 1977, pp. 178–224.

18. Resnick D, Niwayama G: Diagnosis of Bone and Joint Disorders. Philadelphia, W. B. Saunders Company, 1981.

19. Robinson RA: The problem of neck pain. J Med Assoc State Ala 33:1–14, 1963.

20. Robinson RA: Anterior cervical fusion in cervical spine degenerative disease. In Gurdjian ES, Thomas LM (eds.): Neckache and Backache. Springfield, Illinois, Charles C Thomas, 1970.

21. Robinson RA: Cervical spine. In Milch RA (ed.): Surgery of Arthritis. Baltimore, Williams & Wilkins, 1964.

22. Hinck VC, Sachdev NS: Developmental stenosis of the cervical spine canal. Brain 89:27–36, 1966.

23. Munrone I: The importance of the sagittal diameters of the cervical spinal canal in relation to spondylosis and myelopathy. J Bone Joint Surg 56B:30–36, 1974.

24. Wilkinson HA, LeMay ML, Ferris EJ: Clinical radiologic correlations in cervical spondylosis. J Neurosurg 30:213–218, 1969.

25. Wolf BS, Khilnani M, Malis LI: The sagittal diameter of the bony cervical spinal canal and its significance in cervical spondylosis. J Mt Sinai Hosp 23:283–292, 1956.

26. Lipson SJ, Muir H: Vertebral osteophyte formation in experimental disc degeneration. Morphologic and proteoglycan changes over time. Arthritis Rheum 23:319–324, 1980.

27. Bohlman HH: Degenerative arthrosis of the lower cervical spine. In Evarts C (ed.): Surgery of the Musculoskeletal System. New York, Churchill Livingstone, 1983, pp. 22–55.

28. Bohlman HH, Goodfellow D: The treatment of cervical disc disease with Robinson anterior cervical discectomy and fusion. A review of 103 consecutive cases with long-term follow-up. Presented at the Annual Meeting of the Cervical Spine Research Society, New York, December 1982.

29. Riley LH: Cervical disc surgery: Its role and indications. Orthop Clin North Am 2:443–452, 1971.

30. Robinson RA, Smith GW: Anterolateral cervical disc removal and interbody fusion for cervical disc syndrome. Bull Johns Hopkins Hosp 96:223–224, 1955.

31. Riley LH, Robinson RA, Johnson KA, Walker AE: The results of anterior interbody fusion of the cervical spine: Review of 93 consecutive cases. J Neurosurg 30:127–133, 1969.

32. Brain RW, Northfield D, Wilkinson M: The neurologic manifestations of cervical spondylosis. Brain 75:187–225, 1952.

33. Brain L, Wilkinson M: Cervical Spondylosis and Other Disorders of the Cervical Spine. 1st ed. Philadelphia, W. B. Saunders Company, 1967, p. 226.

34. Clarke E, Robinson PK: Cervical myelopathy: A complication of cervical spondylosis. Brain 79:483–510, 1956.

35. Bohlman HH: Cervical spondylosis with moderate to severe myelopathy: A report of 17 cases treated by Robinson anterior cervical discectomy and fusion. Spine 2:151–162, 1977.

36. Gregorious FK, Estin TE, Crandall PH: Cervical spondylotic radiculopathy and myelopathy. Arch Neurol 33:618–625, 1976.

37. Bohlman HH, Riley L Jr, Robinson RA: Anterolateral approaches to the cervical spine. In Wiltse LL, Ruge D (eds.): Spinal Disorders: Diagnosis and Treatment. Philadelphia, Lea & Febiger, 1977, pp. 125–131.

38. White HA, Panjabi MM: Clinical Biomechanics of the Spine. Philadelphia, J. B. Lippincott, 1978.

27

Osteoarthritis of the Thoracic Spine

Thomas K. F. Taylor, M.D.

A perusal of the literature might suggest that the thoracic spine is relatively immune to the diseases and disorders that affect the cervical and lumbar regions of the spine, but this is far from true. Quite a number of conditions, especially osteoarthritis (spondylosis), are not at all uncommon and, moreover, may produce unique and often puzzling clinical syndromes.

ANATOMIC CONSIDERATIONS

The gross morphology of the thoracic spine is well described in standard anatomy texts. Nevertheless, several aspects warrant detailed consideration in the context of this chapter.

The Costovertebral and Costotransverse Joints

The first, eleventh, and twelfth ribs have unifacet articulations on the corresponding vertebral bodies, whereas the remainder are bifacetal. Comparative anatomic studies have demonstrated that this arrangement is independent of the size of the thorax, the number of ribs, and posture.[1] Accordingly, the space for the emerging and relatively large first thoracic nerve is small in comparison with that available for those located more caudally. Furthermore, the first nerve courses obliquely upward and laterally to cross the inner margin of the neck of the corresponding rib, which may have a sharp margin.

Movement of the thoracic cage is an expression of the integrated motion at the costovertebral and costotransverse joints. The capsule of the former is reinforced by the triradiate ligament, the middle limb of which is a vestige of the original hypochordal bow. A flimsy intra-articular ligament connects the rib to the articulating intervertebral disk.

The Thoracic Nerve Roots and Intercostal Nerves

The thoracic nerve roots leave the thecal sac more posteriorly than they do in either the cervical or the lumbar region, and the roots are also located more proximally in the intervertebral foramina. Because of these factors, the roots do not come into direct contact with either the intervertebral disk or the costovertebral joint. The distance between these structures and the segmental neural elements will be reduced as a disk space narrows. The intercostal nerves (anterior primary rami [APR]) pass laterally immediately beneath the costotransverse joints on their way to the undersurface of the rib and here are liable to irritation and/or compression by degenerative spurs and periarticular inflammation. They are joined by the segmental vessels lateral to the joint and are covered anteriorly by the pleura. The dorsal root ganglion lies in the foramen surrounded by a venous plexus and rather tenacious but loose fibrous tissue that connects it to the bony foraminal margins.

The first six thoracic nerves are distributed to the first six intercostal spaces, but nerves T7 to T12 also supply the abdominal wall musculature in a segmental fashion. Each has a lateral branch with anterior and posterior divisions, and the terminal cutaneous twig passes anterior to the segmental arteries. The same arrangement holds in the thoracic region, with the internal mammary artery having an intersegmental value. The twelfth thoracic (subcostal) nerve sends its lateral branch to the superolateral aspect of the buttock, an important consideration in the differential diagnosis of buttock pain.

The posterior primary ramus (PPR) of each thoracic nerve passes backward between the two limbs of the superior costotransverse ligament. This stout structure joins the crest on the neck of the rib below to the lower margin of the transverse process above. The rami are liable to irritation from osteoarthritic costotransverse joints or to entrapment between the limbs of the aforementioned ligament.

The distribution of the PPR is irregular compared with that of the APR. The motor supply is limited to the extensor compartment of the trunk, and there are no branches to any limb musculature in any primate. Laterally, the cutaneous supply does not extend beyond the posterior axillary line. The cutaneous distribution is quite irregular with considerable overlapping of the areas served. The rami course obliquely downward and laterally, particularly the more caudal ones. In clinical examination, assignment of a given cutaneous area to a particular ramus is, at best, only an approximation. On several occasions, when I have purposefully divided a ramus, there has been no observable sensory deficit.

The Autonomic Nervous System

The sympathetic trunk has an intimate relation to various parts of the thoracic spine. In the upper region, it passes across the necks of the ribs. It is in close contact with the rib heads and the costovertebral joints in the middle thorax; distally, the more anterior aspects of the vertebral bodies are reached. The splanchnic nerves run a steep, oblique course over the lower thoracic vertebrae. Nathan[2] has described the distortion, attenuation, and fibrosis of the sympathetic trunk (cord and ganglia) that occurs with lumbar syndesmophytes, and as expected, these changes were less marked at the T12–L1 level. Distribution of branches to the anterior longitudinal ligament and the anterior aspect of the intervertebral disk was observed. Comparable morphologic studies of the sympathetic nervous system in the thorax have not been reported, but in view of the

frequency of spondylotic changes in the adult, they could throw some light on the more puzzling features of the autonomic concomitants of pain in thoracic spondylosis. Sympathetic dysfunction and even inhibition might reasonably be expected as sequelae to irritation and compression. This is a rich but uncertain field for morphologic and neurophysiologic research.

THORACIC PAIN

Without doubt, the least well understood feature of osteoarthritis (OA) is the mechanism of pain production from the joint involved, and the thoracic spine is no exception to this enigma. Because neurologic symptoms are frequently seen with spondylosis in its various forms, a review of what is known about thoracic pain and radiculopathy is germane to this discussion.

The nociceptive system consists of plexuses and free endings of unmyelinated fibers from peripheral nerves. Wyke[3] has identified these in apophyseal joint capsules, the longitudinal ligaments, the ligamentum flavum, interspinous ligaments, vertebral periosteum, dura mater and epidural adipose tissue, and the walls of arteries and veins supplying the various connective tissues of the spine.

Intrinsic (Somatic) Spinal Pain

Pain that arises in the thoracic spine has the qualities of somatic pain to which may be added features of pain associated with inflammation, mechanical insufficiency, and an increase in tissue tension, according to the nature of the pathology. Reflex muscle contraction (spasm) can occur. Wyke[3] has stated that there are fewer intersegmental connections between the neural elements in the thoracic spine than between those in the lumbar and cervical regions, so that intrinsic pain tends to be more accurately localized to the area of the pathology. Clinical observation tends to support this contention.

Referred Somatic Pain

A feature of referred somatic pain is that it tends to be appreciated in an approximately dermatomal distribution. Patients find difficulty in describing the qualities of the pain but not the intensity. Words such as "dull," "aching," "boring," "dragging," and "gnawing" are frequently used. It is felt deeply in the tissues and may be accompanied by muscle tenderness with "trigger spots" of more acute tenderness. The latter can be abolished by local anesthesia. Muscle spasm, tenderness, and "trigger spots" may persist long after the primary stimulus has acted. They can recur with trivial incidents. Possibly, the recrudescence of these reflex phenomena is facilitated by the persistence of a subliminal excitatory state that has a central biasing control.

Cutaneous hyperesthesia and hypoesthesia may also be seen with referred somatic pain, with the former occurring more frequently. They are by no means constant features, and both may be present at the same time. These, too, have an approximately dermatomal distribution but never completely occupy the dermatome or produce pronounced changes. The alterations in cutaneous sensibility are patchy and tend to vary somewhat on repetitive testing. If not sought carefully, they will be missed. When more than one spinal cord segment becomes recruited, as is often the case, the sensory changes will be found over quite wide areas. The described features of referred pain have been reproduced in human subjects by injections of hypertonic saline solution into a variety of spinal connective tissues.[4] Autonomic concomitants with visceral symptoms (e.g., nausea, vomiting, and so on) may be part of the response with induced referred somatic pain.

Root and Nerve Pain in the Thoracic Spine

Thoracic root pain has a sharp quality often described as "burning" or "pricking." In its classic radiating girdle form, it is readily recognizable, but very often it presents differently. As with lumbar root pain, thoracic radiculopathy may result in pain being felt only in a distal part of the dermatome with no intervening discomfort. Paresthesias are variable companions to thoracic root pain, and only rarely are they the single evidence of radiculopathy. When they are prominent, peripheral neuritis should be suspected.

Neck flexion may increase or precipitate root pain when impingement is at or proximal to the foramen by transmission of tension through the thecal sac; when the pathology is just distal to the intervertebral foramen, trunk rotation may augment it.

An intercostal nerve may be irritated by osteoarthritic costovertebral and costotrans-

verse joints, but it is not possible on clinical grounds alone to decide which is primarily responsible. Presumably, in some patients, both contribute to the neuropathy. There are no costotransverse joints at the T11 and T12 levels. Because the pathology is distal to the ganglion, the resultant pain is nerve pain, not root pain, and it has similar characteristics to the pain of entrapment neuropathies elsewhere in the body. Direct compression by osteophytes is probably not a major factor, because pain is not a prominent feature in compression of a peripheral nerve. When nonspecific inflammation associated with degenerative changes in connective tissue occurs and irritative neuropathy ensues, pain tends to be the dominant symptom. This explanation accounts well for the favorable response to local infiltration with corticosteroid preparations.

Another feature of root and nerve pain is that tenderness may be present along the course of the nerve, particularly where the lateral and anterior terminal branches pass through the overlying muscles. In the upper thorax, this tenderness is often mistaken as indicative of local pathology, and the condition is frequently mislabeled as Teitze's syndrome. Tenderness along the course of a peripheral nerve when the pathology is at the root level is not peculiar to the thoracic spine and is frequently seen in acute radiculopathy from lumbar disk prolapse.

Although root and referred pain have been described separately, the two may occur together. In such a case, a detailed history and clinical evaluation are required to determine the nature of the pain. Not uncommonly, no firm conclusion can be reached.

Referred Visceral Pain

The back pain that can occur with disease of thoracic and abdominal viscera is well appreciated by clinicians. This is a reflex phenomenon mediated through the thoracic segmental innervation of the visceral structures. Reflex muscle spasm can take place, setting the stage for diagnostic errors. When spinal symptoms dominate the clinical picture, taking a careful history is vital. This applies more when chronic pain is the presenting symptom.

THORACIC SPONDYLOSIS

The development of secondary degenerative changes during middle age in a kyphotic or scoliotic spine is an expected sequel to the prolonged, uneven distribution of stresses on the intervertebral disks. These bear the roentgenographic hallmarks of spondylosis as seen elsewhere in the spine, namely reduced disk space, osteophyte production, and vertebral body sclerosis (Fig. 27–1). They are invariably more marked on the concavity of a curvature, and even when quite pronounced, the convexity most often shows no evidence of a similar hypertrophic response. Spontaneous fusion may take place between bridging osteophytes. It has been suggested that these degradative changes result from impairment of intervertebral disk nutrition,[5] but the ability of this structure to withstand abnormal physical forces is quite remarkable when one considers the latent period between the initiation of curvature and clear roentgenographic evidence of a degenerative process, let alone the onset of symptoms. This is often in the order of 25 years or even longer (Fig. 27–2)! Morphologic observations strongly suggest that lumbar spondylosis is the sequel to disk degeneration.[6] Furthermore, my own studies and those of others[7] suggest that a significant proportion of patients who present in middle age with symptomatic lumbar spondylosis have had silent osteochondritis in the lumbar spine. It seems quite probable that the same process not productive of a kyphosis is involved in the pathogenesis of thoracic spondylosis in a significant proportion of cases. The high incidence of osteophytes has been established by cadaver studies.[8] These have been observed to be both more frequent and more prominent on the right side (Fig. 27–1), and the inhibitory effect of aortic pulsations has been invoked for this distribution. Lack of osteophytes on the right with their presence on the left in transposition of the aorta has been put forward as evidence for this hypothesis.[9, 10] Bony bridges have been observed to disappear in a patient with Forestier's disease who developed an aortic aneurysm.[11] Recent studies using computer-assisted tomography, which delineates clearly the relationship between the osteophytes and the descending thoracic aorta, lend weight to this explanation for the distribution of the reactive marginal changes.[12]

Clinical Features

The pain and stiffness that characterize lumbar and cervical spondylosis have their parallels in the symptomatic spondylotic thoracic spine, but it is decidedly unusual for the intrinsic spinal pain to be severe or disabling. The

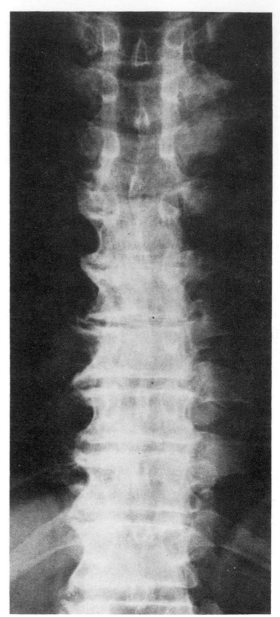

Figure 27–1. Anteroposterior roentgenogram of the thoracic spine of a 70-year-old male who had symptoms compatible with spondylosis throughout his spinal axis. The right side shows prominent osteophytes, but the left side is noticeably free of them.

distal thoracic spine is the most common site of symptoms, but here, the demands of movement and other physical stresses are greater. Pain is often triggered by a minor accident or incident. As with spondylosis at either extreme of the spine the clinical course is one of exacerbations and remissions. Symptoms may be overshadowed by those from the cervical or lumbar regions. Patients seem to accept their thoracic pains more readily, often blithely attributing them to "rheumatism."

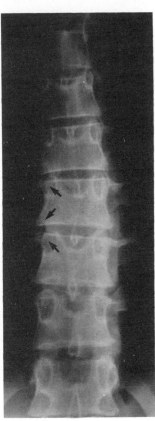

Figure 27–2. Anteroposterior roentgenogram of the thoracic spine of a 35-year-old female with minimal scoliosis. Osteophyte production is slight on the concavity of this curvature (arrows).

Management

It is fortunate that the symptoms of thoracic spondylosis are rarely disabling and do not tend to obtrude markedly on the patient's life style. Management is along empiric lines, with due attention to the general health of the patient, reassuring him, and, in particular, explaining the nature of the problem. According to age and physical fitness, the patient may be able to undertake an exercise program to strengthen the spinal musculature. Emphasis is placed on instruction as to ways and means of avoiding unnecessary strain on the spine by means of postural bracing. Swimming is encouraged. Mild analgesics are prescribed as required. Unfortunately, there is a widespread tendency to administer nonsteroidal anti-inflammatory drugs for spondylosis, whatever region of the spine is affected, but it is extraordinary that the place of these agents in the management of spondylosis has not been established by appropriate clinical trials.[13, 14] This practice has no sound basis, and indeed, the disorder is not an inflammatory one, although focal inflammatory changes may occur from time to time. The analgesic effect of nonsteroidal anti-inflammatory agents is more safely obtained with other medication, and their potential deleterious side effects are not to be dismissed lightly.

Acute severe back pain in the thoracolumbar junction without radicular symptoms is sometimes seen as a demanding problem, with the episode being brought on by an unusual movement, or a sudden unexpected strain. Here, the response to gentle manipulation is often spectacular, with nearly instantaneous relief, provided it is performed shortly after onset of the pain. If manipulation is delayed, the response is less complete. Extension is an important element of the manipulation in this situation. Patients who are prone to recurrent attacks frequently find their own way to chiropractors.

It is *quite exceptional for the apophyseal articulations to be the site of pronounced osteoarthritic change, but when this does occur,* spinal cord compression may ensue.[15]

THE COSTOVERTEBRAL AND COSTOTRANSVERSE JOINTS

These joints are frequently the site of osteoarthritic changes without detectable etiologic factors. In a study of 346 skeletons, Nathan and coworkers[16] found that the changes were more common at the unifacet articulations at the extremes of the thoracic spine. These observations have inexplicable mechanical implications. Ankylosis was occasionally seen. Histologic studies have demonstrated that the histopathology in these joints is similar to that of OA elsewhere in the body.[17] The relationship between OA of the rib articulations and the spondylotic process has not been established.

Clinical Features

Neuropathy in its various manifestations is the usual reason why these problems come to the orthopedic surgeon's attention, and most importantly, they may come under the guise of obscure abdominal or chest pain. The condition, although quite common, is poorly described in the literature.

Females are affected twice as often as males, and the age of the majority of patients ranges from 40 to 60 years. A history of minor trauma is obtained in approximately half the patients.

Back pain is usually not severe. Peripheral pain may be in the distribution of the anterior primary rami or the posterior primary rami, or both, with their features as already described. Entrapment syndromes appear to be somewhat more common on the right side than on the left one. Aggravation of pain may occur on lying down and is often reported as disturbing sleep. Almost invariably, patients note that lifting their arms above their heads, as well as rotation of the torso, either precipitates or increases their pain. It is uncommon for pain to be augmented by deep respiration, as might be expected, but presumably, reflex splinting prevents the aggravating movement.

The clinical course tends to be a fluctuating one, with acute exacerbations often triggered by minor twists, strains, unusually bumpy car rides, and so on. The length of the history is variable, but in more than 50% of patients, it is greater than 6 months, and a history of several years' standing is by no means uncommon.

Physical Examination

Restriction of rotation is best demonstrated with the examiner seated on a low stool behind the patient, steadying the patient's pelvis on both sides. Reproduction of pain on trunk rotation is an important diagnostic sign.[18]

Spinal movement is reduced, particularly extension and rotation. The bulk and tone of the extensor musculature are reduced. Even though these differences cannot be quantitated, they are readily appreciated. Tenderness over the costotransverse joint is sought with the patient in the prone position. It is uncommon for pressure here to reproduce root pain, even from the offending joint or joints.

Sensory defects should be mapped carefully, particularly in relation to the posterior primary rami, as this will give evidence of multiple-level involvement. It has been found useful to use two safety pins, bent at right angles, in the search for abnormalities of cutaneous sensation, comparing both sides of the trunk, because the changes are so often quite subtle. Hypersensitivity is often best demonstrated by pinching a fold of skin and subcutaneous tissue. Occasionally, hyperesthesia may be sufficiently marked for patients to find their clothing quite irritating.

Management

This is demanding for the patient as well as for the attending physician. The long history,

lack of effective treatment, and, particularly, a positive diagnosis take an expected toll on the patient and the family. The complex psychologic reaction to chronic pain is commonly present. Multiple opinions will usually have been sought from a wide variety of disciplines, producing a lengthy series of expensive and negative investigations. The pain, disability, and a marked disturbance of life style remain. The patient's confidence in the medical profession is low and must be restored.

Experience has shown that it is often prudent to hospitalize the patient to start treatment. This is the best environment for the development of a good patient/doctor relationship and, perhaps more importantly, an understanding between the physiotherapist and the patient. All three must have comparable enthusiasm for the program.

The first aim is to mobilize the thoracic spine and rib joints. If these are extremely stiff, manipulation entailing extension and rotation is helpful. Mobilizing therapy techniques are used while the patient is on a motorized traction table. As mobility improves, pain lessens, and extension exercises and postural bracing maneuvers are commenced on a graduated basis. The former should be performed in a manner so as not to increase the lumbar lordosis. Swimming and other forms of hydrotherapy are used whenever possible. For the first week, the patient should spend a prolonged period daily receiving physiotherapy.

Most patients will have had large amounts of medication prior to admission, and the use of narcotics is not exceptional. Dependence on pain medication requires firm decisions with which the patients will comply only if they have confidence in their doctor. The nature of the problem must be fully explained to the patient. The initial therapy sessions may be painful, and medication is sometimes required. The approach adopted is essentially that of a modified operant conditioning program. At all stages, positive reinforcement by the physical therapist is most important, and verbal rewards by all those concerned in the patient's care gradually replace analgesics.

If progress in the first week is not rapid, the costotransverse joints are injected with a local anesthetic and a local steroid. If the disk spaces are very narrow and the costovertebral joints are suspect, these, too, are injected. This maneuver is both diagnostic and therapeutic. On the morning of the injection, the patient works with the therapist to increase the pain by performing an activity that he or she knows will exacerbate it. The injection is done under two-plane fluoroscopic control. Clinical judgment as to the spinal levels is quite unreliable, despite the protestations of some anesthetists. The tender joint or joints are identified by palpation, and a clinically suspect joint is the first one to be injected. A 15-gauge needle is then introduced approximately 1 cm lateral to the tip of the transverse process and angled forward toward the lower margin of the costotransverse joint, according to the fluoroscopic image (Fig. 27–3). When the correct placement and direction of the needle have been confirmed, a 22-gauge needle is inserted through the first needle to the costotransverse joint. A positive response is aggravation of the patient's pain and abolition of it by injection of 2 ml of 1% lidocaine; 1 ml of steroid is then injected periarticularly. The first needle is left in place as a direction guide while needles are inserted in the same manner at the levels above and below. Even when one joint is clearly responsible for the symptoms, it has become my practice to inject adjacent levels, because experience has shown that they frequently contribute to the clinical picture. The technique is simple to master with practice, and no significant complications have been encountered. Rarely, a small pneumothorax of no conse-

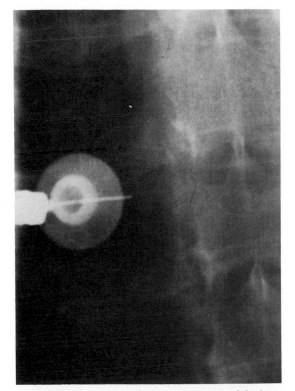

Figure 27–3. Anteroposterior roentgenogram of the lower thoracic spine made at the time of a diagnostic therapeutic block. The needle is placed below the rib adjacent to the costotransverse joint, the ideal location for periarticular infiltration.

quence may occur. This has been seen most often when root irritation has been present on the concave side of a scoliotic curvature. Here, accurate needle placement may be quite difficult. Painful trigger spots in the paraspinal musculature are also injected with local anesthetic.

Relief of pain has a decidedly beneficial effect on the patient's attitude to the overall program, and approximately half of the patients require only one injection series. The patient remains in the hospital for a further week of intensive therapy and is then followed regularly on an outpatient basis by both the orthopedist and the physical therapist. Forty per cent of patients require at least two injections, and if indicated, the second one is given 10 days after the first. In one in 10 patients, there is no improvement at all by this approach, and for them, transcutaneous electrical stimulation (TCNS) may be very helpful. This technique has also been used with good effect in the early stages of the inpatient program.

The former practice of injecting alcohol or phenol into an intercostal nerve for this condition has rightly been discarded, because intractable pain from peripheral neuritis can be the result. Similarly, sensory rhizotomy over multiple levels should not be considered. It is a major surgical operation with very uncertain results.

Electromyographic and nerve conduction studies have been claimed by some workers[19] to be of particular use in the diagnosis of thoracic radiculopathy but this has not been the author's experience. Evaluation of the data is qualitative and diagnostic block is far more reliable. On a number of occasions, however, electromyographic studies have been most useful in establishing that a patient's thoracic pain was due to peripheral neuritis.

Specialized roentgenographic studies have not been found useful in the assessment of these problems. Oblique films, the so-called Williams' views, are required to demonstrate the articulations, and they have not been found to be of assistance in making clinical decisions.

The first thoracic root is particularly susceptible to irritation from an osteoarthritic first costotransverse joint because of the anatomic factors described earlier. This possibility should be kept in mind in the differential diagnosis of the thoracic outlet syndrome. Firm pressure over the joint posteriorly may reproduce pain and, occasionally, so will lateral neck flexion to the opposite side. Nerve irritation in the proximal thoracic spine may simulate cardiac or pulmonary disease. The important clue in diagnosis is that often patients will have noticed that movement, particularly rotation, either precipitates or increases their pain. Tenderness is usually present over the joints and in the intercostal spaces. Minor alterations in cutaneous sensation should be carefully sought.

Irritative neuropathy at T1 responds particularly well to periarticular injections of local steroid and a mobilizing exercise program. Parallel experience has been recorded by other workers.[20]

When all of the described measures fail to produce a favorable response, the question of removal of the proximal end of the rib arises, although this has not been necessary at the T1 level. In recent years, I have advised surgery far less frequently than formerly. The reason for this is not that the results of surgery are unsatisfactory, but that the nonoperative program has evolved to a point at which a high percentage of excellent and good results can be obtained. A contraindication to operation is failure of the diagnostic block to relieve the patient's pain. Because the operation is not mentioned in the text on surgery, it is described briefly.

Technique

The patient is positioned on a Hall-Relton frame, which facilitates roentgenographic localization. A slight lateral tilt of the operating table improves the view of the operative field. A slightly curved, 10-cm-long incision is made just medial to the angle of the ribs and the interval between the iliocostalis and longissimus muscles is developed. The rib to be resected is stripped subperiosteally to the level of the tip of the transverse process, and 3 cm of rib distal to this point are removed. This permits the underlying pleura to be mobilized gently with a cottonoid pledget, and it readily strips well down onto the vertebral body. The transverse process is freed of its soft tissue attachment; a small Cobb elevator is ideal for this purpose. The process is divided at its base with an angled bone cutter and removed. The free end of the rib is then held with bone holders and rotated as the elevator is used to continue the subperiosteal stripping. The costovertebral joint offers little resistance to the maneuver, and the proximal end of the rib is easily resected. The intercostal nerve is then dissected free from the vascular bundle laterally and is mobilized medially. The posterior primary ramus is identified and preserved. The medial end of the intercostal musculature is excised together with the levator costarum.

The nerve is connected by a loose mesh of fibrous tissue to the margins of the intervertebral foramen; small veins in this area can give troublesome bleeding. Mobilization of the nerve is more safely completed at the bony foraminal margin to include the attached connective tissue. Bipolar cautery is useful in obtaining hemostasis. This technique does not entail a precise display of the pathology, hence the need for accurate localization by the diagnostic blocks and the intraoperative roentgenographic control.

The proximal ends of the ribs above and below are excised in a comparable fashion, and access is facilitated after the first rib has been removed. A small dead space is inevitable, and this is reduced by Gelfoam strips. A Hemovac drain is routinely used. Patients are encouraged to move as soon as their wound pain permits, which is usually within 2 to 3 days. Sutures are removed on the eleventh postoperative day. The scar that results from the incision is cosmetically very satisfactory.

DIFFERENTIAL DIAGNOSIS

Although it is not intended to include in this chapter an exhaustive discussion of the differential diagnosis of thoracic pain with and without root involvement, it may be of interest for the reader to peruse the list of diagnoses I have made during the course of the 20-year period in which I have had a particular interest in patients with thoracic disorders. The spectrum of pathology is wide and varied:

1. A mechanical and degenerative condition affecting the costotransverse and costovertebral joints.

2. Thoracic disk prolapse, calcified and noncalcified. Calcification confined to the nucleus pulposus in children and adults.

3. Thoracic spondylosis.

4. Scoliosis and kyphoscoliosis. During rapid progression of curvature and associated with secondary degenerative changes.

5. Scheuermann's disease. During the active phase of the disease and in middle age associated with spondylotic changes.

6. Referred pain from cervical spondylosis.

7. After fracture and fracture-dislocation of the thoracic spine.

8. Metabolic bone disease; osteoporosis with and without demonstrable fracture; osteomalacia, Paget's disease.

9. Postural disorders—principally seen in younger females.

10. Disturbed spinal mechanics occurring in pregnancy.

11. Primary and secondary tumors involving the vertebral column; tumors of the spinal cord and nerve roots; neoplasms of the chest wall and pleura.

12. Vertebral osteomyelitis and disk space infections in children and adults.

13. Ankylosing spondylitis and rheumatoid arthritis.

14. Diabetic peripheral neuropathy.

15. Visceral disease in the chest and abdomen; coronary insufficiency; pleurisy; hiatus hernia; renal disease; penetrating peptic ulcer; biliary disorders; pancreatitis.

16. Aortic aneurysm with vertebral column involvement.

17. Malignant tumors involving the upper posterior abdominal wall, especially from the pancreas.

18. Post-thoracotomy syndrome in adults.

19. Postherpetic neuralgia.

20. After rib fracture; "slipping rib" syndromes and allied mechanical disorders; Teitze's syndrome; avulsion of a lower costochondral junction.

21. Avulsion fractures of spinous processes—clay shoveler's fracture.

22. Subscapular bursitis.

23. Serratus anterior palsy.

24. Intrinsic spinal cord disease; focal arachnoiditis in the thoracic spinal cord; arachnoid cyst; radiation necrosis of the spinal cord.

25. Postnephrectomy syndromes; entrapment of the twelfth thoracic intercostal nerve in scar tissue.

26. Intercostal neuralgia, without definable etiology.

27. Bornholm disease.

A number of these diseases and disorders warrant particular comment.

Thoracic Intervertebral Disk Prolapse

Thoracic disk prolapse is far more common than the orthopedic literature would suggest, and most patients, because of the neurologic complications, are managed by neurosurgeons. It occurs in two forms, calcified and noncalcified. In the former, the calcified nucleus pulposus extrudes into the spinal canal; the latter is similar in type to the common lumbar lesion.[21] The etiology of the calcification is not known, and it is best termed dystrophic calcification.[5] Both types of prolapse occur most frequently in the fifth decade of life and are twice as common in males as in females. Cal-

cified lesions occur most frequently at T9–T10 and noncalcified prolapses occur at T11–T12, which suggests a mechanical factor is at least involved in pathogenesis. There are no data to suggest that noncalcified lesions are in any way linked with the spondylotic process.

Spinal cord compression is an expected manifestation of prolapse in the thoracic region, as this is the narrowest part of the spinal canal. It tends to run a slowly progressive course. Spontaneous remissions, which are so characteristic of lumbar disk prolapse, are less commonly seen. There is no typical clinical picture of the myelopathy. Early surgery is mandatory, and diskectomy is most safely achieved by the transthoracic or posterolateral approach. The results of surgery are most satisfactory, provided the cord deficit is not pronounced. Lateral prolapse may present as a radicular syndrome with its attendant difficulties in diagnosis.[22]

Ankylosing Hyperostosis of the Spine (AHS)

This fascinating disorder of unknown etiology has come to be associated with the name of Forestier[23] (see Chapter 13). It is characterized by ossification of the anterior longitudinal ligament with spontaneous fusion over multiple levels. The posterior ligamentous structures are unaffected. The thoracic spine is more frequently involved than the cervical or lumbar regions. Disk degeneration with narrowing is not present, a crucial point in the differential diagnosis of spondylosis.

The epidemiology of AHS has been studied extensively in Finland by Julkunen and co-workers.[24] In a sample of 8993 subjects over 15 years of age, they found the standardized rates to be 3.8% for men and 2.6% for women. Age-matched controls were employed. One of the more interesting aspects was its link to carbohydrate metabolism and obesity.

There was an age-dependent increase in prevalence, and some regional differences in incidence were found. No evidence was detected to suggest that there was an increase of locomotor symptoms in patients with AHS or that prior spinal trauma was related to the malady. Because spontaneous fusion is the natural history of AHS in the thoracic region, it would be surprising if pain were a feature, and there is no evidence to indicate a primary inflammatory disorder. The multisegmental spinal fusion in the thoracic region produces no disability and minimal stiffness. Giant bridging osteophytes in the cervical region may result in pressure effects, with tracheal and esophageal obstruction. The ossification in the anterior longitudinal ligament seen in ankylosing spondylitis is much flatter, and exuberant hyperostosis is not seen. Spontaneous fusion may also occur in Scheuermann's disease,[25] but the other hallmarks of this condition bespeak the nature of the disorder.

Thoracic Spine Involvement in Arthropathy

The clinical features of ankylosing spondylitis and rheumatoid arthritis are such that they need no expanded discussion in this chapter, and thoracic spinal pain is frequently seen with both. Curiously enough, spinal gout is a clinical entity that remains something of an enigma. On one hand, autopsy studies on patients with gout have shown that the vertebral axis may be extensively involved by tophaceous deposits,[26] but on the other hand, as pointed out by Tkach,[27] there are few guidelines to permit an accurate clinical diagnosis of spinal gout. The reader is referred to Tkach's paper, which highlights the near bewildering complexity of the clinical puzzle.

Obscure Abdominal and Chest Pain

It has long been recognized that the spinal axis can be responsible for abdominal and chest pain. Carnett[28, 29] introduced the term intercostal neuralgia and clearly described how this could mimic a variety of intra-abdominal disorders. He drew attention to the vital physical sign in diagnosis, namely the importance of palpating the abdomen first with the musculature relaxed and then with it contracted. Persistence of tenderness with the musculature contracted was believed to be indicative of neuralgia. I have found this to be a most reliable maneuver, but it may be difficult to interpret if the abdominal muscles are weak and atrophic, as they sometimes are in older subjects. Irritation of the parietal peritoneum can also result in persistence of tenderness with the musculature contracted, and this is well exemplified by the right iliac fossa signs of acute appendicitis with peritoneal spread.

Ashby[30] recently prospectively studied a series of 53 patients seen in the course of 1 year in a general surgical practice and in whom abdominal pain was considered to have a "neurologic" basis. The precise cause of the neuropathy was not determined, but patients with coexistent back pain were excluded from the study. Two thirds of the patients responded to intercostal block with complete and lasting relief from their symptoms. In a further 25% of patients, pain was significantly reduced. The age of most of Ashby's patients was 50 to 60 years, and two thirds of them were females. The eleventh thoracic nerve was the most common site of involvement. In view of these data, it seems probable that degenerative changes in the costotransverse joints were the likely basis of the patients' symptoms in a high percentage of cases. It is relevant that Ashby performed the intercostal nerve blocks lateral to the sacrospinalis musculature and that this led him to conclude that a vicious circle of pain and reflex phenomena was responsible, frequently with depression, tension, and preoccupation with symptoms enhancing the patients' responses. The opinion was expressed that summation may occur with facilitation from multiple minor stimuli. He attributed his good results to interruption of pain synapse-facilitating efferent barrage. It is worthy of note that Ashby saw one patient per week with this syndrome, and this is certainly an important entity in general surgical practice that does not receive the attention it warrants.

A most interesting study on patients with suspected renal pain has been done by Fox and Saunders,[31] who evaluated 100 consecutive females referred with this diagnosis to an outpatient clinic in Sheffield, England. The group constituted one fifth of all new patient referrals. A subsequent diagnosis of "fibromuscular or musculoskeletal pain" was made in 56 patients, but eight of these were later shown to have an upper renal tract abnormality. It was considered that 18 patients had been unnecessarily referred. Further management of the patients was not discussed, but the message concerning the importance of history taking and physical examination in the patient with "loin pain" is quite clear.

A wide variety of diseases affecting the vertebral column can result in root or referred pain, and clinical evaluation needs to be thorough. Reflex phenomena from visceral disease and reflex visceral manifestations of somatic pain can be quite difficult to differentiate. The possible presence of two pathologic entities must always be kept in mind. Nevertheless, if a patient presents with abdominal or chest pain of obscure origin and there are no reasonable clinical clues to pursue, nerve blocks are an attractive alternative to lengthy investigations, especially exploratory laparotomy.

Even if a good response is obtained, patients should be followed regularly, because nerve blocks are not specific therapy in the strictest sense. Malignant invasion of an intercostal nerve may occur by a tumor of the posterior abdominal wall. However, the symptoms of serious disease do not remain stationary, and other signs shortly surface.

SPINAL BRACING IN DISORDERS OF THE THORACIC SPINE

In my experience, patients who would benefit from the use of an orthosis frequently are not supplied with an appropriate brace. The older patient finds the conventional thoracic brace, such as the Taylor or Boston brace, a cumbersome and restrictive burden, and unless it is specifically contoured for the individual, the brace may be decidedly uncomfortable and quickly find its way to the back of the family wardrobe. A far more satisfactory form of orthosis is one of polypropylene manufactured from a torso mould (Fig. 27–4). Furthermore, an orthosis of this type is far less obvious through the patient's clothing than a conventional brace and is much more acceptable to women. A moulded torso orthosis has been found particularly useful in the management of painful adult scoliosis. Patients are not instructed to wear the orthosis at all times but rather to use it to allow them to undertake activities that would otherwise precipitate pain. In hot climates, a cotton singlet worn beneath the orthosis helps to absorb perspiration, which can result in troublesome skin irritation.

ACKNOWLEDGMENTS

The assistance of Miss S. Tandy-Cockram and Mrs. J. Mitchell in the preparation of this chapter is gratefully acknowledged.

References

1. Gloobe H, Nathan H: The costovertebral joint. Anatomical observation in various mammals. Anat Anz 127:22–31, 1970.
2. Nathan H: Compression of the sympathetic trunk by osteophytes of the vertebral column in the abdomen; an anatomical study with pathological and clinical considerations. Surgery 63:609–625, 1968.
3. Wyke BD: The neurological basis for thoracic spinal pain. Rheumatol Rehabil 10:356–367, 1970.
4. Feinstein B, Langton NJK, Jamieson RM: Experiments on pain referred from deep somatic structures. J Bone Joint Surg 36A:981–997, 1954.
5. Taylor TKF, Akeson WH: Intervertebral disc prolapse. A review of morphological and biochemical knowledge concerning the nature of prolapse. Clin Orthop 76:54–80, 1970.
6. Vernon-Roberts B, Pirie CJ: Degenerative changes in

Figure 27–4. Front *(A)* and side *(B)* views of a polypropylene jacket constructed from a torso mould, in this case from a patient with moderately severe scoliosis. The shoulder straps are carefully placed to prevent the top edge of the brace from becoming prominent through clothing.

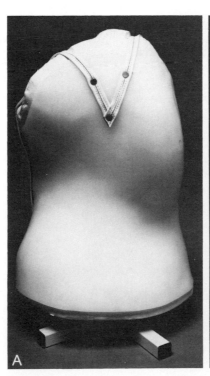
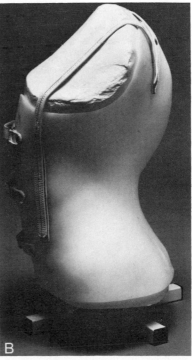

the intervertebral discs of the lumbar spine and their sequelae. Rheumatol Rehabil 16:13–21, 1977.

7. Stoddard A, Osborn JF: Scheuermann's disease or spinal osteochondrosis; its frequency and relationship with spondylosis. J Bone Joint Surg 61B:56–58, 1979.

8. Nathan H: Osteophytes of the vertebral column. An anatomical study of their development according to age, race, and sex with considerations as to their etiology and significance. J Bone Joint Surg 44A:243–268, 1962.

9. Culver GJ, Pirson HS: Preventive effect of aortic pulsations on osteophyte formation in the thoracic spine. Am J Rheumatol 84:937–940, 1960.

10. Shapiro R, Batt HD: Unilateral thoracic spondylosis. Am J Rheumatol 83:660–662, 1960.

11. Chaiton A, Fam A, Charles B: Disappearing lumbar hyperostosis in a patient with Forestier's disease. Arthritis Rheum 22:799–802, 1979.

12. Goldberg RP, Carter BL: Absence of thoracic osteophytes in the area adjacent to the aorta; computed tomography demonstration. J Comput Assist Tomogr 2:173–175, 1978.

13. Ghosh P, Taylor TKF, Meachim D: A double blind crossover trial of indomethacin, flurbiprofen, and placebo in the management of lumbar spondylosis. Curr Ther Res in press.

14. Taylor TKF, Ghosh P: Anti-inflammatory drugs in the management of spondylosis. Br Med J 283:951, 1981.

15. Marzluff JM, Hungerford GD, Kempe LG, et al.: Thoracic myelopathy caused by osteophytes of the articular processes. J Neurosurg 50:779–783, 1979.

16. Nathan H, Weinberg H, Robin GC, Aviad I: The costovertebral joints. Anatomical-clinical observations in arthritis. Arthritis Rheum 7:228–240, 1964.

17. Rocca Rossetti S, Bisogno EM: Studio anatomico-istologico delle articolazioni. Costo-transversarie e cost-vertebrali dell'individuo sano e quello artrosico. Rassegna Medicale Sarda 65:1009, 1960.

18. Taylor TKF: Thoracic and abdominal pain originating in the vertebral axis. Some aspects of physical diagnosis. Northwest Med 69:679–685, 1970.

19. Johnson ER, Powell J, Caldwell J, Crane L: Intercostal nerve conduction and posterior rhizotomy in the diagnosis and treatment of thoracic radiculopathy. J Neurol Neurosurg Psychiatry 37:330–332, 1974.

20. Weinberg H, Nathan H, Magora F, et al.: Arthritis of the first costotransverse joint as a cause of thoracic outlet syndrome. Clin Orthop 86:159–163, 1972.

21. Taylor TKF, Ghosh P, Bushell GR, Stephens RW: The scientific basis for the treatment of intervertebral disc disorders. *In* Owen R, Goodfellow JG, Bullough PG: Scientific Foundations of Orthopaedics and Traumatology. London, Heinemann Medical Books Ltd., 1980, pp. 387–406.

22. Epstein JA: The syndrome of herniation of the lower thoracic intervertebral discs with nerve root and spinal cord compression. A presentation of 4 cases with a review of the literature, methods of diagnosis and treatment. J. Neurosurg 2:528–548, 1944.

23. Forestier J, Rotes-Querol J: Senile ankylosing hyperostosis of the spine. Ann Rheum Dis 9:321–330, 1950.

24. Julkunen H, Heinonen OP, Knekt P, Maatela J: The epidemiology of hyperostosis of the spine together with its symptoms and related mortality in a general population. Scand J Rheumatol 4:23–27, 1975.

25. Butler HW: Spontaneous anterior fusion of vertebral bodies. J Bone Joint Surg 53B:231–235, 1971.

26. Lichtenstein L, Wayne Scott H, Levin MH: Pathological changes in gout; survey of seven necropsied cases. Am J Pathol 32:871–895, 1956.

27. Tkach S: Gouty arthritis of the spine. Clin Orthop 71:81–86, 1970.

28. Carnett JB: Intercostal neuralgia as a cause of abdominal pain and tenderness. Surg Gynecol Obstet 42:625–632, 1926.

29. Carnett JB: Simulation of gallbladder disease by intercostal neuralgia of the abdominal wall. Ann Surg 86:747–757, 1927.

30. Ashby EC: Abdominal pain of spinal origin. Value of intercostal block. Ann R Coll Surg Eng 59:3–7, 1977.

31. Fox M, Saunders NR: Significance of loin pain in women. A study of 100 consecutive cases referred to a urological clinic. Lancet 1:115–116, 1978.

28

Osteoarthritis of the Lumbar Spine, Disk Disease

Robert E. Booth, Jr., M.D.
Richard H. Rothman, M.D., Ph.D.

Back pain may well be one of the most significant penalties that man has paid for the adoption of the erect posture that has freed his prehensile hands and allowed him to outstrip his quadrupedal ancestors. Lumbago and sciatica have plagued mankind for thousands of years, and their descriptions can be found in the Bible and in the writings of Hippocrates. Since the original description of the intervertebral disk by Vesalius in 1543,[1] many anatomic, biochemical, and molecular explanations have been extended to explain the pathophysiology of these complaints. No satisfactory explanation was to emerge until the publication of the classic paper by Mixter and Barr in 1934.[2] Their indictment of the herniation of nuclear material into the spinal canal as a cause of back pain and sciatica opened a new era of understanding and treatment of these complaints. The significance of a degenerative disease process lies in its production of either death or disability in the afflicted individual. Because degenerative disease of the intervertebral disk is largely a nonlethal entity, its importance to our population is best reflected in the discomfort and disability that it appears to produce.

INCIDENCE

Precise and accurate evaluations of the epidemiology of low back pain syndromes have been compromised by the multifactorial components of degenerative disk disease symptoms and the even greater range of diagnostic terms applied to them. Nonetheless, some feeling for the incidence and impact of degenerative disk disease can be gleaned from the well-documented experience in the industrial setting. Nachemson has estimated that approximately 80% of the population will experience symptoms of back pain at some point in their lives.[3] Approximately half of the adult population will at some time be significantly disabled by low back pain.[4] The average age of onset of low back pain is approximately 27 years, and approximately one third of those individuals will develop sciatica within the succeeding 10 years.[5] Although sciatica is not a necessary sequela of disk degeneration, there does exist a broad spectrum of symptoms, ranging from idiopathic low back pain at one extreme to symptoms associated with frank nuclear herniation at the other. Sciatica alone will strike approximately 3% of the population,[6] and disk herniation appears to be the pathologic event in approximately half of these individuals.[7]

It was found that significant spinal symptomatology appeared nearly a decade later in females than in their male counterparts. Nonetheless, after the subsidence of the original attack of low back pain, 90% had a recurrence.[8, 9] There appears to be no significant sexual predilection for back pain and sciatica due to disk disease, yet Kelsey[8] found that males underwent surgical procedures more often than females. No racial differences in the incidence of low back pain and sciatica from disk disease have been substantiated.

Aside from its impact on the individual, low back pain has a significant influence on the population as a whole. Data from the United States National Health Survey, published in 1975, indicate that disorders of the back and spine had an estimated incidence of 8 million in the United States in 1971.[10] This statistic incorporates a prevalence rate of 52 per 1000 people, a disability rate of 18 per 1000 people, and a severe disability rate of 4 per 1000 people. Overall, disorders of the back and spine are the third leading cause of disability in individuals in the working years, ranking behind only arthritis and rheumatism, and heart disease.

In Sweden, where a highly organized system of health care evaluation exists, excellent statistics are readily available for population analysis. In his Munkfors investigation, Hult reported that 53% of persons engaged in light work and 64% of those involved in heavy work suffered from low back pain.[11] This not only indicates a high percentage of spinal symptomatology in the working population but also suggests that light activity does not necessarily protect against spinal disease.

The economic impact of the painful low back is also impressive. Benn and Wood[12] reviewed the medical statistics from the National Insurance in the United Kingdom and found that more than 13 million days were lost annually because of back pain. This accounted for more lost time from work in the United Kingdom in 1970 than even labor strikes.

In the United States, Rowe[13] reported a 10-year study of workers at the Eastman Kodak plant in Rochester, New York. He found that approximately 45% of workers involved in heavy activities and 35% of workers involved in sedentary activities visited the infirmary annually because of low back pain. This represented a work loss of 4 hours per person per year and ranked second only to acute upper respiratory illness in terms of time lost. Rowe reported that disk degeneration was the cause of back pain in approximately half of the individuals treated.

It has been reported that the annual rate of low back pain among workers in the United States is approximately 2%.[10] In 1976, this represented a cost to industry of 14 billion dollars for treatment and compensation.[14] Temporary disability (22%) and permanent disability (45%) accounted for the majority of workers compensation costs, with medical costs representing only 33%.[15] Of the total medical costs involved, hospitalization accounted for one third; physicians' fees accounted for an additional one third; and diagnostic tests, physical therapy, medications, and appliances accounted for the remaining one third. It has been estimated that approximately 260,000 laminectomies were performed in the United States in 1976,[16] and it is highly likely that a significant percentage of these were required because of work-related injuries.

NATURAL HISTORY

It is difficult to overestimate the importance of a clear understanding of the natural history of lumbar disk disease to both the physician and the patient. As with any disease process, the treatment modalities that are recommended and undertaken must constantly be weighed against the expected course and the severity of the patient's symptoms. Otherwise, many ineffective but expensive treatments may seem miraculous when applied to a short-lived problem, and others may seem ineffectual when employed against situations that demand more aggressive treatment. Certainly, this is nowhere more important than in lumbar disk disease, for which a host of therapeutic modalities as well as medical and paramedical subspecialties have sprung forth to arrest or deter the symptoms. Most importantly, the relative merits of surgical intervention must constantly be balanced against the true level of disability and the likelihood of spontaneous recovery with only time and conservative measures.

Most attacks of low back pain begin as a single acute episode, often unrelated to specific trauma. These events, although they may produce disabling pain, are usually self-limited. In general, 70% of individuals will have recovered from these attacks within 3 weeks, and 90% will be improved within 2 months, regardless of treatment.[13] Although the initial episode of back pain may be acute, subsequent recurrences are more likely to surface insidiously.[5, 17] Radicular pain may be a component of the initial attack, but the peripheral symptoms of this disease usually follow the attacks of back pain by 6 to 10 years. Recurrences of sciatic symptoms occur with less traumatic provocation and, in general, continue to increase in severity relative to the discomfort of the back pain itself.[5] Ultimately, sciatica may be the only manifestation of nuclear protrusion, when a decompressed annulus fibrosus is no longer producing significant discomfort.

An excellent overview of the natural history of degenerative disk disease was provided by Hakelius, who studied a group of 583 patients who had had an initial attack of sciatica.[18] The average follow-up was 7 years, with 28% of the patients undergoing surgery and the rest being treated conservatively. Hakelius found that the acute episodes of sciatica ran a relatively brief course in most instances, independent of whether treatment was surgical or conservative. The appendicular symptoms tended to resolve with time, whereas the more axial and chronic symptoms of disk degeneration were prolonged and continued to affect the patient's activity and level of function. At the termination of the evaluation, almost 15% of the group treated with conservative measures continued to have some restriction of their lives, particularly leisure activities and work capacity, and had sleep disturbance. Only 20% of them had sciatica of symptomatic proportions.

Weber reported a long-term review of 280 patients with myelographically proven lumbar disk herniations followed in a well-controlled and well-documented prospective evaluation.[5] After an initial 2-week hospitalization for conservative management, those individuals who failed to improve and who demonstrated relative indications for surgical intervention were randomly assigned to either conservative or surgical treatment groups. Those who did improve were released from the study, and those who had progressive neurologic deficits or sphincter disorders were treated rapidly and also excused from assessment. At the 1-year follow-up examination of the randomized study group, surgical intervention was found to be significantly superior to a conservative regimen in regard to both low back pain and radicular pain produced by the disk herniation. However, after 4 years, no significant difference was observed between the surgical and conservative treatment groups. Similar findings have been suggested previously in both the lumbar[19] and cervical regions of the spine.[20]

It would appear from these reports that the role of surgery is greatest in the early phases of sciatica and in situations in which progressive motor weakness or sphincter dysfunction is imminent. Lesser forms of disability may be treated effectively with only conservative measures with the full expectation that an identical result will ultimately ensue. Further review of these studies would also suggest that there is little to be lost from a 3-month program of conservative therapy. The surgical result was not at all impaired by this length of delay. Conversely, delay of surgical intervention for more than 1 year seems to produce an inferior result. It is unknown whether this represents irreversible damage to sensitive neural tissues despite an adequate decompression, or whether it merely reflects the altered psychologic and functional patterns of behavior that an individual may assimilate during that prolonged period of discomfort.

In the absence of bowel and bladder dysfunction or progressive motor weakness, it would seem appropriate to observe the patient with a radiculopathy for as long as 3 months, allowing the efficacy of conservative treatment as well as natural processes of healing to become evident. Residual weakness in muscle groups, sensory deficits, and reflex abnormalities are helpful diagnostically. They are not uniformly altered by surgical intervention, which should be reserved in most instances for the treatment of pain.[18] Bowel and bladder dysfunction, however, seems to affect a very small proportion of patients with disk disease but assumes greater significance in terms of surgical urgency.

Armed with this information, the physician can better interpret the role of surgery and other treatment modalities for the individual patient with lumbar disk disease. Only through constant recollection of the relative natural history of the disease process can honest and effective decision making occur in the management of this disorder.

PATHOLOGY

The biochemical and microscopic phenomena attendant to the process of disk degeneration currently receive the greatest attention in active research, because they hold the greatest promise for a true understanding of the precipitating factors in this degenerative disease. Nonetheless, some review of the well-delineated gross anatomic changes in lumbar disk disease is appropriate for our comprehension of the broad spectrum of clinical symptoms that may develop in any individual.

It is currently popular and, indeed, appropriate to consider the intervertebral articulations as a "three-joint complex," a concept popularized by Farfan.[21] Nevertheless, it must be remembered that the posterior "two joints" are represented by the facet joints of the posterior spinous elements. These are true diarthrodial synovial articulations and, as such, are subject to all the true degenerative changes described more completely in earlier sections of this text. The primary intervertebral articulation is represented by the fibrocartilaginous disk. In itself, it consists of three principal parts: the cartilaginous endplates, the nucleus pulposus, and the annulus fibrosus, all secured by ligamentous supports. The intervertebral disks constitute approximately 25% of the entire length of the vertebral column. Perhaps because of the increased stresses in the lower levels of the lumbar spine, the lumbar intervertebral disks contribute more to the overall length of the lumbar spine than the cervical and thoracic intervertebral disks contribute to their respective regions. The cartilaginous vertebral endplate is the limiting structure composed of hyaline cartilage that covers the vertebral body and is surrounded by an epiphyseal ring. Its primary contributions are to the nutrition of the nucleus and to the stress transference of axial loads to the disk itself.[22] Macnab has likened the structure of the intervertebral disk to that of a car tire, with the annulus fibrosus being analogous to the inner tube.[23] The nucleus pulposus consists of collagen fibers imbedded within a mucopolysaccharide gel, and it constitutes approximately 40% of the cross-sectional area of the disk. It is located eccentrically toward the posterior aspect of the intervertebral disk, in an area closer to the center of rotation of the motion segment.

The structure of the annulus fibrosus has generated a great deal of interest. It is composed of three lamellae of fibers, the most peripheral of which pass over the edge of the cartilaginous endplates and attach to the vertebral body as Sharpey's fibers.[23] The annulus is somewhat less substantial in its posterior dimension, and this, coupled with the presence of the relatively weak adjacent posterior longitudinal ligament, may help to explain the pathologic preference leading to the predominance of posterior nuclear protrusions.

Although the peak incidence of the clinical appearance of symptoms of degenerative disk disease is approximately the third decade of life, the pathologic sequence of events probably begins even earlier. In late adolescence, the nucleus pulposus tends to lose its gel-like resiliency and to become more fibrotic. It begins to take on a dull, yellowish appearance and to become less distinct from the surrounding inner layers of the annulus fibrosus. With advancing age, the nucleus will slowly lose its ability to bulge, thus reflecting the progressive process of dehydration and desiccation. By the later decades of life, the nucleus has the consistency of wet cardboard, offering little resistance to compression and little hydraulic diffusion of applied stress (Fig. 28–1).

As the annulus itself begins to degenerate, visible fissures and clefts become apparent. The inner layer of the annulus tends to coalesce with the nucleus, and both structures become progressively more disorganized. Osteophytes and traction spurs may develop at the attachment of the outermost fibers of the annulus (Fig. 28–2).[23] These osteophytes are circumferential bony excrescences beginning at the margins of the vertebral body and extending horizontally to diffuse the forces of weight bearing over a wider surface. They should be distinguished from the traction spurs popularized by Macnab,[24] which are also hor-

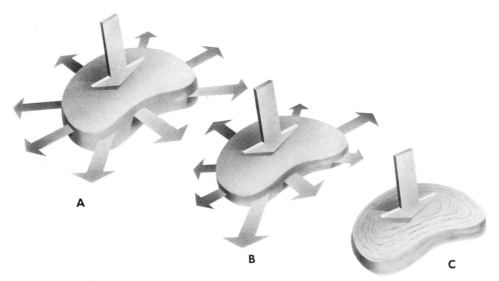

Figure 28–1. The desiccation and degradation of the intervertebral disk produce irregular distribution of forces, as well as compression of the intervertebral disk itself. Thus, true herniations are most common in middle-aged individuals, whereas stenotic problems are more common in the elderly. (From Rothman RH, Simeone FA (eds.): The Spine. 2nd ed. Philadelphia, W. B. Saunders Company, 1982.)

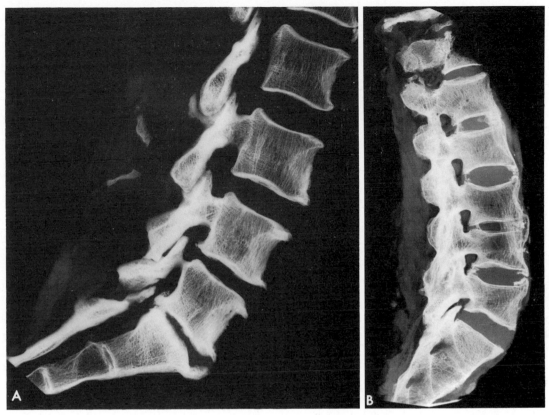

Figure 28–2. A and *B*, Lateral pathologic roentgenograms show narrowing of the disk spaces, osteophyte as well as traction spur formation, and vertical syndesmophytes *(B)*. (From Rothman RH, Simeone FA (eds.): The Spine. 2nd ed. Philadelphia, W. B. Saunders Company, 1982.)

izontal bony protuberances but located 1 or 2 mm away from the edge of the vertebral body and generally smaller in size. Furthermore, it is important to distinguish these degenerative phenomena from the marginal and nonmarginal syndesmophytes that are characteristic of the inflammatory spondylopathies. While these bony growths originate from the margins of the vertebral body, they also extend vertically to join with similar prominences from adjacent vertebral bodies.

As further deterioration of the intervertebral disk occurs, the cartilaginous endplates develop progressive signs of wearing, which are characterized by longitudinal fissures, thinning of the cartilage, and loss of distinction from the nucleus pulposus. When osteoporotic conditions coexist, ballooning of the endplates may occur. Protrusions of the nuclear material into the substance of the vertebral body are also occasionally seen, producing an irregular defect within the vertebral bone surrounded by a small rim of bony sclerosis. The adjacent disk spaces frequently display some thinning from the loss of nuclear material. When these vertical herniations occur during periods of

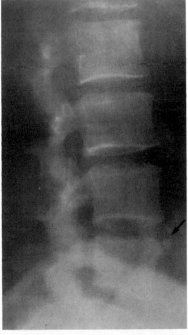

Figure 28–3. A limbus vertebra, marked by sequestration of a fragment of the vertebral body (arrow) and often accompanied by enlargement of that vertebral body itself.

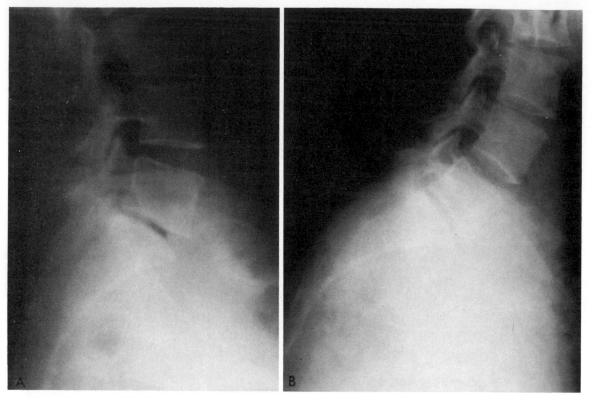

Figure 28–4. *A* and *B*, Lateral roentgenograms demonstrate a narrowed disk space with vacuum phenomenon.

spinal growth, small areas of the ring epiphysis may be isolated and continue to grow independently. This produces a defect known as a limbus vertebra (Fig. 28–3), in which the vertebral body is sometimes slightly enlarged and marked by irregularities, usually of the proximal anterior rim. These should not be mistaken for avulsion fractures, because they bespeak no acute injury or instability.

The overall gross appearance of a degenerated intervertebral disk is that of a desiccated and disorganized structure in which the individual components become indistinct from the adjacent structures. Roentgenologically, one frequently sees a narrowed disk space with osteophytes, traction spurs, violations of the vertebral body by nuclear material, and even gas shadows or vacuum phenomena (Fig. 28–4).[25] Narrowed disk spaces at the L5–S1 level are frequently overinterpreted, however, and may represent only congenital underdevelopment of the intervertebral disk in association with a transitional vertebra. These situations are usually marked by broad transverse processes that may be incorporated either unilaterally or bilaterally into the superior margin of the sacrum.[26]

Disk Protrusion

Nuclear herniation and annular protrusion are thus acute events that are potentiated by a prior pattern of chronic degenerative changes. Indeed, compressive loading of normal youthful spines will result more commonly in compression fractures of the vertebral bodies than in nuclear herniation. It appears that some element of degenerative disease is necessary to precipitate a disk rupture in the average situation.[27]

The pathologic cycle of disk degeneration and nuclear herniation has been described in detail by Armstrong[28] and others. The radiating fissures that develop in the central lamellae of the annulus and gradually extend toward the periphery weaken its resistance to nuclear herniation. With progressive mechanical loading of the disk, nuclear material may begin to insinuate its way into these fissures, transiently distending the disk itself. For reasons that are as yet unclear, this typically occurs in the posterior aspect of the annulus. Frank herniation is most likely to occur in the younger individual, between the third and fifth decades of life, when relative turgor of the nucleus is still present. As the intervertebral disk ages, loss of nuclear turgor diminishes the chance of herniation. This is thought to explain the relative paucity of acute nuclear protrusions in elderly individuals.

There are several patterns of posterior displacement of the nucleus pulposus that should be understood. In the most extreme case, a massive extrusion of the majority of the nuclear contents directly posteriorly into the spinal canal may occur, producing a profound neurologic picture known as the cauda equina syndrome. A more typical pattern is gradual protrusion of the nuclear fragments through the rent in the annulus, constrained only by the posterior longitudinal ligament. This ligament may be stretched and even stripped from its insertion to the posterior surface of the vertebral bodies by the migrating nuclear material.

The posterior longitudinal ligament is an hourglass structure, however, with a rather narrow profile over the vertebral bodies themselves and lateral expansions at each disk space. Thus, the nuclear herniations may be contained for some period and ultimately influenced to protrude in a posterolateral direction by the conformation of the posterior longitudinal ligament. In an extreme example, if the ultimate point of extrusion is located sufficiently far laterally, it may even produce intraforaminal herniation of the nucleus (Fig. 28–5).

Occasionally, the posterior constraints may be totally disrupted, and nuclear material may escape freely into the canal in the form of an extruded fragment. This sequestrum may then migrate cephalad, caudad, or out into the neural foramen. Thus, it is not only the size of the nuclear herniation that determines the relative proportions of symptomatology but also the direction in which it may occur.

Another factor to be considered in the production of symptoms is the shape of the spinal canal (Fig. 28–6). In the lumbar region, most individuals have a spinal canal that is circular or, more commonly, oval in cross section. There are those individuals who have a more triangular or trefoil shape to their canal, with consequent narrowing of the lateral recesses where the nerve roots reside. This pattern is, of course, accentuated by degenerative changes within the facet joints of the posterior spine. Nonetheless, a small nuclear herniation in an individual with short pedicles or a trefoil canal is more likely to be symptomatic than a herniation of similar size in a canal that is more capacious. Failure to remember the differential aspects of the normal anatomy of the spinal canal may lead to confusion about the variety of symptoms that a disk herniation may produce. Certainly, the inflammatory component of disk disease is also predicated on the available space within the spinal canal. Whether the enlargement of sensitive neurologic structures is the result of the ingrowth of inflammatory granulation tissue, an autoimmune mechanism, vascular engorgement, or simple edema of bruised tissues, the symptom complex produced and the efficacy of anti-inflammatory treatments are unquestionably compromised by anatomic narrowing of the neural spaces. It has been dramatically demonstrated by Falconer that myelographic defects remain unchanged after successful conservative treatment of sciatica.[29] Thus, mechanical factors alone do not adequately explain the symptoms of nerve root compression.

Spinal Stenosis

Surgeons have long been comfortable with the concept of "the soft disk" herniation in the cervical and lumbar regions of the spine. We also have no difficulty with the concept of the "hard disk" in the cervical spine, where degenerative burs and osteophytes have been known for decades to produce symptoms of axial and appendicular pain. For some reason, the analogous concept of spinal stenosis or degenerative narrowing of the neural spaces in the lumbar spine has been regarded as a new entity since its popularization in the last two decades. As has just been discussed and as Porter and colleagues[30] have shown, those individuals who suffer from back pain are more apt to have small spinal canals than patients who have been asymptomatic. Because disk degeneration is a natural concomitant of the aging process, we are not surprised to see the natural evolution of pathologic changes within the intervertebral joint leading to a subsequent stiffening of the spine in that area. This is accentuated by the natural processes of healing and osteophyte formation that we term spondylosis. We know from our demographic studies that the roentgenographic stigmata of disk degeneration increase longitudinally with age, whereas the back pain symptoms that we frequently attribute to those changes appear to

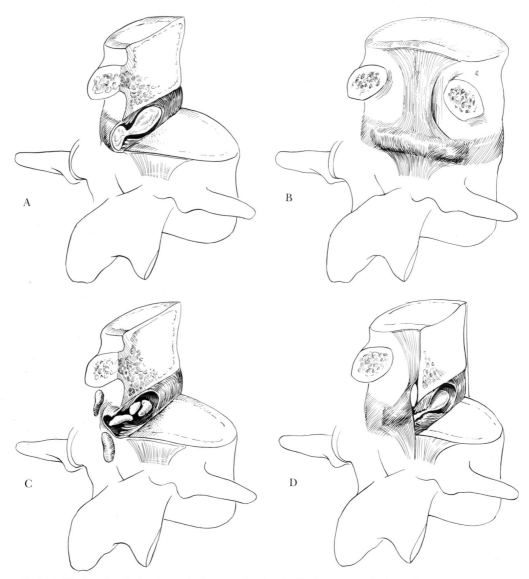

Figure 28–5. *A*, Nuclear herniation beneath the posterior longitudinal ligament. *B*, Central nuclear herniation beneath the most substantial portion of the posterior longitudinal ligament. *C*, Complete extrusion of the nuclear material through an annular rupture, with free fragments in the spinal canal. *D*, Cephalad migration of extruded fragments beneath the ligamentous structures. (From DePalma AF, Rothman RH: The Intervertebral Disc. Philadelphia, W. B. Saunders Company, 1970.)

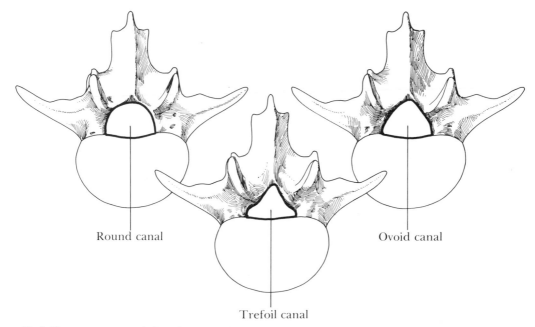

Round canal

Trefoil canal

Ovoid canal

Figure 28–6. Three common variations in the configuration of the spinal canal, with the trefoil canal being the most susceptible to symptomatic herniations and spinal stenosis. (From DePalma AF, Rothman RH: The Intervertebral Disc. Philadelphia, W. B. Saunders Company, 1970.)

peak between the ages of 30 and 50 years and subside to some degree as the individual reaches the later decades of life.

The many facets of the pathology of spinal stenosis have been enunciated by many authors, but they have been best summarized and interrelated by Kirkaldy-Willis and co-workers.[25] The common denominator of almost all forms of spinal stenosis is some element of disk degeneration and disk space narrowing. In its earliest stages, this produces a subclinical mechanical instability with subsequent acceleration of the degenerative process within the disk itself. Laxity of the annulus

fibrosus and supporting ligaments accelerates the annular tears and outstrips the normal healing efforts of the ligaments. The resultant hypermobility at the intervertebral joint produces annular bulging, narrowing of the disk space, and osteophyte formation, all of which serve to encroach upon the space available for the neural elements (Fig. 28–7).

Next, the facet joints are allowed to subluxate because of the laxity of the disk space, generally moving in the axial, sagittal, and frontal planes. This places new stresses on the posterior portion of the intervertebral disk, further accelerating its deterioration. The facet

Figure 28–7. Hypertrophy of the facet joints with disk degeneration produces entrapment of the nerve root in the narrowed lateral recess of the spinal canal. (From Rothman RH, Simeone FA (eds.): The Spine. 2nd ed. Philadelphia, W. B. Saunders Company, 1982.)

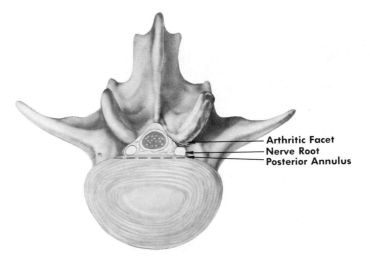

Arthritic Facet
Nerve Root
Posterior Annulus

joints, being diarthrodial synovial joints, undergo erosive, effusive, and degenerative changes themselves, with subsequent osteophyte formation. There is a rotatory component to the subluxation as well, further accentuating the degenerative changes in the anteromedial aspect of the superior vertebral facet (Fig. 28–8). Indeed, this rotational subluxation is usually asymmetric, involving the inferior facet on one side and the superior facet on the contralateral side, allowing both to intrude on the spinal canal from a posterolateral orientation.

Finally, the ligamentum flavum, a passive elastic ligament, is functionally shortened with narrowing of the disk and subluxation of the facet joint. This allows the ligament to thicken in an accordion fashion, and it is passively extruded into the spinal canal, further narrowing this critical passage. These changes can be represented diagrammatically, inferred from myelographic changes, and now clearly delineated with transverse axial tomography.

The neurologic implications of these degenerative changes must also be understood and articulated, particularly as they affect the L4–L5 disk space—the most common level of involvement. At this level, it is common to see the L5 nerve root compressed between the superior facet of L5 and the bulging disk and osteophyte of L4. The L5 nerve root may be displaced medially, and even the L4 nerve root can be caught between the bulging disk and the superior pedicle. Posteriorly, the thickened ligamentum flavum is passively displaced into the neural space. Rotation of the facets will displace them into the neural foramen as well (Fig. 28–8).

Another consequence of joint laxity is the passive subluxation of the vertebral bodies upon one another. These degenerative spondylolistheses, as they are termed, usually involve an anterior subluxation of the superior vertebra upon the inferior one. Retrospondylolisthesis may occur, and the direction of slip is determined by the degree of lordosis in the involved area as well as the tropism of the associated facet joints. The spondylolisthesis is rarely greater than one third of the width of the vertebral body, and it does not usually represent a severe instability because of the advanced age and generalized tissue stiffness of most individuals who display this deformity. Nonetheless, this further contributes to neural compression by the asymmetric settling of the spinal canal. Angular and translational degenerative spondylolistheses may also occur. In degenerative scoliosis of this nature, neural compression may occur on either the convex or the concave side of the curve, but in our experience, it is more common in the latter.

In addition, it must be remembered that spinal stenosis is not necessarily a static problem. As will be discussed in subsequent sections, the symptoms of spinal stenosis frequently are related to ambulation and activity and are eliminated by rest. Just as it may be necessary to produce some hyperextension of the lumbar spine to produce the symptoms, so some hyperextension may be necessary on roentgenographic examination to demonstrate the neural compression or spinal canal narrowing (Fig. 28–9). Spinal stenosis is a dynamic state, and its examination and documentation must reflect this. Finally, there has been much discussion about the role of the pedicle in producing a spinal stenosis syndrome. As Farfan has pointed out,[31] few would argue that the nerve root may be tethered about the pedicle in rotatory deformities. Enthusiasm for an earlier concept of kinking of the nerve root with axial settling, the "guillotine effect," described by MacNab,[32] is waning because the neural elements are also placed under less tension with vertical migration. When spinal stenosis was first popularized as a diagnostic entity to explain the many symptom complexes for which it is responsible, more attention than is probably now appropriate was given to delineating the relative proportions of central and lateral stenosis. Although it would now appear that the vast majority of stenoses do involve the lateral recess primarily, there are still situations, such as congenitally or developmentally short pedicles, severe subluxations, and shingling and hypertrophy of the laminae, which prevent them from accepting the stresses that normally apply to the facet joints, in which a central stenosis may play a prominent role. The best approach, both conceptually and certainly surgically, is to think about the nerves themselves and to be sure that they are adequately decompressed, regardless of the anatomic aberrations responsible for the stenosis.

CLINICAL SYNDROME

Although lumbar disk disease is unequivocally the most common cause of back and leg pain in our society, there remain a wide variety of vascular, infectious, and space-occupying lesions whose symptoms can mimic and whose implications exceed those of disk degeneration. When considering the diagnosis of disk degeneration, one must constantly keep in

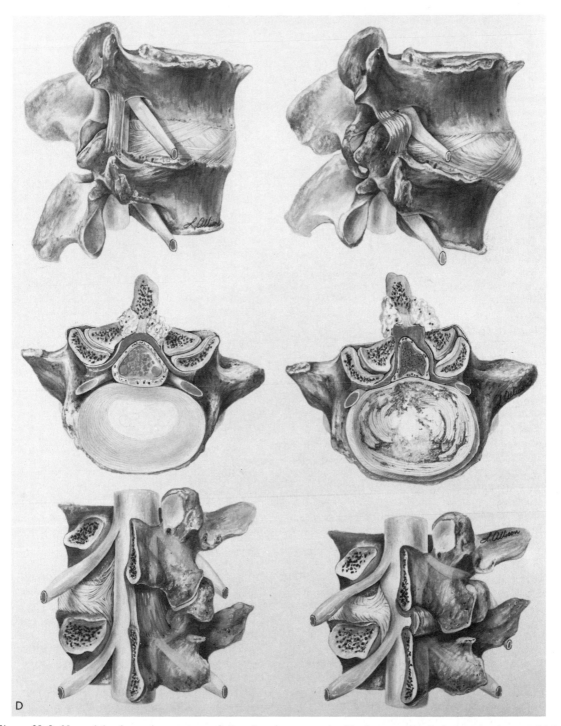

Figure 28–8. Normal lumbar spine anatomy (left column) compared with degenerative and stenotic changes (right column). (From Rothman RH, Simeone FA (eds.): The Spine. 2nd ed. Philadelphia, W. B. Saunders Company, 1982.)

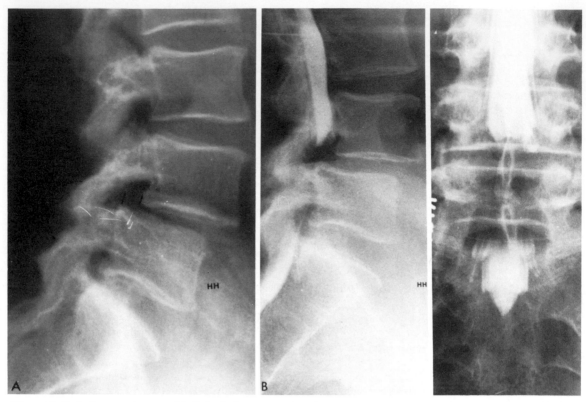

Figure 28–9. A degenerative spondylolisthesis demonstrated both roentgenographically *(A)* and on the myelogram *(B)*. A 4-mm anterior degenerative spondylolisthesis may produce an extensive block on myelographic studies.

mind that this is a multifaceted syndrome on a pathophysiologic basis alone, without even considering the numerous sociologic and psychologic situations that modify its presentation. Just as it is common to dismiss the possibility of the diagnosis of disk degeneration because of an atypical or unusual presentation, so is it necessary to be alert to other possibilities and not attribute all cases of back and leg pain to disk degeneration.

We have reviewed the progressive and interrelated deteriorative processes that are felt to produce pain and deformity in association with disk degeneration. These range from simple desiccation and thinning of the disk to complex deformities with translational and rotatory components. Similarly, there is a wide spectrum of symptoms and presentations in disk degeneration, ranging from simple backache with or without referred pain, through radicular pain, to the sometimes confusing presentations of neurogenic claudication. Our ability to visualize in our mind's eye the pathophysiologic disturbance responsible for our patient's complaint is enhanced by an understanding of the typical historical pattern and the subjective information conveyed to us by our patient. We must constantly keep an open mind when eliciting this information, because many conditions—most notably spinal stenosis—are often most easily diagnosed by a careful historical interrogation.

Low Back Pain

The vast majority of patients who ultimately come to treatment for degenerative disk disease will report episodes of low back pain as their earliest symptoms. Weber, at the Oslo City Hospital, showed that almost all his patients who ultimately suffered a herniated nucleus pulposus had nearly 10 years of episodic low back pain prior to the onset of their radicular symptoms.[5] Spangfort also demonstrated that his patients had over 5 years of low back pain prior to surgical intervention for disk herniation and that the back pain preceded the onset of leg pain by nearly 2 years.[33] Most patients will recall minor episodes of low back pain, usually without any antecedent trauma, which last for only a few hours or days and subside with rest and restricted activities. The pain at this interval is typically mechanical, being exacerbated by activities involving spinal motion and relieved by recumbency. The pain usually extends no farther than the buttock and is frequently symmetric. It is quite probable that discomfort of this sort represents intrusion of the nuclear material into the annular ring as part of the pattern of disk degeneration. Certainly, the onset of these symptoms coincides with the anatomic changes occurring in the disk, and the mechanical nature of the symptoms underscores Nachemson's pressure studies for the postural stress on the disk structures.[34]

Despite the increasing sophistication of diagnostic techniques such as computerized axial tomography, it will probably require even more sensitive methods, such as nuclear magnetic resonance, to explain the true pathophysiology of these frequent attacks of back pain. It has been popular for some time to refer to these attacks as episodes of "acute lumbosacral strain," without any anatomic substantiation for that diagnosis. Certainly, disk degeneration cannot yet be clearly differentiated from certain other common causes of low back pain, such as neural arch defects, postural strains, and unstable lumbosacral mechanisms. Nonetheless, it is our opinion that mechanical degenerative changes within the disk are a more reasonable explanation of low back pain attacks, with the discomfort being mediated through the sinuvertebral nerves that supply the supporting structures of the lumbar spine.

In any event, the typical history is one of episodes of pain that last for a few hours to a few days but gradually occur more frequently and become more intense. As the individual moves on into the middle years, attacks occur more often, and the time for recuperation becomes extended. Lumbosacral range of motion may slowly decrease, either from true pathologic stiffness at the intervertebral articulations or from psychologic restrictions prompted by the fear of further attacks.

The discomfort of a degenerating disk is usually exacerbated by standing and even more by prolonged sitting or riding in motor vehicles. It is nevertheless episodic and is practically never constant. Thus, an individual who complains of unremitting pain, even during bedrest, or of pain that is sufficient to awaken him from sleep during the night should be carefully scrutinized for infectious or neoplastic processes more typical of this symptomatology.

The role of trauma in disk degeneration is always of interest. Weber has shown that more than half of the patients who ultimately develop a disk herniation had some traumatic episode initiating their primary attack.[5] However, these traumatic events had an enormous range of severity, from falling, to lifting heavy objects, to simple abrupt motion. The previously cited work of Jayson and associates[27] clearly showed that compressive loads applied to a healthy young spine will result in vertebral failure prior to disk failure. Only those intervertebral disks with some element of preexisting degeneration were prone to posterolateral nuclear herniations. Although the loads applied were simple compressive forces, the obvious importance of premorbid nucleus pulposus and annulus fibrosus health is apparent. Thus, the most reasonable interpretation of cause and effect that a physician can supply to a curious patient or attorney is to suggest that trauma is a precipitating rather than a causative factor in nuclear herniation.

Other sources of mechanical low back pain must not be overlooked, although they include such difficult diagnoses as facet joint arthritis and vertebral trabecular fractures without roentgenographic collapse. Visceral abnormalities such as abdominal aneurysms, pancreatitis, and perforating ulcers may occasionally elude early diagnosis. Low back pain is such a ubiquitous complaint, however, that all such possibilities should be considered.

Referred Pain

The distention of structures of similar mesodermal origin, such as ligaments, periosteum, joint capsule, and annulus, may produce discomfort characterized as deep, dull, and aching in nature. This is usually felt in the areas of the lumbosacral joints, sacroiliac joints, buttocks, groin, and upper thighs.[35, 36] These areas of referred pain are termed sclerotomes, indicating their common embryonic mesodermal origin. Pains of this nature correspond as well to the meridians of Oriental acupuncture as to the dermatomes of occidental neuroanatomy. Indeed, Melzack and colleagues[37] and others have demonstrated a 71% correspondence between the typical areas of pain referral in these two very different neurologic philosophies. Kellgren[35] has concluded that the distribution of referred pain depends as much on the severity and extent of the discomfort as on the local segmental innervation. Perhaps the most common area for pain referral from discogenic disease of the lumbar spine is the iliolumbar ligaments connecting the transverse processes of the L5 and L4 vertebrae to the pelvis. Many individuals describe counterpressure in this area that relieves or diminishes their discomfort. Referred pain usually coexists with more severe and sharp radicular pain, and the two are far from mutually exclusive. In addition, the signs and symptoms of sympathetic dystrophies from prolonged nerve root embarrassment may further confuse the presentation.

Radicular Symptoms

We have seen that there are many potential mechanisms of neural compression within the spectrum of anatomic changes attendant to disk degeneration. Pressure on an inflamed nerve from a fragment of the disk, a bulging annulus, or a narrow lateral recess may produce a great variety of pain and sensory or motor signs and symptoms in the lower extremities. Certainly, inflammation is a necessary component of this phenomenon, because it has long been known that compression of a normal nerve root will produce only paresthesias, whereas compression of an inflamed nerve root produces pain. This was first demonstrated by Smyth and Wright[38] and later by Macnab[23] and others.

Tension on the spinal nerves is also a significant contributing factor. There is a normal excursion of spinal nerves within their neural foramina when the spine and extremities are flexed or extended. Tethering of the nerve root by subarticular ligaments or by the direct compression of bony or nuclear material may enhance the symptomatic response. Whether this situation represents mere entrapment or some intrinsic structural compromise of the nerve and its supporting vasculature is still uncertain.[39]

The exact etiology of neural inflammation in the production of radicular pain is also unclear. Some authors have indicted an autoimmune mechanism when the privileged tissue of the avascular nucleus pulposus is exposed to the neural canal.[40] Elevation of the titers of IgM and IgG antibodies in patients with disk herniation has encouraged the support for a humoral mechanism.[41, 42] Nonetheless, no immunoglobulins have been found in disk tissue removed at the time of surgery.

Despite the fact that our most effective methods of conservative treatment of disk degeneration with nerve root irritation are directed toward the inflammatory component of the process, we still have a very incomplete understanding of even the rudiments of neural inflammation and its etiology.

Leg Pain

The discomfort of nerve root compression is experienced in the limb as a sharp, lancinating pain, beginning proximally in the back or buttock and extending down the limb in a dermatomal distribution. Although this pain may begin insidiously in more minor attacks of back pain, Weber has established that a popping or tearing sensation may accompany both the initial attack of sciatica and the terminal one, that is, the attack preceding surgical intervention.[5]

Sciatica is usually accompanied by a significant spastic component in the paraspinous musculature. It is said that an individual will typically list away from the side of the common lateral protrusion and toward the side of an axillary disk protrusion (Fig. 28–10). This spasm therefore would appear to be a protective mechanism that diminishes the tension on the nerve root and alleviates both pain and the possibility of further injury.

Most individuals will clearly state that their symptoms are exacerbated by any activity that increases their intra-abdominal pressure. The L5 and S1 nerve roots are the ones most frequently involved in these acute attacks of sciatica, because they are the levels where most herniations occur. In individuals with L4 radiculopathy, less spasm may be present. Many patients will present in a "frozen" position, usually in flexion with some element of lateral listing. This is most common in adolescents, in whom spasm is often a more prominent feature than peripheral reflex or motor abnormalities.[43, 44] There is frequently an hysterical component to this behavior, and the patient's "paralysis" reflects more the fear of future pain than true motor weakness. Nevertheless, some individuals may feel the need to lie immobile on the floor or in bed, resisting all attempts at even passive motion.

Finally, some individuals may observe that the relative proportion of back pain to leg pain is reduced at the time of the sciatic attack. The probable explanation for this phenomenon is that once the annulus has ruptured and the nuclear contents have become extruded, there is little further distention of the paradiskal nerves to create back pain or even local referred discomfort. This, however, is an ominous sign, because in these individuals, there is frequently an increased likelihood that surgical intervention will be required.

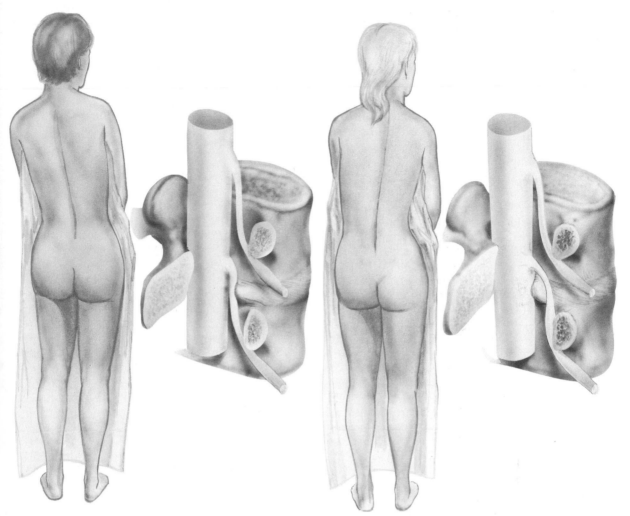

Figure 28–10. *A*, Patient listing away from the side of a lateral disk herniation. *B*, Patient listing toward the side of an axillary disk herniation. (From Rothman RH, Simeone FA (eds.): The Spine. 2nd ed. Philadelphia, W. B. Saunders Company, 1982.)

Motor Symptoms

Occasionally, individuals may be seen whose primary complaint is motor weakness rather than pain or dysesthesias. This is particularly true with involvement of the fourth and fifth lumbar nerves. When the fourth nerve is involved, the patient may complain of knee discomfort and buckling of the leg rather than a more classic radicular pattern. If the fifth nerve is compromised, the patient may present with weakness on dorsiflexion of the foot and toes and, occasionally, a complete footdrop. In this instance, it is helpful to differentiate an L5 nerve root syndrome from peroneal nerve involvement by observing the occasional weakness of the abductor musculature of the hip.

This will often produce an abductor lurch associated with a positive Trendelenburg's sign. Caution must be used in ascribing a painless monoradiculopathy to lumbar disk disease alone, because metabolic, neoplastic, and infectious diseases frequently share this presentation. Finally, one must be aware that in certain individuals the pain from a nuclear herniation is confined to small, isolated anatomic areas, with no linear extension of symptoms from the source in the lumbar spine. Friis and associates have found that approximately 10% of patients with an L5 or S1 lesion had asymptomatic areas of the dermatome between painful foci.[45] Thus, the unwary examiner confronted with an S1 radiculopathy may find himself unsuccessfully treating Achilles tendinitis or calcaneal bursitis, and one confronted with an L5 radiculopathy may misdiagnose it as a painful bunion or gout of the great toe.

Neurogenic Claudication

Perhaps the primary reason that it took so long for spinal stenosis to be included in the family of other disk syndromes was the bizarre and varied nature of its symptoms, particularly that of neurogenic claudication. First appreciated by Verbiest in 1954,[46] this form of claudicatory discomfort is composed of vague leg pain, dysesthesias, and paresthesias over the thighs and calves, classically precipitated by spinal postures that narrowed the neural canal. There remains a controversy as to whether these symptoms are indeed truly ischemic after all, representing a compromise of the supporting vasculature of the peripheral nerve roots. The manifestations of neurogenic claudication are almost identical to those of true vascular insufficiency, at least in the nature and distribution of the discomfort.

The typical presentation is now well known. The patients are usually beyond the age typically associated with nuclear herniations, and their claudicatory symptoms are exacerbated more by walking and standing than by sitting or recumbency. Some are sufficiently alert to relate that their cramping is worse when descending a grade rather than when climbing it, and this fact alone is extremely suggestive. The "bicycle test" of van Gelderen[47] attempts to reproduce the lordotic posture productive of symptoms by having the patient ride a bicycle in a flexed position. Here, claudicatory symptoms would suggest a true vascular insufficiency. If the handlebars are raised and the patient is asked to peddle the bicycle with his spine extended, neurogenic symptoms are more likely to be precipitated. Individuals under suspicion should be carefully examined for variations in the peripheral pulses and the classic skin markings of vascular disease.

Some patients will relate that their claudicatory symptoms progress from the spine down into the limbs, whereas those with true vascular insufficiency feel their calves cramping before their thighs and buttocks. As the symptoms progress, muscle weakness and atrophy as well as asymmetric reflex changes may make the diagnosis more obvious. In earlier-stage cases, it is sometimes necessary to "stress test" the patient by asking him to ambulate until his symptoms appear. At that interval, reflex and motor patterns may develop that were absent at rest.

The inability of patients with spinal stenosis to sleep in a prone position is well known, because it enforces a hyperlordotic posture on their spine. This form of night pain should be carefully defined before extensive evaluations for infectious or neoplastic diseases are undertaken.

The Cauda Equina Syndrome

A relatively rare presentation of acute lumbar disk herniation involves a large midline protrusion of nuclear material. This is known as the cauda equina syndrome and produces severe compression of multiple sensory and motor nerve roots (Fig. 28–11). Pain is largely confined to the buttocks and the back of the thighs and legs, and numbness is widespread from the buttocks to the soles of the feet. There is frequently diffuse weakness or even early paralysis in the lower extremities, and bowel and bladder dysfunction is also quite common.

Raaf[48] reported a 2% incidence of cauda equina syndrome in 624 patients with protruded disks. Spangfort similarly reported a 1.2% incidence of the cauda equina syndrome among 2504 cases, and he found the level of the L4 and L5 disks to be the one most commonly involved.[33] Even more rare are the intradural disk herniations. Although these are relatively rare (0.2% of all disk herniations) and are confined to the upper levels of the lumbar spine, they have been reported to be associated with an extremely high incidence of the cauda equina syndrome, approaching 65%.[49]

The cauda equina syndrome represents a true neurologic emergency. Many times, these lesions are difficult to differentiate from an intraspinal tumor, particularly if they progress slowly. Frequently, back and perianal pain predominates, masking the radicular symptoms. Urinary problems, consisting primarily of frequency or overflow incontinence, may develop relatively early in the syndrome, while impotence may be a later finding. Perianal numbness and a loss of the anal reflex or bulbocavernosus reflex characterize advanced cauda equina syndrome. Sensory deficits are the rule and are frequently situated higher than the motor levels.

As with a progressive motor deficit, the cauda equina syndrome requires prompt sur-

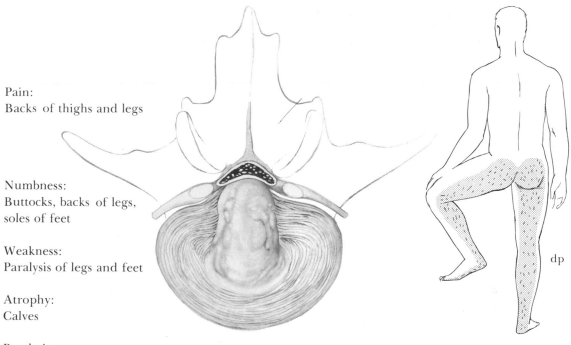

Pain:
Backs of thighs and legs

Numbness:
Buttocks, backs of legs,
soles of feet

Weakness:
Paralysis of legs and feet

Atrophy:
Calves

Paralysis:
Bladder and bowel

Figure 28–11. Massive herniation of nuclear material producing compression of multiple nerve roots in the cauda equina syndrome. (From DePalma AF, Rothman RH: The Intervertebral Disc. Philadelphia, W. B. Saunders Company, 1970.)

gical decompression to prevent persistent paresis or paraplegia. The urinary symptoms are least responsive to decompression, and urgent diagnosis and treatment are mandatory.

Bladder Symptoms

In the absence of infection or other pelvic abnormalities, young adults who develop problems of urinary retention, vesicle irritability, or incontinence, despite the absence of significant back pain or sciatica, may well be suffering from a disk protrusion. This has been clearly demonstrated by several authors.[50, 51] Four specific syndromes have been described in regard to the bladder abnormalities associated with disk disease: (1) total urinary retention, (2) chronic long-standing partial retention, (3) vesicle irritability, and (4) loss of the desire to void associated with an awareness of the necessity to void.

Sharr and coworkers have emphasized the association of bladder dysfunction and spinal stenosis, particularly the degenerative variety.[52] As with other manifestations of spinal stenosis, the urinary symptoms can be intermittent and evanescent.

In these individuals, a cystometrogram and cystoscopic examination, in conjunction with a myelogram, are helpful in confirming the diagnosis. Again, lack of awareness of the syndrome is the primary cause of failure to make the diagnosis.

PHYSICAL EXAMINATION

Inspection and Palpation

Restriction of spinal motion is probably the most common physical finding in the symptomatic phase of lumbar disk disease. Although some of this may be the result of the degenerative changes within the spine itself, much of it represents acute discomfort and muscle spasm. Restriction is present not only in forward and lateral flexion but also in rotation. In younger individuals, particularly adolescents, limitation of spinal motion may be the most dramatic finding. In older individuals, the radicular findings frequently overshadow limitation of motion. Inability to reverse the lumbar lordosis on forward flexion is quite characteristic. It is often interesting to note that patients with a disk herniation will experience a reproduction of their sciatica and an increase in their back pain on forward flexion, whereas individuals with spinal stenosis will become more symptomatic on hyperextension of the spine. This correlates reasonably well with our understanding of the pathologic abnormalities.

When there is acute sciatica, it is typical that the patient will list away from the side of the radicular pain, producing a "sciatic scoliosis." Because most disk herniations are indeed lateral to the affected nerve root, this is the most typical pattern. It is thought that this represents an attempt to create more space for the impinged nerve, thus reducing inflammation and symptoms. In patients with a very lateral or even foraminal encroachment of the nerve, further bending to the affected side will often increase their symptoms and reproduce their sciatica.

In contradistinction to this picture, the posture of an individual with an axillary disk herniation and sciatica usually involves a list toward the side of the affected nerve (Fig. 28–10). Again, this posture appears to decompress the nerve root slightly.

It is helpful to observe the posture of the individual complaining of an acute disk syndrome. Most of these individuals will prefer not to sit, and if they do sit down, they will tend to put most of their weight on the contralateral buttock. When standing, the affected leg is often held in a slightly flexed position, with incomplete weight bearing. Presumably, the flexion of the leg and the spine relaxes the sciatic nerve and is an involuntary effort at decompression of the root. When walking, many of these individuals will affect an antalgic gait, rapidly transferring their weight to the opposite side and creating a short stance phase on the affected limb. This, again, is most typical of adolescents with disk herniations, in whom axial findings sometimes exceed appendicular signs.

The loss of the lumbar lordosis and contracture of paraspinous musculature are also quite typical of the acute phase of lumbar disk disease. These abnormalities are readily appreciated on simple inspection, particularly the contracted and spastic masses of paravertebral muscle, which can be made more pronounced by flexion of the spine. Nonetheless, they are difficult to quantify and are not always reproducible from one examiner to another.

Palpation of these muscle masses will usually reveal firmness and frequently tenderness, particularly if the contraction has been present for some time. Indeed, prolonged contraction of paraspinous muscles may create a sort of myofascial compartment syndrome or just plain overuse ischemia.

Palpation of the bony prominences of the spine is very important. The spinous processes at the level of acute disk disease may well be uncomfortable, further reinforcing a presumptive diagnosis. It is also extremely unusual for infectious or neoplastic processes not to produce tenderness on palpation of the spinous processes posteriorly. Even the facet joints, located 2 to 3 cm from the midline of the spine, will be tender in those patients slim enough to compress in this area. This discomfort is usually exacerbated by pressure and extension of the spine, thus loading the painful facets.

A particularly productive area for palpation is along the iliac crest, the sacroiliac joints, and the iliolumbar ligament. As mentioned previously, this last structure is the most common site of referred pain from lumbar disk disease. Although these areas are not usually diseased in the true sense, they do acquire an associated hyperesthesia from underlying disk pathology.

Palpation lower along the course of the sciatic nerve and down into the sciatic notch may produce not only pain but also radicular phenomena down into the leg. Again, specific areas of referred pain and even trigger points are highly associated with the radiculopathy of a compressed nerve.[53]

From a prognostic standpoint, patients with back pain who do not have radicular signs but who nonetheless display tender motor points in the lower back and legs are likely to remain disabled nearly three times as long as patients without local tenderness. If a radiculopathy is also present, disability is nearly four times as long.[53]

Neurologic Examination

The classic patterns of neurologic supply to the lower extremities are well known and well substantiated. A meticulous evaluation of the lower extremities for these physical findings is imperative, because it has an extremely high correlation with the true pathologic abnormalities determined at surgery. The most common levels of disk herniation are L4–L5 and L5–S1, followed by L3–L4. Nonetheless, variations of the typical pattern frequently occur. Double nerve roots, a prefixed or postfixed lumbar plexus, and transitional vertebrae confuse the issue.

It is the most typical pattern that an L4–L5 disk herniation will involve the L5 nerve root. Because most nuclear herniations are slightly lateral, the L4 nerve root has usually passed safely beneath its pedicle by the time the disk material is encountered. Nevertheless, an even more lateral proximal herniation can entrap the L4 nerve root as it enters the foramen, or a very medial herniation may be seen to involve the S1 nerve root, which passes medially and more ventrally. Combinations of these patterns are also seen, and one must retain the mental flexibility to analyze the neurologic pattern and correlate it with contrast studies. Lastly, frank extrusions of nuclear material may migrate within the spinal canal, producing neurologic patterns that are not typical of any one level.

Motor Findings. Varying degrees of compromise of the muscle strength in a limb from compression of the motor fibers of the nerve root may be seen. In most instances, the patient may not be aware of the muscular weakness until it is demonstrated by the examiner. Compression of the fourth lumbar nerve root produces quadriceps weakness; incomplete strength in extension of the knee or difficulty climbing stairs is usually the first finding. Because of the great bulk of the quadriceps muscle, atrophy is more apparent in this monoradiculopathy than in others.

Compression of the fifth lumbar nerve root produces weakness primarily of the great toe and common toe extensors, with less common involvement of the evertors and dorsiflexors of the foot. There will be atrophy of the anterolateral compartments of the lower leg after prolonged compression, but a frank footdrop is seen uncommonly.

Compromise of the first sacral nerve root produces little motor weakness except for occasional loss of strength in foot and great toe flexion. Shortening of the stride or inability to push off effectively are seen occasionally in severe instances.

In evaluating muscle weakness, one must be particularly careful not to confuse a compressive monoradiculopathy with a metabolic peripheral neuropathy. Diabetes is the most common disease to create this mixed pattern, particularly in the L4 nerve distribution. When there is weakness of dorsiflexion of the foot, it is important to segregate true peroneal nerve symptoms from L5 nerve root symptoms. This is most easily done by testing the hip abductors and checking for a Trendelenburg sign due to gluteus medius denervation from a fifth lumbar radiculopathy.

Sensory Changes. The dermatomes of the lower extremity are fairly clearly delineated, although there is often significant overlap from one to another. This is most specific at the more distal reaches of the lower limb and is least helpful in the thigh and buttock. Compression of the fourth lumbar nerve will produce sensory abnormalities on the anteromedial aspect of the leg. Compression of the fifth lumbar nerve produces sensory changes along the anterolateral portion of the leg, the medial aspect of the foot, and the great toe. An S1 radiculopathy will typically involve the posterior aspect of the calf, the heel, and the sole and the lateral aspect of the foot.

Reflex Changes. It is common to see reflex abnormalities in compression syndromes associated with lumbar disk disease. These, however, are more typical in the older individual and may be unimpressive or even absent in the adolescent. Thus, the relative importance of the neurologic findings is distinctly age-related. Compression of the first sacral nerve root will produce diminution or even absence of the Achilles tendon reflex, with absence of the reflex being more highly associated with disk herniation.[54] It must be remembered that elderly individuals frequently have diminished or absent Achilles tendon reflexes without any overt cause.

Compression of the fifth lumbar nerve root produces reflex change in the posterior tibial tendons, but this is difficult to elicit. Again, this reflex abnormality must be asymmetric to be clinically significant, particularly in the elderly individual. Depression of the patellar tendon reflex is typically classically related to compression of the fourth lumbar nerve root, although large L4–L5 disk herniations may produce an identical pattern. A reflex arc may actually be stress tested to demonstrate earlier fatigue on the involved side by repeated tapping of the specific tendon. This is somewhat analogous to stress testing reflexes in spinal stenosis by asking the patient to ambulate or extend the spine until the radicular symptoms appear.

Tension Signs. When the lower leg is flexed at the hip and extended at the knee and ankle or when the spine is flexed forward, the nerve roots normally move 2 to 6 mm at the level of the foramina (Fig. 28–12).[55] There exists some debate as to whether this represents true sliding of the nerve within the neural canal, pas-

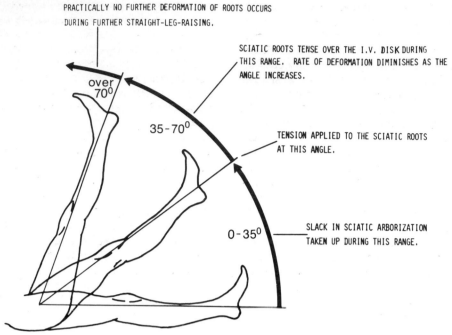

PRACTICALLY NO FURTHER DEFORMATION OF ROOTS OCCURS
DURING FURTHER STRAIGHT-LEG-RAISING.

SCIATIC ROOTS TENSE OVER THE I.V. DISK DURING
THIS RANGE. RATE OF DEFORMATION DIMINISHES AS THE
ANGLE INCREASES.

over 70°

35-70°

TENSION APPLIED TO THE SCIATIC ROOTS
AT THIS ANGLE.

0-35°

SLACK IN SCIATIC ARBORIZATION
TAKEN UP DURING THIS RANGE.

Figure 28–12. The relative degrees of freedom in the straight-leg–raising test. (Modified from Farni WH: Can J Surg 9:44, 1966.)

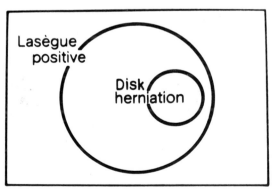

Lasègue positive

Disk herniation

Age: under 30 years

Figure 28–13. These Venn diagrams demonstrate the extremely high association of a positive Lasègue test with disk herniation in individuals under the age of 30 and the degradation of that sensitivity in individuals over that age. (From Spangfort E: Acta Orthop Scand 42:459, 1971.)

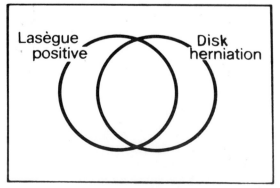

Lasègue positive

Disk herniation

Age: over 30 years

sive deformation of the nerve root, or thinning of the root as its excursion is resisted by paraforaminal ligaments. Nonetheless, clinical maneuvers that reproduce this motion will also reproduce radicular symptoms in affected individuals. The L4 nerve root has a smaller excursion and a different spinal path of exit, and a reverse straight-leg–raising test may be necessary to demonstrate its compression. Many maneuvers have been described, including the classic straight-leg–raising test, the La-sègue test, the Fajersztajn sign, the Cram test, the sitting root test, medial hip rotation test, and so on. An excellent and comprehensive review of these tests has been presented by Scham and Taylor.[55]

It is important to note that a "positive" tension sign should reproduce the patient's sciatic complaints, preferably below the knee. Mere low back pain or buttock pain, although suggestive, lacks the specificity of a more peripheral radiation of the symptoms.

Figure 28–14. A–C, The entrapment of a nerve root by an axillary herniation may explain the positivity of a contralateral straight-leg–raising test, as diagrammed here. (From DePalma AF, Rothman RH: The Intervertebral Disc. Philadelphia, W. B. Saunders Company, 1970.)

Perhaps the greatest significance of the tension sign lies in its high association with disk herniations, making it perhaps our best clinical diagnostic tool. Spangfort, in a review of more than 2000 patients with operatively proven disk herniations, showed a straight-leg–raising test to be positive in 90%[56] (Fig. 28–13). In individuals below the age of 30 years, the test was almost pathognomonic of a nuclear herniation, whereas in older individuals, the specificity of a tension sign diminished. Hudgins supported this observation, reporting positive tension signs in 97% of patients with surgically confirmed disk herniations.[57] Finally, individuals will occasionally be seen in whom a tension sign performed on the limb opposite the one with the sciatica will produce radicular pain in the symptomatic distribution. This is called a "contralateral tension sign" and is said to reflect either an axillary herniation of the nucleus (Fig. 28–14) or a large herniation in a narrow spinal canal. In both of these situa-

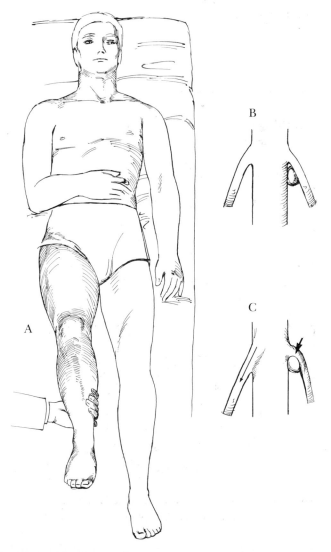

tions, the likelihood that surgical intervention will be required is increased.

General Examination

Obviously, all patients with radicular pain should be evaluated for clonus, pathologic reflexes, and impoverished circulation. The last is probably the most common cause of confusion between disease processes such as a vascular insufficiency and spinal stenosis, which frequently coexist in the elderly population.

Examination of the abdomen for visceral pathology and a thorough rectal examination are critical components of the back examination. Although their yield may be low, pathologic entities uncovered are usually far more significant than the disk degeneration they may be imitating.

Finally, the hip joint must be routinely examined in patients with back, buttock, and leg pain. The complaint of anterior thigh discomfort is very common in the elderly population, and differentiating L4 nerve root compression from spinal stenosis, diabetic L4 mononeuropathy, infiltrating tumors such as lymphoma, and occult arthritis of the hip may sometimes be difficult. Nonetheless, these differential diagnoses include the overwhelming majority of pathologic problems producing anterior thigh discomfort. Simple range of motion with the hip and knee in flexion should not reproduce neurogenic symptoms. If the patient's pain is reproduced by this maneuver, further thought should be given to the diagnosis of hip arthritis.

DIAGNOSTIC STUDIES

Routine Roentgenography

The role of roentgenography in the diagnosis and treatment of lumbar disk disease is obviously enormous, because it is the primary tool by which we attempt to objectify our clinical suspicions and findings. However, it has been the experience of the past several decades that the routine roentgenogram, despite its clear depiction of the many stigmata of degenerative disk disease, correlates better with the aging process than with the disease process.

The many stigmata of lumbar disk deterioration include thinning of the disk space, sclerosis of the endplate, facet arthritis and hypertrophy, ballooning of the endplate, degenerative spondylolistheses, Schmorl's nodes, motion and vacuum phenomena, and the common osteophyte and traction spurs, which were discussed previously (Fig. 28–15). Nonetheless, none of these stigmata corresponds closely with the predictability or even the presence of back pain or sciatica.[58–66] Even such popularly emphasized problems as increased lumbar lordosis, sacralization and lumbarization of the lower vertebrae, spina bifida occulta, tropism of the facets, minor lumbosacral tilts, and leg-length discrepancies have no statistical support as correlates of lumbar disk disease symptoms.[3, 6, 11, 26, 58, 67, 68] Perhaps the most important role of the routine roentgenogram is to preclude more ominous or occult pathologic entities, such as fractures, tumors, and infections of the spine. At least in the early stages of disease, this task is better performed by a technetium diphosphonate bone scan.

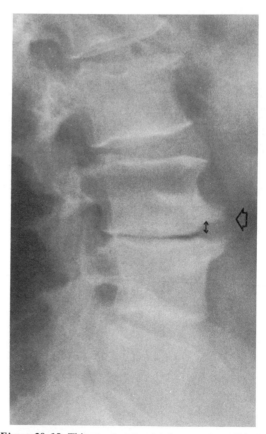

Figure 28–15. This roentgenogram demonstrates disk degeneration with scleritis of the endplates (fine arrow), disk space narrowing, and a traction osteophyte (wide arrow). (From Rothman RH, Simeone FA (eds.): The Spine. 2nd ed. Philadelphia, W. B. Saunders Company, 1982.)

Myelography

For the past 40 years, myelography has been the definitive study in the diagnosis of lumbar disk disease. A review of the literature has revealed an overall accuracy with Pantopaque myelography (Fig. 28–16) of approximately 85%.[69] The 15% error rate is reflected more in the sensitivity (false negative) than in the specificity (false positive).[69–71] The rationale for the use of lumbar myelography is reinforced by the necessity to exclude tumors of the lumbar or thoracic spine, which may mimic or coexist with disk herniations. Cerebral spinal fluid protein should always be obtained at the time of the myelographic assessment.[72] Anatomic abnormalities may confuse or condemn to failure even the best surgical exploration, and the precise localization of spinal nerve compromise should precede any operation. Edgar and Park, for instance, found that they could accurately predict the horizontal location (either central, posterolateral, or lateral) of a disk herniation in 80% of cases by using the tension signs.[73] Nonetheless, they were only 50% accurate in predicting the vertical level of herniation without myelography. Hakelius and Hindmarsh found only a 46% correlation using multiple neurologic signs and symptoms.[74]

Because of the relationship of symptomatic arachnoiditis and oil-base myelography in association with surgical intervention,[75] a variety of other contrast media have been developed. In 1969, Ahlgren[76] reported the use of meglumine iothalamate (Conray) for lumbar radiculopathy. The greater safety and tolerance of this agent enhance the popularity as well as the use of other similar substances. Metrizamide (Amipaque), a water-soluble triionate contrast medium, is the current preference in many institutions (Figs. 28–17 and 28–18). Unlike other water-soluble dyes, metrizamide is nonionic, does not dissociate, and has fewer side effects—particularly for arachnoiditis—than other contrast agents.[77, 78] The low viscosity of the water-soluble contrast media provides very high accuracy in defining lumbar lesions, even in the wide L5–S1 area of the spinal canal or in the lateral recesses. Its use in these instances has been substantiated in several studies.[79]

Epidural Venography

The significant false-negative rate of conventional Pantopaque myelography prompted the development of other techniques to define the spinal canal, particularly at the L5–S1 level

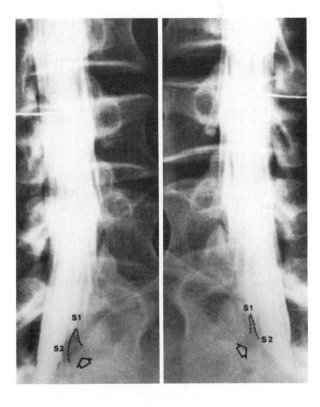

Figure 28–16. Pantopaque myelogram demonstrating the typical impression of a lateral disk herniation (arrows). (From Rothman RH, Simeone FA (eds.): The Spine. 2nd ed. Philadelphia, W. B. Saunders Company, 1982.)

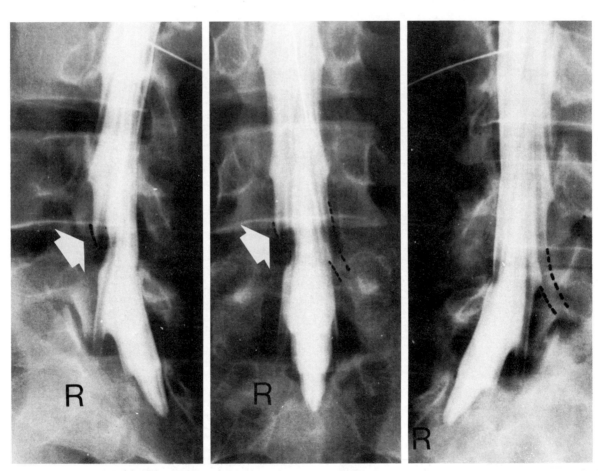

Figure 28–17. Metrizamide myelogram demonstrating lateral disk herniation at L4–L5 (arrows). (From Rothman RH, Simeone FA (eds.): The Spine. 2nd ed. Philadelphia, W. B. Saunders Company, 1982.)

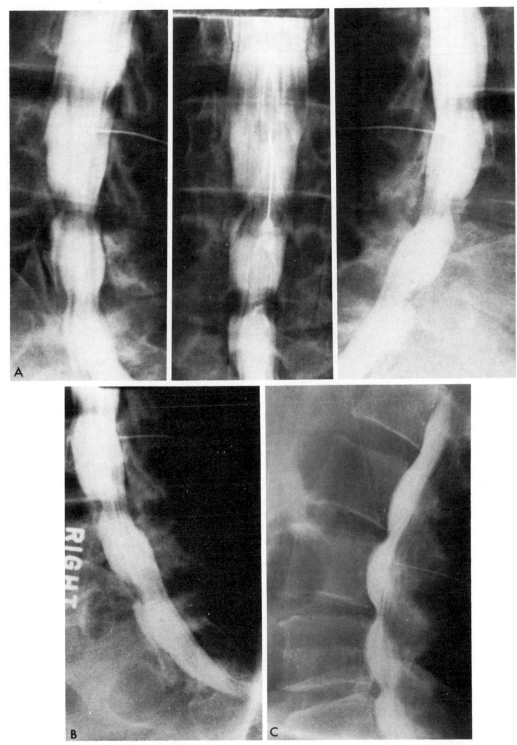

Figure 28–18. *A–C*, Metrizamide myelogram representing the multi-level waisting or hourglass deformities typical of spinal stenosis. (From Rothman RH, Simeone FA (eds.): The Spine. 2nd ed. Philadelphia, W. B. Saunders Company, 1982.)

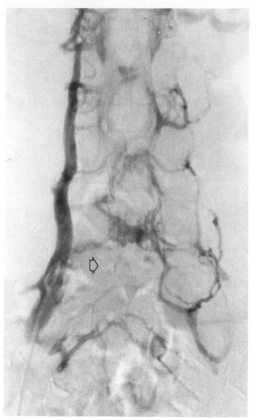

Figure 28–19. Epidural venogram, with arrow pointing to interruption of the anterior intervertebral vein at L5–S1 on the right. (From Rothman RH, Simeone FA (eds.): The Spine. 2nd ed. Philadelphia, W. B. Saunders Company, 1982.)

and in the lateral recesses. Epidural venography was introduced in 1961[80] and has undergone many changes since that time, with the current technique best described by Gargano and associates.[69] Catheterization of the ascending lumbar veins provides a view of the reliable lattice of vessels that surround and accompany the lumbosacral nerve roots (Fig. 28–19). Disruption of this normal anatomy has been shown to coincide with lumbar disk disease, and several authors have demonstrated greater sensitivity with epidural venography than with Pantopaque myelography.[69, 70, 81] The disadvantages of this technique are that it is invasive, technically demanding, contraindicated in the face of prior surgery, and probably less accurate than metrizamide myelography.[82]

Computerized Axial Tomography

One of the newest and certainly the most promising roentgenographic techniques for de-

fining degenerative disease in the lumbar spine is the computerized axial tomogram (CAT scan). The application of transverse axial tomography to spinal disorders really began only a decade ago,[83] but its enhancement by the use of sophisticated computer technology has provided a whole new dimension to the understanding of spinal disease. Perhaps the primary benefit of the CAT scan is that it is noninvasive, and the many concerns about myelographic side effects have now been obviated. The transverse view of the spine has created a better understanding of and orientation toward the disease processes because of the three-dimensional information provided when combined with more routine studies (Fig. 28–20). This is particularly true in the area of spinal fractures, in which the relative proportions of anterior and posterior pathology can be appreciated as never before and surgery appropriately directed toward the area of disease. The CAT scan has been particularly beneficial in the diagnosis of spinal stenosis, because it reveals in similar fashion the relative proportions of disk pathology, facet arthritis, and developmental spinal canal encroachment (Fig. 28–21). Other diagnostic possibilities, such as bony and soft tissue tumors mimicking disk disease, may now be seen on the peripheral portions of the CAT scan, thus providing a greater spectrum of diagnostic power than is enjoyed by myelography. In brief, the various components of degenerative disk disease compromising the neural elements can now be seen in a visual mode very relevant to the surgeon, who can plan his treatment with the three

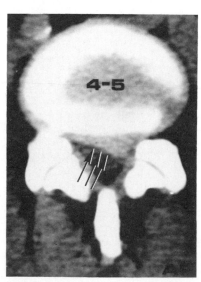

Figure 28–20. A computerized axial tomogram representing a large lateral nuclear herniation (arrows).

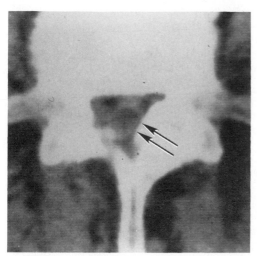

Figure 28–21. A computerized axial tomogram showing lateral recess narrowing in spinal stenosis (arrows).

dimensional aspects of the spinal canal firmly in mind.

Nonetheless, the CAT scan is still a tool very much in the process of development and suffering from several flaws. First, it is too sensitive. We are now able to see on the CAT scan many structures and spinal abnormalities that, just as with the early irregularities seen on routine roentgenograms and myelograms, are not necessarily correlated with spinal disease. Facet arthritis, slight narrowing of the spinal canal, posterior intrusion of the ligamentum flavum, hypertrophy of the laminae, and, most particularly, the omnipresent diffuse bulging of a degenerated disk are more frightening on a CAT scan than their pathologic significance would merit (Fig. 28–22). Furthermore, one must not be misled by such abnormalities as very lateral disk protrusions, however discrete, beyond the margins of the neural canal, or by hypertrophy of the epidural veins (Fig. 28–23). These entities are frequently mistaken for disk pathology, and their pursuit will yield negative spinal explorations. Thus, we must be careful not to allow the excessive sensitivity of the CAT scan to lure us into aggressive treatment of symptomatic complaints.

Another difficulty is that the CAT scan remains too inaccurate. Certainly, there are technical problems that even the current fourth generation of CAT scanners have yet to overcome. Poor photographic resolution, a high degree of sensitivity to the cut or angulation of the gantry, scolioses and other deformities, and the presence of metal and foreign bodies will obscure the results of all but the most

sophisticated techniques available today. The diagnostic accuracy of the CAT scan is also subject to controversy, with an enormous range of reliability being reported in studies with surgical confirmation of the pathology. Weinstein and associates, for example, reported the CAT scan to be absolutely correct in only 48% of the diagnoses of herniated nucleus pulposus when strict criteria were used. However, when no significant proportion of spinal stenosis was present and when the radiologist was "sure" of his diagnosis, the CAT scan was correct in 96%.[84] Tchang, Kirkaldy-Willis, and coworkers compared myelography and computerized axial tomography in individuals with surgically proven disk herniations and found a myelographic accuracy of 87% and a CAT scan accuracy of 94%.[85] Our own studies at Pennsylvania Hospital are less optimistic when strict diagnostic criteria are applied. If the interpreter of the roentgenologic study is asked to be absolutely precise as to both the level of the pathology and the exclusive diagnosis of either herniation or stenosis, the CAT scan can claim only two-thirds the accuracy of a metrizamide myelogram.[86]

Thus, our current concept of the role of the CAT scan is dependent on the presumptive clinical diagnosis. If a herniated nucleus pulposus is suspected, we feel that the CAT scan should be obtained first at the levels of clinical concern. If the diagnosis is firm and if it correlates precisely with neurologic findings,

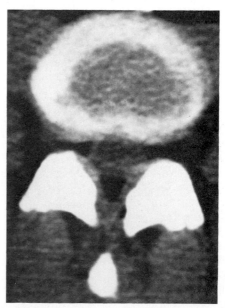

Figure 28–22. A computerized axial tomogram showing diffuse bulging of the intervertebral disk.

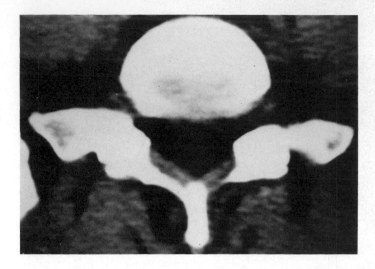

Figure 28–23. A computerized axial tomogram demonstrating engorged epidural veins, not to be confused with nuclear herniation.

myelography is probably not necessary. If there is any uncertainty or confusion in the elements of the diagnosis, myelography should be done in addition to the CAT scan before surgical intervention.

If, however, the suspected diagnosis is spinal stenosis, we feel that myelography is still the definitive procedure and that the CAT scan is a secondary test to be added for confirmation of the myelogram and for planning of the surgical approach. Certainly, in cases of prior surgery, recurrent herniations, or possible arachnoiditis, the combined use of CAT scan, myelography, and intravenous contrast material may be quite helpful in differentiating the relative proportions of scarring, stenosis, and new disk herniation. This technique is still developmental as well and may prove to be of great benefit in the future.

A final concern about the CAT scan is its great accessibility. It is becoming popular to order a CAT scan of the lumbar spine very early in the treatment of the patient, when symptoms have been present for only a short time. This creates difficulty for the treating physician with what has been termed "information overload." Too much information too early in the disease process is almost as difficult to manage as too little information, too late. Our usual therapeutic recommendations may be modified toward a more aggressive approach when we are fully aware of the nature of the pathology. Both the individual with a disk herniation and his physician may be less patient about pursuing appropriate conservative treatment when the knowledge of a disk herniation has been revealed. Just as with all

other diagnostic studies, we face a problem of patient selection that is accentuated by the noninvasive and readily accessible CAT scan. Perhaps the best way to retain an appropriate threshold for diagnostic studies is to recall that none should be ordered unless its outcome will alter the current treatment regimen.

Electromyography

Electromyography is a very useful diagnostic technique that documents the functional integrity of the motor unit, specifically the anterior horn cell, the axon, the neuromuscular junctions, and the muscle fibers innervated by the spinal nerve. When muscle groups of either anterior or posterior ramus innervation demonstrate excessive irritability (fibrillations), increased motor unit action potentials, or an excessive number of polyphasic motor unit action potentials, acute or chronic abnormal neural function is implied.

However, since the electromyogram (EMG) does not precisely define the altered anatomy producing the neural dysfunction, it is of greatest use in differentiating intraspinal pathology from the metabolic, ischemic, or peripheral neuropathies that may mimic lumbar disk disease.

The great increase in sophistication of other diagnostic techniques such as water-soluble myelography, epidural venography, and CAT scanning has minimized the role of electromyography in the diagnosis of lumbar disk syndromes.

Diskography

Diskography is a technique in which spinal needles are placed into disk spaces under image intensification, with the subsequent injection of radiopaque dye. Information is then recorded concerning the reproduction of the patient's pain, the configuration of the opaque material within the disk space, and the pressure and amount of dye accepted by the intervertebral disk. It was hoped that this test would confirm the presence of symptomatic disk degeneration. However, diskography has not proved to be either essential or reliable in our experience or in that of other investigators because of the relatively high incidence of age-related asymptomatic disk degeneration.[87, 88]

Therefore, a normal diskogram may be helpful in ruling out disk degeneration, but abnormalities compatible with multiple degenerative disks are so common that insufficient reliability can be invested in a positive diskogram to make this study a reliable predictor of surgical result. Currently, diskography retains its greatest use in the treatment of disk disease with chymopapain injections.

TREATMENT: AN ALGORITHM

The challenge to the physician treating a patient with lumbar disk disease is to return that individual as rapidly as possible to a normal functional existence. His ability to accomplish this task is determined less by the potency of his medications or surgical skill than by his effectiveness in decision making. The algorithm presented in Figure 28–24 is then a set of suggested rules for solving the particular problems that lumbar disk disease may present. It represents a logical and well-founded sequence of diagnostic and therapeutic techniques whose rational application will, it is hoped, obviate the "shotgun" approach to low back pain and sciatica.

Let us begin with the broad spectrum of patients who present with various combinations of low back pain and sciatica. Assume that the treating physician has examined these individuals and has concluded that their symptoms are the result of lumbar disk degeneration. Presuming that these individuals have not had extensive prior treatment, the overwhelming majority should then be instructed to begin a course of conservative therapy. Only those individuals with a frank cauda equina syndrome or unequivocal progressive motor weakness should proceed along the pathway to immediate myelography and spinal decompression. These two entities, previously discussed, represent a true emergency situation, the prognosis of which is distinctly dependent on the rapidity of diagnosis and neural decompression.

The components of the early conservative therapy of lumbar disk disease are relatively simple. They consist of bed rest, anti-inflammatory medications, and time. We have discussed earlier the high rate of cure that mere observation and conservative measures may effect, and we would thus continue with this conservative treatment for an average of 6 weeks with a high expectation of improvement.

Bed rest is perhaps the most significant modality in the treatment of acute back pain or sciatica. Matched controlled studies such as that by Wiesel and Rothman[89] have shown that individuals treated with bed rest had 50% less pain and were returned to function 50% faster than those treated in ambulatory or supported fashion. This can be accomplished at home and does not necessitate hospitalization. Pillows and other supports under the lower extremities will encourage a position of lumbar flexion, which reduces disk pressures and provides greater comfort. Traction and other modalities have been evaluated in controlled studies, and only an unusual kind of autotraction has shown any significant benefit over bed rest alone.[90, 91]

Anti-inflammatory medications are also appropriate to reduce the inflammatory component of lumbar disk disease, which, indeed, may be the primary treatable aspect of the entire pathologic process. Salicylates remain the definitive drug in this category, despite the necessity for encouragement and caution in their prescription. Despite the host of nonsteroidal anti-inflammatory drugs available for the treatment of back syndromes, there are very few controlled, randomized, and blind studies reflecting the use of these medications in this particular disease process. If a physician feels obliged to use medications other than salicylates for the treatment of inflammation, only naproxen[92] and diflunisal[93] seem to have substantiation in the literature.

Although analgesics may be helpful in the control of pain, they are generally superfluous if the individual is truly at bed rest and on a good regimen of anti-inflammatory medication. In general, we would recommend that non-narcotic analgesics be employed at this stage of treatment.

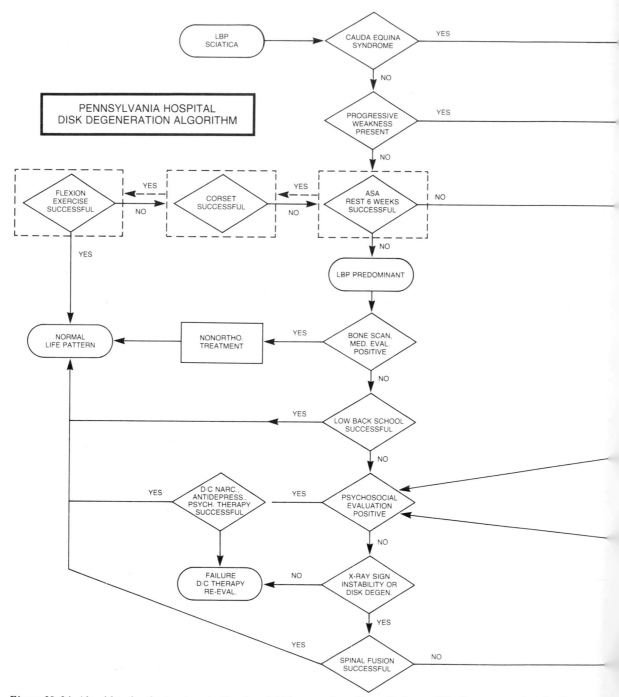

Figure 28–24. Algorithm for the treatment of lumbar disk degeneration. (From Rothman RH, Simeone FA (eds.): The Spine. 2nd ed. Philadelphia, W. B. Saunders Company, 1982.)

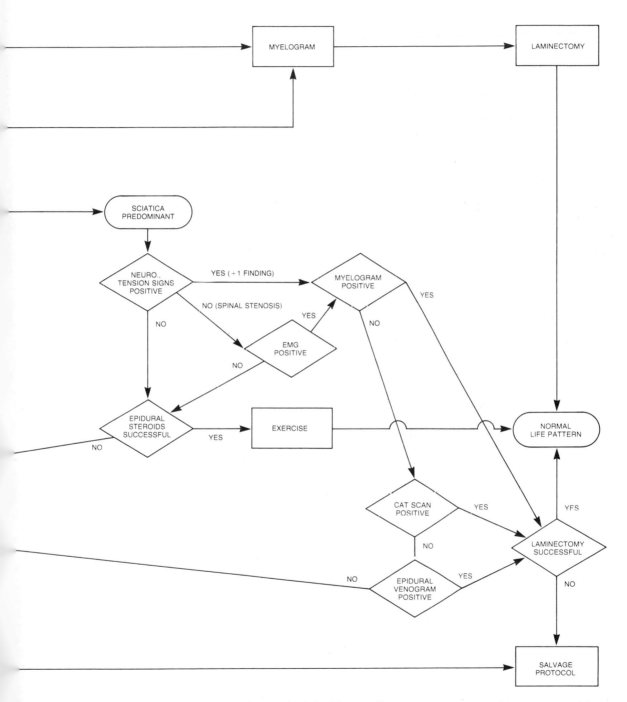

Figure 28–24 (Continued).

The use of muscle relaxants or antispasmodics represents another controversial area of therapy. Some feel that these medications are contraindicated, because the muscle spasm associated with lumbar disk disease is usually either ischemic or protective. These aspects are better treated with heat and bed rest or external support than with medications. Furthermore, the antispasmodics generally share a central site of action, producing more sedation and depression than true muscle relaxation. Certainly, this is the case with diazepam, the use of which we feel is counterproductive.

Those individuals who respond to conservative treatment should be gradually mobilized with the use of a lightweight flexible corset when they have attained approximately 80% relief of their symptoms. Once they are relatively comfortable and are able to return to normal functions, we would recommend the inception of a program of lumbar flexion exercises based on thc theory expounded by Williams.[94] Although a wide variety of exercise programs have been espoused in the past, the best evidence of efficacy exists for the use of isometric flexion exercises as described by Kendall and Jenkins.[95] Thereafter, it is imperative that the individual return to an active life style, keeping his weight and psychologic restriction low and his flexibility and endorphin levels high through daily exercise and light activity. Following this regimen, the vast majority of individuals will be able to return to an active life style within 2 weeks to 2 months from the onset of their symptoms, with usual subsequent resolution of the pain syndrome.

The remaining and relatively small group of patients who have failed to improve from this conservative regimen should then be carefully evaluated and sorted into two groups: those in whom low back pain is the predominant complaint and those in whom sciatica is the major disabling feature. In the latter group, the patients must now be carefully scrutinized for neurologic findings and tension signs. If they are absent, we would recommend the administration of epidural steroids in a further attempt to reduce the inflammatory component of lumbar disk disease. Although the efficiency of this treatment is only approximately 70% in our hands, we prefer it to the systemic administration of steroid medication because of the obvious side effects of the latter. If the epidural steroid treatment is successful, the patient is encouraged to return to an exercise program and a normal life style. We would allow 6 weeks to pass before considering epidural steroids a failure.

Those individuals who do have a positive tension sign or neurologic deficit would at this juncture be considered for a confirmatory roentgenographic study, either a myelogram or a CAT scan, as discussed previously. If this is positive, surgical intervention may then be considered at this time with a high expectation of a good result. If the patient persistently complains of sciatica but has no confirmatory phyical findings, an EMG may be a helpful diagnostic adjunct to differentiate patients with sciatica due to mechanical nerve compression from those with sciatica of other etiology.

If a contrast study and subsequent spinal decompression produce the expected good result, the patient would again be encouraged to return to an active life style and to an exercise program to minimize the possibility of future episodes of lumbar disk disease. As mentioned previously, the roentgenographic procedure of choice depends somewhat on the patient's presumptive diagnosis. If the individual's age, physical findings, and historical information suggest a nuclear herniation, a CAT scan alone may be adequate for diagnostic and surgical purposes. If there is any suspicion about the pathology, a myelogram or epidural venogram would also be appropriate.

If the patient's pathology is thought to be spinal stenosis by virtue of greater age, more chronic history, and less impressive physical examination, myelography remains the diagnostic procedure of choice, supplemented by a CAT scan. In patients who have a positive neurologic deficit, a positive tension sign, and a positive roentgenographic study, 95% should be expected to have a good or excellent surgical result.

Let us now return to those patients who were originally classified as predominantly having back pain and who failed to respond to the initial program of conservative treatment. We feel that these individuals should now undergo a technetium diphosphonate bone scan and a thorough evaluation by an internist. The bone scan is an excellent survey test, far more effective than routine roentgenograms in precluding the possibility of occult disease from tumors or infection. An internist's thorough search may reveal problems such as penetrating ulcer, pancreatitis, or abdominal aneurysms that have been masquerading as persistent low back pain. If such problems are found, the patient is appropriately referred for nonorthopedic treatment. If no abnormality is found, we would currently recommend that the individual attend a Low Back School, where an intensive educational effort will be made to enhance his understanding of his disease process and the techniques of self-administered conservative therapy to manage it. Ergonomics, the proper and efficient use of the body in work and recreation, is stressed. This type of schooling is both inexpensive and effective and frequently allows individuals with chronic low back pain to return to a normal life.

If, however, the Low Back School is ineffective, these individuals should probably begin an intensive psychosocial evaluation. We are all aware of the tremendous interplay between psychologic and organic factors in low back pain syndromes. The patient's pathologic anatomy may be a relatively minor part of his disability, which may be related more to his perception of the pain and his stability in relationship to his sociologic environment. In some individuals, it is simply the fear of further episodes of back pain that is disabling. Often, the physician's mere suggestion that every hurt does not imply harm or bodily damage is sufficient to return the patient to activity. Sometimes, a more thorough interrogation concerning the patient's daily functions, such as sleep, sex, appetite, and activity, will reveal a more profound disturbance. Depression, substance abuse, and compensation/litigation entanglements are the most commonly observed factors. The role of these problems in the development and perpetuation of symptoms of back disease is well known and well documented. Routine therapeutic techniques will remain ineffective until these disturbances have been identified and treated. Individuals who are depressed may be appropriately referred to psychiatrists, psychologists, group therapists, or psychiatric social workers, depending on the nature of the depression and their resources. Facilities for the detoxification of those addicted to alcohol or drugs do exist, and it is critical that the individual purge himself of those addictions so that the true degree of his discomfort can be determined and so that treatment can be effective. Finally, it is frequently in the best interest of the patient that a physician may recommend that legal and compensatory entanglements be terminated as rapidly as possible so that the business of getting well may go forward.

If an individual, with the help of his physician and other facilities, is able to eliminate these psychosocial influences, his back pain will frequently become easily manageable or will even disappear. If the patient is unwilling or unable to follow the programs outlined, continues to use narcotics, or rejects and fails to respond to the recommended treatment,

discontinuation of medical therapy would be advocated at that time. To continue random measures of treatment for these individuals and their back pain without correcting the underlying abnormality is inefficient and inappropriate. We would discharge them from the treatment protocol, with the offer to re-evaluate them after 6 months to 1 year if they should wish to re-enter the program.

Returning to those individuals who have persistent back or leg pain with no demonstrable abnormality on routine studies, we would recommend at this juncture an extensive evaluation for the development of insidious spinal instability. The criteria for lumbar instability are less clear than those in the cervical spine, but for our purposes, these would include to-and-fro motion with flexion-extension, reversal of the normal lordotic position of the motion segment, or presence of traction osteophytes at one level. Spinal fusion may be of assistance to these individuals, although not with the high level of confidence of success associated with decompression procedures. Nonetheless, if success is achieved with a lumbar spinal fusion, the patient must again return to normal life and activity.

If the patients fail to improve after either a lumbar decompression or lumbar fusion, they must be referred to a separate salvage protocol. The details of this complex analysis exceed the scope of this chapter, but it is clearly described in other texts.[20]

Surgical Treatment

Selection of the Patient

In the most simplistic view, there are really only two things that a spinal surgeon can offer a patient with lumbar disk disease: the decompression of compromised nerves and the stabilization of a hypermobile spine. Perhaps the most significant factor in predicting a good result from either of these procedures would be the clear preoperative demonstration that either neural compression or spinal instability does indeed exist. In the treatment of mere disk degeneration, lumbar laminectomy and/or fusion adds nothing to the patient's treatment other than the risks associated with anesthesia and the complications of surgery.

The indications for immediate intervention in a lumbar spine are the cauda equina syndrome, which was discussed previously, and progressive demonstrable motor weakness. In particular, the rarity of spontaneous recovery of sexual and sphincter function make myelographic definition and spinal decompression a true emergency.[96] Lesser forms of motor nerve dysfunction require good clinical judgment, because minor disturbances that do not severely compromise the total function of the limb may not merit surgery.

Because 80% of Weber's patients who did not undergo surgery showed good or fair results within 3 months, observation appears justified for this period of time.[5] Thereafter, persistent sciatica or recurrent episodes of sciatica with substantiating clinical and roentgenographic findings should be the basis for consideration of surgical decompression. The quality of the surgical result also seems to deteriorate when more than a year has elapsed since the onset of symptoms. Whether this represents neural scarring and irritation or merely learned patterns of pain behavior is as yet unclear.

There is little question that the overwhelming indication for lumbar disk surgery is pain. Sensory and reflex changes may be useful in terms of diagnosis, but they are not in themselves indications for surgical intervention and they are of no prognostic value in predicting the ultimate outcome of the disease. Weber[5] found sensory dysfunction in nearly half of his total series of patients after 4 years, and reflex abnormalities may persist in 25% of patients despite a successful lumbar decompression. The presence or absence of a reflex deficit does not in any way predict the success of the operation.

We now know that the degenerated disk is a poor target for the surgeon. The results of lumbar decompression correspond almost linearly to the degree of disk herniation discovered at operation; that is, in patients with a true herniation or extrusion of nuclear material and subsequent nerve compromise, the surgical results are excellent, whereas in those with "negative explorations" the prognosis is gloomy. Thus, the success of surgery depends heavily on the ability to predict neural compromise. In a review of 3000 lumbar spine operations, Hirsch[97] found that the most significant preoperative factors in the determination of mechanical nerve compression were a positive tension sign, a well-defined neurologic deficit, and a positive myelogram. When all three factors are present, a surgeon may expect to relieve all of the patient's leg pain and most of his back pain at a 95% confidence level with a well-performed surgical procedure. If one of these factors is absent, the chance of a good result drops more than 10 percentage points.

If two factors are absent, surgery should probably be avoided, because the rate of improvement seldom exceeds the natural history of the disease. This represents a slight oversimplification of the problem, because some of these predictive factors must be weighed in relation to the age of the patient to place them in proper perspective. For example, many elderly patients with spinal stenosis will not have a positive tension sign, but they will usually demonstrate a neurologic deficit, particularly under stress testing. In contrast, adolescents and young adults may suffer large nuclear extrusions without sufficient neural damage to produce a reflex deficit, although they invariably show a tension sign at a very high confidence level. The absence of a true tension sign in a young adult almost precludes the diagnosis of a nuclear herniation.

Patients with persistent symptoms of back pain or sciatica without confirmatory physical or roentgenographic findings should be carefully scrutinized for psychosocial disturbances prior to any surgical intervention. Even the best operation is likely to fail in the face of depression, substance abuse, or compensatory and legal entanglement.

Selection of the Operation

The procedure of choice in symptomatic lumbar disk disease should be determined by the pathologic entity predicted from the patient's preoperative evaluation and also by the situation uncovered at the time of the procedure itself. With thorough historical, clinical, and roentgenographic evaluations, however, surprises should be uncommon and the procedure should be predictable in advance.

In acute disk herniations, a simple limited laminotomy or hemilaminectomy that is adequate to identify the level of the lumbar spine in question and to remove the nuclear prolapse without damaging the neural elements is sufficient. Indeed, in cases with a wide interlaminar space, little or no bone may need to be removed. The approach should be confined to the side of symptoms, and asymptomatic levels of roentgenographic abnormalities should not be disturbed, in order to avoid creating pathology where it did not previously exist.

When the preoperative diagnosis suggests chronic disk degeneration or spinal stenosis, a bilateral approach with complete laminectomy at the affected levels is most appropriate, to prevent contralateral symptomatology in the future. On the symptomatic side, as much dissection must be performed as is necessary to free the nerve roots. This will usually not necessitate more than a hemifacetectomy and thus will not precipitate spinal instability. The disk space seldom needs to be entered. The symptomatic nerve roots must be examined and decompressed, occasionally as far out as the pedicle. It is best to focus attention on the nerve in question rather than on the structural elements surrounding and compressing it. Whatever dissection is necessary to free that nerve should be performed. If the individual is young, has a high proportion of back pain to leg pain, or has had more than the sum total of one facet sacrificed at any level, a concurrent lumbar fusion would also be indicated. The necessity for lumbar fusion diminishes with age, as the general stiffening of the spine confers some structural integrity even in the case of generous decompression. In most patients with chronic disk degeneration, at least two levels of decompression are appropriate, but often three or more may be necessary.

With a diagnosis of chronic disk degeneration or spinal stenosis, patients with predominant back pain can usually be managed conservatively. It is rare that these individuals may come to require spinal fusion, but in certain isolated circumstances, a bilateral fusion to the sacrum from the affected level may diminish the back pain complaint.

The indications for fusion of the lumbar spine are still controversial, with good articles supporting disk excision alone[98] and disk excision plus fusion.[99] Further studies of a prospective and randomized nature are needed to help settle this issue. It is our opinion that in the vast majority of cases, the addition of a fusion to a disk excision in no way improves the quality of the result.

Our current recommended indications for lumbar fusion are confined to those individuals with acute or chronic disk degeneration with a very high proportion of back pain, the presence of neural arch defects coincident with disk disease, symptomatic and roentgenographically demonstrable segmental instability, or iatrogenic surgical instability created during decompression of the neural elements.

Surgical Technique

Lumbar decompression for an acute soft disk herniation may be performed under a wide variety of anesthetic techniques, from local to general endotracheal anesthesia. We prefer spinal anesthesia with light sedation. The patient is placed in a kneeling position on a laminectomy frame with the abdomen hanging free. This minimizes the intra-abdominal pressure and subsequent epidural bleeding. Prophylactic measures such as elastic stockings, antibiotics, and preoperative skin preparation are recommended.

A midline skin incision approximately 4 cm long is made directly over the affected disk. Clinical confirmation of the appropriate level is aided by observing the level of the iliac crest on plain spine films, spinous process irregularities and abnormalities seen on lateral spine films, notation of the skin mark from the myelographic needle with roentgenologic correlation, observation of the decussation of fascial fibers at the L5–S1 level, and palpation of the last spinous process with toggling of the free disk space. Using these elements of supportive evidence, it is uncommon that an incorrect disk space will be entered, even in the situation of transitional vertebrae. A subperiosteal dissection of the spinous processes and laminae is performed, with retraction of the intact muscle mass with a Taylor retractor just beyond the facet joints (Figs. 28–25 to 28–30).

Residual muscle is debrided from the laminae with a rongeur, and a curette is used to identify and free the inferior surface of the lamina in question. From this stage on, visual magnification is quite helpful. The lamina is dissected in a cephalad direction using a Schlessinger or Kerrison punch rongeur. This dissection is terminated when the proximal extent of the ligamentum flavum has been reached. The dura is gently freed from the overlying ligamentum flavum by blunt dissection, and a scalpel is used to excise a large window of ligamentum flavum down to the superior surface of the lamina below. The dissection is then extended laterally using rongeurs and punches until the lateral margin of the nerve root is identified. Attempts to retract or dissect more anterior structures should be postponed until the nerve root is clearly seen, because a thinned or splayed nerve root may be damaged if its location is not clearly observed. Cottonoid patties are used to provide gentle retraction of the neural elements toward the midline, both above and below the disk space. Gentle longitudinal dissection with a Penfield dissector will usually reveal the bulging disk just lateral to the nerve root at the intervertebral disk space.

If free fragments are found, they are gently teased from the wound with a pituitary ron-

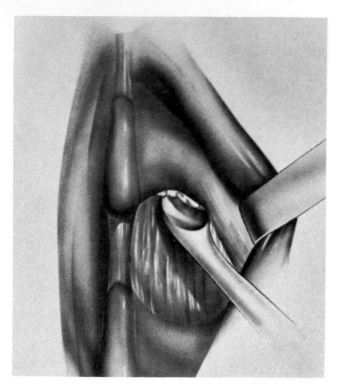

Figure 28–25. The undersurface of the lamina is cleared of soft tissue to free and expose the ligamentum flavum. (From Rothman RH, Simeone FA (eds.): The Spine. 2nd ed. Philadelphia, W. B. Saunders Company, 1982.)

Figure 28–26. A rongeur is used to excise the distal margin of the lamina up to the exposed end of the ligamentum flavum. (From Rothman RH, Simeone FA (eds.): The Spine. 2nd ed. Philadelphia, W. B. Saunders Company, 1982.)

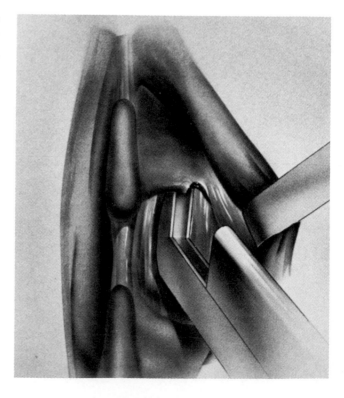

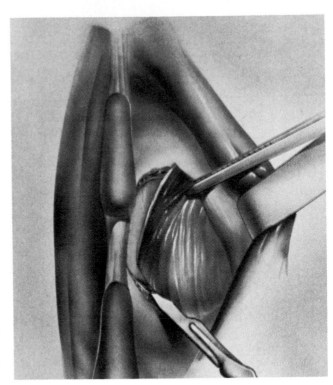

Figure 28–27. The ligamentum flavum is excised sharply under direct vision with a small scalpel. (From Rothman RH, Simeone FA (eds.): The Spine. 2nd ed. Philadelphia, W. B. Saunders Company, 1982.)

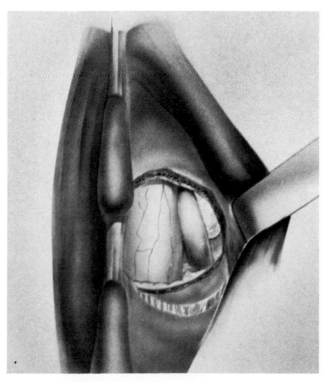

Figure 28–28. The lateral resection is extended toward the foramen until the nerve root is clearly identified. No retraction should be performed until the anatomy is apparent. (From Rothman RH, Simeone FA (eds.): The Spine. 2nd ed. Philadelphia, W. B. Saunders Company, 1982.)

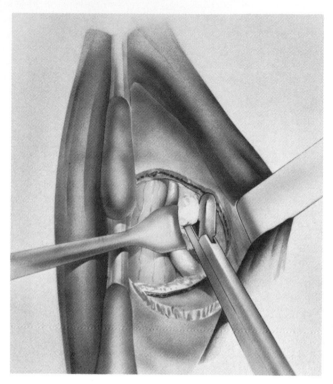

Figure 28–29. With gentle retraction of the nerve root, the nuclear extrusion is removed with a pituitary rongeur. (From Rothman RH, Simeone FA (eds.): The Spine. 2nd ed. Philadelphia, W. B. Saunders Company, 1982.)

Figure 28–30. After removal of the disk material, the neural foramen is explored to ensure that no further extruded material is present. (From Rothman RH, Simeone FA (eds.): The Spine. 2nd ed. Philadelphia, W. B. Saunders Company, 1982.)

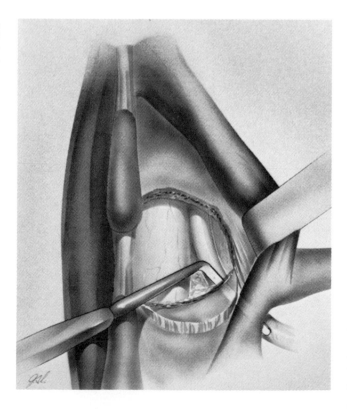

geur. A 5-mm square window of annulus is then created with a No. 15 knife blade, and pituitary rongeurs of various configuration are used to evacuate the disk space. Great care is taken to avoid excessive penetration or plunging, and the endplates of the vertebral body should be palpated with every pass of the instrument.

Thorough examination of the foramen, epidural space, and general tension on the nerve root should now be performed, using a Fraser or malleable uterine probe. Only when the nerve root is completely free should the dissection be terminated and a thin membrane of fat be applied to the neural tissues. Some drainage is helpful to prevent hematoma formation, and we employ this technique uniformly unless a durotomy was performed.

In spinal stenosis, a bilateral approach is used, with early excision of the spinous processes with a bone cutter. After careful dissection of the ligamentum flavum, large rongeurs are used to remove the laminae. Lateral foraminotomies and facetectomies can be performed with an angled Kerrison punch rongeur with relative safety, particularly when the instrument is used in an orientation parallel to the nerve root in question (Figs. 28–31 to 28–37).

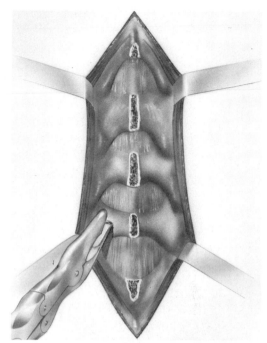

Figure 28–32. A rongeur is used to remove the lamina up to the level of the free ligamentum flavum. (From Rothman RH, Simeone FA (eds.): The Spine. 2nd ed. Philadelphia, W. B. Saunders Company, 1982.)

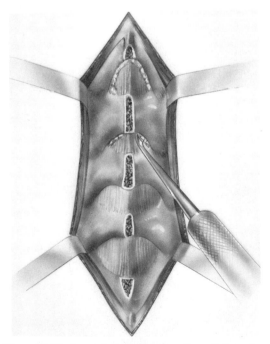

Figure 28–31. A curette is used to free the soft tissue from the laminar undersurface above the ligamentum flavum. (From Rothman RH, Simeone FA (eds.): The Spine. 2nd ed. Philadelphia, W. B. Saunders Company, 1982.)

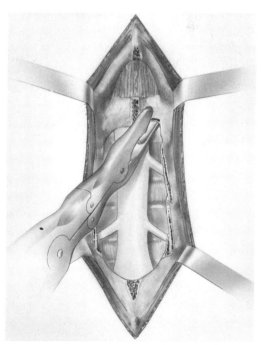

Figure 28–33. The lamina and ligamentum flavum are excised completely out to the level of the facet joint. (From Rothman RH, Simeone FA (eds.): The Spine, 2nd ed. Philadelphia, W. B. Saunders Company, 1982.)

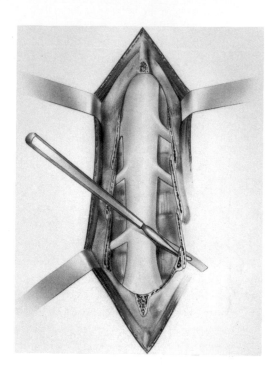

Figure 28–34. An instrument is used to explore the neural foramen and to test the degree of freedom of the nerve root under compression. (From Rothman RH, Simeone FA (eds.): The Spine. 2nd ed. Philadelphia, W. B. Saunders Company, 1982.)

Figure 28–35. A foraminotomy may be performed, with emphasis on removing the superior facet of the vertebra composing the foramen. It is safest to use the instrument in the direction of the spinal nerve under examination. (From Rothman RH, Simeone FA (eds.): The Spine. 2nd ed. Philadelphia, W. B. Saunders Company, 1982.)

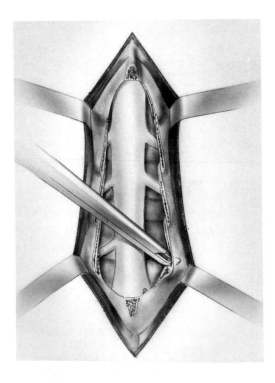

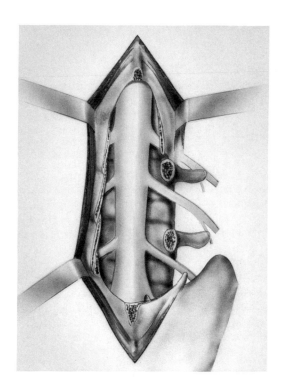

Figure 28-36. A complete foraminotomy has been performed on the right, unroofing the L4 and L5 spinal nerves. The facet joints on the left have been preserved to avoid instability. (From Rothman RH, Simeone FA (eds.): The Spine. 2nd ed. Philadelphia, W. B. Saunders Company, 1982.)

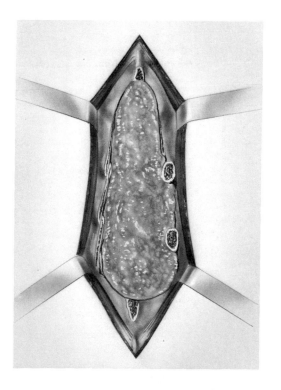

Figure 28-37. An autogenous fat graft is placed on the exposed neural material to prevent scar tissue adhesions. (From Rothman RH, Simeone FA (eds.): The Spine. 2nd ed. Philadelphia, W. B. Saunders Company, 1982.)

When arthrodesis of the spine is indicated, we favor a bilateral lateral fusion. This technique has the advantages of greater biomechanical integrity, a higher fusion rate, good utility despite the absence of posterior elements, and the avoidance of iatrogenic spinal stenosis. The preoperative precautions and positioning that are employed are identical to those just described. A midline incision with a hockey-stick deviation toward the side where the iliac graft will be obtained is commonly used if a decompression is performed as well. If a fusion alone is indicated, bilateral lateral incisions 3 to 4 cm from the midline may be employed. In the latter instance, blunt dissection through the paraspinous muscles and thoracodorsal fascia allows direct visualization and exposure of the transverse processes of the vertebra. The paraspinous muscles are stripped from the bone, and the laminae and lateral gutters of the vertebrae are decorticated with a curette. If the fusion is to incorporate the sacrum, the alae are similarly decorticated on the superior and posterior surfaces. Bone graft material removed from the iliac crest in standard fashion is cut into thin strips and is applied across the transverse processes into the gutters of the lateral vertebral bodies and over the top of the sacrum (Fig. 28–38).

The wounds are closed over deep suction drains after all devitalized tissue has been debrided. The patients are allowed to be mobilized on the second or third day, and generally, no external support is indicated. This program of early mobilization has not been shown to lower the rate of successful fusion.

Complications of Lumbar Disk Surgery

Perhaps the most feared complications of the common procedures for lumbar disk disease involve damage to the great vessels, particularly the aorta, inferior vena cava, and iliac vessels. The aorta and vena cava lie in proximity to the L3–L4 and L4–L5 disk spaces, and the iliac vessels reside just anterior to the L5–S1 disk spaces. Injuries to these vessels from excessive penetration or laceration with

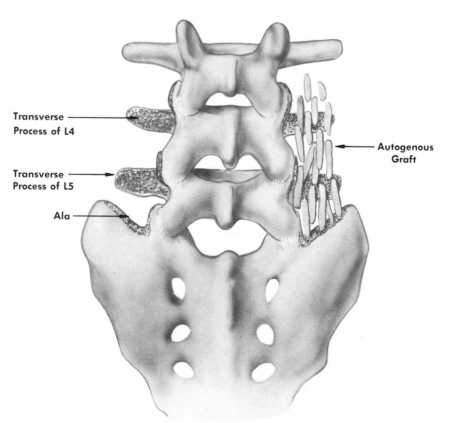

Transverse Process of L4

Transverse Process of L5

Ala

Autogenous Graft

Figure 28–38. The sacral ala and transverse processes have been decorticated, and an autogenous graft is placed bilaterally to perform a lateral fusion. (From Rothman RH, Simeone FA (eds.): The Spine. 2nd ed. Philadelphia, W. B. Saunders Company, 1982.)

sharp instruments are frequently not appreciated at the time of surgery.[100] The arteriovenous fistulas that form can present some months later as high-output cardiac decompensation. If a fistula does not form, these injuries carry mortality rates of up to 78% for arterial compromise and 89% for venous injury.[101] The use of the kneeling position for surgery, the constant attention to keeping grasping and cutting instruments on bone or the vertebral endplates, the use of adequate exposure and good hemostasis, and care to insure that the instruments employed do not penetrate the disk space more than 1⅛ inches should minimize the chance that this dreaded type of complication will occur.

Injuries to the neural elements themselves are not as uncommon. Tears of the dura may occur, particularly in cases of spinal stenosis, in which the dura may be thin, or in previously operated spines, in which the dura may be enclosed in scar tissue. Repair of these injuries is crucial and consists of using continuous fine-silk sutures on a noncutting needle.

More insidious are the effects of blunt trauma to the nerve root from excessive or rough retraction, laceration, or stripping of the vascular supply. This occasionally produces the "battered root syndrome," with a disastrous postoperative result.[102]

Of the common postoperative surgical complications, urinary retention is seen more frequently after spinal surgery. This may be the result of anxiety, pain when lying supine on the surgical incision, or nerve root irritation preceding and during the surgical procedure itself. Fortunately, most patients may stand at the bedside or use a commode shortly after surgery, and bethanechol chloride (Urecholine) is helpful in restoring bladder function. The aggressive use of urethral catheters should be avoided because the danger of infection.

Wound infections themselves are another concern, and preoperative and postoperative administration of antibiotics seems prudent in spinal surgery. Spangfort reported a 2.9% incidence of postlaminectomy infections in a review of 10,000 surgical procedures.[33] This is many times higher than that in our current experience, and new antibiotics and sterile techniques should make spinal infection an uncommon occurrence.

Of great concern is the postoperative cauda equina syndrome. Although the exact mechanism is uncertain, mechanical trauma to the nerve roots, hematoma formation, and compromise of the vascular supply to the spinal cord have been implicated. The artery of Adamkowitz (arteria radicularis anteria magna) usually enters the spinal cord from the left side between T9 and T11; however, it may occasionally be on the opposite side and has been reported entering the canal as low as L4.[103] Inadvertent damage to this vessel during spinal decompression is usually catastrophic, with only 40% of the patients recovering.[33]

Perhaps the most common late complication of a spinal decompression is inadequate release of the nerve roots. The persistence of sciatic symptoms even after sufficient pathology has been removed often relates to undiscovered extruded fragments, unrecognized lateral recess syndromes in addition to a disk herniation, foraminal encroachment, tethering of the nerve root about a pedicle, or anomalous nerve root anatomy. The opportunity for this complication to occur is minimized by a wide exposure and by thorough exploration and palpation of the neural elements prior to closure. Although it is fashionable in some areas to employ "keyhole" or microscopic diskectomy techniques, there is no apparent additional morbidity or mortality from a wide laminectomy.[104]

Even in the most gentle hands, it is routine to discover scar formation about the dura and nerve roots after surgical exploration. This does not commonly cause symptoms, despite the obvious nerve root adhesions that develop. Many techniques have been employed to diminish scarring about the nerve roots, including the use of Gelfoam membrane and more recently a free fat graft or pedicle fat graft.[105-107] Persistent pain from intradural scarring or arachnoiditis is a very difficult and serious complication, because there is no apparent therapy that is effective for reversing this problem. In fact, surgical attempts to remove scar and to free nerve roots from adhesions of the arachnoid membrane usually produce more symptoms.

Spinal instability may occasionally be the result of an aggressive decompression, particularly in the younger individual, or may take place when more than the sum total of one facet joint has been removed at any single spinal level. If this occurs and can be demonstrated roentgenographically, a lateral spine fusion may be undertaken to reduce these symptoms. The criteria for a combined procedure have been discussed previously.

With respect to the complications of spinal fusion, pseudarthrosis can occasionally occur and be the focus of the patient's persistent

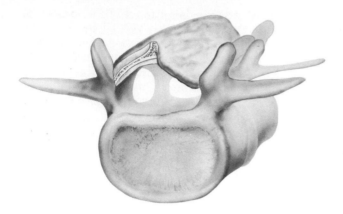

Figure 28–39. A hypertrophied midline fusion will occasionally produce an iatrogenic spinal stenosis. (From Rothman RH, Simeone FA (eds.): The Spine. 2nd ed. Philadelphia, W. B. Saunders Company, 1982.)

pain. It is worth recalling, however, that studies of pseudarthroses have suggested that only 15% to 20% of the cases may indeed be symptomatic.[108] Pseudarthroses are usually related to inadequacies of surgical technique, postoperative restriction or immobilization, or treatment of postoperative anemia.[109] An iatrogenic spinal stenosis can also be responsible for pain after a lumbar fusion, particularly when it is of the midline variety (Figs. 28–39 and 28–40). Not only will the bone graft material hypertrophy, but also periosteal stripping of the laminae and other structural elements will frequently precipitate their hypertrophy. This entity is usually apparent on the computerized axial tomograms that are now available.

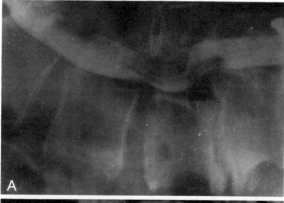

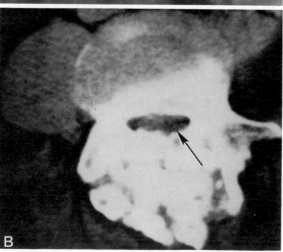

Figure 28–40. *A* and *B*, Myelogram and CAT scan demonstrate neural compression and spinal canal encroachment (arrow) from a midline fusion for spondylolisthesis.

Finally, disk space infection should be considered when there is a rapid recurrence of severe back pain 1 to 6 weeks after the excision of an intervertebral disk. Neurologic findings such as a positive tension sign may frequently return, and the patient's back pain will nonetheless usually exceed his sciatica. General malaise and nocturnal discomfort are the hallmarks of this problem, but temperature elevations and laboratory abnormalities may not become apparent until late in the disease process. Routine roentgenograms may also be far less revealing than the clinical picture, and the diagnosis must necessarily be made by aspiration or biopsy of the suspected disk space.

Results

It has been more than five decades since Mixter and Barr[2] introduced the era of the operative treatment of lumbar disk disease. Surprisingly, there are relatively few long-term studies that adequately assess our experience.[61, 99]

One of the most helpful studies is the report by DePalma and Rothman of their experience with 1500 patients over twenty years.[61] The average follow-up was between 8 and 10 years, and the average age of the individual at surgery was approximately 40 years. A summary of their results reveals that approximately 15% of patients had persistent back pain, 7% had persistent sciatica, and 14% had both back pain and sciatica after procedures done for the criteria mentioned earlier in this section. The more proximal the disk disease, the less the relief of symptomatology in general. Negative tension signs correlated closely with poor results postoperatively.

When interrogated as to the overall relief of their pain, approximately 60% of the patients had obtained complete relief of back and leg pain, approximately 30% considered themselves partially relieved, and only 3% were unimproved. Overall, almost 90% of the patients felt that the surgery was worthwhile.

It is of interest that physical findings such as muscle spasm, tenderness, limitation of motion, and tension signs disappeared in 90% of those patients who demonstrated them preoperatively. Neurologic deficits were less likely to return, and motor and sensory deficits disappeared in only 50% of the patients. This is consistent with other reports in the literature.[110]

In those individuals who had a lumbar fusion, either with or without concomitant spinal decompression, the rate of development of pseudarthrosis was only 8%. This has been reduced to 6% in those individuals who had the more modern lateral fusion technique.[108] As discussed earlier, the occurrence of a pseudarthrosis does not necessarily predict or coincide with persistent pain. Of those patients who had a pseudarthrosis, 82% felt that their surgery was worthwhile, as opposed to 90% of the patients with solid fusion. However, only 56% of patients with a pseudarthrosis and 61% of patients with a solid fusion had total relief of their back pain.

Thus, spinal decompression remains a very effective technique for the early treatment of lumbar disk disease, particularly the appendicular symptoms as opposed to the axial symptoms. Fusions, with or without decompression, are a more complex consideration, with a much lower success rate. With either approach, the necessity for the development of and adherence to strict criteria for surgical intervention should be obvious to all those who treat diseases of the spine.

CHEMONUCLEOLYSIS

The injection of chymopapain, the proteolytic component of the papaya plant, into the nucleus of a diseased intervertebral disk is another technique for the decompression of symptomatic nerve roots. First described in humans by Lyman Smith,[111–113] the chymopapain acts on the noncollagenous portion of the diskal structures, reducing the viscosity of the water-soluble nucleus pulposus. This in turn reduces the height of the disk space, diminishes the turgor of the annular protrusion, relaxes Hoffman's ligaments, and effects a chemical decompression of compromised neural tissues.

Despite much early enthusiasm and reports of "marked" relief in nearly 70% of 16,985 patients treated with chymopapain in the 10 years following Smith's initial report, the drug was withdrawn from general use by the Food and Drug Administration. Early studies of the drug's efficacy were not objective or double-blind.[114] The first good study in myelographically confirmed lumbar disk herniations by Schwetschenau and associates[115, 116] showed no statistical difference between treated and control groups. More recent randomized double-blind studies organized by Smith Laboratories[117, 118] showed between 82% and 90% success at 6 months. Long-term follow-up showed less striking results, with 70% achieving satisfactory results and 80% achieving "definite improvement."[119] Chymopapain was again approved for general use on November 10, 1982.

The selection of the appropriate candidate for chemonucleolysis remains the critical issue in the clinical setting. As will be discussed, the risks of chymopapain instillation are equal to those of surgery, and it should not be undertaken as a "lesser procedure" or for lesser indications than surgical decompression itself. Thus, all the presurgical predictive criteria reviewed in preceding sections apply to chemonucleolysis patients as well. Although chymopapain injection may well help patients with a relatively high proportion of back-to-leg pain or with a "protruding" rather than a truly herniated disk, it should not be used for back pain alone. At the other end of the spectrum, it would seem illogical that those patients with a fully extruded and sequestered disk fragment should obtain relief from this treatment. Thus, a patient should, as recommended by the American Academy of Orthopaedic Surgeons and the American Association of Neurological Surgeons, undergo both CT scanning and myelography to define the spinal pathology as precisely as possible. Furthermore, the value of diskography during chemonucleolysis may be debated, but it should certainly suggest normal disk levels even better than abnormal ones.

The contraindications for chemonucleolysis include patients with progressive motor weakness, cauda equina syndromes, extensive spondylosis or spinal stenosis, and some forms of spondylolisthesis. Pregnancy, prior chymopapain injections, or allergy to papaya extracts are also obvious contraindications. The failure of prior surgery at the symptomatic level is a strong negative predictor from both the standpoint of further scar formation and the validity of the initial diagnosis of diskogenic disease. Finally, those patients with complicating factors such as psychiatric disturbances, litigation, and compensation claims should be expected to fare no better from chemonucleolysis than from spinal surgery.

The technique of chemonucleolysis is relatively simple and has changed little from its inception. Under radiographic control, a needle is placed into the nucleus of a suspected intervertebral disk, and the pathologic state is confirmed by injection of contrast material— usually Conray (iothalamate meglumine) or Renografin (diatrizoate meglumine). Once the needle is correctly positioned and no allergic reponse to the contrast material or a 0.3-ml test dose of chymopapain has been seen after 10 minutes, the remaining 1.2 ml of chymopapain are injected. If there is no untoward reaction after close observation for 30 minutes, transfer to the recovery area is allowed.

The primary complication of chymopapain injection is an allergic reaction, ranging from a feeling of malaise to fatal anaphylactic shock. For this reason, many prefer to perform the procedure under general anesthesia. The delayed awareness of the reaction is offset by the security of central intravenous lines and endotracheal ventilation. Other recent reports[120] have endorsed the use of local anesthesia, citing as its primary advantage the early awareness and treatment of serious reactions. The reported incidence of anaphylactic shock has varied from zero[117] to 0.35%[10] to 1%.[118] All studies show a predilection for allergic attacks in females. The mortality rate from the procedure compares favorably with that from surgical laminectomy, being 0.1%.[121] Several preoperative tests for identifying IgE antibodies to chymopapain have become available, but their specificity and sensitivity are as yet uncertain. The use of H_1 and H_2 receptor blockers such as Benadryl (diphenhydramine) and Tagamet (cimetadine) may reduce the severity but not the incidence of allergic response.[122]

Other seldom-mentioned complications, occurring in over a third of patients, include severe back pain and spasm, lasting several days to several weeks and often requiring rehospitalization.[117] The relief of radicular pain is not as immediate as with surgical decompression, requiring as long as 6 weeks to resolve in some studies. Other problems such as radiation exposure and hemorrhagic responses are rare and difficult to evaluate. Repeat injections are currently forbidden, but failure of chemonucleolysis does not adversely affect the results of subsequent surgery.[118]

Therefore, chemonucleolysis has evolved as a viable technique in the treatment of degenerative disk disease. Although it is at least 10% less successful than surgical decompression, is limited to problems of nuclear herniation without full extrusion or secondary spinal stenosis, has a considerable incidence of severe back pain and slow resolution of radicular symptoms, shares an anesthetic risk and overall mortality equivalent to those of surgery, and can be administered only once under current guidelines, there is an enlarging body of information to support its use. It remains the responsibility of the treating physician to temper the enthusiasm for a panacea for back pain of diverse etiologies and to be clear in the indications and risks of chemonucleolysis before advocating its use.

References

1. Vesalius A: De Humani Corporis Fabrici Libri Septum. Basileae, Ex Officina Ioannis Oporini, 1543.
2. Mixter WJ, Barr JS: Ruptures of the intervertebral disc with involvement of the spinal canal. N Engl J Med 211:210–215, 1934.
3. Nachemson AL: The lumbar spine: An orthopaedic challenge. Spine 1:59–71, 1976.
4. Rothman RH: The pathophysiology of degeneration. *In* Wilkins RH (ed.): Clinical Neurosurgery, Vol. 20. The Congress of Neurological Surgeons. Baltimore, Williams and Wilkins, 1973, pp. 174–182.
5. Weber H: Lumbar disc herniations: A prospective study of prognostic factors including a controlled trial. J Oslo City Hosp 28:33–64, 1978.
6. Horal J: The clinical appearance of low back disorders. Acta Orthop Scand (Suppl) 118:7–109, 1969.
7. Nachemson AL: The natural course of low back pain. *In* White AA, Gordon SL (eds.): AAOS Symposium on Low Back Pain. St. Louis, C.V. Mosby Co., 1982.
8. Kelsey JL: Demographic characteristics of persons with acute herniated lumbar intervertebral disc. J Chronic Dis 28:37–50, 1975.
9. Kelsey JL: An epidemiological study of the relationship between occupations and acute herniated lumbar intervertebral discs. Int J Epidemiol 4:197–204, 1975.
10. Kelsey JL, White AA, Bisbee QE: The impact of musculoskeletal disorders on the population of the United States. J Bone Joint Surg 61A:954–964, 1979.
11. Hult L: The Munkfors investigation. Acta Orthop Scand (Suppl) 16:5–102, 1954.
12. Benn RT, Wood PHN: Pain in the back: An attempt to estimate the size of the problem. Rheumatol Rehabil 14:121–128, 1975.
13. Rowe ML: Low back pain in industry. A position paper. J Occup Med 11:161–169, 1969.
14. Akeson WH, Murphy RW: Editorial comment: Low back pain. Clin Orthop 129:2–3, 1977.
15. Leavitt SS, Johnston TL, Beyer RD: The process of recovery; patterns in industrial back injury: Part 1. Costs and other quantitative measures of effort. Ind Med Surg 40:7–14, 1971.
16. Krempen JR, Silver RA, Hadley J: An analysis of differential epidural spinal anesthesia and pentothal: Pain study in the differential diagnosis of back pain. Spine 2:452–459, 1979.
17. Gulliver J: Acute low back pain in industry. Acta Orthop Scand (Suppl) 170:9–17, 1977.
18. Hakelius A: Prognosis in sciatica. Acta Orthop Scand 129:6–76, 1970.
19. Pearce J, Moll J: Conservative treatment and natural history of acute lumbar disc lesions. J Neurol Neurosurg Psychiatry 30:13–17, 1967.
20. Rothman RH, Simeone FA: The Spine. Philadelphia, WB Saunders Company, 1975, p. 437.
21. Farfan HS: Mechanical Disorders of the Low Back. Philadelphia, Lea and Febiger, 1973.
22. Ogab K, Whiteside LA: Nutritional pathways of the intervertebral disc. Spine 6:211–216, 1981.
23. Macnab I: Backache. Baltimore, Williams and Wilkins, 1977.
24. Macnab I: The traction spur. J Bone Joint Surg 53A:663–670, 1971.
25. Kirkaldy-Willis WH, Wedge JH, Yong-Hing K, Reilly J: Pathology and pathogenesis of lumbar spondylosis and stenosis. Spine 3:319–328, 1978.
26. Timmi PG, Wieser C, Zinn WM: The transitional vertebra of the lumbosacral spine: Its radiological classification, incidence, prevalence, and clinical significance. Rheumatol Rehabil 16:180–185, 1977.
27. Jayson MI, Herbert CM, Barks JS: Intervertebral discs: Nuclear morphology and bursting pressures. Ann Rheum Dis 32:308–315, 1973.
28. Armstrong JR: Lumbar Disc Lesions. Baltimore, Williams and Wilkins, 1965.
29. Falconer MA, et al: Observations on the causes and mechanics of symptom production in low back pain and sciatica. J Neurol Neurosurg Psychiatry 11:13–26, 1948.
30. Porter PW, Hibbert CS, Wicks M: The spinal canal in symptomatic lumbar disc disease. J Bone Joint Surg 60B:485–487, 1978.
31. Farfan HF: A reorientation in the surgical approach to degenerative lumbar intervertebral joint disease. Orthop Clin North Am 8:9–21, 1977.
32. Macnab I : Negative disc exploration: An analysis of the causes of nerve root involvement in sixty-eight patients. J Bone Joint Surg 53A:891–903, 1971.
33. Spangfort EV: The lumbar disc herniation. A computer-aided analysis of 2504 operations. Acta Orthop Scand (Suppl) 142:61–77, 1972.
34. Nachemson A: The load on lumbar disks in different positions of the body. Acta Orthop Scand 136:426, 1965.
35. Kellgren JH: The anatomical source of back pain. Rheumatol Rehabil 16:3–11, 1977.
36. Mooney V, Robertson J: The facet syndrome. Clin Orthop 115:149–156, 1976.
37. Melzack R, Stillwell DM, Fox EJ: Trigger points and acupuncture points for pain: Correlations and implications. Pain 3:3–23, 1977.
38. Smyth MJ, Wright VJ: Sciatica and the intervertebral disc. An experimental study. J Bone Joint Surg 40A:1401, 1958.
39. Murphy RW: Nerve roots and spinal nerves in degenerative disk disease. Clin Orthop 129:46–60, 1977.
40. Bobechko WT, Hirsch C: Auto-immune response to nucleus pulposus in the rabbit. J Bone Joint Surg 47B:574, 1965.
41. Bisla RS, Marchisello PJ, Lockshin MD, et al: Autoimmunological basis of disk degeneration. Clin Orthop 121:205–211, 1976.
42. Naylor A: Intervertebral disc prolapse and degeneration. The biochemical and biophysical approach. Spine 1:108–114, 1976.
43. Bulos S: Herniated intervertebral lumbar disc in the teenager. J Bone Joint Surg 55B:273–278, 1973.
44. Bradford DS, Garcia A: Lumbar intervertebral disk herniations in children and adolescents. Orthop Clin North Am 2:583–592, 1971.
45. Friis ML, Gulliksen GC, Rasmussen P, Husby J: Pain and spinal root compression. Acta Neurochir 39:241–249, 1977.
46. Verbiest H: Radicular syndrome from developmental narrowing of the lumbar vertebral canal. J Bone Joint Surg 36B:230–237, 1954.

47. Dyck P, Doyle JB: "Bicycle test" of van Gelderen in diagnosis of intermittent cauda equina compression syndrome. J Neurosurg 46:667–670, 1977.

48. Raaf J: Some observations regarding 905 patients operated upon for protruded lumbar intervertebral disc. Am J Surg 97:388–399, 1959.

49. Peyser E, Harari A: Intradural rupture of lumbar intervertebral disk: Report of two cases with review of the literature. Surg Neurol 8:95–98, 1977.

50. Emmett J, Love J: Vesical dysfunction caused by protruded lumbar disc. J Urol 105:80–91, 1971.

51. Ross JC, Jackson RM: Vesical dysfunction due to prolapsed disc. Br Med J 3:752–754, 1971.

52. Sharr MM, Garfield JS, Jenkins JD: The association of bladder dysfunction with degenerative lumbar spondylosis. Br J Urol 45:616–620, 1973.

53. Gunn CC, Chir B, Milgrand WE: Tenderness at motor points: A diagnostic and prognostic aid to low back injury. J Bone Joint Surg 58A:815–825, 1976.

54. Hakelius A, Hindmarsh J: The significance of neurological signs and myelography findings in the diagnosis of lumbar root compression. Acta Orthop Scand 43:234–238, 1972.

55. Scham S, Taylor T: Tension signs in lumbar disc prolapse. Clin Orthop 44:163–170, 1966.

56. Spangfort E: Lasègue's sign in patients with lumbar disc herniation. Acta Orthop Scand 42:459, 1971.

57. Hudgins WR: The cross-straight-leg-raising test. N Engl J Med 297:1127, 1977.

58. Magora A, Schwartz A: Relation between the low back pain syndrome and x-ray findings. Scand J Rehabil Med 8:115–125, 1976.

59. Torgerson WR, Dotter WE: Comparative roentgenographic study of the asymptomatic and symptomatic lumbar spine. J Bone Joint Surg 58A:850–853, 1976.

60. Fitzgerald JAW, Newman PH: Degenerative spondylolisthesis. J Bone Joint Surg 58A:184–192, 1976.

61. DePalma W, Rothman R: Surgery of the lumbar spine. Clin Orthop 63:162–170, 1969.

62. LaRocca H, Macnab I: Value of pre-employment radiographic assessment of the lumbar spine. R Ind Med 39:253–258, 1970.

63. Ericksen MF: Some aspects of aging in the lumbar spine. Am J Phys Anthropol 45:575–580, 1976.

64. Ericksen MF: Aging in the lumbar spine (L1 and L2). Am J Phys Anthropol 48:241–246, 1978.

65. Harris R, Macnab I: Structural changes in the lumbar vertebral discs. J Bone Joint Surg 35B:304, 1954.

66. Resnick D, Niwayama G: Intervertebral disk herniations: Cartilaginous (Schmorl's) nodes. Radiology 126:57–65, 1978.

67. Splitoff C: Roentgenographic comparison of patients with or without backache. JAMA 152:1610, 1953.

68. Roche MD, Rowe GG: The incidence of separate neural arch in coincident bone variations. J Bone Joint Surg 34A:491, 1952.

69. Gargano FP, Meyer JD, Sheldon JJ: Transfemoral ascending lumbar catheterization of the epidural veins in lumbar disk disease. Radiology 111:329–335, 1974.

70. Macnab I, St. Louis EL, Grabias SL, et al.: Selective ascending lumbosacral venography in the assessment of lumbar disc herniations. J Bone Joint Surg 58A:1093–1098, 1976.

71. Magnussen W: Über die bedingunden des herror-tretons der werklukekh gelenkspatte auf rontgenbilde. Acta Radiol 18:733–741, 1937.

72. Wiesel S, Ignatius P, Marvel JP, et al.: Intradural neurofibroma simulating lumbar disc disease. J Bone Joint Surg 58A:1040–1042, 1976.

73. Edgar MA, Park WM: Induced pain patterns on passive straight leg raising in lower lumbar disc protrusion. J Bone Joint Surg 56B:658–668, 1974.

74. Hakelius A, Hindmarsh J: The comparative reliability of preoperative diagnostic methods in lumbar disc surgery. Acta Orthop Scand 43:234–238, 1972.

75. Symposium: Lumbar arachnoiditis: Nomenclature, etiology and pathology. Spine 3:21–92, 1978.

76. Ahlgren P: Lumbale myographie mit conray meglumine 282. Fortschr Rontgenstr 111:270–276, 1969.

77. Grainger RG, Kendall BE, Wylie IG: Lumbar myelography with metrizamide—a new nonionic contrast medium. Br J Radiol 49:996–1003, 1976.

78. Post MJ, Gargano FP, Vining DQ, Rosomoff HL: A comparison of radiographic methods of diagnosing constrictive lesions of the spinal canal. J Neurosurg 48:360–368, 1978.

79. Rothman RH, et al.: Metrizamide myelography and the identification of anomalous lumbosacral nerve roots. J Bone Joint Surg 62A:1203–1208, 1980.

80. Schobinger RA, Krueger E, Sobel G: Comparison of intraosseous vertebral venography and Pantopaque myelography in the diagnosis of surgical conditions of the lumbar spine and nerve roots. Radiology 77:397, 1961.

81. Gershater R, St. Louis EL: Lumbar epidural venography. Radiology 131:409–421, 1979.

82. Rothman RH, et al.: Metrizamide myelography and epidural venography. Spine 7:55–64, 1982.

83. Gargano FP, Meyer J, Houdek PV, Charyulu KN: Transverse axial tomography of the cervical spine. Radiology 113:363, 1974.

84. Weinstein MA, Moufarrij NA, Hardy RW: Computed tomographic, myelographic and operative findings in patients with suspected herniated lumbar discs. Neurosurgery 12:184–188, 1983.

85. Tchang SPK, Howie JL, Kirkaldy-Willis WH, et al.: Computed tomography versus myelography in diagnosis of lumbar disc herniation. J Can Assoc Radiol 33:15–20, 1982.

86. Rothman RH: Personal communication, 1983.

87. Holt E: The question of lumbar discography. J Bone Joint Surg 50A:720–726, 1968.

88. Patrick BS: Lumbar discography: A five year study. Surg Neurol 1:267–273, 1973.

89. Wiesel SW, Rothman RH: Acute low back pain. An objective analysis of conservative therapy. Clin Orthop 143:290, 1979.

90. Larsson U, Choler U, Lindstrom A, et al.: Autotraction for the treatment of lumbago-sciatica: A multicentre controlled investigation. Acta Orthop Scand 51:791–798, 1980.

91. Weber H: Traction therapy in sciatica due to disc prolapse. J Oslo City Hosp 23:167–179, 1973.

92. Berry H, Bloom B, Hamilton EBD, Swinson DR: Naproxen sodium, diflunisal, and placebo in the treatment of chronic back pain. Ann Rheum Dis 41:129–132, 1982.

93. Hickey RFJ: Chronic low back pain. A comparison of diflunisal with paracetamol. N Z Med J 95:312–314, 1982.

94. Williams SJ: Back school. Physiotherapy 63:590, 1977.

95. Kendall PH, Jenkins JM: Exercises for backache: A double-blind controlled trial. Physiotherapy 54:154–157, 1968.

96. Maury M, Francois N, Skoda A: About the neurological sequelae of herniated intervertebral disc. Paraplegia 11:221–227, 1976.

97. Hirsch C: Efficiency of surgery in low back disorders. J Bone Joint Surg 47A:991, 1965.

98. Semmes E: Ruptures of the Lumbar Intervertebral Disc. Springfield, Illinois, Charles C Thomas, 1964.

99. Young H, Love J: End results of removal of protruded lumbar intervertebral discs with and without fusion. AAOS Instructional Course Lecture 16:213–216, 1959.

100. Jartsfer BS, Rich NM: The challenge of arteriovenous fistula formation following disk surgery: A collective review. J Trauma 16:726–733, 1976.

101. Desausseure RL: Vascular injuries coincident to disc surgery. J Neurosurg 16:222–229, 1959.

102. Bertrand G: The "battered" root problem. Orthop Clin North Am 6:305–309, 1975.

103. Domisse GF: The blood supply of the spinal cord. J Bone Joint Surg 56B:225–235, 1974.

104. Jackson RK: The long term effects of wide laminectomy for lumbar disc excision. J Bone Joint Surg 53B:609–616, 1971.

105. LaRocca H, Macnab I: The laminectomy membrane. J Bone Joint Surg 56B:545–550, 1974.

106. Langenskiöld A, Kiviluoto O: Prevention of epidural scar formation after operations on the lumbar spine by means of free fat transplants. Clin Orthop 115:92–95, 1976.

107. Gill GC, Sakovich L, Thompson E: Pedicle fat graft for the prevention of scar formation after laminectomy: An experimental study in dogs. Proceedings of the 5th Annual Meetings of the International Society for the Study of the Lumbar Spine, San Francisco, 1978.

108. DePalma A, Rothman R: The nature of pseudarthrosis. Clin Orthop 59:113–118, 1968.

109. Rothman R, et al.: The effect of iron deficiency anemia on fracture healing. Clin Orthop 77:276–283, 1971.

110. Knutsson B: Aspects of the neurogenic electromyographic records of voluntary contraction in cases of nerve root compression. Electromyography 2:238–242, 1962.

111. Smith L, Garvin PJ, Gesler RM, Jennings RB: Enzyme dissolution of the nucleus pulposus. Nature 198:1311, 1963.

112. Smith L: Enzyme dissolution of the nucleus pulposus in humans. JAMA 187:137, 1964.

113. Smith L: Chemonucleolysis. Clin Orthop 67:72–80, 1969.

114. Schneider RC: Statement from the American Association of Neurological Surgeons. (Position statement on chymopapain.) J Neurosurg 42:373, 1975.

115. Martins AN, Ramierz A, Johnson J, Schwetschenau PR: Double blind evaluation of chemonucleolysis for herniated lumbar discs. J Neurosurg. 49:816–827, 1978.

116. Schwetschenau PR, Ramierz A, Johnson J, et al.: Double blind evaluation of intradiscal chymopapain for the herniated lumbar discs. J Neurosurg 45:622–627, 1976.

117. Javid MJ, Nordby EJ, Ford LT, et al.: Safety and efficacy of chymopapain (Chymodiactin) in herniated nucleus pulposus with sciatica. Results of a randomized, double-blind study. JAMA, 249:2489–2494, 1983.

118. Nordby EJ: Chymopapain in intradiscal therapy. J Bone Joint Surg 65A:1350–1353, 1983.

119. Nordby EJ: Eight to thirteen year follow-up of chemonucleolysis patients. Clin Orthop, in press.

120. Hall BB, McCulloch JA: Anaphylactic reactions following the intradiscal injection of chymopapain under local anesthesia. J Bone Joint Surg 65A:1215–1219, 1983.

121. Spangfort EV: The lumbar disc herniation. A computer-aided analysis of 2,504 operations. Acta Orthop Scand Suppl 142, 1972.

122. Philbin DM, Moss J, Atkins CW, et al.: The use of H_1 and H_2 histamine antagonists with morphine anesthesia: A double-blind study. Anesthesiology 55:292–296, 1981.

29

Osteoarthritis of the Temporomandibular Joint

Walter Guralnick, D.M.D.
David A. Keith, B.D.S., F.D.S.R.C.S.

In contrast to rheumatoid arthritis, osteoarthritis (degenerative arthritis or degenerative joint disease) is a common noninflammatory disease that usually occurs in individual joints, including the temporomandibular joint.[1-3] In this joint, it is characterized by a unique biologic process in which there is deterioration of the articular surfaces and simultaneous remodeling of the underlying bone. Understanding the remodeling process as it occurs in the temporomandibular joint is essential if one is to interpret clinical signs and symptoms accurately and recommend treatment to the patient with osteoarthritis. Therefore, the biologic basis of remodeling will be discussed first.

BIOLOGIC BASIS OF REMODELING

In its mature state, the mandibular condyle (Fig. 29–1) is covered by an articular layer of fibrocartilage consisting of collagen fibers interspersed with some elastic fibers. Between this surface layer and the subchondral plate of bone lies a diminutive layer of cartilage cells that is all that remains of the condylar cartilage of the fetus and young child. This layer is a constant feature of adult specimens and retains the capacity to respond to physical forces by way of remodeling.[4-8]

Progressive remodeling has the effect of moving the articular surface toward the joint cavity (Figs. 29–2 and 29–3). The stimulus causes the cartilaginous zone to increase in size and lay down cartilaginous matrix, and this is accompanied by an increase in vascularization

of the area. The cartilage becomes calcified, and subsequently bone is formed. The result is that the articular surface layer, which has taken no active part in the process, is advanced.[6]

Regressive remodeling has the reverse effect (Figs. 29–4 and 29–5), in that the articular

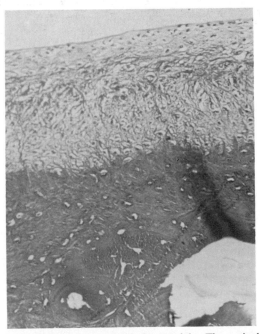

Figure 29–1. Mature mandibular condyle. The articular surface consists of a basket-weave of collagen fibers. Below this is a more cellular layer, the remains of the condylar cartilage of the growing jaw. The subchondral plate of bone is completely formed. (H & E stain, × 60.)

523

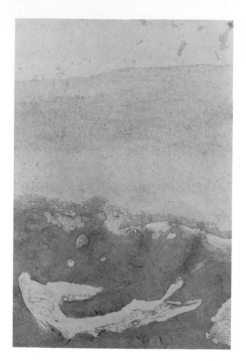

Figure 29–2. Progressive remodeling. The cartilaginous zone proliferates, and there is an increase in vascularity. The surface layer remains intact and does not appear to actively participate in the process. (H & E stain, × 60.)

Figure 29–3. Progressive remodeling—high power. The cartilage matrix calcifies, thus advancing the subchondral plate of bone in this local area. (Verhoeff's stain, × 150.)

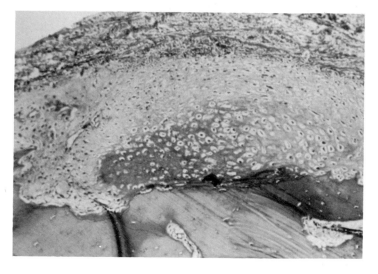

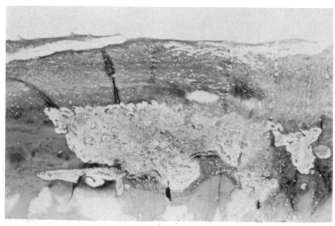

Figure 29–4. Regressive remodeling. The subchondral plate of bone is resorbed and replaced with a vascular corrective tissue. Although showing some artifactual changes, the articular layer remains intact. (Verhoeff's stain, × 60.)

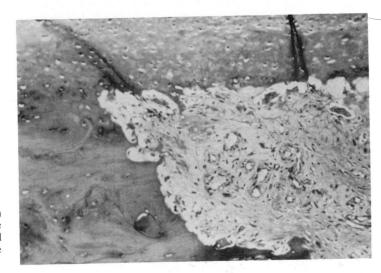

Figure 29–5. Regressive remodeling—high power. Note the highly vascular connective tissue replacing the subchondral bone and osteoclasts in lacunae resorbing the bone edge. (Verhoeff's stain, × 150.)

surface moves away from the joint cavity. The cartilaginous zone is activated, and osteoclasts resorb the subchondral plate of bone. Again, there is an increase in vascularity of the area. As a result of the resorption of the underlying bone, the articular layer is removed from the joint space.[6]

In both types of remodeling the process involves the subarticular tissues only, and the articular surface layer appears to remain unaffected. Although these processes have been described as separate entities, they can and frequently do occur in closely adjacent areas (Fig. 29–6). Typically, regressive changes are noted in the superoanterior aspect of the condyle and in the posterior aspect of the articular eminence, whereas progressive changes are seen in the posterior aspect of the condyle.[5]

DEGENERATIVE CHANGE

The previous section has indicated that extensive changes can occur in the shape and size of the mandibular condyle. When the limit of these changes is exceeded, degenerative changes occur, leading to the destruction of the articulating surfaces. In these cases, the changes take place in the surface layer, although evidence of previous remodeling is invariably present.

The process of degeneration (Figs. 29–7 and 29–8) has been described histologically in much the same terms as osteoarthritis of other joints, although the tissues involved, fibrocartilage in the temporomandibular joint and hyaline cartilage in other joints, are fundamentally different in their structure and properties. The

Figure 29–6. Progressive and regressive remodeling. Both types of remodeling are seen in adjacent areas. Two triangular areas of progressive remodeling are noted. A resorption cavity is seen to the extreme left of the field; the surface layer is intact. (Verhoeff's stain, × 150.)

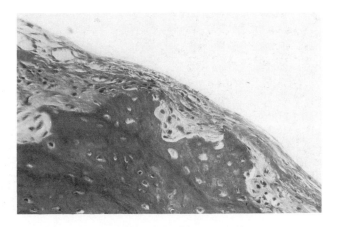

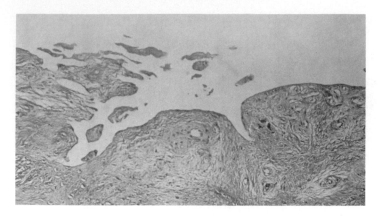

Figure 29–7. Osteoarthritis—early stage. The articular surface demonstrates splitting of the fibrous layer. (Verhoeff's stain, × 150.)

initial change is a disorganization of the cells of the surface layer, with clumping and an increased affinity for basophilic dyes. Fissuring in the vertical or horizontal plane occurs next, with subsequent loss of the surface layer until bone is exposed.[1, 4] These processes may, in fact, be seen in different parts of the same specimen, with end-stage degenerative change being represented by bare bone on one aspect of the condyle and active progressive remodeling occurring on the opposite aspect.

ANIMAL MODEL

Very little experimental work has been done on degenerative change in the temporomandibular joint. In one study[9] of the age-related changes in the mouse mandibular joint, in which degenerative disease occurs relatively early in adult life, the initial stages were considered to be a form of chondromalacia with considerable decrease in the cell-to-matrix ratio and a tendency toward cell clustering. The transition from chondromalacia to osteoarthrosis was demonstrated by ankylosis, cell necrosis, splitting and fraying of the matrix, osteophyte formation, bone eburnation, and osteosclerosis.

CLINICAL FEATURES

Because the symptoms of degenerative arthritis are so similar to those of functional temporomandibular joint disorders (e.g., myofascial pain-dysfunction syndrome, mandibular dysfunction), it is difficult to cite its incidence. Clinical experience, however, suggests that it is common.[10]

The patient may complain of joint noise and pain, masticatory muscle tenderness, limited motion, deviation of the jaw to the affected side, and pain with movement as well as ten-

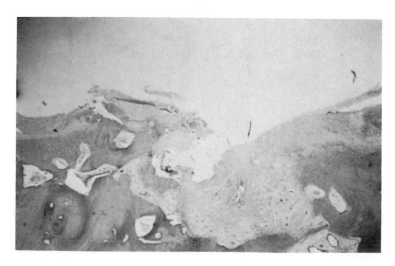

Figure 29–8. Osteoarthritis—end stage. The articular layer is entirely destroyed, exposing bare bone and vascular marrow spaces. (Verhoeff's stain, × 60.)

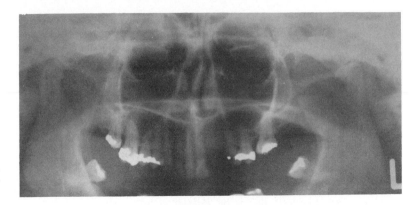

Figure 29–9. Panoramic jaw film. Condyles are particularly well visualized in the open mouth position.

derness on palpation over the condyle. All symptoms are not necessarily present in every case, but the majority usually are. The distinction between degenerative arthritis and mandibular dysfunction is primarily established by objective findings. In degenerative arthritis, there is roentgenographic evidence of joint abnormality, whereas in mandibular dysfunction, there is no change found in the temporomandibular joint.[11]

Some comment about roentgenography of the temporomandibular joint is appropriate. There are numerous diagnostic roentgenographic techniques presently available, and several can be recommended. The panoramic jaw film (Fig. 29–9) is very useful, particularly for initial screening and, occasionally, for definitive diagnosis. Two views should be used: the first is with the mouth closed; the second is with the mouth open, so that condylar motion can be assessed. In most instances, pathology suggested by the panoramic films will demand the detail obtained from polytomography (Fig. 29–10). In some cases, in which information about the meniscus is desired, arthrograms should be obtained.[12–14] Arthrography has now progressed to the point of being both available and reliable and should be done

to assess internal derangements, particularly displacement of the meniscus (Fig. 29–11).

It is just as important to appreciate the limitations of roentgenographic findings as it is to appreciate their benefits. Changes characteristic of degenerative arthritis are bony spurs (osteophytes) (Fig. 29–12), generalized irregularity of the condylar surface, and cyst-like areas within the condyle (Fig. 29–13). Because remodeling of this joint is a continuing process, the abnormalities noted on the films may be temporally related to either regressive or progressive remodeling. They can be considered pathologic only when they are correlated with clinical symptoms (Fig. 29–14).

Radin and associates'[15] orthopedic studies of osteoarthritis, suggesting that repetitive impulse loading of a joint produces bone changes, is applicable to degenerative arthritis of the temporomandibular joint as well. Occlusion, or bite, is the loading agent of the temporomandibular joint and is believed to be a primary cause of some temporomandibular joint problems.[16] A similar thesis was suggested many years ago by Costen[17] and is still the basis for the importance many practitioners place on occlusal adjustment, restoration, equilibration, and bite alteration in treating

Figure 29–10. Polytomogram of the condyle.

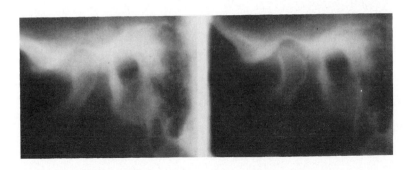

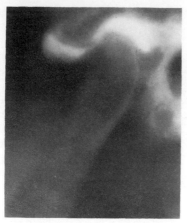

Figure 29–11. Arthrogram of the temporomandibular joint. Semilunar appearance of the dye anterior to the condyle indicates a displaced meniscus.

patients with temporomandibular joint symptoms.

Tension habits, such as clenching or grinding the teeth, place undue stress on the joints and also create muscle spasm. They are a variant of the basic "loading" mechanism. What may begin as a minor assault on the joint by an oral expression of tension (e.g., clenching) has been shown to produce osteoarthritis of the temporomandibular joint if continued over time.[18, 19]

Toller[1] demonstrated the genesis of degenerative arthritis in patients with mandibular dysfunction whose tension habits were uncontrolled. He also provided equally important evidence of the beneficial effects of the joint's remodeling ability, because unlike degenerative arthritis in other joints, the symptoms of osteoarthritis of the temporomandibular joint decrease after the age of 40 years. He postu-

lated that patients with degenerative arthritis who are symptomatic between the ages of 20 and 40 years, may be "cured" by physiologic remodeling of the condyle if the cause of the joint condition (e.g., clenching or grinding) is eliminated.

TREATMENT

The treatment of degenerative joint disease is dependent on the patient's degree of discomfort and/or disability and the extent of demonstrable joint pathology. Patients with minimal condylar change are often amenable to the same measures applicable to the management of those with pain-dysfunction syndrome.[20] Essentially, treatment is aimed at controlling pain, alleviating tension and stress, and correcting any existing occlusal disharmony. Teeth that are broken down should be restored, and missing teeth should be replaced, particularly posterior ones. However, extensive dental work is best deferred until acute discomfort is relieved. The simplest and least traumatic way of balancing the bite is to have an occlusal splint made that will provide a flat plane of occlusion without interference to free jaw movement (Fig. 29–15). This is customarily worn at night to relieve the temporomandibular joints from the trauma of bruxism (night grinding). It is also useful during the day for patients who are habitual "clenchers."

Analgesics, aspirin, and other nonsteroidal anti-inflammatory drugs are useful, and diazepam utilized as a muscle relaxant can be helpful when the condition is acute and muscle spasm is present. In addition, psychologic counseling is often important in reducing the

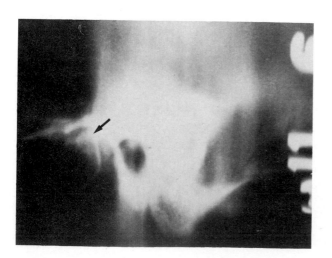

Figure 29–12. Degenerative joint disease. Osteophyte of condyle.

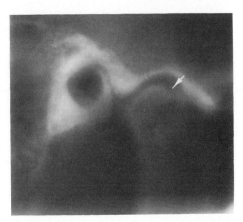

Figure 29–13. Degenerative joint disease. Cystic change in condyle (arrow).

tension habits that so often precipitated the impairment.

Other ancillary measures that will help in the nonsurgical management of degenerative arthritis are rest and the application of heat. The temporomandibular joint is a more difficult joint to put at rest than most others. Fortunately, it need not be immobilized; in fact, it should not be immobilized to achieve satisfactory relief of pain and improvement. A soft diet, carefully adhered to for 7 to 10 days, is sufficient. In addition, the application of moist heat to the joint area several times a day is comforting and is more readily obtained than mechanical techniques such as short-wave diathermy or ultrasound treatment. One other nonsurgical treatment modality, although invasive, is occasionally useful. It is the instillation of steroids into the joint spaces.[21] Some patients with demonstrable, but minimal, persistent regressive changes of the condylar surface and continued discomfort can be treated by injection. A corticosteroid, 0.5 to 1 ml, is injected into the joint; if discomfort persists,

the procedure is repeated once (and only once) 2 weeks later. Poswillo terms the effect of corticosteroids "chemocondylectomy."[21] It is what Toller similarly described as pharmacologically achieved arthroplasty.[1] Roentgenographic evidence of remodeling may occur after steroid injections, but the condyle can be expected to be slightly reduced in size.

Because osteoarthritis of the temporomandibular joint usually follows a course of spontaneous repair (through the physiologic process of remodeling), most patients with this disease will not require surgery. However, some patients have irreparable joint damage and will require surgical intervention. The operation that is recommended is a high condylectomy.[18, 22] The term "high" is used advisedly to stress the removal of only the surface of the condyle and not the entire condyle (condylectomy). It is done through a preauricular approach, by which the joint is readily exposed. Using an oscillating saw, the roughened superior surface of the condyle is removed, and the wound is then closed in layers.

Several points should be emphasized. Following a high condylectomy, remodeling will take place by normal healing. It is therefore unnecessary and unwise to place any material, either organic or alloplastic, over the cut, bony surface. In addition, the patient's jaws should not be immobilized. Normal function is important for both healing and patient comfort. Normal postoperative discomfort and edema will provide the only necessary limitation of jaw motion. When the patient is able to eat normally, he will do so, and this can be anticipated about 2 weeks postoperatively.

The cosmetic result of the preauricular approach to the joint is eminently satisfactory and makes consideration of other incisions unnecessary.

The recognition and treatment of degener-

Figure 29–14. Markedly changed condylar morphology in an asymptomatic patient.

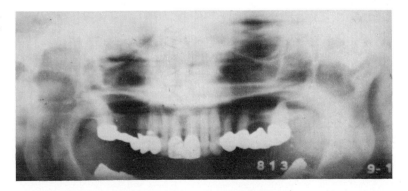

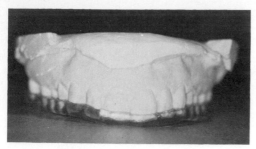

Figure 29–15. Occlusal splint.

ative arthritis of the temporomandibular joint have been reviewed. There are several noteworthy aspects of the disease in this particular joint. Its differentiation from temporomandibular joint dysfunction is difficult, because symptoms of the two conditions are often similar. However, in degenerative joint disease, unlike its functional counterpart, there are demonstrable roentgenographic changes. Stress and tension habits are important factors in dysfunction. If they are not eliminated, temporomandibular joint dysfunction may evolve into degenerative joint disease. Fortunately, degenerative joint disease is often self-limiting and spontaneously repaired by normal remodeling of the joint. It is for this reason that the treatment of osteoarthritis of the temporomandibular joint is more often nonsurgical than surgical, with surgery reserved for those patients with intractable pain and irreversible destructive disease of the condyle.

References

1. Toller PA: Osteoarthritis of the mandibular condyle. Br Dent J 134:223–231, 1973.
2. Toller PA: Ultrastructure of the condylar articular surface in severe mandibular pain dysfunction syndrome. Int J Oral Surg 6:297–312, 1977.
3. Zarb GA, Carlsson GE: Temporomandibular Joint Function and Dysfunction. St. Louis, C.V. Mosby Co., 1979.
4. Blackwood HJ: Arthritis of the mandibular joint. Br Dent J 115:317–326, 1963.
5. Blackwood HJ: Adaptive changes in mandibular joints with function. Dent Clin North Am 10:559–566, 1966.
6. Johnson LC: Joint remodelling as a basis for osteoarthritis. J Am Vet Med Assoc 141:1237–1241, 1962.
7. Moffett BC Jr, Lent CJ, McCabe JB, et al.: Articular remodelling in the adult human temporomandibular joint. Am J Anat 115:119–142, 1964.
8. Sharpe CJ, Gee EJ, Griffen CJ: The osteogenic potential of the human condyle. Aust Dent J 10:287–291, 1965.
9. Silbermann M, Livne E: Age-related degenerative changes in the mouse mandibular joint. J Anat 129:507–520, 1979.
10. Ogus H: Rheumatoid arthritis of the temporomandibular joint. Br J Oral Surg 12:275–284, 1975.
11. Laskin DM: Etiology of the pain-dysfunction syndrome. J Am Dent Assoc 79:147–153, 1969.
12. Blaschke DD, Solberg WK, Sanders B: Arthrography of temporomandibular joint: Review of current status. J Am Dent Assoc 10:388–395, 1980.
13. Katzberg RW, Dolwick MF, Helms CA, et al.: Arthrotomography of the temporomandibular joint. Am J Radiol 134:995–1003, 1980.
14. Katzberg RW, Dolwick MD, Keith DA, et al.: New observations with routine and CT-assisted arthrography in suspected internal derangements of the temporomandibular joint. Oral Surg. 51:569–574, 1981.
15. Radin EL, Paul IL, Rose RM: Role of mechanical factors in the pathogenesis of primary osteoarthrosis. Lancet 1:519, 1972.
16. Schwartz L: Disorders of the Temporomandibular Joint: Diagnosis, Management, Relation to Occlusion of Teeth. Philadelphia, W. B. Saunders Company, 1959, pp. 3–44.
17. Costen JB: Some features of the mandibular articulation as it pertains to medical diagnosis, especially in otolaryngology. J Am Dent Assoc 24:1507–1511, 1937.
18. Guralnick W, Kaban LB, Merrill RB: Temporomandibular-joint afflictions. N Engl J Med 299:123–129, 1978.
19. Moulton RE: Oral and dental manifestations of anxiety. Psychiatry 18:261–273, 1955.
20. Greene CS, Laskin DM: Long-term evaluation of conservative treatment for myofascial pain-dysfunction syndrome. J Am Dent Assoc 89:1365–1368, 1983.
21. Poswillo DE: Experimental investigation of the effects of intra-articular hydrocortisone and high condylectomy on the mandibular condyle. Oral Surg 30:161–173, 1970.
22. Henny FA, Baldridge OL: Condylectomy for the persistently painful temporomandibular joint. J Oral Surg 15:24–31, 1957.

OTHER CONSIDERATIONS

Roland W. Moskowitz, M.D.
Section Editor

SECTION
5

30

Industrial Considerations

George Ehrlich, M.D.

Many contemporary architects subscribe to the dictum "form follows function." This dictum is true for joints as well, and it seems clear that osteoarthritis occurs in joints that are used more extensively than others, used under specific circumstances that favor certain movements, and both abused and overused. In this sense, the form taken by the joint in osteoarthritis, with osteophytes increasing the surface area and splinting the joints at the same time to reduce their motion, can be said to reflect the function to which these joints had been put.

The major questions to be asked include the following: Can osteoarthritis be a consequence of what one does? Is osteoarthritis responsible for the many symptoms that rank rheumatic diseases among the chief causes of total and partial disability? Is osteoarthritis in itself disabling and enough to disqualify an otherwise willing individual from joining or rejoining the work force in general or in a specific job?

ARTHRITIS AND THE WORKER

A flyer issued by the Arthritis Foundation claims that

. . . one out of every seven of your employees probably has arthritis . . . arthritis afflicts every age and can be costing your company many dollars—unnecessarily. Arthritis ranks first as the cause of absenteeism. Twenty-seven million working days were lost last year because of it. No one knows how many costly industrial accidents and production line breakdowns occurred daily because of workers who have become weakened or crippled because of arthritis. Accidents and breakdowns mean untold dollars lost in down time, defective products, and damaged equipment. Arthritis means higher Work-

men's Compensation and other health insurance premiums. Every day, thousands of American wage earners are forced to quit their jobs prematurely. They can no longer cope with the pain and crippling. Too often, these are highly skilled employees who represent years of experience and training. Another loss to business.[1]

Of course, this brochure has several purposes besides drawing attention to the problem, but its message is supported by facts. It points to the importance of musculoskeletal disorders, and arthritis in particular, in interfering or seeming to interfere with the ability of workers to continue to be productive.[1] Osteoarthritis remains the most prevalent type of arthritis and probably the most important from an industrial standpoint.[2] Although it takes years to develop and therefore occurs in an older population than initial rheumatoid arthritis or other inflammatory disorders generally do, osteoarthritis nevertheless afflicts the worker during the working years and may be the cause of disability. A feeling of hopelessness, that nothing much can be done to alleviate the problem, leads many patients who have osteoarthritis to accept disability pensions and to "learn to live with it," in contrast to many of the people who have inflammatory joint diseases and who seek remedial help from physicians and other health professionals. Even when osteoarthritis can be treated successfully, disability pensions are not difficult to come by.[3]

Anecdotal linkage between work and play and the subsequent development of osteoarthritis is prevalent, not only in medicine but also in popular concepts (e.g., housemaid's knee). The relationship of usage to subsequent osteoarthritis can be documented, but whether usage accelerates cartilage degeneration[4] or

533

constitutes the primary insult[5] remains to be determined. A major study of hand structure and function in an industrial setting therefore assumes great importance.[6] This study attempted to address the null hypothesis that there is no clinically detectable difference in the structure and function of the hands in groups of subjects, each with distinct and different patterns of usage. Such groups of subjects were identified in an industrial setting in which occupations that called for stereotypic (but presumed to be atraumatic) patterns of hand usage were continued by workers for decade after decade. A worsted mill in a small rural Virginia town provided the setting. Because the rural community had a stable population and many of its members worked for the mill, it proved ideal for this assessment. Only female employees working continuously in their respective tasks for at least 20 years were considered eligible. Volunteers were chosen from among the eligible employees, and in the three different groups, each doing a different type of work, that were the target of the study, the majority volunteered. There was no evidence that those missing, that is, not volunteering, were in any way different from those included. Ultimately, 29 of 39 eligible burlers, 16 of 16 winders, and 19 of 20 spinners were included in the study.

Burlers need to use a five-finger precision grip. Spinners use the thumb, the forefinger, and the middle finger, but not the ring finger or little finger. Winders employ a power grip, need predominantly wrist motion, and have little need for the fine motions of the fingers. In the analysis of the workers, the right hand was found more impaired than the left, regardless of the task. (This means the dominant hand, because only one burler, one winder, and two spinners were left-handed.) Analysis of the structure and function detected impairment of a bimanual nature at the wrist of winders, and such impairment was not found in either burlers or spinners. In contrast, winders had less finger impairment than burlers and spinners did. The burlers and the spinners were found to have osteoarthritic lesions of the second and third fingers of the right hand, exactly the digits used in precision gripping. No impairment of the right fifth digit was found in spinners, who, as noted, utilized a three-finger precision grip that spared digits four and five. Thus, osteoarthritic involvement was found to parallel the use to which the hand was put in the industrial setting.

Because it was a retrospective study, no comment could be made on the loss from the cohort employed at the same time as the respondents. Nevertheless, the authors of the study were able to conclude that the null hypothesis could be rejected, because causes for attrition from the initial cohort almost certainly would be multifactorial and would not skew the statistics. The patterns of Heberden's node distribution commented on by others[7, 8] tend to emphasize the dominant over the nondominant hand, and thus suggest that factors similar to those in this study might be operative. In fact, the precision grip is more commonly employed by women than by men and tends to transduce more force across the distal joints, perhaps leading to earlier development of Heberden's nodes in those affected.

Other surveys have focused on carpal tunnel syndrome and on tendinitis and tenosynovitis at various upper-extremity sites. Several of these conditions seem to be related to industrial influences, but the development of osteoarthritis in the appropriate area (i.e., elbows, shoulders, and smaller adjacent joints) is relatively uncommon. Why this should be so is not entirely clear, but it may have to do with weight bearing and specific power transduction. Inevitably, elbows and shoulders do not bear weight except when assistive walking devices, such as canes and crutches, are used. Wrists, like the tarsi of the feet, appear to be mosaic joints, in which the placement of the various bones is such as to transmit forces across a number of joints and surfaces rather than concentrating them on a single joint and two opposing surfaces. However, repetitive wringing motions are very likely to result in osteoarthritis of the scaphotrapezoid joints.[9] In the lower extremities, most of the lesions are very obviously related to various activities that require weight bearing or reflect patterns of use. There is often more pain associated with osteoarthritis of the lower extremities, perhaps because the forces of weight bearing increase pressures or otherwise elicit this pain. Although the roentgenographic picture of an osteoarthritic lesion in a lower- and an upper-extremity joint may be very similar, involvement of the lower-extremity joint is far more often attended by pain. Secondary synovitis also is more commonly seen, and radicular pain and disability are also more likely.

At the hip, osteoarthritis tends to develop on the longer side more commonly than on the shorter one.[10] This has obvious pathogenic implications, especially in laborers who carry weights and in drivers who use the right lower extremity for driving and braking and the left lower extremity to engage the clutch. For reasons not fully understood, men develop osteoarthritis of the hips more commonly than women do, and women develop osteoarthritis of the knees more commonly than men do. However, when the occupational exposure has been athletic, especially contact sports, knee involvement is more common in men.[11] In football, injuries to the knees are extremely common, as they are in other sports in which spiked shoes are worn that can catch in turf or artificial surfaces, in which trauma through pivoting or through contact with another player approaching from the side is common, or in which excessive stress is applied (running and kicking at the same time, as in soccer, for example). In some sports, meniscal injuries are common and surgical removal of menisci is routinely practiced. Numerous investigators have now confirmed that removal of menisci leads to earlier development of osteoarthritis than does nonsurgical treatment of the meniscal injury.[12] Osteoarthritis as a consequence of sports-incurred injuries is nevertheless of industrial importance, because not only has professional sports become an important industry in its own right but also many large industries, and small ones, too, have company teams or have workers who participate in contact sports in their free time. Thus, the possibility of sports-incurred injury always exists, and when the joint is involved by this injury, osteoarthritis is an almost inevitable (if sometimes remote) consequence.

Back pain is a leading cause of disability.[13] Although the peak incidence of back injury appears to be in individuals between the ages of 30 and 40 years and seems to be associated with tasks that require the handling and lifting of materials, Hadler rightly points out that this need not imply a primary pathogenic influence for this mode of usage but merely a setting in which underlying disease becomes manifested.[13] The important aspect of disability resulting from injury, however, is not so much the development of osteoarthritic lesions subsequently, but how the patient identifies the risk for continued disability and recurrence of precipitating factors in the job.[14–16] Low back pain is obviously not a new symptom and probably has accompanied man throughout his assumption of the erect posture. Sociopolitical considerations and legal aspects, subjects of another chapter, have led to more frequent identification of back pain in the industrial setting. Improvement in working conditions, compensation, and excuse for lesser performance become attributes of back pain in the contemporary setting. In the past, when such

complaints availed one nothing and failed to result in any improvement of conditions, the afflicted individual just did not register his complaint, even if he was unable to continue to work as a result of the problem. Thus, if the pains were not reported or documented, we can only assume they existed but have little contemporary evidence. Because of the current system of compensation law, however, a better appreciation of the prevalence of back pain has resulted. The type of work that leads to back pain is more likely to be identified, and cost effectiveness has become an important issue.

Laborers who have to carry heavy loads are quite obviously at risk. The osteoligamentous lumbar spine is most at risk in the lordotic posture and when bending forward. Sustained lordotic posture can produce abnormal loading of the apophyseal joints, and the forward bending wedges the lumbar disks. This makes them vulnerable to fatigue injuries if this posture is maintained during the performance of heavy labor. Posterior ligamentous damage results from excessive flexion at any spinal level, and prolapse of an intervertebral disk can result from strong contraction of back muscles.[17] Miners and others who use their backs in their work and often must work in a crouched position are more likely to report difficulties than executives who work behind a desk, even though the sitting posture also promotes increased pressure and osteoarthritis in apophyseal joints. Thus, although the sedentary occupation may aggravate back problems, the worker's view of this occupation colors the complaints and the disability. Various surveys suggest that back pain is as common in bank clerks, bus drivers, post office clerks, and nurses, as it is in workers involved in heavy labor.[18] Nevertheless, most of the patients with back disease who can be identified appear to be involved in the handling and lifting of materials.[13]

Osteoarthritic changes of the spine increase with age, so that in later years, they are seen in just about everyone. However, there appears to be little relationship between the roentgenographically determined changes and symptoms, back pain being complained of by both those with few changes and those with many. A study performed by Lawrence[19] in 1955 is instructive in this regard. British coal miners were thought of as a group at high risk for occupationally induced back pain. Thus, the study included seven groups, miners and others, each employed in different tasks, to compare prevalence of back pain in these groups. All groups had a similar incidence of symptoms and of incapacity. Lesser roentgenologic changes were found among heavy laborers than among the miners, but the most extensive changes were found in office workers. Some environmental characteristics, including the height of the seam in relation to the miner and the usage pattern, appear to be involved in the production of some of the lesions in that subgroup. Criteria of diagnosis and type of population may also play a role in the definition. However, obviously, some other factors are at work, and no criteria have yet been determined to anticipate who is likely to develop back problems. The discrepancy between symptoms and roentgenographic findings suggests that multivariate factors are responsible. Some studies by industrial engineers lauded by Hadler[13] show that the more discordant the worker and the task, the higher the incidence of back pain. It was dramatic, says Hadler, for the weaker, less fit worker performing demanding tasks. At the same time, the more fit worker, performing less demanding tasks, also showed a trend toward a higher incidence of back pain. The role of prior back pain and the decision for compensation for renewed back pain vary from state to state and from court to court. Therefore, such compensation decisions depend more on legal factors and local custom than they do on medical criteria.[16] Disk degeneration seems to play little part in the development of osteoarthritis in the spine.[14] Low back pain, but not osteoarthritis, appeared significantly more frequently in those who considered their work to be harder in another study.[18] Contrary to popular belief, correlation with lifting of heavy loads could not be confirmed. Interestingly, prolonged sitting frequently resulted in back pain.

Studies of cadaveric lumbar intervertebral joints loaded to simulate the erect standing and erect sitting postures showed that sustained loading reduced the intervertebral disk height and permitted greater resistance to intervertebral compressive forces in the standing position but not in the erect sitting position.[20] The phenomenon of excessive stress on the apophyseal joints occurs particularly in the unsupported sitting position in chairs. Intervertebral disk degeneration may be promoted by the Western style of sitting and can perhaps be avoided by sitting in an Oriental fashion, cross-legged or on one's heels.

Osteoarthritis is promoted by chronic overloading of the articular cartilages. Nachemson and colleagues have reported a number of studies on this subject.[20, 21] These studies have concluded that standing is preferable to unsupported sitting. A back rest is advisable when sitting, with the knees and hips fully flexed. Lumbar support is necessary in the chair to preserve lumbar lordosis. Anterior sitting in the unsupported seat is the most disadvantageous sitting position and is perilous to the back. Use of a typewriter increases the intradiskal pressure and thus suggests that there is more stress to the back than when one is merely writing or resting. The height of a table on which the typewriter sits should be lower than the corresponding height of the table for writing. Intradiskal pressure can be reduced by the use of arm rests. Adjusting the height and position of the worker is always desirable in most household tasks, to avoid forward bending and flexion, both of which are responsible for increased back problems. One should never lift if at all avoidable. However, if it is necessary to lift, flexion of the back must be avoided, and the knees must be flexed, with the spine kept as straight as possible and the object held as close to the body as possible. Coughing, straining, and jumping produce more pressure than bending to the side, twisting, and walking.

Hadler points out that the various studies are of individuals, not of industries themselves, and that industry need have no fear of these.[15, 16] As a matter of fact, the identification of risk factors should help in prophylaxis and should reduce the financial burden associated with compensation payments and loss of employees through absenteeism, disability, resignation, and premature retirement. Because the majority of studies have been retrospective, cohort loss may have influenced the results, or some preselection may have been at work. It would be important to do these studies prospectively in order to identify additional risk factors and to determine the validity of job-induced osteoarthritic lesions. Personal attitudes and motivation play a considerable role, despite the presence of osteoarthritic lesions.[22]

EMPLOYMENT OF THE OSTEOARTHRITIC WORKER

Rehabilitation in all its aspects can retain a number of workers at their jobs and return others to the work force. The longer the functional disability, however, the more difficult this is.[23] Return to work appears to be easier and more motivated if the job is remunerative, prestigious, and satisfying than if the job is low paying and not highly regarded. It is the task of the physician to identify the problem and to develop teams—not merely ad hoc teams, constituted for the purpose at that time, but teams that effectively work together and are regularly constituted in a hospital, clinic, or other health facility setting—to deal with the total concept of work rehabilitation.[24] In the best-developed systems, the referral by the physician results in an interview by a patient advocate. A clear assessment of future working prospects is made, and an assessment of the patient's motivation to return to work is attempted. The place of employment is then assessed, and both management and union are engaged in a dialogue. This interview takes place soon after the patient is admitted to the program, so that it places the health care facility and its team in a position to help with the problems of the employer's employee and the union's member. Too long a delay results in attempting to place the health facility's patient in employment, and here, resistance by employer and union is likely.[25] Time and motion studies of the job, the height of benches and space, and the dimensions of the spaces, the distance from the parking area, and the accessibility all need to be assessed. Increased accessibility, preferred parking, use of restricted elevators in some instances, and redesigning of tools or spaces may be necessary to return a patient to the job. In the instances in which this is impossible, retraining may have to be done, and here, the cooperation of the employer and the union is all-important.[25]

In a study of complaints in a large industrial plant, osteoarthritis was found to account for most of the arthritic complaints of workers claiming disability.[26] There was some correlation with the length of service to the company, but this probably reflected the increasing time for development of lesions rather than some other factor. However, soft tissue problems thought to be rheumatic were more common, and these ultimately could give rise to osteoarthritic changes because they alter the habitus, posture, and working positions and promote factors that may be pathogenic to osteoarthritic change. Many attempts have been made to counteract this, with redesigning of spaces and equipment being among them.[27]

Employability and employment both are influenced by the perceptions of the work potential of the patient. These have been studied more for rheumatoid arthritis than for osteoarthritis.[28] However, social and work factors seem to have a greater effect on the probability of disability at work than do disease factors.

In the study by Yelin and coworkers,[28] those factors that measured autonomy within work rather than demographic background and physical characteristics of the worker had the strongest effect on disability. In that connection, leisure satisfaction and morale seem to be substantially related in an analysis of older individuals, a factor of importance in determining whether an individual wishes to enter or re-enter the job market or to continue at work.[29] The obvious emphasis on psychologic factors in the assessment of osteoarthritic complaints and in the ability of workers to return to or remain at their jobs has been well established and plays an important role. Appropriate studies still need to be done, and the majority of factors involved are legal, socioeconomic, and political, the subject of a later chapter. The consequences of the Rehabilitation Act of 1973, most particularly Section 504, are yet to be felt.[30] This section determines that no one may be denied employment solely because of disability. When one speaks of heavy laborers, a man in his 50's or 60's who already suffers from osteoarthritis might well be denied employment because he might be considered potentially too disabled or too likely to have a short working span. This problem is even more accentuated with respect to women. However, a large number of jobs today require less physical activity than formerly, and then, the question whether such lesions inhibit employment obviously becomes a difficult one. Return to the job market in the older age group is difficult enough, but for the physically disabled, it is made even more uncertain because of a number of barriers. First, there are architectural barriers. Access to many spaces is by stairs, and it may well be that no elevator is available or that there is only a freight elevator or an executive elevator. The solution to the latter problem, worked out at the Royal National Orthopaedic Hospital in England,[25] is to convince the employer to make the executive elevator available to a disabled employee. This succeeded only when the employee had already worked for the employer and when labor representatives were also present, so that the negotiation was enhanced by being bilateral. It is unlikely to be successful when special dispensation is required for someone unknown to the employer and about whom the union cares little.

If access to the building is not a problem, access to individual spaces often is. Moreover, refurnishing of the spaces may be required so as to avoid improper positions at work. All this entails expense, and ways will be sought to avoid putting someone in this position for whom such expenses are required. Assuming all these can be arranged, however, access to toilets is often difficult. The stalls may be too shallow or too narrow, the toilet too low, and the space itself too convoluted for someone with motion difficulties to get into. Many individuals might provide themselves with raised toilet seats to obviate one of these problems, but that is not always feasible or likely. Assuming that all other conditions are met, however, it may be that access to the building is difficult for someone who has locomotor difficulties. For example, the parking lot for the business may be large or there may be only on-the-street parking, and thus, a spot may be available only some distance from the building. The distance to be traversed to and from work might itself be a problem. There are ways around it, such as to designate certain space as reserved for disabled individuals. Designation decals are often ignored by the public, however, and in the absence of rigid enforcement and education of the public, the disabled individual suffers handicaps that would not otherwise be his. Thus, legislation such as the Rehabilitation Act of 1973 can supply legal justification for employment but cannot prevent the various problems that still make such employment unlikely.[30]

Other factors militate against employment of individuals in their 50's and 60's. The retirement plans many companies have developed require a number of years of consecutive employment before the individual becomes vested. The purpose is clearly to develop a skilled work force, but in practice, such plans make it less likely that an older individual will be hired, even if no disability or arthritic disorder is present. Moreover, many tasks, especially those requiring only unskilled labor, may prove too difficult for someone in these age groups, given the loss of reserve and of muscular tone that attends aging. In addition, the compensation and health plans of many companies, part of the fringe benefits offered, would be taxed severely by someone more likely to require the appropriate services. In some of the larger companies, these plans were developed on the basis of actuarial data that predicted the likelihood of the need for medical care, and an individual is usually vested in such a plan relatively quickly. According to probabilities, a young, healthy individual will require less medical care, and by the time more medical care is required, when chronic illnesses are more likely, the individual may have given many years of service to the com-

pany to justify the investment. If someone who already has some chronic problem or disability were to be hired, the likelihood of needing compensation and the health plans much earlier and to a greater degree is obviously greater. Before the Rehabilitation Act of 1973, such individuals could be refused employment, but since then, the chronic illness or disability can no longer be used as sole justification for rejecting an application for employment. Some companies have therefore actually given up their excellent plans because they have become actuarially unsound.

Examples abound. A milkman in his late 50's who develops an arthritic disorder and draws benefits through company and union health and compensation plans and through Social Security disability provisions is unlikely to return to a low-paying and arduous job that causes him to leave the house in the dark, early morning and to work physically for many hours, encountering hazards and bad weather, when he can earn just about as much by staying home and doing nothing. The reward of the job, the physical problems the job entails as seen by the employee, and the benefits to be derived in most developed industrial countries militate against re-employment.

How is one, then, to facilitate re-employment or employment for the person who already has osteoarthritis, especially considering that such an individual is likely to be middle-aged or older? Comprehensive outpatient and inpatient management may be part of the answer, and it becomes the responsibility of the health establishment to facilitate such re-employment, whenever possible, by eliminating factors that work against it.

Of paramount importance in assisting individuals to work is a comprehensive arthritis management program.[31] These programs rarely function well if they are ad hoc. Rather, they require a team of health professionals accustomed to working together on such problems. Such a team needs to feature medical, surgical, and rehabilitative approaches to arthritis. The scope and complement of personnel are such that they fall under the halfway technology described by Lewis Thomas.[32] This means that considerable expense will be necessary to achieve something short of a cure, a system replaced by a far less expensive one as soon as cures are available. In the case of osteoarthritis, the time for the latter has not yet come. The team features a medically oriented physician, usually a rheumatologist, working in concert with an orthopedic surgeon interested in arthritis, and a rehabilitation team.[31] The last is usually composed of a physiatrist, a physical therapist, and an occupational therapist, all of whom deal with motion. The physical therapist is particularly concerned with muscle power and range of motion; the occupational therapist is especially concerned with fine movement, with a particular emphasis on the capability of the upper extremities. Vocational rehabilitation is best handled by an assessment team that includes a vocational guidance counselor and, if necessary, an occupational therapist, who can work through time and motion studies of the kinds of work the individual has done previously and can assess, with the assistance of psychologists, the work potential of the patient in this or other jobs. Rarely, teams will also include a patient advocate, similar to the position developed at the Royal National Orthopaedic Hospital in England, who works to bring together the disparate forces of labor and management to assure the individual the opportunity to work in that particular concern.[25] Transportation assessment and counseling are all-important and, unfortunately, not commonly available.[33] The stock car is difficult to get into, especially for someone encumbered by arthritic lesions, and an assessment of the ability to drive and the ability to be a passenger in the car and teaching the tasks necessary to achieve these goals are problems for a transportation counselor. Moreover, where public transportation is available, assessment of the ability to use it and teaching the skills necessary also come under the purview of a transportation advisor.[33]

Social service workers can often assist in assessing the home situation and other environmental factors that play important roles. In other words, the lesion itself is not the problem. The response of the person to that lesion, how it is viewed—whether as a disease or merely as an encumbrance—and what one wishes to do to overcome it, and the relationship to the family, work situation, and the community are all important and need to be assessed and dealt with. Environmental manipulation is therefore at least as important as medical control.

Surgical remedies are quite successful but raise new problems. In the past, an individual who developed osteoarthritic involvement of the hip or the knee, in particular, could look forward only to gradual crippling; there was little alternative to premature retirement from the vocational competition. Today, with advances in reconstructive surgery, such individuals can be returned to full function, although

with some precautions. Under those circumstances, they again will become competitive for jobs at precisely the time that it would normally be harder for them to obtain employment, owing to a number of non–disease-related factors, such as age, education, and various constraints of health and compensation and retirement plans. This raises new social issues that legislation attempts to address. Although many of these are not medical issues, they become problems for the medical profession, and failure to find solutions to social issues is often placed squarely at the feet of the medical profession, who are really only tangential to the issue.

Thus, osteoarthritis, which is a condition of a joint or of several joints, leaves the individual relatively unencumbered except for the involved joints. It becomes a particular problem when it is identified as a disease, an infirmity, a disability, or a source of handicap, or if the individual is identified as "arthritic," whereas it is merely the joint that has undergone some changes. Osteoarthritis is often blamed for symptoms to which it contributes little and is used as an excuse for not working or not employing an individual, when that is merely a subterfuge to disguise the real reasons for lack of work or employment. The discrepancy between the roentgenogram and the clinical presentation has set up adverse sociopolitical responses that are inappropriate from a medical point of view.

The problem of osteoarthritis in industry is as yet unresolved. As stated, some osteoarthritis appears to be the consequence of what one does at work. The evidence for much of this is anecdotal, although retrospective studies are beginning to accrue respectable data that provide confirmation for such suppositions; anticipated prospective studies should, in the future, provide further supporting evidence. Employment of someone who has arthritis requires a definitive statement from the physician, when decisions are based more on legal and sociopolitical grounds.

Finally, the development of arthritis in someone at work raises additional issues, such as those of compensation, retirement, and disability. Clearly, industry is reluctant to recognize that osteoarthritis may derive from types of work. If this were an accepted premise, most osteoarthritis could then fall under compensation laws and be costly to industry itself. In contrast, and of greater attraction to employers, is identification of osteoarthritis as an intercurrent event not related to the job. Early retirement and Social Security disability can.

then be initiated, and the direct cost to industry can be significantly reduced. These economic considerations and implications of responsibility accordingly make the subject of osteoarthritis of a worker an industrial "hot potato." If it is accepted, for example, that sitting in a chair, leaning forward in an unsupported position, such as is done when typing, might give rise to osteoarthritic change in the involved joints, including the spine, it becomes obvious that this pathogenesis may occur in countless numbers of secretaries and clerks who work under such conditions. Because almost every condition is multifactorial, many more studies will need to be done before the final answer on osteoarthritis and its industrial consequences and relationships is obtained.

References

1. Arthritis Foundation: One Out of Every Seven . . . of Your Employees. 1979.
2. Rubenstein HM: A review of arthritic diseases. Ind Med Surg 42:4–22, 1973.
3. Barton EM: Prognosis of patients with arthritis. Ind Med Surg 42:23–24, 1973.
4. Sokoloff L: The Biomechanics of Osteoarthritis. The Biology of Degenerative Joint Disease. Chicago, University of Chicago Press, 1969, p. 69.
5. Radin EL: Mechanical aspects of osteoarthrosis. Bull Rheum Dis 26:862–865, 1976.
6. Hadler HM, Gillings DB, Imbus HR, et al.: Hand structure and function in an industrial setting. Influence of three patterns of stereotyped, repetitive usage. Arthritis Rheum 21:210–220, 1978.
7. Radin EL, Parker HG, Paul IL: Pattern of degenerative arthritis. Preferential involvement of distal finger joints. Lancet 1:377–379, 1971.
8. Ehrlich GE: Inflammatory osteoarthritis. I. The clinical syndrome. J Chronic Dis 25:317–328, 1972.
9. Fitton JM, Shey FW, Goldie W: Lesions of the flexor carpi radialis sheath causing pain at the wrist. J Bone Joint Surg 50B:359–363, 1968.
10. Gofton JP: Unilateral osteoarthritis of the hip. Arthritis Rheum 10:281, 1967.
11. Ehrlich GE: Pathogenesis and treatment of osteoarthritis. Comp Ther 5:36–40, 1979.
12. McGinty JB: Arthroscopy. *In* Kelley WN, Harris ED, Ruddy S, Sledge CB (eds.): Textbook of Rheumatology. Philadelphia, W. B. Saunders Company, 1981, p. 657.
13. Hadler NM: Industrial rheumatology. Clinical investigations into the influence of the pattern of usage on the pattern of regional musculoskeletal disease. Arthritis Rheum 20:1019–1025, 1977.
14. Quinet RJ, Hadler NM: Diagnosis and treatment of back ache. Semin Arthritis Rheum 8:261–287, 1979.
15. Hadler NM: The sociopolitical climates surrounding low back pain (LBP). J Occup Med 21:681–682, 1979.
16. Hadler NM: Legal ramifications of the medical definition of back disease. Ann Intern Med 89:992–999, 1978.
17. Adams, MA, Hutton WC: The effect of posture on the role of the apophyseal joints in resisting intervertebral compressive forces. J Bone Joint Surg 62B:358–362, 1980.
18. Magora A: Investigation of the relation between low back pain and occupation. Scand J Rehabil Med 6:81–88, 1974.
19. Lawrence JS: Rheumatism in coal miners. III. Occupational factors. Br J Ind Med 12:249–261, 1955.
20. Nachemson A, Elfström G: Intravital dynamic pressure measurements in lumbar discs. A study of common movements, maneuvers, and exercises. Scand J Rehabil Med 2 (Suppl 1):1–40, 1970.
21. Andersson BJG, Ortengren R: Lumbar disc pressure and myoelectric back muscle activity during sitting. 2. Studies on an office chair. Scand J Rehabil Med 6:115–121, 1974.
22. Wolff BB: Personal attitudes and motivation. Penn Med 72:68–70, 1969.
23. Robinson HS: The rehabilitation specialist. Penn Med 72:70–73, 1969.
24. Brewerton DA: The physician. Penn Med 72:74–75, 1969.
25. Daniel JW: Labor. Penn Med 72:75–79, 1969.
26. Harley WJ: The industrial physician. Penn Med 72:85–88, 1969.
27. Ehrlich GE: The rheumatologist. Penn Med 72:89–91, 1969.
28. Yelin E, Menan R, Nevitt M, Epstein M: Work disability in rheumatoid arthritis: Effects of disease, social, and work factors. Ann Intern Med 93:551–556, 1980.
29. Mancini JA, Orthner DK: Situational influences on leisure satisfaction and morale in old age. J Am Geriatr Soc 28:466–471, 1980.
30. Abrams S: Section 504 of the Rehabilitation Act of 1973. Appendix 1. *In* Ehrlich GE (ed.): Rehabilitation Management of Rheumatic Conditions. Baltimore, Williams and Wilkins, 1980, pp. 296–303.
31. Ehrlich GE: Referral resources. *In* Ehrlich GE (ed.): Total Management of the Arthritic Patient. Philadelphia, J. B. Lippincott, 1973, pp. 209–222.
32. Thomas L: The technology of medicine. *In* The Lives of a Cell. New York, Viking Press, 1974, p. 35.
33. Boblitz M: Transportation evaluation, counseling, and training. *In* Ehrlich GE (ed.): Rehabilitation Management of Rheumatic Conditions. Baltimore, Williams and Wilkins, 1981, pp. 201–233.

31

Medicolegal Considerations

George J. Annas, J.D., M.P.H.

Unfortunately, there is no law limited to osteoarthritis, any more than there is a law of kidney disease or a law of stroke. Indeed, one can argue quite persuasively that there is no such thing as "health law" either. The law applies to all individuals, natural and corporate, and governmental bodies. The United States Constitution, for example, applies to all citizens, irrespective of whether they suffer from osteoarthritis and irrespective of their profession. Nevertheless, there are some problems that are unique to the health care field that make knowledge of it essential for the provision of reasonable legal advice; and there are legal principles, although general, that have special significance to physicians dealing with osteoarthritis.

Accordingly, this chapter will provide an overview summarizing "health law," i.e., the law as it affects the health care industry, with special use of osteoarthritis examples where possible. Before discussing any specific situations, some understanding of the legal system is required. The information in this chapter should prove useful to all physicians dealing with arthritis problems. The material related to informed consent and human experimentation has high relevance given the increased availability of accepted beneficial surgical approaches to therapy and exciting advances in research therapeutic modalities. Similarly, increased awareness of judicial review of recommendations of disability determination predicates a better understanding of this evaluation process.

INTRODUCTION TO THE LAW

Like other citizens, almost everything the physician does in the practice of medicine is governed by the legal system. The law defines "the practice of medicine" and provides a system of licensing those engaged in this profession. It defines the physician's relationship with his patients in terms of both explicit and implied contract and defines his duties to his patients in terms of such things as consent and confidentiality. It governs the use of prescription drugs, the parameters of staff privileges, the limits of human experimentation, the terms of insurance policies, reimbursement from Medicare and Medicaid, and procedures for documenting disability assessments, to name only a few. Knowledge of the law can make a physician much more effective in terms of patient care, and can allow him to be much better equipped to obtain consent, use drugs for unapproved indications, maintain confidentiality, process disability applications, and so on. Ignorance of the law can lead to much counterproductive work and worry in the name of "defensive medicine."[1]

The law can be found in a number of places, and the source of the law usually determines its applicability to the physician's practice, the potential penalties involved in ignoring it, and the methods by which it can be changed. The most important sources of the law are (1) the Constitution; (2) state and federal statutes; (3) state and federal regulations; (4) case law or "judge-made" law; and (5) private law.[2] Although all are important, this chapter will deal primarily with health law as it has developed in cases decided by appellate judges and regulations interpreted by appellate judges. The Constitution, of course, applies to all citizens, and its Bill of Rights specifically sets forth the limits of governmental intervention in the lives of citizens. It prohibits, for example, governmental interference in religious establishments, religious exercise, free speech, and free

541

assembly. By recent judicial decision, it also sets forth a citizen's "right to privacy" and forbids governmental interference with certain "personal" decisions that affect health care, such as contraception and abortion.[3] Private law can be seen as equally pervasive, because it covers all agreements or contracts between two private individuals or corporations. It is "private" because it is made by private agreement; it is "law" because unless the agreement is against the public policy (e.g., slavery), it will be enforced by a court if one party breaks the agreement to the other's detriment.

As a basic introduction to the legal system for physicians involved in caring for patients with osteoarthritis, this chapter will focus on four topics: (1) informed consent and the doctor-patient relationship; (2) human experimentation; (3) confidentiality; and (4) administrative law involving disability evaluations. These are selected because of their intrinsic importance and because they are the legal issues most likely to accompany the diagnosis and treatment of osteoarthritis.

INFORMED CONSENT AND THE DOCTOR-PATIENT RELATIONSHIP

One of the most critical and controversial issues in the provider-patient relationship involves consent. Recent court actions have caused many providers to fear that the legal system has set up burdensome and arbitrary standards for obtaining a patient's consent to undergo medical procedures. However, the issue of consent is not new. It is based on the common-law enforcement of the concept of personal autonomy and self-determination. In 1905, an Illinois court wrote:

Under a free government at least, the free citizen's first and greatest right which underlies all others—the right to the inviolability of his person, in other words, his right to himself, is the subject of universal acquiescence and this right necessarily forbids a physician . . . to violate without permission the bodily integrity of his patient by a major or capital operation.[4]

Consent can be obtained orally or in writing or can be implied by actions of the patient. In the hospital setting, consent has traditionally been obtained through the use of "blanket" consent forms. A typical form might read as follows:

I hereby authorize the performance of any medical or surgical procedure, either major or minor, including the administration of local or general anesthesia, which may be deemed necessary by the attending physician or surgeon during my stay at any hospital.

Such a form technically meets the consent requirement. However, it is so vague and broadly worded as to give the patient almost no information about what he is consenting to. For this reason, such forms should not be used and, indeed, are generally found legally ineffectual by the courts. Because of the use of such forms and the lack of communication of more detailed information about treatment to patients, the courts have created the doctrine of informed consent, which requires that before a patient is asked to consent to a procedure he be given certain information: (1) a description of the procedure; (2) any reasonable alternatives; (3) the risks of death or serious disability; (4) problems of recuperation; and (5) whatever information other physicians usually disclose.[5] Arguably, the cost of the recommended procedure and the success rates must also be disclosed.

Physicians are required to disclose this information for two fundamental reasons: (1) it promotes the patient's right of self-determination, to make the ultimate decision about what is to be done with his body; and (2) it promotes rational decision making, requiring that certain material information be disclosed by the person who has it to the person who is ignorant of it. Some courts have actually founded the requirement on the "fiduciary" nature of the doctor-patient relationship. The notion is that the doctor has the patient's trust, and the patient is not knowledgeable about medicine. These two facts combine to create a duty of disclosure on the part of the physician.[5]

Decisions as to what specific pieces of information should be disclosed are often troublesome. Perhaps the best way to think about it is to ask this question: Might knowing this piece of information influence the patient's decision? If the answer is affirmative, the information should be disclosed, because, as mentioned before, promoting self-determination is the primary purpose of the disclosures. Thus, for example, if you sincerely believe that your patient's osteoarthritis can be best managed by intra-articular steroids, you still have an obligation to explain to him that there are other possibly effective treatments (if this is true) such as other drug therapy, physical therapy, and surgery. You must also discuss these alternatives in detail, or refer the patient to someone who can do so if he wants further information about them.

Consent need not be in writing, but it should be documented. Consent is a *process* of information exchange, not a form. A form serves only as evidence that the process took place. If a form sets forth the details of the specific procedure consented to, such as alternatives and risks, it can be quite useful, because it can provide the patient another opportunity to review the matter and can provide the physician with a written record of the information disclosed. On the other hand, a contemporaneous note in the chart summarizing the content of the conversation or conversations with the patient may be even better evidence of what actually took place, because it will be specific to the patient and the physician involved.

There are times when treatment can be administered without consent, but these are unlikely to occur in the management of osteoarthritis. For example, in a frank emergency, the rule is "treat first and ask legal questions later."[6] If the procedure is simple, with remote dangers that are commonly understood, no disclosure need be made. A patient may also "waive" his right to the information. Finally, there may be rare cases in which disclosure of alternatives or risks may so upset the patient that he will be unable to make a rational decision. Because this would undercut the very idea of self-determination, the law has carved out a "therapeutic exception" in this case. Physicians, however, should use this only when absolutely necessary and should document in the chart the reasons why this particular patient cannot be given certain information.

Approximately 20 states have statutes dealing with informed consent. Almost all of these statutes were enacted in 1975 and 1976 as a result of the medical malpractice insurance "crisis." All make it more difficult for a patient to will a suit based on failure to obtain informed consent.[7] Statutes in 9 states,* for example, provide that a patient's signature on a consent form shall be conclusive evidence that the information was provided to the patient and that the consent was valid. Unfortunately, this emphasis on the form rather than on the process tends to undercut the doctrine's rationale. Only by going through the sometimes difficult task of tailoring information to fit the procedure and the individual patient is it likely that either self-determination or rational decision making will be promoted. If neither of these functions is furthered, the

informed consent process becomes a hollow exercise.

A few words on tangential consent matters are in order. First, the family need have no role in the consent of a competent person. Although competence is a legal matter, all adults are presumed to be competent unless declared otherwise in a court of law. The general test of competence is whether or not the individual can understand and appreciate the nature and consequences of his decision. In a medical setting, this usually means whether the patient can understand what the doctor is recommending and what the consequences of accepting or rejecting the recommendation will be. If he does understand, he has the legal capacity to either accept or reject the proposed treatment. If, on the other hand, the patient is incompetent, it is usual to have a court appoint a guardian to make treatment decisions for the patient. In these cases, the guardian has all the rights to information that the patient would have had. Likewise, parents can consent to beneficial medical treatment for their children and are entitled to all the information necessary to make an informed decision. In some cases, children can also consent to their own care. If they are found to be "mature minors," i.e., able to understand the nature and consequences of their decisions, they may consent on their own. Although this is a matter of state law, no physician has ever been successfully sued for treating a consenting minor over the age of 14. Likewise, emancipated minors, those no longer under the care, custody, and control of their parents, may also consent to their own medical care.[7]

HUMAN EXPERIMENTATION

Advances in the treatment of osteoarthritis, like those in other diseases, depend on innovation and, ultimately, human experimentation with new treatment modalities. In this regard, the law's attitude toward human experimentation in medicine has changed radically over the past four decades. Prior to World War II, courts tended to view experimentation as quackery and often held physicians absolutely liable for the injuries suffered by patients. Any major deviation from standard medical practice was considered malpractice—physicians experimented at their own peril.[8] Now, however, courts generally support the medical profession's research enterprises as both legitimate and necessary for medical progress.

---

*Colorado, Florida, Iowa, Idaho, Nevada, North Carolina, Ohio, Utah, and Washington.

As in most areas of medicine, the law has been reactive rather than prospective; reaction has been to atrocities rather than to "standard medical activity." Thus, one finds the most comprehensive and authoritative legal statement on human experimentation embodied in the Nuremberg Code, which was articulated in a court opinion concerning the trial of 23 Nazi physicians for "war crimes and crimes against humanity" during World War II. The court rejected the defendants' contention that their experiments with both prisoners of war and civilians were consistent with the ethics of the medical profession as evidenced by previously published experiments on venereal diseases, plague, and malaria, among others. Instead, the court found that only "certain types of medical experiments on human beings, when *kept within reasonably well-defined bounds,* conform to the ethics of the medical profession generally."

The basis of the Code is a type of natural law reasoning. In the court's words: "All agree . . . that certain basic principles must be observed in order to satisfy moral, ethical, and legal concepts." Principle 1 demonstrates the primacy the court placed on the concept of consent:

1. The voluntary consent of the human subject is absolutely the essential.

This means that the person involved should have *legal capacity to give consent*; should be so situated as to be able to exercise *free power of choice,* without the intervention of any element of force, fraud, deceit, duress, over-reaching, or other ulterior form of constraint or coercion; and should have *sufficient knowledge* and *comprehension* of the elements of the subject matter involved as to enable him to make an understanding and enlightened decision. This latter element requires that before the acceptance of an affirmative decision by the experimental subject there should be made known to him the nature, duration and purpose of the experiment; the method and means by which it is to be conducted; all inconveniences and hazards reasonably to be expected; and the effects upon his health or person which may *possibly* come from his participation in the experiment.

The duty and responsibility for ascertaining the quality of the consent rest upon each individual who initiates, directs, or engages in the experiment. It is a personal duty and responsibility which may not be delegated to another with impunity. (Emphasis supplied.)

The Nuremberg Code thus requires that the consent of the experimental subject have at least four characteristics: it must be competent, voluntary, informed, and comprehending. The Code has been adopted by the United Nations and has been used as the basis for other international documents, such as the Declaration of Helsinki. It is a part of international common law and can properly be viewed as both a criminal and a civil basis for liability in the United States.[8]

The principles of the Code have been articulated in specific federal regulations governing human experimentation in the United States. As reformulated in 1981, these regulations specify that the subjects must be given the following information about a proposed experiment:

1. A statement that the study involves research, an explanation of its purposes and expected duration, and a description of the procedures to be followed, identifying which are experimental.

2. A description of reasonably foreseeable risks or discomforts.

3. A description of any reasonably expected benefits to the subject or others.

4. A disclosure of appropriate alternative procedures or courses of treatment that might be advantageous to the subject.

5. A statement describing the extent to which confidentiality of records identifying the subject will be maintained.

6. For research involving more than minimal risk, an explanation about any compensation or medical treatment available if injury occurs.

7. An explanation of who to contact for answers to questions or in the event of injury.

8. A statement that participation is voluntary, that refusal to participate will involve no penalty or loss of benefits, and that the subject may discontinue participation at any time without prejudice.[9]

Although informed consent is a necessary precondition for lawful experimentation, it is not sufficient. Other requirements, such as the reasonableness of the experiment, review by an institutional review board, and compensation for harm, may also be necessary under certain circumstances. Institutional Review Boards (IRBs) are committees required by federal regulations to review all projects before they are funded by the federal government. Their mandate is to insure that the risks of the experiment to subjects is outweighed by the potential benefits, that the subjects' welfare is adequately protected, that informed consent is obtained, and that the experiment is reviewed at timely intervals. IRBs are the classic form of governmental regulation—the use of public incentives to induce self-regulation on the part of powerful institutions. Functioning properly, they can protect not only the research subject but also the researcher and the institution.[10]

Although there are stringent requirements for engaging in human experimentation designed to test a hypothesis, a physician may deviate from the labeled recommendations of a drug in the treatment of an individual patient because this is not the type of experimentation the regulations are designed to deal with; the FDA's enabling legislation does not permit it to interfere with the practice of medicine. Put another way, the FDA is responsible for judging safety and efficacy and for accurate labeling. Once a drug is on the market, a physician may exercise his professional judgment as to how it should be used in therapy.[6, 11] Thus, in the treatment of osteoarthritis, for example, a physician may legally prescribe a drug whose labeling does not indicate its use for this condition or may prescribe higher doses than are indicated if he believes that such deviation is appropriate for this individual patient. The physician should, of course, obtain the patient's consent for this deviation and be prepared to explain why the deviation is medically indicated.

CONFIDENTIALITY

The more dependent society becomes upon the maintenance of a galaxy of information systems, the more defined two conflicting trends become. The first, exemplified by state and federal "freedom of information" or "sunshine" acts, aims at providing the public access to all information held by governmental agencies. The premise is that public knowledge of the most intimate details of how government works is likely to make government more responsive to the will of the people and also prevent official wrongdoing. The second is exemplified by state and federal laws aimed at protecting information about individual citizens from public disclosure. Although details remain to be worked out in many areas, the consensus is that with all forms of personal data-keeping systems—credit, insurance, education, taxation, criminal, and medical, to name some of the most important—individuals have or should have a right of "privacy" broad enough to enable them to examine and correct

the information and to prevent the release of this information without their express consent.

Medical records have been the last to come under public scrutiny, perhaps because medicine has a tradition of "keeping confidences." Nevertheless, as the solo practitioner-patient relationship becomes an endangered species, record keeping in medicine comes to resemble other massive recordkeeping systems. Accordingly, the rules applied to these systems are likely to become applicable to medical records as well. As to medical records specifically, only about two dozen cases have reached the appellate courts. The law in this area must therefore be considered to be in its infancy, and resort must often be made to public policy and arguments by analogy.[12] The maintenance of confidentiality is both a legal and an ethical obligation of health-care providers.

The reason for the rule is that health-care providers need to know the most personal and possibly embarrassing details of the patient's life to help the patient, and patients are not likely to freely disclose these details unless they are certain that no one who is not directly involved in their care will learn of them. As one court described the patient's dilemma:

Since a layman is unfamiliar with the road to recovery, he cannot sift the circumstances of his life and habits to determine what information is pertinent to his health. As a consequence, he must disclose all information in his consultations with his doctor—even that which is embarrassing, disgraceful, or incriminating. To promote full disclosure, the medical profession extends the promise of secrecy. The candor which this promise elicits is necessary to the effective pursuit of health; there can be no reticence, no reservation, no reluctance when patients discuss their problems with their doctors.[13]

Even though the law is quite explicit, it is notable that there are few reported cases involving breaches of confidentality. This can mean that such violations are rare, that patients never learn of violations when they do occur, that patients do not think it is appropriate to sue for such violations (because of the cost, uncertain damages, and possible further publicity of the confidential information), or that almost all such cases are settled before they reach an appellate court.

Those cases that have been appealed have most often alleged violation of confidences by physicians in one of the following situations: disclosure to a spouse (involving either a disease related to the marriage or a condition relevant to a divorce, alimony, or custody action), disclosure to an insurance company, or disclosure to an employer.* The last two situations are the ones most likely to arise in osteoarthritis cases. Physicians can, of course, disclose confidential medical information to others with the patient's consent. In this regard, there have been some recent attempts to make sure that the patient's consent to disclosure is an informed one. For example, the American Psychiatric Association has made the following recommendations regarding release forms:

Whenever an individual's authorization is required before a medical-care provider may disclose information it collects or maintains about him, the medical-care provider should not accept as valid any authorization which is not:
(a) in writing;
(b) signed by the individual on a date specified or by someone authorized in fact to act in his behalf;
(c) clear as to the fact that the medical-care provider is among those either specifically named or generally designated by the individual as being authorized to disclose information about him;
(d) specific as to the nature of the information the individual is authorizing to be disclosed;
(e) specific as to the institutions or other persons to whom the individual is authorizing information to be disclosed;
(f) specific as to the purpose(s) for which the information may be used by any of the parties named in (e) both at the time of the disclosure and at any time in the future;
(g) specific as to its expiration date, which should be for a reasonable time not to exceed one year. . . .[14]

---

*In Curry v. Corn, 227 N.Y.S. 2d 470 (1966), for example, the physician disclosed information to his patient's husband, who was contemplating a divorce action. In Schaffer vs. Spicer, 215 N.W. 2d 134 (S.D. 1974), the wife's psychiatrist disclosed information to the husband's attorney to aid him in a child custody case. Representative of the insurance cases are Hague v. Williams, 181 A. 2d (N.J. 1962), in which the pediatrician of an infant informed a life insurance company of a congenital heart defect that he had not informed the child's parents of; and Hammonds v. Aetna, in which the physician revealed information to an insurance company when the insurance company falsely represented to him that his patient was suing him for malpractice. Cases involving reporting to employers include Beatty vs. Baston, 13 Ohio L. Abs. 481 (Ohio App. 1932), in which the physician revealed to a patient's employer during a woman's compensation action that the patient had a venereal disease; Clark v. Geraci, 208 N.Y.S. 2d 564 (S. Ct. N.Y. 1960), in which a civilian employee of the Air Force asked his doctor to make an incomplete disclosure to his employer to explain absences, but the doctor made a complete disclosure, including the patient's alcoholism; and the more recent case of Horne v. Patton, 287 So. 2d 824 (Ala. 1973), which involved the disclosure of a nervous condition to the patient's employer.

These recommendations are not limited to psychiatric information: Any information that could be used by someone else to the patient's detriment (e.g., to deny him benefits or employment) should not be released unless these provisions are followed. Furthermore, medical information regarding a patient cannot be disclosed to his spouse or other family members without his consent.[6]

Finally, it is worth noting the recommendations of the Privacy Protection Study Commission, which was set up by Congress in 1974 to study individual privacy rights and record-keeping practices. Its 1977 report on medical records recommended the following:

—that each State enact a statute creating individual rights of access to, and correction of medical records, and an enforceable expectation of confidentiality for medical records;
—that federal and state penal codes be amended to make it a criminal offense for any individual knowingly to request or obtain medical record information from a medical-care provider under false pretenses or through deception;
—that upon request, an individual who is the subject of a medical record maintained by a medical-care provider, or another responsible person designated by the individual, be allowed to have access to that medical record, including the opportunity to see and copy it; and have the opportunity to correct or amend the record;
—that each medical-care provider be required to take affirmative measures to assure that the medical records it maintains are made available only to authorized recipients and on a "need-to-know" basis;
—that any disclosure of medical-record information by a medical-care provider be limited only to information necessary to accomplish the purpose for which the disclosure is made;
—that each medical-care provider be required to notify an individual on whom it maintains a medical record of the disclosures that may be made of information in the record without the individual's express authorization.

These recommendations set the tone for protection of confidential medical information and are useful guides for individual practitioners until the legal changes called for are made.

ADMINISTRATIVE LAW INVOLVING DISABILITY EVALUATION

The term "administrative law" generally refers to those aspects of the law dealing with administrative or regulatory agencies—agencies set up by Congress to perform specific governmental functions. Here, we will examine only one aspect of one agency: the court's review of a determination by a Social Security Administrative Law Judge (ALJ) that a person has not submitted sufficient evidence of disability based on osteoarthritis to qualify for disability benefits.

It should first be emphasized that a disability determination is primarily an issue of medical fact to be decided by physicians. Nevertheless, the definition of disability entitled to benefits is set forth in statutes, and courts have the authority to review the medical evidence to make sure that it is sufficient to meet the statutory and regulatory mandates. In this regard, it is essential for the protection of the patient that the reviewing physician be familiar with the legal requirements and that he document medical findings sufficiently to permit a review of them by a judge at a later date. Judges will almost never reverse a finding of fact made by a medical panel, unless they find the conclusion arbitrary or an abuse of discretion. A recent case in which an unusual reversal did occur provides an illustration of some major administrative law rules.[15]

In October 1978, a patient filed an application for disability insurance benefits with the Social Security Administration on the basis of a condition that he claimed had prevented him from working since August 30, 1975. He complained of shoulder, hip, ankle, and neck problems involving osteoarthritis, which prohibited him from engaging in any type of gainful employment. Medical reports indicated that he also suffered from ulcers and gout. After this application was denied, he requested a hearing on his claim. This hearing was conducted before an ALJ, who denied disability benefits. The judge determined that evidence of disability before his first application in 1975 was not sufficiently new to warrant reopening his case and that evidence after 1975 did not prove he was disabled. Instead, the ALJ found that the patient had a "residual capacity to work in a sedentary job." The U.S. District Court affirmed this determination. The U.S. Court of Appeals for the Fifth Circuit reversed this decision and ruled in favor of the claimant.

The court first examined the facts that indicated that the claimant traced his disability back to World War II and that the Veteran's Administration had given him a 40% disability rating in 1945. He voluntarily renounced these benefits in 1955 and engaged in a variety of occupations, primarily auto and real estate sales, until 1972. From 1972 to 1975, he worked sporadically and had not been able to work since. On review, the court could legally consider only one question: Was the Social Security Administration's denial of his benefits "supported by substantial evidence"? This is generally an easy test for the Social Security Administration to meet. Courts will almost never critically review the facts and medical history on appeal, because they believe that fact finders who have seen and heard the claimant personally are better able to judge the merits of his case.

The burden of proving the disability, of course, rests squarely on the claimant. As defined in the Social Security Act, a "disability" is "an inability to engage in any substantial gainful activity by reason of any medically determinable physical or mental impairment which can be expected to last for a continuous period of not less than 12 months."[16] The question is not whether the claimant can actually obtain work, but whether he is able to work.

In reviewing some of the evidence that was presented, the court gave us some insights into how courts are likely to treat certain types of information, and this can be very useful for examining physicians. For example, the court found that the ALJ's conclusion that the claimant was not in severe pain was not supported. The claimant had been seen by an officer in the Motor Vehicles Office when he went to have the address on his license changed. Subsequently, the officer took steps to have his license to drive revoked on the grounds that he could not operate a vehicle safely. Although the ALJ did not consider this important (because he found that there were jobs available that did not require driving), the court found that "the claimant must have been suffering badly for the officer to have noticed him initially." The court also took notice that "pain itself may be enough to justify an award of disability benefits." Although the ALJ did note the fact that claimant was "not on narcotics" in finding he was not in severe pain, he overlooked the report of claimant's physician, who had noted that the claimant was "allergic to morphine, Demerol, codeine and penicillin, and . . . sensitive to all medications except Tylenol." On this point, the court decided that the ALJ had misinterpreted the medical records sufficiently to justify reversal of his decision.

Similarly, although the ALJ had concluded that there were many jobs for which the claimant was still qualified, the Social Security Administration's own vocational consultant had testified that an individual with periodic attacks of severe arthritis would not be qualified for these jobs. In overruling the ALJ's decision on this issue, the court summarized the law on job availability:

> Once a claimant has met his burden, an ALJ may not suggest narrow areas of possible employment and assert that the claimant can perform them without some support in the record, either through medical testimony, or reports, or some type of vocational testimony.[17]

The court concluded with some useful comments on the claimant's osteoarthritis. It noted that his condition was "not constant" and that he had "some days on which he will feel fairly well" but that, nevertheless, his claim of osteoarthritis was "clearly shown." The court found that the claimant had been penalized by the ALJ for not being "in severe pain every day" and made it clear that this was *not* a legal requirement for disability benefits. It concluded that the claimant was, in fact, disabled and qualified for benefits. The court stressed the fact that his physician had indicated in his notes that the claimant was "unable to work" and that his conclusion had been ignored by the ALJ.

A number of things should be noted about this opinion. First, osteoarthritis that is severe enough to cause the individual to be unable to work on a regular basis can be a disabling condition under the Social Security Act, even if the patient has some good days. Second, medical records documenting this condition and indicating the relief, if any, that pain medication provides can be critical to a claimant's case. Third, courts will give very heavy weight to physicians' opinions that are clearly set forth and well documented; unless these opinions are refuted by other evidence, courts are likely to accept them as sufficient evidence in themselves of the claimant's disability. Finally, it is important for examining physicians to know what the relevant legal criteria are for the benefits their patients are seeking. Unless the physician is aware of them, he may not do a complete enough report or examination, and the result may be that the patient is denied benefits that he both desperately needs and is legally entitled to.

SUMMARY

This chapter has presented a brief overview of some of the areas of the law that a physician dealing with patients suffering from osteoarthritis may encounter. It is hoped that it will encourage thought and discussion and that it may even change some practice patterns where indicated. The references may be consulted for additional readings, but when a legal problem is identified, expert advice should be sought from hospital counsel or your own attorney.

References

1. Annas GJ: Law and medicine: Myths and realities in the medical school classroom. Am J Law Med 1:195–208, 1975.
2. Wing K: Law and the People's Health. St. Louis, C.V. Mosby, 1976.
3. Roe v. Wade 410 U.S. 113, 1973.
4. Pratt v. Davis, 118 Ill. App. 161, 1905, affd, 224 Ill. 30, 79 N.E. 562, 1906.
5. Cobbs v. Grant, 8 Cal. 3d 229, 502 P. 2d 1, 1972.
6. Annas GJ, Glantz LH, Katz BK: The Rights of Doctors, Nurses and Allied Health Professionals. Cambridge, Massachusetts, Ballinger Books, 1981, pp. 91–95, 98, 123, 184.
7. Annas GJ: Informed consent. Ann Rev Med 29:9–14, 1978.
8. Annas GJ, Glantz LH, Katz BK: Informed Consent to Human Experimentation: The Subject's Dilemma. Cambridge, Massachusetts, Ballinger Books, 1977.
9. 45 CFR 46.116 (promulgated January 26, 1981).
10. Robertson J: The law of institutional review boards. UCLA L Rev 26:484–504, 1979.
11. Gibson: Medication, Law and Behavior. New York, John Wiley and Sons, 1976.
12. Annas GJ: Medical privacy and confidentiality. In Day SB, Bradejs JF (eds.): Computers for Medical Office and Patient Management. New York, Van Nostrand Reinhold Co., 1981, pp. 102–123.
13. Hammonds v. Aetna Cas. & Sr. Co., 243 F. Supp. 793 (N.D. Ohio 1965).
14. American Psychiatric Association: Confidentiality and Third Parties. Washington, D.C., American Psychiatric Association, 1975, p. 13.
15. Olson v. Schweiker, 663 F.2d. 593 (1981) (5th Cir. 1981).
16. 42 U.S.C. sec. 423 (D) (1) (A).
17. Rodriguez v. Schweiker, 640 F.2d 682, 686 (5th Cir. 1981).

32

Experimental Modes of Therapy in Osteoarthritis

Rose Spitz Fife, M.D.
Kenneth D. Brandt, M.D.

Osteoarthritis is a very common condition for which no definitive specific medical treatment currently exists. Multiple modes of therapy have been proposed and tried over the years. Several of the agents discussed below appear to hold some promise as potential modifiers of this disease process. It is obvious, however, that any agent promoted as beneficial in osteoarthritis must be evaluated with carefully controlled human studies before such claims can be substantiated. It is evident that there is a very large component of placebo response in patients with osteoarthritis when either systemic or intra-articular compounds are administered, and this must be taken into account before a drug can be considered effective in the treatment of this disorder.

SUPEROXIDE DISMUTASE

Superoxide dismutase is an enzyme found in all mammalian cells studied that catalyzes the reaction:

$$O \cdot_2^- + O \cdot_2^- + 2H^+ \xrightarrow{\text{superoxide dismutase}} H_2O_2 + O_2$$

It also suppresses the reaction:

$$O \cdot_2^- + H_2O_2 \longrightarrow OH \cdot + OH^- + O_2$$

It therefore removes superoxide and hydroxyl radicals from the cell. These radicals, which are produced by activated polymorphonuclear leukocytes and other cells and released into the extracellular environment, have been implicated by some in the pathogenesis of joint damage.[1, 2]

Orgotein is the generic name of a bovine liver metalloprotein extract with Cu-Zn superoxide dismutase activity.[1] It has been used in mostly uncontrolled studies for the treatment of inflammatory and traumatic arthritides in horses and dogs. In one study, 60 of 70 horses receiving intra-articular injections of orgotein for various rheumatic conditions showed rapid improvement, with a prompt return to racing. No adverse side effects were noted.[3] In another study, 134 horses with traumatic arthritis were treated with intra-articular orgotein. Ninety-four per cent of those that had symptoms for less than 2 months recovered their pre-injury function, whereas only 49% of those whose symptoms had lasted for more than 2 months recovered completely.[4] In a small, double-blind, controlled trial, injection of orgotein into the digital cushion for treatment of navicular disease in horses resulted in improvement in three of seven horses, whereas none of seven horses receiving placebo responded. Subsequently, three of the seven placebo-treated horses improved when they were given orgotein.[5]

Rosner and associates reported on the effect of intra-articular orgotein in an experimental model of osteoarthritis in the rabbit.[2] The results of multiple injections of orgotein in two doses were compared with those seen with a saline-sucrose placebo, and with no injections. Severe synovitis occurred in normal and osteoarthritic knees injected with either orgotein or placebo. No difference was noted between the severity of developing osteoarthritis in the orgotein groups and controls. However, incorporation of labeled sulfate in proteoglycans, a measure of proteoglycan synthesis, was diminished in osteoarthritic knees injected with either orgotein or placebo.[2, 6]

In an uncontrolled Danish study, orgotein was administered intra-articularly to 22 elderly patients with osteoarthritis of the knee or hip.[7] Clinical improvement was thought to have occurred in 20 joints in 16 patients, and benefits in some patients lasted for more than 3 months after the drug was discontinued. No adverse side effects were noted. Three of these patients received an intra-articular injection of corticosteroid in the contralateral knee, and it was felt that the response to orgotein was greater than that to the steroid.

In six double-blind, controlled trials with a combined total of 157 patients with osteoarthritis, intra-articular orgotein was reported to produce greater, longer-lasting improvement than placebo, but a significant beneficial effect of placebo was also noted.[1]

At present, the only conclusion that can be drawn about orgotein is that there is some suggestion from the veterinary literature that it may be useful in inflammatory or traumatic arthritis in animals. Intra-articular injection of orgotein in an experimental rabbit model of osteoarthritis was not beneficial and, indeed, produced severe synovitis; nonspecific response to components in the vehicle could not be totally excluded. In contrast, however, in the Danish study in humans,[7] clinical evidence of synovitis was not present, and patients seemed to experience a subjective improvement. This study was neither double-blind nor placebo-controlled, and the results are therefore difficult to interpret. In the controlled trials, orgotein appeared beneficial, but this is difficult to evaluate because of the similar response to placebo. Furthermore, carefully controlled animal and clinical studies are needed before final judgment can be passed on the role, if any, of orgotein in the treatment of osteoarthritis.

ASCORBIC ACID

It has been proposed that degradative enzymes, including arylsulfatases, acid phosphatases, and other lysosomal enzymes, may be involved in the pathogenesis of human osteoarthritis.[8–10] Elevated levels of many of these enzymes can be found in human osteoarthritic cartilage.[10, 11] It is unclear, however, whether this represents a primary insult in osteoarthritis or only a secondary phenomenon. As a result of such enzyme elevations, attempts have been made to modulate enzymatic activity in articular cartilage, with the hope that this will reduce cartilage damage.

Schwartz and Adamy have shown that ascorbic acid decreases arylsulfatase A and B levels in cultures of normal and osteoarthritic chondrocytes.[12] EDTA reversed this effect of ascorbic acid. In contrast to its effect on the arylsulfatases, ascorbate led to an increase in acid phosphatase activity in the cell cultures. Ascorbate also caused a marked increase in the synthesis of sulfated proteoglycans, as measured by labeled sulfate incorporation, in normal and osteoarthritic cell lines. A higher proportion of the newly synthesized proteoglycans were found extracellularly in the presence of ascorbate than in its absence. The authors interpreted their data as evidence that ascorbic acid caused an increased synthesis and decreased catabolism of proteoglycans in tissue culture, as well as increased stabilization of the extracellular environment.[12]

Schwartz and colleagues have also recently examined the effect of ascorbic acid in an experimental model of osteoarthritis in guinea pigs.[13] Pathologic changes in osteoarthritic cartilage from animals on a high–vitamin C diet were less severe than those seen in animals on a low–vitamin C diet.[13] In accord with data from tissue culture studies,[12] lower levels of arylsulfatase A and B activity and higher acid phosphatase activity were noted in the arthritic cartilage from animals on the high–vitamin C diet. Furthermore, an increase was noted in the weight of the cartilage from normal joints in the vitamin C–supplemented group, which the authors felt was the result of increased synthesis of collagen and proteoglycans. An increase in DNA synthesis was noted in the osteoarthritic cartilage from both groups and did not appear to be affected by the dietary ascorbate intake. The authors concluded that ascorbic acid modulated the development of osteoarthritis in this in vivo model.[13]

Subsequently, the same group examined the effect of vitamin C on the structure and synthesis of sulfated proteoglycans in osteoarthritic cartilage.[14] An increase in labeled sulfate incorporation into osteoarthritic guinea pig cartilage was noted regardless of the ascorbate content of the diet. However, a vitamin C–dependent increase in sulfate incorporation was observed in normal guinea pig cartilage. No structural changes were found in the sulfated proteoglycans from the arthritic cartilage.[14] These studies lend credence to the thesis that ascorbic acid may have a modifying effect on the cartilage breakdown occurring in osteoarthritis. Work on such studies needs to be extended to other animal models. Furthermore, more data are necessary to elucidate the action of vitamin C on cartilage.

HORMONES

In 1952, Kellgren and Moore described a subset of primary osteoarthritis that was generalized and associated with Heberden's nodes and occurred mainly in women.[15] Although they found no correlation between this condition and menopause, they conducted a blind trial of estrogen therapy in 20 middle-aged women with this disorder. Their results provided no subjective or objective evidence of benefit.[15]

Observations such as these and the fact that male mice are known to develop osteoarthritis earlier than females have prompted speculation that estrogen may play a protective role in osteoarthritis.[16] Estrogen is involved in the mineralization of bone, prevention of linear growth, rapid skeletal development, bone condensation, and chondrocyte maturation.[17]

The effect of sex hormones on the in vivo and in vitro incorporation of labeled sulfate into hyaline costal cartilage and the aorta has been examined in Sprague-Dawley rats. In costal cartilage from estradiol-treated rats, the incorporation of sulfate was reduced to 34% of normal, although no significant change occurred in sulfate incorporation into the aorta. Testosterone, in contrast, did not affect sulfate incorporation in female mice.[18]

Further studies on the effects of estrogen and testosterone on the development and progression of osteoarthritis have been performed in mice that were selected as the experimental model because of the observed naturally occurring increase in osteoarthritis in the males. Results of such studies, however, have produced conflicting results. Silberberg and Silberberg found an increased incidence of osteoarthritis in female C57BL JAX/6 mice that had been oophorectomized at 1 or 6 months of age and then treated with testosterone until old age.[16] An increased incidence of osteoarthritis occurred in animals receiving testosterone, regardless of the age at castration. Less osteoarthritis was noted in untreated castrated females than in untreated noncastrated controls.[16] In another study, the same authors

treated male C57BL JAX/6 mice with estradiol at three different ages and noted that this compound, when given between the ages of 1 and 6 months or between 6 and 11 months, retarded the development of osteoarthritis.[19]

Notably, these effects do not appear to be generalizable to all strains of mice. Thus, testosterone did not increase the incidence of osteoarthritis in spayed female DBA/2JN mice. Two of three estrogen-treated castrated male STR/1N mice had severe osteoarthritis, as did five testosterone-treated castrated females. These numbers are small but there appear to be significant strain-dependent differences in the responses of murine joints to hormonal manipulation.[20]

Estradiol was shown to inhibit proteoglycan synthesis in an experimental rabbit model of osteoarthritis.[6] Testosterone had no effect on the lesions in this model of osteoarthritis. Notably, tamoxifen, an anti-estrogenic compound, was given to female rabbits after oophorectomy and diminished femoral ulceration and pitting in the same model of osteoarthritis.[6]

In a carefully controlled study in an experimentally induced model of osteoarthritis in the rabbit, estrogen at low and high dosages was found to have no beneficial effect in modifying the disease process.[21] However, a statistically significant reduction in sulfate incorporation into glycosaminoglycans by the cartilage was found in the estrogen-treated animals. Because there was no decrease in safranin-O staining, it was felt that estrogen suppressed both proteoglycan synthesis and catabolism. Because a 3-day lag period was noted between the administration of estrogen and the suppression of sulfate incorporation, it was postulated that its effect on cartilage may occur through an intermediary substance.[21] Subsequent studies demonstrated a statistically significant worsening of osteoarthritis pathology in rabbits given supplemental estradiol.[21a]

It would appear from these studies that the effects of the various sex hormones vary from species to species, and even from strain to strain, so that experimental results in one type of animal cannot necessarily be generalized to others.

Several investigators have postulated a role for growth hormone in the synthesis of cartilage as a result of observations in hypophysectomized animals in which loss of linear growth was restored by administration of growth hormone. However, a direct effect on cartilage could not be shown in tissue culture systems.[22, 23] It has been demonstrated subsequently that growth hormone stimulates the production by the liver of somatomedin, the so-called "sulfation factor," which, in turn, is directly responsible for mediating the increases in the synthesis of proteoglycans and collagen noted when growth hormone is given in vivo.[24, 25]

In a rabbit model of chondromalacia, growth hormone led to an increase in toluidine-blue staining, an indicator of the proteoglycan content of the cartilage, compared with controls. In an experimental rabbit model of osteoarthritis, growth hormone–treated animals showed a greater tendency toward healing of their lesions and more proteoglycan synthesis than controls. Collagen formation was also increased.[26]

These studies suggest that growth hormone might have a beneficial effect when administered to osteoarthritic individuals, but the lack of large quantities of human growth hormone make clinical trials impossible at present. These studies also raise important questions as to the role of growth hormone and somatomedin in the metabolism and degeneration of cartilage.

INTRA-ARTICULAR CORTICOSTEROID INJECTION

Intra-articular corticosteroid injections are often beneficial in the treatment of rheumatoid arthritis. Because of the occasional inflammatory component in osteoarthritis, they have been used for many years in this condition as well. However, many studies over the years have failed to demonstrate any lasting benefit of these agents in osteoarthritis, and indeed, some harmful effects of steroids on cartilage have been identified, as will be discussed later.

In an experimental model of osteoarthritis in rabbits, produced by partial meniscectomy, Moskowitz and associates found that intra-articular administration of triamcinolone acetonide suppressed osteophyte formation.[27] In an in vitro model using pig costal cartilage disks, very low doses of hydrocortisone stimulated sulfate incorporation into glycosaminoglycans, and higher doses suppressed sulfate incorporation.[28]

In a double-blind, cross-over study of patients with osteoarthritis of the knee, Wright and coworkers found evidence of symptomatic improvement in patients receiving intra-articular steroid injections at 2 weeks after the injection, but not later.[29] In another study, intra-articular triamcinolone hexacetonide was found to reduce pain more than placebo, but the effect was small and short-lived.[30] In a double-blind, randomized study of patients with osteoarthritis of the knee, Friedman and Moore found that intra-articular corticosteroids caused more reduction in pain at 1 week than placebo, but after 1 week, the effects of both were the same.[31] Indeed, Wright demonstrated the existence of a significant placebo effect after intra-articular injections of saline solution.[32]

The placebo effect was confirmed by Miller and co-workers, who compared the efficacy of five types of intra-articular injections in osteoarthritis of the knee in 181 patients. The five injections were lactic acid, novocaine, hydrocortisone, normal saline solution, and mock injections. No significant difference in response was noted among the five groups, indicating a marked placebo response.[33]

More recently, Steinetz and colleagues reported a reduction of degenerative lesions in a lateral meniscectomy model of osteoarthritis in rabbits in response to orally or intra-articularly administered corticosteroids.[34] They noted that although corticosteroids cause glycosaminoglycan synthesis, they also inhibit proteoglycan destruction by intrinsic or extrinsic proteases. They postulated that glucocorticoids in physiologic concentrations might be required for, or actually stimulate, synthesis of protease inhibitors by chondrocytes.

At present, no good clinical evidence exists to support the claim that intra-articular corticosteroids are of any more than very transient benefit in osteoarthritis, and indeed, even this short-lived benefit is frequently not significantly greater than the improvement occurring after injection of placebo. In addition, there are data suggesting that repeated intra-articular administration of corticosteroids may be harmful. In 1959, Chandler and coworkers reported on a case of Charcot-like arthropathy occurring after multiple steroid injections into an osteoarthritic hip.[35] Moskowitz and associates produced cartilage damage in rabbit knees by intra-articular triamcinolone acetonide injections.[36]

CHLOROQUINE

Chloroquine, an antimalarial agent with known efficacy in the treatment of rheumatoid arthritis, prevents the release of lysosomal enzymes in vitro.[37] Because of the possible role of such enzymes in osteoarthritis, the effect of chloroquine on a rabbit model of chondromalacia has been studied.[38] When chloroquine was administered intraperitoneally, there was microscopic evidence of healing of the experimental cartilage lesion and more toluidine-blue staining was seen than in controls. Decreased cathepsin activity was also found. However, when chloroquine was given intra-articularly, marked joint destruction occurred. After six injections, the knees showed evidence of severe synovitis. One of three animals developed a Charcot-like arthropathy. Microscopically, all three knees demonstrated frank necrosis, with polymorphonuclear leukocyte infiltration and absence of toluidine-blue staining of the cartilage. Interestingly, the contralateral knee, which had been subjected to the same surgical procedure to induce chondromalacia but had not received the intra-articular injections, showed healing similar to the knees of animals treated with intraperitoneal chloroquine.[38]

The effect of chloroquine on the action of various proteolytic enzymes has been studied in vitro. Chloroquine has no effect on the action of hyaluronidase, papain, or trypsin but partially inhibits the bacterial collagenase clostridiopeptidase A from *Clostridium histolyticum*.[39] Chloroquine also inhibits endogenous collagenase activity of bovine nasal cartilage and rat skin. A chloroquine-sensitive endogenous chondromucoprotease was identified in bovine tracheal and nasal cartilage.[39] Incubation of canine cartilage with chloroquine reduced endogenous proteolytic activity, as evidenced by diminished glycosaminoglycan release.[40]

In a partial meniscectomy model of osteoarthritis in rabbits, Moskowitz and colleagues showed that chloroquine feeding reduced femoral ulceration from 40% to 14% at 6 weeks but not at 12 weeks. No effect on osteophyte formation was observed.[6]

These studies raise the possibility that oral chloroquine therapy may promote healing in damaged cartilage, possibly by the inhibition of protease activity. There would appear to be no place for the use of intra-articular chloroquine, which induced a severe chemical synovitis with joint destruction. Further studies on the effect of chloroquine on experimental and human osteoarthritis are indicated.

SALICYLATES

Early work by Chrisman and coworkers suggested that salicylates inhibited proteoglycan degradation in vitro and in vivo in a rabbit model, using scarification of the femoral and patellar cartilage. Histologically, cartilage from salicylate-treated animals was less abnormal than that from controls. It was postulated that the salicylates inhibited catabolic enzyme activity.[41] Ginsberg and associates reported that salicylate administration reduced the severity of histologic changes and decreased the losses of hydroxyproline and hexosamine in another rabbit model of cartilage degeneration.[42]

In an uncontrolled study of patients with recurrent lateral patellar dislocation and chondromalacia patellae, Chrisman and Snook reported that, at surgery, knees from those given salicylates had less fibrillation than controls.[43] These investigators then attempted a controlled study of aspirin in patients with this disorder. The patients then underwent surgery, at which time the cartilage was examined grossly. In the control group, 21 of 23 knees showed evidence of chondromalacia, whereas only 3 of 16 knees in the treated group did. However, none of these knees was examined prior to the institution of salicylates, so that one cannot safely attribute this difference between the two groups to aspirin alone.[44]

In a more recent study, 29 patients with arthroscopically proved chondromalacia patellae were randomized to receive aspirin or placebo for 3 months, at which time arthroscopy was repeated. At arthroscopy, no significant change in the cartilage was found in either group, and the patients did not note any subjective improvement.[45]

Palmoski and Brandt have shown that addition to the culture medium of 10^{-3} M sodium salicylate (which approximates 16 mg/dl) decreases proteoglycan synthesis in organ cultures of normal canine articular cartilage but does not alter glycosaminoglycan catabolism.[46] In other in vitro studies, salicylates suppressed proteoglycan synthesis to a greater extent in osteoarthritic canine cartilage than in normal cartilage.[47] The uptake of radiolabeled acetylsalicylic acid by osteoarthritic cartilage was greater than that by normal cartilage, suggesting that salicylates permeated the abnormal cartilage more readily than they did normal cartilage.[47] In vivo studies have shown that feeding aspirin to dogs in amounts sufficient to maintain a serum salicylate concentration of 20 to 25 mg/dl worsens the degeneration of canine knee cartilage induced by immobilization of the leg.[48] Similarly, when dogs that had undergone transection of the anterior cruciate ligament were fed aspirin, the uronic acid content of the osteoarthritic cartilage was lower than that seen in cartilage from the unstable osteoarthritic knees of dogs that did not receive aspirin, and the augmentation of proteoglycan synthesis in the osteoarthritic cartilage (presumably representing repair) was aborted.[49] It has also been found that cartilage degeneration in C57BL mice genetically predisposed to osteoarthritis is worsened by salicylate ingestion.[50]

TRANEXAMIC ACID

Trans-4-(aminomethyl)-cyclohexanecarboxylic acid (tranexamic acid, AMCA, Cyklokapron) is an inhibitor of plasminogen activation. Telhag has studied its effect, when administered orally, on sulfate incorporation into cartilage in a rabbit model of osteoarthritis, using the contralateral unoperated knee as a control.[51] In animals receiving no tranexamic acid, in comparison with the controls, there was a decrease in hexosamine content and an increase in chondroitin sulfate synthesis in the operated knees. In the treated group, neither the hexosamine content nor the synthesis of chondroitin sulfate was significantly altered in the operated or control knees. The author concluded that tranexamic acid may prevent degeneration of cartilage in this animal model.[51] No studies have been performed in humans.

ARTEPARON

Several groups have studied the effect of Arteparon, a glycosaminoglycan polysulfate, on cartilage degeneration in animal models and in vitro. Ueno administered this compound to dogs in which osteoarthritis had been experimentally induced and found that the treated dogs exhibited less thinning and loss of cartilage than controls.[52] In a rabbit model of cartilage degeneration, Dustmann and associates found that animals treated with intra-articular Arteparon demonstrated less decrease in glycosaminoglycans and no alteration in chondrocyte number compared with controls.[53] Walton and coworkers, using labeled proteoglycan as substrate, studied the effect of Arteparon on the activity of polymorphonuclear leukocyte elastase and cathepsin G in an in vitro system.[54] They found that Arteparon had a marked inhibitory influence on these enzymes at very low concentrations. Baici and colleagues also showed that Arteparon inhibited human lysosomal elastase from polymorphonuclear leukocytes.[55] Stancikova and associates demonstrated that Arteparon inhibited the collagenolytic activity of cathepsin B$_1$ in vitro.[56] Recently, Carrero and associates demonstrated that Anteparon, administered intra-articularly, reduced osteoarthritic lesions of the knee in experimentally induced osteoarthritis in rabbits following partial meniscectomy.[56a] Neutral protease activity was correspondingly reduced. Further studies of this agent would appear to be indicated.

RUMALON

An extract of calf costal cartilage or cartilage and bone marrow, marketed in Europe for many years under the name of Rumalon, has been claimed to be of experimental and clinical benefit in the treatment of osteoarthritis.[57-65]

Rumalon is an unpurified preparation whose components have not been well characterized. The extract has been found to contain "low–molecular-weight" and "high–molecular-weight" fractions. The so-called low–molecular-weight fraction, consisting of amino acids, nucleic acid derivatives, sugars, and salts, stimulated sulfate incorporation into cartilage. The high–molecular-weight fraction, called DAK-16, stimulated mucopolysaccharide synthesis by embryonic fibroblast monolayers. The average molecular weight of this fraction was 55,000 daltons. Compositional analysis suggested that DAK-16 was a mucopolysaccharide-peptide complex.[57]

Bollet studied the effects of Rumalon on cartilage preparations in vitro.[58] He found that it increased ^{35}S incorporation by costal cartilage from young rats and also by human articular cartilage from normal and osteoarthritic joints.[58] Increased incorporation of ^{3}H-uridine into RNA and increased uptake of ^{3}H-serine were also noted in the presence of Rumalon.[58] When injected into 13-day-old chick embryos, the preparation stimulated ^{14}C-proline incorporation, an indicator of collagen synthesis.[59]

In a partial meniscectomy model in rabbits, Rumalon decreased femoral ulceration at 6 weeks, but not at 12 weeks, and did not have an effect on osteophytes.[6] In mice, Rumalon stimulated the growth of epiphyseal chondrocytes. In C57BL mice, but not in STR/1N mice, Rumalon appeared initially to increase cartilage degeneration, but with continued treatment this change disappeared.[60]

A plethora of human trials have been conducted with Rumalon. In a double-blind, controlled trial, the effects of Rumalon on osteoarthritis in the knee was studied in 106 patients.[61]

Sixty-four per cent of patients receiving intramuscular Rumalon improved subjectively and/or objectively, compared with 29% of the placebo-treated group. This was a statistically significant difference.

In a multicenter, double-blind, controlled trial, 150 patients with osteoarthritis of the hip were given Rumalon by intramuscular injection three times a week for 12 weeks.[62] Twelve weeks after completion of therapy, no difference was found between the Rumalon- and placebo-treated groups, but at 36 weeks the Rumalon-treated group had less pain. No statistical analysis was performed.[62] In another multicenter, controlled trial of 107 patients, no difference was found between the Rumalon-treated and control groups at 3 and 6 months, but more roentgenographic deterioration was found in the controls at 6 months.[62]

In a small, uncontrolled trial of intramuscular Rumalon given to 20 patients with osteoarthritis of the hip, Denko reported clinical improvement in 15 patients and actual roentgenographic improvement, with an increase in the joint space, in four patients.[63–65] No other group, however, has reported roentgenographic improvement with this agent.

An activated acid-pepsin–digested bovine tracheal cartilage of calf origin (Catrix-S) administered subcutaneously has also been evaluated in the treatment of osteoarthritis.[66] Although the investigation noted encouraging results, studies were uncontrolled. The efficacy of this agent, if any, remains to be demonstrated.

At present, more controlled trials are required to support the claim that cartilage–bone marrow extracts are beneficial in the treatment of osteoarthritis.

INTRA-ARTICULAR LUBRICANTS

Because of the observation that osteoarthritic joints are frequently crepitant, a search has been made by many groups for the so-called "ideal lubricant," in the hope that improved lubrication would favorably affect joint function.[67] Wright and coworkers have described a set of criteria to define the ideal artificial lubricant, including resemblance in frictional behavior to the normally occurring hyaluronic acid–protein complex found in joints, ability to resist various forms of degradation, and lack of adverse effects when instilled in the joint space. Such an agent should also be inexpensive and easily manufactured.[68]

Using a cartilage-on-glass frictional system,

Gvozdanovic and colleagues studied the lubricating properties of molecular monolayers.[69] They compared various synthetic substances with synovial mucin and found that sodium dodecyl sulfate in the pH range of 7 to 10 behaved like mucin, whereas cetyl-3-methyl ammonium bromide, a cationic surfactant, was less effective.[69]

Early workers studied silicone oil as a possible lubricant. In one study, a chemical synovitis was produced in rabbit knees by injection of 10% phenol. Knees treated with silicone showed "some reduction in adhesion formation." Silicone was then injected into the knees of patients with osteoarthritis or rheumatoid arthritis who were scheduled for knee surgery. No systemic side effects were noted, and 75% of the patients improved so much that surgery could be postponed. Notably, no control group was included.[67]

Corbett and associates compared the results of injection of silicone oil, hydrocortisone acetate, and hydrocortisone acetate diluted with normal saline solution into the knees of 22 osteoarthritic patients.[70] No statistically significant difference was observed in responses among the groups. In both a controlled clinical trial involving 40 osteoarthritic knees from 25 patients and an experimental model of rabbit osteoarthritis, Wright and coworkers found no evidence that silicone was beneficial either as a lubricant or in the prevention of cartilage damage.[68]

Hyaluronic acid has also been proposed as a lubricant for injection into joints. Weibkin and Muir found that hyaluronic acid in concentrations greater than 5×10^{-2} μg/ml inhibited incorporation of $^{35}SO_4$ into proteoglycans by laryngeal chondrocytes in vitro.[71] Wigren and colleagues found that injection of high–molecular-weight hyaluronic acid into normal rabbit knees produced diffuse infiltration of mononuclear, and occasional polymorphonuclear, cells into the synovial membrane and subsynovial tissue but did not affect normal cartilage or subchondral bone.[72]

In the treatment of osteoarthritis in horses, intra-articular injection of hyaluronic acid led to marked clinical improvement, although the histologic specimens showed obvious osteoarthritic changes. In a group of horses with naturally occurring front-limb lameness, hyaluronic acid also produced a good clinical response.[73] In racehorses with traumatic arthritis, Rydell and Balazs noted less swelling after injection of hyaluronic acid with cortisone than after injection of cortisone alone.[74] In another study, horses with traumatic arthritis that were shown to have abnormally low–molecular-weight hyaluronate in their joints received intra-articular injection of highly purified, high–molecular-weight sodium hyaluronate (Healon). Within 6 weeks after the injection, the limiting viscosity number of sodium hyaluronate in the joints, a measure of molecular size, normalized and symptoms diminished.[75]

Weiss and associates injected Healon into 16 osteoarthritic human knees and performed a sham injection in another 16.[76] A statistically significant improvement was found in the knees that received Healon. The same authors then compared the injection of Healon with intra-articular administration of balanced saline solution in another 42 patients and again found significant improvement with Healon.[76]

Attempts have been made to increase the production of endogenous hyaluronic acid in the joint by injecting Arteparon, an oversulfated heparinoid (see previous discussion), as a possible enzyme inhibitor. The rationale for this maneuver is the observation that human synovial cells in culture can be stimulated by exogenous glycosaminoglycans. In a clinical trial, 18 patients with a multitude of rheumatic conditions received either intra-articular Arteparon or normal saline solution.[77] The concentration of hyaluronic acid in the joints treated with Arteparon was significantly increased 4 days after the injection but returned to the baseline concentration 6 days later. The clinical response was not analyzed.[77]

None of the studies just described has demonstrated an impressive benefit from the use of existing materials presumed to be lubricants. If diminished lubrication is indeed an important aspect of osteoarthritis, it would appear that the ideal lubricant has not yet been found.

GLUCOSAMINE SULFATE

Glucosamine has been called "the building block of the ground substance of the articular cartilage, the proteoglycans"[78] and has therefore been proposed as a treatment for osteoarthritis.

Several small inconclusive trials with glucosamine sulfate have been conducted in Europe. In one double-blind study of 30 patients with osteoarthritis, half the patients received glucosamine sulfate and half received placebo. Treatment was administered by daily intramuscular injection for 1 week and was then given orally for 2 weeks. Piperazine and chlorobutanol were used as placebos. The difference in response between the two groups was

not statistically significant.[79] In another double-blind trial, 20 patients were studied; 50% of these patients received glucosamine sulfate, and the others were given placebo. The drugs were given orally. All patients receiving glucosamine and six of those taking placebo experienced some symptomatic relief. No drug toxicity was noted in either of these reports.[80] In a third study of 30 patients with osteoarthritis, 15 patients received glucosamine sulfate and 15 received placebo. It was claimed that "significantly" more improved when given glucosamine sulfate, but no statistical analysis of the data was provided.[78] At this time, based on these studies, no conclusions can be drawn about any possible efficacy of glucosamine sulfate in osteoarthritis.

TRIBENOSIDE

Tribenoside is a glucofuranoside that purportedly has anti-inflammatory and analgesic effects and may inhibit the release of cathepsin D. Oral tribenoside was compared with olive oil placebo in male and female C57BL mice. High doses of tribenoside were found to cause a statistically significant decrease in the incidence of osteoarthritis in these animals.[81] In a model of chemically induced osteoarthritis in adult hens, tribenoside ameliorated the cartilage degeneration.[82] Systemic tribenoside administration also reduced osteoarthritic joint pathology following partial meniscectomy in rabbits.[82a]

MISCELLANEOUS AGENTS

A variety of miscellaneous agents have also been reported to be useful in the treatment of osteoarthritis. For most of them, there is very little documentation for their claims of efficacy.

Some patients with osteoarthritis have been found to have low plasma levels of pantothenic acid.[83] This prompted an uncontrolled therapeutic trial in 1966 that claimed success for this agent.[84] However, a subsequent double-blind, controlled study by Haslock and Wright, comparing pantothenic acid with placebo in patients with osteoarthritis of the knee, demonstrated no significant difference in response between the two groups.[85]

Rhein, a compound found in Chinese rhubarb, is a quinone that has redox properties and the ability to chelate bivalent metals. Its diacetyl derivative, diacetylrhein, is more absorbable from the gastrointestinal tract than the parent compound. Claims have been made that it has analgesic, antipyretic, and anti-inflammatory properties in animal models of inflammation. In a single-blind, placebo-controlled study, a sequence of placebo, diacetylrhein, and placebo was given to 12 patients with osteoarthritis of the hip or the knee. The results of this study were inconclusive.[86]

In a double-blind, controlled study, 38 patients with osteoarthritis received either placebo or an extract of *Perna canaliculus*, the New Zealand green-lipped mussel, in capsule form for 3 months.[87] All patients then received the extract for the next 3 months. During the first 3-month period, 6 of 16 patients receiving the extract exhibited symptomatic improvement, as did 3 of 22 patients taking placebo. During the next 3 months, six additional patients receiving the extract improved. No change in joint function was noted, however.[87]

Studies of the etiopathogenesis and pathophysiology of osteoarthritis have advanced sufficiently to allow more intelligent trials of specific agents to retard, reverse, or prevent this disorder based on reasonable hypothetical concepts. Although no specific agent capable of interrupting the basic disease process has been defined to date, trials of various agents using experimental models and clinical investigations in humans provide encouragement that such agents may someday prove effective and practical.

References

1. Huber W, Menander-Huber KB: Orgotein. Clin Rheum Dis 6:465–498, 1980.
2. Rosner IA, Goldberg VM, Getzy L, Moskowitz RW: A trial of intraarticular orgotein, a superoxide dismutase, in experimentally-induced osteoarthritis. J. Rheumatol 7:24–29, 1980.
3. Decker WE, Edmondson AH, Hill HE, Holmes RA, Padmore CL, Warren HH, Wood WC: Local administration of orgotein in horses. Mod Vet Pract 55:773–774, 1974.
4. Ahlengard S, Tufvesson G, Pettersson H, Andersson T: Treatment of traumatic arthritis in the horse with intra-articular orgotein (Palosein). Equine Vet J 10:122–124, 1978.
5. Coffman JR, Johnson JH, Tritschler LG, Garner HE, Scrutchfield WL: Orgotein in equine navicular disease: A double blind study. J Am Vet Med Assoc 174:261–264, 1979.
6. Moskowitz RW, Goldberg VM, Rosner IA, Getzy L, Malemud CJ: Specific drug therapy of experimental osteoarthritis. Semin Arthritis Rheum 11(Suppl 1): 127–129, 1981.
7. Lund-Olesen K, Menander KB: Orgotein: A new anti-inflammatory metalloprotein drug: Preliminary evaluation of clinical efficacy and safety in degenerative joint disease. Curr Ther Res 16:607–717, 1974.

8. Bollet AJ: Connective tissue polysaccharide metabolism and the pathogenesis of osteoarthritis. Adv Intern Med 13:33–60, 1967.
9. Mankin HJ, Dorfman H, Lippiello L, Zarins A: Biochemical and metabolic abnormalities in articular cartilage from osteoarthritic human hips. J Bone Joint Surg 53A:523–527, 1971.
10. Schwartz ER, Ogle RC, Thompson RC: Arylsulfatase activities in normal and pathologic human articular cartilage. Arthritis Rheum 17:455–467, 1974.
11. Ehrlich MG, Mankin HJ, Treadwell BV: Acid hydrolase activity in osteoarthritic and normal human cartilage. J Bone Joint Surg 55A:1068–1076, 1973.
12. Schwartz ER, Adamy L: Effect of ascorbic acid on arylsulfatase activities and sulfated proteoglycan metabolism in chondrocyte cultures. J Clin Invest 60:96–106, 1977.
13. Schwartz ER, Oh WH, Leveille CR: Experimentally induced osteoarthritis in guinea pigs: Metabolic responses in articular cartilage to developing pathology. Arthritis Rheum 24:1345–1355, 1981.
14. Schwartz ER, Leveille CR, Stevens JW, Oh WH: Proteoglycan structure and metabolism in normal and osteoarthritic cartilage of guinea pigs. Arthritis Rheum 24:1528–1539, 1981.
15. Kellgren JH, Moore R: Generalized osteoarthritis and Heberden's nodes. Br Med J 1:181–187, 1952.
16. Silberberg M, Silberberg R: Role of sex hormone in the pathogenesis of osteoarthrosis of mice. Lab Invest 12:285–289, 1963.
17. Silberberg M, Silberberg R: Steroid hormones and bone. *In* Bourne GH (ed.): The Biochemistry and Physiology of Bone. Vol. 3. 2nd ed. New York, Academic Press, 1972, pp. 406–442.
18. Priest RE, Koplitz RM, Benditt EP: Estradiol reduces incorporation of radioactive sulfate into cartilage and aortas of rats. J Exp. Med 112:225–236, 1960.
19. Silberberg M, Silberberg R: Modifying action of estrogen on the evolution of osteoarthrosis in mice of different ages. Endocrinology 72:449–451, 1963.
20. Sokoloff L, Varney DA, Scott JF: Sex hormones, bone changes and osteoarthritis in DBA/2JN mice. Arthritis Rheum 8:1027–1038, 1965.
21. Rosner IA, Goldberg VM, Getzy L, Moskowitz RW: Effects of estrogen on cartilage and experimentally induced osteoarthritis. Arthritis Rheum 22:52–58, 1979.
21a. Rosner IA, Malemud CJ, Goldberg VM, et al.: Pathologic and metabolic responses of experimental osteoarthritis to estradiol and an estradiol antagonist. Clin Orthop 171:280–286, 1982.
22. Sledge CD: Growth hormone and articular cartilage. Fed Proc 32:1503–1505, 1973.
23. Salmon WD Jr, Daughaday WH: The importance of amino acids as dialyzable components of rat serum which promote sulfate uptake by cartilage from hypophysectomized rats *in vitro*. J Lab Clin Med 51:167–173, 1958.
24. McConaghey P, Sledge CB: Production of "sulphation factor" by the perfused liver. Nature 225:1249–1250, 1970.
25. Daughaday WH, Hall K, Raben MS, Salmon WD Jr, Van den Brande JL, Van Wyk JJ: Somatomedin: Proposed designation for sulphation factor. Nature 235:107, 1972.
26. Chrisman OD: The effect of growth hormone on established cartilage lesions. Clin Orthop 107:232–238, 1975.
27. Moskowitz RW, Goldberg VM, Schwab W, Berman L: Effects of intraarticular corticosteroids and exercise in experimental models of inflammatory and

degenerative arthritis. (Abstract.) Arthritis Rheum 18:417, 1975.

28. Dekel S, Falconer J, Francis MJO: The effect of anti-inflammatory drugs on glycosaminoglycan sulphation in pig cartilage. Prostaglandins Med 4:133–140, 1980.

29. Wright V, Chadler GN, Morison RAH, Hartfall SJ: Intra-articular therapy in osteo-arthritis: Comparison of hydrocortisone acetate and hydrocortisone *tertiary*-butylacetate. Ann Rheum Dis 19:257–261, 1960.

30. Dieppe PA, Sathapatayavongs B, Jones HE, Bacon PA, Ring EFJ: Intra-articular steroids in osteoarthritis. Rheum Rehabil 19:212–217, 1980.

31. Friedman DM, Moore ME: The efficacy of intraarticular steroids in osteoarthritis: A double-blind study. J Rheumatol 7:850–856, 1980.

32. Wright V: Treatment of osteo-arthritis of the knees. Ann Rheum Dis 23:389–391, 1964.

33. Miller JH, White J, Norton TN: The value of intra-articular injections in osteoarthritis of the knee. J Bone Joint Surg 40B:636-643, 1958.

34. Steinetz BG, Colombo C, Butler MC, O'Byrne E, Steele RE: Animal models of osteoarthritis: Possible applications in a drug development program. Curr Ther Res 30:S61–S75, 1981.

35. Chandler GN, Jones DT, Wright V, Hartfall SJ: Charcot's arthropathy following intra-articular hydrocortisone. Br Med J 1:952–953, 1959.

36. Moskowitz RW, Davis W, Sammarco J, Mast W, Chase SW: Experimentally induced corticosteroid arthropathy. Arthritis Rheum 13:236–243, 1970.

37. Weissmann G: Labilization and stabilization of lysosomes. Fed Proc 23:1038–1044, 1964.

38. Volastro PS, Malawista SE, Chrisman OD: Chloroquine: Protective and destructive effects on injured rabbit cartilage *in vivo*. Clin Orthop 91:243–248, 1973.

39. Cowey FK, Whitehouse MW: Biochemical properties of anti-inflammatory drugs: VII. Inhibition of proteolytic enzymes in connective tissue by chloroquine (resochin) and related antimalarial/antirheumatic drugs. Biochem Pharmacol 15:1071–1084, 1966.

40. Chrisman OD, Ladenbauer-Bellis IM, Fulkerson JP: The osteoarthritic cascade and associated drug actions. Semin Arthritis Rheum 11(Suppl 1):145, 1981.

41. Simmons DP, Chrisman OD: Salicylate inhibition of cartilage degeneration. Arthritis Rheum 8:960–969, 1965.

42. Ginsberg JM, Eyring EJ, Lacy S, Tomblin W: Inhibition of cartilage degeneration by intermittent salicylate. (Abstract.) Arthritis Rheum 11:824, 1968.

43. Chrisman OD, Snook GA: Studies on the protective effect of aspirin against degeneration of human articular cartilage: A preliminary report. Clin Orthop 56:77–82, 1968.

44. Chrisman OD, Snook GA, Wilson TC: The protective effect of aspirin against degeneration of human articular cartilage. Clin Orthop 84:193–196, 1972.

45. Bentley G, Leslie IJ, Fischer D: Effect of aspirin treatment on chondromalacia patellae. Ann Rheum Dis 40:37–41, 1981.

46. Palmoski MJ, Brandt KD: Effect of salicylate on proteoglycan metabolism in normal canine articular cartilage *in vitro*. Arthritis Rheum 22:746–754, 1979.

47. Palmoski MJ, Colyer RA, Brandt KD: Marked

48. suppression by salicylate of the augmented proteoglycan synthesis in osteoarthritic cartilage. Arthritis Rheum 23:83–91, 1980.

48. Palmoski MJ, Brandt KD: Aspirin aggravates the degeneration of canine joint cartilage caused by immobilization. Arthritis Rheum 25:1333–1342, 1982.

49. Palmoski MJ, Brandt KD: In vivo effect of aspirin on canine osteoarthritic cartilage. Arthritis Rheum 26:994–1001, 1983.

50. Wilhelmi VG: Fordernde und hemmende Einflusse ven Tribenosid und Acetylsalicylsaure auf die spontane Arthrose der Maus. Arzneimittelforsch 28:1724–1726, 1978.

51. Telhag H: Effect of tranexamic acid (Cyklokapron) on the synthesis of chondroitin sulfate and the content of hexosamine in the same fraction on normal and degenerated joint cartilage in the rabbit. Clin Orthop Scand 44:249–255, 1973.

52. Ueno R: Ergebnisse der Behandlung mit einem Mucopolysaccharid-polyschwefelsaureester bei der experimentellen Arthrose des Kniegelenks. Z Orthop 111:886–892, 1973.

53. Dustmann HO, Puhl W, Martin K: Der Einflub intraartikulärer Arteparoninjektionen bei Arthrose. Z Orthop 112:1188–1196, 1974.

54. Walton EA, Stevens RW, Fhosh P, Taylor TKF: Nonsteroidal antiinflammatory drugs (NSAIDs) and articular cartilage integrity. Semin Arthritis Rheum 11(Suppl 1):147–149, 1981.

55. Baici A, Salgam P, Fehr K, Boni A: Inhibition of human elastase from polymorphonuclear leucocytes by a glycosaminoglycan polysulfate (Arteparon). Biochem Pharmacol 29:1723–1727, 1980.

56. Stancikova M, Trnavsky K, Keilova H: The effect of antirheumatic drugs on collagenolytic activity of cathepsin B1. Biochem Pharmacol 26:2121–2124, 1977.

56a. Carrero MR, Muniz OE, Torrero G, Howell DS: Effect of a neutral protease inhibitor, Anteparon, on lesions in a rabbit model of osteoarthritis. Presented at the Southeastern Region meeting of the American Rheumatology Association. Lake Buena Vista, Florida, December 9, 1983.

57. Kalbhen DA, Karzel K, Domenjoz R: A high molecular mucopolysaccharide peptide complex stimulating connective tissue metabolism. Pharmacology 1:33–42, 1968.

58. Bollet AJ: Stimulation of protein–chondroitin sulfate synthesis by normal and osteoarthritic articular cartilage. Arthritis Rheum 11:663–673, 1968.

59. Ada M, Brettschneider I, Musilova J, Praus R: Effect of cartilage bone-marrow extract on articular cartilage collagen formation. Pharmacology 16:49–53, 1978.

60. Silberberg M, Silberberg R, Ruttner J: Effects of a cartilage bone-marrow extract on growing cartilage of mice. Exp Med Surg 21:241–250, 1964.

61. Adler E, Wolf E, Taustein I: A double blind trial with cartilage and bone marrow extract in degenerative gonarthrosis. Acta Rheum Scand 16:6–11, 1970.

62. Dixon A St J, Kersley GD, Mercer R, Thompson M, Mason RM, Barnes C, Wenley G: A double-blind controlled trial of Rumalon in the treatment of painful osteoarthrosis of the hip. Ann Rheum Dis 29:193–194, 1970.

63. Denko CW: Restorative chemotherapy in degenera-

tive joint disease (DJD) of the hip. Presented at the Seventh Pan-American Congress of Rheumatology, Bogota, Colombia, June 1978, pp. 1–7.

64. Denko CW: Restorative chemotherapy in degenerative hip disease. Agents Actions 8:268–279, 1978.

65. Denko CW: Treatment of osteoarthritis with Rumalon R. Arthritis Rheum 21:494–496, 1978.

66. Prudden JF, Balassa LL: The biological activity of bovine cartilage preparations. Semin Arthritis Rheum 3:287–321, 1974.

67. Helal B, Karadi BS: Artificial lubrication of joints: Use of silicone oil. Ann Phys Med 9:334–340, 1968.

68. Wright V, Haslock DI, Dowson D, Seller PC, Reeves B: Evaluation of silicone as an artificial lubricant in osteoarthritic joints. Br Med J 2:370–373, 1971.

69. Gvozdanovic D, Wright V, Dowson D: Formation of lubricating monolayers at the cartilage surface. Ann Rheum Dis 34(Suppl 2):100–101, 1975.

70. Corbett M, Seifert MH, Hacking C, Webb S: Comparison between local injections of silicone oil and hydrocortisone acetate in chronic arthritis. Br Med J 1:24–25, 1970.

71. Wiebkin OW, Muir H: The inhibition of sulphate incorporation in isolated adult chondrocytes by hyaluronic acid. FEBS Lett 37:42–46, 1973.

72. Wigren A, Wik O, Falk J: Intra-articular injection of high-molecular hyaluronic acid: An experimental study on normal adult rabbit knee joints. Acta Orthop Scand 47:480–485, 1976.

73. Auer JA, Fackelman GE, Gingerich DA, Fetter AW: Effect of hyaluronic acid in naturally occurring and experimentally induced osteoarthritis. Am J Vet Res 41:568–574, 1980.

74. Rydell N, Balazs EA: Effect of intra-articular injection of hyaluronic acid on the clinical symptoms of osteoarthritis and on granulation tissue formation. Clin Orthop 80:25–32, 1971.

75. Balazs EA, Briller SO, Denlinger JL: Na-hyaluronate molecular size variations in equine and human arthritic synovial fluids and the effect on phagocytic cells. Semin Arthritis Rheum 11(Suppl 1):141–143, 1981.

76. Weiss C, Balazs EA, St Onge R, Denlinger JL: Clinical studies of the intraarticular injection of Healon (sodium hyaluronate) in the treatment of osteoarthritis of human knees. Semin Arthritis Rheum 11(Suppl 1):143–144, 1981.

77. Verbruggen G, Veys EM: Influence of an oversulphated heparinoid upon hyaluronate metabolism of the human synovial cell *in vivo*. J. Rheumatol 6:554–561, 1979.

78. D'Ambrosio E, Casa B, Bompani R, Scali G, Scali M: Glucosamine sulphate: A controlled clinical investigation in arthrosis. Pharmatherapeutica 2:504–508, 1981.

79. Crolle G, D'Este E: Glucosamine sulphate for the management of arthrosis: A controlled clinical investigation. Curr Med Res Opin 7:104–109, 1980.

80. Pujalte JM, Llavore EP, Ylescupidez FR: Double-blind clinical evaluation of oral glucosamine sulphate in the basic treatment of osteoarthrosis. Curr Med Res Opin 7:110–114, 1980.

81. Wilhelmi G, Faust R: Suitability of the C57 black mouse as an experimental animal for the study of skeletal changes due to ageing, with special reference to osteo-arthrosis and its response to tribenoside. Pharmacology 14:289–296, 1976.

82. Kalbhen DA, Felten K: Effects of tribenoside (Glyvenol) on experimental osteoarthrosis. Pharmacology 19:68–74, 1979.

82a. Colombo C, Butler, M, Hickman L, et al.: A new model of osteoarthritis: Evaluation of anti-osteoarthritic effects of selected antirheumatic drugs administered systemically. Arthritis Rheum 26:1132–1139, 1983.

83. Barton-Wright EC, Elliott WA: The pantothenic acid metabolism of rheumatoid arthritis. Lancet 2:862–863, 1963.

84. World Medicine, September 20, 1966, p. 29.

85. Haslock DI, Wright V: Pantothenic acid in the treatment of osteoarthrosis. Rheum Phys Med 11:10–13, 1971.

86. Kay AGL, Griffiths LG, Volans GN, Grahame R: Preliminary experience with diacetylrhein in the treatment of osteoarthritis. Curr Med Res Opin 6:548–551, 1980.

87. Gibson RG, Gibson SLM, Conway V, Chappell D: *Perna canaliculus* in the treatment of arthritis. Practitioner 224:995–960, 1980.

33

Exercise and Osteoarthritis

S. David Stulberg, M.D.
Cary S. Keller, M.D.

During the last 10 years, exercise and athletic competition have become increasingly popular among an expanding segment of society. The general population has come to recognize exercise as being healthful as well as socially desirable and has begun to engage regularly in a great variety of individual and team sports activities. Convinced that exercise improves productivity, decreases absenteeism due to illness, and promotes longevity, employers are providing financial incentives for individuals to exercise.

Traditional team sports involving all segments of the population are receiving increasingly enthusiastic support. The passage of Title XIII has led to a dramatic increase in the number of women participating in organized athletic programs. National, state, and local programs to encourage the participation of preadolescents and teenagers in sports are flourishing. There are currently one million high school students playing football annually.

The growth of individual sports activities such as jogging, tennis, racquetball, weight training, cycling, swimming, aerobic dance, and roller skating has proved to be more than a passing fad and truly represents a social phenomenon affecting all age groups. Twenty-five million men, women, and children in the United States are regular joggers, and another 12 million are competitive marathoners.[1, 2]

In this climate of changing social and medical attitudes toward exercise, the physician is increasingly called upon to weigh the potential benefits against the risks and disadvantages of exercise to the individual. An increasing amount of information has become available concerning the cardiovascular benefits of exercise. Moreover, guidelines have been developed to aid the physician in prescribing exercise to individuals who wish to either optimize the cardiovascular benefits of exercise or recover from a cardiovascular illness. However, very little information is available regarding the effect of regular exercise on the musculoskeletal system in general or the joints specifically. Athletes, patients, and physicians have become concerned that regular intensive physical exercise may provoke future degenerative joint disease. Physicians, parents, and coaches have feared that participation by preadolescents in contact sports presents risk of epiphyseal injury and the subsequent development of growth abnormalities or arthritis. Information concerning the quantity of exercise that can be safely prescribed for individuals with joint deformities (e.g., hip dysplasia) or arthritic joints has not been available to physicians caring for patients who wish to exercise or participate in sports.

There are a number of explanations for the relative paucity of data on the effects of exercise on joints. Several problems are encountered when prospective or retrospective studies are performed to evaluate the effects of exercise. For example, the type and extent of stress on joints must be known. The stress on various joints differs with, among other things, the sport, the position played, the intensity and duration of participation, and the type of protective equipment used. There is very little information about the magnitude of the stress that is placed on the joints of individuals who exercise. Moreover, joints may vary in their reaction to a given stress. Normal, injured, and arthritic joints function differently and can be expected to respond differently to exercise. This chapter will review the information that is available on the effects of exercise on joints. It will examine the different ways in which exercise exerts an effect on joints. The consequences of exercise on normal joints will be compared with and contrasted to the potential implications of exercise for joints that have been injured or have become arthritic. This chapter will also attempt to stimulate clinicians and investigators interested in joint diseases to consider the ways in which exercise might be healthful or harmful to joints.

THE RESPONSE OF THE MUSCULOSKELETAL SYSTEM TO EXERCISE

The bones, muscles, ligaments, menisci, and articular surfaces work together to withstand the stress imposed on the musculoskeletal system by physical activity. The response of bone to exercise is, perhaps, better understood than the response of the joints. Lanyon and co-workers,[3] for example, have measured in vivo the stress on the human anterior tibia during walking and jogging. Although the magnitude of compressive stress experienced by the tibia is approximately the same during the two activities, tensile stresses are three to four times greater during jogging. These increased stresses within bone that occur during running have been shown, in laboratory animals, to result in hypertrophy of the bone that is proportional to the duration of the running activity.[4] This response of bone to the increased stresses produced by exercise has also been observed in humans. A comparison of 64 male Olympic and professional athletes with age-matched controls demonstrated significantly higher distal femoral bone density in the athletes. Furthermore, among the controls, those who regularly exercised had greater bone density than those who did not.[5] The bone response of middle-aged female marathon runners has been compared with that of age-matched controls. The controls were found to have undergone the usual involutional bone loss associated with menopause; the marathoners, however, had maintained or increased their bone mass in both the upper and lower extremities.[6]

The response of normal joints to stress is less well understood. The magnitude of the compressive force on various joints that occurs during walking has been studied. For example, the forces during a normal gait cycle approach seven times body weight in the hip,[7] four times body weight in the tibiofemoral and patellofemoral joints,[8, 9] and five times body weight

in the ankle.[10] Running increases these forces across the joints.[11–13] Moreover, a runner's foot strikes the ground 800 to 2000 times per mile or 50 to 70 times per minute,[13] causing the joints of the lower extremity to respond to the increased compressive forces much more often in a given time period than is necessary during walking. The prospect of increased compressive loads being repetitively imposed on the joints of the lower extremity has led many conscientious physicians to express concern that running may accelerate the degeneration of joints.

However, repetitious increased compressive loads across joints, as may occur during running, are only one type of stress that articular cartilage must withstand during physical activity. Angular, torsional, and tensile stresses are also applied to joints during many athletic activities, such as football, racquet sports, skiing, and bicycling. There is very little experimental information on the magnitudes that these types of stresses reach within joints during exercise. Moreover, it is not known whether a given joint is better able to tolerate repetitive compressive loads, as might be generated during jogging, or intense, momentary angular or torsional loads, as may be produced during a game of tennis. However, an ever-increasing clinical experience is beginning to suggest how normal joints respond to various types of stress.

Although joint symptoms, especially of the knee, are very common in long-distance runners, very few serious joint injuries occur.[14] This reflects the fact that running, unlike sports that require twisting of a joint, places very little stress on the supporting structures, i.e., ligaments, capsule, menisci. However, the repetitive motion that jogging imposes on joints is responsible for the high incidence of periarticular symptoms seen in runners. Although no evidence exists to suggest that the occurrence of these symptoms in runners with normal joints leads to arthritis, it has been estimated that 60% of runners experience periarticular symptoms severe enough to require temporary discontinuation of running.[13] The periarticular symptoms that occur in sports such as jogging resolve almost uniformly with rest, anti-inflammatory medication, attention to details of conditioning, training, and equipment, and efforts to control the environment, e.g., running surface, in which the sport is played. Periarticular symptoms do not imply articular injury, and there is no evidence that they have any long-term effect on joint function or health.

Sports, such as football, in which joints are often exposed to large torsional and bending stresses are associated with a high incidence of potentially serious joint injuries. Moreover, less violent sports in which such stresses are also applied to joints (e.g., tennis) are associated with intra-articular injuries (e.g., meniscal tears) of potentially serious consequence much more frequently than occurs in sports in which these types of stresses do not occur (e.g., running, bicycling). Even swimming, a sport commonly thought to produce very little stress on joints, may be associated, as is the case in "breast stroker's knee," with a markedly increased incidence of significant joint damage if high torsional stresses are applied to the joints.[15]

Thus, in considering the potential effect of exercise on the development of degenerative joint disease, one must develop an understanding of how joints carry load and which joint stresses adversely affect articular cartilage and periarticular joint structures. The information currently available suggests that the ultimate health of articular cartilage is best protected if the integrity of the joint and its supporting structures is maintained.

THE EFFECTS OF EXERCISE ON UNINJURED JOINTS

A large number of roentgenographic studies have been performed to assess the relationship of exercise to the development of degenerative joint disease. The interpretation of these studies requires an awareness of the ways that stresses on joints that occur during exercise are manifested roentgenographically.

The diagnosis of osteoarthritis in athletes is often based on the presence of periarticular osteophytes alone. Many investigators have questioned the relationship of the presence of these osteophytes to the existence of significant articular cartilage disease.[16-24] A study of 384 cadaver hips concluded that osteophytes were ubiquitous and age-related and that their presence did not imply articular cartilage destruction.[21] A 10-year review of patients diagnosed roentgenographically as having osteoarthritis of the hip showed that the presence of osteophytes is not correlated with clinical evidence of osteoarthritis or subsequent roentgenologically demonstrable alteration of the articular cartilage.[20] Similarly, in a 14- to 18-year follow-up of 2195 knees in which osteoarthritis had been roentgenographically diagnosed on the basis of osteophytes, two-thirds showed no

evidence of articular cartilage changes based on history, physical examination, or roentgenographic study, and osteophytes of the patella alone were rarely found to be associated with subsequent structural changes within the joint.[19] Studies that report osteoarthritis in athletes based on the presence of osteophytes are therefore difficult to interpret.

Studies in which the presence of osteophytes is the primary criterion for the existence of osteoarthritis are numerous, however. These studies suggest that the distribution of osteoarthritis is related to the specific sports activity: the hands in boxing,[25] the fingers in cricket,[26] the shoulders, elbows, and wrists in gymnastics,[27] the shoulders and elbows in baseball pitching,[28-32] the elbows, spine, and knees in wrestling,[33] the spine in judo,[34] the knees and ankles in English football (soccer),[35-45] the knees and ankles in parachute jumping,[46] and the knee in American football.[47]

The presence of osteophytes as an indication of the presence of osteoarthritis has led many investigators to conclude that the disease is particularly commonly associated with participation in English football (soccer). A roentgenologic examination of 34 English football players whose average age was 27 years revealed osteoarthrosis of the ankle in 33, with bilateral involvement in 27.[41] A clinical and roentgenographic examination of 36 English football players whose average age was 26 years revealed peripatellar osteophytes in 28%, as compared with 21% of the matched control group. Osteoarthrosis of the ankle, as evidenced by osteophytes, was diagnosed in 92% of the football players and 20% of the controls.[43] When 56 professional football players and 10 former professional players were examined roentgenologically, osteoarthritic changes of the knees, ankles, or feet were found in all players, with the most severe changes reported to be in the ankles and feet.[45] A survey of the long-term effects of American football on the knee was conducted by roentgenologic examination of 205 present and former players. Half of these reported previous knee injury of some kind, and 40% had persistent symptoms. The incidence of osteoarthritis in these knees was 84%.

The Ahlback criteria for the roentgenologic diagnosis of osteoarthritis are based on destruction of the articular cartilage as evidenced by loss of roentgenographic joint space. When these criteria are used to evaluate athletes' joints, there is little evidence that exercise is deleterious to joints that have not been injured. For example, the examination of the hip joints of 74 former Finnish track record holders whose average age was 55 years and who had competed for an average of 21 years revealed a 4% incidence of osteoarthritis, as compared with an 8.7% incidence in an age-matched control group.[48] Similarly, the clinical and roentgenologic examination of 51 professional and ex-professional football players aged 37 to 76 with an average of 14 years of professional football experience revealed a 3% incidence of osteoarthritis of the knee.[35] Therefore, there is little evidence to confirm that regular exercise of normal, uninjured joints leads to the development of osteoarthritis.

There is, however, a high incidence of osteophytes in joints that have been subjected to exercise. Cabot[49] noted this association of periarticular bone changes accompanied by normal joint space in athletes and referred to this finding as "periarthropathie sportive." This phenomenon has been reported in the lower and upper extremities of athletes participating in a variety of activities. For example, "footballer's ankle" has been repeatedly reported as anterior osteophytes of the distal tibia accompanying a normal joint space and is thought to represent a response to repeated ligament strain experienced while kicking in the equinus position.[39, 40] Moreover, the periarticular osteophytes found in the ankles and knees of 66 English football players[45] showed no evidence of change in roentgenographic appearance with increasing years of play, suggesting that periarthropathie sportive is not a progressive or destructive process.

In the knee, the appearance of mild osteophytes on the intercondylar eminences of the tibia (Felsenreich's sign)[50] is frequently interpreted as an early sign of osteoarthritis. However, "tibial spiking" accompanied by a normal joint space is a common finding in the athletic knee. In a study of 205 American football players, for example, osteoarthritis was diagnosed roentgenologically in 84% of the knees examined, usually based on the presence of osteophytes alone. Similarly, a study[35] of 51 English football players aged 37 to 76 revealed tibial spiking in 86%, although Ahlback's criteria for osteoarthritis of the knee were met by only 3%. Therefore, tibial spiking represents another site of periarthropathie sportive, implying not osteoarthritis but rather a response to repeated stress at the insertion of the cruciate ligaments.[23]

Periarthropathie sportive does not require weight bearing and can develop in the joints of the upper extremity as well. Numerous reports describe changes in the shoulders and elbows of athletes engaged in gymnastics[27] and throwing sports.[29–32, 51] Occasionally, destructive changes in the articular cartilage have been reported, and these probably represent injured joints.[28] The majority of changes noted, however, are spurring or osteophytes, most commonly occurring at the humeral epicondyles, olecranon, and other points of muscle origin and insertion. These changes constitute periarthropathie sportive of the upper extremity and are thought to represent a response to repeated stress at the myo-osseous or osseotendinous junction.[31]

The roentgenographic response of normal joints to regular exercise is "periarthropathie sportive," the formation of osteophytes at the site of periarticular soft tissue attachments in the upper and lower extremities. There is no evidence that regular exercise of normal joints produces progressive, destructive changes of the articular cartilage.

THE EFFECT OF EXERCISE ON INJURED JOINTS

When abnormal stress is applied to a joint, injury to one or more of its components can occur and potentially permanent disruption of the normal joint biomechanics can result. Intra-articular fractures, meniscal tears, and ligament injuries result in the most serious alterations of joint biomechanics. Fractures of the articular surface may produce incongruous joint surfaces or defects that predispose to articular cartilage degeneration. Local stress concentration in abnormal joints can reach high levels and may be the initiating event leading to the fatigue failure that manifests itself as osteoarthritis.[43, 52] As the articular cartilage receives negligible blood supply, the chondrocyte response to chondral injury is limited and partial-thickness chondral injuries are not spontaneously repaired.[53] Full-thickness osteochondral injuries do provoke a full healing response as blood supply from the subchondral bone is available. Thus, full-thickness articular cartilage defects are repaired by replacement with fibrocartilage. However, the extent to which fibrocartilage can act as a substitute for hyaline articular cartilage remains unknown.

The menisci transfer and distribute load as well as contribute to the stability of the joint. Menisci carry load by virtue of the hoop stress developed when the centrifugal spread of the meniscus under load is resisted by the principally circumferential orientation of the meniscal collagen fibers. In this way, the menisci significantly decrease load and stress transmission across the joint.[54] Thirty to 60% of load applied across a joint is carried by the menisci.[54–61] Tearing or resection of a meniscus interrupts the circumferential collagen fibers and prevents the normal development of hoop stress, resulting in a twofold to threefold increase in the stress transmitted across the joint with load.[54] Furthermore, meniscal tears and resection alter the path of the instant center of joint motion and result in joint instability.[52] This abnormal joint motion produces abnormal articular surface motion with increased articular surface friction and high local surface stresses that encourage mechanical wear and fatigue. These factors combine, making the development of degenerative joint disease more likely.[52, 61–65]

Degenerative changes consisting of articular cartilage erosion and osteophyte formation have been observed to develop rapidly following meniscectomy in animals,[66–69] with lesions primarily noted in the overlying femoral condyle. The incidence of osteoarthritis following meniscectomy in man ranges from 1% to 92% and depends on the duration of follow-up and the criteria used for the diagnosis of osteoarthritis.[23, 63, 65, 66, 70–78] For example, when 107 meniscectomies were followed for 3 months to 14 years, it was found that roentgenographic abnormalities consisting of ridging, joint space narrowing, or femoral condylar flattening occurred with an incidence of 67% following medial meniscectomy and 50% following lateral meniscectomy. However, when 99 meniscectomies were followed for an average 17.5 years and analyzed using Ahlback's[79] criteria, the incidence of osteoarthritis was 39%.[72] In this study, increased duration and frequency of meniscal symptoms preoperatively, such as locking, clicking, giving way, and effusion, were associated with an increased incidence of osteoarthritis.

Disruption of the anterior cruciate ligament has been referred to as "the beginning of the end for the knee,"[80] for it can be followed by progressive deterioration of knee function, characterized by anterior and rotational instability, meniscal tears, and progressive articular cartilage degeneration.[81, 82] A torn anterior cruciate ligament alters the path of the instant center of joint motion, producing abnormal articular surface motion that results in increased articular surface friction and high local surface stresses, which encourage wear and fatigue of the menisci and articular cartilage.[52] Insufficiency of the anterior cruciate liga-

ment has been observed to result in both proliferative and degenerative articular changes in animals.[83–90] In dogs, proliferative marginal osteophyte formation begins soon after surgical ablation of the anterior cruciate ligament[86] and progresses despite only occasional early evidence of articular cartilage degeneration,[85] perhaps reflecting the increased stress being borne by the secondary stabilizing structures of the knee. With increasing length of follow-up, articular cartilage degeneration is more common and is related to the degree of joint laxity. In an up-to-4-year follow-up of dogs that had undergone primary repair or reconstruction following section of the anterior cruciate ligament, for example, the incidence of osteoarthritis was 80% in knees with severe instability and 30% in knees with slight or moderate instability.[91]

The development of osteoarthritis following anterior cruciate ligament injury has been noted in humans as well[71, 72, 92–95] and is associated with a high incidence of meniscal tears.[92, 93, 96–100] The incidence of osteoarthritis associated with insufficiency of the anterior cruciate ligament varies with the length of follow-up, the existence of other ligamentous or meniscal injuries, and the criteria for diagnosis of osteoarthritis. At a 2- to 12-year follow-up of one group of 50 patients with tears of the anterior cruciate ligament, the incidence of roentgenologic evidence of osteoarthritis was 16%, and an additional 11% also underwent arthrotomy, which confirmed osteoarthritis.[100] By comparison, 48 patients, almost all of whom were younger than 40 years old and who had had a tear of the anterior cruciate ligament 6 months to 21 years previously, were examined by roentgenogram and arthrotomy. Fifty-six per cent had pathologic evidence of osteoarthritis at arthrotomy using Collins' criteria,[101] and 15% showed severe articular changes at arthrotomy and signifiant bony changes such as cysts or sclerosis on roentgenogram.[94] The incidence and severity of osteoarthritis and the incidence of meniscal tears increase with time after an anterior cruciate tear,[94] and osteoarthritis develops more rapidly when other ligamentous or meniscal injuries accompany the anterior cruciate tear.[94, 100]

The response of injured upper-extremity joints to exercise is analogous to that observed in the lower extremity. When abnormal motion or load is forced on an upper-extremity joint, injury to one or more of its components can occur and can result in permanent disruption of normal joint biomechanics. Although not functionally weight-bearing joints, the elbow and shoulder experience joint reaction forces that approach body weight under static conditions and that can greatly exceed body weight under dynamic conditions.[102–105] Therefore, the abnormal motion accompanying exercise following injury can significantly alter joint friction and stress distribution. As in the lower extremity, this process encourages the biomaterial fatigue and failure that can lead to degenerative joint disease. For example, injury and laxity of the medial collateral ligament of the elbow are experienced by both skeletally immature and adult baseball pitchers and are considered to result from repeated valgus stress associated with curve-ball and side-arm pitching. Continued pitching motion in the presence of medial ligamentous insufficiency is associated with progressive articular cartilage degeneration and osteochondritis, especially of the lateral compartment.[28, 106, 107]

CONCLUSION

Normal joints in individuals of all ages appear to tolerate prolonged and vigorous exercise without adverse consequences. However, joints that are injured in sports, improperly treated, and continually stressed may rapidly develop significant and disabling osteoarthritis. Lowering the incidence of degenerative joint disease associated with some sports may result not from curtailing participation in such activities, but from identifying the factors that result in injuries to vulnerable joints and thus preventing the injuries. The effects of exercise on the natural history of degenerative joint disease may be analogous to its role in cardiovascular disease. Vigorous exercise of the normal joint and normal heart does not lead to and may well prevent their deterioration. The injured joint and the injured heart are susceptible to further injury and deterioration with continued exercise, but one may be able to safely engage in activity following proper treatment and full rehabilitation.

References

1. Haycock CE: Sports medicine. JAMA 247:2984, 1982.
2. Gudas CJ: Patterns of lower extremity injury in 224 runners. Compr Ther 6:50–59, 1980.
3. Lanyon LE, Hampson WGJ, Goodship AE, et al.: Bone deformation recorded in vivo from strain gauges attached to the human tibial shaft. Acta Orthop Scand 46:256–268, 1975.
4. Saville PD, Whyte MP: Muscle and bone hypertrophy—positive effect of running exercise in the rat. Clin Orthop 65:81, 1969.
5. Nilsson BE, Westlin NE: Bone density in athletes. Clin Orthop 77:179–182, 1971.
6. Brewer V, Meyer B, Upton J, Hagan RD: Role of exercise in prevention of involutional bone loss. Med Sci Sports Exerc 14:106, 1982.
7. Paul JP: Forces at the Human Hip. Ph.D. Thesis, University of Chicago, 1967.
8. Morrison JB: The mechanics of the knee joint in relation to normal walking. J Biomech 3:51, 1970.
9. Reilly DT, Martens M: Experimental analysis of the quadriceps muscle force and patello-femoral joint reaction force for various activities. Acta Orthop Scand 43:126–137, 1972.
10. Stauffer RN, Chad EYS, Brewster RC: Force and motion analysis of the normal, diseased, and prosthetic ankle joint. Clin Orthop 127:189, 1977.
11. Root ML, Orien WP, Weid JW: Normal and abnormal function of the foot. Clin Biomech 2:154, 1977.
12. Pearson K: The control of walking. Sci Am 235:72–74, 79–82, 83–86, 1976.
13. Brody DM: Running injuries. Clin Symp 32:1–36, 1980.
14. Leach RE, Baumgard S, Broom J: Obesity: Its relationship to osteoarthritis of the knee. Clin Orthop 93:271–273, 1973.
15. Stulberg SD: Sports injuries and arthritis. Compr Ther 6:8–11, 1980.
16. Jacqueline F, Arlet J, Laporte C: La coxite densifiante et l'evolution benigne. Rev Rhum 17:114–120, 1950.
17. Brailsford EF: Osteoarthritis of the hip joint. Br J Radiol 25:76–84, 1952.
18. Jacqueline F, Veraguth P: Étude radiologique de la tête fémorale de sujet âgé. Rev Rhum 21:237–242, 1954.
19. Danielsson L, Hernborg J: Clinical and roentgenologic study of knee joints with osteophytes. Clin Orthop 69:302–321, 1970.
20. Danielsson LG: Incidence and prognosis of coxarthrosis. Acta Orthop Scand Suppl 66:1–114, 1964.
21. Byers PD, Contepomi CA, Farkas TA: A post mortem study of the hip joint. Ann Rheum Dis 29:15–31, 1970.
22. Adams ID: Osteoarthrosis and sport. Clin Rheum Dis 2:523–531, 1976.
23. Smillie IS: Injuries of the Knee Joint. 3rd ed. Baltimore, Williams and Wilkins, 1962, pp. 161–164.
24. Tobin WJ: The relationship of trauma to arthritis. Am Surg 25:332, 1959.
25. Iselin M: Importance de l'arthrose dans le syndrome "main fragile" des boxeurs. Rev Rhum 7-8:242, 1960.
26. Vere Hodge N: Chronic injury—cricket. In Larson LA (ed.): Encyclopedia of Sports Sciences and Medicine. New York, Macmillan, 1971, p. 606.
27. Bozdech Z: Chronic injury—gymnastics. In Larson LA (ed.): Encyclopedia of Sports Sciences and Medicine. New York, Macmillan, 1971, p. 616.
28. Adams JE: Injury to the throwing arm: A study of traumatic changes in the elbow joint of boy baseball players. Calif Med 102:127–132, 1965.
29. Bennett GE: Shoulder and elbow lesions distinctive of baseball players. Ann Surg 126:107–110, 1947.
30. Diveley RL, Meyer PW: Baseball shoulder. JAMA 171:1659–1661, 1959.
31. Bateman JE: AAOS Symposium on Sports Medicine. St. Louis, C.V. Mosby, 1969.

32. Brewer B: Chronic injury—baseball. *In* Larson LA (ed.): Encyclopedia of Sports Sciences and Medicine. New York, Macmillan, 1971, p. 616.

33. Layani F, Roeser J, Naddud M: Les Lésions ostéoarticulaires des catcheursit. Rev Rhum 7-8:244–248, 1960.

34. Rubens-Duval A, Belin A, Ficheuxs JM, et al.: Les rachis des ceintures noir. Rev Rhum 7-8:233–241, 1960.

35. Adams ID: Osteoarthrosis of the knee joint in sportsmen. M.D. Thesis, University of Leeds, 1973.

36. Klunder KB, Rud B, Hansen J: Osteoarthritis of the hip and knee joint in retired football players. Acta Orthop Scand 51:925–927, 1980.

37. Pelissier M, Bruschet J, Levere F, Leenhardt P: Le pied des footballers. J Radiol Electrol 35:403, 1952.

38. Bourel M, Cormier M, Dagorne J, Delahaye D: Complications locomotrices du football. Rev Rhum 7-8:297–303, 1960.

39. Morris LH: Case reports. J Bone Joint Surg 25:220, 1943.

40. McMurray TP: Footballer's ankle. J Bone Joint Surg 32B:68–69, 1950.

41. Brodelius A: Osteoarthrosis of the talar joints in footballers and ballet dancers. Acta Orthop Scand 30:309–314, 1961.

42. Arens W: Zur frage der arthrose als mechanischer uberlastungsproblem. Sportarzt 5:95, 1963.

43. Solonen KA: The joints of the lower extremities of football players. Ann Chir Gynaecol Fenn 55:176, 1966.

44. Bagneres H: Lésion ostéo-articulaires chroniques des sportifs. Rheum Halneol Allergol 19:27–34, 1967.

45. Pelligrini P, Nibbio N, Piffanelli A: Artropatie croniche da attivate sportiva: il piede e il ginocchio del calciatore professionista. Archispedale S Anna di Ferrara 17:879, 1964.

46. Murray-Leslie CF, Lintott DJ, Wright V: The knees and ankles in sport and veteran miliary parachutists. Ann Rheum Dis 36:327–331, 1977.

47. Rall KL, McElroy GL, Keats TE: A study of long-term effects of football injury to the knee. Missouri Med 61:435–438, 1964.

48. Puranen J, Ala-Ketola L, Peltokallio P, et al.: Running and primary osteoarthrosis of the hip. Br Med J 2:424–425, 1975.

49. Cabot JR: Lésions chroniques dans le sport au niveau des extrémités inférieures. Médicine, Éducation Physique et Sport 4:277, 1964.

50. Felsenreich F: Die rontgendiagnose der veralteten kreuzbandlasion des kniegelenks. Fortschr Rontgenstr 49:341, 1934.

51. Peltokallio P: Chronic injury—baseball. *In* Larson LA (ed.): Encyclopedia of Sports Sciences and Medicine. New York, Macmillan, 1971, p. 567.

52. Frankel VH, Burstein AH, Brooks DB: Biomechanics of internal derangement of the knee. Pathomechanics as determined by analysis of the instant centers of motion. J Bone Joint Surg 53A:945–962, 1971.

53. Mankin HJ: Response of articular cartilage to mechanical injuries. J Bone Joint Surg 64A:460–466, 1982.

54. Krause W, Pope M, Johnson R, Wilder D: Mechanical changes in the knee after meniscectomy. J Bone Joint Surg 58A:599–604, 1976.

55. Shrive N: The weight-bearing role of the menisci of the knee. J Bone Joint Surg 56B:381, 1974.

56. Seedhom BB, Dowson D, Wright V: Proceedings: Function of the menisci—a preliminary study. Ann Rheum Dis 33:111, 1974.

57. Walker PS, Erkman MJ: The role of menisci in force transmission across the knee. Clin Orthop 109:184–192, 1975.

58. Brantigan OC, Voshell AF: The mechanics of the ligaments and menisci of the knee joint. J Bone Joint Surg 23A:44–66, 1941.

59. Bruce J, Walmsley R: Replacement of the semilunar cartilages of the knee after operative excision. Br J Surg 25:17–28, 1937.

60. Kettelkamp DB, Jacobs AW: Tibiofemoral contact area—determination and implications. J Bone Joint Surg 54A:349–356, 1972.

61. King D: The function of the semilunar cartilages. J Bone Joint Surg 18:1069–1076, 1936.

62. Bullough PG, Munuera L, Murphy J, Weinstein A: The strength of the menisci of the knee as it relates to their fine structure. J Bone Joint Surg 52B:564–570, 1970.

62a. MacConaill MA: The function of intra-articular fibro-cartilages with special reference to the knee and inferior radio-ulnar joints. J Anat 66:210–227, 1932.

63. Fairbank TJ: Knee joint changes after meniscectomy. J Bone Joint Surg 30B:664–670, 1948.

64. Keyes EL: Erosions of the articular surfaces of the knee joint. J Bone Joint Surg 15:369–371, 1933.

65. Tapper EM, Hoover NW: Late results after meniscectomy. J Bone Joint Surg 51A:517–526, 1969.

66. Cox JS, Nye CE, Schaefer WW, Woodstein IJ: The degenerative effects of partial and total resection of the medial meniscus in dogs' knees. Clin Orthop 109:178–183, 1975.

67. Pfab B: Weitere experimentelle studien zur pathologie der binnenverletzungen des kniegelenkes. Dtsch Chir 211:339–345, 1928.

68. Dieterich H: Die regeneration des meniscus. Dtsch Chir 230:251–260, 1931.

69. King D: Regeneration of semilunar cartilage. Surg Gynecol Obstet 62:167–170, 1936.

70. Appel H: Late results after meniscectomy in the knee joint. A clinical and roentgenologic follow-up investigation. Acta Orthop Scand Suppl 133:1, 1970.

71. Jackson JP: Degenerative changes in the knee after meniscectomy. Br Med J 2:525–527, 1968.

72. Johnson RJ, Kettelkamp DB, Clark W, Leaverton P: Factors affecting late results after meniscectomy. J Bone Joint Surg 56A:719–729, 1974.

73. Aarstrand T: Treatment of meniscal rupture of the knee joint. A follow-up examination of material where only the ruptured part of the meniscus has been removed. Acta Chir Scand 107:146–157, 1954.

74. Ferguson LK, Thompson WD: Internal derangements of the knee joint: An analysis of one hundred cases with follow-up study. Ann Surg 112:454–470, 1940.

75. Huckell JR: Is meniscectomy a benign procedure? A long-term follow-up study. Can J Surg 8:254–260, 1969.

76. Lagergren K-A: Meniscus operations and secondary arthrosis deformans. Acta Orthop Scand 14:280–283, 1953.

77. Neviaser JS: Division of the tibial collateral ligament for removal of the medial meniscus. A long-term follow-up study. Clin Orthop 55:105–116, 1967.

78. Woodyard JE: A long-term survey after meniscectomy. Orthopaedics, 1:29, 1968.

79. Ahlback S: Osteoarthrosis of the knee: A radiographic investigation. Acta Radiol Suppl 277:7–72, 1968.

80. Allman FL, cited in Torg JS, Conrad W, Kalen V: Clinical diagnosis of anterior cruciate ligament instability in the athlete. Am J Sports Med 4:84–93, 1976.

81. Drez D: Modified Eriksson procedure for chronic anterior cruciate instability. Orthopedics 1:30, 1978.

82. Marshall JL, Rubin RM, Wang JB, et al.: The anterior cruciate ligament. The diagnosis and treatment of its injuries and their serious prognostic implications. Orthop Rev 7:35, 1978.

83. Nilsson F: Meniscal injuries in dogs. North Am Vet 30:504, 1948.

84. McDevitt CA, Muir H: Biochemical changes in the cartilage of the knee in experimental and natural osteoarthritis in the dog. J Bone Joint Surg 58B:94–101, 1976.

85. Marshall JL, Olsson SE: Instability of the knee: A long-term experimental study in dogs. J Bone Joint Surg 53A:1561–1570, 1971.

86. Marshall JL, Warren RF, Wickiewicz T: Primary surgical treatment of anterior cruciate ligament lesions. Am J Sports Med 10:103, 1982.

87. Paatsama S: Ligament Injuries in the Canine Stifle Joint: A Clinical and Experimental Study. Helsinki, 1952.

88. Bohr H: Experimental osteoarthritis in the rabbit knee joint. Acta Orthop Scand 47:558–565, 1976.

89. Magnuson PB: Joint debridement. Surgical treatment of degenerative arthritis. Surg Gynecol Obstet 73:1, 1941.

90. Hulth A, Lindberg L, Telhag H: Experimental osteoarthritis in rabbits. Acta Orthop Scand 41:522–530, 1970.

91. O'Donoghue DH, Frank GR, Jeter GL, et al.: Repair and reconstruction of the anterior cruciate ligament in dogs—factors influencing long-term results. J Bone Joint Surg 53A:710–718, 1971.

92. Slocum DB, James SL, Larson RL, et al.: Clinical test for anterolateral rotatory instability of the knee. Clin. Orthop 118:63–69, 1976.

93. Losee RE, in personal communication with Clancey WG, et al.: Anterior cruciate ligament reconstruction using one-third of the patellar ligament, aug-mented by extra-articular tendon transfers. J Bone Joint Surg 64A:352, 1982.

94. Jacobsen K: Osteoarthrosis following insufficiency of the cruciate ligaments in man. Acta Orthop Scand 48:520–526, 1977.

95. Liljedahl S-O, Lindvall N, Wetterfors J: Early diagnosis and treatment of acute ruptures of the anterior cruciate ligament. J Bone Joint Surg 47A:1503–1513, 1965.

96. Torg JS, Conrad W, Kalen V: Clinical diagnosis of anterior cruciate ligament instability in the athlete. Am J Sports Med 4:84, 1976.

97. Kennedy JC, Weinberg HW, Wilson AS: The anatomy and function of the anterior cruciate ligament. As determined by clinical and morphological studies. J Bone Joint Surg 56A:223–235, 1974.

98. Kennedy JC, Stewart R, Walker DM: Anterolateral rotary instability of the knee joint. An early analysis of the Ellison procedure. J Bone Joint Surg 60A:1031–1039, 1978.

99. Ellison AE: Distal iliotibial band transfer for anterolateral rotatory instability of the knee. J Bone Joint Surg 61A:330–337, 1979.

100. McDaniel WJ, Dameron TB: Untreated ruptures of the anterior cruciate ligament. J Bone Joint Surg 62A:696–705, 1980.

101. Collins DH: The Pathology of Articular and Spinal Diseases. London, Arnold, 1949.

102. Inman VT, Saunders JE deC M, Abbott LC: Observations on the function of the shoulder joint. J Bone Joint Surg 26A:1–30, 1944.

103. Poppen NK, Walker PS: Forces at the glenohumeral joint in abduction. Clin Orthop 135:165–170, 1978.

104. Nicol AC, Berme N, Paul JP: A biomechanical analysis of elbow joint function. In Institution of Mechanical Engineers Conference Publications, 1977–5, London, pp. 45–51.

105. Matsen FA: Biomechanics of the elbow. In Frankel VH, Nordin M (eds.): Basic Biomechanics of the Skeletal System. Philadelphia, Lea and Febiger, 1980, pp. 250–252.

106. Dehaven KE, Evarts CM: Throwing injuries of the elbow in athletes. Orthop Clin North Am 4:801, 1973.

107. Brown R, Blazina ME, Kerlan RK, et al.: Osteochondritis of the capitellum. J Sports Med 2:27, 1974.

INDEX

Note: Page numbers in *italic* type indicate illustrations; page numbers followed by t refer to tables.

Acetabulum, collapse of, in late-stage osteoarthritis, *160*
Eggers' cyst of, 162, *162*
Acetaminophen, 319
Acid phosphatase, in osteoarthritic articular cartilage, 67, *68*
Acromegaly, 243–244
laboratory assessment of, 186t
secondary osteoarthritis in, 243–244
Acromioclavicular joint, arthroplasty of, 384
osteoarthritis of, 382–384
treatment of, 383–384
surgical, 384
steroid injection into, 341, *341*
Activities of daily living (ADL), in rehabilitative assessment, 288
Acupuncture, 293
Adrenocorticosteroids, systemic. See *Steroids.*
Age, as factor in osteoarthritis, 1, 10t, 11–12, *11,* 11t, 12t
Aging, and pathophysiology of osteoarthritis, 12–14
Alkaline phosphatase, in articular cartilage, 64
serum, in osteoarthritis, 185–186
Alkaptonuric ochronosis, 64, 238
Analgesic drugs, 319–320, 319t
centrally acting, 319–320
addiction to, 320
combination (centrally and peripherally acting), 320
local, 320
narcotic. See *Analgesic drugs, centrally acting.*
peripherally acting, 319
Animal models, of osteoarthritis. See *Experimental models of osteoarthritis.*
Ankle, and foot, anatomic aspects of, 389–391
orthosis for, 393, *393*
osteoarthritis of, 389–402
diagnosis of, 391
arthrodesis of, 393–394, *393*
biomechanics of, 96
"footballer's," 564
location of axes from, *97*

Ankle (*Continued*)
malrotation of, adverse effects of, 290
orthosis for, 297, *298, 393, 393*
osteoarthritis of, 392–394
positioning for, 296
roentgenogram of, *392*
treatment of, 393
surgical, 393–394
steroid therapy for, 345–346, *346*
stretching exercises for, 296
total replacement of, 394
Ankylosing hyperostosis (Forestier's disease), 175–178. See also *Diffuse idiopathic skeletal hyperostosis (DISH).*
of some (AHS), 469–470
roentgenographic appearance of, 175, *175–177*
Ankylosis, interphalangeal, in erosive inflammatory osteoarthritis, 202
Annulus fibrosus, structure of, 476
Antibodies, 81
assays of, 85
classes of, 82
Antigenicity, of chondrocytes, 87–88
of collagen, 87
of proteoglycan, 86
Anti-inflammatory drugs, 320–323
adverse effects of, 321–322, 322t
types of, 321t
contraindications for, 322
in osteoarthritis, responses to, 21
nonsteroidal, dosage of, 321t
generic and trade names for, 321t
precautions for, 322
rationale for use of, 320–321
recent proliferation of, 322, 323t
role of, in etiology of osteoarthritis, 142
Antirheumatic drugs, 330
Apatite crystals, electron microscopic appearance of, *252*
Apatite crystal deposition disease, 251–253
secondary osteoarthritis in, 251–253, *252*
Aponeurosis, plantar, function of, 391, *392*
Apophysitis, in diagnosis of knee pain, 215–216

Aristocort Forte. See *Triamcinolone diacetate.*

Aristospan. See *Triamcinolone hexacetonide.*

Arteparon, in treatment of osteoarthritis, investigation of, 554, 556

Arthralgia, patellofemoral, 211. See also *Chondromalacia patellae.*

Arthritis, chronic infective, specific, differential diagnosis of, 283
  fungal, differential diagnosis of, 283
  gouty, of great toe, differential diagnosis of, 282, *282*
  psoriatic, differential diagnosis of, 283
  rheumatoid, differential diagnosis of, 283
  tuberculous, differential diagnosis of, 283

Arthrocentesis. See also *Steroid therapy, intraarticular.*
  nonsteroidal, 346–347
  of ankle, technique of, 345–346, *346*
  of elbow, technique of, 341–342, *342*
  of finger joints, technique of, 342–344
  of foot joints, technique of, 342–344
  of hip, technique of, 344–345, *344*
  of knee, technique of, 338–340, *339*
  of shoulder, technique of, 340–341
  of temporomandibular joint, technique of, 345, *345*

Arthrodesis, of carpometacarpal joints, 369
  of distal interphalangeal joint of hand, 365
  of elbow, 386
  of hip, 433–434
    conversion to total hip replacement of, 438
  of knee, 416–417, *417*
  of metatarsophalangeal joints, 400
  of proximal interphalangeal joint, 366
  of spine, in intervertebral disk disease, 514, *514*
  of subtalar joint, 395, *395*
  of talonavicular joint, 396
  of tarsometatarsal joints, 398
  of wrist, 374, *374, 375*
  role of, in osteoarthritis, 355
  trapeziometacarpal, 369

Arthro-ophthalmopathy, progressive hereditary (Stickler's syndrome), secondary osteoarthritis in, 247

Arthropathy, cuff tear, 379, *379*
  neuropathic, frequency of joints affected in, 170
    roentogenologic diagnosis of, 169, *170, 170–172, 171*
    vs. osteoarthritis, 170
  of rheumatic syndromes, differential diagnosis of, 282–284
  osteoarthritis-like, laboratory assessment of, 186t
  "steroid," 336

Arthroplasty, loosening as complication in, 356
  mold, of hip, 430–431
  of acromioclavicular joint, 384
  of distal interphalangeal joint of hand, 365
  of elbow, 386
  of hip, total. See *Hip joint, osteoarthritis of, total replacement in.*
  of knee, total, 414–416, *416*
    complications of, 415
    indications for, 415
    types of implants available for, 415
  of proximal interphalangeal joint, 366
  of trapeziometacarpal joint, 370, *371*
  role of, in osteoarthritis, 355–358
  unicompartmental, in osteoarthritis of knee, 413–414, *414*

Ascorbic acid, in treatment of osteoarthritis, 550–551

Ashworth-Blatt implant, 370

Aspirin, 319, 323–324
  adverse reactions to, 324
  dosage of, 323
  drug interactions with, 324
  in treatment of osteoarthritis, investigations of, 553
  pharmacokinetics of, 323
  therapeutic applications of, 323–324
  toxicity of, 319, 324

Athletes, incidence of osteoarthritis in, 15, 16, 563

Athletic injuries, secondary osteoarthritis due to, 257, 535

Atlantoaxial joint, osteoarthritis of, 452, *454, 455, 456*

Atrophy, cutaneous, as complication of steroid therapy, 336

Auricular stimulation, 293

Auto, grab bars for, 305, *306*

Autoimmunity, 86

Azolid. See *Phenylbutazone.*

B cells, 81

Back pain, lower, syndromes of, 473. See also *Low back pain.*

Bathtub seat, *305*

Betamethasone acetate, and disodium phosphate, dosage of, 337t

Biomaterial failure, in etiopathogenesis of osteoarthritis, 131–133

Biomechanics, in rehabilitative assessment, 288
  principles of, 289–290
  of foot and ankle, 389–391
  of hand, 97
  of joints, 93–107

Blacks, vs. whites and American Indians, incidence of osteoarthritis in, 10t, 19

Bladder, symptoms of, in intervertebral disk disease, 489

Blood, cellular constituents of, in osteoarthritis, 185
  laboratory values for, in osteoarthritis, 185–187

Bone, density of, correlation to osteoarthritis of, 16–17
  dysplasias of, secondary osteoarthritis in, 245–248
  fragments of, intra-articular injection of, in experimental models of osteoarthritis, 111
  infarct of, in femoral head, 40, *40*
  necrosis of, avascular (nonseptic), 40
  osteoarthritic, exposed surface of, histologic appearance of, 33, *33*
    subarticular, osteoblastic and osteoclastic activity in, 33, *33, 34, 35*
  remodeling of, mechanism of, 36
  subchondral, biomechanical aspects of, 100, *100*
    change in resilience of, 30
    microfractures of, in theory of etiology of osteoarthritis, 132
    trabecular microfractures in, 104

Bone scanning, in osteoarthritis, 194, *194*

Bouchard's nodes, as sign of osteoarthritis, 151, *152,* 201 365–367

Bouchard's osteoarthritis, 365–367

Bowleg deformity, as sign of osteoarthritis, *152*

Brushes, long-handled, *306*

Bruxism, in osteoarthritis of temporomandibular joint, 528

Bursa, trochanteric, steroid injection of, 345

Bursitis, anserine, steroid injection for, 340
    calcaneal, with spur, steroid injection for, 346
    of knee, diagnosis of, 215
    prepatellar, steroid injection for, 339–340
    suprapatellar, steroid injection for, 340
    trochanteric, steroid therapy for, 345

Butazolidin. See *Phenylbutazone.*

Button hook, *307*

Calcaneocuboid joint, function of, 390, *391*
    osteoarthritis of, 397

Calcification, capsular, as complication of steroid therapy, 336
    incidence of, in osteoarthritis, 22

Calcium, serum, in osteoarthritis, 185–186

Calcium crystal deposition diseases, secondary osteoarthritis in, 248–253

Calcium pyrophosphate, deposition of, 22
    in articular cartilage, 249, *250*
    in chondrocalcinosis, 137
    in knee, 281, *282*
    steroid injection for, 346

Calcium pyrophosphate deposition disease 248–251
    differential diagnosis of, 284
    laboratory assessment of, 186t
    secondary osteoarthritis in, 248–251

Cane(s), 304
    for osteoarthritis of hip, 427
    Lumex, *304*
    quad, *304*

Capsular changes, in late osteoarthritis, 36–37

Car, grab bars for, 305, *306*

Car door opener, 302, *303*

Carpal tunnel syndrome, occupational aspects of, 534

Carpometacarpal joint, first, osteoarthritis of, differential diagnosis of, 278–279
    roentgenogram of, in erosive inflammatory osteoarthritis, *202*
    steroid injection of, 342, *342*
    osteoarthritis of, 368–370
    pattern of involvement in, 18
    post-traumatic, 369
    signs of, 152
    treatment of, 369–370
    reduction of deforming force at, 290

Cartilage, articular, aging of, resistance wear in, 133
    atrophy of, in joint immobility, 44
    biochemical changes in, age-related, 13
    biochemical composition of, 45t
    biochemistry of, in osteoarthritis, 43–79
    biomechanical aspects of, 97–100
    changes in, in pathogenesis of osteoarthritis, 67–68
    chemical effects of aging on, 58–59
    chemistry of, 44–51
    collagen framework of, early changes in, 29–30
    crystal deposition in, 30
    degeneration of, cycle of changes in, *31*
    role of site in, 31
    degradation and repair of, in etiology of osteoarthritis, 133–135

Cartilage (*Continued*)
    articular, degradation enzymes of 30, 56–57, 134–135
    degradation rate of ³H glycine in, *54*
    destruction of, forms of, *32*
    in intermediate stage, 32–33
    physical forces and chondrocyte responses in, *130*
    fatigue failure in, age-related, 13
    focal defects in, in experimental models of osteoarthritis, 112–113
    freezing of, in experimental models of osteoarthritis, 113
    immature, biochemistry of, 57–59
    cell replication in, 58, *58*
    histologic appearance of, 57, *57*
    immunogenicity of, 86–88
    immunology of, 81–92
    in osteoarthritis, biochemical alterations in, 59–64
    loss of proteoglycans in, 61, *61*
    metabolism of, 51–57
    in osteoarthritis, 64–66
    degradative enzymes in, 66–67
    nutrition of, 43–44
    of hip, natural history of, 423
    patellar, blister lesion of, 219, *221*
    pathology of, 219–221
    shaving of, in chondromalacia patellae, 222
    stages in degeneration of, *220*
    repair of, role of cellular intervention in, 134
    mechanisms of, in etiology of osteoarthritis, 133–134
    scarification of, in experimental models of osteoarthritis, 113
    shearing damage to, 32
    splitting of, in intermediate stage, 32, *32*
    structural changes in, age-related, 13
    structure of, 97–100
    thinning of, by abrasion, 32, *33*
    bovine, therapeutic use of, 330
    homogenous, intra-articular injection of, in experimental models of osteoarthritis, 111

Cartilage-bone interface, disturbance at, in joint degeneration, 30

Cathepsin(s), in degradation of articular cartilage, 56, 67

Cauda equine syndrome, 488–489
    nerve root compression in, 488, *489*
    postoperative, 515

Cavalryman's disease, 340

Celestone Soluspan. See *Betamethasone acetate.*

Center-edge angle of Wiburg, 156

Cerebral palsy, athetoid, osteoarthritis of cervical spine in, 456, *456*

Ceruloplasmin, serum, in Wilson's disease, 186t, 187

Chair blocks, 305, *305*

Charcot joints (neuropathic arthropathy), 170, 253–254
    treatment of, 254

Cheilectomy, for hallux rigidus, 400, *400*

Chemonucleolysis, in intervertebral disk disease, 517–519

Chest pain, obscure, 470. See also *Thoracic pain.*

Chloroquine, in treatment of osteoarthritis, 552–553

Cholesterol, crystals of, in synovial fluid, 190

Chondrectomy, in chondromalacia patellae, 222

Chondrocalcinosis, calcium pyrophosphate dihydrate in, 137
    in generalized osteoarthritis, 205

Chondrocalcinosis (*Continued*)
  in incidence of osteoarthritis, 22
  of knee, *282*
  role of mineral deposits in, 139
Chondrocytes, antigenicity of, 87–88
  in proteoglycan synthesis, 51, *52*
  lysosomes in, 56, *56*
Chondrodysplasia punctata (Conradi's disease),
    secondary osteoarthritis in, 248
Chondroectodermal dysplasia, secondary osteoar-
    thritis in, 248
Chondroitin, sulfation of, metabolic pathway in,
    52, *54*
  synthesis of, metabolic pathways in, 52, *53*
Chondroitin sulfate, in articular cartilage, 46
  in osteoarthritis, concentrations of, 62, *62*
Chondroitin 4-sulfate, chemical structure of, *46*
Chondroitin 6-sulfate, chemical structure of, *46*
Chondromalacia patellae, 211–223
  arthrography in, 214–215
  clinical history in, 212
  conservative management of, 221
  definition of, 211
  diagnosis of, 212–219
  diagnostic arthroscopy in, 215
  differential diagnosis of, 215–219
  distal realignment in, 222
  lateral patellar release in, 222
  pathology of, 219–221
  physical examination in, 212–213
  post-traumatic, 217, *217*
  proximal realignment in, 222
  roentgenography in, 213–214, *213, 214*
  tibial tubercle elevation in, 223
  treatment of, 221–223
Chondronectin, in articular cartilage, 50
Chymopapain, injection of, intervertebral disk
    disease, 517–519
Claudication, neurogenic, in intervertebral disk
    disease, 488
Climate, as factor in osteoarthritis, 2
  in epidemiology of osteoarthritis, 18
Clinoril. See *Sulindac.*
Cold, therapeutic, 293
Collagen, antigenicity of, 87
  biochemical changes in, age-related, 13
  immune response to, in osteoarthritis, 90
  immunogenicity of, 87
  in articular cartilage, chemistry of, 49–50
    electron micrograph of, *49*
    in osteoarthritis, biochemistry of, 63–64
    synthesis of, 55–56
      in osteoarthritis, 66, *66*
      pathway of, *55*
  Type I, in cartilage, 50
  Type II, in cartilage, 50
Collagen framework, of cartilage, early changes
    in, 29–30
  tight and loose, in theory of etiology of osteoar-
    thritis, 132
Collagenase, in degradation of articular cartilage,
    57
  in synovial fluid, 192
Collar, cervical, *301*
  Philadelphia, *301*
Complement, in synovial fluid, 193
  serum, in osteoarthritis, 187
Compression-immobilization, in experimental
    models of osteoarthrititis, 117–119, *119*

Computerized axial tomography (CAT), in inter-
    vertebral disk disease, 498–500, *498–500*
Condylectomy, in osteoarthritis of temporoman-
    dibular joint, 529
Confidentiality, in doctor-patient relationship,
    545–546
Connective tissue diseases, hereditary, incidence
    of osteoarthritis in, 21
Conradi's disease, secondary osteoarthritis in, 248
Copper, in synovial fluid, 192
  serum, in Wilson's disease, 187t, 187
Coracoacromial ligament syndrome, 378
Corset, lumbosacral, *300*
Cortex, of bone, buttressing of, in osteoarthritis,
    163–164, *164*
Corticosteroids. See *Steroids.*
Costotransverse joints, anatomy of, 461
  diagnostic and therapeutic injection of, 466,
    467
  osteoarthritis of, 465–468
    clinical features of, 465–466
    management of, 466–468
      surgical, 468
    physical examination in, 466
Costovertebral joints, anatomy of, 461
  osteoarthritis of, 465–468
    clinical features of, 465–466
    management of, 466–468
      surgical, 468
    physical examination in, 466
Coxarthropathy, Postel's destructive, roentgeno-
    logic diagnosis of, 169, *169*
Coxarthrosis. See also *Hip joint, osteoarthritis of.*
  developmental hip abnormalities in, 266
  differential diagnosis of, 279–280
  epidemiology of, 265–266
  etiology of, 265–273
  immunologic mechanisms in, 270
  mechanical factors in, 266–269
  metabolic factors in, 269–270
  natural course of, 265–273
  racial incidence of, 266
  rehabilitative management of, 295
  systemic factors in, 270
Crepitus, as symptom of osteoarthritis, 151
Crutch(es), for osteoarthritic hip, 299–300, 427
  forearm, 304, *304*
Crystals, in synovial fluid, 190
Crystal deposition disease, differential diagnosis
    of, 283–284
Cuff tear arthropathy, 379, *379*
Cup arthroplasty, for hip, 430
Curbs, dropped, for ease of ambulation, 306
Cutaneous atrophy, as complication of steroid
    therapy, 336
Cyst(s), degenerative, roentgenologic appearance
    of, 160–162, *160–162*
  Egger's, of acetabulum, 162, *162*
  interphalangeal, as sign of osteoarthritis, 151
  mucoid (synovial), 200, *200*
  osteoarthritic, aspiration of, 364
  subarticular bone, 33, *34, 35*
  synovial, 200, *200*
Cytoplasmic inclusions, in synovial fluid, 189, *189*

Debridement, in osteoarthritis of knee, 408–409
  role of, in osteoarthritis, 354–355

Deformity, as factor in choice of therapy, 352
    as sign of osteoarthritis, 151, 152
Denervation, limb, in experimental models of
    osteoarthritis, 115
Depo-Medrol. See *Methylprednisolone acetate.*
de Quervain's disease, symptoms of, 152
Diabetes mellitus, and diffuse idiopathic skeletal
        hyperostosis (DISH), 231
    Charcot joints in, 253, *254*
    osteoarthritis in, 245
Diagnosis, differential, of osteoarthritis, 275–284
    laboratory, in osteoarthritis, 185–197
Diathermy, 292
Diet, role of, in etiology of osteoarthritis, 141–142
Diffuse idiopathic skeletal hyperostosis (DISH),
        225–233
    age and sex of patients with, 228t
    clinical features of, 227–230
    coexistent diseases with, 230
    diagnostic criteria for, 176, 226–227
    etiology of, 231–232
    genetic factors in, 231
    historical aspects of, 225
    iliac and sacroiliac osteophytosis in, *227*
    laboratory aspects of, 229–230
    manubriosternal excrescences in, *226*
    metabolic factors in, 231
    pathogenesis of, 231–232
    physical signs of, 229
    postsurgical ossification in, 230
    primary clinical clues to, 228t
    racial distribution of, 228t
    roentgenographic abnormalities in, 228,
        229, 456, 457
    special clinical problems of, 230
    spinal ankylosis in, *226*
    spinal ossification in, *226*
    symptoms of, 228, 228t
    synonyms for, 227t
    toxic factors in, 232
    treatment of, 230–231
Diflunisal, dosage of, 323
Disability, evaluation of, administrative law in-
        volving, 546–548
    by Social Security Administration, 546–548
Disk, intervertebral. See *Intervertebral disk.*
Diskectomy, and fusion, for osteoarthritis of cer-
        vical spine, 450, *452*
Diskography, in intervertebral disk disease, 501
Dislocation, patellar, in experimental models of
        osteoarthritis, 119–120
DNA, in articular cartilage, in osteoarthritis,
        59–60, *60*
    synthesis of, 66, *67*
Dolobid. See *Diflunisal.*
Door openers, 307, *308*
Drugs, adverse reactions to, in elderly, 318
    analgesic. See *Analgesic drugs.*
    anti-inflammatory. See *Anti-inflammatory
        drugs.*
    interactions of, in elderly, 318
Drug therapy, choice of drugs in, 318–319
    for elderly patients, 318
    outline of, 317t
    principles of, 317–332
Drug use, excessive, in etiology of osteoarthritis,
        142
Dysplasia, multiple epiphyseal, secondary os-
        teoarthritis in, 245–246

Dysplasia (*Continued*)
    spondyloepiphyseal (SED), secondary osteoar-
        thritis in, 246

Ehlers-Danlos syndrome, 242–243
    secondary osteoarthritis in, 242–243
Elbow, arthrodesis of, 386
    biomechanics of, 95
    design of, 95, *95*
    injury of, in baseball pitchers, 566
    osteoarthritis of, 384–386
        intra-articular steroid therapy for, 341–342
        secondary, 385
        treatment of, 385–386
    total replacement of, 386
Elderly patient, drug therapy for, 318
Electrical nerve stimulation, transcutaneous
        (TENS), 293
Electromyography, in intervertebral disk disease,
        500
Electrophoresis, rocket, 85
Ellis-van Creveld syndrome, secondary osteoar-
        thritis in, 248
Employment, of osteoarthritic worker, 536–540
Endocrine diseases, secondary osteoarthritis in,
        243–245
Energy, conservation of, recommendations for,
        311–312
Enthesopathies, spinal, roentgenologic diagnosis
        of, 175–181
Environmental design, for osteoarthritis patients,
        305–307
Enzymes, lysosomal, in synovial fluid, 192
    neuroregulatory, in synovial fluid, 192
    role of, in degradation of cartilage, 134–135
    synovial, in etiology of osteoarthritis, 136
Epidemiology, of coxarthrosis, 265–266
    of osteoarthritis, 1–2, 9–27
        heredity in, 19–21
        history and methods in, 9–10
        protective factors in, 22–23
        systemic factors in, 17–18
Epiphyses, diseases involving, secondary osteoar-
        thritis in, 247–248
Erythrocyte sedimentation rate (ESR), in os-
        teoarthritis, 185
Esophagus, impingement of, by osteophytosis,
        456, *457*
Estradiol, in treatment of osteoarthritis, 551
Estrogens, role of, in etiology of osteoarthritis,
        141
    in incidence of osteoarthritis, 14
    in treatment of osteoarthritis, 551
Ethnic groups, epidemiology of osteoarthritis in,
        10, 10t, 19
Ethoheptazine citrate, 319
Etiologic agent, definition of, 129
Etiology, of osteoarthritis, 155
Etiopathogenesis, of osteoarthritis, 129–146
    factors in, *130, 131*
    hypothesis of, 129–130, *130*
    interrelationships of factors in, *131*
Excessive lateral pressure syndrome (ELPS), of
        knee, 217–218, *218*
Exercise(s), active vs. passive, 294
    and osteoarthritis, 561–568
    effect on injured joints of, 564–566

Exercise(s) (*Continued*)
  effect on uninjured joints of, 563–564
  excessive, signs of, 295
  for flexion deformity of knee, 408
  isokinetic (dynamic), 294
  isometric, 294
    for osteoarthritis of knee, 407–408
  isotonic, 294
  response of musculoskeletal system to, 562–563
  strengthening, 295
  stretching, 294
  therapeutic, 294–297
Experimental models of osteoarthritis, 109–128
  alteration of joint forces in, 113–115
  compression-immobilization in, 117–119, *119*
  degenerative changes after release of joint contact in, 116–117
  endocrine manipulation in, 110–111
  immobilization in, 117–119
  induction of focal cartilage defects in, 112–113
  joint injections in, 111–112
  limb denervation in, 115
  meniscectomy in, 122–124
    degenerative changes following, *122–124*
  metabolic manipulation in, 110–111
  section of cruciate ligaments in, 120–121, *121*
  spontaneously occurring, 115–116
  surgical manipulation of joints in, 124–126
Experimentation, human, legal aspects of, 543–545

Farmers, incidence of osteoarthritis in, 15
Fasciitis, plantar, steroid injection for, 346
Fatigue, avoidance of, recommendations for, 312
Fatigue failure, in collagen framework damage, 29
Feldens. See *Pyroxicam.*
Felsenreich's sign, in athletes, 564
Femoral hemiarthroplasty, for osteoarthritis of hip, 433
Femur, erosion of cortex of, in osteoarthritis of knee, 167, *167, 168*
  head of. See also *Hip joint.*
    aseptic necrosis of, osteoarthritis due to, 258
    bone infarct in, 40, *40*
    bone remodeling in, *36*
    deformity of, in Perthes' disease, *268*
    destructive loss of bony height in, *36*
    giant "cysts" of, roentgenologic appearance of, *161*
    hemiarthroplasty for, 433
    roentgenologic appearance of, 158
    subarticular bone cyst in, *35*
    "tilt" deformity of, *268*
  neck of, cortical buttressing of, 163–164, *164*
Fenoprofen calcium, 319, 328
  adverse effects of, 328
  dosage of, 321t, 328
  drug interactions with, 328–329
Ferrokinetics, serum, in osteoarthritis, 186
Fibrillation, of articular cartilage, in intermediate stage, 32, *32*
  in senescent joint, roentgenologic appearance of, *157*
Fibrinogen, in synovial fluid, 192
Filipin, intra-articular injection of, in experimental models of osteoarthritis, 112

Fingers. See also specific joints.
  joints of, steroid therapy for, 342–344
    interphalangeal, osteoarthritis of, differential diagnosis of, 277–278
  osteoarthritis of, 363–368
Foot, and ankle, anatomic aspects of, 389–391
  biomechanics of, 389–391
  osteoarthritis of, 389–402
    diagnosis of, 391
      primary vs. secondary, 391
  biomechanics of, 96
  joints of, section of, in walking, *98*
    location of axes of, *97*
    steroid therapy for, 342–344, 346
  misalignment in, effect on other joints of, 290
  orthoses for, 297–299
  pressure distribution in, 96
  strengthening exercises for, 296
  stretching exercises for, 296
Foraminotomy, *512, 513*
Forearm crutch, 304, *304*
Forefoot, orthoses for, 297–299
Forestier's disease (ankylosing hyperostosis), 175–178
  roentgenographic appearance of, 175, *175–177*
Fractures, in etiology of neuropathic arthropathy, 171
Frostbite, 257
  secondary osteoarthritis due to, 257, *258*
Fusion (arthrodesis), role of, in oseoarthritis, 355. See also *Arthrodesis.*

Gaucher's disease, 240
  diagnosis of, 240
  roentgenographic changes in, 240
  secondary osteoarthritis in, 240
Genu valgum, 410
  femoral osteotomy for, 411, *411*
  tibial osteotomy for, 413
Genu varum, abnormal stress due to, 404
  as sign of osteoarthritis, 151, *152*
  barrel-vault osteotomy for, 411, *412*
  closing wedge osteotomy for, 411, *411*
  progression of osteoarthritis in, 404
  tibial osteotomy for, 410, *410, 411*
Girdlestone hip procedure, conversion to total hip replacement of, 438
Glenohumeral joint, Neer replacement of, 380
  osteoarthritis of, 379–384
    treatment of, 380–382
      surgical, 380–382
Glenoid, replacement of, 381, *381*
Glucosamine sulfate, in treatment of osteoarthritis, investigation of, 556
Glucose, serum, in osteoarthritis, 185
Glycolysis, and energy production, in articular cartilage, 51
Glycoprotein, in articular cartilage, 51
Glycosaminoglycans, in articular cartilage, 46
  chemical structure of, *46*
Glycosaminoglycan chains, sulfation of, metabolic pathway for, *54*
Gold, radioactive, intra-articular injection of, 347
"Golfer's boss," 368
Goniometry, in rehabilitative assessment, 288
Gout, differential diagnosis of, 283–284
  of great toe, differential diagnosis of, 282

Growth hormone, in treatment of osteoarthritis, 551
  role of, in etiology of secondary osteoarthritis, 140–141

Hallux rigidus, cheilectomy for, 400, *400*
Hammer toe, 401
  repair of, technique of, 401, *402*
Hand. See also specific joints.
  and wrist, osteoarthritis of, 363–376
  biomechanics of, 97
    osteoarthritis of, erosive, roentgenogram of, *203*
    in textile workers, 534
    positioning for, 297
    splints for, 301–302
  stretching exercises for, 297
Heat, deep, therapeutic use of, 292–293
  moist, 292
  superficial, therapeutic use of, 292
  therapeutic, 291–293
    methods of application of, 292t
Heberden, William, 199
Heberden's nodes, 199, 363–365
  as sign of osteoarthritis, 151, *152*
  excision of, 364
  hereditary occurrence of, 20
  roentgenographic appearance of, *364*
  steroid injection of, 343
  treatment of, 364–365
Heel, SACH, 393
Heel spurs, steroid injection for, 346
Hemiarthroplasty, femoral, for osteoarthritis of hip, 433
    conversion to total hip replacement of, 438
  role of, in osteoarthritis, 356
Hemochromatosis, 235–237
  laboratory assessment of, 186t
  phalangeal joint enlargement in, *236*
  roentgenogram of hands in, *236, 237*
  secondary osteoarthritis in, 235–237
  synovial histology in, 194
  treatment of, 236–237
Hemoglobinopathies, secondary osteoarthritis in, 240–242
Hepatolenticular degeneration. See *Wilson's disease.*
Heredity, in incidence of osteoarthritis, 19–21
  animal studies of, 20–21
Heuter-Volkmann principle, 424
Hip joint. See also *Femur, head of.*
  arthroplasty of, roentgenogram of, *357, 358*
  articular cartilage of, natural history of, 423
  assistive devices for, 299–300
  avascular necrosis of, 279, *280*
  axial migration of, roentgenologic appearance of, *159*
  biomechanical forces acting on, 427, *428*
  biomechanical reduction of pain in, 290
  biomechanics of, 94
  developmental abnormalities of, coxarthrosis in, 266–269
  "destructive coxarthropathy" of, roentgenologic diagnosis of, 169, *169*
  displacement of, by osteophyte, roentgenologic appearance of, *159*
  dysplasia of, measurement of, *267*
    congenital, coxarthrosis in, 266–269
  general design of, 94

Hip joint (*Continued*)
  joint space narrowing in, as roentgenologic sign of osteoarthritis, 156–158
  mold arthroplasty for, 430–431
  muscle forces around, *94*
  normal, biomechanical homeostasis of, 423–424
    increased forces on, 269
  osteoarthritis of, 423–442. See also *Coxarthrosis.*
    abnormal stress in, 424–425
    advanced stage of, 425–426
    arthrodesis for, 433–434
    articular surface repair in, 37, *38*
    assistive devices for, 427
    clinical manifestations of, 425–426
    differential diagnosis of, 279–280
    early stages of, 425
    etiology of, 423
    femoral hemiarthroplasty for, 433
    intermediate stage of, 425
    management of, 426–440
      influence of osteoarthritic process on, 426
      nonoperative, 426–427
      patient factors in, 426
      surgical, 427–440
        choice of, 428, 440
        feasibility of, 428, *429*
        indications for, 427–429, *430*
        patient factors in, 429
        procedures for, 430–440
        role of, 427
    medications for, 426–427
    natural history of, 424
    occupational aspects of, 534
    osteotomy for, 431–433, *431*
    physical therapy for, 427
    positioning for, 295
    rehabilitative management of, 295
    rest and activity in, 427
    roentgenographic appearance of, *153*
    roentgenologic evaluation of, *163*
    secondary, 39
      incidence of pre-existing conditions in, 156t
      pathogenesis of, 39
    symptoms of, 153
    synovial changes in, 37
    total hip replacement in, 434–438, *435*
      complications in, 434
        pathophysiologic factors in, 436
      conventional, 434–438, *435*
        vs. resurfacing, *435*
      conversion of arthrodesis to, 438
      conversion of Girdlestone procedure to, 438
      conversion of hemiarthropathy to, 438
      dislocation in, 437
      failures in, 356
      heterotopic bone in, 437
      medical complications in, 437–438
      operative revision in, 438
      nerve palsy in, 437
      prosthetic design and materials for, 434–435
      sepsis in, 436
      trochanteric problems in, 437
    weight reduction in, 427
  osteonecrosis of, roentgenogram of, *358*
  periarticular pain points in, steroid injection of, 345

Hip joint (*Continued*)
  resurfacing of, *435,* 439–440
    complications in, 439
  steroid therapy for, 344–345
  strengthening exercises for, 295
  stretching exercises for, 295
  structural changes in, osteoarthritis in, 425
HLA, association of, with diffuse idiopathic skeletal hyperostosis (DISH), 231
Hormones, gonadotropic, in incidence of osteoarthritis, 14
  growth, in incidence of osteoarthritis, 14
  in treatment of osteoarthritis, 551–552
  role of, in etiology of secondary osteoarthritis, 140–141
  sex, role of, in prevalence of osteoarthritis, 14
"Housemaid's knee," 339
Hubbard tank, in hydrotherapy, 292
Humeroradial joint, design of, *95*
Humeroulnar joint, design of, *95*
  steroid injection into, 341–342, *342*
Humerus, head of, replacement of, 381, *381*
Hyaluronate, in articular cartilage, 47
  in osteoarthritis, 63
  in joint lubrication, 101
Hyaluronate therapy, intra-articular, 347
Hyaluronic acid, as lubricant in osteoarthritis, 555
  chemical structure of, 46
Hyaluronidase, in degradation of articular cartilage, 56
  in synovial fluid, 192
Hydeltra-TBA. See *Prednisolone tebutate.*
Hydrocortisone tebutate, dosage of, 337t
Hydrocortone-TBA. See *Hydrocortisone tebutate.*
Hydrotherapy, Hubbard tank in, 292
Hydroxyapatite, possible role of, in etiology of osteoarthritis, 137–138
  hypothetical scheme of, *138*
Hydroxyapatite crystals, in osteoarthritis, steroid injection for, 346
Hydroxyproline, in synovial fluid, 193
Hyperglycemia, in osteoarthritis, 185
Hypermobility joint, in incidence of osteoarthritis, 14–15
Hyperostosis, ankylosing. See *Diffuse idiopathic skeletal hyperostosis (DISH).*
Hyperparathyroidism, secondary osteoarthritis in, 244–245
Hypertension, correlation to osteoarthritis of, 18
Hypothyroidism, secondary osteoarthritis in, 244

Ibuprofen, 319, 238
  adverse effects of, 328
  dosage of 321t, 328
  drug interactions with, 328–329
Immobilization, in experimental models of osteoarthritis, 117–119
Immune response, 83–85
  antibody-mediated, outline of, *84*
  cell-mediated, outline of, *84*
  in osteoarthritis, demonstration of, 89–90
  origins of, *82*
  roles of, in etiology of osteoarthritis, 136–137
Immune system, characteristics of, 82t, *84*
Immunity, cell-mediated, characteristics of, 82t, *84*
  in osteoarthritis, 187
  in vitro tests of, 85

Immunity (*Continued*)
  humoral, characteristics of, 82t, *84*
    in osteoarthritis, 187
    in vitro tests of, 85
  role of, in osteoarthritis, 88–90
Immunobiology, principles of, 81–85
Immunodiffusion, Ouchterlony method of, 85, *85*
  single radial, 85
Immunoelectrophoresis, 85, *85*
Immunofluorescence, 85
Immunogenicity, of cartilage, 86–88
Immunoglobulins, 81
  structure of, 82, *83*
Immunology, laboratory studies of, in osteoarthritis, 187
  of articular cartilage, 81–92
  of synovial fluid, 192–193
Impingement syndrome, 378–379
  treatment of, 378–379
Indians, American, incidence of osteoarthritis in, 10t, 19
Indocin. See *Indomethacin.*
Indomethacin, 325–326
  dosage of, 321t, 326
  drug interactions with, 326
  side effects of, 326
  therapeutic application of, 325–326
Infection, as complication of steroid therapy, 335
Inflammation, and osteoarthritis, relationships of, 21–22
  synovial enzymes due to, in etiology of osteoarthritis, 136
Inflammatory response, in osteoarthritis, 88
  in synovial membrane, 88, *88*
Informed consent, and doctor-patient relationship, 542–543
  recording of, 542
  role of family or guardian in, 543
  statutes dealing with, 543
Injections, intra-articular, nonsteroidal, 346–347
  osteoarthritis due to, 259
  steroid. See *Steroid therapy, intra-articular.*
  local, for pain relief, 294
Intercarpal joint, arthrodesis of, 374, *375*
Intercostal nerves, anatomy of, 461–462
Intercostal neuralgia, 470
Interphalangeal joints, distal, of hand, arthrodesis for, 365
    arthroplasty for, 365
    osteoarthritis of, 363–365
      differential diagnosis of, 277–278
      roentgenographic appearance of, *364*
      treatment of, 364–365
    secondary osteoarthritis of, 363
  of hand, osteoarthritis of, definition of, 200
    pattern of involvement in, 18
    signs of, 151
    steroid injection of, 342–343, *343*
  of toes, osteoarthritis of, 401–402
    treatment of, 401–402
  proximal, of hand, osteoarthritis of, 365–367
    differential diagnosis of, 278–279
    roentgenographic appearance of, 365, *366*
    treatment of, 365–367
    secondary osteoarthritis of, 365
    treatment of, 367
Intertarsal joints, function of, 391
  osteoarthritis of, 397

Intervertebral disk(s), anatomy of, 475
  cervical, herniation of, 444, *448, 449*
  degeneration of, 476, *476*
    clinical syndromes of, 482–489
    vacuum phenomenon in, 478, *478*
  degenerative disease of. See *Intervertebral disk disease.*
  herniation of, 478–479, *480, 481*
    CAT scan of, *498*
    in cauda equina syndrome, 488, *489*
    myelogram of, *495, 496*
    surgical technique for, 507–514, *508–514*
  lumbar, degenerative disease of, 473–521
    natural history of, 474–475
    pathology of, 475–482
    role of surgery in, 475
    spinal stenosis in, 479–482
  osteophytosis of, 476, *477*
  thoracic, prolapse of, 469
Intervertebral disk disease, arthrodesis for, 514, *514*
  bladder symptoms in, 489
  cauda equina syndrome in, 488, *489*
  chemonucleolysis in, 517
  diagnostic studies in, 494–501
  general examination in, 494
  industrial aspects of, 535
  leg pain in, 486
  motor symptoms in, 487–488, 491
  neurogenic claudication in, 488
  neurologic examination in, 490–494
  palpation in, 489–490
  physical examination in, 489–490
  posture in, 486, *487*, 490
  radicular symptoms in, 486
  referred pain in, 485–486
  reflex changes in, 491
  sensory changes in, 491
  tension signs in, 491, *492, 493*
  treatment of, 501–519
    algorithm for, 501, *502–503*
    nonsurgical, 501
    surgical, 505–517
      choice of operation in, 506–507
      complications of, 514–517
      results of, 517
      selection of patient for, 505–506
      technique in, 507–514
Iron, serum, in osteoarthritis, 186
  synovial deposition of, in hemochromatosis, 236

Joint(s). See also specific joints.
  anatomic changes in, with aging, 12–14
  anatomy of, 97–102
  biomechanics of, 93–107
  boundary lubrication of, *102*
  composition of, 97–102
  destruction of, early-stage, roentgenologic appearance of, 158
    late-stage, roentgenologic appearance of, 159–160, *160*
    stages of, 162t
  effect of abnormal biomechanical stresses on, 104
  effect of exercise on, 562
  enlargement of, as sign of osteoarthritis, 151

Joint(s) (*Continued*)
  function of, as factor in choice of therapy, 352
    effect of wear and tear on, 102–103
  general design of, 93–97
  hyperlaxity of, in incidence of osteoarthritis, 14–15
  hypermobility of, in Ehlers-Danlos syndrome, 242, *242*
    without Ehlers-Danlos syndrome, 243
  injured, effect of exercise on, 564–566
  interphalangeal. See *Interphalangeal joints.*
  lubrication of, 101–102
  most frequent involvement of, in osteoarthritis, 149, 164
  multiple involvement of, in osteoarthritis, patterns of, 18–19
    roentgenologic diagnosis of, 164–165, *165*
  protection of, patient education for, 308
    recommendations for, 311–312
  range of motion in, as factor in choice of therapy, 352
    limitation of, as symptom of osteoarthritis, 151
  release of contact in, in experimental models, 116–117
  repair of, 103–104
    early-stage, roentgenologic appearance of, 158–159, *159*
    late-stage, roentgenologic appearance of, 162–163
    stages of, 162t
  senescent vs. osteoarthritic, roentgenologic diagnosis of, 157, *157*
  shock-absorbing mechanisms of, 103
  specific, age correlation of osteoarthritis in, 12
  stiffness of, as symptoms of osteoarthritis, 151
  surgical manipulation of, in experimental models of osteoarthritis, 124–126
  total reconstruction of, role of, in osteoarthritis, 356
  typical structure of, *99*
  uninjured, effects of exercise on, 563–564
Joint disease, inflammatory, of nonspecific etiology, differential diagnosis of, 283
Joint scanning, radionuclide, in osteoarthritis, 194
Joint space narrowing, as roentgenologic sign of osteoarthritis, 156–158

Kashin-Beck disease, secondary osteoarthritis in, 248
Kayser-Fleischer ring, in Wilson's disease, 237
Kenalog-40. See *Triamcinolone acetonide.*
Keratan sulfate, chemical structure of, *46*
  in articular cartilage, 46
  in osteoarthritis, concentrations of, 62, *62*
Key ignition piece, *303*
Kienböck's disease, 371
  osteoarthritis following, *372*
  treatment of, 372
Knee. See also *Patella* and *Chondromalacia patellae.*
  arthroplasty of, total, 414–416, *416*
    contraindications for, 415
    failures in, 356
    indications for, 415
    types of implants available for, 415
  biomechanics of, 95

Knee (*Continued*)
  bracing for, 299
    hinged, *299*
  "carpet cutter's," 339
  design of, 95, *95, 96*
  excessive lateral pressure syndrome (ELPS) of, 217–218, *218*
  flexion deformity of, 404
    exercises for, 408
    osteoarthritis in, 408
  flexion of, patellofemoral joint contact range in, *214*
  "housemaid's," 339
  injury of anterior cruciate ligament of, 565
  intra-articular steroid therapy for, 338–340
  malalignment of, 216–217
    roentgenogram of, *216*
  meniscectomy in, in experimental animal models, 122–124
  "nun's," 339
  orthoses for, 299
  osteoarthritis of, 403–421
    arthrodesis in, 416–417, *417*
    biomechanics of, 403–404
    clinical examination in, 405–406
    debridement in, 408–409
    differential diagnosis of, 280–281
    erosion of femoral cortex in, 167, *167, 168*
    form for evaluation of function in, *352*
    history and symptoms of, 404–405
    incidence of, 10
    isometric exercises for, 407–408
    joint narrowing in, 166
    loose bodies in, 409
    osteophyte repair in, *166*
    osteotomy in, 409–413
    positioning for, 296
    rehabilitative management of, 295–296
    roentgenologic diagnosis of, 165–168, 406, *406, 407*
    symptoms of, 152
    treatment of, 407–419
      nonoperative, 407–408
      operative, 408–419
        results in, 413
    unicompartmental, arthroplasty in, 413–414, *414*
  osteophytes in, excision of, 409
  periarthritis of, steroid injection for, 340
  reflex sympathetic dystrophy of, 218–219, *219*
    thermography in, 219, *220*
  section of cruciate ligaments in, in experimental animal models, 120–121
  stretching exercises for, 296
  synovial osteochondromatosis of, *281*
  trauma of, in chondromalacia patellae, 212
  valgus deformity of, femoral osteotomy for, 411, *411*
    tibial osteotomy for, 413
  varus deformity of, barrel-vault osteotomy for, 411, *412*
    closing wedge osteotomy for, 411, *411*
    tibial osteotomy for, 410, *410, 411*
Knee cap, "squinting," 212
Knee cage, Swedish, *299*
Kniest syndrome, secondary osteoarthritis in, 247

Laboratory findings, in osteoarthritis, 185–197
Lactic dehydrogenase, in synovial fluid, 191

"Lamina splendens," 43, *44*
Lasegue test, in intervertebral disk herniation, *492*, 493
Leg(s), length discrepancies in, orthoses for, 298–299
Leg pain, in degenerative disk disease 486
Legal aspects, of osteoarthritis, 541–548
Leukocytes, in synovial fluid, 189
Ligament(s), anterior cruciate, of knee, injury of, 565
  cruciate, section of, in experimental animal models, 120–121, *121*
  of vertebral arch, ossification of (OVAL), 180–181, *179–181*
  posterior longitudinal, ossification of (OPLL), 178, *179*
  role of, in joint function, 100–101
Limb denervation, in experimental models of osteoarthritis, 115
Limbus vertebra, *477, 478*
Link proteins, in articular cartilage, 47
Lipids, in articular cartilage, 50
  in synovial fluid, 191
Lipoproteins, in synovial fluid, 191
Low back pain, 484–485
  industrial aspects of, 535
  syndromes of, 473
    incidence of, 473–474
Lower extremity, mechanical axis vs. anatomical axis in, 404, *405*
Lubrication, intra-articular, in treatment of osteoarthritis, 555–556
  mechanism of, 101–102
Lumbar disk disease. See *Intervertebral disk disease.*
Lumex cane, *304*
Lunate, aseptic necrosis of (Kienböck's disease), 371
  dislocation of, unreduced, osteoarthritis following, *374*
Lupus erythematosus, systemic (SLE), differential diagnosis of, 283
Lymphokines, role of, in osteoarthritis, 89
Lysosomes, in chondrocytes, 56, *56*
Lysozyme, in articular cartilage, 51
  in synovial fluid, 192

Mafucci's syndrome, secondary osteoarthritis in, 248
Mallet toe, 401
Mandibular condyle, histologic appearance of, *523*
  polytomogram of, *527*
  remodeling of, biologic basis of, 523–525, *524, 525*
Massage, 294
Mechanical factors, in incidence of osteoarthritis, 14–17
Mechanical overuse, in incidence of osteoarthritis, 15–16
Meclofenamate sodium, 329
  dosage of, 321t, 329
  drug interactions with, 329
  precautions for, 329
  therapeutic role for, 329
Meclomen. See *Meclofenamate sodium.*
Meniscectomy, degenerative changes following, 565
  for meniscal tears, 409

Meniscectomy (*Continued*)
  in experimental models of osteoarthritis, 122–124
    degenerative changes following, *122–124*
Meniscus, displacement of, in temporomandibular joint, 527, *528*
  role of, in joint function, 101
Metabolic diseases, secondary osteoarthritis in, 235–243
Metabolism, role of, in etiology of osteoarthritis, 142
"Metacarpal boss," 368
Metacarpal-hamate joint, post-traumatic osteoarthritis of, 369
Metacarpal-trapezial joint, osteoarthritis of, 369
Metacarpophalangeal joints, osteoarthritis of, 367–368
  treatment of, 368
Metatarsal bar, *298*
Metatarsal pads, *298*
Metatarsocuneiform joints, osteoarthritis of, 398
Metatarsophalangeal joint(s), arthrodesis of, 400
  function of, 391
  of great toe, osteoarthritis of, differential diagnosis of, 281–282
    roentgenogram of, *399*
  osteoarthritis of, 398–401
    differential diagnosis of, 399
    pattern of involvement in, 18
    treatment of, 399–401
      surgical, 400–401
  steroid injection of, 343–344, *343*
  tuberculous infection of, *284*
Methylprednisolone acetate, dosage of, 337t
Midtarsal joints, function of, 391
  osteoarthritis of, 397
Milwaukee shoulder, 253
"Milwaukee shoulder" syndrome, role of synovial enzymes in, 136
Miners, incidence of osteoarthritis in, 15
Mineral salts, possible role of, in etiology of osteoarthritis, 137–139
Mold arthroplasty, of hip, 430–431
Moniliform hyperostosis. See *Diffuse idiopathic skeletal hyperostosis (DISH)*.
Motrin. See *Ibuprofen*.
Mucin, in synovial fluid, 189
Mucoid (synovial) cyst, 200, *200*
Multiple epiphyseal dysplasia (MED), secondary osteoarthritis in, 245–246
Muscles, atrophy of, as sign of osteoarthritis, 151
Muscle spasm, in altered joint kinematics, 290
Muscle strength, in maintaining joint alignment, 290
Muscle strength testing, in rehabilitative assessment, 288
Muscle strengthening, recommendations for, 311
Myelography, in intervertebral disk disease, 495, *495, 496, 497*

Nail-patella syndrome (osteo-onychodystrophy), secondary osteoarthritis in, 246–247
Nalfon. See *Fenoprofen calcium*.
Naprosyn. See *Naproxen*.
Naproxen, 328
  adverse effects of, 328
  dosage of, 321t, 328
  drug interactions with, 328–329

Naproxen sodium, 319
Narcotic drugs. See *Analgesic drugs, centrally acting*.
Neck. See also *Spine, cervical*.
  osteoarthritis of, positioning for, 296
    rehabilitative management of, 296
  pain in, in osteoarthritis of spine, 444
  strengthening exercises for, 296
Neer glenohumeral joint replacement, 380
Nerve(s), intercostal, anatomy of, 461–462
  sectioning of, in experimental models of osteoarthritis, 115
  thoracic, anatomy of, 461–462
Nerve roots, compression of, in cauda equina syndrome, 488, *489*
  thoracic, anatomy of, 461–462
Nervous system, autonomic, anatomy of, 462
Neuralgia, intercostal, 470
Neuropathic arthropathy (Charcot joints), 253–254
  secondary osteoarthritis in, 253–254
  treatment of, 254
Nuremberg Code, human experimentation and, 544

Obesity, 256–257
  as factor in osteoarthritis, 2
  correlation to osteoarthritis of, 17
  in osteoarthritis of knee, 408
  secondary osteoarthritis in, 256–257
Occupation, as factor in osteoarthritis, 2, 15–16
Ochronosis, 238–240
  alkaptonuric, 64
  blackened knee meniscus in, *239*
  cartilage embedded in synovium in, *239*
  intervertebral disk ossification in, *239*
  laboratory assessment of, 186t
  secondary osteoarthritis in, 238–240
  synovial histology in, 194
  treatment of, 239
OPLL (ossification of posterior longitudinal ligament), 456, *458*
Orgotein, in treatment of osteoarthritis, 549
Orthoses, and assistive devices, 297–305
  ankle, 393, *393*
  lower-extremity, 297–301
  upper-extremity, 301–302
Osgood-Schlatter disease, 216
Osmic acid, intra-articular injection of, 347
Ossification, of posterior longitudinal ligament (OPLL), 178
  roentgenologic appearance of, *179*
  of vertebral arch ligaments (OVAL), 180–181, *179–181*
Osteitis deformans. See *Paget's disease*.
Osteoarthritis, and osteonecrosis, roentgenologic diagnosis of, 168–169, *169*
  articular surface repair in, 37–39
  as occupational illness, 533
  classification of, 2, 3t
    in Atlas of Standard Radiographs, 9
  definition of, 2, 129
  diagnosis of, introduction to, 3–4
  differential diagnosis of, 275–284
    difficult examples in, 276–277
  drug therapy for. See *Drug therapy* and names of specific drugs.

Osteoarthritis (*Continued*)
epidemiology of, 1–2, 9–27. See also *Epidemiology, of osteoarthritis.*
erosive inflammatory, 201–204
etiologic theories of, 139–140
interphalangeal joints in, 201, *201*
prognosis in, 206
treatment of, 206–207
etiology of, 155
etiopathogenesis of. See *Etiopathogenesis.*
experimental models. See *Experimental models of osteoarthritis.*
general prevalence of, 10–11
"generalized," definition of, 10
hereditary aspects of, 20
pattern of joint involvement in, 18–19
histologic-histochemical grading system for, 62t
industrial considerations of, 533–540
intermediate stage of, pathologic changes in, 31–33
interphalangeal, definition of, 200
laboratory findings in, 185–197
late stage of, pathologic changes in, 33–37
location of, correlation of pathogenetic factors to, 23t
mechanical factors in, 14–17
medicolegal considerations of, 541–548
morphologic changes in, correlation with clinical features of, 40
myths about, 1
of hip. See *Coxarthrosis* and *Hip joint, osteoarthritis of.*
of spine, 443–521. See also *Spine, osteoarthritis of.*
pathogenesis of, biochemical, 67–68
stages of, 162t
pathology of, 2–3, 29–42. See also *Pathology.*
pathophysiology of, aging and, 12–14
preclinical stage of, 29–31
pathologic changes in, 29–31
primary, vs. secondary, 2
definition of, 129
roentgenologic diagnosis of, 155–156
primary generalized, 204–207
definition of, 199
differential diagnosis of, 205
etiologic theories of, 139–140
prognosis in, 206
treatment of, 206–207
regional, differential diagnosis of, 277–282
rehabilitation in, 287–315
research in, 4–5
roentgenologic characteristics of, 156–165
roentgenologic diagnosis of, 155–184
roentgenologic grading system for, 9
role of immunity in, 88–90
role of surgery in, 351–359
secondary, 235–264
causes of, 39t
etiology of, 140–142, 141t
mechanical factors in, 257–259
occupational aspects of, 257
pathology of, 39–40
symptoms and signs of, 149–154, 150t, 151t
spontaneously occurring, in animal models, 115–116
treatment of, experimental models of, 549–559
introduction to, 4
worker with, 533–536

Osteoarthritis (*Continued*)
worker with, architectural barriers to, 537
employment of, 536–540
Osteoarthropathy, hypertrophic pulmonary, 280, *282*
Osteoarthrosis. See *Osteoarthritis.*
Osteochondritis, in metatarsal head, roentgenogram of, *399*
Osteochondritis dissecans, 280, *281*
Osteochondromatosis, of elbow, 385
synovial, of knee, *281*
Osteochondrophytes, in osteoarthritic process, 2
Osteonecrosis, and osteoarthritis, roentgenologic diagnosis of, 168–169, *169*
Osteo-onychodystrophy (nail-patella syndrome), secondary osteoarthritis in, 246–247
Osteopetrosis, 255–256
secondary osteoarthritis in, 255–256
Osteophytes, excision of, in osteoarthritis of proximal interphalangeal joints, 365–366
in generalized osteoarthritis, 205
in osteoarthritic process, 2
on femoral head, in senescent joint, roentgenologic appearance of, *157*
Osteophytosis, significance of, 35
Osteoporosis, incidence of coxarthrosis in, 269
Osteosclerosis, with cysts, in subarticular bone, 33, *34, 35*
Osteotomy, articular surface repair following, 37, *38*
in osteoarthritis of hip, 37, 431–433, *431*
indications for, 432
results of, 432
in osteoarthritis of knee, 409–413
indications for, 419
role of, in osteoarthritis, 354
Ouchterlony immunodiffusion method, *85, 85*
Oxalid. See *Oxyphenbutazone.*
Oxyphenbutazone, 324–325
dosage of, 321t
drug interactions with, 325
side effects of, 325
therapeutic limitations of, 325

Paget's disease (osteitis deformans), 255
secondary osteoarthritis in, 255
serum alkaline phosphatase in, 186
treatment of, 255
Pain, abdominal, obscure, 470
as factor in choice of therapy, 351, *352*
as potentiator of joint abnormalities, 290
as symptom of osteoarthritis, 150
as symptom of hip osteoarthritis, 153
as symptom of knee osteoarthritis, 152
as symptom of spinal osteoarthritis, 153
assessment of, in rehabilitative evaluation, 289
control of, specific recommendations for, 310–311
in chest, obscure, 470
in leg, in degenerative disk disease, 486
in lower back, syndromes of, 473. See also *Low back pain.*
in osteoarthritis of cervical spine, 444
on passive motion, as sign of osteoarthritis, 151
referred, in degenerative disk disease, 485–486
root and nerve, in thoracic spine, 463
thoracic, 462–463
differential diagnosis of, 468–471

Pain (*Continued*)
   thoracic, intrinsic (somatic) spinal, 462
     referred somatic, 462–463
     referred visceral, 463
Pantothenic acid, in treatment of osteoarthritis, investigation of, 556
Papain, intra-articular injection of, in experimental models of osteoarthritis, 111
Paraffin wax, hot, as hand bath, 292
Patella. See also *Chondromalacia patellae.*
   dislocation of, in experimental models of osteoarthritis, 119–120
   medial, 222, *222*
   fissure formation in, 219, *221*
   "play" in, 213, *213*
   shaving of articular cartilage of, 222
   subluxation of, in osteoarthritis, 167, *167*, 216–217, *216*, 418, *418*
Patellectomy, for osteoarthritis of patellofemoral joint, 416
   in experimental models of osteoarthritis, 119–120, *120*
Patellofemoral joint, contact range of, *214*
   malalignment of, 216–217
   osteoarthritis of, operative procedures for, 417–419
     patellectomy for, 416
     tibial tubercleplasty for, 418, *419*
     with patellar subluxation, *418*
Pathogenesis, of osteoarthritis, biochemical, 67–68
   stages of, 162t
Pathogenic mechanism, definition of, 129
Pathology, of osteoarthritis, 29–42
   intermediate stage of, 31–33
   late stage of, 33–37
   preclinical stage of, 29–31
   of secondary osteoarthritis, 39–40
Pathophysiology, of osteoarthritis, aging and, 12–14
Pellegrini-Stieda syndrome, 340
Pentazocine, 320
Periarthritis, of knee, steroid injection for, 340
Periarthropathie sportive, 564
Perna canaliculus, extract of, in treatment of osteoarthritis, 557
Perthes' disease, hip deformity in, *268*
Phenylbutazone, 324–325
   dosage of, 321t
   drug interactions with, 325
   side effects of, 325
   therapeutic limitations of, 325
Phlebography, intraosseous, in osteoarthritis, 194–195
Phospholipids, in articular cartilage, 50
Phosphorus, serum, in osteoarthritis, 185–186
Physical factors, role of, in etiology of osteoarthritis, 142
Piroxicam, 329–330
   adverse reactions to, 329–330
   dosage of, 321t, 329
   drug interactions with, 330
Plasminogen, in synovial fluid, 192
Plica synovialis, in diagnosis of knee pain, 215
Postel's destructive coxarthropathy, roentgenologic diagnosis of, 169, *169*
"Postinjection flare," after intra-articular steroid injection, 336
Posture, patient education for, 308
Prednisolone tebutate, dosage of, 337t

Preiser's disease, 371
Pressure, intraosseous, measurement of, 194
Procaine, 330
Procollagen, in synthesis of collagen, 55
Progesterone, role of, in incidence of osteoarthritis, 14
Propionic acid derivatives, 327–329
   drug interactions with, 328–329
   toxicity of, 328
Propoxyphene hydrochloride, 319
   withdrawal from 320
Proteins, in synovial fluid, 192
   link, in articular cartilage, 47
Proteoglycan(s), age-related changes in, 13
   antigenicity of, 86
   chemistry of, 45–49
   electron micrograph of, *46*
   in articular cartilage, in osteoarthritis, 61–63
     synthesis of, 65, *65*
     "turnover" of, 52, *54*
   structure of, *45, 48*
   synthesis of, 51–55
     changes in, 30
Proteoglycan aggregate, model of, *48*
Proteoglycan antigens, sensitivity to, in osteoarthritis, 187
Pseudocysts, degenerative, roentgenologic appearance of, 160–162, *160–162*
Psychosocial measurements, in rehabilitative assessment, 289
Psychosocial problems, 309–310
Pyrophosphate, in articular cartilage, 64
   inorganic, in synovial fluid, 193

Q angle, in osteoarthritis of knee, 405
Quad cane, *304*
Quadriceps wasting, 295

Race, as factor in osteoarthritis, 2, 10t
Radiocarpal joint, osteoarthritis of, 370
Radiocarpal osteoarthritis, *373*
   secondary, *374*
Radiohumeral joint, degeneration of, 385
Radioisotopes, intra-articular injection of, 347
Radioisotopic assays, antibody, 85
Radioscaphoid osteoarthritis, *373*
Radius, head of, osteoarthritis of, 385
   replacement of, 386
Ramps, and inclines, for ease of ambulation, 306
Range of motion, maintaining or increasing, specific recommendations for, 311
Recordkeeping, medical, legal aspects of, 545
Reflex sympathetic dystrophy (RSD), of knee, 218–219, *219*
   thermography in, 219, *220*
Refractory arc syndrome, 378
Rehabilitation, in osteoarthritis, 287–315
   employment aspects of, 538
   goals in, 287, 291
   organization of treatment plan for, 291
   patient assessments used in, 288–289
   patient education in, 307–310
     planning for, 312
   patient reply format for, 289t
   postoperative, 310

Rehabilitation (*Continued*)
  in osteoarthritis, specific treatments in, 291–293
    techniques of, 293–297
  vocational, 538
Rehabilitation Act of 1973, 537, 538
Reiter's syndrome, differential diagnosis of, 283
Research, in osteoarthritis, 4–5
Retrolisthesis, spondylotic, in spinal osteoarthritis, 452, *454*
Rhein, in treatment of osteoarthritis, investigation of, 556
Rheumatoid arthritis, secondary osteoarthritis due to, vs. idiopathic, 40
Rhizarthrosis, 202
Right hand, vs. left, incidence of osteoarthritis in, 16
Ring splints, 301–302, *302*
Roentgenography, in intervertebral disk disease, 494, *494*
Roentgenologic diagnosis, 155–184
Rotator cuff, impingement of, 378
  tear of, 379, *379*
Rufen. See *Ibuprofen*.
Rumalon, in treatment of osteoarthritis, investigation of, 554–555
Runners, incidence of osteoarthritis in, 16

SACH heel, 393
Salicylates, 319, 323–324
  adverse reactions to, 324, 324t
  dosage of, 323
  drug interactions with, 324, 324t
  in treatment of osteoarthritis, investigations of, 553–554
  pharmacokinetics of, 323
  therapeutic applications of, 323–324
  toxicity of, 324
Scaphoid, aseptic necrosis of (Preiser's disease), 371
    treatment of, 373
  fracture of, radiocarpal arthritis following, *373*
Scapulohumeral joint, steroid injection into, 340–341, *341*
Sciatica, incidence of, 473
  in degenerative disk disease, 486
Scissors, Stirex, *307*
Sclerosis, subchondral, in osteoarthritis of knee, 167, *167*
Scoliosis, torso orthosis for, 471, *471*
Seat, toilet, elevated, 305, *305*
  tub, 305, *305*
Semimembranosus tenosynovitis, steroid injection for, 340
Serum chemistry, in osteoarthritis, 185–186
Sex, and hormones, role of, in prevalence of osteoarthritis, 14
  distribution of, in osteoarthritis, 10t, 11t, 12t, 14
Sexual counseling, 309
Shelf sign, 152
Shoe(s), orthotic, 297–298
  biomechanical effects of, 290
  for osteoarthritis of hip, 427
  UCBL inserts for, *397*
  wide toe-box, *298*
  with rocker sole, *298*
Shoehorn, long-handled, *306*

Shoe support, for osteoarthritis of talonavicular joint, 396
Shoulder. See also *Acromioclavicular joint; Scapulohumeral joint; Sternoclavicular joint*.
  biomechanics of, 93
  destruction of, in neuropathic arthropathy, *173*
  "frozen," roentgenologic appearance of, *168*
  general design of, 93
  osteoarthritis of, 377–384. See also *Impingement syndrome*.
    etiology of, 377
    intra-articular steroid therapy for, 340–341
    roentgenologic diagnosis of, 168
  pain in, causes of, 377
  rotation of, following total shoulder replacement, *382, 383*
  therapeutic exercise for, 297
  total replacement of, 380, *380, 381*
    roentgenogram following, *382*
  vs. hip joint, bony constraints of, *94*
Sickle cell disease, 240–241
  marrow infarctions of shoulder in, *241*
  secondary osteoarthritis in, 240–241
Silicone oil, as lubricant in osteoarthritis, 555
Sinding-Larsen-Johansson disease, 216
Sitting, as cause of intervertebral disk disease, 536
Skeletal hyperostosis, diffuse idiopathic (DISH). See *Diffuse idiopathic skeletal hyperostosis*.
Social Security Administration, evaluation of disability by, 546–548
Sodium hyaluronate, as joint lubricant in osteoarthritis, 556
  intra-articular injection of, 347
Sodium iodoacetate, intra-articular injection of, in experimental models of osteoarthritis, 112
Spinal canal, anatomic variations in, 479, *481*
Spinal cord, compression of, 447
Spinal nerve roots, symptoms of, in degenerative disk disease, 486
Spine(s). See also *Intervertebral disk(s)* and *Low back pain*.
  ankylosing hyperostosis of (AHS), 469–470
  bracing for, 300
  cervical, collar for, *301*
    osteoarthritis of, 443–459
      differential diagnosis of, 277
      diskectomy and fusion for, 450, *452*
      etiology of, 443
      neck pain in, 444
      rare forms of, 456–458
      roentgenographic appearance of, *153, 445, 446*
      subluxations in, 452, *453, 454*
      symptoms and signs of, 444–448
      treatment of, 448–458
        nonsurgical, 448
        surgical, 450
  decompression of, surgery for, 505–517
  degenerative disease of. See *Spondylosis deformans*.
  enthesopathies of, roentgenologic diagnosis of, 175–181
  hyperostosis of. See *Diffuse idiopathic skeletal hyperostosis (DISH)*.
  "kissing," in generalized osteoarthritis, 205, *205*
  lumbar, fusion of, spinal stenosis following, 516, *516*

Spine(s) (*Continued*)
lumbar, normal anatomy of, vs. degenerative changes in, 482, *483*
osteoarthritis of, 473–521
roentgenogram of, in generalized osteoarthritis, *205*
lumbosacral, osteoarthritis of, differential diagnosis of, 277
therapeutic exercises for, 296–297
orthoses for, 300–301
osteoarthritis of, 443–521. See also *Spondylosis deformans.*
neurologic symptoms of, 154
symptoms of, 153
thoracic spondylosis in, 463–465
senile ankylosing hyperostosis of. See *Diffuse idiopathic skeletal hyperostosis (DISH).*
stenosis of, in intervertebral disk disease, 479–482
CAT scan of, *499, 500*
myelogram of, *497*
surgical technique for, 511, *511–513*
thoracic, anatomic aspects of, 461–462
arthropathy of, 470
osteoarthritis of, 461–472
management of, 466–468
thoracic pain in, 462–463
root and nerve pain in, 463
spinal bracing for, 471, *471*
Spinner bar, for steering wheel, 302, *302*
Splint(s), functional wrist, 301, *301*
ring, 301–302, *302*
thumb post, 301, *302*
Spondylarthritis, vs. spondylosis deformans, 172
Spondylitis, ankylosing, differential diagnosis of, 283
Spondylitis ossificans ligamentosa. See *Diffuse idiopathic skeletal hyperostosis (DISH).*
Spondyloepiphyseal dysplasia (SED), secondary osteoarthritis in, 246
Spondylolisthesis, degenerative, 482, *484*
Spondylosis, cervical, in osteoarthritis of spine, *447–449, 450, 451, 453*
hyperostotic. See *Diffuse idiopathic skeletal hyperostosis (DISH).*
thoracic, 463–465
clinical features of, 464
management of, 465
roentgenogram of, *464, 465*
Spondylosis deformans, intervertebral osteophytes in, 172, *173*
roentgenologic diagnosis of, 172–174
Sports activities, and osteoarthritis, 561
Spray can, assistive device for, *308*
"Squinting knee cap," 212
Stairs, and slopes, design problems of, 306
Steering wheel, spinner bar for, 302, *302*
Sternoclavicular joint, osteoarthritis of, 384
treatment of, 384
steroid injection into, 341
Steroids, effect of, in experimental models of osteoarthritis, 110
injectable, brand names of, 337t
dosages of, 337t
role of, in etiology of osteoarthritis, 142
systemic, 330
Steroid therapy, intra-articular, 333–349, 552. See also names of specific steroids.

Steroid therapy (*Continued*)
intra-articular, choice of drug for, 336
clinical efficacy of, 334–335
complications of, 335–336, 335t
contraindications for, 335–336, 335t
dosage and administration of, 336–337
factors affecting response to, 337t
indications for, 334, 334t
investigations of, 552
preparation of site for, 337
rationale for, 333–334
role of, 333
techniques of, 337–346
Stickler's syndrome, secondary osteoarthritis in, 247
Stiffness, of joints, as symptom of osteoarthritis, 151
Strength, increasing, recommendations for, 311
Stress, abnormal, as etiologic factor, in osteoarthritis of hip, 424–425
in experimental models of osteoarthritis, 113
chronic, as factor in osteoarthritis, 2
in osteoarthritis of hip, 424
Subluxation, as sign of osteoarthritis, 151
Subtalar joint, arthrodesis of, 395, *395*
function of, 389, *390*
osteoarthritis of, 394–395
differential diagnosis of, 394
roentgenogram of, *394, 395*
treatment of, 395
Sugars, in synovial fluid, 191
Sulindac, 326, 327
adverse effects of, 327
dosage of, 321t, 327
Superoxide dismutase, in treatment of osteoarthritis, 549–550
Supraspinatus syndrome, 378
Surgery, in osteoarthritis, 351–359
cost vs. benefit ratio in, 353
indications for, 351–354
postoperative rehabilitation following, 310
risk vs. benefit ratio in, 353
types of, 354–358
"Swiss cheese cartilage" syndrome, secondary osteoarthritis in, 247
Symptoms, of osteoarthritis, 150–151, 150t
Synovial changes, in late osteoarthritis, 36–37, *36*
Synovial (mucoid) cyst, 200, *200*
Synovial fluid, appearance of, in osteoarthritis, 188, 188t
as source of nutrition for cartilage, 44
biomechanical role of, 101–102
bone and cartilage metabolic studies of, 193
bone cells in, 190
calcium hydroxyapatite crystals in, 190
cartilage fragments in, 190
cholesterol crystals in, 190
clotting factors in, 192
collagen fibrils in, 190, *190*
copper in, 192
cytoplasmic inclusions in, 189, *189*
defect in, 30
electrolytes in, 191
enzymes in, 191–192
immunologic studies of, 192–193
laboratory assessment of, in osteoarthritis, 187–193
lipids in, 191
mucin in, 189

Synovial fluid (*Continued*)
  normal vs. osteoarthritic, 188t
  oxygen tension in, 191
  pH of, 191
  proteins in, 192
  sugars in, 191
  synovial lining cells in, 190, *190*
  viscosity of, 188–189, *189*
  volume of, 188
Synovial membrane, role of, in etiology of os-
    teoarthritis, 135–136
Synovitis, crystal, and osteoarthritis, steroid in-
    jection for, 346
  following steroid injection, 336, 346
  due to hydroxyapatite, 137
  in idiopathic osteoarthritis, 37
  secondary, occupational aspects of, 534
Synovium, biopsy of, 193, *193*
  histologic examination of, 193–194, *193*
Syringomyelia, Charcot joints in, 253, *254*

T cells, 81
Tabes dorsalis, Charcot joints in, 253
Talocalcaneal joint, function of, 389, *390*
Talonavicular joint, arthrodesis of, 396
  function of, 390, *391*
  osteoarthritis of, 396
    roentgenogram of, *396*
    treatment of, 396
Tandearil. See *Oxyphenbutazone.*
TARA prosthesis, for hip, 439
Tarsal coalition, roentgenogram of, 395
Tarsal joint, transverse, function of, 390, *391*
Tarsometatarsal joints, arthrodesis of, 398
  function of, 391
  osteoarthritis of, 397–398
    roentgenogram of, *398*
    treatment of, 398
Teeth, grinding of, in osteoarthritis of temporo-
    mandibular joint, 528
Temporomandibular joint, degenerative changes
    in, 525–526, *528, 529*
  animal models of, 526
  displaced meniscus in, arthrogram of, 527, *528*
  osteoarthritis of, 523–530
    clinical features of, 526–528
    early stage of, histologic appearance of, *526*
    end stage of, histologic appearance of, *526*
    high condylectomy for, 529
    occlusal splint for, 528, *530*
    treatment of, 528–530
  panoramic jaw film of, *527*
  remodeling in, biologic basis of, 523–525, *524,
    525*
  steroid injection of, 345, *345*
Tenderness, as sign of osteoarthritis, 151
Tendinitis, occupational aspects of, 534
  of knee, 216
Tenosynovitis, occupational aspects of, 534
  "popliteal," steroid injection for, 340
  semimembranosus, steroid injection for, 340
Testosterone, in treatment of osteoarthritis, 551
  role of, in incidence of osteoarthritis, 14
Thalassemia, 241–242
  secondary osteoarthritis in, 241–242
THARIES hip resurfacing technique, 439
Thermography, in osteoarthritis, 195

Thiemann's disease, secondary osteoarthritis in,
    248
Thoracic nerves, anatomy of, 461–462
Thoracic pain. See *Pain, thoracic.*
Thumb, metacarpophalangeal joint of, arthro-
    desis of, 368
  pain at base of, as sign of osteoarthritis, 152
Thumb post splint, 301, *302*
Tibia, fractures of, abnormal knee stress due to,
    404
  tubercle of, elevation of, in patellofemoral os-
    teoarthritis, 418, *419*
Tibiotalar joint, steroid injection of, 345–346, *346*
Toe(s). See also names of specific joints.
  interphalangeal joints of, osteoarthritis of,
    401–402
  great, first metatarsophalangeal joint of, os-
    teoarthritis of, differential diagnosis of, 281
  gouty arthritis of, differential diagnosis of,
    282
  joints of, steroid therapy for, 342–344
Toilet paper holder, *307*
Toilet seat, elevated, 305, *305*
Tolectin. See *Tolmetin sodium.*
Tolerance, immunologic, 86
Tolmetin sodium, 319, 326–327
  adverse effects of, 327
  dosage of, 321t, 327
Traction, 293–294
Tranexamic acid, in treatment of osteoarthritis,
    investigation of, 554
Transcutaneous electrical nerve stimulation
    (TENS), 293
Transfer, adaptive devices for, 305
Trapeziometacarpal joint, arthroplasty of, 370,
    371
  osteoarthritis of, 369
    roentgenographic appearance of, *370*
Trapezium, replacement of, 370
Trauma, in pathogenesis of secondary osteoar-
    thritis, 39
  secondary osteoarthritis due to, 257
Treatment. See also *Drug therapy, Surgery,* and
    under specific disease entities.
  patient education in, 317–318
  patient motivation in, 317–318
Triamcinolone acetonide, dosage of, 337t
  effect of, in experimental models of osteoar-
    thritis, 110, *110*
Triamcinolone diacetate, dosage of, 337t
Triamcinolone hexacetonide, dosage of, 337t
Tribenoside, in treatment of osteoarthritis, inves-
    tigation of, 556
Trichorhinophalangeal syndrome, secondary os-
    teoarthritis in, 247
Trochanteric bursa, steroid injection of, 345
Tropocollagen, molecular structure of, 49
Tub seat, 305, *305*
Tubercleplasty, tibial, in patellofemoral osteoar-
    thritis, 418, *419*
Turner's syndrome, secondary osteoarthritis in,
    248

UCBL inserts, *397*
Ultrasound, therapeutic, 292–293

Upper extremity, osteoarthritis of, 363, 387
Uric acid, increased levels of, correlation to osteoarthritis of, 17
Urine, laboratory assessment of, in osteoarthritis, 187
  tests of, in ochronosis, 186t, 187
Utensils, eating, large-handled, *307*

"Vacuum sign," in late osteoarthritis, 167
Valgus deformity, at knee, hip osteotomy for, 432
Varus deformity, at knee, hip osteotomy for, 432
Venography, epidural, in intervertebral disk disease, 495–498, *498*
Vertebra(e), fusion of, in Forestier's disease, 176, *177*
  limbus, *477, 478*
  lumbar, subluxation of, 482
Vertebral arch, ligaments of, ossification of (OVAL), 180–181, *179–181*
Vertebral ligamentous calcification, physiologic. See *Diffuse idiopathic skeletal hyperostosis (DISH).*
Vitamin A, and diffuse idiopathic skeletal hyperostosis (DISH), 232
  intra-articular injection of, in experimental models of osteoarthritis, 111
Vitamin C, in treatment of osteoarthritis, 550–551

Walking, action of foot joints in, *98*
  ankle dorsiflexion and plantar flexion in, 389, *390*
  biomechanics of, 389
Ward's triangle, 158, *158*
Water, in articular cartilage, 45
  in osteoarthritis, 60–61, *60*
  role of, in etiology of osteoarthritis, 132
Wheelchair, 302
  Amigo, *303*
Wiburg, center-edge angle of, 156
Wilson's disease (hepatolenticular degeneration), 237–238
  laboratory assessment of, 186t, 187
  secondary osteoarthritis in, 237–238
  treatment of, 238
Wrist, and hand, osteoarthritis of, 363–376
  arthrodesis of, 374, *374, 375*
  biomechanics of, 96
  functional splint for, 301, *301*
  osteoarthritis of, 370–375
  pain in, as sign of osteoarthritis, 152

Yttrium, intra-articular injection of, 347

Zipper hook, *307*